Pediatric Dentistry

Pediatric Dentistry: Infancy Through Adolescence

SIXTH EDITION

Arthur J. Nowak, DMD, MA

Professor Emeritus
Pediatric Dentistry and Pediatrics
University of Iowa
Iowa City, Iowa

Associate Editors:

John R. Christensen, DDS, MS (Ped Dent), MS (Ortho)

Adjunct Associate Professor
Department of Pediatric Dentistry
University of North Carolina at Chapel Hill School of
    Dentistry
Chapel Hill, North Carolina;
Durham Pediatric Dentistry and Orthodontics
Durham, North Carolina

Tad R. Mabry, DDS, MS

Clinical Professor
Department of Pediatric Dentistry
University of Iowa College of Dentistry
Iowa City, Iowa

Janice A. Townsend, DDS, MS

Associate Professor and Chair
Division of Pediatric Dentistry
The Ohio State University College of Dentistry;
Chief, Department of Dentistry
Nationwide Children's Hospital
Columbus, Ohio;
Clinical Associate Professor
Louisiana State University Health Sciences Center School of
    Dentistry
New Orleans, Louisiana

Martha H. Wells, DMD, MS

Associate Professor and Program Director
Department of Pediatric Dentistry
The University of Tennessee Health Science Center
Memphis, Tennessee

ELSEVIER

ELSEVIER

1600 John F. Kennedy Blvd.
Ste 1800
Philadelphia, PA 19103-2899

Previous editions copyrighted 2013, 2005, 1999, 1994, 1988 by Saunders, an imprint of Elsevier Inc.

Library of Congress Cataloging-in-Publication Data

Names: Nowak, Arthur J., 1937- editor. | Christensen, John R. (Pediatric dentist and orthodontist), editor. |
　　Mabry, Tad R., editor. | Townsend, Janice A., editor. | Wells, Martha H., editor.
Title: Pediatric dentistry : infancy through adolescence / [edited by] Arthur J. Nowak ; associate editors:
　　John R. Christensen, Tad R. Mabry, Janice A. Townsend, Martha H. Wells.
Other titles: Pediatric dentistry (Pinkham)
Description: Sixth edition. | Philadelphia, PA : Elsevier, [2019] | Preceded by Pediatric dentistry / [edited by]
　　Paul S. Casamassimo. 5th ed. c2013. | Includes bibliographical references and index.
Identifiers: LCCN 2018006375 | ISBN 9780323608268 (hardcover : alk. paper)
Subjects: | MESH: Dental Care for Children | Pediatric Dentistry
Classification: LCC RK55.C5 | NLM WU 480 | DDC 617.6/45–dc23 LC record available at
　　https://lccn.loc.gov/2018006375

Senior Content Strategist: Jennifer Flynn-Briggs
Senior Content Development Specialist: Rae Robertson
Publishing Services Manager: Catherine Jackson
Book Production Specialist: Kristine Feeherty
Design Direction: Brian Salisbury

Working together
to grow libraries in
developing countries

www.elsevier.com • www.bookaid.org

Printed in India

Last digit is the print number:　9　8　7　6　5　4

Contributors

Bhavini Acharya, BDS, MPH
Associate Professor/Program Director
Pediatric Dentistry
University of Texas Health Science Center at Houston
Houston, Texas
Chapter 5 Case Study

Abimbola O. Adewumi, BDS, MPed Dent RCS (Eng)
Clinical Associate Professor and Residency Program Director
Department of Pediatric Dentistry
University of Florida College of Dentistry
Gainesville, Florida
Chapter 29

Ola B. Al-Batayneh, BDS, MDSc, JDB
Associate Professor in Pediatric Dentistry
Department of Preventive Dentistry
Faculty of Dentistry
Jordan University of Science and Technology;
Consultant in Pediatric Dentistry
Head, Special Surgery-Pediatric Dental Surgery Division
King Abdullah University Teaching Hospital
Irbid, Jordan
Chapter 13 Case Study

Alexander Alcaraz, DMD
Assistant Professor of Clinical Dentistry
Pediatric Dentistry
Herman Ostrow School of Dentistry of USC;
Director of Clinical Education
Division of Dentistry
Children's Hospital Los Angeles
Los Angeles, California
Chapter 25 Case Study

Veerasathpurush Allareddy, BDS MBA, MHA, PhD, MMSc
Professor
Department of Orthodontics
Collegiate Director of Clinical Research
College of Dentistry and Dental Clinics
University of Iowa
Iowa City, Iowa
Chapter 5

Sahar M. Alrayyes, DDS, MS
Clinical Associate Professor and Clinic Director
Department of Pediatric Dentistry
University of Illinois at Chicago College of Dentistry
Chicago, Illinois
Chapter 41 Case Study

Homa Amini, DDS, MPH, MS
Professor of Clinical Dentistry and Program Director
Division of Pediatric Dentistry
The Ohio State University College of Dentistry
Columbus, Ohio
Chapter 11

Paul Andrews, DDS, MSc
Assistant Professor
Faculty of Dentistry
University of Toronto
Toronto, Ontario, Canada
Chapter 24 Case Study

Kay S. Beavers, DDS, RDH
Professor
Department of Diagnosis and Preventive Services
University of Oklahoma Health Sciences Center College of
    Dentistry
Oklahoma City, Oklahoma
Chapter 15

Erica Brecher, DMD, MS
Assistant Professor
Pediatric Dentistry
Virginia Commonwealth University
Richmond, Virginia
Chapter 38

R. John Brewer, EMT-P
Dental Education, Inc.
Bethel Park, Pennsylvania
Chapter 10

Jeffrey N. Brownstein, DDS
Clinical Instructor
Midwestern University College of Dental Medicine-Arizona
Glendale, Arizona;
Clinical Instructor
Department of Dental Anesthesiology
NYU Langone Medical Center
Brooklyn, New York;
Private Practice
Peoria, Arizona
Chapter 6

Paul S. Casamassimo, DDS, MS
Professor Emeritus
Pediatric Dentistry
The Ohio State University;
Department of Dentistry
Nationwide Children's Hospital
Columbus, Ohio
Chapter 1

Zafer C. Cehreli, DDS, PhD
Professor
Department of Pediatric Dentistry
Faculty of Dentistry
Hacettepe University
Ankara, Turkey
Chapter 39 Case Study
Chapter 40 Case Study

Donald L. Chi, DDS, PhD
Associate Professor, Department of Oral Health Sciences, School
    of Dentistry
Adjunct Associate Professor, Department of Pediatric Dentistry,
    School of Dentistry
Adjunct Associate Professor, Department of Pediatrics, School of
    Medicine
Adjunct Associate Professor, Department of Health Services,
    School of Public Health
University of Washington
Seattle, Washington
Chapter 11

John R. Christensen, DDS, MS (Ped Dent), MS (Ortho)
Adjunct Associate Professor
Department of Pediatric Dentistry
University of North Carolina at Chapel Hill School of Dentistry
Chapel Hill, North Carolina;
Durham Pediatric Dentistry and Orthodontics
Durham, North Carolina
Chapter 19
Chapter 27
Chapter 28
Chapter 28 Case Study
Chapter 31
Chapter 36
Chapter 38

Samuel J. Christensen, DDS, MS
Private Practice
Ankeny, Iowa
Chapter 27 Case Study

Matthew Cooke, DDS, MD, MPH
Associate Professor
Departments of Anesthesiology and Pediatric Dentistry
School of Dental Medicine
University of Pittsburgh
Pittsburgh, Pennsylvania;
Adjunct Clinical Assistant Professor
Department of Oral and Maxillofacial Surgery
School of Dentistry
Virginia Commonwealth University
Richmond, Virginia
Chapter 10

Marcio A. da Fonseca, DDS, MS
Chicago Dental Society Associate Professor and Head
Department of Pediatric Dentistry
University of Illinois at Chicago College of Dentistry
Chicago, Illinois
Chapter 4

William O. Dahlke, Jr., DMD
Associate Professor and Chair
Department of Pediatric Dentistry
Virginia Commonwealth University School of Dentistry
Richmond, Virginia
Chapter 33 Case Study

Kevin J. Donly, DDS, MS
Professor and Chair
Department of Developmental Dentistry
Professor
Department of Pediatrics
University of Texas Health Science Center at San Antonio
San Antonio, Texas
Chapter 21

Zameera Fida, DMD
Department of Dentistry
Boston Children's Hospital
Instructor, Developmental Biology
Harvard School of Dental Medicine
Boston, Massachusetts
Chapter 30

Henry Fields, DDS, MS, MSD
Professor and Division Chair
Orthodontics
The Ohio State University College of Dentistry;
Chief, Section of Orthodontics
Department of Dentistry
Nationwide Children's Hospital
Columbus, Ohio
Chapter 19
Chapter 26
Chapter 27
Chapter 28
Chapter 30
Chapter 31
Chapter 35 (boxed material)
Chapter 36
Chapter 38

Catherine M. Flaitz, DDS, MS
Professor
Pediatric Dentistry
The Ohio State University College of Dentistry;
Associate Chief of Dentistry
Department of Dentistry
Nationwide Children's Hospital
Columbus, Ohio
Chapter 2

Fernando L. Esteban Florez, DDS, MS, PhD
Assistant Professor
Department of Dental Materials
University of Oklahoma College of Dentistry
Oklahoma City, Oklahoma
Chapter 21 (boxed material)

Suzanne Fournier, DDS
Postgraduate Program Director
Department of Pediatric Dentistry
Louisiana State University
New Orleans, Louisiana
Chapter 11 Case Study
Chapter 11 (boxed material)

Anna B. Fuks, DDS
Department of Pediatric Dentistry
Hadassah School of Dental Medicine
Hebrew University
Jerusalem, Israel;
Professor Emeritus
The Maurice and Gabriela Goldschleger School of Dental
    Medicine
Department of Pediatric Dentistry
Tel Aviv University
Tel Aviv, Israel
Chapter 23
Chapter 34

Matthew K. Geneser, DDS
Clinical Associate Professor
Department of Pediatric Dentistry
University of Iowa College of Dentistry
Iowa City, Iowa
Chapter 5

Gayle J. Gilbaugh, RDH
Specialized Care Coordinator/Dental Hygienist
Department of Pediatric Dentistry
University of Iowa College of Dentistry
Iowa City, Iowa
Chapter 20 (boxed material)

Elizabeth S. Gosnell, DMD, MS
Assistant Professor
Division of Pediatric Dentistry and Orthodontics
Cincinnati Children's Hospital Medical Center
Cincinnati, Ohio
Chapter 7
Chapter 8

Erin L. Gross, DDS, PhD, MS
Assistant Professor-Clinical
Division of Pediatric Dentistry
College of Dentistry
The Ohio State University
Columbus, Ohio
Chapter 13
Chapter 18

Steven H. Gross, CDT
President
SML Space Maintainers Laboratories
Headquarters
Chatsworth, California
Chapter 26 (boxed material)

Marcio Guelmann, DDS
Professor and Chair
Department of Pediatric Dentistry
University of Florida
Gainesville, Florida
Chapter 23

Kerrod B. Hallett, MDSc, MPH
Paediatric Dentist
Director, Department of Dentistry
Research Fellow, Clinical Sciences, Murdoch Children's Research
    Institute
Clinical Associate Professor, University of Melbourne
Melbourne, Victoria, Australia
Chapter 4 Case Study

Kimberly J. Hammersmith, DDS, MPH, MS
Nationwide Children's Hospital
Adjunct Assistant Professor
Division of Pediatric Dentistry
College of Dentistry
The Ohio State University
Columbus, Ohio
Chapter 3 Case Study
Chapter 18 Case Study

Kevin L. Haney, DDS, MS
Professor
Pediatric Dentistry
University of Oklahoma College of Dentistry
Oklahoma City, Oklahoma
Chapter 15

Brian D. Hodgson, DDS
Associate Professor, Program in Pediatric Dentistry
Department of Developmental Sciences
Marquette University School of Dentistry
Milwaukee, Wisconsin
Chapter 23 Case Study

Gideon Holan, DMD
Clinical Associate Professor
Pediatric Dentistry
The Hebrew University-Hadassah School of Dental Medicine
Jerusalem, Israel
Chapter 16

Cody C. Hughes, DMD, MSD
Program Director
Advanced Education Program in Pediatric Dentistry
UNLV School of Dental Medicine
Las Vegas, Nevada;
Pediatric Dentist
Valley Pediatric Dental
Mesquite, Nevada
Chapter 22 Case Study

Michael A. Ignelzi, Jr., DDS, PhD
Adjunct Professor
Department of Pediatric Dentistry
University of North Carolina at Chapel Hill
Chapel Hill, North Carolina;
Lake Jeanette Orthodontics and Pediatric Dentistry
Greensboro, North Carolina
Chapter 36 Case Study

Janice G. Jackson, DMD
Professor and Program Director
Department of Pediatric Dentistry
University of Alabama at Birmingham
Birmingham, Alabama
Chapter 35 Case Study

Faris Jamjoom, BDS, MS
Advanced Implantology Program
Department of Restorative and Biomaterial Sciences
Harvard School of Dental Medicine
Boston, Massachusetts
Chapter 3 Case Study

Michael J. Kanellis, DDS, MS
Associate Dean and Professor
Department of Pediatric Dentistry
University of Iowa College of Dentistry
Iowa City, Iowa
Chapter 22 (boxed material)

Piranit Nik Kantaputra, DDS, MS
Center of Excellence in Medical Genetics Research
Division of Pediatric Dentistry
Department of Orthodontics and Pediatric Dentistry
Chiang Mai University
Chiang Mai, Thailand
Chapter 17

Sharukh S. Khajotia, BDS, MS, PhD
Associate Dean for Research
Professor and Chair, Department of Dental Materials
University of Oklahoma College of Dentistry
Affiliate Associate Professor of Chemical, Biological, and
   Materials Engineering
University of Oklahoma College of Engineering
Oklahoma City, Oklahoma
Chapter 21 (boxed material)

Lisa Knobloch, DDS, MS
Professor
Division of Restorative Science and Prosthodontics
The Ohio State University College of Dentistry
Columbus, Ohio
Chapter 3 Case Study

Ari Kupietzky, DMD, MSc
Visiting Professor
Department of Pediatric Dentistry
Rutgers School of Dental Medicine
Newark, New Jersey;
Faculty Member
Department of Pediatric Dentistry
The Hebrew University-Hadassah School of Dental Medicine
Jerusalem, Israel
Chapter 23

Clarice S. Law, DMD, MS
Associate Clinical Professor
Sections of Pediatric Dentistry and Orthodontics
Division of Growth and Development
UCLA School of Dentistry
Los Angeles, California
Chapter 26
Chapter 27

Kecia S. Leary, DDS, MS
Associate Professor
Department of Pediatric Dentistry
University of Iowa College of Dentistry
Iowa City, Iowa
Chapter 32

Tad R. Mabry, DDS, MS
Clinical Professor
Department of Pediatric Dentistry
University of Iowa College of Dentistry
Iowa City, Iowa
Chapter 39

Cindy L. Marek, PharmD
Clinical Associate Professor
Department of Oral Pathology, Radiology, and Medicine
University of Iowa College of Dentistry
Department of Pharmacy Practice and Science
University of Iowa College of Pharmacy
Iowa City, Iowa
Chapter 9

Dennis J. McTigue, DDS, MS
Professor Emeritus
Pediatric Dentistry
The Ohio State University College of Dentistry
Columbus, Ohio
Chapter 16
Chapter 35

Beau D. Meyer, DDS, MPH
Research Assistant Professor
Pediatric Dentistry
University of North Carolina at Chapel Hill
Chapel Hill, North Carolina
Chapter 3
Chapter 31 Case Study

Travis Nelson, DDS, MSD, MPH
Clinical Associate Professor
Department of Pediatric Dentistry
University of Washington
Seattle, Washington
Chapter 22

Man Wai Ng, DDS, MPH
Associate Professor, Developmental Biology (Pediatric Dentistry)
Harvard School of Dental Medicine
Chief, Department of Dentistry
Boston Children's Hospital
Boston, Massachusetts
Chapter 30
Chapter 30 Case Study

Arthur J. Nowak, DMD, MA
Professor Emeritus
Pediatric Dentistry and Pediatrics
University of Iowa
Iowa City, Iowa
Chapter 13
Chapter 18
Chapter 20
Chapter 32

Eyal Nuni, DMD
Endodontist, Senior Member
Department of Endodontics
The Hebrew University-Hadassah School of Dental Medicine
Jerusalem, Israel
Chapter 34

Arwa I. Owais, BDS, MS
Associate Professor
Department of Pediatric Dentistry
University of Iowa School of Dentistry
Iowa City, Iowa
Chapter 20

Bhavna T. Pahel, BDS, DDS, MPH, PhD
Adjunct Assistant Professor
University of North Carolina at Chapel Hill
Chapel Hill, North Carolina;
Private Practice
Village Family Dental
Fayetteville, North Carolina
Chapter 19 Case Study

Rocio B. Quinonez, DMD, MS, MPH
Professor and Associate Dean of Educational Leadership and Innovation
Pediatric Dentistry and Academic Affairs
University of North Carolina at Chapel Hill
Chapel Hill, North Carolina
Chapter 19

Diana Ram, DMD
Associate Professor
Chair of the Department of Pediatric Dentistry
School of Dental Medicine
The Hebrew University-Hadassah School of Dental Medicine
Jerusalem, Israel
Chapter 7 Case Study

Steve K. Rayes, DDS, MS
Associate Director, Advanced Training in Pediatric Dentistry
Pediatric Dentistry
NYU-Lutheran;
Chief of Pediatric Dentistry
Department of Dentistry
Southcentral Foundation
Anchorage, Alaska
Chapter 14 Case Study

Issa S. Sasa, BDS, MS
Associate Clinical Professor
Developmental Dentistry
University of Texas Health Science Center at San Antonio
San Antonio, Texas
Chapter 21

Scott B. Schwartz, DDS, MPH
Assistant Professor
Division of Pediatric Dentistry and Orthodontics
Cincinnati Children's Hospital Medical Center
Cincinnati, Ohio
Chapter 31
Chapter 37 Case Study

N. Sue Seale, DDS, MSD
Clinical Professor
Department of Orthodontics and Pediatric Dentistry
University of Maryland School of Dentistry
Baltimore, Maryland
Chapter 22 (boxed material)

Rose D. Sheats, DMD, MPH
Adjunct Associate Professor
School of Dentistry
University of North Carolina at Chapel Hill
Chapel Hill, North Carolina
Chapter 36
Chapter 38

Jonathan D. Shenkin, DDS, MPH
Clinical Associate Professor
Health Policy, Health Services Research, and Pediatric Dentistry
Boston University School of Dental Medicine
Boston, Massachusetts;
Private Practice
Augusta, Maine
Chapter 11

Sujatha S. Sivaraman, BDS, DMD, MPH
Director of Pediatric Dentistry
Family Dental Center East
Columbia, Missouri
Chapter 20 Case Study

M. Catherine Skotowski, RDH, MS
Clinical Assistant Professor
Department of Pediatric Dentistry
College of Dentistry
University of Iowa
Iowa City, Iowa
Chapter 15 (boxed material)
Chapter 32 (boxed material)

Rebecca L. Slayton, DDS, PhD
Professor Emeritus
Department of Pediatric Dentistry
University of Washington School of Dentistry
Seattle, Washington
Chapter 17
Chapter 17 Case Study

Andrew Spadinger, DDS
Pediatric Dentist
Private Practice
Children's Dentistry and Orthodontics
Bridgeport, Connecticut
Chapter 41

Thomas R. Stark, DDS
Pediatric Dentistry and Orofacial Pain
Assistant Professor at Uniform Service Health Science University
Comprehensive Dentistry Program
Schofield Barracks, Hawaii
Chapter 38
Chapter 38 Case Study

William V. Stenberg, Jr., DDS, MPH, MS
Clinical Assistant Professor
Periodontics
Texas A&M University
Dallas, Texas
Chapter 25

Deborah Studen-Pavlovich, DMD
Professor and Graduate Program Director
Department of Pediatric Dentistry
University of Pittsburgh School of Dental Medicine
Pittsburgh, Pennsylvania
Chapter 37

Rosalyn M. Sulyanto, DMD, MS
Instructor of Developmental Biology (Pediatric Dentistry)
Harvard School of Dental Medicine
Associate in Dentistry
Boston Children's Hospital
Boston, Massachusetts
Chapter 30 Case Study

Thomas Tanbonliong, Jr., DDS
Associate Professor of Clinical Dentistry and Clinic Director
Division of Pediatric Dentistry and Dental Public Health
Herman Ostrow School of Dentistry of USC
Los Angeles, California
Chapter 8 Case Study

S. Thikkurissy, DDS, MS
Professor and Division Director
Director, Residency Program
Division of Pediatric Dentistry
Cincinnati Children's Hospital
University of Cincinnati
Cincinnati, Ohio
Chapter 7
Chapter 8

Sherry R. Timmons, DDS, PhD
Clinical Associate Professor
Department of Oral Pathology, Radiology, and Medicine
University of Iowa College of Dentistry
Iowa City, Iowa
Chapter 9

Norman Tinanoff, DDS, MS
Professor
Department of Orthodontics and Pediatric Dentistry
University of Maryland School of Dentistry
Baltimore, Maryland
Chapter 12

Janice A. Townsend, DDS, MS
Associate Professor and Chair
Division of Pediatric Dentistry
The Ohio State University College of Dentistry;
Chief, Department of Dentistry
Nationwide Children's Hospital
Columbus, Ohio;
Clinical Associate Professor
Louisiana State University Health Sciences Center School of
    Dentistry
New Orleans, Louisiana
Chapter 1
Chapter 24

Elizabeth Velan, DMD, MSD
Pediatric Dentist
Dental Department
Seattle Children's Hospital;
Affiliate Assistant Professor
Department of Pediatric Dentistry
University of Washington School of Dentistry
Seattle, Washington
Chapter 40

Adriana Modesto Vieira, DDS, MS, PhD, DMD
Professor and Chair
Department of Pediatric Dentistry
University of Pittsburgh School of Dental Medicine
Pittsburgh, Pennsylvania
Chapter 37

Craig V. Vinall, DDS, MDS
Predoctoral Program Director
Department of Pediatric Dentistry and Community Oral Health
The University of Tennessee Health Science Center
Memphis, Tennessee
Chapter 40 Case Study

William F. Waggoner, DDS, MS
Private Practice
Las Vegas, Nevada
Chapter 22

Jillian Wallen, BDS, MS
Associate Professor and Chair
Growth and Development
University of Nebraska Medical Center College of Dentistry
Omaha, Nebraska
Chapter 29 Case Study

Karin Weber-Gasparoni, DDS, MS, PhD
Professor
Department of Pediatric Dentistry
University of Iowa College of Dentistry
Iowa City, Iowa
Chapter 14

Martha H. Wells, DMD, MS
Associate Professor and Program Director
Department of Pediatric Dentistry
The University of Tennessee Health Science Center
Memphis, Tennessee
Chapter 24
Chapter 33

A. Jeffrey Wood, DDS
Professor and Chair
Department of Pediatric Dentistry
University of the Pacific Arthur A. Dugoni School of Dentistry
San Francisco, California
Chapter 37 Case Study

J. Timothy Wright, DDS, MS
Bawden Distinguished Professor
Department of Pediatric Dentistry
University of North Carolina at Chapel Hill
Chapel Hill, North Carolina
Chapter 3

Vajahat Yar Khan, BDS
Practicing Pediatric Dentist and Principal
Texas Family Dentistry, PLLC
DBA Creative Smiles and Kidzone Dental
Houston, Texas
Chapter 6 Case Study

Juan F. Yepes, DDS, MD, MPH, MS, DrPH
Associate Professor of Pediatric Dentistry
Department of Pediatric Dentistry
James Whitcomb Riley Hospital for Children
Indiana University School of Dentistry
Indianapolis, Indiana
Chapter 2 Case Study

Audrey Jung-Sun Yoon, DDS, MS
Lecturer, Clinical Faculty
Pediatric Dentistry and Orthodontics
UCLA School of Dentistry
Los Angeles, California
Chapter 26 Case Study

Feda Zawaideh, BDS, ADC (Vic), GradDipClinDent, DClinDent (Melb)
Assistant Professor in Paediatric Dentistry
Jordan University of Science and Technology;
Consultant in Pediatric Dentistry
King Abdullah University Hospital
Al Rabieh-Amman, Jordan
Chapter 9 Case Study

Pediatric Dentistry: Infancy Through Adolescence was first published in 1988, has been translated into multiple foreign languages, and is now proceeding into another edition. When honored to write a foreword for this edition, I reviewed what was written in 1988 and realized that what was offered then was still applicable today. Citing some of the language of that preface:

> This book exists because the editors believe that a reference textbook on dentistry for children was needed that was, by design, developmentally organized. This book has been written in the belief that age is so incredibly relevant to pediatric dentistry that by presenting information according to a developmental organization, a student's appreciation of the science and techniques needed to effectively practice dentistry for children will be enlarged.

Those words are still critical for this new edition. In 1988 they seemed almost pioneering in that they allowed the book to use the word "infancy" in its title. It was felt by the editors that the next refinement in preventive dentistry for children had to embrace all children as early in age as possible. Prevention should not wait for the child's linguistic maturity. This customary age of 3 just did not make sense in terms of diet, home care, fluoride needs, habits, and other preventive dentistry concerns. Infancy has to be embraced by the contemporary dentist who values the prevention of dental disease in his or her child patients. Having a dental home cannot come too early for any child.

The developmental design also allows for a focus on the adolescent patient whose needs are unique when compared with children age 12 years and younger. Issues like periodontal disease, trauma, and esthetic dentistry, though important for children of all ages, often become pivotal concerns for these maturing patients.

The other two developmental divisions of the book are the primary dentition years (3 to 6) and the transitional years (6 to 12). All four age-related divisions have their own diagnoses and treatment planning as well as prevention chapters. This allows for the age-related focus that parallels the realities of clinical pediatric dental care.

At some point in the maturity of the clinician who treats children there is an appreciation of how dynamic the world of pediatric dentistry is when assessed by age. The 3-year-old presents an entirely different dentition than the 15-year-old. The panoramic x-ray of a 5-year-old is an image very different from that of a 10-year-old. The behavior of children changes from one recall appointment to the next. Their treatment needs tend to fit into different age zones. This dynamism of change is one of the challenges of pediatric dentistry and for many practitioners one of the joys of this area of clinical practice. This book honors that dynamic.

Jimmy R. Pinkham, DDS, MS
Emeritus Professor of Pediatric Dentistry
University of Iowa

Preface

Why a new edition now?

We live in a world of change. New information is constantly being reported. With the explosion of the internet into every office, home, and pocket, we are inundated with information on new discoveries, new drugs, and new procedures. Time-honored treatments are challenged and replaced with new evidence-based possibilities. And so it is in pediatric dentistry.

Since the 2013 edition, our understanding of the importance of oral health in systemic health has grown; children can grow and develop without cavities; the caries process is preventable; early stress in the infant's life can have profound effects on the child's growth, development, and behavior; common risk factors have been identified that lead to both obesity and cavities; we know more about the contribution of genetics to susceptibility or resistance to dental caries; infant oral health is embraced by many primary care providers, dentists, and parents; the importance of caries risk assessment early in the baby's life during the well-baby visits by primary care providers is now understood; fluoride content of community waters has been updated; fluoride varnish applications have become standard practice; use of esthetic crowns to restore badly destroyed primary teeth is now a common treatment option; use of medicinal agents to arrest the caries process is common; new treatments for vital and necrotic primary pulps are now available; retention of traumatized teeth has been extended; regenerative endodontic techniques for luxated teeth with open apices hold promise; and adolescent health, risky behaviors including smoking/vaping, bullying, and suicide, and transition from pediatric to adult dental supervision have become a part of our practice.

This sixth edition is intended for all audiences from the undergraduate dental student, to residents in training, and, finally, to seasoned practitioners. In addition, those in the allied health professions will also find the text an excellent reference for understanding the oral health needs of all children.

With this edition, we introduce four new associate editors whose enthusiasm and creativity were greatly appreciated by the senior editor. In addition, 35 new contributors have been invited to continue the work contributed by 57 colleagues in the first five editions.

The support this textbook receives is greatly appreciated. The text is recognized by educational programs throughout the world. All chapters have been comprehensively reviewed and updated with evidence-based references and guideline-supported recommendations.

What else is new? The text is now available electronically through the Expert Consult platform. Many chapters are accompanied by case studies and videos to enhance the learning experience.

Thirty years ago the first edition of the textbook was designed around developmental stages of childhood, whereby most textbooks were disease oriented. This format highlights the dramatic changes in the patients we treat as they develop from infancy through adolescence and has proven its benefit to learners.

The foundation for a lifetime of good oral health is established early in the child's life, maybe even before a child is born. We hope this new edition of *Pediatric Dentistry: Infancy Through Adolescence* will provide you with information and tools to provide optimal oral health care for all your pediatric patients.

Lastly, I would like to acknowledge the following individuals from Elsevier who helped produce this edition: Jennifer Flynn-Briggs, Senior Content Strategist; Kelly Skelton and Angie Breckon, Content Development Specialists; Rae Robertson, Senior Content Development Specialist; Brian Salisbury, Book Designer; and Kristine Feeherty, Book Production Specialist.

Arthur J. Nowak

Contents

Video Contents

Fundamentals of Pediatric Dentistry

Children are not small adults. Children have unique needs based on their ethnicity, stage of development, family composition, medical history, temperament, and mental well-being. Therefore this first part with 12 chapters provides information and themes pertinent to children of all ages. Unfortunately, children continue to be vulnerable to dental and oral diseases, and those from poor and minority families are the most at risk. This first part will further your understanding of children and set the stage for the remaining four age-related parts.

1

The Importance of Pediatric Dentistry

PAUL S. CASAMASSIMO AND JANICE A. TOWNSEND

The world continues to change around us, and since the last edition of this textbook, changing social mores in this country and events around the world have shown that children, now more than ever, are vulnerable to oral disease and its complications. The dentist unquestionably has the responsibility to educate and advocate for a childhood free of pain and dental disease for all children regardless of nationality, ethnicity, or socioeconomic background. Fortunately science and technology have improved our ability to care for these children. This chapter attempts to place the changes affecting the oral health of children into a clearer picture for the general practitioner and pediatric dental specialist and create a broader concept of the dental home to best serve the interests of children.

Table 1.1 provides a timeline that depicts the evolution of dentistry for children. The historic mission of pediatric dentistry was threefold: stop the advance of early childhood caries (ECC) with restoration, pulp therapy, and extraction; establish prevention to stop recurrence of disease; and develop a regular care seeker to help ensure oral health into adulthood. In truth, the mission differed little from that for adults. It was not until the turn of the last century that the dental profession recognized the continuing epidemic of ECC and its disparate effect on the poor and under-served minority communities and a broader view of pediatric dentistry began to emerge.[1,2] Overlaying this continued epidemic was a changing social matrix that altered traditional doctor-directed care into a more complex mosaic that still accounted for management of dental caries but within a more complicated set of expectations and conditions.[3] Parents, society, the media, other professionals, and a host of environmental and scientific variables emerged to challenge traditional approaches to the tripartite mission of pediatric dentistry.[4] In Table 1.2, we attempt to lay out these changes, using the multidimensional model of Fisher-Owens et al.[5] The remainder of this chapter explains how these new variables impact the delivery of care to children and preview much of what will follow in more detail on current therapies used in pediatric dentistry.

Prevention and Diagnosis

For decades, our preventive arsenal remained the same, with a four-part message of drink fluoridated water, brush teeth with fluoridated dentifrice, eat wisely (which meant low sugar intake), and see a dentist twice a year. We have moved from a general blanket preventive message to one that is keyed to the individual child and the family's characteristics based on caries risk assessment (CRA), better diagnosis of caries, and an ever-increasing choice of preventive agents, including fluoride varnish and silver diamine fluoride (SDF).[6] Digital radiography and other electronic diagnostic tools offer better assessment of caries progression, adding to our ability to more conservatively and individually manage this disease.[7] Dental sealants have withstood critical review and achieved universal acceptance as a caries preventive technique promising a significant reduction in the lifelong caries experience of many Americans.[8] Also gaining universal acceptance is CRA, which promises to be a useful chairside diagnostic also supporting individualized, patient-centered care. More research is needed to achieve the sensitivity and specificity of a truly useful clinical tool. When CRA is matched with early intervention, the promise of a "cavity-free generation" may finally be realized.[9]

Behavior Guidance

Along with advances in dental science are changes in how children and families engage the dental profession in oral health care. Longstanding beliefs on how best to manage a child's in-office behavior and communicate with families have been reassessed as society changes and views on the value of oral health, acceptance of advice and trust of health professionals, and parental involvement in direct provision of care evolve. No doubt, the generational changes that affect both providers and parents have made interaction with children at chairside more challenging.[10,11] Similarly, the concentration of ECC in the poor and minority child populations and the emergence of cultural subgroups needing care have complicated a hierarchical approach to child behavior.[12,13] The application of basic behavior guidance techniques advocated by the American Academy of Pediatric Dentistry (AAPD) now must be meshed with our deeper understanding of adverse childhood experiences (ACEs) in the lives of those most affected with dental caries and, even more simply, the cultural overlays that, for example, limit touch and gender interactions in a clinical setting.[14] Parents

TABLE 1.1	Milestones in Dentistry for Children in the United States
1900	Few children are treated in dental offices. Little or no instruction in the care of "baby teeth" is given in the 50 dental schools in the United States.
1924	First comprehensive textbook on dentistry for children is published.
1926	The Gies Report on dental education notes that only 5 of the 43 dental schools in the United States have facilities especially designed for treating children.
1927	After almost a decade of frustration in getting a group organized to promote dentistry for children, the American Society for the Promotion of Dentistry for Children is established at the meeting of the American Dental Association (ADA) in Detroit.
1932	A report of the College Committee of the American Society for the Promotion of Dentistry for Children states that in 1928, 15 dental schools provided no clinical experience with children and 22 schools had no didactic information in this area.
1935	Six graduate programs and eight postgraduate programs exist in pedodontics.
1940	The American Society for the Promotion of Dentistry for Children changes its name to the American Society of Dentistry for Children.
1941	Children's Dental Health Day is observed in Cleveland, Ohio, and Children's Dental Health Week is observed in Akron, Ohio.
1942	The effectiveness of topical fluoride applications at preventing caries is described. The Council on Dental Education recommends that all dental schools have pedodontics as part of their curriculum.
1945	First artificial water fluoridation plant is begun at Grand Rapids, Michigan.
1947	The American Academy of Pedodontics is formed. (To a large degree, the start of the Academy was prompted by the need for a more scientifically focused organization concerned with the dental health of children.)
1948	The American Board of Pedodontics, a group formulated to certify candidates in the practice of dentistry for children, is formally recognized by the Council on Dental Education of the ADA.
1949	The first full week of February is designated National Children's Dental Health Week.
1955	The acid-etch technique is described.
1960	Eighteen graduate programs and 17 postgraduate programs in pedodontics exist.
1964	Crest becomes the first ADA-approved fluoridated toothpaste.
1974	The International Workshop on Fluorides and Dental Caries Reductions recommends that appropriate fluoride supplementation begin as soon after birth as possible. (This recommendation was later modified by authorities to start at 6 months of age.)
1981	February is designated National Children's Dental Health Month.
1983	A Consensus Development Conference held at the National Institutes of Dental Health endorses the effectiveness and usefulness of sealants.
1984	The American Academy of Pedodontics changes its name to the American Academy of Pediatric Dentistry.
1995	A new definition is adopted for the specialty of pediatric dentistry by the ADA's House of Delegates: *Pediatric dentistry* is an age-defined specialty that provides both primary and comprehensive preventive and therapeutic oral health care for infants and children through adolescence, including those with special health care needs.
2003	The AAP establishes "Policy Statement on Oral Health Risk Assessment Timing and Establishment of a Dental Home," and issuance of this policy statement will be manifested in several outcomes, including the need to identify effective means for rapid screening in pediatricians' offices, and the mechanisms for swift referral and intervention for high-risk children.
2011	The AAPD establishes the Pediatric Oral Health Research and Policy Center to inform and advance research and policy analysis to promote optimal oral health care for children.
2017	Pediatric Dentistry MATCH results show 676 applicants for 408 positions, which exceeds all other specialties.

AAP, American Academy of Pediatrics; *AAPD*, American Academy of Pediatric Dentistry.

want to be present during treatment and will seek providers who will commit to that practice.[15]

Pharmacologic management of behavior continues to be a major consideration in pediatric dental care but has also seen dramatic change. Sedation deaths have prompted new guidelines, better training, and better patient monitoring and, of course, greater scrutiny of how this service is delivered.[16,17] Drugs such as chloral hydrate, long a staple of pediatric sedation, have largely been replaced by medications thought to be safer and reversible.[18] General anesthesia for dental care has seen a dramatic increase, in part due to the epidemic of ECC. In spite of that pharmacologic option being the top choice of parents, it too is challenged by cost, availability of surgical sites, and growing research on possible effects of anesthetics on early brain development.[19] Also driving the changes in behavior guidance is a greater recognition of the role of pain in behaviors, both chairside and in care seeking.[20]

TABLE 1.2   **A Cross-Millennium View of the Changing Character of Pediatric Dentistry**

Traditional Elements of Pediatric Oral Care for Children	Current and Future Directions and Their Drivers
Prevention	
• Diagnosis with traditional radiography and caries diagnostics	• Digital radiography and electronic caries detection
• A preventive arsenal composed largely of fluoride options including water fluoridation, fluoride dentifrice, office fluoride, fluoride supplements, and at home over-the-counter (OTC) fluoride rinses	• Prevention continues to emphasize most traditional modalities but now includes fluoride varnish, silver diamine fluoride (SDF), and a caries risk paradigm to the application of fluoride and other techniques, discontinuing supplementation
• Dental sealants to prevent occlusal and pit and fissure caries selectively applied	• Dental sealants now evidence-based and accepted universally as a primary preventive technique and may have therapeutic implications
• Caries risk assessment not considered essential to provision of preventive services	• Caries risk assessment now considered integral to preventive therapeutic plans and compensation for preventive services
Behavioral Guidance	
• Simplistic application of communicative and more advanced techniques based on chairside behaviors and special needs with dentist directing choice	• More sophisticated application of techniques with attention to chairside and other aspects of behavior with a strong parental advisement component
• Parental separation from clinical aspects of care	• Recognition of the changing parental attitudes toward restraint, pharmacologic management, and parental presence
• All children managed with the same paradigm and hierarchy of behavior techniques without regard to systemic, emotional, and other mitigating factors	• Recognition of the effects of poverty on child behavior from toxic stress and adverse childhood experiences (ACEs)
• Pain and anxiety addressed primarily as preoperative treatment need	• Greater understanding and subsequent management of pain and anxiety as factors in care avoidance, social and developmental behaviors, and intraoperative outcomes during dental treatment
• Largely office-based nonpharmacologic management of behavior	• Newer models of advanced behavior guidance using sedation, general anesthesia in-office with dental and medical anesthesiologists and surgery centers
• Simplistic vision of behavior in the dental office based on traditional family structure, majority social characteristics, and middle-class value system	• Recognition of the contribution of culture, poverty, and other nontraditional factors on behavior in the dental office
Treatment of ECC	
• Simplistic armamentarium of composite, amalgam, stainless steel crowns	• Fuller integration of preveneered crowns, zirconia crowns, resin infiltration
• Pulpotomy as a preferred therapy using formocresol, ferric sulfate	• Pulp therapy with fuller range options, including indirect techniques, mineral trioxide aggregate (MTA)
• Emphasis on immediate and primary tooth lifespan success in choice of materials and techniques	• Addition of safety and toxicity concerns in choices of restorative care
• Definitive treatment (restoration or extraction) in most cases of ECC	• Consideration of a range of treatment options including deferral of treatment, use of fluoride and other caries-static agents like SDF teamed with more frequent interventions
Dental Diseases Emphasis	
• Dental caries as the preeminent singular driver of care for children	• Greater recognition of esthetic concerns (fluorosis, tooth whiteness) in pediatric dentistry • Emergence of new conditions such as molar-incisal hypocalcification (MIH) and dental erosion as treatment considerations
Systemic Disease and Conditions and Oral Health	
• Traditional disease entities occurring in predictable patterns allowing application of consistent management	• New disease entities such as obesity and its management considerations; other eating disorders; increase in autism spectrum
• Predictable dental outcomes based on disease progression in special needs patients	• Lifespan elongation with complications of end-organ damage, effects of new medication and growing technology dependence to support life and function

TABLE 1.2	A Cross-Millennium View of the Changing Character of Pediatric Dentistry—cont'd	
Traditional Elements of Pediatric Oral Care for Children	**Current and Future Directions and Their Drivers**
Practice Considerations	
• Paper-based records and office management	• Digitalization of records, billing, imaging, and laboratory procedures
• Simplistic safety orientation (OSHA, NIOSH, CDC)	• Office safety including risk mitigation, growing concerns about radiation exposure with introduction of CBCT and other digital advances; HIPAA changes, waterline management
• Global dental consent procedures	• Changing consent requirements based on procedures
• Regional and training-based care patterns	• Emergence of evidence-based guidelines for pediatric dental care

CBCT, Cone-beam computed tomography; *CDC*, Centers for Disease Control and Prevention; *ECC*, early childhood caries; *HIPAA*, Health Insurance Portability and Accountability Act of 1996; *NIOSH*, National Institute for Occupational Safety and Health; *OSHA*, Occupational Safety and Health Administration.

We more often confront a very young child who has been in pain from dental caries for many days, challenging the simple notion that pain control is confined to administration of local anesthesia.[21]

The science and clinical translation of anxiety, pain, and pharmacologic behavior guidance will likely continue. Our tools will also change as we add more powerful local anesthetics, such as articaine and intranasally administered local anesthesia, and as reversal agents like phentolamine sodium gain acceptance.[22,23] The subsequent chapters in this text address both longstanding and new approaches to management of pain, anxiety, and chairside behavior.

Treatment Options

The treatment of ECC continues to change with the science of materials and understanding of biology of the oral cavity and teeth. Today, clinicians can approach pulpal therapy with more choices and better outcomes. Mineral trioxide aggregate (MTA) and bioactive glass stand to revolutionize both permanent and primary teeth pulpal therapy.[24] Indirect pulp caps with various agents, including traditional calcium hydroxide and more recent glass ionomer cements, have challenged traditional thinking that a primary tooth with a large carious lesion is doomed to invasive pulp therapy.[25,26] Traumatic injuries now benefit from larger and longer studies that direct clinicians to better outcomes. Autotransplantation is now an accepted technique for hopeless permanent teeth due to caries or trauma.[27,28] Advances in regeneration techniques can now add vitality to immature teeth that traditionally had a poor long-term prognosis and may lead to full tooth regeneration in the future, as well as other systemic therapies.[29]

Restorative choices for primary teeth continue to increase. The strip crown, long a stalwart of anterior primary tooth restoration, has been joined by the preveneered stainless steel crown. Zirconia crowns, offering better esthetics, strength, and technique ease, are gaining favor, especially for posterior primary teeth.[30] The open-faced stainless steel crown has joined its less esthetic stainless steel crown in the annals of pediatric history. Bioactive restorative materials may lead to a class of restorative materials with intrinsic reparative abilities.[31]

Perhaps the most exciting advance in care of ECC, especially for very young children, is the expansion of our thinking about treatment urgency, restoration longevity, and adjunctive nonrestorative care. Restoration or extraction once dominated treatment of ECC, and application was often immediate, with accompanying use of behavioral techniques to accomplish care. Today, clinicians can reliably use nonrestorative techniques to stop ECC's advance, such as fluoride varnish and SDF, and avoid a costly general anesthetic that too often is just a precursor to another one later on.[32,33] A Hall technique crown can also be reliably and safely placed to stop caries and restore function, requiring minimal cooperation by the child.[34] The advances in treatment of ECC have made care safer, more effective, and more palatable to many families.

Dental Disease Emphasis and Systemic Disease

ECC has long been and remains the driver of attendance in a dental home, but other conditions have emerged as considerations in pediatric dental care, such as fluorosis, esthetic challenges, and management of molar-incisor hypocalcification.[35] Dental erosion has moved from an isolated condition suggestive of an eating disorder to a more widespread condition of children.[36] These conditions join inherited disorders of the dentition, such as amelogenesis imperfecta, intrinsic staining, and tooth number irregularities, as important intersection points in childhood oral assessment.

Systemic diseases affecting children fall into the purview of dentists caring for children by default. Caring for those children with special needs requires a working knowledge of medical, functional, and social and programming aspects of the lives of these children. Medical advances have prolonged life in many conditions but brought into play technology dependence, such as cerebral shunts and implanted devices, and organ effects from drugs, surgery, or the continued onslaught of the original condition. Care of these children requires the dentist to understand the disease, its treatment, and the effects on oral physiology and function, but more so today, the social and programmatic aspects of the lives of these children.[37] Although pediatric dentists continue to take the lead in caring for the very young with special needs, the intent of our health care system is to transition them to adult care as their dental needs grow outside the usual concerns of pediatric dentistry.[38,39]

Contemporary Practice and Care of Children

As all dental practice moves along the path of growing sophistication and digitalization, those areas addressing care of children follow. Paper-based offices are a thing of the past, and movement to the full electronic office means systems that can track caries risk, health histories, referrals, and serial disease manifestations and treatment. Models, radiographs, and analyses of the developing dentition are now electronic files.[40] As treatment techniques advance using lasers and other approaches, consent procedures for children become more complicated, especially with changing family structures. Office design, toys, and other aspects of dental offices have special considerations when children are a part of the patient family.

The concern of parents about safety of their children requires a more detailed attention to safety considerations, regulations, and office environment. Basic infection control remains a keystone of patient safety, but waterline safety, chemicals in dental materials, and radiation have emerged as special considerations in the dental care of children.[41] A growing area is interprofessional care, which suggests that dentists treating children need to heed obesity, immunizations, and other areas not necessarily considered in the realm of dentistry. Child abuse continues to be a required safety consideration for those treating children.

This Edition

Many of these topics are dealt with in depth in this latest edition. New chapters on management of patients with cleft lip and palate and cariology have been added to address the changing nature of oral health care for children. New online content has been added to enhance the understanding of basic principles and to address advanced topics in pediatric dentistry. The textbook retains its developmental view of pediatric dentistry, validating its changing science, including the benefits of early intervention and new age-related conditions and treatments. The text continues to offer in-depth chapters on many techniques and its age epoch diagnostic sections. Welcome to this sixth edition!

References

1. U.S. Department of Health and Human Services. Oral Health in America: A Report of the Surgeon General. Rockville, MD: U.S. Department of Health and Human Services, National Institute of Dental and Craniofacial Research, National Institutes of Health, 2000.
2. Fisher-Owens S. Broadening perspectives on pediatric oral health care provision: social determinants of health and behavioral management. *Pediatr Dent.* 2014;36(2):115–120.
3. Sheller B. Challenges of managing child behavior in the 21st century dental setting. *Pediatr Dent.* 2004;26(2):111–113.
4. Stange DM. The evolution of behavior guidance: a history of professional, practice, corporate and societal influences. *Pediatr Dent.* 2014;36(2):128–131.
5. Fisher-Owens SA, Gansky SA, Platt LJ, et al. Influences on children's oral health: a conceptual model. *Pediatrics.* 2017;120(3):e510–e520.
6. Slayton RL. Clinical decision-making for caries management in children: an update. *Pediatr Dent.* 2015;37(2):106–110.
7. Berg J. Caries detection tools keep making progress. *Compendium Contin Educ Dent.* 2012;33(9):696.
8. Wright JT, Crall JJ, Fontana M, et al. Evidence-based clinical practice guideline for the use of pit-and-fissure sealants: a report of the American Dental Association and the American Academy of Pediatric Dentistry. *J Am Dent Assoc.* 2016;147(8):672–682.
9. Fontana M. The clinical, environmental, and behavioral factors that foster early childhood caries: evidence for caries risk assessment. *Pediatr Dent.* 2015;37(3):217–225.
10. Wells M, McTigue DJ, Casmassio PS, et al. Gender shifts and effects on behavior guidance. *Pediatr Dent.* 2014;36(2):138–144.
11. Juntgen LM, Sanders BJ, Walker LA, et al. Factors influencing behavior guidance: a survey of practicing pediatric dentists. *Pediatr Dent.* 2013;35(7):539–545.
12. da Fonseca MA. Eat or heat? The effects of poverty on children's behavior. *Pediatr Dent.* 2014;36(2):132–137.
13. Goleman J. Cultural factors affecting behavior guidance and family compliance. *Pediatr Dent.* 2014;36(2):121–127.
14. Boyce WT. The lifelong effects of early childhood adversity and toxic stress. *Pediatr Dent.* 2014;36(2):102–108.
15. Shroff S, Hughes C, Mobley C. Attitudes and preferences of parents about being present in the dental operatory. *Pediatr Dent.* 2015;37(1):51–55.
16. Lee HH, Milgrom P, Starks H, et al. Trends in death associated with pediatric dental sedation and general anesthesia. *Paediatr Anaesth.* 2013;23(8):741–746.
17. American Academy of Pediatric Dentistry. Guideline for monitoring and management of pediatric patients before, during, and after sedation for diagnostic and therapeutic procedures: update 2016. *Pediatr Dent.* 2016;38(6):216–245.
18. Wilson S, Houpt M. Project USAP 2010: use of sedative agents in pediatric dentistry—a 25-year follow-up survey. *Pediatr Dent.* 2016;38(2):127–133.
19. SmartTots. Consensus statement regarding anesthesia safety in children. Available at: http://smarttots.org/smarttots-releases-consensus-statement-regarding-anesthesia-safety-in-young-children/. Accessed April 17, 2017.
20. Nutter DP. Good clinical pain practice for pediatric procedure pain: target considerations. *J Calif Dent Assoc.* 2009;37(10):719–722.
21. Thikkurissy S, Allen PH, Smiley MK, et al. Waiting for the pain to get worse: characteristics of a pediatric population with acute dental pain. *Pediatr Dent.* 2012;34(4):289–294.
22. Malamed S. What's new in local anaesthesia? *SAAD Dig.* 2009;25:4–14.
23. Hersh EV, Pinto A, Saraghi M, et al. Double-masked, randomized, placebo-controlled study to evaluate the efficacy and tolerability of intranasal K305 (3% tetracaine plus 0.05% oxymetazoline) in anesthetizing maxillary teeth. *J Am Dent Assoc.* 2016;147(4):278–287.
24. Smaïl-Faugeron V, Courson F, Durieux P, et al. Pulp treatment for extensive decay in primary teeth. *Cochrane Database Syst Rev.* 2014;(8):CD003220.
25. Hoefler V, Nagaoka H, Miller CS. Long-term survival and vitality outcomes of permanent teeth following deep caries treatment with step-wise and partial-caries-removal: a systematic review. *J Dent.* 2016;54:25–32.
26. Smaïl-Faugeron V, Porot A, Muller-Bolla M, et al. Indirect pulp capping versus pulpotomy for treating deep carious lesions approaching the pulp in primary teeth: a systematic review. *Eur J Paediatr Dent.* 2016;17(2):107–112.
27. Yu HJ, Jia P, Lv Z, et al. Autotransplantation of third molars with completely formed roots into surgically created sockets and fresh extraction sockets: a 10-year comparative study. *Int J Oral Maxillofac Surg.* 2017;46(4):531–538.
28. Waldon K, Barber SK, Spencer RJ, et al. Indications for the use of auto-transplantation of teeth in the child and adolescent. *Eur Arch Paediatr Dent.* 2012;13(4):210–216.
29. Rombouts C, Giraud T, Jeanneau C, et al. Pulp vascularization during tooth development, regeneration, and therapy. *J Dent Res.* 2017;96(2):137–144.
30. Waggoner WF. Restoring primary anterior teeth: updated for 2014. *Pediatr Dent.* 2015;37(2):163–170.
31. Croll TP, Berg JH, Donly KJ. Dental repair material: a resin-modified glass-ionomer bioactive ionic resin-based composite. *Compend Contin Educ Dent.* 2015;36(1):60–65.

32. Milgrom P, Zero DT, Tanzer JM. An examination of the advances in science and technology of prevention of tooth decay in young children since the Surgeon General's Report on Oral Health. *Acad Pediatr.* 2009;9(6):404–409.

33. Horst JA, Ellenikjotis H, Milgrom PL. UCSF protocol for caries arrest using silver diamine fluoride: rationale, indications and consent. *J Calif Dent Assoc.* 2016;44(1):16–28.

34. Innes NP, Ricketts D, Chong LY, et al. Preformed crowns for decayed primary molar teeth. *Cochrane Database Syst Rev.* 2015;(12):CD005512.

35. Elhennawy K, Schwendicke F. Managing molar-incisor hypomineralization: a systematic review. *J Dent.* 2016;55:16–24.

36. Corica A, Caprioglio A. Meta-analysis of the prevalence of tooth wear in primary dentition. *Eur J Paediatr Dent.* 2014;15(4):385–388.

37. American Academy of Pediatric Dentistry. Policy on the ethical responsibilities in the oral health care management of infants, children, adolescents, and individuals with special health care needs. *Pediatr Dent.* 2016;38(6):124–125.

38. Cruz S, Neff J, Chi DL. Transitioning from pediatric to adult dental care for adolescents with special health care needs: adolescent and parent perspectives—part one. *Pediatr Dent.* 2015;37(5):442–446.

39. Bayarsaikhan Z, Cruz S, Neff J, et al. Transitioning from pediatric to adult dental care for adolescents with special health care needs: dentist perspectives—part two. *Pediatr Dent.* 2015;37(5):447–451.

40. Fleming PS, Marinho V, Johal A. Orthodontic measurements on digital study models compared with plaster models: a systematic review. *Orthod Craniofac Res.* 2011;14(1):1–16.

41. Wirthlin MR, Roth M. Dental unit waterline contamination: a review of research and findings from a clinic setting. *Compend Contin Educ Dent.* 2015;36(3):216–219.

2

Differential Diagnosis of Oral Lesions and Developmental Anomalies

CATHERINE M. FLAITZ

A wide variety of oral lesions and soft tissue anomalies are detected in children, but the low frequency at which many of these entities occur makes them challenging to clinically diagnose. The purpose of this chapter is to highlight selected oral lesions that are most commonly found in children and pathologic entities that primarily develop in this age group. In addition, oral lesions associated with several genetic disorders and specific malignancies, which may mimic benign or inflammatory conditions, are included to broaden the disease scope. The material is outlined in tables to make this comprehensive subject more succinct and easier to review. The brief description for each entity summarizes the most important clinical information that is relevant to the child patient. Representative examples of these conditions are included to illustrate the characteristic clinical or radiographic features.

Each oral lesion is described according to key points: (1) the most common pediatric age group affected and the gender predilection, (2) the characteristic clinical and radiographic findings of the lesion, (3) the most frequent location for the lesion, (4) the pediatric significance of the lesion, (5) the treatment and prognosis for the lesion, and (6) the differential diagnosis that is pertinent to this age group.

Except for the first table on selected developmental anomalies, the other tables are arranged to capture the primary clinical or radiographic characteristics for the purpose of comparison. The sequential headings for each of the tables include the following disease categories:

Developmental anomalies (Table 2.1, Fig. 2.1)
White soft tissue lesions (Table 2.2, Fig. 2.2)
 White surface thickening lesions
 White surface material lesions
 White subsurface lesions
Dark soft tissue lesions (Table 2.3, Fig. 2.3)
 Red or purple-blue lesions
 Brown-black lesions
Ulcerative lesions (Table 2.4, Fig. 2.4)
Soft tissue enlargements (Table 2.5, Fig. 2.5)
 Papillary lesions
 Acute inflammatory lesions
 Tumor and tumorlike lesions
Radiolucent lesions of bone (Table 2.6, Fig. 2.6)
Mixed radiolucent and radiopaque lesions of bone (Table 2.7, Fig. 2.7)
Radiopaque lesions of bone (Table 2.8, Fig. 2.8)

Bibliography

American Academy of Pediatric Dentistry Reference Manual. Useful medications for oral conditions. *Pediatr Dent.* 2016;38(6):443–450.

Greer RO, Marx RE, Said S, et al. *Pediatric Head and Neck Pathology.* New York: Cambridge University Press; 2017.

Hennekam R, Krantz I, Allanson J. *Gorlin's Syndromes of the Head and Neck.* 5th ed. New York: Oxford University Press; 2010.

Kolokythas A, Miloro M. Pediatric oral and maxillofacial pathology. *Oral Maxillofac Surg Clin North Am.* 2016;28(1):ix–x.

Neville BW, Damm DD, Allen CM, et al. *Oral & Maxillofacial Pathology.* 4th ed. St Louis: Elsevier; 2016.

Philipone E, Yoon AJ. *Oral Pathology in the Pediatric Patient. A Clinical Guide to the Diagnosis and Treatment of Mucosal Lesions.* Heidelberg: Springer; 2017.

Scully C, Welbury R, Flaitz C, et al. *A Color Atlas of Orofacial Health and Disease in Children and Adolescents.* 2nd ed. London: Martin Dunitz; 2002.

Woo S-B. *Oral Pathology: A Comprehensive Atlas and Text.* New York: Elsevier; 2012.

TABLE 2.1   Developmental Anomalies (see Fig. 2.1)

Condition	Pediatric Age and Gender	Clinical Findings	Location	Pediatric Significance	Treatment and Prognosis	Differential Diagnosis
Fissured tongue (scrotal tongue)	First and second decades No gender predilection	Deep central groove; multiple, short furrows; tender, if irritated; may occur with *erythema migrans*	Dorsal and lateral tongue	Polygenic or autosomal dominant trait; occurs in *Down syndrome*, dry mouths, diabetes; detected in 1% of children; source of halitosis	Brush tongue; becomes more prominent with age	Erythema migrans Macroglossia with crenations Hemihyperplasia of tongue Orofacial granulomatosis
Ankyloglossia (tongue-tie)	Present at birth Male predilection	Short, thick lingual frenum or attachment to tip of tongue; may cause slight cleft at tip	Ventral tongue and floor of mouth	Occurs in 2%–11% of infants; rarely causes speech, feeding, swallowing or periodontal problems; multiple frenula associated with *oral-facial-digital* syndrome	Infrequently frenectomy is indicated; many self-correct with age	Bifid tongue Microglossia Palatoglossal adhesion (ankyloglossia superior) Tongue scar
Lingual thyroid	Second decade Female predilection	Nodular mass with pink or red, smooth surface; may cause dysphagia, dysphonia, or dyspnea	Midline base of tongue; *thyroglossal duct cyst* is variant that occurs in midline neck	Symptoms develop during puberty or pregnancy; normal thyroid absent in 70%; important cause of infantile hypothyroidism	Thyroid hormone therapy, excision or radioactive iodine ablation; carcinomas arise in <1%	Lymphoid hyperplasia Hemangioma Lymphangioma Epiglottis
Commissural lip pits	Second decade Male predilection	Unilateral or bilateral depressions or fistulas; fluid may be expressed	Corners of mouth	Occurs in <1% of children; an association with preauricular pits	None required	Paramedian lip pits Angular cheilitis
Paramedian lip pits (congenital lip pits)	Present at birth No gender predilection	Bilateral and symmetric depressions or swellings; fluid may be expressed	Adjacent to the midline of the lower lip vermilion	Autosomal dominant trait; associated with cleft lip and palate; van der Woude and other syndromes	None required; surgery, if cosmetic problem	Mucocele Soft tissue abscess Median lip fissure Double lip Lip piercing
Retrocuspid papilla	First and second decades Female predilection	Asymptomatic, pink, sessile papule or nodule; usually bilateral	Lingual attached gingiva, adjacent to mandibular canines	Very common in children and regresses with age	None required; normal anatomic variation	Irritation fibroma Giant cell fibroma Soft tissue abscess
Bifid uvula	Present at birth No gender predilection	Midline groove or splitting of uvula; may have speech impairment	Midline, posterior soft palate	Minimal expression of cleft palate; marker for submucous palatal cleft; associated with *Loeys-Dietz syndrome* and others	None required; genetic counseling may be indicated	Traumatic defect

Continued

Developmental Anomalies (see Fig. 2.1)—cont'd

Condition	Pediatric Age and Gender	Clinical Findings	Location	Pediatric Significance	Treatment and Prognosis	Differential Diagnosis
Hyperplastic labial frenum	Present at birth No gender predilection	Thick triangular band of pink soft tissue; may be associated with gingival recession or diastema	Midline labial mucosa and gingiva; both maxillary and mandibular lip	Bleeds freely when lacerated; multiple frenula associated with *oral-facial-digital syndrome;* rare breastfeeding problems	None required; frenectomy for some large diastemas, gingival recession or lip mobility problems	Traumatic scar Frenal tag
Torus palatinus (palatal torus)	Second decade Female predilection	Bony hard mass that varies in size and shape; asymptomatic, unless traumatized; rarely seen as radiopacity on radiographs	Midline hard palate	Most tori in this age group are slightly elevated with a smooth surface; autosomal dominant inheritance or multifactorial influence	None required; will continue to grow during adulthood	Prominent median palatal raphe Palatal exostosis Median palatal cyst
Torus mandibularis (mandibular torus)	Second decade Male predilection	Bony hard mass that varies in size and shape; asymptomatic, unless traumatized; radiopacity may be superimposed over roots of teeth	Bilateral, lingual mandible	Less common than torus palatinus; genetic and environmental influence	None required; will continue to grow during adulthood	Exostosis Peripheral osteoma Proliferative periostitis Fibrous dysplasia Condensing osteitis Idiopathic osteosclerosis
Exostosis	Second decade No gender predilection	Single or multiple bony hard nodules; asymptomatic, unless traumatized; radiopacity may be superimposed over roots of teeth	Maxillary and mandibular alveolar ridge on the facial aspect; usually bilateral; may occur on the palate	Exostoses that are traumatized mimic odontogenic infection because of the location; may be tender to palpation in children	None required; will continue to grow during adulthood	Peripheral osteoma Proliferative periostitis Ectopic tooth eruption Condensing osteitis Idiopathic osteosclerosis

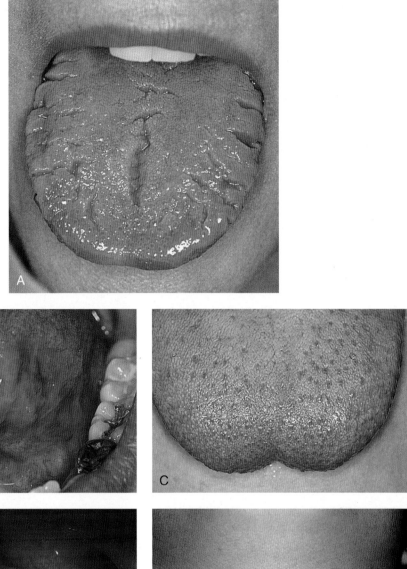

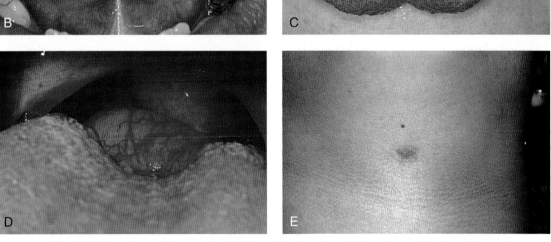

• **Figure 2.1** Developmental anomalies. (A) Fissured tongue. (B and C) Partial ankyloglossia with lingual frenum attachment at the tip of the tongue (B). Note the restricted mobility of the tongue with extension (C). (D) Lingual thyroid of the midline base of the tongue. (E) Thyroglossal duct cyst with sinus tract, midline neck.   *Continued*

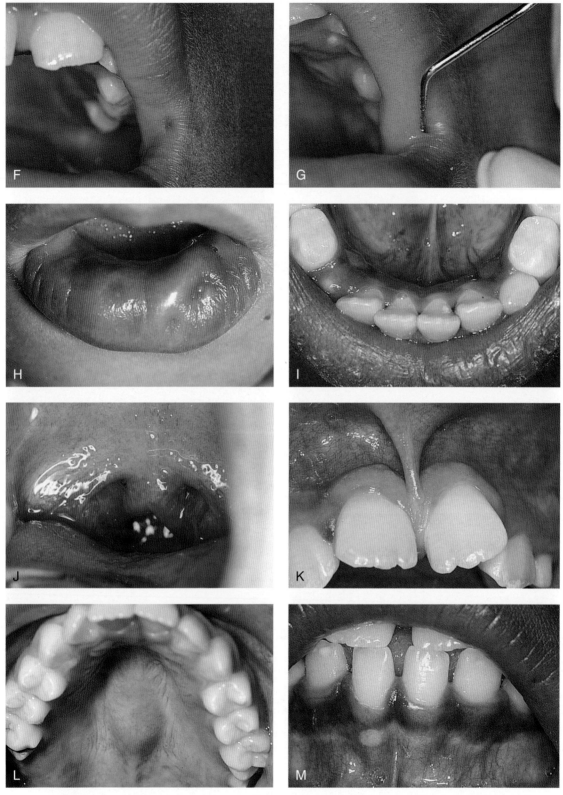

• **Figure 2.1, cont'd** (F and G) Commissural lip pit (F) with depth illustrated by periodontal probe (G). (H) Paramedian lip pits. (I) Retrocuspid papilla of the lingual mandibular gingiva. (J) Bifid uvula. (K) Hyperplastic maxillary labial frenum. (L) Torus palatinus of the midline hard palate. (M) Small exostosis of the anterior mandibular alveolus, facial aspect. ([D] Courtesy Dr. G.E. Lilly, University of Iowa College of Dentistry.)

TABLE 2.2 White Soft Tissue Lesions (see Fig. 2.2)

Lesion	Pediatric Age and Gender	Clinical Findings	Location	Pediatric Significance	Treatment and Prognosis	Differential Diagnosis
White Surface Thickening Lesions						
Frictional keratosis and Morsicatio mucosae oris	First and second decades No gender predilection	Localized to diffuse, white, rough or shredded patches; adherent; asymptomatic	Mucosa adjacent to occlusal plane, including buccal, labial mucosa, lateral tongue; attached gingiva	Caused by chronic nibbling habits *(morsicatio)*, irritation from orthodontic appliances, fractured teeth, and improper tooth brushing	Elimination of cause; lesion regresses; acrylic splint therapy for severe cases of *morsicatio*	Leukoedema Linea alba Smokeless tobacco keratosis Cinnamon contact stomatitis Lupus erythematosus Hyperplastic candidiasis
Smokeless tobacco keratosis (tobacco pouch keratosis)	Second decade Male predilection	Diffuse, white, wrinkled patch; adherent; asymptomatic; gingival recession; tooth staining; caused by snuff or chewing tobacco	Vestibular, labial and buccal mucosa; usually mandibular site	Highly addictive habit; lesions develop after 1–5 years of use; increased risk for periodontal disease, dental caries, tooth sensitivity, and halitosis	Discontinuation of habit results in lesion reversal; biopsy of persistent lesions; low risk for malignant transformation	Leukoedema Frictional keratosis Cinnamon contact stomatitis Chronic hyperplastic candidiasis
Leukoedema	First and second decades No gender predilection	Widespread, filmy white, wrinkled mucosa; adherent; disappears when stretched	Bilateral buccal, labial mucosa and soft palate	Most prominent in black children; condition increases with age; more pronounced in cigarette smokers	None required; common variant of normal mucosa	Frictional keratosis Linea alba White sponge nevus
Cinnamon contact stomatitis	Second decade No gender predilection	Oblong to broadly linear, white plaques with a shaggy, thickened surface; diffuse erythema; tender	Gingiva, mucosa adjacent to occlusal plane, including buccal mucosa and lateral tongue	Cinnamon flavoring in candy, chewing gum, toothpaste, mouth rinses	Identify and discontinue use of offending product; lesions resolve within 1 week	Morsicatio mucosae oris Hyperplastic candidiasis Smokeless tobacco keratosis Hairy leukoplakia

Continued

TABLE
2.2   **White Soft Tissue Lesions (see Fig. 2.2)—cont'd**

Lesion	Pediatric Age and Gender	Clinical Findings	Location	Pediatric Significance	Treatment and Prognosis	Differential Diagnosis
Linea alba	Any age following the eruption of teeth; female predilection	Smooth or shaggy white line; may be scalloped; asymptomatic	Bilateral buccal mucosa, along occlusal plane	Associated with biting irritation or sucking habit; may be associated with leukoedema	None required; may spontaneously regress	Cinnamon contact stomatitis Scar formation Morsicatio mucosae oris
Hairy tongue	Second decade No gender predilection	Cream to brown discoloration; diffuse elongation of filiform papillae	Dorsal tongue	Contributes to halitosis; associated with cigarette smoking, poor oral hygiene, antibiotics, dry mouth, overuse of mouth rinses; coated tongue is more common in children	Eliminate cause; brush tongue	Coated tongue Frictional keratosis Hyperplastic candidiasis
White sponge nevus	First decade, may be present at birth No gender predilection	Diffuse, symmetric, corrugated, or velvety white plaques: adherent; asymptomatic; persistent	Bilateral buccal mucosa is most common; also found on labial mucosa, ventral tongue, floor of mouth, and soft palate	Autosomal dominant skin disorder; defect in *keratin 4* and *keratin 13*; extraoral sites may be involved; reaches full expression during adolescence	None required; condition stabilizes in young adulthood	Leukoedema Hereditary benign intraepithelial dyskeratosis Frictional keratosis Hyperplastic candidiasis Syndrome-related leukoplakia
White Surface Material Lesions						
Pseudomembranous candidiasis (thrush)	Any age, especially infancy No gender predilection	Widespread, white plaques that wipe off leaving a normal or red, raw base; mild burning	Any mucosal site but common on buccal mucosa, tongue, and palate	Caused by *Candida albicans* and other species; contributing factors are antibiotics, steroids, immune suppression; infants may have diaper rash; pacifiers, orthodontic appliances, and toothbrushes may harbor fungus	Antifungal medication and proper oral hygiene; may recur if cause is not eliminated	Plaque Chemical burn Coated tongue Oral mucosal peeling Morsicatio mucosae oris Koplik spots of rubeola

Chemical burn	First and second decades No gender predilection	Localized or widespread, white nonadherent plaques, erosions or ulcers; tender to painful; sudden onset	Any site but common on lips, tongue, buccal mucosa, and gingiva	Multiple chemicals and drugs may cause this reaction, including those used in dentistry—inappropriate use of mouth rinses, topical anesthetics, phenol, formocresol	Identify and remove cause; ask about homeopathic remedies; symptomatic relief management	Thermal burn Pseudomembranous candidiasis Coated tongue Oral mucosal peeling Mucous patch of syphilis
Coated tongue (furred tongue)	First and second decades No gender predilection	White or yellow nonadherent coating on tongue; asymptomatic; may be source of halitosis	Dorsal tongue	Common condition associated with mouth breathing, febrile illnesses, dehydration, poor oral hygiene; source of halitosis	Brushing tongue and adequate hydration; tends to recur	Pseudomembranous candidiasis Hairy tongue White strawberry tongue
Oral mucosal peeling	Second decade No gender predilection	Translucent to white strips of mucosa that peel off; stringy and slimy in texture; may burn	Buccal and labial mucosa, tongue	Associated with detergents and other ingredients in toothpastes and mouth rinses	Identify and discontinue the oral hygiene product; resolves spontaneously	Plaque Pseudomembranous candidiasis Allergic contact stomatitis Thermal/chemical burn
White Subsurface Lesions						
Scar formation (cicatrix)	First and second decades No gender predilection	White or pale pink line or irregular patch with smooth surface; cross-hatch or starburst pattern; asymptomatic	Any site but common on labial mucosa, lip vermilion, tongue	History of oral trauma or surgery; may represent child abuse or self-mutilation	None required; scar revision if cosmetic concern or if restricts function	Linea alba Mucosal graft Lichen planus
Fordyce granules	Second decade Male predilection	Small, yellow-white, multifocal papules; discrete or clustered; asymptomatic	Bilateral buccal mucosa, retromolar pad and upper lip vermilion	Oral sebaceous glands occur in 20%–30% of children; puberty stimulates development	No treatment is necessary; may increase in size; laser treatment for cosmetics	Frictional keratosis Scar formation Pustules Milia

Continued

TABLE 2.2   White Soft Tissue Lesions (see Fig. 2.2)—cont'd

Lesion	Pediatric Age and Gender	Clinical Findings	Location	Pediatric Significance	Treatment and Prognosis	Differential Diagnosis
Oral lymphoepithelial cyst	Second decade No gender predilection	Solitary, soft, pinkish white nodule with superficial fine vascular pattern; usually nontender	Posterior lateral tongue, floor of mouth, soft palate	Mimics an abscess because it may fluctuate in size and discharge contents	Excisional biopsy; does not recur	Soft tissue abscess Lipoma Sialolith Tonsillolith Hyperplastic lymphoid aggregate
Sialolithiasis	Second decade No gender predilection	Solitary or multiple, hard, yellowish white globular mass; episodic pain and swelling when eating; obstructive disease of the duct	Usually floor of mouth within Wharton duct, submandibular gland	Occlusal or panoramic radiograph may assist with diagnosis; circular calcified mass	Massage of gland, surgical removal of stone and sometimes the gland; lithotripsy; stone may recur	Soft tissue abscess Oral lymphoepithelial cyst Epidermoid cyst Calcified lymph nodes
Palatal cysts of the newborn	Neonates No gender predilection	Solitary or multiple, discrete or clustered papules with a smooth pearly white surface; usually 1–3 mm in size, asymptomatic	*Epstein pearls:* median palatal raphe *Bohn nodules:* lateral hard and soft palate and junction	Cysts occur in up to 85% of neonates	None required; keratin-filled cysts that spontaneously rupture within first month	Soft tissue abscess Oral lymphoepithelial cyst
Gingival cysts of the newborn (dental lamina cysts)	Neonates No gender predilection	Solitary or multiple, discrete or clustered papules with a smooth translucent to pearly white surface; usually 1–3 mm in size, asymptomatic	Alveolar mucosa, especially maxillary mucosa	Cysts occur in up to 50% of neonates	None required; spontaneously rupture within first 3 months	Natal/neonatal teeth Soft tissue abscess Neonatal alveolar lymphangioma

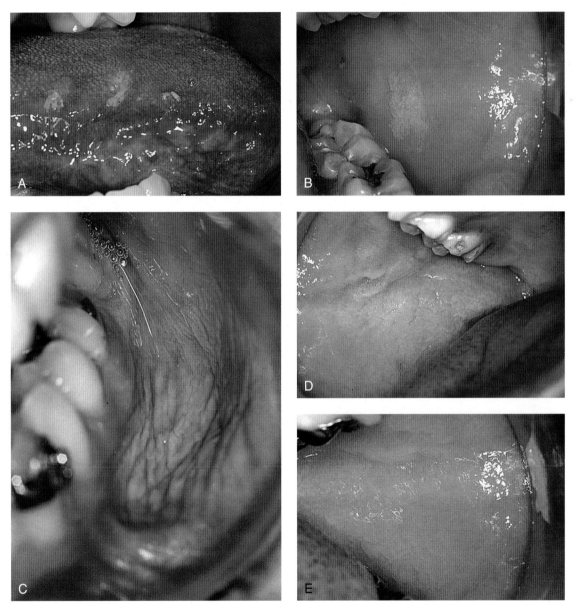

• **Figure 2.2** White soft tissue lesions. (A and B) Frictional keratosis of the lateral tongue (A) and buccal mucosa (B) from chronic biting of the tissues. (C) Smokeless tobacco keratosis of the posterior mandibular vestibule. (D and E) Leukoedema of the buccal mucosa, bilaterally.   *Continued*

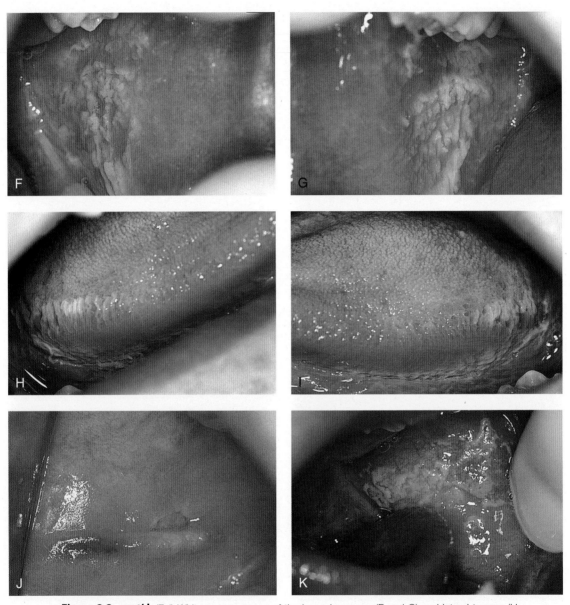

• **Figure 2.2, cont'd** (F–I) White sponge nevus of the buccal mucosa (F and G) and lateral tongue (H and I). (J) Ulcerated linea alba from aggressive sucking habit. (K) Pseudomembranous candidiasis of the buccal mucosa.

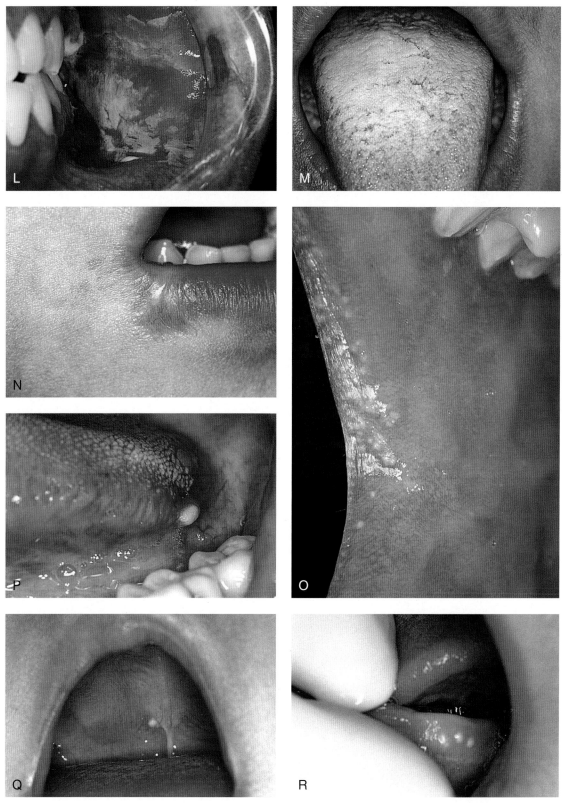

• **Figure 2.2, cont'd** (L) Chemical burn from overuse of a topical anesthetic. (M) Coated tongue in a child who is mouth breathing. (N) Fan-shaped scar at the corners of the mouth due to an electrical burn. (O) Cluster of Fordyce granules of the anterior buccal mucosa. (P) Oral lymphoepithelial cyst of the posterior lateral tongue. (Q) Single palatal cyst of the newborn on the midline hard palate. (R) Cluster of gingival cysts of the newborn on the mandibular alveolar mucosa.

TABLE 2.3   Dark Soft Tissue Lesions (see Fig. 2.3)

Lesion	Pediatric Age and Gender	Clinical Findings	Location	Pediatric Significance	Treatment and Prognosis	Differential Diagnosis
Red or Purple-Blue Lesions						
Port-wine stain (capillary vascular malformation)	Infancy No gender predilection	Localized to diffuse, red to purple macular lesions; variable blanching; bleeds freely; gingival and bony enlargement; grows with child	Face, along distribution of trigeminal nerve, is most common site; may have lip and oral mucosal involvement	Occurs in approximately 1% of newborns; may be sign of *Sturge-Weber syndrome*; bleeding is complication; possible neurologic disease; gingival lesion mimics *pyogenic granuloma*	Laser treatment; persistent lesion that may become darker in color and nodular with age	Hemangioma Venous and arteriovenous malformation Ecchymosis Hereditary hemorrhagic telangiectasia
Submucosal hemorrhage, including petechiae, ecchymosis, and hematoma	First and second decades No gender predilection	Localized to diffuse, pinpoint spots, patches or swellings with smooth surface; early lesions are red; late lesions are blue-black; may be tender	Buccal mucosa, lips, lateral tongue, and soft palate; may develop concurrently on skin	If multiple lesions, need to exclude child abuse, factitial injury, infectious diseases, such as infectious mononucleosis, and blood disorders including leukemia, thrombocytopenia, anemia, and hemophilia	Identify the cause; no treatment for lesions; spontaneously resolve	Amalgam/graphite tattoo Blue nevus Hemangioma Vascular malformation Erythematous candidiasis Blood dyscrasia
Erythematous candidiasis	First and second decades No gender predilection	Multiple red macules to diffuse red patches; depapillation of tongue; burning sensation; may have *angular cheilitis*	Palate, buccal mucosa, dorsal tongue	Caused by *Candida albicans* and other species; contributing factors are antibiotics, immunosuppression, xerostomia, pacifier, and palatal coverage appliances	Antifungal medication and proper oral hygiene; may recur if cause is not eliminated or managed	Contact allergy Traumatic erythema Erythema migrans Thermal burn Palatal petechiae Anemia Scarlet fever (strawberry tongue)
Median rhomboid glossitis	First and second decades No gender predilection	Localized red, depapillated patch; oval to rhomboid in shape with smooth or lobulated surface; asymptomatic	Midline posterior dorsal tongue	Caused by candidal infection; ocalized palatal erythema or "kissing lesion" may be present	Antifungal medication and proper oral hygiene	Erythema migrans Traumatic erosion Contact allergy Hemangioma Vascular malformation Lingual thyroid
Erythema migrans (benign migratory glossitis)	First and second decades Female predilection	Multiple oval or circular red patches with white scalloped borders; loss of filiform papillae; pattern changes; may burn	Dorsal and ventrolateral tongue; rarely at other mucosal sites	More common in children than adults; increased risk in atopic children; may occur with *fissured tongue* and *transient lingual papillitis*	None required; avoidance of hot, spicy, or acidic foods; topical coating agents or steroids in symptomatic cases	Median rhomboid glossitis Contact allergy Erythematous candidiasis Transient lingual papillitis Lichen planus

Condition	Age/Gender	Clinical Features	Location	Comments	Treatment	Differential Diagnosis
Eruption hematoma and cyst	First and second decades; No gender predilection	Localized patch or swelling; amber, red, or blue in color; overlying an erupting tooth; usually nontender	Alveolar mucosa	Eruption cyst is soft tissue counterpart of *dentigerous cyst*; infrequently delays tooth eruption; minimal bleeding may occur at this site	No treatment is usually necessary; resolves with tooth eruption; uncover tooth if symptomatic	Hemangioma; Neonatal alveolar lymphangioma; Pyogenic granuloma; Amalgam tattoo
Brown-Black Lesions						
Physiologic (racial) pigmentation	First and second decades; No gender predilection	Gray, brown, or black patches with smooth surface; patchy to generalized distribution	Any location but attached gingiva is most common	Pigmentation increases with age of child; common in dark-complexioned skin types	None required; common variant of normal mucosa	Postinflammatory pigmentation; Drug-induced pigmentation; Smoker's melanosis; Lead poisoning
Amalgam tattoo	Second decade; No gender predilection	Gray-blue, black macule with smooth surface and well-defined to irregular margins; radiographs may show opaque fragments	Gingiva, alveolar mucosa, buccal mucosa	Graphite tattoo is found on palate from self-inflicted wound; intentional tattooing rarely observed on lower labial mucosa	None required unless melanocytic neoplasm cannot be excluded; permanent discoloration	Melanotic macule; Graphite tattoo; Melanocytic nevus; Varix; Late ecchymosis
Oral melanotic macule (focal melanosis)	First and second decades; Female predilection	Brown, gray, or black oval macule with smooth surface, well-defined margins; single or multiple	Lower lip vermilion, buccal mucosa, gingiva	Most common oral pigmentation of fair-complexioned children; multiple lip macules in *Peutz-Jeghers syndrome*	None required unless a melanocytic neoplasm cannot be excluded; no malignant transformation	Amalgam tattoo; Graphite tattoo; Melanocytic nevus; Smoker's melanosis; Late ecchymosis; Drug-induced melanosis
Melanocytic nevus	Second decade; Female predilection	Brown, blue, or black well-defined nodule or macule with smooth surface	Lip vermilion, palate, gingiva	Oral lesions are uncommon but head and neck skin is frequently involved	Excisional biopsy; low risk of malignant transformation on skin but uncertain risk on oral mucosa	Amalgam tattoo; Graphite tattoo; Oral melanotic macule; Melanoacanthoma; Melanoma

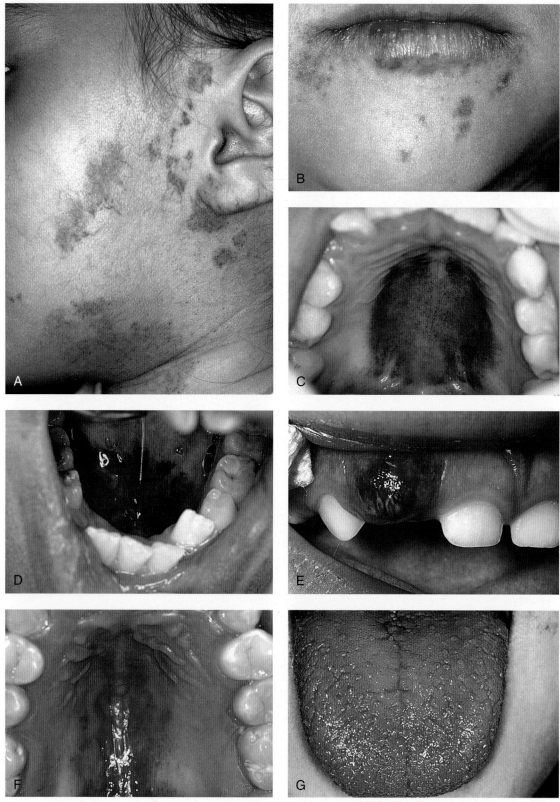

• **Figure 2.3** Dark soft tissue lesions. (A and B) Vascular malformation on the side of the face (A) and around the lips (B). (C) Ecchymosis of the hard palatal mucosa from sucking aggressively on a lollipop. (D) Hematoma of the floor of the mouth following trauma to the chin, which is frequently associated with fracture of the condyles. (E) Eruption hematoma of the maxillary alveolar mucosa. (F and G) Erythematous candidiasis of the hard palatal mucosa (F) and dorsal tongue (G).

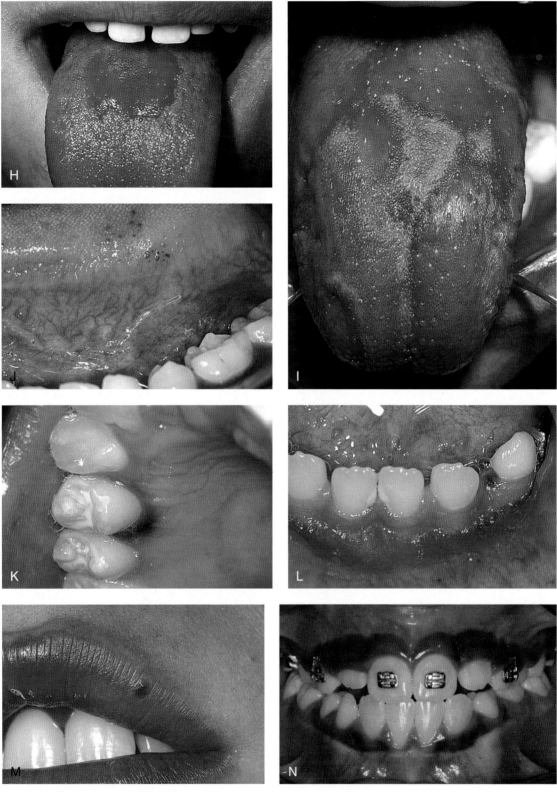

• **Figure 2.3, cont'd** (H) Median rhomboid glossitis of the dorsal tongue. (I) Erythema migrans of the dorsal tongue. (J) Postinflammatory pigmentation of fungiform papillae on the lateral tongue (papillary tip melanosis). (K) Amalgam tattoo of the maxillary palatal gingiva adjacent to the first premolar. (L) Oral melanotic macule of the mandibular gingiva in a child with a history of oral melanoma. (M) Compound nevus on the vermilion of the maxillary lip. (N) Physiologic pigmentation of the attached gingiva.

TABLE 2.4   Ulcerative Lesions (see Fig. 2.4)

Lesion	Pediatric Age and Gender	Clinical Findings	Location	Pediatric Significance	Treatment and Prognosis	Differential Diagnosis
Aphthous ulcer	First and second decades; Female predilection	Recurrent, painful ulcers; *Minor variant:* 1–5 superficial oval ulcers <1 cm; resolves in 7–10 days; *Major variant:* multiple, deep ulcers >1 cm; resolves in 2–6 weeks; *Herpetiform variant:* showers of multiple small ulcers	Buccal, labial mucosa, and ventral tongue are most common; primarily occurs on nonkeratinized mucosa	Occurs in 20%–30% of children; T cell–mediated immune reaction; trauma and orthodontic appliances are important factors in children; genetic predisposition; associated with several systemic diseases, food sensitivities, nutritional deficiencies	Topical anesthetics and coating agents for symptomatic relief; topical and systemic steroids, chlorhexidine oral rinse, laser treatment, nutritional supplements; Major variant heals with scarring	Traumatic ulcer; Secondary herpetic ulcer; Transient lingual papillitis; Crohn disease; Behçet syndrome; Celiac disease; Neutropenic ulcer; PFAPA syndrome; Gastroesophageal reflux disease
Secondary herpetic ulcer	First and second decades; No gender predilection	Multiple, recurrent, small ulcers; painful; preceded by vesicles; clustered pattern; prodromal burning sensation; heals in 7–14 days	Herpes labialis on lip vermilion and perioral skin; intraoral herpetic ulcers on hard palate, attached gingiva; herpetic whitlow on fingers, especially with digit sucking habit	Reactivation of HSV; occurs in one-third of children; ultraviolet light, systemic diseases, trauma, stress, menses are triggering factors	Sunscreen for prevention; topical anesthetics for symptomatic relief; topical antiviral agents, systemic acyclovir, valacyclovir; immunocompromised children should be treated	Traumatic erosion; Aphthous ulcer; Angular cheilitis; Impetigo; Contact allergy; Transient lingual papillitis; Herpes zoster
Angular cheilitis	First and second decades; No gender predilection	Red fissures that bleed and may ulcerate; scaling and crusted surface; burning sensation; may be recurrent	Commissures of mouth; may be associated with concurrent oral candidal infection	Caused by *Candida* species and staphylococci; lip incompetence, licking of lips and drooling are aggravating factors	Lubrication of lips, antifungal, antifungal/steroid ointments; recurring lesions may require oral antifungal treatment	Secondary herpetic ulcer; Impetigo; Exfoliative cheilitis; Traumatic erosions; Contact allergy; Anemia

	Age/Gender	Clinical Features	Location	Etiology	Treatment	Differential Diagnosis
Traumatic ulcer	First and second decades; No gender predilection	Usually single ulcer; variable shape with irregular margins; shallow or deep; painful; typically heals in 1–3 weeks	Lateral tongue, buccal mucosa, lips and gingival; *Riga-Fede disease* occurs in infants on ventral tongue from rubbing against lower incisors	Most common oral ulcer; may indicate child abuse, neurologic impairment, or factitial injuries when persistent and recurrent	Symptomatic relief; eliminate cause; factitial ulcers are diagnostic problem; may heal with scarring	Aphthous ulcer; Mucosal burn; Secondary herpetic ulcer; Contact allergy
Contact allergy	First and second decades; No gender predilection	Focal or widespread erythema, vesicles, and ulcers; swelling, burning sensation and pain; if chronic, then white plaques may develop	Any mucosal site that comes in contact with allergen, especially lips, buccal mucosa, and gingiva	Wide variety of allergens including foods, dental materials, oral hygiene products, topical medications, cosmetic products	Identify and eliminate allergen; patch testing helpful in older children; topical steroids to reduce symptoms; lesions recur with reexposure to allergen	Mucosal burn; Secondary herpetic ulcer; Aphthous ulcer; Angular cheilitis; Erythema multiforme
Erythema multiforme	Second decade; Male predilection	Widespread, painful, red macules, vesicles, bullae, and ulcers; blood-crusted lesions on lips; target lesions on skin; acute onset; fever, malaise	Oral lesions on lips, tongue, buccal mucosa, and soft palate; Skin lesions on extremities and head and neck region	Common precipitating factors include HSV and medications; minor and major forms of the disease	Withdrawal of medication; lubrication of lips, symptomatic relief; hospitalization if severe; recurrences are common if triggered by HSV	Primary herpetic gingivostomatitis; Necrotizing ulcerative gingivitis; Hand, foot, and mouth disease; Chemical burn
Primary herpetic gingivostomatitis	Usually first decade; No gender predilection	Fever, irritability, pain, lymphadenopathy, drooling, multiple vesicles, and ulcers; diffuse erythema; sudden onset; resolves in 7–10 days	Widespread oral and perioral involvement; gingival lesions are usually chief complaint; pharyngeal involvement in adolescents	Caused by HSV; high fever and dehydration are serious complications in children; digital and ocular lesions may occur	Supportive care includes antipyretics, analgesics, palliative oral rinses, hydration; systemic acyclovir may be indicated	Necrotizing ulcerative gingivitis; Erythema multiforme; Herpangina; Hand, foot, and mouth disease

HSV, Herpes simplex virus; *PFAPA,* periodic fever, aphthous-stomatitis, pharyngitis, adenitis syndrome.

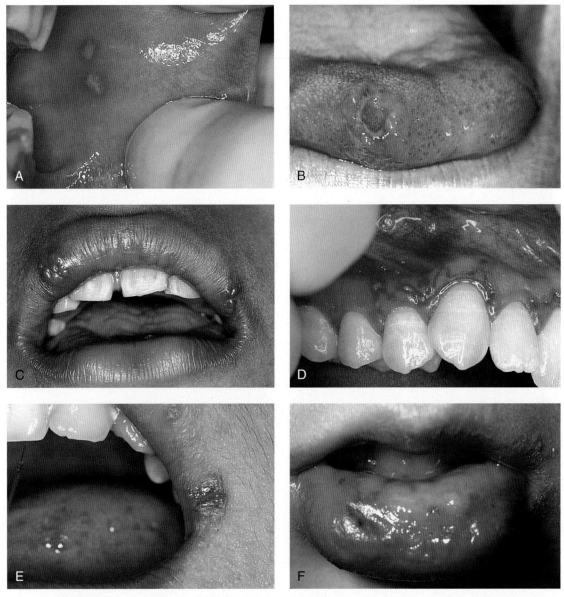

• **Figure 2.4** Ulcerative lesions. (A) Aphthous minor ulcer of the posterior buccal mucosa. (B) Aphthous major ulcer of the anterior dorsal tongue. (C) Herpes labialis of the vermilion of the maxillary lip. (D) Secondary herpetic ulcers of the maxillary attached gingiva. (E) Angular cheilitis. (F) Diffuse traumatic ulcer from biting the lip following local anesthesia for restorative treatment.

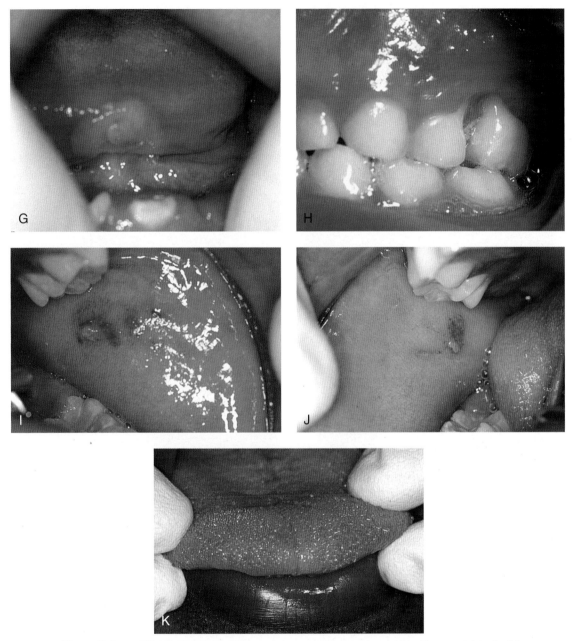

• **Figure 2.4, cont'd** (G) Riga-Fede disease of the ventral tongue in a child with neonatal teeth. (H) Erythema and recession of the attached gingiva between the primary first and second maxillary molars from picking the tissues with the fingernails. (I and J) Bilateral erosions of the buccal mucosa (I and J) and tenderness of the fungiform papillae at the tip of the tongue (K) from a toothpaste hypersensitivity.

Continued

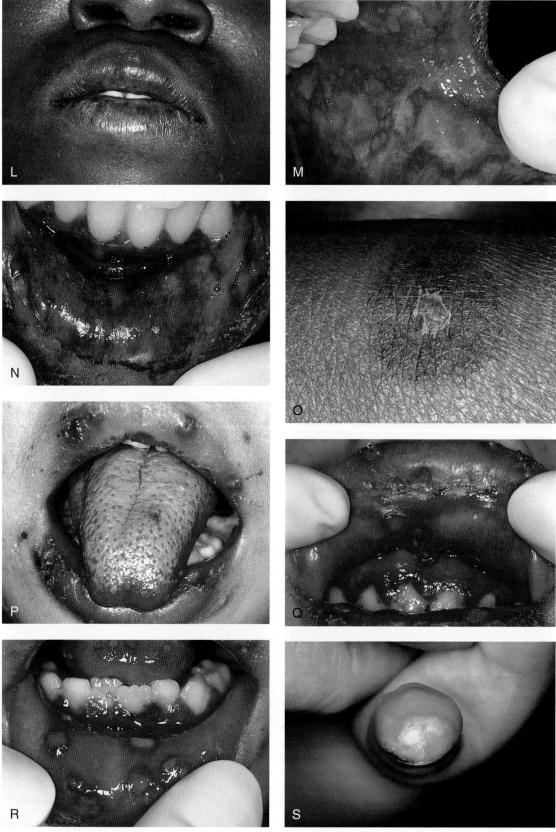

• **Figure 2.4, cont'd** (L–O) Drug-induced erythema multiforme with swelling of the lips (L), erythema and ulcerations of the buccal mucosa (M) and labial mucosa (N), and target lesions on the skin (O). (P–S) Primary herpetic gingivostomatitis of the tongue and lips (P), maxillary gingiva and labial mucosa (Q) and mandibular gingiva and labial mucosa (R), and vesicles on the thumb (S).

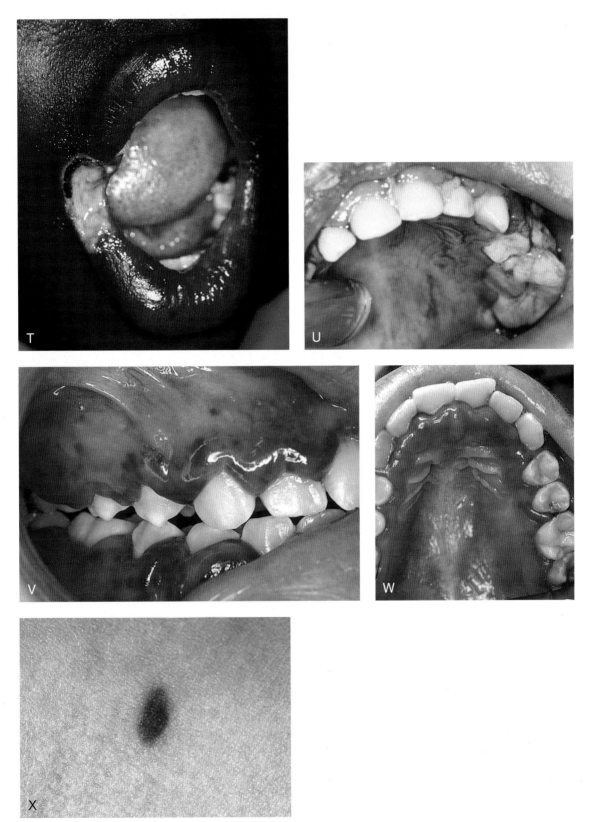

• **Figure 2.4, cont'd**   (T) Electrical burn of the lip. (U) Necrotizing gingival ulcer with a thick pseudomembrane in a child with acute lymphoblastic leukemia. (V–X) Red-purple enlargements of the buccal gingiva (V), palatal mucosa (W), and skin (X) that represent leukemic infiltrates in a child with acute myeloid leukemia.

TABLE 2.5 Soft Tissue Enlargements (see Fig. 2.5)

Lesion	Pediatric Age and Gender	Clinical Findings	Location	Pediatric Significance	Treatment and Prognosis	Differential Diagnosis
Papillary Lesions						
Squamous papilloma	Second decade No gender predilection	Single, pedunculated nodule with fingerlike projections; pink to white; soft and nontender	Any oral site but predilection for the tongue, lips, and soft palate	Caused by HPV, especially types 6, 11; low virulence and infectivity rate	Excisional biopsy; recurrence is rare; no evidence of malignant transformation	Verruca vulgaris Condyloma acuminatum Giant cell fibroma Localized juvenile spongiotic gingival hyperplasia
Verruca vulgaris (common wart)	First and second decades No gender predilection	Multiple sessile or pedunculated papules and nodules with rough, pebbly or papillary surface; white; nontender	Common on skin of hands and face; infrequently found on the lip vermilion, labial mucosa, and anterior tongue	Caused by HPV, especially type 2; spread by autoinoculation to oral site by sucking on fingers or nail biting	Excisional biopsy of oral warts; low risk for recurrence for oral lesions; spontaneous resolution may occur for skin lesion; no risk for malignant transformation	Squamous papilloma Verruca plana Condyloma acuminatum Giant cell fibroma Molluscum contagiosum Frictional keratosis
Condyloma acuminatum (venereal wart)	Second decade No gender predilection	Multiple, discrete, sessile nodules with blunted papillary surface; pink; nontender	Usually anogenital lesions; oral sites include labial mucosa, soft palate, and ventral tongue	Oral lesions caused by HPV 6, 11, 16, 18; oncogenic HPV types 16, 18; autoinoculation, vertical or sexual transmission; may indicate child abuse	Excisional biopsy, laser ablation of oral warts; highly contagious; frequently recur; oral HPV 16, 18 associated with oropharyngeal carcinoma; HPV vaccine available	Squamous papilloma Multifocal epithelial hyperplasia Inflammatory papillary hyperplasia Giant cell fibroma Superficial lymphangioma Linear epidermal nevus Focal dermal hypoplasia
Giant cell fibroma	Second decade Female predilection	Solitary, sessile, or pedunculated nodule with a pebbly surface; pink; nontender	Attached gingiva, dorsal tongue, and hard palate	Fibrous lesion of unknown cause that has a predilection for children	Excisional biopsy; recurrence is rare	Squamous papilloma Retrocuspid papilla Irritation fibroma
Multifocal epithelial hyperplasia (Heck disease)	First and second decades No gender predilection	Multifocal, sessile, papules and nodules with pink grainy to stippled surface; lesions coalesce, display cobblestone appearance; nontender	Usually located on labial and buccal mucosa and tongue	Caused by HPV 13, 32; familial tendency, genetic susceptibility Other risk factors include poor oral hygiene, crowded living conditions, nutritional deficiencies	Excisional biopsy; laser ablation; recurrence is common; spontaneous regression may occur; no malignant transformation potential	Verruca vulgaris Condyloma acuminata Multiple hamartoma syndrome Multiple endocrine neoplasia syndrome 2B

Continued

Localized juvenile spongiotic gingival hyperplasia	Second decade; Female predilection	Isolated red, velvety to papillary patch or enlargement; bleeds freely; persistent; does not respond to oral hygiene measures	Anterior facial gingiva, usually maxillary gingiva; represents transplanted crevicular or junctional epithelium	Contributing factors appear to be mouth breathing, anterior crowding, orthodontic appliances; used to be diagnosed as puberty gingivitis	Excisional biopsy; may spontaneously resolve; recurs up to 16%	Pyogenic granuloma; Inflamed squamous papilloma; Giant cell fibroma; Superficial gingival lymphangioma
Inflammatory papillary hyperplasia	Second decade; No gender predilection	Multiple, clustered papules and nodules with pink to red granular surface; cobblestone appearance; nontender	Hard palatal mucosa	Caused by continuous wear of palatal coverage appliance; other factors include mouth breathing and high palatal vault; candidal infection may be present	Remove and clean appliance; reline appliance if needed; antifungal therapy; excisional biopsy of persistent lesions	Condyloma acuminata; Multifocal epithelial hyperplasia; Erythematous candidiasis; Early nicotine stomatitis

Acute Inflammatory Lesions

Soft tissue abscess (parulis)	First and second decades; No gender predilection	Solitary pinkish white or deep red nodule; purulence; fluctuates in size; tender to painful; may progress to cellulitis	Gingiva and alveolar mucosa are most common sites	Usually caused by odontogenic infection or entrapped foreign body; *pericoronitis* is a gingival abscess associated with erupting molars	Manage source of infection; local debridement; usually antibiotics are not indicated; recurs if infection is not eliminated	Pyogenic granuloma; Oral lymphoepithelial cyst; Sialolithiasis; Tonsilithiasis; Gingival cysts of newborn
Cellulitis	First and second decades; No gender predilection	Diffuse erythematous swelling of sudden onset; soft to board-like; warm and painful tissues; fever, headache, airway obstruction, and leukocytosis may be present	Upper or lower face and neck	Caused by odontogenic infection, facial or oral lacerations, insect bites, peritonsillar abscesses, jaw fractures, sialadenitis, sinusitis, and bacteremia	Manage source of infection; antibiotic therapy; incision and drainage in severe cases *Ludwig angina* and *cavernous sinus thrombosis* may be life threatening	Facial hematoma; Plunging ranula; Emphysema; Obstructive sialadenitis; Angioedema; Acute sinusitis; Acute lymphadenitis
Angioedema	First and second decades; No gender predilection	Diffuse swelling of sudden onset; soft and nontender; may be associated with respiratory and gastrointestinal problems	Lips, tongue, soft palate and face, and other cutaneous sites	Acquired form is caused by allergic reaction to foods, plants, drugs, insect bites, cold, heat, latex, pressure, stress, and infections; most hereditary forms are caused by C1-INH deficiency	Allergic forms are treated by antihistamines, steroids, or epinephrine; other drugs are used for the hereditary forms; may be life threatening	Cellulitis; Emphysema; Traumatic edema; Contact allergy; Orofacial granulomatosis

TABLE 2.5 Soft Tissue Enlargements (see Fig. 2.5)—cont'd

Lesion	Pediatric Age and Gender	Clinical Findings	Location	Pediatric Significance	Treatment and Prognosis	Differential Diagnosis
Mucocele	First and second decades No gender predilection	Fluid-filled nodule with a smooth, translucent, red or blue surface; sudden onset; fluctuates in size; tender if traumatized; periodically drains	Lower labial mucosa, buccal mucosa, and anterior ventral tongue	Most common lip swelling in children; may be associated with trauma and orthodontic appliances; rare cases are congenital	Excisional biopsy with removal of underlying minor salivary glands; may recur with incomplete removal or repeated trauma	Lymphangioma Hemangioma Hematoma Soft fibroma Soft tissue abscess Salivary duct cyst
Ranula	First and second decades No gender predilection	Fluid-filled swelling with smooth, translucent to blue surface of recent onset; fluctuates in size; mildly tender; periodically drains; may elevate tongue	Floor of mouth, lateral to midline; plunging variant results in diffuse swelling of the submandibular region and neck	Usually associated with sublingual gland; rare cases are congenital and caused by aplasia of submandibular excretory duct	Excisional biopsy of sublingual gland or marsupialization; recurrences are common with marsupialization	Lymphangioma Hemangioma Mucoepidermoid carcinoma Obstructive sialadenitis Salivary duct cyst Dermoid cyst
Tumor and Tumorlike Lesions						
Irritation fibroma	First and second decades No gender predilection	Nodule with pink smooth surface; firm and nontender; limited growth potential	Buccal and labial mucosa, tongue, and attached gingiva	Common reactive hyperplastic lesion caused by chronic trauma and mimics a tumor	Conservative excisional biopsy; may recur if irritation continues	Fibrosing mucocele Giant cell fibroma Fibrosing pyogenic granuloma Benign submucosal neoplasm
Peripheral ossifying fibroma	Second decade Female predilection	Nodule with pink to red surface; frequently ulcerated; firm and nontender; may resorb alveolar bone; limited growth potential	Emanates from interdental papilla of attached gingiva; most common site is anterior region	Reactive hyperplastic lesion with mineralized product from cells of periosteum or periodontal ligament; may displace teeth	Excisional biopsy down to periosteum and remove local irritation; 16% recurrence rate	Irritation fibroma Peripheral giant cell granuloma Giant cell fibroma Pyogenic granuloma Peripheral odontogenic fibroma
Peripheral giant cell granuloma	Second decade Female predilection	Nodule with red or purple-blue surface; may be ulcerated; firm and nontender; resorb alveolar bone; limited growth potential	Attached gingiva or alveolar mucosa	Reactive hyperplastic lesion caused by irritation; may displace teeth	Excisional biopsy to periosteum and remove local irritation; 10%–18% recurrence rate	Pyogenic granuloma Ulcerated irritation fibroma Peripheral ossifying fibroma Hemangioma Foreign body granuloma

Lesion	Age/Gender	Clinical Features	Location	Comments	Treatment	Differential Diagnosis
Pyogenic granuloma	First and second decades; Female predilection	Nodule with smooth to irregular, red surface; usually ulcerated; bleeds freely; soft and friable; nontender; limited growth potential	Most occur on attached gingiva; other sites include lip, tongue, and buccal mucosa; also occurs on skin	Reactive hyperplastic lesion caused by irritation and poor oral hygiene; may be associated with pregnancy (pregnancy tumor) or may develop at extraction site because of bony sequestra (epulis granulomatosa)	Excisional biopsy and remove local irritation; recurrence rate is 3%–15%	Ulcerated irritation fibroma; Peripheral ossifying fibroma; Peripheral giant cell granuloma; Soft tissue abscess; Hemangioma; Localized, juvenile spongiotic gingival hyperplasia
Gingival fibromatosis	First and second decades; No gender predilection	Localized or generalized gingival enlargements; pink, smooth to stippled surfaces; firm and nontender; affects both dentitions	Attached gingiva and maxillary tuberosity	May be familial or idiopathic; associated with several syndromes; interferes with eruption of teeth; displacement of teeth	Gingivectomy and good oral hygiene; high recurrence rate	Drug-induced gingival overgrowth; Mouth breathing gingivitis; Chronic hyperplastic gingivitis; Leukemic gingival infiltrates; Scorbutic gingivitis
Hemangioma	Infancy; Female predilection	Localized to diffuse, red, blue, or purple lesion, flat or nodular, soft and compressible; may blanch; bleeds freely; 20% are multiple	60% occur in head and neck region; lips, tongue, and buccal mucosa are most common sites; rarely occurs in jaws	Hemorrhage is potential complication; may cause malocclusion; scarring is common with involution	Involution of lesion within first decade; surgery for select cases and scar revision, laser ablation, corticosteroids, propranolol; does not recur	Vascular malformation; Pyogenic granuloma; Lymphangioma; Eruption cyst/hematoma; Mucocele
Lymphangioma (lymphatic malformation)	Infancy; most detected by 2 years; No gender predilection	Localized to diffuse, translucent to red or purple swelling; smooth or pebbly surface; soft and compressible; crepitus may be palpated	Up to 75% occur in head and neck; common oral sites include the tongue, lip, and buccal mucosa	May cause malocclusion, dysphagia, and respiratory problems; cystic hygroma and neonatal alveolar lymphangioma are variants	Surgical excision; recurrences are common; airway obstruction and death may occur with large neck or tongue lesions	Hemangioma; Squamous papilloma; Lingual papillitis; Mucocele; Plunging ranula; Parotitis; Branchial cleft cyst
Congenital epulis	Infancy; Female predilection	Pedunculated or sessile nodule; pink to red smooth surface; may be ulcerated; 10% are multiple	Anterior alveolar ridge; usually maxilla	May cause feeding problems; usually reaches maximum size at birth	Surgical excision; occasional spontaneous regression; no recurrence; normal tooth development	Hemangioma; Pyogenic granuloma; Neonatal alveolar lymphangioma; Neuroectodermal tumor of infancy

Continued

TABLE 2.5   Soft Tissue Enlargements (see Fig. 2.5)—cont'd

Lesion	Pediatric Age and Gender	Clinical Findings	Location	Pediatric Significance	Treatment and Prognosis	Differential Diagnosis
Neurofibroma	Second decade No gender predilection	Single or multiple nodules with smooth surface; discrete or diffuse; soft to firm on palpation; nontender	Tongue, buccal mucosa, and palate; rarely within mandible; syndromic lesions occur at any site, especially skin	*Neurofibromatosis* is autosomal dominant condition with neurofibromas, café-au-lait macules, axillary freckling, and Lisch nodules on iris	Surgical excision if solitary lesion; selective excision of syndrome type; 5% malignant transformation of syndrome type	Schwannoma Mucosal neuroma Irritation fibroma Benign submucosal neoplasm Salivary gland neoplasm
Mucosal neuromas (multiple endocrine neoplasia syndrome, type 2B)	First decade No gender predilection	Multiple, pink papules and nodules; soft and nontender; marfanoid body type; narrow face with full lips	Labial and buccal mucosa, anterior tongue, gingiva; also on conjunctiva and eyelid	Autosomal dominant syndrome; other stigmata include pheochromocytoma and medullary carcinoma of thyroid gland	Surgical excision of neuromas for cosmetics; aggressive thyroid cancer develops in second decade	Neurofibromatosis Multifocal epithelial hyperplasia Multiple hamartoma syndrome
Pleomorphic adenoma (benign mixed tumor)	Second decade Slight female predilection	Pink, dome-shaped enlargement with smooth surface; slowly growing; firm and nontender	Parotid gland is most common site; palate is most common oral site	Most common benign salivary gland neoplasm; *mucoepidermoid carcinoma* is most common malignant salivary gland tumor in this age group	Surgical excision with adequate margins; recurrence is low; malignant transformation rate of <4%	Neurofibroma Schwannoma Mucoepidermoid carcinoma Irritation fibroma
Juvenile aggressive fibromatosis	First and second decades No gender predilection	Rapidly growing, pink, firm mass with an irregular surface; may be ulcerated; painless; large in size; facial disfigurement; destruction of adjacent bone	Head and neck region; paramandibular soft tissues are common intraoral sites	Rare, locally aggressive and destructive lesion that mimics a malignancy; associated with *familial adenomatous polyposis, Gardner syndrome*	Surgical excision with wide margins; adjunctive chemotherapy and radiotherapy may be indicated; high recurrence rate	Large pyogenic granuloma Fibrosarcoma Rhabdomyosarcoma Metastatic disease
Rhabdomyosarcoma	First and second decades Male predilection	Rapidly growing, infiltrative and destructive mass; painless	Head and neck region is the most common site; face, orbit, nasal cavity, maxillary sinus, palate	Skeletal muscle malignancy; one of the most common sarcomas in children	Surgical excision, multiagent chemotherapy with or without radiation therapy Pediatric prognosis is 70% 5-year survival rate	Desmoidlike fibromatosis Lymphoma Neuroblastoma Malignant salivary gland tumor Retinoblastoma Juvenile nasopharyngeal angiofibroma

C1-INH, C1-esterase inhibitor; *HPV*, human papillomavirus.

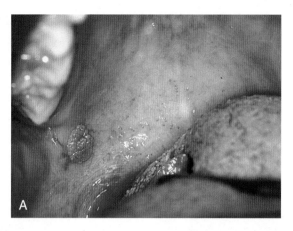

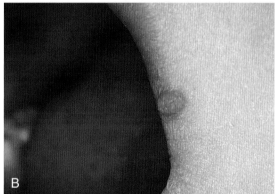

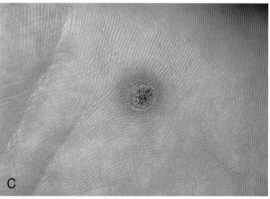

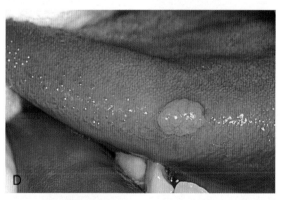

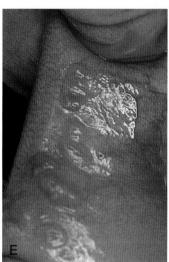

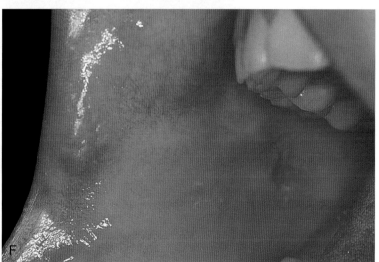

• **Figure 2.5** Soft tissue enlargements. (A) Squamous papilloma of the soft palate. (B and C) Verruca vulgaris of the lip vermilion (B) and hand (C). (D) Giant cell fibroma of the lateral tongue. (E and F) Focal epithelial hyperplasia of the buccal mucosa displaying a cobblestone appearance (E) or a small clustered pattern (F).

Continued

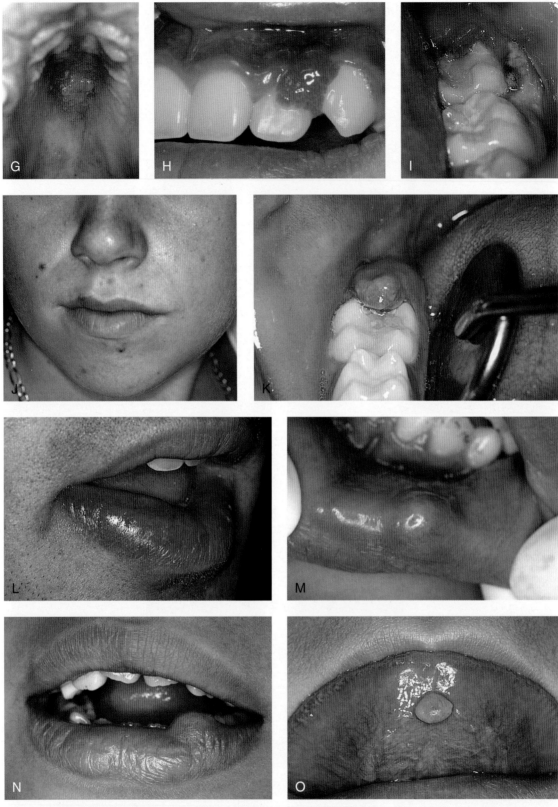

• **Figure 2.5, cont'd** (G) Inflammatory papillary hyperplasia of the hard palatal mucosa. (H) Localized juvenile spongiotic gingival hyperplasia. (I and J) Pericoronitis associated with an erupting mandibular molar (I) and a lower face cellulitis (J). (K) Inflamed operculum associated with an erupting mandibular molar. (L) Angioedema of the lips due to a latex allergy. (M and N) Mucocele of the mandibular labial mucosa (M). The lesion was obvious when the child's lips were at rest (N). (O) Mucocele at the anterior midline ventral tongue.

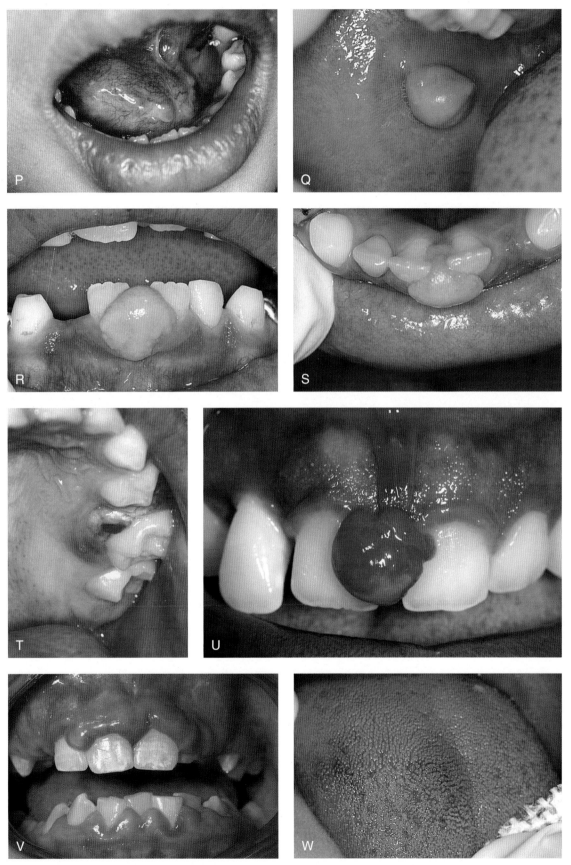

• **Figure 2.5, cont'd** (P) Ranula resulting in a diffuse swelling of the floor of the mouth. (Q) Irritation fibroma of the buccal mucosa. (R and S) Peripheral ossifying fibroma of the mandibular anterior gingiva (R). Note the separation of the incisors (S). (T) Peripheral giant cell granuloma of the palatal gingiva between the primary molars. (U) Pyogenic granuloma and physiologic pigmentation of the maxillary gingiva. (V) Hereditary gingival fibromatosis. (W) Hemangioma of the dorsal tongue.   *Continued*

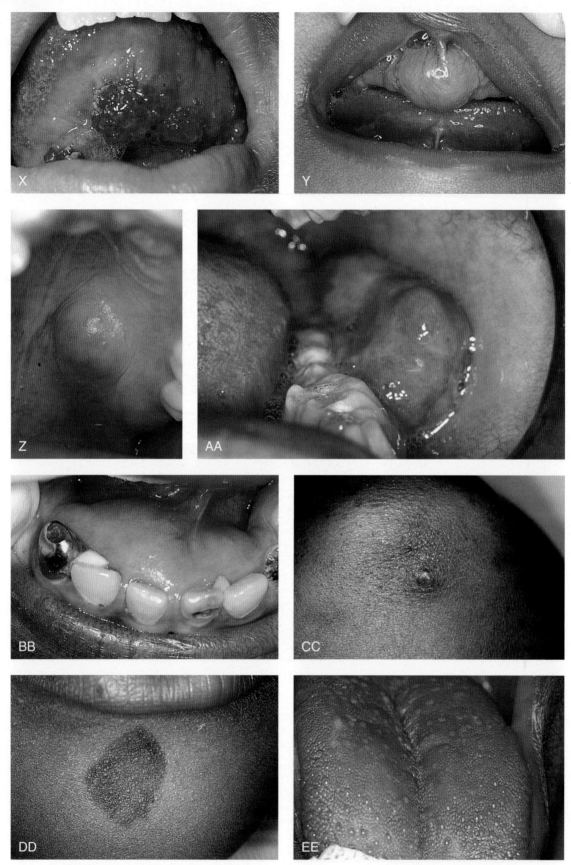

• **Figure 2.5, cont'd** (X) Lymphangioma of the ventral tongue. (Y) Congenital epulis of the anterior maxillary alveolar mucosa. (Z) Pleomorphic adenoma of the posterior hard palate. (AA) Juvenile fibromatosis of the posterior mandibular vestibule and gingiva. (BB–EE) Child with neurofibromatosis including neurofibroma of the floor of the mouth (BB), skin of the neck (CC), café-au-lait macule on the chin (DD), and enlarged fungiform papillae (EE).

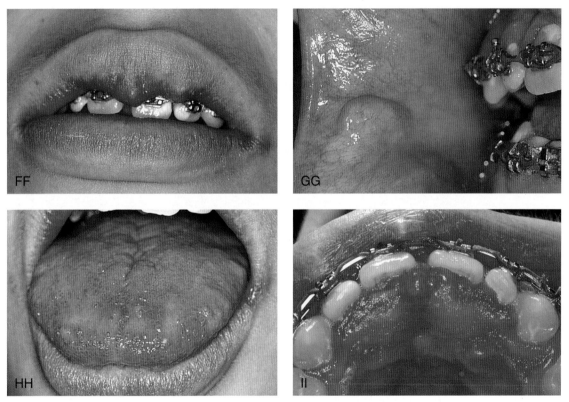

• **Figure 2.5, cont'd** (FF–II) Child with multiple endocrine neoplasia syndrome, type 2B, including mucosal neuromas of the lips (FF), buccal mucosa (GG), tongue (HH), and palatal gingiva (II).

TABLE 2.6 Radiolucent Lesions of Bone (see Fig. 2.6)

Lesion	Pediatric Age and Gender	Clinical and Radiographic Findings	Location	Pediatric Significance	Treatment and Prognosis	Differential Diagnosis
Dentigerous cyst	Second decade Slight male predilection	Well-defined, unilocular, radiolucency around crown of unerupted tooth; may displace teeth, cause cortical expansion and root resorption; asymptomatic unless infected	Mandibular and maxillary third molar and canine regions	Common odontogenic cyst in children; growth may be rapid; may involve primary or supernumerary teeth; *eruption cyst* is soft tissue analogue	Enucleation; marsupialization if extensive; orthodontic treatment to assist tooth eruption; seldom recur; ameloblastoma and carcinoma are rare complications	Hyperplastic dental follicle Periapical cyst Ameloblastic fibroma Unicystic ameloblastoma Odontogenic keratocyst Adenomatoid odontogenic tumor Buccal bifurcation cyst
Odontogenic keratocyst (keratocystic odontogenic tumor)	Second decade Slight male predilection	Well-defined, unilocular or multilocular radiolucency with corticated margins; expansile; 25%–40% associated with unerupted tooth; may resorb and displace teeth; may be painful	Posterior body and ramus of mandible; maxillary third molar and canine regions	Multiple cysts are consistent with *nevoid basal cell carcinoma syndrome* and includes jaw cysts, basal cell carcinomas, palmar-plantar pits, bifid ribs, epidermal cysts, and calcified falx cerebri	Surgical excision; may include peripheral ostectomy or chemical cautery; may treat by decompression of cyst; recurrence rate of 30%	Dentigerous cyst Unicystic ameloblastoma Ameloblastic fibroma Odontogenic myxoma Central vascular malformation Central giant cell granuloma
Ameloblastic fibroma	First and second decades Slight male predilection	Well-defined unilocular or multilocular lesion with sclerotic margins; expansile; 75% associated with unerupted tooth	Posterior mandible (70%)	Rare malignant counterpart, *ameloblastic fibrosarcoma* arises de novo or from preexisting or recurrent tumor	Surgical excision; recurrences are common (18%); long-term follow-up is recommended	Dentigerous cyst Odontogenic keratocyst Central vascular malformation Central giant cell granuloma Ameloblastoma
Ameloblastoma	Second decade No gender predilection	Well-defined, unilocular or multilocular radiolucency; cortical perforation; expansile; slow growing; root displacement and resorption; usually asymptomatic	Mandibular molar and ramus areas	*Unicystic ameloblastoma* is most common variant in children; associated with unerupted molar; treatment varies from enucleation to resection; less aggressive than conventional tumor	Aggressive odontogenic tumor requires marginal or en bloc resection; 50%–90% recurs with curettage; rarely undergoes malignant transformation	Dentigerous cyst Odontogenic keratocyst Odontogenic myxoma Central giant cell granuloma Ameloblastic fibroma
Melanotic neuroectodermal tumor of infancy	Infancy, may be present at birth Slight male predilection	Rapidly expanding bony lesion; may exhibit blue-black pigmented surface; ill-defined, unilocular radiolucency; displacement of tooth buds; "floating tooth" appearance	Anterior maxilla	Lesion mimics malignancy with destructive, rapid growth rate; dental abnormalities due to surgery; high urinary levels of vanillylmandelic acid	Surgical excision or curettage; 20% recurrence rate; reported cases of metastasis	Metastatic sarcoma Central vascular malformation Large eruption cyst Large congenital epulis

Lesion	Age/Gender	Clinical/Radiographic Features	Location	Comments	Treatment	Differential Diagnosis
Central giant cell granuloma	First and second decades; Female predilection	Well-defined, unilocular or multilocular radiolucency with scalloped border; expansile; may displace teeth and cause root resorption; pain and paresthesia may be noted	Most frequently in mandible; anterior to first molar; may cross midline	Aggressive form exists; need to rule out *hyperparathyroidism*, *cherubism*, and other syndromes, especially with multiple lesions	Thorough curettage; alternative treatments include intralesional corticosteroids, calcitonin, interferon, bisphosphonates; recurrence rate of 20%	Periapical cyst; Odontogenic keratocyst; Simple bone cyst; Odontogenic myxoma; Central vascular malformation; Aneurysmal bone cyst; Ameloblastic fibroma
Cherubism	First decade; usually by 5 years; Male predilection	Chubby face appearance; bilateral, symmetric, painless enlargement of jaws; extensive, multiple, well-defined, multilocular radiolucencies	Maxilla and mandible; in particular, angles of mandible; all four quadrants frequently involved	Autosomal dominant condition; causes premature exfoliation of primary teeth; displacement of tooth buds, severe malocclusion, and malformed teeth	Treatment is controversial; spontaneous regression with onset of puberty; surgery may improve function and cosmetics	Nevoid basal cell carcinoma syndrome; Hyperparathyroidism; Noonan-like syndrome; Ramon syndrome; Neurofibromatosis, type 1
Simple bone cyst (traumatic bone cyst)	Second decade; No gender predilection for jaw lesions	Well to poorly delineated, unilocular radiolucency with thin, sclerotic border; scalloping between roots of teeth; 20% are expansile; teeth are vital	Posterior and anterior body of mandible and ramus; bilateral lesions are uncommon	Cause is uncertain but may be associated with trauma; extensive, expansile lesions may occur; may be seen with fibro-osseous lesions	Surgical exploration and curettage; low recurrence rate of 1%–2%	Central giant cell granuloma; Periapical cyst; Odontogenic keratocyst; Developing tooth bud
Aneurysmal bone cyst	First and second decades; No gender predilection	Painful swelling with rapid growth; unilocular or multilocular radiolucency with ballooning distention of buccal cortex; may be painful; tooth displacement	Posterior mandibular region	Blood-filled pseudocyst; 20% associated with preexisting lesion, including *central giant cell granuloma, fibrous dysplasia, ossifying fibroma*	Curettage or enucleation; hemorrhage control; 2-year recurrence rate is approximately 13%; incomplete removal is common	Ameloblastic fibroma; Ameloblastoma; Central giant cell granuloma; Central vascular malformation; Odontogenic keratocyst; Odontogenic myxoma
Periapical abscess	First and second decades; No gender predilection	Nonvital, mobile tooth; soft tissue swelling with purulence; sinus tract may be present; painful; widening of periodontal ligament space or poorly defined radiolucency	Alveolus; primary dentition is most frequently affected in children	May progress to cellulitis; may result in aborted development or enamel hypoplasia of succedaneous tooth	Endodontic treatment or tooth extraction; antibiotics and analgesics may be needed; serious complications include *cavernous sinus thrombosis* and *Ludwig angina*	Incomplete apexification of erupted tooth; Periodontal abscess; Periapical granuloma or cyst; Buccal bifurcation cyst; Langerhans cell histiocytosis

Continued

TABLE 2.6 Radiolucent Lesions of Bone (see Fig. 2.6)—cont'd

Lesion	Pediatric Age and Gender	Clinical and Radiographic Findings	Location	Pediatric Significance	Treatment and Prognosis	Differential Diagnosis
Periapical granuloma and cyst	First and second decades No gender predilection	Nonvital tooth; usually asymptomatic unless acute exacerbation of the lesion; well or poorly defined radiolucency at the root apex; loss of lamina dura; root resorption	Alveolar bone adjacent to root apex and bifurcation	May displace succedaneous teeth and cause dental abnormalities; large lesions in primary dentition resemble a *dentigerous cyst* when a succedaneous tooth is present	Endodontic treatment or tooth extraction and gentle curettage to avoid disturbing permanent tooth bud, if present	Dentigerous cyst Developing tooth bud Solitary bone cyst Central giant cell granuloma Langerhans cell histiocytosis
Acute osteomyelitis	First and second decades Male predilection	Diffuse radiolucency with poorly defined margins; sequestra; fever, swelling, pain, lymphadenopathy, leukocytosis, and draining sinus tracts	Posterior mandible in children; anterior maxilla in infants	Most cases are due to odontogenic infections or jaw fractures; occasionally caused by bacteremia	Incision and drainage with culture and sensitivity testing; antibiotic coverage; may develop into *chronic osteomyelitis*	Jaw fracture Ewing sarcoma Burkitt lymphoma Langerhans cell histiocytosis Osteosarcoma
Langerhans cell histiocytosis (histiocytosis X)	*Disseminated form:* first decade *Localized form:* second decade Male predilection	Lymphadenopathy, rash, oral pain, gingivitis, ulcers, mobile teeth, multiple punched-out radiolucencies with "floating tooth" appearance; premature tooth loss	Skull, mandible, ribs and vertebrae are most often involved; jaws affected in 20% of cases	Neoplastic disease of myeloid cells; chronic disseminated form includes lytic bone lesions, exophthalmos, diabetes insipidus; all forms mimic periodontal disease or multifocal odontogenic infection	Multiagent chemotherapy, low-dose radiotherapy, surgical curettage, and stem cell transplantation are used, depending on form of disease and location; children younger than 2 years have worst prognosis	Cyclic neutropenia Burkitt lymphoma Leukemia Aggressive periodontitis Periapical abscess or granuloma Acute osteomyelitis
Burkitt lymphoma	First and second decades Male predilection	Lymphadenopathy, facial swelling, tenderness, tooth mobility, extrusion and premature loss; patchy loss of lamina dura, irregular radiolucencies, "floating tooth" appearance	Posterior mandible is most common site; may involve all four quadrants; African (endemic) form affects the jaws in 50%–70% of cases	Most jaw lesions are misdiagnosed as odontogenic infection; associated with Epstein-Barr virus and chromosomal translocation	Treatment includes multiagent chemotherapy; aggressive malignancy with 5-year survival rate of 75%–95%, depending on disease stage	Acute osteomyelitis Langerhans cell histiocytosis Periapical abscess or granuloma Acute leukemia Aggressive periodontitis

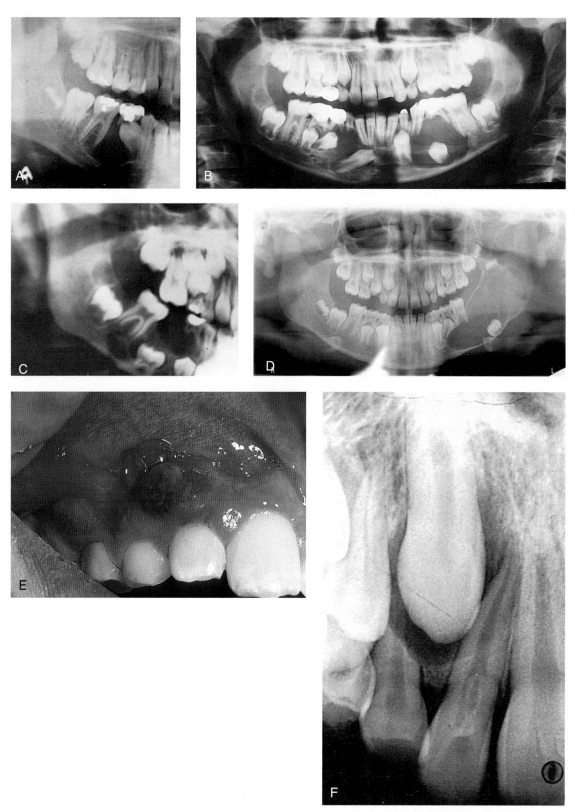

• **Figure 2.6** Radiolucent lesions of bone. (A) Dentigerous cyst of the posterior mandible. (B) Bilateral odontogenic keratocysts of the mandible associated with nevoid basal cell carcinoma syndrome. (C) Ameloblastic fibroma of the posterior mandible. (D) Ameloblastoma of the posterior mandible. (E and F) Periapical abscess of the maxillary lateral incisor due to dens invaginatus, parulis (E), and radiographic findings (F). Note the hyperplastic dental follicle surrounding the crown of the permanent canine.

Continued

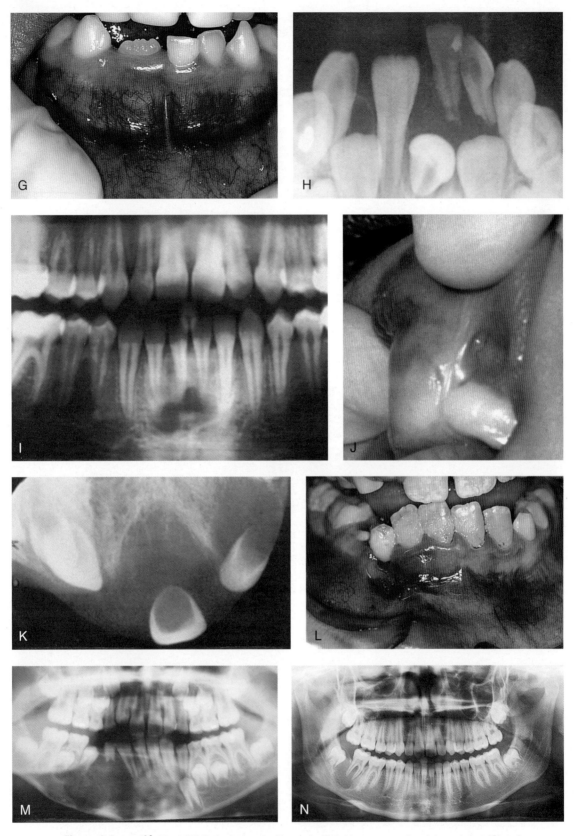

• **Figure 2.6, cont'd**   (G and H) Periapical cyst with no significant bony expansion, intraoral view (G) and radiographic view (H). (I) Simple bone cysts of the anterior and posterior mandible. (J and K) Melanotic neuroectodermal tumor of infancy of the anterior maxilla, clinical view (J) and radiographic view (K). (L and M) Central giant cell granuloma of the mandible, clinical view (L) and radiographic view (M). (N) Buccal bifurcation cyst, panoramic radiographic view.

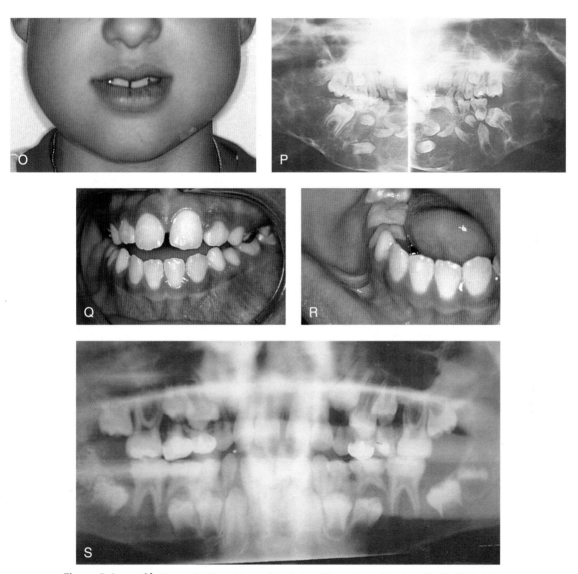

• **Figure 2.6, cont'd** (O and P) Cherubism, clinical view (O), radiographic view (P). (Q–S) Burkitt lymphoma, open bite due to extrusion of posterior teeth (Q), mandibular buccal expansion (R), and panoramic radiographic view (S).

TABLE 2.7   Mixed Radiolucent and Radiopaque Lesions of Bone (see Fig. 2.7)

Lesion	Pediatric Age and Gender	Clinical and Radiographic Findings	Location	Pediatric Significance	Treatment and Prognosis	Differential Diagnosis
Calcifying odontogenic cyst (Gorlin cyst)	Second decade No gender predilection	Well-defined, unilocular radiolucency with irregular calcifications or toothlike structures; expansile; 33% associated with unerupted teeth; asymptomatic	Most develop in incisor-canine region of maxilla and mandible; may occur as gingival lesion	In this age group, this odontogenic cyst is often associated with *odontoma*	Enucleation; minimal risk of recurrence; rarely manifests aggressive or malignant behavior	Odontoma Adenomatoid odontogenic tumor Ameloblastic fibro-odontoma Calcifying epithelial odontogenic tumor Central ossifying fibroma
Adenomatoid odontogenic tumor	Second decade Female predilection	Well-defined, unilocular radiolucency with fine snowflake calcifications; most associated with unerupted tooth (canine); root divergence; asymptomatic expansion	Anterior maxilla is most common site, followed by the anterior mandible	Most lesions occur between 10 and 20 years of age; rarely occurs as gingival lesion	Enucleation; does not recur	Dentigerous cyst Calcifying odontogenic cyst Developing odontoma Odontogenic keratocyst
Ameloblastic fibro-odontoma	First and second decades No gender predilection	Well-defined unilocular radiolucency with calcified material and toothlike structures; expansile; often associated with unerupted tooth	Mandibular molar and premolar regions	Odontogenic tumor is frequently diagnosed because tooth fails to erupt	Conservative curettage; rarely recurs	Developing odontoma Calcifying odontogenic cyst Calcifying epithelial odontogenic tumor Central ossifying fibroma Osteoblastoma
Ossifying fibroma (cemento-ossifying fibroma)	Second decade Female predilection	Painless swelling; circular growth pattern; well-defined, unilocular lesion with sclerotic borders; downward bowing of inferior cortex of mandible; may be radiolucent, mixed, or radiopaque	Premolar and molar region; usually occurs in mandible	*Juvenile ossifying fibroma* is aggressive variant that usually occurs in maxilla and frequently recurs	Enucleation or resection; rarely recurs	Calcifying odontogenic cyst Ameloblastic fibro-odontoma Fibrous dysplasia Idiopathic osteosclerosis Focal cemento-osseous dysplasia Osteoblastoma Cementoblastoma
Osteomyelitis with proliferative periostitis (Garré osteomyelitis)	First and second decades No gender predilection	Diffuse, poorly defined, mixed radiolucent and opaque lesion; expansile; cortical bone duplication with laminated or onion skin pattern; mild tenderness	Posterior mandible; usually involves first permanent molar	Usually carious molar is noted; occlusal radiograph is helpful for demonstrating cortical laminations	Endodontic treatment or tooth extraction; if necessary, antibiotic therapy; expanded bone usually remodels without surgical recontouring	Fibrous dysplasia Fracture callus Buccal bifurcation cyst Ewing sarcoma Infantile cortical hyperostosis Osteosarcoma

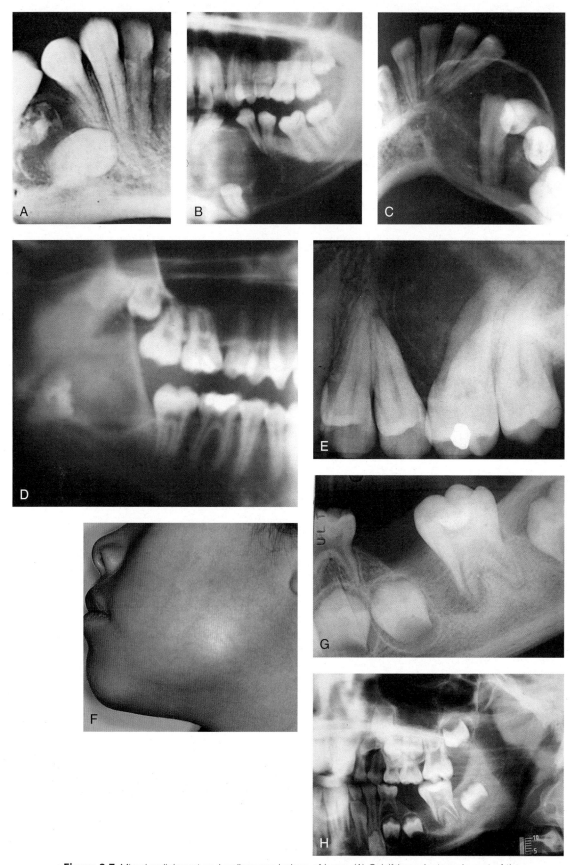

• **Figure 2.7** Mixed radiolucent and radiopaque lesions of bone. (A) Calcifying odontogenic cyst of the mandible with displacement of the unerupted premolar. (B and C) Adenomatoid odontogenic cyst of the mandible with displacement of the unerupted canine, cropped panoramic view (B), occlusal radiographic view (C). (D) Ameloblastic fibro-odontoma of the posterior mandible and ramus. (E) Ossifying fibroma of the posterior maxilla. (F–H) Osteomyelitis with proliferative periostitis, clinical view (F), periapical radiographic view (G), and cropped panoramic view (H).

TABLE 2.8   Radiopaque Lesions of Bone (see Fig. 2.8)

Lesion	Pediatric Age and Gender	Clinical and Radiographic Findings	Location	Pediatric Significance	Treatment and Prognosis	Differential Diagnosis
Odontoma, compound and complex	First and second decades No gender predilection	Well-defined radiopacity surrounded by narrow radiolucent rim; develop in pericoronal or radicular areas *Compound type* resembles miniature teeth; *complex type* is amorphous opaque mass	*Compound type:* anterior maxilla *Complex type:* posterior mandible Rarely occurs in gingiva	Represents a hamartoma; most common odontogenic tumorlike lesion; frequent cause of isolated delayed tooth eruption	Local excision; recurrence is rare	Eruption sequestrum Ameloblastic fibro-odontoma Cementoblastoma Calcifying odontogenic cyst Calcifying epithelial odontogenic tumor
Osteoma	Second decade No gender predilection	Usually solitary, well-defined, spherical radiopacity; slow growing, may be expansile and result in facial deformity	Body of mandible and condyle are most common sites; endosteal or periosteal location	*Gardner syndrome,* autosomal dominant: characterized by osteomas, intestinal polyposis, supernumerary teeth, odontomas, and skin lesions; malignant polyps	Surgical excision; periodically evaluate small lesions; no recurrence	Torus/exostosis Complex odontoma Fibrous dysplasia Condensing osteitis Familial gigantiform cementoma Idiopathic osteosclerosis
Fibrous dysplasia	Second decade No gender predilection	Unilateral, fusiform enlargement; ground-glass radiopacity with ill-defined borders; may displace teeth and delay eruption; slow growing and asymptomatic; facial asymmetry	Maxilla is more frequently affected than mandible; buccal and lingual cortical expansion	*McCune-Albright syndrome* includes polyostotic fibrous dysplasia, café-au-lait macules, and endocrine abnormalities	Osseous recontouring for cosmetic and functional problems; stabilizes after completion of skeletal development; rare malignant transformation	Chronic sclerosing osteomyelitis Ossifying fibroma Osteoma Segmental odontomaxillary dysplasia
Condensing osteitis (focal sclerosing osteomyelitis)	First and second decades No gender predilection	Localized radiopacity at root apices of pulpally involved tooth; margins blend into surrounding bone; usually asymptomatic	Most cases are in mandibular premolar and molar region	Most common periapical radiopacity; sclerotic bone may impede eruption of succedaneous tooth	No treatment of bony lesion; manage odontogenic infection; may regress after treatment or cause a bone scar	Cementoblastoma Idiopathic osteosclerosis Complex odontoma Exostosis/torus
Cementoblastoma	First and second decades No gender predilection	Radiopaque mass surrounded by thin radiolucent rim; may be mixed radiolucent-radiopaque; fused to root of vital tooth; pain and swelling are common	Posterior mandible in molar and premolar region	Rarely involves primary teeth	Surgical extraction of tooth with attached tumor or endodontic treatment with root amputation	Condensing osteitis Osteoblastoma Complex odontoma Hypercementosis
Idiopathic osteosclerosis (bone scar)	First and second decades No gender predilection	Asymptomatic, nonexpansile, uniformly radiopaque lesion that blends into surrounding bone; round or elliptical in shape; adjacent teeth are vital	Molar-premolar mandible; usually by root apices	Rare cases reach >2 cm in size and may interfere with tooth eruption	No treatment is necessary; tend to stabilize in size in young adulthood	Condensing osteitis Residual root tip Exostosis Osteoma

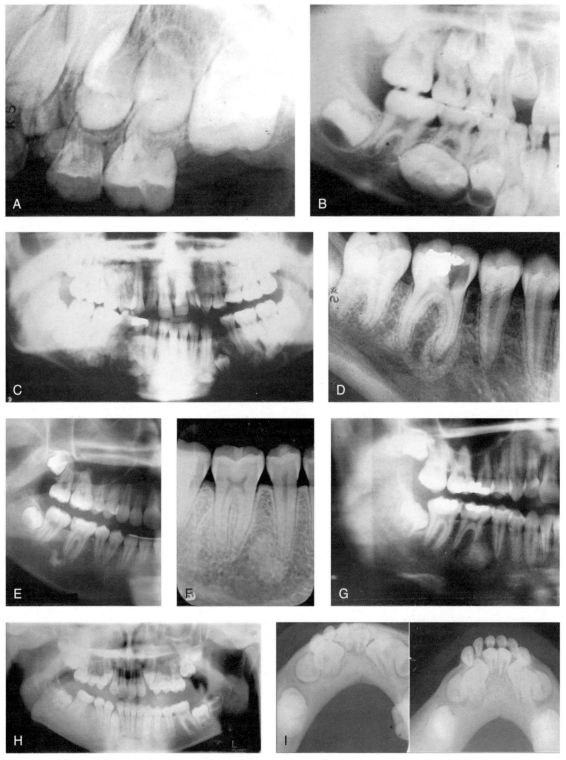

• **Figure 2.8** Radiopaque lesions of bone. (A) Compound odontoma of the maxilla. (B) Complex odontoma of the mandible. (C) Multiple osteomas associated with Gardner syndrome. (D) Condensing osteitis associated with carious mandibular molar. (E and F) Idiopathic osteosclerosis of the posterior mandible, cropped panoramic radiographic view (E), periapical example that mimics condensing osteitis (F). (G) Cementoblastoma associated with the mandibular molar. (H–I) Fibrous dysplasia of the mandible, panoramic radiographic view (H), and occlusal radiographic view (I). ([H and I] Courtesy Dr. J.F. Yepes, Indiana University School of Dentistry.)

3

Anomalies of the Developing Dentition

J. TIMOTHY WRIGHT AND BEAU D. MEYER

Developmental Controls and Environmental Interactions

Developmental defects of teeth are clinically heterogeneous in their phenotypes, and as a result they present diverse challenges in their clinical management. Tooth formation involves a complex series of tightly orchestrated events that are highly regulated at the molecular level, with thousands of genes involved.[1,2] Many of these genes are now known to be associated with developmental defects of teeth.[3] The cellular events and processes are sensitive to environmental stressors that can alter cell and tissue function and result in developmental dental defects. The clinician is faced with diagnosing these defects, identifying their underlying etiology (genetic, environmental, combined), understanding how the dental tissues are affected, and then managing these conditions. The goal of this chapter is to review some of the more common conditions that are likely to present to clinicians who provide oral health care for the pediatric population.

Making an accurate diagnosis for many hereditary conditions can now be confirmed with molecular testing. The dentist should establish if the patient's presenting condition is likely to have a hereditary basis through evaluation of family history of the trait and, when indicated, referral to the child's pediatrician or a geneticist for further evaluation and any indicated laboratory or genetic tests (such as the family history and pedigree development tutorial found at https://www.genome.gov/pages/education/modules/yourfamilyhealthhistory.pdf). This is becoming increasingly important because new therapies are now available that can effectively treat a variety of conditions (e.g., hypophosphatasia).[4] Being able to optimally treat individuals is predicated on obtaining an accurate and timely diagnosis so that available therapeutics and treatments can be provided. Clinicians should become accustomed to searching databases that provide current information on known hereditary conditions, clinical phenotypes or clinical manifestations, and the molecular basis that causes the condition, such as the Online Mendelian Inheritance in Man (OMIM) website (http://www.omim.org) that provides an electronic catalog of hereditary conditions and their causes. In this chapter we include the OMIM number that is used to designate specific conditions to facilitate the reader who wants to further investigate specific hereditary dental traits.

Anomalies of Tooth Number

Developmental dental defects involving tooth number can be classified a number of ways, but for simplicity we will use hypodontia to denote any number of missing teeth and hyperdontia as any number of extra teeth. Other commonly used terms include oligodontia, which is defined as missing more than six teeth excluding third molars, and anodontia, the complete absence of teeth. Developmental anomalies of tooth number are relatively common, with missing teeth being more prevalent than having extra or supernumerary teeth. Alterations in tooth number often result from abnormalities in the genetic and molecular regulation of tooth development, but any number of environmental stressors can also arrest tooth bud development at later developmental stages.[5]

Environmental stressors such as infection, radiation, and trauma can be associated with changes in tooth number, size, and shape. The effects will depend largely on the magnitude, duration, and timing of the stressor in relation to tooth development. Radiation and chemotherapy can be associated with hypodontia, small teeth, or teeth with only rudimentary root formation, depending upon the dose and timing of treatment and the concomitant stage of dental development. Two of the most commonly implicated chemotherapeutic agents are vincristine and the alkylating agent cyclophosphamide.[6,7] If these agents are administered during tooth formation, the pediatric patient is at risk for developing dental

TABLE 3.1	Syndromes Demonstrating Hyperdontia			
Condition	Mode of Inheritance	Phenotype	OMIM #	Gene
Apert syndrome	Autosomal dominant	Scaphocephaly, craniosynostosis, bilateral syndactyly, midface hypoplasia	101200	FGFR2
Cleidocranial dysplasia	Autosomal dominant	Aplastic clavicles, frontal bossing, hypoplastic midface	119600	RUNX2
Gardner syndrome	Autosomal dominant	Osteomas, epidermoid cysts, odontomas, intestinal polyps	175100	APC
Down syndrome	Trisomy 21	Brachycephaly, mental retardation, epicanthal folds	190685	Many
Crouzon syndrome	Autosomal dominant	Craniosynostosis, exophthalmos, hypoplastic midface	123500	FGFR2
Sturge-Weber syndrome	(In progress)	Angiomatosis and calcification of leptomeninges, seizures, port-wine nevi of face	185300	GNAQ
Oral-facial-digital syndrome	X-linked dominant (in progress)	Hypoplastic alar cartilage, cleft tongue, clinodactyly	311200	OFD1
Oculodentodigital dysplasia	Autosomal recessive (in progress)	Maxillary hypoplasia, micrognathia, enamel hypoplasia	257850	GJA1

OMIM, Online Mendelian Inheritance in Man.

anomalies, including hypodontia.[8] Radiation doses of 30 Gray (Gy) and 10 Gy can arrest tooth development and amelogenesis, respectively.[8,9]

Hyperdontia

The presence of supernumerary teeth can be an isolated trait or be associated with a syndrome (Table 3.1). The most commonly occurring supernumerary teeth are called *mesiodens,* with a prevalence of approximately 1% in the population (reports vary from 0.15% to 4%).[10] Mesiodens develop in the anterior midline of the maxillary arch. Ninety percent to 98% of supernumerary teeth occur in the maxilla, with the permanent dentition being more frequently affected than the primary dentition. The extra tooth or teeth are often diagnosed during routine radiographic examination or due to asymmetric tooth eruption of a central incisor whose eruption is being impeded by the supernumerary tooth (Fig. 3.1). There may be one or two extra teeth present; they frequently have a conical or abnormal morphology, can be oriented to either erupt normally or be inverted, and are most often positioned palatal to the permanent incisors. Mesiodens are thought to be an isolated developmental anomaly and are not known to be associated with syndromes or to be hereditary with an increased familial occurrence.

Supernumerary teeth can be classified as supplemental or rudimentary. Supplemental supernumerary teeth duplicate the typical anatomy of posterior and anterior teeth. Rudimentary supernumerary teeth are dysmorphic and can assume conical forms, tuberculate forms, or shapes that duplicate molar anatomy. From a clinical standpoint, the tuberculate, or barrel-shaped, supernumeraries generate the most severe complications with respect to difficulty of removal and adverse effects on adjacent teeth, such as impaction or ectopic eruption. Additional complications associated with supernumeraries include dentigerous cyst formation, diastema, and crown resorption.[11] The presence of supernumerary teeth has a similar radiographic and clinical presentation as an odontoma, given the similar morphologic characteristics of a compound odontoma.[12]

Supernumerary teeth can occur in nonsyndromic and syndromic cleft lip with or without cleft palate, further complicating

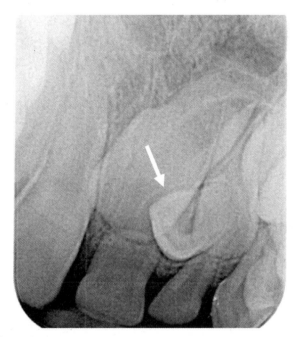

• **Figure 3.1** This 8-year-old shows asymmetric eruption of the maxillary incisors leading to diagnosis of this mesiodens (arrow) that was just lingual to teeth #9 and #10.

management of these patients. Patients with cleft lip and palate have been reported to have an increased incidence of hyperdontia, with reports indicating an incidence of up to 5%.[13] Careful evaluation by the craniofacial team to determine which teeth are best kept and which will require extraction and the timing of treatment is essential.

There are multiple syndromes associated with supernumerary teeth that are caused by a variety of genetic mutations involving diverse development pathways (see Table 3.1).[14] Gardner syndrome (OMIM #175100) is caused by mutations in the APC gene that is involved in the beta catenin pathway (as is the AXIN2 gene that is associated with congenitally missing teeth).[15] Individuals with this condition are at increased risk for developing intestinal cancer

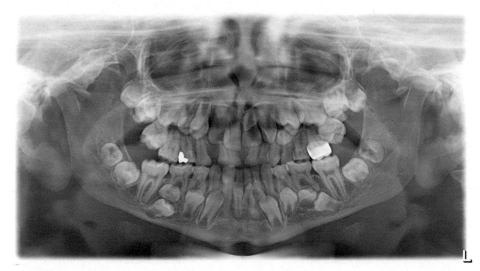

• **Figure 3.2** This 10-year-old with cleidocranial dysplasia demonstrates failed eruption of the succedaneous teeth and multiple supernumerary visible in this panoramic radiograph.

(adenopolyposis carcinoma), making it critical to evaluate the family history for this associated clinical feature.

Cleidocranial dysplasia (OMIM #119600) is a syndrome caused by mutations in the *RUNX2* gene that is important in the development of bone and teeth.[16] Individuals having this condition are typically short in stature and can exhibit the following: frontal bossing and delayed suture closure, multiple supernumerary teeth, and failure of the succedaneous teeth to erupt (Fig. 3.2). Although cleidocranial dysplasia is inherited as an autosomal dominant trait, there often is no family history because the affected individual's condition is caused by a de novo mutation in the *RUNX2* gene. Managing the dental manifestations of this condition can be quite challenging, often requiring a team approach.[17]

Hypodontia

Approximately 6% of the white population is missing a tooth other than third permanent molars, and there is racial variance regarding the prevalence of missing teeth. The most frequently occurring congenitally absent permanent tooth, excluding the third molars, tends to be the mandibular second bicuspid (3.4%), followed by the maxillary lateral incisor (2.2%).[18] Missing primary teeth is much less common compared with permanent teeth, with a prevalence of approximately 1%. However, there is a high correlation between having a missing primary tooth and absence of its permanent tooth successor. The greater the number of teeth a person is missing, the more likely they are to have a syndrome such as an ectodermal dysplasia. Family history will often reveal that the missing tooth trait is present in multiple generations of family members and often demonstrates an autosomal dominant mode of inheritance.

Like hyperdontia, mentioned previously, hypodontia is also seen in nonsyndromic and syndromic cleft lip with or without cleft palate. Patients with cleft lip and palate have been reported to have an increased incidence of hypodontia, with reports indicating an incidence of up to 47% in patients with a cleft diagnosis.[19] In cases of hypodontia associated with cleft lip and palate, there is approximately a 30% incidence of hypodontia outside the cleft site. Multiple genes have been identified as being causative of congenitally missing teeth in the absence of a syndrome including

TABLE 3.2	Hereditary Traits Associated With Hypodontia		
Condition	**Inheritance**	**OMIM #**	**Gene**
Hypodontia			
Hypodontia: premolar, third molar	Autosomal dominant	106600	MSX1
Oligodontia: incisor, molar	Autosomal dominant	604625	PAX9
Oligodontia	Autosomal dominant		WNT10A
Syndrome/Hypodontia			
Hypohidrotic ectodermal dysplasia	X-linked recessive	305100	EDA
Hypohidrotic ectodermal dysplasia	Autosomal dominant–recessive	129490–224900	DL
Incontinentia pigmenti	X-linked dominant	308300	NEMO
Witkop/tooth and nail syndrome	Autosomal dominant	189500	MSX1
Reiger syndrome type I	Autosomal dominant	180500	RIEG1
Ellis–van Creveld syndrome	Autosomal recessive	225500	EVG
Ectodermal dysplasia, cleft, syndactyly	Autosomal recessive	225000	PVRL1

OMIM, Online Mendelian Inheritance in Man.

MSX1, PAX9, WNT10A, AXIN2, and *EDA* (Table 3.2). Mutations in the *WNT10A* gene appear to be the most prevalent cause of nonsyndromic hypodontia.

In addition to nonsyndromic hypodontia, there are many syndromes that have missing teeth as a common feature.

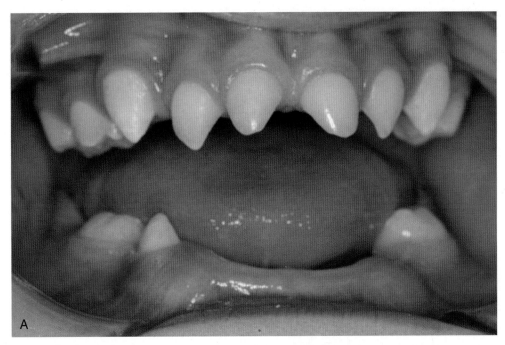

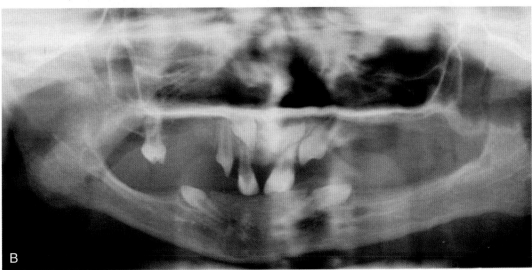

• **Figure 3.3** (A and B) Conical-shaped incisors and missing teeth are common clinical features of X-linked hypohidrotic ectodermal dysplasia, as seen in these two affected males.

Ectodermal dysplasia is a term used to described conditions with two or more tissues of ectodermal derivation (e.g., teeth, hair, sweat glands, mammary glands, salivary glands, fingernails) that demonstrate abnormal development due to genetic causes (Fig. 3.3). There are nearly 200 conditions that can be considered as ectodermal dysplasias, with the X-linked hypohidrotic ecto-dermal dysplasia (OMIM #305100) being the most common type.[20] Numerous other conditions display hypodontia as part of their phenotype. For example, Down syndrome is frequently (20% to 40%) associated with conical-shaped incisors and missing teeth.[21]

Anomalies of Size

Abnormalities in tooth size can be localized affecting one or several teeth or generalized affecting all the teeth. A reduction in tooth size is called *microdontia* and is more common than an increase in tooth size termed *macrodontia*. The peg-shaped maxillary lateral incisor is an example of localized microdontia and has been linked to mutations in the *WNT10A* gene (OMIM #150400). It is often transmitted as an autosomal dominant trait with variable expressivity and incomplete penetrance. In some cases, patients develop one maxillary lateral incisor that is peg-shaped and one that fails to form and is missing.

Not surprisingly, reduced tooth size and conical-shaped teeth are features of many of the ectodermal dysplasias (e.g., OMIM #305100, 604292, 224900, 129490), oculodentodigital dysplasia (OMIM #164200), and many other syndromes, including Down syndrome (OMIM #190685). Furthermore, environmental stressors such as chemotherapy and radiation as part of cancer treatment can interfere with the normal development of tooth size, with many cases resulting in microdontia.[8,22]

Microdontia

Diminished tooth size can result from a change in the overall tooth size or can occur secondary to reduction in the enamel thickness or both. Conditions demonstrating microdontia include many of the ectodermal dysplasias and the tricho-dento-osseous syndrome (OMIM #190320) that can have generally small teeth with thin enamel (Fig. 3.4; also see Fig. 3.3). A decrease in dental crown size occurs due to generalized thin enamel (e.g., generalized thin hypoplastic amelogenesis imperfecta) despite the dentin morphology and dimension being normal. The overall tooth size in individuals affected with dentinogenesis imperfecta is typically reduced as well.

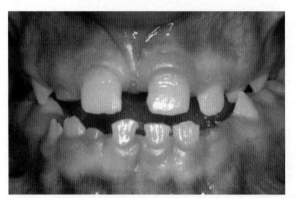

• **Figure 3.4** Generalized microdontia is seen in the late transitional dentition (permanent incisors) of this child affected with the tricho-dento-osseous syndrome.

Macrodontia

Macrodontia can occur as a localized trait, and most commonly occurs as gemination. Gemination is the incomplete twining of primary or permanent teeth and is not known to have any genetic predilection or heritable etiology. This developmental disturbance can result in teeth that are almost twice the width of the normal nontwinned tooth (Fig. 3.5). Fusion of developing teeth also can result in an enlarged tooth, but there will be one less individual tooth in the affected area, whereas gemination manifests with the normal number of teeth present. Gemination and fusion are both relatively rare, with a prevalence of approximately 0.5%.[23] Fusion is more common in the primary dentition compared with the permanent dentition.

Hereditary conditions with macrodontia include otodental syndrome (OMIM #166750) and the rare but quite remarkable Ekman-Westborg and Julin trait.[24] Otodental syndrome/otodental dysplasia (OMIM #166750) is an autosomal dominant condition caused by microdeletion at *FGF3* gene on chromosome 11q13. It is characterized by grossly enlarged canines and molars and is frequently associated with sensorineural hearing loss and ocular coloboma.

Anomalies of Tooth Morphology

Developmental abnormalities in crown and/or root morphology or shape are collectively relatively common and are diverse in both their clinical presentation and apparent etiology. These developmental variances can involve one or more teeth and can affect any portion or component of the tooth (e.g., crown, root, pulp).

Environmental stressors can have a profound influence on tooth shape as well. Infectious conditions such as congenital syphilis,

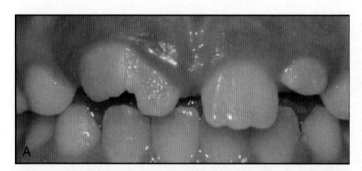

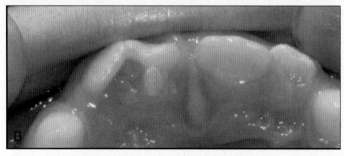

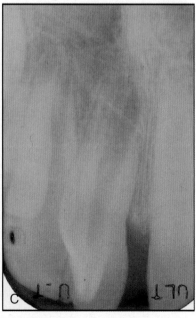

• **Figure 3.5** As seen in this patient, gemination can produce localized macrodontia (A) and other developmental abnormalities such as a talon cusp in the lingual-cingulum area (B). Discerning whether there is communication between the different dental segments can be difficult using traditional radiography as illustrated in this periapicle radiograph (C). Cone beam computed tomography can help to determine pulp and root communication status.

which is caused by the spirochete *Treponema pallidum,* produce classic patterns of hypoplastic and dysmorphic permanent teeth. The tapered and notched incisal edges of anterior teeth with screwdriver shapes are called *Hutchinson incisors,* and the irregular and accentuated occlusal patterns of posterior teeth known as mulberry molars are classic clinical findings for prenatal syphilis infection.[25]

Regional odontodysplasia affects all three tissues and typically is localized to one or more teeth in a specific area or developmental field. The affected teeth show marked dysplasia of the crown, root, and pulp morphology and are most often not compatible with a functioning tooth. The prognosis and management for each of these conditions also can be quite variable and should be investigated by further research when clinicians are managing patients with one of these developmental variances.[26]

Crown Size and Morphology

Tooth crown size and morphology are highly regulated at the genetic level, producing quite predictable dental morphologies for each specific primary and permanent tooth. Despite this regulation, a variety of developmental defects present as abnormal crown development, including variable cuspal patterns (talon, dens evaginatus, dens invaginatus, cusp of Carabelli), or more globally, crown shape, such as the marked cervical constriction seen in teeth (especially the posterior teeth) of individuals with dentinogenesis imperfecta.

Dens Evaginatus/Invaginatus

Dens evaginatus (OMIM #125280) describes an outfolding of the enamel organ that results in an extra cusp, usually in the central groove or ridge of posterior teeth and in the cingulum area of the anterior teeth, sometimes called a talon cusp (see Fig. 3.5). It occurs with a frequency of 1% to 4% and results from the evagination of inner enamel epithelium cells, which are the precursors of ameloblasts. The extra cusp contains enamel, dentin, and pulp tissue; therefore pulp exposure is possible by radically equilibrating the occlusion. Management of this anomaly includes careful enameloplasty or preventive resin restorations.[27]

Dens invaginatus, or dens in dente (OMIM #125300), is a condition resulting from invagination of the inner enamel epithelium producing the appearance of a tooth within a tooth (Fig. 3.6). The prevalence ranges from 0.25% to 3%, with the maxillary lateral incisors being most frequently affected.[28] The clinical significance of this anomaly is the high likelihood of carious and/or pulpal involvement through the communication of the invaginated portion of the lingual surface of the tooth with the outside environment. Therefore prompt diagnosis and preventive care (e.g., sealant, restoration) are crucial in cases of dens in dente.

Root Size and Morphology

Root morphology can be affected by environmental stressors (e.g., trauma to a developing tooth bud resulting in root dilacerations), can be caused by genetic factors that affect only root development, or can be associated with a syndrome. Severe infections such as that which occur in Stevens-Johnson syndrome or meningococcemia can lead to abnormal root formation.[29] Chemotherapy and radiation can lead to V-shaped or stunted roots if administered while tooth roots are developing (Fig. 3.7).[8,22]

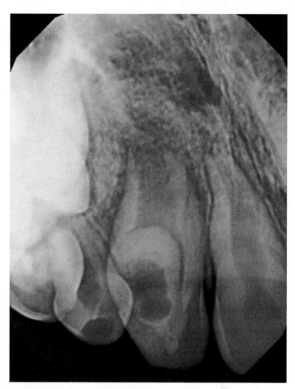

• **Figure 3.6** This maxillary incisor has undergone pulpal necrosis as a result of dens in dente and presumably communication between the dental pulp and the oral environment.

Genetic causes of abnormal root formation include truncated root formation caused by mutations in the *IFIH1* gene that is associated with the Singleton-Merten syndrome 1 (OMIM #182250).[30] Individuals with tumoral calcinosis (OMIM #211900) can have short bulbous roots and is caused by mutations in the *GALNT3* gene.[31] Short dental roots are also seen with sponastrime dysplasia (OMIM #271510) and Bardet-Biedl syndrome 1 (OMIM #209900).[32,33]

Molar Incisor Root Malformation

A novel dental phenotype has recently been described that is characterized by diminished and dysplastic root formation of the first permanent molars and a narrow abnormal pulp chamber (Fig. 3.8).[34] This molar dysmorphology is the cardinal or primary feature of this trait. The second primary molars and other primary and permanent teeth are affected in some cases with developmental changes that appear similar to those seen in the affected first permanent molars. The permanent anterior teeth can be involved and exhibit cervical crown constrictions and changes in the pulp chamber morphology. These phenotypic features have led to this condition being referred to as molar incisor root malformation (MIRM).[35] The etiology remains unclear; however, the majority of affected individuals have a history of systemic illness or neonatal conditions, such meningomyelocele or sacral dimple, meningitis, preterm birth, or chronic renal disease to name a few. Clinicians identifying cases of MIRM should carefully evaluate them due to the increased potential of ectopic eruption, pulp necrosis, and permanent incisor malformations.[35]

Short Root Anomaly

First described in the 1970s, short root anomaly is still a poorly understood phenomenon. Central incisors and premolars are the

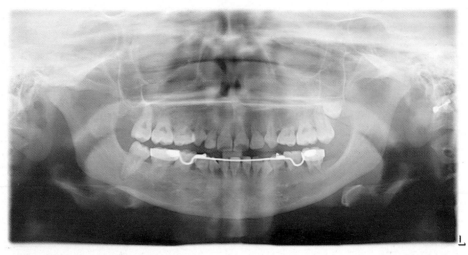

• **Figure 3.7** This panoramic radiograph of this 18-year-old cancer survivor's dentition displays numerous developmentally missing permanent teeth and marked disruption of the normal root development secondary to aggressive chemotherapy between age 1 and 2 years.

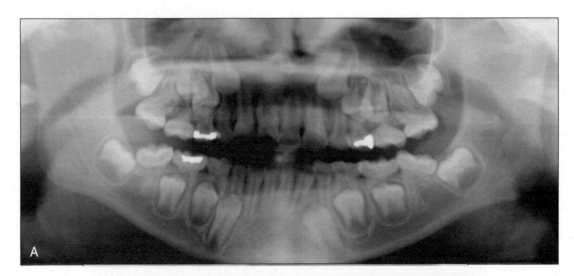

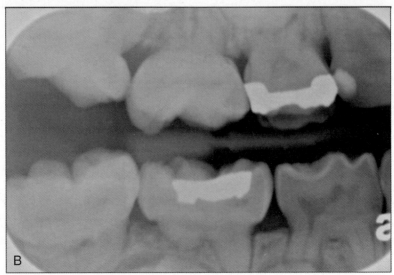

• **Figure 3.8** Molar incisor root malformation affects the first permanent molars root and pulp morphology, as seen in the panoramic radiograph as well as incisors (A). (B) The periapical radiograph of this same child shows the second primary molar, and, to less extent, the first primary molar also are affected.

most commonly affected teeth, frequently presenting with shortened, wide, and round roots. Although few epidemiologic studies exist, it is estimated that short root anomaly has a prevalence of 1.3%.[36] The etiology remains unclear, but it is suspected to be of genetic origin and transmitted as an autosomal dominant trait.[37] In syndromic cases of short root anomaly, such as Rothmund-Thomson syndrome (OMIM #268400), specific genes have been associated with the dental anomaly.[38] Many clinicians often misdiagnose this condition as a pathologic resorption, when the two conditions are distinctly different. Correctly diagnosing this condition has major implications for treatment planning decisions because treatment options for an abnormal variant differ from options for a pathologic condition with root resorption. In contrast to short root anomaly, there have been reports of elongated roots in oculofaciocardiodental syndrome (OMIM #300166) due to mutations in the *BCOR* gene that lead to increased periodontal ligament (PDL) cell proliferation and uncontrolled root growth, particularly of the permanent canines.[39,40]

Hypercementosis

Hypercementosis is the increase in cementum deposition on a root surface resulting in an abnormal root shape, frequently a bulbous tip at the root apex. The prevalence of hypercementosis is estimated to be 1.3%.[41] The etiology can include a reactive response to periapical inflammation, dental trauma to the PDL, or an abnormal developmental process. Several systemic conditions have been related to hypercementosis including atherosclerosis, acromegaly, and Paget disease.

Taurodontism

Taurodontism affects multirooted teeth and is characterized by an elongated pulp chamber due to apical displacement of the pulpal floor. Thus the root furcation moves apically leaving the individual roots greatly shortened even though the overall root length may be normal. The prevalence in the general population reportedly ranges from 0.5% to 5%, with the permanent molar most often affected. The condition can be classified according to the extent of the pulp chamber elongation.[42] Because root furcation results from invagination of Hertwig's epithelial root sheath, many of the ectodermal dysplasias exhibit taurodontism. Individuals with tricho-dento-osseous syndrome (OMIM #190320) often have quite pronounced taurodontism (Fig. 3.9).[43] Taurodontism has also been associated with a variety of syndromes and has an increased prevalence in individuals with sex chromosome aneuploidy (Table 3.3).

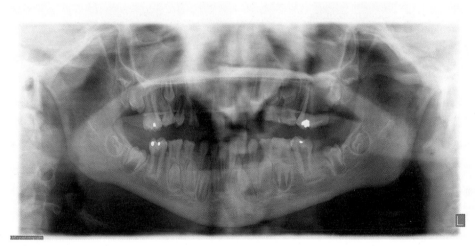

• **Figure 3.9** This patient with tricho-dento-osseous syndrome demonstrates marked taurodontism of both the first permanent and second primary molars, as seen in this panoramic radiograph of their mixed dentition.

TABLE 3.3 Conditions Demonstrating Taurodontism

Condition	Characteristics	OMIM #	Gene	Mode of Inheritance
Klinefelter syndrome	Aspermatogenesis, mental retardation	400045	46,XX	—
Tricho-dento-osseous syndrome	Sclerotic bones, coarse gnarled hair, enamel defects	190320	*DLX3*	Autosomal dominant
Oral-facial-digital syndrome type 2	Dystrophic nails, hyperplastic frenum, lobed tongue	252100	*OFD2*	Autosomal recessive
Ectodermal dysplasia (hypohidrotic)	Hypotrichosis, aplasia of sweat/sebaceous glands	305100	*EDA*	X-linked recessive
Amelogenesis imperfecta type 4	Enamel hypoplasia and hypomaturation, mottled yellow teeth	104510	*DLX3*	Autosomal dominant
Down syndrome	Brachycephaly, mental retardation, epicanthal fold	190685	Many	Trisomy 21

OMIM, Online Mendelian Inheritance in Man.

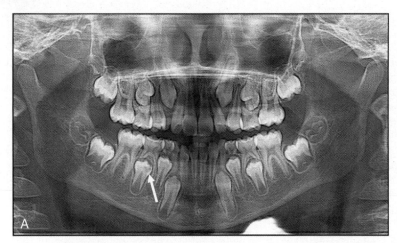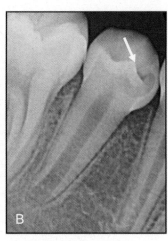

• **Figure 3.10** This child had showed an approximately 0.5-cm radiolucency just below the dentin enamel junction on this panoramic radiograph *(arrow)* (A). This well-circumscribed lesion *(arrow)* that does not extend through the proximal enamel can be appreciated after the tooth erupted in this periapical radiograph (B).

Dental Tissue Composition and Structural Defects

The composition and structure of the dental tissues are unique and highly specialized, giving each tissue the requisite properties related to wear, flexure, fracture resistance, and attachment (tissue to tissue and tooth to bone) to have a viable dentition that can withstand the rigors of oral function. The etiologies of defects involving the composition and/or structure of the dental tissues can be either environmental or hereditary. However, in certain teeth the etiology is not well understood. For example, preeruptive dentinal radiolucencies can be seen on radiographs (Fig. 3.10), and, although no prevalence studies exist for this condition, case reports and case series do document its presence. The etiology is unclear, but the most likely explanation seems to be a combination of developmental anomaly, internal, and/or external resorption.[44] Some have posited that the developmental anomaly is a type of hypoplasia or the inclusion of a noncalcified enamel matrix in dentin.[44,45] The processes involved in development of the dental tissues are highly specialized so it is not surprising that there are so many different etiologies and clinical presentations of dental defects involving composition and structure.

Environmental Defects Altering Tooth Color

Enamel development, or amelogenesis, is an exquisitely regulated process at the molecular level but can be disrupted by many environmental factors, such as fever, infection, trauma, changes in oxygen saturation, antibiotics, and many other factors (Table 3.4). In general, the resulting enamel defects can be classified as defects in the amount of enamel (hypoplasia) or deficiencies in the mineral content (hypomineralization). Changes in enamel mineralization result in altered enamel translucency and color. Because enamel is translucent, changes in dentin can result in tooth color changes even when the enamel is relatively unchanged (e.g., tetracycline staining). Enamel hypoplasia or hypomineralization can be generalized throughout the dentition or it can be localized. Environmental stressors that are of short duration often cause localized defects (e.g., fever), whereas chronic stressors are more likely to be associated with generalized defects (e.g., fluorosis).

TABLE 3.4	Environmental Influences on Enamel and/or Tooth Color
Condition	**Phenotype**
Fever	Hypomineralization to marked enamel hypoplasia
Starvation	Enamel hypoplasia
Excess fluoride exposure	Enamel hypomineralization
Trauma	Hypomineralization to marked enamel hypoplasia, blue-gray to yellow-brown color
Hypoxia (e.g., severe cardiac defect)	Hypomineralization to marked enamel hypoplasia
Infection (e.g., congenital syphilis, cytomegalovirus, congenital rubella)	Hypomineralization to marked enamel hypoplasia
Tetracycline	Blue-gray color, dentin staining possible enamel hypoplasia
Low birth weight	Enamel hypoplasia
Hyperbilirubinemia	Green discoloration

Enamel defects are common in the general population, with reports suggesting that between 20% and 80% of people will have an enamel defect.[46,47] The broad range of reported enamel defect prevalence is largely due to what was classified as an enamel defect (actual hypoplasia versus color change indicating hypomineralization). Not all teeth are affected equally, with anterior teeth being more affected than premolars in the permanent dentition. Children who have more frequent and serious illnesses are more likely to have enamel defects. Common causes of intrinsic stains include blood-borne pigments, drug administration, and hypoplastic-hypocalcified disease states (see Table 3.4). Congenital porphyria, bile duct defects, anemias, and transfusion-reaction hemolysis are examples of conditions with characteristic blood-borne pigments.

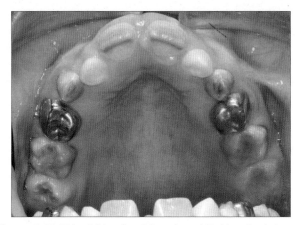

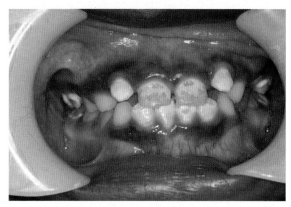

• **Figure 3.11** This child suffered from hyperbilirubinemia during early development of the primary and permanent dentitions. Note the staining in both primary and some permanent teeth.

• **Figure 3.12** This child demonstrates severe fluorosis of the permanent incisors and molars while the primary dentition appears unaffected as a consequence of reduced fetal fluoride exposure resulting from fluid dynamics and fluoride uptake differentials in the mother and infant.

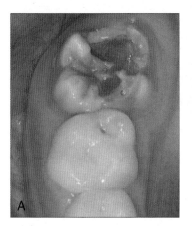

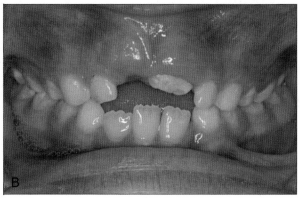

• **Figure 3.13** Molar incisor hypomineralization is highly variable in its presentation and in severe cases (A) can be associated with early enamel loss and dental sensitivity. Involvement of other teeth is variable as well but often involves the incisors as seen in this partially erupted maxillary central incisor (B).

For example, biliary atresia and the resultant hyperbilirubinemia often cause green teeth (Fig. 3.11).

A classic example of drug-induced intrinsic staining occurs from the tetracycline group of antibiotics. Both dentitions can have severe discoloration from this antibiotic when given over as brief a period as 3 days. Tetracycline hydrochloride has the greatest potential for staining among the cycline antibiotics. The agent forms an orthocalcium phosphate complex with dentin and enamel, which is then oxidized by ultraviolet light. The oxidation process results in pigments that stain the hard tissues. The critical period for initiation of primary and permanent tooth staining is that of intrauterine development through 8 years of age. Tetracycline administration must be especially avoided during this time. The International Association of Dental Traumatology (IADT) does recommend systemic doxycycline twice a day for 7 days for avulsion injuries but includes a caution that clearly states tetracycline administration may result in discoloration.[48] Doxycycline is present in significant levels within gingival crevicular fluid.

Fluorosis

Dental fluorosis is a pathologic condition characterized by hypomineralization of the enamel due to excessive exposure to fluoride during enamel mineralization. The level of hypomineralization and clinical appearance of the fluorotic enamel varies from mild to severe (Fig. 3.12) and is partially determined by the amount of fluoride in the individual's serum during amelogenesis. Individuals have differing risk and resistance to developing dental fluorosis based on their genetic makeup and health. Studies suggest a number of genes are important in defining the population's variance for dental fluorosis risk.[49] Fluoride has a variety of actions that contribute to the development of dental fluorosis, including direct effects on the ameloblasts, the developing matrix, and processing of the matrix.[50]

Molar-Incisor Hypomineralization

Molar-incisor hypomineralization (MIH) is a developmental defect of the human dentition that primarily affects the enamel of the first permanent molars and can involve the incisors. Typically the second permanent molars and premolars are not involved. This condition has been recognized since approximately 1970 and has been described using a variety of terms (e.g., cheese molars, idiopathic hypomineralization of enamel). The term *molar-incisor hypomineralization* was adopted by leaders in the field that convened at the European Academy of Pediatric Dentistry Annual Meeting in 2000.[51] The clinical characteristics vary from case to case and between teeth in the same individual. The more severely affected the first permanent molars, the more likely it is that there will be incisor involvement. The defects vary from small well-demarcated areas of color change to extensive hypomineralization that includes the entire dental crown (Fig. 3.13). Affected teeth form with a normal thickness of enamel with the abnormal areas of enamel having a decreased mineral content and increased protein and water content. Thus the defects are not hypoplastic in that the full thickness of enamel develops. Once the tooth begins to erupt and comes into function, rapid enamel loss can make the crown appear hypoplastic, but this is typically the result of enamel fracturing, wear, and dental caries.[52]

Hereditary Enamel Defects

There are thousands of genes expressed by ameloblasts, and there are more than 100 different hereditary conditions associated with an enamel phenotype.[53] Most hereditary conditions affecting enamel formation are syndromes and have clinical manifestations and phenotypes that extend beyond the dental enamel. Genes with known ameloblastic function cause many of these conditions. The most common resulting enamel phenotype is hypoplasia. For example, junctional epidermolysis bullosa (OMIM #226700) is caused by mutations in genes that are expressed by ameloblasts and are important in cell-to-cell adhesion. The abnormal proteins produced from these genes (e.g., *COL17A1, LAM3, IGbeta6*) result in fragility of the skin that blisters. Abnormal function of these proteins results in ameloblasts that do not adhere to each other or the stratum intermedium cells, resulting in cell separation and enamel hypoplasia.

Hereditary conditions affecting primarily the enamel have been referred to as amelogenesis imperfecta (AI) (Table 3.5).[54] The prevalence of AI varies around world and is thought to occur in approximately 1 out of 8000 people, although there has only been one epidemiologic study ever conducted in the United States.[54] These disorders have been classified based on their clinical phenotype and mode of inheritance. The AI types were also classified based on the perceived mechanism leading to the enamel defect (i.e., deficient matrix formation leading to hypoplasia, deficient crystal growth and mineralization during the maturation stage of enamel development causing hypomaturation, and abnormal initiation of the enamel crystallites with subsequent abnormal mineralization or hypocalcification). Both hypomaturation and hypocalcification are characterized by deficient enamel mineral or hypomineralization (Fig. 3.14). Hypomineralized AI enamel has greater amounts of protein present compared with normal enamel and will thus have

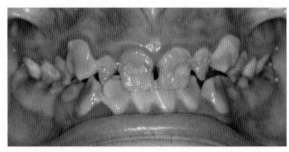

• **Figure 3.14** This individual with autosomal recessive hypomaturation amelogenesis imperfecta has marked discoloration of her teeth due to the lack of mineral and therefore limited insulating capacity of the enamel.

TABLE 3.5	Hereditary Enamel Defects		
AI Type and Inheritance	**Phenotype**	**OMIM #**	**Gene/Loci**
X-linked type IE	Hypoplasia/hypomaturation	301200	*AMELX*
X-linked hypoplastic: hypomaturation	Hypoplasia/hypomaturation	301201	*Xq22–q28*
Autosomal dominant type IB	Localized to generalized hypoplastic	104500	*ENAM*
Autosomal dominant type III	Hypocalcified	130900	*FAM83H*
Autosomal dominant type IV	Hypoplastic hypomaturation	104510	*DLX3*
Autosomal dominant	Hypomineralized	Not Listed	*AMTN*
Autosomal recessive type IC	Hypoplastic	204650	*ENAM*
Autosomal recessive type IIA1	Hypomaturation	204700	*KLK4*
Autosomal recessive type IIA2	Hypomaturation	612529	*MMP20*
Autosomal recessive type IIA3	Hypomaturation	613211	*WDR72*
Autosomal recessive type 1G (enamel renal syndrome)	Hypoplastic, pulp calcifications, eruption abnormalities	611062 614253	*FAM20A*
Autosomal recessive type IIA4	Hypomaturation	614832	*C4ORF26*
Autosomal recessive type IIA5	Hypomaturation	615887	*SCL24A4*
Autosomal recessive type IF	Hypoplastic	616270	*AMBN*
Autosomal recessive	Hypoplastic	Not listed	*ACPT*
Autosomal recessive	Hypomaturation	Not listed	*GPR68*

Hypomaturation and hypocalcified phenotypes are characterized by a deficiency in enamel mineral content or hypomineralization.
AI, Amelogenesis imperfecta; *OMIM*, Online Mendelian Inheritance in Man.

an altered translucency and can be markedly weakened depending on the decrease in mineral content.

Hereditary Dentin Defects

The process of dentin development, or dentinogenesis, is thought to be relatively resistant to environmental insults or systemic conditions compared with tooth enamel formation. It is the mesenchymally derived dentin that is the most abundant tissue in teeth and the tissue that determines much of the crown and root morphology. Normal dentin development and mineralization requires adequate levels of vitamin D (the active form is 1-25 dihydroxy vitamin D or calcitriol). Inadequate vitamin D levels during tooth development can result in decreased dentin production, resulting in large pulp chambers and a decreased dentin mineral content. Genetic mutations in several genes related to vitamin D can cause similar developmental disturbances such as the X-linked conditions vitamin D resistant (OMIM #307800) and autosomal dominant vitamin D dependent rickets (OMIM #193100).

Dentinogenesis Imperfecta

Hereditary dentin defects have been classified as dentinogenesis imperfectas (DGIs) and dentin dysplasias (DDs) (Table 3.6).[55] These hereditary conditions are associated with abnormal dentin mineralization and varying degrees of changes in tooth morphology. DGI type I (OMIM #166200) is associated with osteogenesis imperfecta, whereas the clinically similar DGI type II (OMIM #125490) is not associated with a syndrome and is caused by mutations in the gene encoding dentin sialophosphoprotein

TABLE 3.6 Hereditary Dentin Anomalies: Shields Classification

Condition	Dental Phenotype	OMIM #	Gene
DI type I	Yellow-brown to blue-gray color, enamel fracturing, diminished tooth size, cervical constriction, enamel fracturing pulp chamber obliteration, typically more severe in primary dentition, short roots	166200	COL1A1 COL1A2
DI type II	Essentially the same as above Primary and permanent frequently affected similarly Risk of periapical abscess	125490	DSPP
DI type III	Generally the same as DI type II except initially have large pulp chambers that obliterate with age	125500	DSPP
DD type I	Normal clinical crown morphology, and color, short or no roots, pulp chamber obliteration	125400	Unknown

DD, Dentin dysplasia; *DI,* dentinogenesis imperfecta; *OMIM,* Online Mendelian Inheritance in Man.

(DSPP).[56] Osteogenesis imperfecta or brittle bone disease is caused by mutations in the genes coding for type I collagen or proteins involved in fibrillogenesis. The DGI tooth phenotype is highly variable and is characterized by an opalescent blue-gray to yellow-brown coloration due to the discolored dentin shining through the relatively normal translucent enamel (enamel is affected in some cases; Fig. 3.15). The teeth can have a pronounced cervical constriction at the cementoenamel junction area that demarcates the junction of the clinical crown and the tooth root. Individuals with DGI often have dental root structures that are diminished in size and can appear sharp and "tent peg-like." The dentin in DGI teeth or in DD type II is poorly organized structurally and is less mineralized than normal dentin. This abnormal structure and lack of mineral result in the dentin inadequately supporting the enamel that often fractures away from the tooth, leaving it susceptible to undergoing rapid attrition due to the poor wear resistance of the hypomineralized DGI dentin. Enamel loss and subsequent rapid attrition is a common but variable feature of DGI. In those cases in which enamel is lost the teeth tend to wear very rapidly. Full coverage crowns are typically the treatment of choice once this process begins.

Dentin Dysplasias

DD type II, or the coronal DD type (OMIM #125420), is an allelic disorder of DGI type II caused by *DSPP* mutations. DD type II is characterized by a DGdI phenotype in the primary dentition and slight or no discernable clinical phenotype in permanent dentition (e.g., there may be slight discoloration of the dental crown).[57] Radiographically, DD type II permanent teeth often have an abnormal pulp morphology that can present as a thistle tube in the anterior teeth and sometimes a bowtie morphology in the molar teeth. Both DGI type II and DD type II are inherited as autosomal dominant traits and are highly penetrant. Interestingly, individuals with DD type II may not remember having affected primary teeth, making determination of a family history more challenging.

The phenotype in DD type I, or radicular DD type (OMIM #125400), is characterized by clinically normal-appearing tooth crowns and markedly altered dentin formation that has a pathognomonic cascading waterfall histologic appearance, pulp chamber obliteration, and abnormal to nearly missing root development. The etiology of this classic DD type I with normal crowns and unique histologic appearance is not known yet.[57]

Hereditary Cementum Defects

Cementum is deposited on the tooth surface by cementoblasts in a process known as cementogenesis. Of the dental hard tissues, cementum is the least mineralized and most cellular with many cementoblasts becoming encased in the developing tooth layer. This cellular cementum is seen more in the apical half of the root, whereas acellular cementum dominates the coronal half.

Hypophosphatasia (OMIM #146300, 241500, 241510) results from mutations in the tissue nonspecific alkaline phosphatase gene. Alkaline phosphatase is essential for normal mineralization and development of tissues including bone, dentin, and cementum. Osteoporosis, bone fragility, and premature loss of primary incisors are classic clinical features (Fig. 3.16). Abnormal development of cementum results in early loss of primary teeth that occurs without root resorption. Children presenting with early tooth loss, especially without evidence of root resorption or systemic illness, should be evaluated for hypophosphatasia. This condition is now treatable

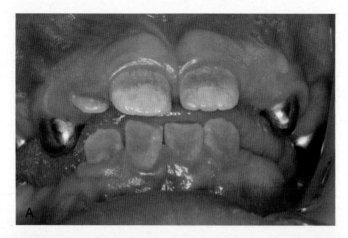

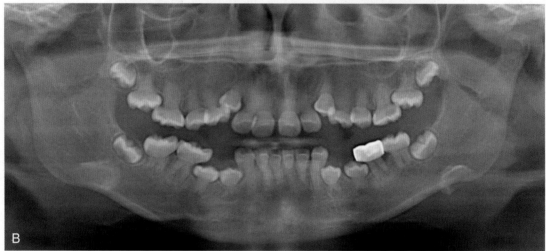

• **Figure 3.15** Dentinogenesis imperfecta is characterized clinically by variable yellow-brown to blue-gray coloration of the dentition (A). Radiographically the teeth often display pulp obliteration, cervical constriction at the cementoenamel junction, and diminished root formation (B). Ectopic eruption due to the marked cervical coronal constriction also can be a feature of dentinogenesis imperfecta as seen in this panoramic radiograph (B).

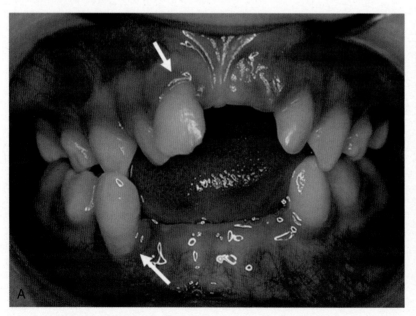

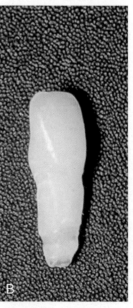

• **Figure 3.16** (A) Premature tooth loss is a hallmark feature of hypophosphatasia, and as seen in this affected child the teeth exfoliate with minimal inflammation despite gingival recession around the maxillary primary incisor and mandibular canine *(arrows)*. Children with teeth exfoliating prematurely without root resorption (B) and soft tissue inflammation should be evaluated for hypophosphatasia.

TABLE 3.7   Conditions With Abnormal Tooth Eruption Phenotype

Condition	Phenotype	OMIM #	Gene	Mode of Inheritance
Cleidocranial dysplasia	Failure of succedaneous tooth to erupt, supernumerary teeth, retention cysts	119600	RUNX2	Autosomal dominant
Primary failure of eruption	Failure of posterior teeth to erupt and not orthodontically movable	125350	PTHRP1	Autosomal dominant
Osteopetrosis	Failure of eruption due to abnormal osteoclast function	259700	TCIRG1	Autosomal recessive
Cherubism	Multilocular cystic changes in the jaws that interfere with tooth eruption and facial growth	11840	SH3BP2	Autosomal dominant
Mucopolysaccharidosis	Defective enzyme results in accumulation of material around dental follicles	309900	IDS	X-linked recessive
Oculodentodigital dysplasia	Small teeth with abnormal eruption	164200 257850	GJA1	Autosomal dominant Autosomal recessive
Autosomal recessive AI and gingival fibromatosis syndrome (enamel renal syndrome)	Hypoplastic enamel, pulp calcifications, eruption abnormalities	614253	FAM20A	Autosomal recessive

AI, Amelogenesis imperfecta; *OMIM,* Online Mendelian Inheritance in Man.

with a fusion protein that replaces the lost alkaline phosphatase protein function.

Anomalies of Tooth Eruption

The process of tooth eruption (particularly of permanent teeth) has been described in several stages, namely preemergent and postemergent eruption. Once root formation begins during the preemergent stage, eruption is thought to begin. This process requires resorption of alveolar bone and primary tooth roots, as well as a propulsive movement in an occlusal direction. Some suggest that hard tissue proliferation at the root apex is the primary mechanism for eruption. However, some teeth, for example intruded or luxated teeth, will show eruption/reeruption without apical proliferation. The mechanisms controlling tooth eruption are complex and likely involve a variety of dental components including the dental follicle and PDL.[58]

The clearance of an eruption path is the primary control for preemergent eruption. In general, so long as a path is cleared, a tooth will erupt into that path and begin its postemergent eruption. However, a blocked eruptive path can lead to eruption anomalies. Inadequate space is thus a common cause of failed tooth eruption. One of the more common eruption anomalies is ectopic eruption, which has a prevalence of approximately 3%, and the most commonly involved teeth are the permanent first molars, lateral incisors, and canines.[59] Aside from ectopic eruption, primary teeth can experience delayed exfoliation and permanent teeth can experience delayed eruption. Table 3.7 lists a few common syndromes associated with eruption anomalies, including cleidocranial dysplasia, cherubism, and enamel-renal syndrome.

Primary Failure of Eruption

Primary failure of eruption (PFE, OMIM #125350), a nonsyndromic condition affecting tooth eruption, is caused in many cases by mutations in the *PTHP1R* gene that is a regulator of bone homeostasis. PFE is characterized by having at least one affected first permanent molar; the teeth distal to the affected first permanent molar also show failed eruption usually with a progressive open bite. The involved teeth tend to have a supracrestal position, meaning they have a completely cleared eruption pathway with no alveolar bone occlusal to the affected tooth.[60] Orthodontic extrusion of affected teeth is unsuccessful and leads to ankylosis.

Summary

Pediatric oral health care providers are challenged with the diagnosis and management of a plethora of developmental defects of the dentition. The etiologies are diverse and can make obtaining an accurate diagnosis challenging. Optimal treatment and patient management are predicated on establishing a diagnosis that then allows prognosis determination and selection of treatment approaches that are based on how the tissues are affected and will respond to different treatment approaches. With new biopharmaceutical therapeutics becoming available, it is increasingly important that clinicians diagnose conditions that affect dental development and know how to search the available databases to help establish or confirm a diagnosis, the need for referral to medial or genetic specialists, and the most current and appropriate treatment options available.

References

1. Hu S, Parker J, Wright JT. Towards unraveling the human tooth transcriptome: the dentome. *PLoS ONE.* 2015;10(4):e0124801.
2. Balic A, Thesleff I. Tissue interactions regulating tooth development and renewal. *Curr Top Dev Biol.* 2015;115:157–186.
3. Cobourne MT, Sharpe PT. Diseases of the tooth: the genetic and molecular basis of inherited anomalies affecting the dentition. *Wiley Interdisc Rev Dev Biol.* 2013;2(2):183–212.
4. Hofmann C, Jakob F, Seefried L, et al. Recombinant enzyme replacement therapy in hypophosphatasia. *Subcell Biochem.* 2015;76:323–341.
5. Yin W, Bian Z. The gene network underlying hypodontia. *J Dent Res.* 2015;94(7):878–885.

6. Maguire A, Craft AW, Evans RG, et al. The long-term effects of treatment on the dental condition of children surviving malignant disease. *Cancer*. 1987;60(10):2570–2575.

7. Owosho AA, Brady P, Wolden SL, et al. Long-term effect of chemotherapy-intensity-modulated radiation therapy (chemo-IMRT) on dentofacial development in head and neck rhabdomyosarcoma patients. *Pediatr Hematol Oncol*. 2016;33(6):383–392.

8. Kaste SC, Goodman P, Leisenring W, et al. Impact of radiation and chemotherapy on risk of dental abnormalities: a report from the Childhood Cancer Survivor Study. *Cancer*. 2009;115(24):5817–5827.

9. Kaste SC, Hopkins KP, Jenkins JJ 3rd. Abnormal odontogenesis in children treated with radiation and chemotherapy: imaging findings. *AJR Am J Roentgenol*. 1994;162(6):1407–1411.

10. Demiriz L, Durmuslar MC, Misir AF. Prevalence and characteristics of supernumerary teeth: a survey on 7348 people. *J Int Soc Prev Community Dent*. 2015;5(suppl 1):S39–S43.

11. Bereket C, Cakir-Ozkan N, Sener I, et al. Analyses of 1100 supernumerary teeth in a nonsyndromic Turkish population: a retrospective multicenter study. *Niger J Clin Pract*. 2015;18(6):731–738.

12. Pippi R. Odontomas and supernumerary teeth: is there a common origin? *Int J Med Sci*. 2014;11(12):1282–1297.

13. Sa J, Mariano LC, Cangucu D, et al. Dental anomalies in a Brazilian cleft population. *Cleft Palate Craniofac J*. 2016;53(6):714–719.

14. Lubinsky M, Kantaputra PN. Syndromes with supernumerary teeth. *Am J Med Genet A*. 2016;170(10):2611–2616.

15. Panjwani S, Bagewadi A, Keluskar V, et al. Gardner's syndrome. *J Clin Imaging Sci*. 2011;1:65.

16. Mundlos S, Otto F, Mundlos JB, et al. Mutations involving the transcription factor CBFA1 cause cleidocranial dysplasia. *Cell*. 1997;89:773–779.

17. Angle AD, Rebellato J. Dental team management for a patient with cleidocranial dysostosis. *Am J Orthod Dentofacial Orthop*. 2005;128(1):110–117.

18. Khalaf K, Miskelly J, Voge E, et al. Prevalence of hypodontia and associated factors: a systematic review and meta-analysis. *J Orthod*. 2014;41(4):299–316.

19. Slayton RL, Williams L, Murray JC, et al. Genetic association studies of cleft lip and/or palate with hypodontia outside the cleft region. *Cleft Palate Craniofac J*. 2003;40(3):274–279.

20. Itin PH. Etiology and pathogenesis of ectodermal dysplasias. *Am J Med Genet A*. 2014;164A(10):2472–2477.

21. Andersson EM, Axelsson S, Austeng ME, et al. Bilateral hypodontia is more common than unilateral hypodontia in children with Down syndrome: a prospective population-based study. *Eur J Orthod*. 2014;36(4):414–418.

22. Maciel JC, de Castro CG Jr, Brunetto AL, et al. Oral health and dental anomalies in patients treated for leukemia in childhood and adolescence. *Pediatr Blood Cancer*. 2009;53(3):361–365.

23. Lochib S, Indushekar KR, Saraf BG, et al. Occlusal characteristics and prevalence of associated dental anomalies in the primary dentition. *J Epidemiol Glob Health*. 2015;5(2):151–157.

24. Ekman-Westborg B, Julin P. Multiple anomalies in dental morphology: macrodontia, multituberculism, central cusps, and pulp invaginations. Report of a case. *Oral Surg Oral Med Oral Pathol*. 1974;38(2):217–222.

25. Nissanka-Jayasuriya EH, Odell EW, Phillips C. Dental stigmata of congenital syphilis: a historic review with present day relevance. *Head Neck Pathol*. 2016;10(3):327–331.

26. Crawford PJM, Aldred MJ. Regional odontodysplasia: a bibliography. *J Oral Pathol Med*. 1989;18:251–263.

27. Sim TP. Management of dens evaginatus: evaluation of two prophylactic treatment methods. *Endod Dent Traumatol*. 1996;12(3):137–140.

28. Hulsmann M. Dens invaginatus: aetiology, classification, prevalence, diagnosis, and treatment considerations. *Int Endod J*. 1997;30(2):79–90.

29. Bajaj N, Madan N, Rathnam A. Cessation in root development: ramifications of 'Stevens-Johnson' syndrome. *J Indian Soc Pedod Prev Dent*. 2012;30(3):267–270.

30. Rutsch F, MacDougall M, Lu C, et al. A specific IFIH1 gain-of-function mutation causes Singleton-Merten syndrome. *Am J Hum Genet*. 2015;96(2):275–282.

31. Lyles KW, Burkes EJ, Ellis GJ, et al. Genetic transmission of tumoral calcinosis: autosomal dominant with variable clinical expressivity. *J Clin Endocrinol Metab*. 1985;60(6):1093–1096.

32. Gripp KW, Johnson C, Scott CI Jr, et al. Expanding the phenotype of SPONASTRIME dysplasia to include short dental roots, hypogammaglobulinemia, and cataracts. *Am J Med Genet A*. 2008;146A(4):468–473.

33. Majumdar U, Arya G, Singh S, et al. Oro-dental findings in Bardet-Biedl syndrome. *BMJ Case Rep*. 2012;2012.

34. Witt CV, Hirt T, Rutz G, et al. Root malformation associated with a cervical mineralized diaphragm—a distinct form of tooth abnormality? *Oral Surg Oral Med Oral Pathol Oral Radiol*. 2014;117(4):e311–e319.

35. Wright JT, Hong SP, Simmons D, et al. DLX3 c.561_562delCT mutation causes attenuated phenotype of tricho-dento-osseous syndrome. *Am J Med Genet A*. 2008;146(3):343–349.

36. Apajalahti S, Holtta P, Turtola L, et al. Prevalence of short-root anomaly in healthy young adults. *Acta Odontol Scand*. 2002;60(1):56–59.

37. Apajalahti S, Arte S, Pirinen S. Short root anomaly in families and its association with other dental anomalies. *Eur J Oral Sci*. 1999;107(2):97–101.

38. Roinioti TD, Stefanopoulos PK. Short root anomaly associated with Rothmund-Thomson syndrome. *Oral Surg Oral Med Oral Pathol Oral Radiol Endod*. 2007;103(1):e19–e22.

39. Surapornsawasd T, Ogawa T, Tsuji M, et al. Oculofaciocardiodental syndrome: novel BCOR mutations and expression in dental cells. *J Hum Genet*. 2014;59(6):314–320.

40. Kantaputra PN. BCOR mutations and unstoppable root growth: a commentary on oculofaciocardiodental syndrome: novel BCOR mutations and expression in dental cells. *J Hum Genet*. 2014;59(6):297–299.

41. Burklein S, Jansen S, Schafer E. Occurrence of hypercementosis in a German population. *J Endod*. 2012;38(12):1610–1612.

42. Jaspers M, Witkop C Jr. Taurodontism, an isolated trait associated with syndromes and x-chromosomal aneuploidy. *Am J Hum Genet*. 1980;32:396–413.

43. Hart T, Hall K, Kula K, et al. Diagnostic criteria of the tricho-dento-osseous syndrome. *Am J Hum Genet*. 1996;59:A95 (Abstract 513).

44. Seow WK. Pre-eruptive intracoronal resorption as an entity of occult caries. *Pediatr Dent*. 2000;22(5):370–376.

45. Ignelzi MA Jr, Fields HW, White RP, et al. Intracoronal radiolucencies within unerupted teeth. Case report and review of literature. *Oral Surg Oral Med Oral Pathol*. 1990;70(2):214–220.

46. Suckling G, Brown R, Herbison G. The prevalence of developmental defects of enamel in 696 nine-year-old New Zealand children participating in a health development study. *Community Dent Health*. 1985;2:303–313.

47. Hall R. The prevalence of developmental defects of tooth enamel (DDE) in a pediatric hospital department of dentistry population. *Adv Dent Res*. 1989;3(2):114–119.

48. Flores MT, Andersson L, Andreasen JO, et al. Guidelines for the management of traumatic dental injuries. II. Avulsion of permanent teeth. *Dent Traumatol*. 2007;23(3):130–136.

49. Everett ET. Fluoride's effects on the formation of teeth and bones, and the influence of genetics. *J Dent Res*. 2011;90(5):552–560.

50. Jiao YZ, Mu LH, Wang YX, et al. [Association between ameloblastin gene polymorphisms and the susceptibility to dental fluorosis]. *Zhonghua Liu Xing Bing Xue Za Zhi*. 2013;34(1):28–32.

51. Weerheijm KL, Jalevik B, Alaluusua S. Molar-incisor hypomineralisation. *Caries Res*. 2001;35(5):390–391.

52. William V, Messer LB, Burrow MF. Molar incisor hypomineralization: review and recommendations for clinical management. *Pediatr Dent*. 2006;28(3):224–232.

53. Wright JT, Carrion IA, Morris C. The molecular basis of hereditary enamel defects in humans. *J Dent Res*. 2015;94(1):52–61.

54. Witkop C. Amelogenesis imperfecta, dentinogenesis imperfecta and dentin dysplasia revisited: problems in classification. *J Oral Pathol.* 1988;17:547–553.
55. Witkop CJ Jr. Amelogenesis imperfecta, dentinogenesis imperfecta and dentin dysplasia revisited: problems in classification. *J Oral Pathol.* 1988;17(9–10):547–553.
56. McKnight DA, Simmer JP, Hart PS, et al. Overlapping DSPP mutations cause dentin dysplasia and dentinogenesis imperfecta. *J Dent Res.* 2008;87(12):1108–1111.
57. Kim JW, Simmer JP. Hereditary dentin defects. *J Dent Res.* 2007;86(5):392–399.
58. Wise GE, King GJ. Mechanisms of tooth eruption and orthodontic tooth movement. *J Dent Res.* 2008;87(5):414–434.
59. Pulver F. The etiology and prevalence of ectopic eruption of the maxillary first permanent molar. *ASDC J Dent Child.* 1968;35(2):138–146.
60. Frazier-Bowers SA, Simmons D, Wright JT, et al. Primary failure of eruption and PTH1R: the importance of a genetic diagnosis for orthodontic treatment planning. *Am J Orthod Dentofacial Orthop.* 2010;137(2):160.e1–160.e7, discussion 60–61.

4

Oral and Dental Care of Local and Systemic Diseases

MARCIO A. DA FONSECA

Sickle Cell Disease

Sickle cell anemia (SCA) is the most common genetic disorder of the blood and is most frequently observed in persons of African, Afro-Caribbean, Middle Eastern, Indian, Central and South American, and Mediterranean ancestry, but now has a worldwide distribution.[1,2] Sickle cell trait has been largely thought to be benign, but this has been recently challenged due to a high incidence of pathology found with the trait.[3] Sickle cell disease (SCD) is caused by a variant of the B-globin gene called *sickle hemoglobin*

(HbS) due to a substitution of valine for glutamic acid at the sixth amino acid in the B-globin protein, which allows HbS to polymerize when deoxygenated.[2] The disease is characterized by hemolysis, chronic organ infarction and damage, acute painful episodes, and unpredictable acute complications that may become life-threatening.[1,2]

The polymerization of deoxygenated HbS leads to a ropelike fiber that aligns with others, forming a bundle and distorting the red blood cell (RBC) into a sickle shape, which interferes with their deformability. The sickled cells are trapped mostly in the slow-flowing venular side of the microcirculation, enhancing their adhesion to the endothelium, forming a heterocellular aggregate that leads to local hypoxia, increased HbS polymerization, and spread of the occlusion to the adjacent vasculature.[2] Thus, HbS produces a problem of RBC "sticking" rather than simply sickling, leading to chronic endothelial damage. The remarkably varied clinical picture is one of a chronic inflammatory vascular disease. Anemia and vasculopathy are the hallmarks of the disease, with symptoms appearing within the first 6 months of life.[2] The mean life span of a sickled RBC is reduced from 120 days to 12 to 17 days, and Hb levels are 6 to 9 g/dL (normal: 12 to 18 g/dL).[4]

Painful crises in early years manifest as dactylitis (hand-foot syndrome) and can be triggered by infection, dehydration, extreme temperatures, hypoxia, physical or emotional stress, and menstruation.[2,4] Bone pain is often excruciating, symmetric, and present in multiple locations, lasting from a few minutes to several days.[2] Splenic sequestration crises are caused by a large number of RBCs becoming trapped in the spleen, which can induce sudden and severe anemia, thrombocytopenia, and reticulocytosis.[5] Life-threatening postsplenectomy sepsis is primarily caused by polysaccharide encapsulated bacteria, particularly *Streptococcus pneumoniae*, which is a leading cause of mortality among infants affected by SCD.[6,7] Other systemic manifestations include cardiovascular problems, osteomyelitis, osteoporosis, growth disturbances, osteonecrosis, acute chest syndrome (ACS), cerebrovascular accidents, chronic renal failure, and priapism.[2]

The most important intervention in SCD is administration of penicillin V potassium 125 mg orally twice daily starting at 2 months of age to prevent pneumococcal infection. The dose is doubled at age 3 years and should be continued until age 5 years. Blood transfusion is crucial for stroke prevention and improved oxygenation in ACS.[2] However, chronic transfusion can lead to iron overload, which can cause organ damage and alloimmunization.[2] Hydroxyurea (HU) is associated with increased fetal hemoglobin levels, which leads to fewer sickling episodes and fewer long-term sequelae.[2,8] Many new therapies have been developed to target vascular adhesion, inflammation, and hemolysis.[8] Hematopoietic stem cell transplantation (HSCT), which should be done at an early age before organ dysfunction develops, is curative for almost all children who have a human leukocyte antigen-matched sibling donor.[2,8,9]

Oral and Dental Manifestations

The oral and dental manifestations seen in SCD are nonspecific to the disease. The mucous membranes may show jaundice, and glossitis and delayed tooth eruption may also be apparent.[10–12] Radiographic findings include decreased radiodensity in the bones, coarse trabecular pattern, thin inferior border of the mandible, loss of alveolar bone height, pronounced lamina dura, dentin hypomineralization, interglobular dentin in the periapical region, calcifications in the pulp chamber, and hypercementosis.[11,12] Craniofacial abnormalities include bimaxillary protrusion with flared incisors, prominent parietal and zygomatic bones ("tower skull"), widening of the diploic space with thinning of the outer table of the calvarium and vertical trabeculations ("hair-on-end" appearance), and fibrotic calvarial lesions with a ringlike appearance ("doughnut lesions").[11,12]

Sickling crises within the microcirculation of the facial bones and dental pulps may cause orofacial pain without any odontogenic pathology.[12] Vasoocclusive episodes near the mental nerve foramen may result in persistent paresthesia of the lower lip.[12] It seems that long-term use of penicillin prophylaxis in these patients prevents the acquisition of mutans streptococci, resulting in significantly lower caries rate in the primary dentition. However, by 8 years of age, once the prophylactic regimen has stopped, children experience the same level of caries as unaffected peers.[13]

Oral and Dental Treatment Concerns

Individuals carrying the trait present no challenges for dental treatment. For patients affected with the disease, a detailed medical history must be taken, including the use of bisphosphonates because of the risk of bisphosphonate-related osteonecrosis of the jaws (BRONJ) following invasive dental procedures. Complaints of pain in healthy teeth must be taken seriously because the possibility of pulpal infarction and necrosis exists with SCD. All oral infections must be treated vigorously and elective surgeries should be avoided.[10] Orthodontic planning should include consideration the bony architecture and physiology.[10,11] All dental care can be safely done in the dental office during noncrisis periods. If the patient is taking HU, a complete blood count is warranted because of the risk of neutropenia and thrombocytopenia.[14] Coagulation factors should also be checked if the liver is involved. The use of local anesthetics with vasoconstrictors in SCD patients and nitrous oxide is safe but care should be taken to avoid hypoxia with the latter. Low-risk patients can be treated in an outpatient surgery center; higher risk individuals need a fully equipped operating room in a hospital facility for adequate medical support.

Bleeding Disorders

Hemophilia A

Hemophilia A is an X-linked recessive disorder resulting in deficiency of plasma factor VIII coagulant activity, occurring in 1 in 5000

male births.[15] It accounts for about 85% of all hemophilia patients and can be classified as severe (plasma has <1% of detectable factor VIII), moderate (only 1% to 5% of the normal factor VIII level is present), and mild (6% to 40% of the factor is present).[15] The condition should be suspected when a male patient presents with unusual bleeding with normal platelet count, bleeding time, thrombin time, and prothrombin time, but a prolonged activated partial thromboplastin time.[16–18] Hemophilia A and B (deficiency of factor IX) are the most common inherited coagulation disorders.[15]

The clinical hallmarks of hemophilia A are muscle and joint hemorrhages (hemarthroses), easy bruising, and prolonged hemorrhage after trauma or surgery, although bleeding can also occur spontaneously.[15] Despite their effectiveness, current prophylactic therapies do not completely prevent joint disease.[19] The knee joint, as a muscle-controlled joint, became more stable with prophylaxis so now the ankle joints are the first to be affected.[19] Intramuscular hematomas can compress vital structures and may cause nerve paralysis, as well as vascular or airway obstruction. Clinical management of hemophilia A is done according to the severity of the condition, type of bleeding present or anticipated, and presence of inhibitors.[16–18,20] Regular infusions of factor VIII should be used in cases of major surgery and life-threatening bleeding. Prophylactic use of clotting factor concentrates is the basis of contemporary treatment of severe hemophilia A.[19] Vasopressin (desmopressin) increases the plasma levels of factor VIII and von Willebrand factor (vWF) and can be used in mild and moderate cases of hemophilia A. Its peak effect occurs in 20 to 60 minutes, with a duration of 4 hours. Less frequently used methods for management include administration of fresh frozen plasma, cryoprecipitate, and lyophilized factor VIII concentrate.[16–18] A challenging situation arises when the patient has developed antibodies to factor VIII, which are present in up to 15% of persons with severe hemophilia.[20]

Von Willebrand Disease

Von Willebrand disease (vWD) is one of the most commonly inherited bleeding disorders, with a prevalence of 1:10,000.[21] It is characterized by abnormal quantity or quality of vWF, and the disease is classified into type 1 and type 3 (mild to moderate and severe quantitative deficiencies of vWF, respectively) and type 2 (qualitative defects of vWF).[21] Desmopressin will provide adequate hemostatic coverage to treat mucocutaneous bleeding and to prevent bleeding after minimally invasive procedures for cases of type 1 and 2 disease.[22] Supportive therapy with antifibrinolytic agents (tranexamic acid) is also important in vWD.[22]

Oral and Dental Treatment Concerns

Oral and dental treatment requires attention to historical and clinical findings and should follow protocols and guidelines. A careful review of the patient's medical and dental histories, as well as a consultation with the hematologist before invasive procedures, is of paramount importance to restore the hemostatic system to avoid bleeding complications. No pretreatment is required for supragingival scaling in mild and moderate cases of hemophilia. However, if subgingival scaling is necessary, pretreatment should be discussed with the hematologist. Block anesthesia and certain infiltration anesthesia in severe hemophiliacs should not be performed until the hemostatic problem is corrected because they can cause deep tissue bleeding and potential airway obstruction. For patients with mild to moderate disease, the risk is low. Use of a rubber dam with a stable clamp is important to protect the soft tissues. Wedges and matrices can be used with gentle handling, and appliances can be cemented if they are atraumatic to the tissues. Pulpotomies, pulpectomies, and root canal therapy usually can be done without significant bleeding, and avoidance of instrumentation and filling beyond the apex is important. The surgical technique should be atraumatic and primary closure should be obtained to protect the blood clot. Orthodontic treatment is not a contraindication, but particular attention should be paid to wires with sharp edges and placement of bands.

Patients with moderate to severe hemophilia require factor VIII concentrate infusion before oral surgery, complemented by local hemostatics (pressure, sutures, gelatin sponge, cellulose materials, thrombin, microfibrillar collagen, fibrin glue, etc.) and oral antifibrinolytics (tranexamic acid mouthwash) to help achieve hemostasis. Vasopressin, ε-aminocaproic acid, and tranexamic acid can also be used systemically after dental extractions.

Pediatric Osteoporosis

Bone fractures are the main reason for hospitalization in children between 10 and 14 years of age.[23,24] Childhood factors such as lifestyle, diet, chronic illness, and medications can have a short-term impact on bone health and a long-term effect on the achievement of peak bone mass. Unmodifiable intrinsic factors (e.g., race, genetics, gender) are responsible for determining 75% to 80% of an individual's peak bone mass, whereas potentially changeable extrinsic factors (e.g., diet, hormones, illness, physical activity) make up a significant component of the variability in ultimate bone mass. Adequate calcium and vitamin D intake and regular physical activity are among the most important extrinsic factors in gaining optimal bone mineral mass and density.[25]

Osteoporosis is characterized by low bone mass and microarchitectural deterioration of bone structure resulting in increased bone fragility.[26] The primary forms of osteoporosis occur in rare inherited conditions (e.g., osteogenesis imperfecta, cleidocranial dysplasia, Marfan syndrome, Ehlers-Danlos syndrome, etc.).[26,27] Secondary osteoporosis is seen in children with chronic systemic diseases due either to the effects of the disease itself on the skeleton or its medical treatment (e.g., leukemia, immobility, inflammatory conditions, glucocorticoid therapy, poor nutrition, etc.).[26,27] Children with symptomatic osteoporosis usually presents with a history of recurrent low impact fractures or moderate to severe backache due to vertebral fracture.[26]

Defining pediatric osteoporosis is challenging because pediatric bone mineral density (BMD) values constantly change with age and depend on many variables such as gender, body size, pubertal stage, skeletal maturation, hormone action, bone size, and ethnicity.[23,25,26] Pediatric BMD is assessed by a Z-score whose reference population is one of ethnicity-, gender-, and age-matched controls, data that are unfortunately limited.[24–26] The Z-score does not account for some of the variables previously mentioned, so it poses a problem of diagnostic accuracy because serial measurements in a single child may be difficult to interpret. Z-score values below −2 are generally considered a serious warning for osteoporosis, but most specialists do not make that diagnosis until at least one fragility fracture has been observed.[25] The term *low bone mass for chronologic age* should be used if the Z-score is −2 or lower; the term *osteopenia* should not be used in pediatric bone reports.[23,24] Fragility fractures constitute the clinical hallmark of osteoporosis.[25] The most widely used tool for diagnosis and management of adult osteoporosis is dual-energy x-ray absorptiometry (DEXA), but it can be particularly deceptive when used in a growing child.[24–26] The most appropriate and reproducible sites for densitometry in children are the posterior/anterior spine and total body, less head.[23,26]

Anticipatory guidance regarding healthy lifestyle habits, such as regular physical activity, a balanced diet, and avoidance of tobacco, alcohol, and illicit drugs, is of great importance to prevent bone loss and should start from an early age. This is an area where the dental professional can make an impact on the patient's health and thus should be addressed at every recall visit. In less severe cases of reduced BMD, correcting poor nutrition and calcium and vitamin D intake along with promoting weight-bearing physical activity provide benefits with minimal risk. Soft drink consumption negatively influences bone mineral accrual in adolescent girls more than in boys.[28] Bisphosphonates are the pharmacologic treatment of choice for both primary and secondary osteoporosis, although the duration and intensity of treatment are still a concern for long-term safety.[26,27] Intravenous pamidronate is most widely used.[26]

Oral and Dental Treatment Concerns

Dental professionals have to be meticulous when taking the medical history of individuals who may have a history of low BMD and osteoporosis. It is important to know:

1. How low the patient's BMD is. Transferring patients from wheelchairs to the dental chair, physical restraint and extractions, especially of permanent teeth, may lead to bone fractures.
2. What the cause of the patient's low BMD or osteoporosis is.
3. What medical treatment is being provided for the bone condition to prevent other complications following invasive dental procedures, such as BRONJ. It is important to be aware of the drug's potential long-term oral complications, given that its half-life may be several years.

Education of the patient and caretakers about the importance of oral health and the potential long-term side effects of the drug with invasive dental procedures is a must. Elimination of all potential sources of odontogenic and mucosal infection must be done before the patient starts therapy with bisphosphonates. Avoiding oral surgical procedures is crucial to decrease the risk of BRONJ; however, no cases have been reported in children to date.[26] One can speculate that extraction of primary teeth may not pose a risk for the development of BRONJ, given the relatively small wound, as well as the increased porosity and vascularity of the jaw bones in young subjects compared to that of adults. Another reason may be the smaller dose given to children. Published studies on the lack of occurrence of BRONJ in pediatric patients present many design flaws (e.g., small numbers of patients, lack of randomization, short follow-up period, differing drugs and doses used). However, as more adolescents and young adults are referred for orthodontically related extractions, removal of impacted teeth and third molars, periodontal surgery, and tissue biopsies, the risk of BRONJ could increase. Bisphosphonates can inhibit tooth movement, posing a problem for orthodontic therapy.[29]

Pediatric Cancer

Cancer is the second most common cause of fatalities in children between 5 and 14 years of age in the United States, after accidents.[30] The incidence of childhood malignancy is greatest in the first year of life, with a second peak at 2 to 3 years of age.[31] Acute leukemias, brain tumors, soft tissue tumors, and renal tumors are the more common malignancies in children.[30] Early diagnosis and advances in medicine have increased the overall 5-year survival rate to 80%.[30]

The multimodal treatment approach uses surgery and radiotherapy to control local disease and chemotherapy to eradicate systemic disease. Chemotherapy interferes with the synthesis or function of the vital nucleic acids in all cells, whereas radiation therapy damages DNA in cancerous cells, with minimal harm to adjacent tissues (critical in pediatric patients). Immunotherapy uses leukocytes, monoclonal antibodies, and cytokines for tumor destruction with the potential for target specificity, which may spare children from the major side effects associated with standard oncology therapies.

Acute lymphoid leukemia (ALL) accounts for about 80% of all childhood leukemias and 56% in adolescence, with a peak incidence at age 4 years and an overall cure rate of 90%.[30] The most common signs and symptoms are anorexia, irritability, lethargy, anemia, bleeding, petechiae, fever, lymphadenopathy, splenomegaly, and hepatomegaly. Bone pain and arthralgias may be caused either by leukemic infiltration of the perichondral bone or joint or by leukemic expansion of the marrow cavity, leading the child to present with a limp or refusal to walk.[32] The most common head, neck, and intraoral manifestations of ALL at the time of diagnosis are lymphadenopathy, sore throat, laryngeal pain, gingival bleeding, and oral ulceration.[33] Patients who relapse during treatment are given intensive chemotherapy followed by HSCT. Management of ALL is based on clinical risk and is usually divided into four phases:[32]

1. Remission induction: generally lasts 28 days and consists of three or four drugs (e.g., vincristine, prednisone, and L-asparaginase), with a 95% success rate.
2. Central nervous system (CNS) preventive therapy/prophylaxis: the CNS can act as a sanctuary for leukemic infiltrates because systemically administered chemotherapeutic drugs cannot cross the blood-brain barrier. Cranial irradiation and/or weekly intrathecal injection of a chemotherapeutic agent, usually methotrexate, can be used. This presymptomatic treatment can be done in each phase as well.
3. Consolidation or intensification: designed to minimize the development of drug cross-resistance through intensified treatment in an attempt to kill any remaining leukemic cells.
4. Maintenance: aimed at suppressing leukemic growth through continuous administration of methotrexate and 6-mercaptopurine. The optimal length of this phase has not been established yet, but it usually lasts 2.5 to 3 years.

The patient's blood counts normally start falling 5 to 7 days after the beginning of each treatment cycle; they stay low for approximately 14 to 21 days before rising again.

Dental and Oral Care Considerations[31]

Treatment with chemotherapy and/or radiation therapy may lead to many acute and long-term sequelae of the oral cavity (Box 4.1). Oral and dental infections may complicate the oncology treatment as well as delay it, leading to morbidity and an inferior quality of life for the child. Early and radical dental intervention minimizes the risk for oral and associated systemic complications (Figs. 4.1–4.3). Trauma associated with oral function and damage to the mucosa increases the risk of bleeding. Therefore, the dental consultation on a newly diagnosed patient should be done at once so that enough time is available for care to be completed before the cancer therapy starts.

Patient's Medical History and Hematologic Status

A thorough review of the patient's history should include information about the underlying disease, time of diagnosis, modalities

---

• BOX 4.1 Oral and Craniofacial Complications of Cancer Therapy

Acute Complications From Chemotherapy and Radiotherapy
Mucositis
Salivary gland dysfunction
Sialadenitis (radiation only)
Xerostomia
Neurotoxicity
Taste dysfunction
Dentinal hypersensitivity
Temporomandibular dysfunction
Oral bleeding
Opportunistic infections (viral, fungal, bacterial)

Long-Term Complications of Radiotherapy to the Face
Mucosal fibrosis and atrophy
Xerostomia
Dental caries
Postradiation osteonecrosis
Taste dysfunction
Mucosal fibrosis
Muscular/cutaneous fibrosis
Fungal and bacterial infections
Dental and craniofacial developmental problems (also with chemotherapy)

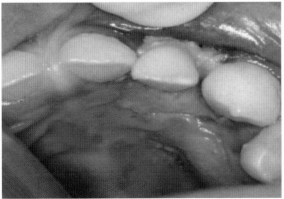

• **Figure 4.1** *Pseudomonas* infections resulting in early loss of primary teeth in a 2-year-old girl with acute lymphoid leukemia.

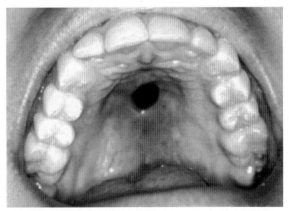

• **Figure 4.2** *Aspergillus* infection on the palate of a 14-year-old girl with acute lymphoid leukemia.

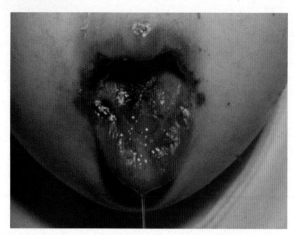

• **Figure 4.3** Moderate mucositis caused by chemotherapy in a 5-year-old patient.

TABLE 4.1	Normal Blood Count Reference Values
Blood Component	**Normal Values**
Hemoglobin (g/dL)	Males: 13.5–17.5; females: 12.3–15.3
Hematocrit (%)	Males: 41.5–50.4; females: 35.9–44.6
White blood cell count	4,000–10,000/mL
Platelet count	150,000–450,000/mm³
Differential	**Normal Values**
Neutrophils (polymorphonuclear leukocytes)	Segmented: 56 Bands: 3
Lymphocytes	34
Monocytes	4
Eosinophils	2.7
Basophils	0.3

Data from McPherson RA, Pincus MR, eds. *Henry's Clinical Diagnosis and Management by Laboratory Methods.* 21st ed. Philadelphia: Saunders; 2007:1404–1418.

of treatment the patient has received since the diagnosis, and complications. Hospitalizations, emergency room visits, infections (both oral and systemic), current hematologic status, allergies, medications, and a review of systems should be noted.

Most patients are given a central line, which is an indwelling catheter inserted into the right atrium of the heart, useful for obtaining blood samples and administering chemotherapeutic agents. There is no scientific evidence for the need of antibiotic prophylaxis before invasive dental procedures for patients who have a central line.[31,34,35]

Prolonged bleeding in childhood cancer may be caused by chemotherapy-induced myelosuppression, some medications, and disorders of clotting and platelets related to the baseline disease. Clinically significant bleeding is unlikely to occur with a platelet count greater than 20,000/mm³ in the absence of other complicating factors. Dental procedures can be done when the platelet count is greater than 40,000/mm³, with attention paid to measures for controlling prolonged bleeding.[31] Other coagulation tests may be appropriate for patients with liver involvement and coagulopathies.

Neutrophils are the body's first line of defense; therefore the incidence and severity of infection are inversely related to their number. When the absolute neutrophil count (ANC) is less than 1000/mm³, elective dental work should be deferred because the risk for development of infections and bacteremia increases greatly. However, many dental teams do elective invasive dental work with an ANC above 500/mm³, without complications for the patient. Table 4.1 shows normal blood count reference values.

Oral Hygiene, Diet, and Caries Prevention[31,36]

Regardless of the child's hematologic status, routine oral hygiene throughout the entire oncology treatment is important to decrease oral complications. Thrombocytopenia should not be the sole determinant of oral hygiene as patients are able to brush without bleeding at widely different levels of platelet count. There is evidence that patients who perform intensive oral care have a reduced risk of developing moderate to severe mucositis, without causing an increase in septicemia and infections in the oral cavity. A regular soft toothbrush or an electric brush used at least twice daily is the most efficient means to reduce the risk of significant bleeding and infection in the gingiva. Sponges, foam brushes, and supersoft brushes cannot provide effective mechanical cleansing because of their softness; therefore they should be used only in cases of severe

mucositis when the patient cannot tolerate a regular brush. Brushes should be air dried between uses, and a toothpaste without heavy flavoring agents should be considered because such agents can irritate the tissues. Patients who have poor oral hygiene or periodontal disease can use aqueous chlorhexidine rinses daily until the gingival health has been restored. When mucositis is present, rinses containing alcohol and flavoring agents should be avoided because they can dehydrate and irritate the mucosa. Periodontal infection is a major concern because colonizing organisms have been shown to cause bacteremias.

The child with cancer may be at high risk for dental caries because of dietary issues, treatment-induced xerostomia, and sucrose-rich pediatric medications. Despite the fact that nystatin is often prescribed, it is not effective at preventing *Candida* infections in immunodepressed patients and should not be recommended.[37] Fluoride supplements, varnish, and neutral rinses or gels are indicated for patients at risk for caries.

Oral and Dental Treatment Concerns[31]

The patient's dental history should be reviewed, and a thorough head, neck, and oral cavity examination should be performed, complemented by radiographs when indicated. Some patients may complain of paresthesias caused by leukemic infiltration of the peripheral nerves. Others may report dental pain mimicking irreversible pulpitis in the absence of a dental/periodontal infection. This can be a side effect of vincristine and vinblastine, two commonly used vinca alkaloid chemotherapeutic agents. In this case, the patient should avoid situations that exacerbate the discomfort (sweets, ice, etc.), and analgesics can be prescribed for pain control. The pain usually disappears within a few days or weeks after the cessation of the causative chemotherapy.

The patient's blood count usually returns to normal or near normal between chemotherapy cycles, and dental care can usually be done then. When time is limited for dental care before the oncologic therapy starts, infections, extractions, periodontal care, and sources of irritation should be given higher treatment priority than carious teeth, root canal therapy for permanent teeth, and replacement of faulty restorations. The risk for pulpal infection and pain should determine which carious lesions are to be treated first, because a pulpal infection during immunosuppression could lead to a life-threatening situation. Temporary restorations can be placed, and nonacute dental treatment can be delayed until the patient's health is stabilized. Platelet transfusions should be considered preoperatively and 24 hours postoperatively when the level is between 40,000 and 75,000/mm³. When the platelet level is below 40,000/mm³, dental care should be deferred. During immunosuppression, all elective dental procedures should be avoided. In cases of emergency, the physician must be consulted before any dental treatment is initiated.

When there is time before the initiation of cancer therapy, dental scaling and prophylaxis should be performed, defective restorations should be repaired, and teeth with sharp edges should be polished. It is prudent to provide a more radical treatment in the form of extraction of primary teeth with pulpal infection to minimize the risk for oral and systemic complications of failed pulp therapy during immunosuppression periods. Teeth that have already been pulpally treated and are clinically and radiographically sound should present no threats. Symptomatic nonvital permanent teeth should receive root canal therapy at least 1 week before initiation of cancer therapy. If that is not possible, extraction is indicated followed by antibiotic therapy for about 1 week. Endodontic treatment of permanent teeth with asymptomatic periapical involvement can be delayed if the patient is neutropenic.[38] During immunosuppression, swelling and purulent exudate may not be present, masking some of the classical signs of odontogenic infections, leaving them clinically undetected.[38] In this situation, radiographs are vital to determine periapical or bifurcation pathologic processes.

Fixed orthodontic appliances and space maintainers should be removed if the patient has poor oral hygiene and/or the treatment protocol carries a risk for the development of moderate to severe mucositis. Appliances can harbor food debris, compromise oral hygiene, and act as mechanical irritants, increasing the risk for secondary infection. Removable appliances and retainers that fit well may be worn as long as tolerated by the patient who shows good oral care.

Partially erupted molars can become a source of infection because of pericoronitis, so the overlying gingival tissue should be excised if the dentist believes it is a potential risk. Loose primary teeth should be left to exfoliate naturally, and to prevent bacteremia, the patient should be counseled to not play with them. If the patient cannot comply with this recommendation, loose teeth should be removed. Impacted teeth, root tips, partially erupted third molars, teeth with periodontal pockets greater than 6 mm, teeth with acute infections, and nonrestorable teeth should be removed ideally 2 weeks before cancer therapy starts to allow adequate healing.[38] If a permanent tooth cannot be extracted for medical reasons at that time, a decoronation can be performed. Antibiotics should be given for 7 to 10 days afterward, with the extraction subsequently done when the patient's hematologic status allows it. Particular attention should be given to extraction of permanent teeth in patients who will receive or have received radiation to the face because of the risk of osteoradionecrosis. Surgical procedures must be as atraumatic as possible, with no sharp bony edges remaining and satisfactory closure of the wounds. Local measures to control bleeding such as pressure packs, sutures, gelatin sponges, topical thrombin, or microfibrillar collagen should be readily available. If local measures fail, the physician must be contacted immediately.

When the patient is in the maintenance phase of the treatment and the overall prognosis is good, it is likely that the hematologic status is close to normal. Dental procedures can be performed routinely but not before checking the blood count. Orthodontic treatment may start or resume after completion of all therapy and after at least a 2-year disease-free survival.[39] By then, the risk of relapse is decreased and the patient is no longer using immunosuppressive drugs. However, the clinician must assess any dental developmental disturbances caused by the cancer therapy, especially in children treated before the age of 6 years (Fig. 4.4).[40,41] Dahllof et al.[42] described the following strategies to provide orthodontic care for patients with dental sequelae: (1) use appliances that minimize the risk of root resorption, (2) use lighter forces, (3) terminate treatment earlier than normal, (4) choose the simplest method for the treatment needs, and (5) do not treat the lower jaw. Pediatric patients with cancer may develop osteoporosis, and many receive bisphosphonates, which leads to additional concerns in the delivery of oral and dental care.

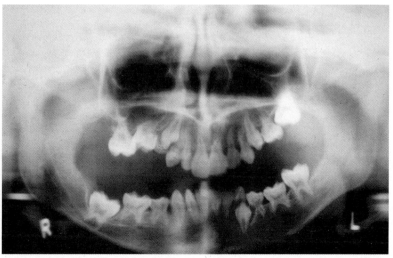

• **Figure 4.4** Long-term effects on dental development in a 14-year-old boy conditioned with chemotherapy and total body irradiation before a hematopoietic stem cell transplant at age 13 months.

Hematopoietic Stem Cell Transplantation[43,44]

HSCT has been used to replace the marrow of patients with hematologic disorders, congenital immunodeficiencies, lipidoses, and inborn errors of metabolism, as well as for marrow support to allow the administration of higher doses of chemotherapy and/or radiotherapy in patients with solid tumors. The stem cells used in HSCT can be obtained from multiple aspirations of bone marrow from the iliac crest and other bones, from the peripheral blood, and from the placenta or umbilical cord blood. The cells can be collected from the patient's own marrow (autologous transplant), from a donor related to the recipient or from an unrelated person (allogeneic transplant), from an identical twin (syngeneic transplant), or from a different species (xenogeneic transplant). Human leukocyte antigen (HLA) tissue typing is done to identify antigens on the short arm of chromosome 6 of potential donors to match as closely as possible those of the recipient (full or partial match). The regimens can be myeloablative (high dose intensity, very toxic), nonmyeloablative (causes minimal cytopenia), or reduced-intensity conditioning (low toxicity with the tumor not always being eradicated until the grafted cells take over). A few days before transplantation, the patient is admitted to receive high-dose chemotherapy alone or in combination with total body irradiation. Evidence of engraftment is usually evident between days 20 and 30, sometimes earlier, by increased peripheral white cell and platelet counts; it is substantiated by the presence of donor cells on marrow aspirations.

Dental and Oral Care Considerations

Most of the principles of dental and oral care for the pediatric patient undergoing HSCT are similar to those discussed in the section on pediatric cancer. The two major differences are as follows: (1) in HSCT, there are no cycles of chemotherapy with periods of rest in between when the blood counts return to normal, as is the case in the management of nontransplant oncology patients; and (2) there will be prolonged immunosuppression following transplantation, with most immune functions probably fully restored by 1 year if chronic graft-versus-host disease or other complications are not present.[31,45] Therefore all dental treatment must be completed before the patient is admitted in order to eliminate disease that could lead to complications during and after transplantation.

Regular dental examinations with radiographs can be done routinely, but elective dental work, including prophylaxis, should be avoided in patients with profound impairment of immune function.[31,45] If a dental emergency arises during that period, the patient's physician must be consulted before any treatment is instituted.

Acute and Chronic Oral Complications of Chemotherapy and Radiotherapy

Cancer therapy can cause extensive morbidity in the oral cavity (see Box 4.1), compromising the child's quality of life and increasing treatment costs. Among all complications, mucositis (see Fig. 4.3) is the most common cause of oral pain in cancer treatment and the most common complication in HSCT.[31,36,46] The agents used in the preparative regimen can largely affect tissues of the gastrointestinal mucosa, inhibiting its basal layers to replace the superficial cells leading to a generalized mucosal inflammation. The occurrence and severity of mucositis show great individual variability, with tissue changes noticeable between 4 and 7 days after the initiation of therapy and generally lasting from 10 to 14 days.[31] Its management is directed at palliation of symptoms and prevention of infection and soft tissue trauma.[31,36]

A long-term issue of particular interest for pediatric dentists is the development of dental and/or craniofacial abnormalities (see Fig. 4.4). The younger the child is at the beginning of therapy (especially before 6 years of age), the greater the risks for craniofacial and dental disturbances such as tooth agenesis; complete or partial arrest of root development with thin, tapered roots; early apical closure; globular and conical crowns; dentin and enamel opacities and defects; microdontia; enlarged pulp chambers; taurodontism; and abnormal occlusion.[40,41,47,48] Vertical growth of the condyles and the alveolar and molar heights may be adversely affected by the oncologic therapies.[40,47]

Patients who have experienced chronic or severe mucositis are at risk for malignant transformation of the oral mucosa and thus should be followed closely.[47] Careful monitoring of chronic xerostomia and oral graft-versus-host disease are also very important issues.[36,45,47,49]

In patients with compromised immune systems, recurrent herpes simplex virus (HSV) ulcerations may be large, progressive, and persistent (Fig. 4.5). The diagnosis is often delayed because of their atypical presentation, which may involve any intraoral site including nonkeratinized areas.[31,50,51] Patients undergoing cancer treatment have a high risk for development of recrudescent HSV infections; thus their management is toward prophylaxis.[50] In this group, lesions that do not heal within 7 to 10 days should be recultured or rebiopsied, and sensitivity testing to acyclovir (ACY) should be performed.[50]

Primary Herpetic Gingivostomatitis

Herpes simplex virus type 1 (HSV-1) is a large DNA virus that causes primary herpetic gingivostomatitis (PHG).[50,52,53] It is mostly acquired through direct skin contact or bodily fluids, which can spread rapidly in closed settings such as daycare centers. The onset is sudden and its clinical manifestations may vary from a mild

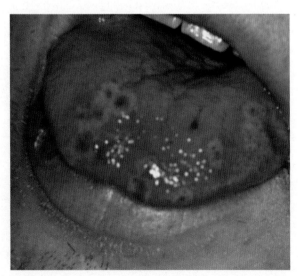

• **Figure 4.5** Herpetic lesions on the tongue of an immunosuppressed patient.

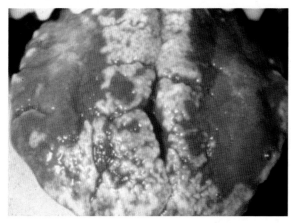

• **Figure 4.6** Pseudomembranous candidiasis.

illness to a severe course requiring hospital admission. Nonspecific symptoms include cervical lymphadenopathy, malaise, irritability, upper respiratory tract infection, and low-grade fever.[54] Oral lesions may start as vesicles on the tongue, buccal mucosa, and gingiva, rapidly rupturing to become ulcers 1 to 3 mm in size, which may subsequently form a large ulcerated area covered by a yellowish-gray membrane.[54] The infection is self-limiting, lasting 10 to 14 days, and healing without scarring.[54] Children may present with severe local pain, which can lead to difficulties with fluid and food intake, putting them at risk for dehydration.[53,54] Excessive drooling, halitosis, and sore throat are frequently present.

Management of PHG is directed at promoting lesion healing, providing palliation, promoting adequate hydration and nutrition, and preventing further spread of the infection through avoiding direct contact with other people and not sharing such items as toys, food, utensils, pacifiers, cups, bottles, toothbrushes, and towels. Drinks and foods with high acid or spice content should be avoided. Cold items such as ice cream, popsicles, and ice chips can soothe affected tissues and help with hydration. Analgesics, topical anesthetics, and coating agents help relieve pain and facilitate food intake, with nutritional supplements added as needed.[52,54] Topical anesthetics should be used with extreme caution because they are rapidly absorbed through ulcerated tissues. Nonalcoholic antimicrobial rinses may help decrease the risk of secondary infections when there is significant gingival involvement and poor oral hygiene. Patients who are at risk for dehydration should be admitted to a hospital. It is important to follow-up the visit with a phone call 48 to 72 hours later to see if the PHG symptoms have subsided. If no improvement has occurred or it has become worse, the patient must be sent for a consultation immediately to rule out systemic disease (malignancy, neutropenia, etc.).

There is weak evidence that ACY can decrease some of the symptoms of PHG and the number of hospitalizations for children under 6 years of age.[54] The dosage for oral acyclovir (ACY) suspension is 15 mg/kg, with a maximum of 80 mg/kg per day to be used every 3 hours when awake or five times a day for 10 days.[53]

Oropharyngeal Candidiasis

Candidiasis is an opportunistic infection caused by the overgrowth of *Candida* species due to antibiotic and/or corticosteroid use, xerostomia, diabetes mellitus, appliances covering the palate, smoking, and/or an immature or compromised immune system.[33,35] The most common forms in children are pseudomembranous (Fig.

4.6) and erythematous candidiasis. It typically occurs on the buccal mucosa, mucobuccal folds, dorsolateral tongue, and oropharynx.[55] The erythematous or atrophic form ranges from a diffuse to patchy redness involving mostly the palate and dorsum of the tongue.[55,56] Patients with oral candidiasis may experience pain, a burning feeling on the mucous membranes and tongue, dysphagia, and difficulty eating or drinking.[56]

It is important to improve oral hygiene, control caries, keep pacifiers and appliances clean, and replace contaminated toothbrushes to control disease.[57] Most available antifungal agents have reasonably broad activity against *Candida* species. Unexplained or frequent relapses should prompt an evaluation of occult systemic disease, conditions that can lead to an immunocompromised state, or maternal breast in breastfeeding infants.[56] Topical antifungal agents include compounded clotrimazole suspension (10 mg/mL) and nystatin oral suspension (100,000 U/mL) to swish for 2 minutes and swallow or expectorate four times daily for 2 weeks, followed by a reevaluation of the oral cavity.[56,57] The patient should not eat or drink for 30 minutes afterward. Adolescents can use one to two pastilles (200,000 U) slowly dissolved in the mouth five times daily.[55] Nystatin solution contains 30% to 50% of sucrose so oral hygiene must be reinforced. Clotrimazole troches (10 mg), also very rich in sucrose, can be used by slowly dissolving one troche in the mouth every 3 hours while awake (five per day) for 14 days.[57] Systemic antifungal drugs are advantageous when other topically delivered medications are administered concurrently. For chronic cases of angular cheilitis, nystatin and triamcinolone acetonide cream (Mycolog-II) are the best choices when applied to the corners of the mouth three times a day for 5 days.[57]

Cystic Fibrosis

Cystic fibrosis (CF) is caused by a defect in the CF transmembrane conductance regulator *(CFTR)* gene, which is located in the long arm of chromosome 7.[58] It is the most common genetic disease (1 in 2500 newborns of Northern European descent) and almost 2000 mutations have been identified, the most common being F508 deletions.[59] A defective *CFTR* causes decreased chloride secretion and increased sodium absorption across the epithelial surface, thus "salty skin" is a hallmark of the disease.[58] This, in turn, results in depletion of the airway surface liquid and impaired mucociliary clearance, leading to early infection and inflammation, increased mucus viscosity, impaired mucus clearance, and decreased bacterial killing.[58,59] The most common symptoms of the CF are progressive lung disease and chronic digestive conditions, but other areas, such as the pancreas, sinuses, heart, kidneys, and reproductive organs, can be affected as well.[59,60] There is a high prevalence of osteopenia and osteoporosis in young adults with CF; therefore bisphosphonates may be part of their treatment. A novel form of treatment is *CFTR* modulator therapies, which are designed to correct the function of the defective protein made by the CF gene. There are currently two US Food and Drug Administration–approved agents: ivacaftor (for children 2 years and older) and lumacaftor/ivacaftor (for those 6 years and older), which are effective only in those with certain mutations.[61] Most patients require a daily routine of inhaled therapies, pancreatic enzyme replacement, and exercise to prevent the progression of lung disease.[59] The most common pathogen in CF is *Pseudomonas aeruginosa*, and the use of inhaled or nebulized antibiotics, such as tobramycin and colomycin, has been useful to prevent infections.[58] Unless they get a lung transplant, 90% of patients will die of respiratory failure.[58]

Oral and Dental Treatment Concerns

Patients with CF present significantly more enamel defects in their permanent teeth, more calculus deposits, and worse gingival health than those with other respiratory disorders.[62] The chronic use of antibiotics and pancreatic enzymes may offer some protection against development of caries in this population.[62] Children with CF may be at lower risk for dental caries but adolescents may not; all studies to date addressing the issue of dental caries in CF have been flawed in their design, thus more research is needed.[63] Although the majority of patients self-reported good or excellent oral health in a study by Patrick et al.,[64] adolescents had a statistically significant poorer oral health-related quality of life than younger patients. Multiple patients with CF should not be scheduled at the same time in the dental office to avoid cross-contamination with *P. aeruginosa*. The use of nitrous oxide, conscious sedation, and general anesthesia must be discussed with the patient's physician due to respiratory compromises. The dental professional must be aware that patients with CF may be using bisphosphonates for the treatment of osteoporosis.[65] Patients may also present with involvement of the liver, which may affect their coagulation abilities.

Crohn Disease

Inflammatory bowel disease (IBD) is a disorder of intestinal inflammation caused by chronic conditions, whose incidence is rising in children.[66] The etiology is unknown but it may be a combination of genetics, host immunity, and environmental factors.[66] IBD encompasses ulcerative colitis (inflammation of the colon and rectum) and Crohn disease (inflammation of the large intestine, small intestine, or both).[66] Diarrhea and abdominal pain are common features of the disorder in children and adults, but some children may not have any laboratory abnormalities (anemia, iron deficiency, elevated inflammation markers, etc.).[66] Malnourishment may be present in children with Crohn disease because of suboptimal dietary intake, increased gastrointestinal losses, or malabsorption, which may lead to growth failure and osteoporosis.[66] Endoscopic evaluation (both upper endoscopy and colonoscopy) is the gold standard in IBD diagnosis.[66] Goals of therapy are mucosal healing and long-lasting remission, but currently there is a lack of therapies approved specifically for children.[66]

Oral Manifestations

The oral cavity can be involved in Crohn disease, with aphthous ulcers, lip swelling, buccal mucosa swelling or cobble stoning, mucogingivitis, deep linear ulceration, and mucosal tags being the most common presentations.[67] Examination of the oral cavity in children for disease manifestations is of value only at initial presentation of Crohn disease because oral activity does not parallel disease activity in the intestine.[67] However, the presence of oral manifestations may be a marker of severity of disease. The oral manifestations are usually subclinical, self-resolving, and do not require specific treatment.[67] Patients whose oral cavity is symptomatic should use a cinnamon- and benzoate-free diet to start. A short course of a steroid rinse (0.5 mg beclamethasone dissolved in water, up to six times a day) can bring relief, and topical tacrolimus can be used on swollen lips.[67] If the patient has persistent pain, swelling, and cosmetic disfigurement, use of immunosuppressors should be discussed with the physician.[67] Thalidomide has been shown to be effective in leading to remission of oral and intestinal symptoms in children.[68]

The term *orofacial granulomatosis* (OFG) describes patients with granulomatous lesions in the orofacial tissues in the absence of intestinal lesions.[67,68] Concurrent Crohn disease is present in about 40% of children with OFG.[69] Lip and facial swelling is the most common sign of OFG.[68] Thus, dental professionals should include Crohn disease in their differential diagnosis when they encounter children with OFG.[67,69]

Celiac Disease

Gluten is the main protein of wheat, but homologous proteins are also found in rye and barley.[70] Gluten-related disorders (celiac disease, wheat allergy, and non-celiac gluten sensitivity) have an estimated prevalence of 5% worldwide.[70] In celiac disease, a T-cell–mediated autoimmune reaction occurs in the small intestine, leading to enteropathy and malabsorption.[70] Diagnosis is based on the patient's clinical history, serology, and duodenal biopsy.[70] Suspicion of celiac disease should be raised when children present with unexplained chronic gastrointestinal symptoms with malabsorption (chronic diarrhea, abdominal pain, distension, and failure to thrive or weight loss).[70,71] Growth retardation, iron deficiency anemia, chronic fatigue, delayed puberty, amenorrhea, dermatitis herpetiformis, osteoporosis, and/or liver function alterations can also be seen.[70,71] A strict, life-long gluten-free diet is currently the only available therapy for the disease, but it is expensive, socially isolating, and not always effective and can lead to nutritional deficiencies.[71] Use of corticosteroids and immune modulators is mostly reserved for refractory celiac disease.[71] Autoimmune thyroid disease and type 1 diabetes mellitus are the most common autoimmune diseases associated with celiac disease.[71] Associations with Sjögren syndrome, Addison disease, parathyroid disorders, and growth hormone deficiency have been reported.[71] Adults with celiac disease are at risk for development of fatal malignancies, most commonly non-Hodgkin lymphoma.[71]

Oral Manifestations

Enamel defects are frequently present in children with the disease, with a low Ca/P ratio observed in their teeth.[72,73] The disease can be protective against dental caries due to its rigid diet, which tends to eliminate many cariogenic foods, but more studies are needed to elucidate the relationship.[72] De Carvalho et al.[72] showed a low caries experience, high occurrence of recurrent aphthous stomatitis, and significantly reduced salivary flow in children with celiac disease. Acar et al.[73] also found a high prevalence of stomatitis and significantly lower levels of cariogenic microflora in young patients with celiac disease compared with healthy individuals. Ferraz et al.[74] presented a comprehensive review of the oral manifestations of the disease. Due to the risk of osteoporosis, patients may be using bisphosphonates.

References

1. Section on Hematology/Oncology Committee on Genetics, American Academy of Pediatrics. Health supervision for children with sickle cell disease. *Pediatrics*. 2002;109(3):526–535.
2. Chavravorty S, Williams TN. Sickle cell disease: a neglected chronic disease of increasing global health importance. *Arch Dis Child*. 2015;100(1):48–53.
3. Kotila TR. Sickle cell trait: a benign state? *Acta Haematol*. 2016;136:147–151.
4. Marchant WA, Walker I. Anesthetic management of the child with sickle cell disease. *Paediatr Anaesth*. 2003;13(6):473–489.

5. Wanko SO, Telen MJ. Transfusion management in sickle cell disease. *Hematol Oncol Clin North Am.* 2005;19(5):803–826.

6. Price VE, Dutta S, Blancette VS, et al. The prevention and treatment of bacterial infections in children with asplenia and hyposplenia: practice considerations at the Hospital for Sick Children, Toronto. *Pediatr Blood Cancer.* 2006;46(5):597–603.

7. Quinn CT, Zogers ZR, Buchanan GR. Survival of children with sickle cell disease. *Blood.* 2004;103(11):4023–4027.

8. Field JJ, Nathan DC. Advances in sickle cell therapies in the hydroxyurea era. *Mol Med.* 2014;20(suppl 1):S37–S42.

9. Walters MC. Update of hematopoietic cell transplantation for sickle cell disease. *Curr Opin Hematol.* 2015;22(3):227–233.

10. Alves PVM, Alves DKM, de Souza MMG, et al. Orthodontic treatment of patients with sickle cell anemia. *Angle Orthod.* 2006;76(2):269–373.

11. Sanger RG, McTigue DJ. Sickle cell anemia: its pathophysiology and management. *J Dent Handicap.* 1978;3(2):9–21.

12. Javed F, Correa FO, Nooh N, et al. Orofacial manifestations in patients with sickle cell disease. *Am J Med Sci.* 2013;345(3):234–237.

13. Fukuda JT, Sonis AL, Platt OS, et al. Acquisition of mutans streptococci and caries prevalence in pediatric sickle cell anemia patients receiving long-term antibiotic therapy. *Pediatr Dent.* 2005;27(3):186–190.

14. da Fonseca MA, Oueis HS, Casamassimo P. Sickle cell anemia: a review for the pediatric dentist. *Pediatr Dent.* 2007;29(2):159–169.

15. Van Herrewegen F, Meijers JCM, Peters M, et al. The bleeding child. Part II: disorders of secondary hemostasis and fibrinolysis. *Eur J Pediatr.* 2012;171:207–214.

16. Brewer A, Correa ME. *Guidelines for dental treatment of patients with inherited bleeding disorders, Treatment of hemophilia monograph no. 40.* Montreal: World Federation of Hemophilia; 2006.

17. Scully C, Dioz PD, Giangrande P. *Oral care for people with hemophilia or a hereditary bleeding tendency, Treatment of hemophilia monograph no. 27.* Montreal: World Federation of Hemophilia; 2008.

18. World Federation of Hemophilia. *Guidelines for the management of hemophilia.* Montreal: World Federation of Hemophilia; 2005.

19. Oldenburg J. Optimal treatment strategies for hemophilia: achievements and limitations of current prophylactic regimens. *Blood.* 2015;125(13):2038–2044.

20. Brewer A. *Dental management of patients with inhibitors to factor VIII or factor IX, Treatment of hemophilia monograph no. 45.* Montreal: World Federation of Hemophilia; 2008.

21. Ng C, Motto DG, Di Paola J. Diagnostic approach to von Willebrand disease. *Blood.* 2015;125(13):2029–2037.

22. Lillicrap D. von Willebrand disease: advances in pathogenic understanding, diagnosis, and therapy. *Blood.* 2013;122(23):3735–3740.

23. Bianch ML, Baim S, Bishop NJ, et al. Official positions of the International Society for Clinical Densitometry (ISCD) on DXA evaluation in children and adolescents. *Pediatr Nephrol.* 2010;25(1):37–47.

24. Bogunovic L, Doyle SM, Vogiatzi MG. Measurement of bone density in the pediatric population. *Curr Opin Pediatr.* 2009;21(1):77–82.

25. Bianchi ML. Osteoporosis in children and adolescents. *Bone.* 2007;41(4):486–495.

26. Saraff V, Hogler W. Endocrinology and adolescence: osteoporosis in children: diagnosis and management. *Eur J Endocrinol.* 2015;173(6):R185–R197.

27. Baroncelli GI, Bertelloni S. The use of bisphosphonates in pediatrics. *Horm Res Paediatr.* 2014;82(5):290–302.

28. McGartland C, Robson PJ, Murray L, et al. Carbonated soft drink consumption and bone mineral density in adolescence: the Northern Ireland young hearts project. *J Bone Miner Res.* 2003;18(9):1563–1569.

29. Zahrowski JJ. Bisphosphonate treatment: an orthodontic concern calling for a proactive approach. *Am J Orthod Dentofacial Orthop.* 2007;131(3):311–320.

30. Ward E, DeSantis C, Robbins A, et al. Childhood and adolescent cancer statistics, 2014. *CA Cancer J Clin.* 2014;64(2):83–103.

31. Hong CH, da Fonseca M. Considerations in the pediatric population with cancer. *Dent Clin North Am.* 2008;52(1):155–181.

32. Rabin KR, Gramatges MM, Margolin JF, et al. Acute lymphoblastic leukemia. In: Pizzo PA, Poplack DG, eds. *Principles and Practice of Pediatric Oncology.* 7th ed. Philadelphia: Wolters Kluwer; 2016:463–497.

33. Hou G-L, Huang J-S, Tsai C-C. Analysis of oral manifestations of leukemia: a retrospective study. *Oral Dis.* 1997;3(1):31–38.

34. Baddour LM, Bettmann MA, Bolger AF, et al. Nonvalvular cardiovascular device-related infections. *Circulation.* 2003;108(16):2015–2031.

35. Hong CHL, Allred R, Napenas JJ, et al. Antibiotic prophylaxis for dental procedures to prevent indwelling catheter-related infections. *Am J Med.* 2010;123(12):1128–1133.

36. Lalla RV, Bowen J, Barasch A, et al. MASCC/ISOO practice guidelines for the management of mucositis secondary to cancer therapy. *Cancer.* 2014;120(10):1453–1461.

37. Gotzche PC, Johansen HK. Nystatin prophylaxis and treatment in severely immunocompromised patients. *Cochrane Database Syst Rev.* 2002;(2):CD002033.

38. Little JW, Falace DA, Miller CS, et al. Cancer and oral care of the cancer patient. In: *Little and Falace's Dental Management of the Medically Compromised Patient.* 8th ed. St Louis: Elsevier; 2013:459–492.

39. Sheller B, Williams B. Orthodontic management of patients with hematologic malignancies. *Am J Orthod Dentofacial Orthop.* 1996;109(6):575–580.

40. Vesterbacka M, Ringden O, Remberger M, et al. Disturbances in dental development and craniofacial growth in children treated with hematopoietic stem cell transplantation. *Orthod Craniofac Res.* 2012;15(1):21–29.

41. Kaste SC, Goodman P, Lesirenring W, et al. Impact of radiation and chemotherapy on risk of dental abnormalities. *Cancer.* 2009;115(24):5817–5827.

42. Dahllof G, Jonsson A, Ulmner M, et al. Orthodontic treatment in long-term survivors after bone marrow transplantation. *Am J Orthod Dentofacial Orthop.* 2001;120(5):459–465.

43. Epstein JB, Raber-Drulacher JE, Wilkins A, et al. Advances in hematologic stem cell transplant: an update for oral health providers. *Oral Surg Oral Med Oral Pathol Oral Radiol Endod.* 2009;107(3):301–312.

44. Juric MK, Ghimire S, Ogonek J, et al. Milestones of hematopoietic stem cell transplantation—from first human studies to current developments. *Front Immunol.* 2016;7:470.

45. da Fonseca MA, Hong C. An overview of chronic graft-versus-host disease following pediatric hematopoietic stem cell transplantation. *Pediatr Dent.* 2008;30(2):98–104.

46. Hong CH, Brennan MT, Lockhart PB. Incidence of acute oral sequelae in pediatric patients undergoing chemotherapy. *Pediatr Dent.* 2009;31(5):420–425.

47. da Fonseca MA. Long-term oral and craniofacial complications following pediatric bone marrow transplantation. *Pediatr Dent.* 2000;22(1):57–62.

48. Goho C. Chemoradiation therapy: effect on dental development. *Pediatr Dent.* 1993;15(1):6–12.

49. Hong HL, Napenas JJ, Hodgson BD, et al. A systematic review of dental disease in patients undergoing cancer therapy. *Support Care Cancer.* 2010;18(8):1007–1021.

50. Woo SB, Challacombe SJ. Management of recurrent oral herpes simplex infections. *Oral Surg Oral Med Oral Pathol Oral Radiol Endod.* 2007;103(suppl 1):S12.e1–S12.e18.

51. Wilson SS, Fakioglu E, Herold BC. Novel approaches in fighting herpes simplex virus infections. *Expert Rev Anti Infect Ther.* 2009;7(5):559–568.

52. Drugge JM, Allen PJ. A nurse practitioner's guide to the management of herpes simplex virus-1 in children. *Pediatr Nurs.* 2008;34(4):310–318.

53. Usatine RP. Tinitigan R: Nongenital herpes simplex virus. *Am Fam Physician.* 2010;82(9):1075–1082.

54. Nasser M, Fedorowicz Z, Khoshnevisan MH, et al. Acyclovir for treating primary herpetic gingivostomatitis. *Cochrane Database Syst Rev*. 2008;(4):CD006700.

55. Flaitz CM, Hicks MJ. Oral candidiasis in children with immune suppression: clinical appearance and therapeutic considerations. *ASDC J Dent Child*. 1999;66(3):161–166.

56. Krol DM, Keels MA. Oral conditions. *Pediatr Rev*. 2007;28(1):15–22.

57. Flaitz CM, Baker KA. Treatment approaches to common symptomatic oral lesions in children. *Dent Clin North Am*. 2000;44(3):671–696.

58. Davies JC, Ebdon AM, Orchard C. Recent advances in the management of cystic fibrosis. *Arch Dis Child*. 2014;99:1033–1036.

59. Ehre C, Ridley C, Thornton DJ. Cystic fibrosis: an inherited disease affecting mucin-producing organs. *Int J Biochem Cell Biol*. 2014;52:136–145.

60. Davies JC, Alton EWFW, Bush A. Cystic fibrosis. *BMJ*. 2007;335:1255–1259.

61. Cystic Fibrosis Foundation. *CFTR* modulator therapies. https://www.cff.org/Life-With-CF/Treatments-and-Therapies/CFTR-Modulator-Therapies/. Accessed August 23, 2017.

62. Narang A, Maguire A, Nunn JH, et al. Oral health and related factors in cystic fibrosis and other chronic respiratory disorders. *Arch Dis Child*. 2003;88(8):702–707.

63. Chi DL. Dental caries prevalence in children and adolescents with cystic fibrosis: a qualitative systematic review and recommendations for future research. *Int J Paediatr Dent*. 2013;23(5):376–386.

64. Patrick JRD, da Fonseca MA, Kaste LM, et al. Oral health-related quality of life in pediatric patients with cystic fibrosis. *Spec Care Dent*. 2016;36(4):187–193.

65. Paccou J, Zeboulon N, Combescure C, et al. The prevalence of osteoporosis, osteopenia, and fractures among adults with cystic fibrosis: a systematic literature review with meta-analysis. *Calcif Tissue Int*. 2010;86(1):1–7.

66. Rabizadeh S, Dubinsky M. Update in pediatric inflammatory bowel disease. *Rheum Dis Clin North Am*. 2013;39(4):789–799.

67. Rowland M, Fleming P, Bourke B. Looking in the mouth for Crohn's disease. *Inflamm Bowel Dis*. 2010;16(2):332–337.

68. Lazzerini M, Martelossi S, Cont G, et al. Orofacial granulomatosis in children: think about Crohn's disease. *Dig Liver Dis*. 2015;47(4):338–341.

69. Lazzerini M, Bramuzzo M, Ventura A. Association between orofacial granulomatosis and Crohn's disease in children: systematic review. *World J Gastroenterol*. 2014;20(23):7497–7504.

70. Elli L, Branchi F, Tomba C, et al. Diagnosis of gluten related disorders: celiac disease, wheat allergy and non-celiac gluten sensitivity. *World J Gastroenterol*. 2015;21(23):7110–7119.

71. Kelly CP, Bai JC, Liu E, et al. Advances in diagnosis and management of celiac disease. *Gastroenterol*. 2015;148(6):1175–1186.

72. de Carvalho FK, de Queiroz AM, da Silva RAB, et al. Oral aspects of celiac disease children: clinical and dental enamel chemical evaluation. *Oral Surg Oral Med Oral Pathol Oral Radiol*. 2015;119(6):636–643.

73. Acar S, Yetkiner AA, Ersin N, et al. Oral findings and salivary parameters in children with celiac disease: a preliminary study. *Med Princ Pract*. 2012;21(2):129–133.

74. Ferraz EG, Campos EJ, Sarmento VA, et al. The oral manifestations of celiac disease: information for the pediatric dentist. *Pediatr Dent*. 2012;34(7):485–488.

5

Cleft Lip and Palate

MATTHEW K. GENESER AND VEERASATHPURUSH ALLAREDDY

CHAPTER OUTLINE

O rofacial clefts are one of the most common head and neck birth defects worldwide, affecting children of all socio-economic and cultural backgrounds. The overall prevalence rate is roughly 1 in 700 live births, but there is much variation depending on geographic location.[1] In the United States, it is estimated that nearly 1 in 1000 babies are born with an orofacial cleft with a slightly higher incidence in babies of Asian or Native American descent.[2] Clefts may involve the lip, alveolus, and palate in various combinations. Half of all orofacial clefts involve both the palate and the lip. Clefts that are isolated to the palate are less common.[2]

Children born with an orofacial cleft often have complex medical and dental conditions, necessitating the need for care from health care teams involving multiple specialists.[3] Common conditions that occur in children with orofacial clefts are hearing difficulty, speech and language disorders, middle ear abnormalities, psychosocial issues, and dental abnormalities. Pediatric dentists serve an important function on these multidisciplinary teams, as they will not only provide a dental home, but will also often coordinate the many aspects of treatment.[4]

Cleft Lip and Palate Team

Typically, a cleft lip and palate team is comprised of members drawn from multiple specialties, as shown in Table 5.1, each of whom plays a pivotal role in the overall care for patients with cleft lip and palate. Key procedures and interventions take place throughout childhood, as shown in Fig. 5.1, although the exact sequence and timing will vary depending on the characteristics of the child's cleft and the philosophy of the cleft lip and palate team members.

Anatomy

The palate is divided into a primary and a secondary palate at the incisive foramen. The primary palate extends anteriorly from the incisive foramen and includes the premaxilla, lip, nasal tip, and columella, as shown in Fig. 5.2. The secondary palate extends posteriorly from the incisive foramen and includes the hard and soft palates as well as the uvula.

Classification of Cleft Lip and Palate

Cleft lip and palate has a long history of varied and sometimes conflicting classification systems.[5] In 1931 Veau grouped palatal clefts into four forms based on anatomical position: clefts of the soft palate, clefts up to the incisive foramen, clefts extending through the alveolus unilaterally, and clefts extending through the alveolus bilaterally.[6] Veau's system is still used today but other systems exist and debate continues regarding how to best classify clefts. Regardless of the system utilized, understanding the anatomy of the oral cavity is the basis for understanding the classification system as shown in Fig. 5.3.

Cleft lip is classified as being complete or incomplete based on the extent of the cleft, as well as unilateral or bilateral depending on whether it affects one or both sides. An incomplete cleft of the lip does not involve the complete thickness of the lip, but has a band of tissue intact across the cleft. Conversely, a complete cleft of the lip involves the entire vertical thickness of the lip and is more often associated with a cleft of the alveolus.

Cleft palate is defined in a similar fashion, as either complete or incomplete as well as unilateral or bilateral, as shown in Fig. 5.4. A complete cleft of the palate involves both the primary and secondary palates as well as the alveolus. There is also the less common possibility of an isolated cleft palate,[7] which usually involves the secondary palate, posterior to the incisive foramen. This occurs in 1 in 1500 live births in the United States.[2]

A less severe form of cleft palate is a submucous cleft, which is a deformity in which there is a defective muscle union across the soft palate but the oral mucosa is intact. Classically, this presents as a bifid uvula, an absent posterior nasal spine, and a transparent band of mucosa at the midline of the palate called the zona pellucida. A submucous cleft often goes undiagnosed until the toddler years, with one of the first signs being hypernasal speech.[8] This abnormal speech pattern is a result of a velopharyngeal dysfunction (VPD),

TABLE 5.1 Members of a Typical Cleft Lip and Palate Team

Member	Role
Plastic surgeon	Early surgical interventions, including lip adhesion and/or primary lip repair as well as esthetic surgical procedures throughout growth to minimize scarring and improve facial features
Pediatric otolaryngologist	Early surgical interventions, including lip adhesion and/or primary lip repair, palate repair, velopharyngeal surgery, and other possible surgical interventions such as ear tubes
Oral and maxillofacial surgeon	Depending on training, may play a role in surgical repair of lip and palate Commonly involved in extractions, bone grafting procedures, as well as distraction osteogenesis
Geneticist	Counsels families on the risk of having future children with CLP Determines if clefting is a part of a syndrome or an isolated event
Pediatric dentist	Provides a dental home for children with CLP or other craniofacial abnormalities May play a role in presurgical molding techniques (e.g., NAM) Prevention of dental disease in high risk populations as well as restorations and interceptive orthodontics
Orthodontist	May play a role in presurgical molding techniques (e.g., NAM or Latham) Early treatment for alignment and expansion of constricted dental arches and comprehensive orthodontic treatment
Prosthodontist	Restoration of dentition to full function and esthetics in adolescence and adulthood
Audiologist	Follows milestones for normal hearing and work with otolaryngologist to determine if ear tubes are needed
Speech pathologist	Follows milestones for speech development Works with local speech therapists to devise a program that will maximize speech development Input is important when the decision has to be made regarding velopharyngeal surgery
Nurse	Provides support and counseling for families Coordinates many aspects of medical care Works with families to develop a program for feeding, particularly early in life
Psychologist	Assesses child's mental and emotional well-being throughout life Helps child adjust to stages of life and offers assistance and support when needed
Social worker	Provides support and assistance to families, helping to overcome barriers, allowing the best possible care to be delivered to the child Financial assistance, transportation, local arrangements, and school programs are a few examples

Makeup of group and roles will vary depending on a number of factors including geographic location, hospital policies, and available specialists.
CLP, Cleft lip and palate; NAM, nasoalveolar molding.

which occurs in roughly half of patients with submucous cleft palate.[9]

Causes of Cleft Lip and Palate

Clefts of the lip and palate may result from isolated mutations, syndromes, as shown in Box 5.1, environmental factors, teratogen exposure (including alcohol and tobacco), or a combination of the above. Genetics plays a strong role in the development of orofacial clefts, both syndromic and nonsyndromic, but it is known that genetics is not the sole determinant of whether or not a child will develop a cleft.

During normal development, the facial prominences appear at the end of the fourth embryonic week. These prominences are derived from the neural crest and consist of maxillary prominences laterally as well as a frontonasal prominence. Nasal placodes, located on either side of the frontonasal prominence, appear during the fifth embryonic week, eventually forming the nasal pits, which are bordered by the lateral and medial nasal prominences. The fusion of the medial nasal prominences forms the nasal tip, columella, and philtrum, as well as a portion of the upper lip. The fusion of the maxillary prominences forms the remainder of

• BOX 5.1 Common Syndromes and Abnormalities Associated With Cleft Lip and Palate

Van der Woude syndrome
Velocardiofacial syndrome
CHARGE syndrome
Beckwith-Wiedemann syndrome
Apert syndrome
DiGeorge syndrome
Pierre Robin sequence
Treacher-Collins syndrome
Kabuki syndrome
Klippel Feil syndrome
Goldenhar syndrome
Stickler syndrome

the upper lip. These fusion events take place during the seventh embryonic week.

The palate begins to form during the 5th embryonic week, continuing through the 12th embryonic week. The primary palate is formed when the medial nasal prominences fuse, only at a deeper level. The secondary palate begins to form soon after the primary palate is fused, around the seventh embryonic week. This results from fusion of the lateral palatine shelves, beginning at the incisive foramen in the 8th week and ending at the uvula in the 12th embryonic week.

Cleft Lip/Palate Team

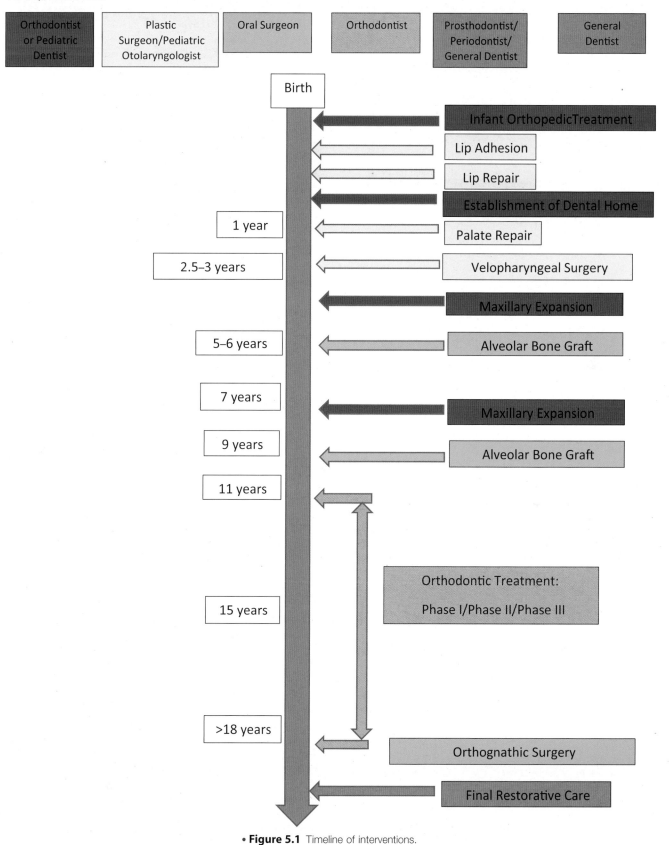

• **Figure 5.1** Timeline of interventions.

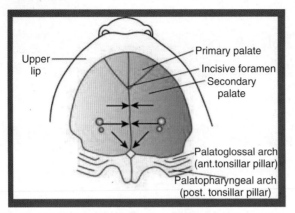

• **Figure 5.2** Primary and secondary palate divided by the incisive papilla. (From Holzman R. Airway management. In: Davis P, Cladis F, eds. *Anesthesia for Infants and Children*. Philadelphia: Elsevier; 2017:349–369.)

Challenges and Anomalies Associated With Cleft Lip and Palate

Children with cleft lip and palate may suffer from a number of other complications and conditions. A common presentation for patients with cleft lip and palate is the concurrent presence of micrognathia and glossoptosis. Together, this triad is commonly referred to as Pierre Robin sequence, as shown in Fig. 5.5, named after Dr. Pierre Robin who described this in the 1920s.[10] This sequence occurs in a number of syndromes and a major concern for these children is airway obstruction due to the malposition of the tongue. It has become common for children with Pierre Robin sequence to have mandibular distraction osteogenesis at a very young age to prevent upper airway obstruction.[11]

Children with cleft lip alone usually have little difficulty feeding and can often nurse or bottle feed normally. Children with cleft palate often struggle to feed due to the limited or absent ability

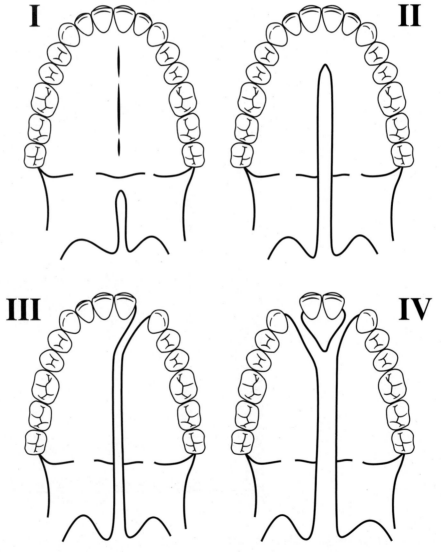

• **Figure 5.3** Classification of cleft palate. *I,* Incomplete cleft of secondary palate. *II,* Complete cleft of the secondary palate. *III,* Unilateral complete cleft of primary and secondary palate. *IV,* Bilateral complete cleft of the primary and secondary palate. (Courtesy Monica Byrne.)

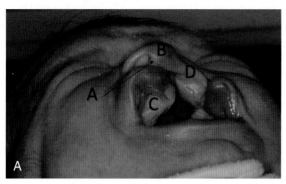
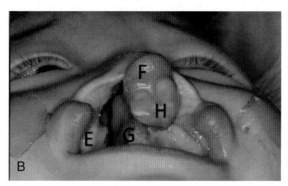

• **Figure 5.4** (A) Unilateral complete cleft lip and palate. *A*, Columella; *B*, Nasal tip; *C*, Greater segment of alveolus; *D*, Alar rim. (B) Bilateral complete cleft lip and palate. *E*, Lateral shelf of alveolus; *F*, Prolabium; *G*, Vomer; *H*, Premaxilla. Note erupting primary tooth on right side of premaxilla.

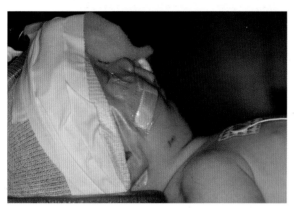

• **Figure 5.5** Child with Pierre Robin sequence (in preparation for surgical placement of distractors to improve mandibular position by distraction osteogenesis).

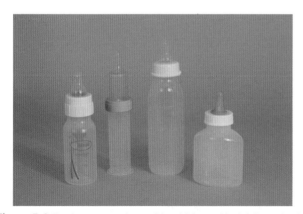

• **Figure 5.6** Bottles commonly used for children with cleft lip and palate.

of the infant to create suction and suck to feed.[12] In order to help families navigate these feeding challenges, nursing professionals will demonstrate unique bottles and feeding methods to determine what works best for each child and family, as shown in Fig. 5.6.

Another common challenge for children with cleft lip and palate is frequent otitis media and other middle ear abnormalities. Studies have shown that a very high percentage of children with cleft palate require ear tubes and often multiple sets of ear tubes during childhood as a result of recurrent infections.[13] It is important to

screen these children for hearing loss and intervene early, as delays in the correction hearing problems can hinder the development of speech.

Individuals with cleft lip and palate have a higher incidence of dental anomalies, particularly in the permanent dentition, than individuals without clefts.[14] These anomalies vary in degree of severity and can include rotation of the teeth near the cleft, hypoplasia of enamel, particularly in teeth adjacent to the cleft, missing teeth, and supernumerary teeth.

Hypodontia, or missing teeth, occurs more commonly in patients with cleft lip and palate and it occurs more frequently in the permanent dentition as compared with the primary dentition. The tooth most likely to be missing is the lateral incisor with the prevalence being higher on the side with the cleft.[15] The prevalence of missing lateral incisors increases as the extent of clefting increases, from cleft lip alone to cleft palate alone to cleft lip and palate.[15]

One question that has proven to be difficult to answer is, "Do children with orofacial clefts have higher rates of dental caries?" Research in this area is contradictory, with numerous studies from around the world showing significantly higher caries rates for children with clefts,[16,17] while other studies show no difference between these populations.[18] It has been shown that the rate of dental caries for children with cleft lip and palate is greater in the maxillary arch and particularly in those teeth adjacent to the cleft.[16] This may be attributable to the hypoplasia and other structural anomalies more commonly found in these teeth.[19]

One likely reason for the discrepancies in caries rates is the complexity of overall health for children with orofacial clefts. Many have syndromes and other conditions that can predispose them to dental caries. There are also physical challenges with accessing the area around the cleft for routine hygiene and plaque removal, as it is common for teeth in and around the cleft to be malposed, making accessibility more difficult and plaque retention more likely. Depending on the child's physical challenges, poor dexterity may be an issue that further complicates the cleaning of the oral cavity. It also must be considered that for children with myriad health concerns, dentistry may not rank as highly on the priority list and routine hygiene may suffer due to more seemingly pressing concerns.

Infant Orthopedics

The use of appliances and forces, in various forms, to mold the alveolus and lessen the severity of the cleft has been around for

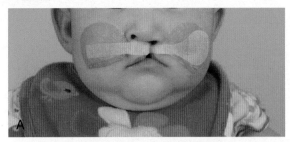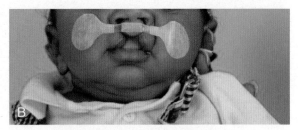

• **Figure 5.7** Elastomeric taping. (A) Child with a unilateral cleft. (B) Child with a bilateral cleft.

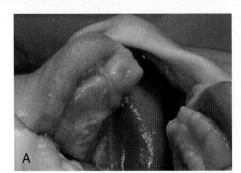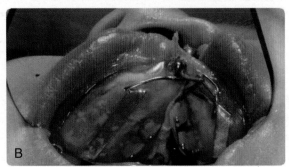

• **Figure 5.8** (A and B) Latham appliance.

decades[20,21] or even longer if you consider Hoffman's head cap and the use of extraoral forces described in the late 1600s.[22]

In its simplest form, the use of elastomeric tape to apply force can cause movement and decrease the width of the alveolar cleft, as shown in Fig. 5.7.[23] Tape has the advantage of being relatively inexpensive and less onerous for families when compared to other molding devices, but it has the disadvantage of applying forces indiscriminately, so palatal constriction may result. Taping can be done alone or in conjunction with other molding techniques such as intraoral appliances.

Intraoral appliances are often more cumbersome to use, but they do maintain the palatal width, since force can be applied in smaller areas and with greater precision. Recently, these intraoral appliances have gained acceptance on many craniofacial teams worldwide and are a hot topic of research. The Latham appliance shown in Fig. 5.8 is an appliance that is surgically placed into a young child's mouth and retained to the palate with a screw.[24] The Latham appliance is adjusted regularly to reduce the cleft size. The advantage of this appliance is that compliance is not required, but the disadvantage is increased surgical interventions in a very young child, both at the time of insertion and at the time of removal.

One less invasive method, pioneered by Dr. Barry Grayson and his team at New York University is nasoalveolar molding or NAM, as shown in Fig. 5.9.[25] This method uses an acrylic plate to mold the bony alveolus, in a similar fashion to the Latham appliance and early appliances like the Hotz plate, but it is removable and uses a nasal stent to shape the cartilage of the nose, in an attempt to improve symmetry and decrease the need for future invasive surgical correction that may cause scarring and hinder growth.

The NAM appliance is worn throughout the day and held in place by tape to the child's cheeks. Changes are made to the plate incrementally by the dental professional and over time the bony segments are slowly moved to a more favorable position, lessening the amount of surgical correction that is needed to bring the lip segments together while simplifying the surgical approach for the nose. NAM has even been shown to decrease the number

of future surgical interventions that are typically performed for esthetics.[26]

An Overview of the Timeline of Interventions

Many procedures are required for children born with cleft lip and palate, as outlined in Fig. 5.1. The earliest intervention is often infant orthopedic treatment (see previous section). The goal of infant orthopedic treatment is to enhance the surgical repair of lip and nose by establishing a proper skeletal base.[27–29] A wide variety of approaches are used, with one of the most popular being NAM, which is initiated within the first few weeks of life.[30]

A cleft lip is repaired between 3 and 6 month of age, following infant orthopedic treatment. A few craniofacial centers may elect to perform another surgery called a naso-labial (lip) adhesion prior to repairing the cleft lip, although this has largely fallen out of favor in the United States. The naso-labial (lip) adhesion procedure is purported to reduce the extent of undermining and minimize labial tension at the time of lip repair.[31] Any surgical intervention in a young child has to be considered carefully, and traditionally cleft repair surgeries have been subject to the "rule of 10s." This rule states that a child must be 10 pounds in weight, have a hemoglobin value greater than 10 g/dL, and be older than 10 weeks of age prior to the surgical intervention.[32] This rule is not an absolute, but one must certainly consider the risk of taking a very young baby under general anesthesia when planning care, and this is one reason that naso-labial (lip) adhesion has fallen out of favor.

A cleft palate is repaired between the ages of 9 and 18 months, most often by age 1. Early repair of the palate has the advantage of better speech development but the downside is that scar tissue can form and inhibit proper maxillary growth, leading to malocclusion (typically class III malocclusions and skeletal pattern) and poor facial esthetics. Conversely, if palate repair is done late, after 18 months, the opposite is true and growth may occur normally but speech will likely be negatively impacted.[33] Determining the

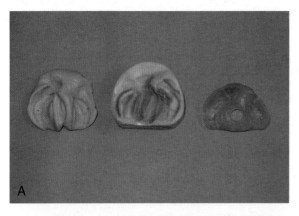
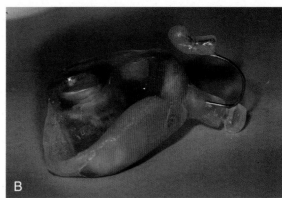
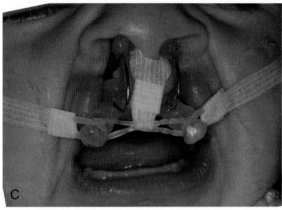

• **Figure 5.9** Nasoalveolar molding (NAM) appliance. (A) Fabrication of NAM appliance. (B) NAM appliance. (C) NAM and taping for presurgical orthopedics.

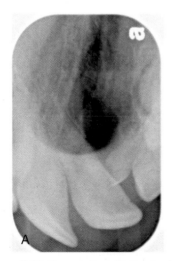
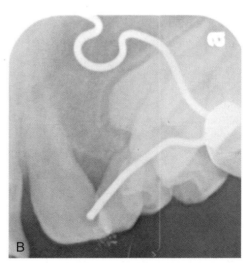

• **Figure 5.10** Bone grafting. (A) Alveolar defect in a patient with complete cleft lip and palate. (B) Alveolar defect repaired with an alveolar bone grafting procedure.

best time for palate repair means taking these competing priorities into consideration and working as a team to develop an optimal surgical plan.

If speech development is suboptimal, a velopharyngeal surgery may be performed between 2.5 and 3 years of age.[34] Repair of the cleft lip and palate and velopharyngeal surgeries are performed by either a plastic surgeon, pediatric otolaryngologist, or an oral and maxillofacial surgeon with advanced training in pediatric cranio-maxillofacial surgery.

Patients with clefts of the alveolus often have collapsed maxillary arches and require alveolar bone grafting, as shown in Fig. 5.10. Alveolar bone grafting enables the surgeon to obtain maxillary arch continuity, provide support for the dentition to erupt, and stabilize the maxillary arch prior to any orthodontic treatment.[35–41]

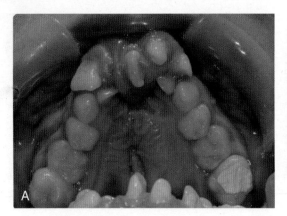
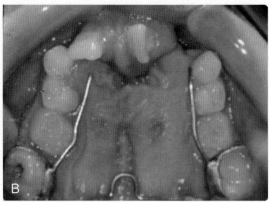

• **Figure 5.11** (A and B) Maxillary arch in a patient with bilateral complete cleft lip and palate. (Note the collapsed anterior segment of the maxillary arch prior to expansion.)

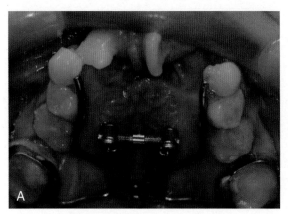
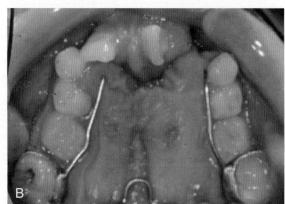

• **Figure 5.12** Palatal expansion. (A) Differential expansion with a fan-shaped expander was needed to address the collapsed maxillary arch. (B) Retain expansion with a transpalatal arch appliance.

The timing of alveolar bone grafting is dependent on the presence of a viable maxillary permanent lateral incisor adjacent to the alveolar cleft area and proximity of the roots of central incisors to the alveolar cleft.[35–41] If a viable permanent lateral incisor is present or if the root of the developing maxillary central incisor is too close to the alveolar cleft, alveolar bone grafting is recommended by 5 to 7 years of age. A number of craniofacial centers elect to perform the alveolar bone grafting at a later time, closer to eruption of the maxillary permanent canines. The most frequently used donor site for alveolar bone grafting is the iliac crest because of ease of access and abundance of bone.[27,40] Alternative donor sites include the mandibular symphysis, rib, cranial bones, and tibia. A few craniofacial centers also use bone morphogenetic protein (BMP).[27,40] This alveolar bone grafting procedure is usually performed by an oral and maxillofacial surgeon.

It is recommended that maxillary arch expansion be performed prior to alveolar bone grafting to establish proper arch form and to address transverse discrepancies, as shown in Fig. 5.11.[27,34] Maxillary arch expansion facilitates better access for alveolar bone graft sites. Maxillary expansion (differential or symmetric) is performed either by the pediatric dentist or by an orthodontist on the cleft lip and palate team and appliances vary, as shown in Fig. 5.12.

Following alveolar bone grafting, the patient is typically followed periodically by the cleft lip and palate team. The eruption pattern of the permanent dentition is closely observed and if indicated, a limited phase of orthodontic treatment (often in the maxillary arch only) is completed during the mixed dentition phase. The goals of limited maxillary arch orthodontic treatment are to align and level the maxillary arch, correct crossbites, create space for facilitating eruption of permanent teeth, and treat impacted or ectopically erupting teeth, as shown in Fig. 5.13.

During the early teenage years, if it is determined that the amount of anterior-posterior skeletal discrepancy is too large, then maxillary distraction osteogenesis is indicated.[42,43] This procedure is performed by an oral and maxillofacial surgeon following eruption of all permanent teeth into the arch. The orthodontist aligns and levels the maxillary arch and prepares the patient to undergo the maxillary distraction osteogenesis procedure. Until a few years ago, maxillary distraction was accomplished by a rigid external distractor (RED) appliance, as shown in Fig. 5.14. Internal distractors, as shown in Fig. 5.15, are being increasingly used by oral and maxillofacial surgeons in place of the more cumbersome extraoral appliances.[43,44]

The patient is followed during the teenage years and the orthodontist determines the timing of a comprehensive phase of orthodontic treatment. If there are no significant skeletal discrepancies to address, the orthodontic treatment can be initiated following eruption of all permanent teeth. If large skeletal discrepancies exist, it is recommended that a comprehensive phase of orthodontic treatment in conjunction with an orthognathic surgery be initiated following completion of growth.

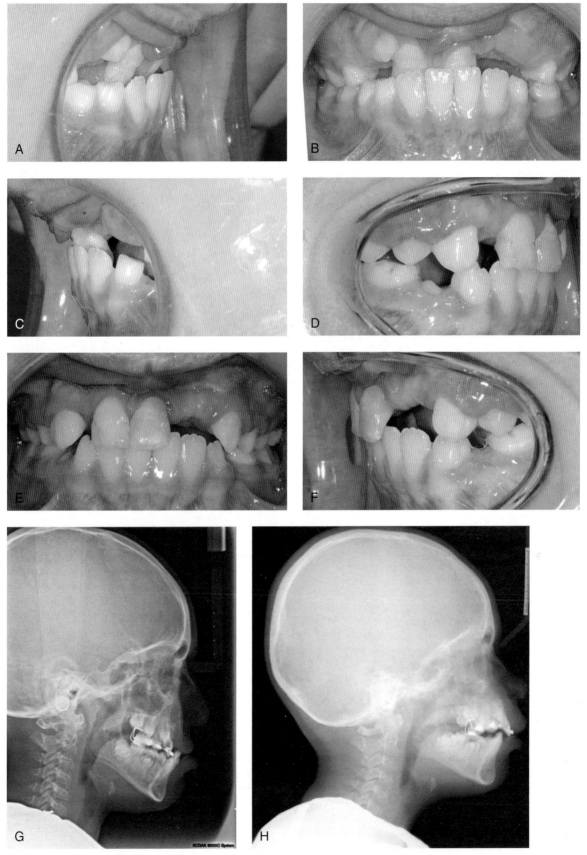

• **Figure 5.13** Orthodontic treatment. (A–C) Pretreatment photographs. (D–F) Posttreatment photographs. (G) Pretreatment cephalometric film. (H) Posttreatment cephalometric film.

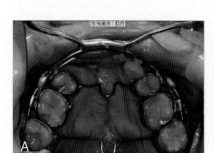
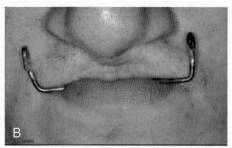

• **Figure 5.14** (A and B) Setup for a rigid external distractors appliance.

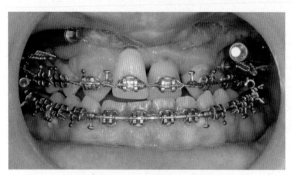

• **Figure 5.15** Internal distractors.

Role of the Dentist

Children born with cleft lip and palate face a long and difficult road through the health care system. They will have many interventions by myriad providers. One must consider the impact this will have on the physical, mental, and emotional well-being of the child and work closely with other members of the health care team to provide the most comprehensive care possible. Even if a dentist is not an active member of a cleft lip and palate team, he or she must have the knowledge to refer to the proper provider at the proper time. A pediatric dentist has a unique opportunity to work with these children and their families from infancy into young adulthood and play a key role in the promotion of optimal oral health as well as ensuring that the family is able to properly navigate the complexities of the health care environment.

References

1. Mossey PA, Castilla E, eds: Global registry and database on craniofacial anomalies. WHO Reports. Human Genetics Programme: International Collaborative Research on Craniofacial Anomalies, Geneva, Switzerland. 2003;WHO.
2. Parker SE, Mai CT, Canfield MA, et al. National Birth Defects Prevention Network, updated national birth prevalence estimates for selected birth defects in the United States, 2004–2006. *Birth Defects Res A Clin Mol Teratol.* 2010;88:1008–1016.
3. Strauss RP. ACPA Team Standards Committee, cleft palate and craniofacial teams in the United States and Canada: a national survey of team organization and standards of care. *Cleft Palate Craniofac J.* 1998;35:473–480.
4. American Academy of Pediatric Dentistry. Policy on management of patients with cleft lip/palate and other craniofacial anomalies. *AAPD Reference Manual.* 2016;38:386–387.
5. Allori AC, Mulliken JB, Meara JG, et al. Classification of cleft lip/palate: then and now. *Cleft Palate Craniofac J.* 2017;54(2):175–188.
6. Venu V. *Division Palatine: Anatomie, Chirugie, Phonetique.* Paris: Masson; 1931.
7. Burg ML, Chai Y, Yao CA, et al. Epidemiology, etiology, and treatment of isolated cleft palate. *Front Physiol.* 2016;7:67.
8. Hocevar-Boltezar I, Jarc A, Kozelj V. Ear, nose and voice problems in children with orofacial clefts. *J Laryngol Otol.* 2006;120(4):276–281.
9. Reiter R, Brosch S, Wefel H, et al. The submucous cleft palate: diagnosis and therapy. *Int J Pediatr Otorhinolaryngol.* 2011;75:85–88.
10. Robin P. La chute de la base de la langue considérée comme une nouvelle cause de gans la respiration naso-pharyngienne. *Bull Acad Natl Med.* 1923;89:37–41.
11. Wittenborn W, Panchal J, Marsh JL, et al. Neonatal distraction surgery for micrognathia reduces obstructive apnea and the need for tracheotomy. *J Craniofac Surg.* 2004;15(4):623–630.
12. Redford-Badwal DA, Mabry K, Frassinelli JD. Impact of cleft lip and/or palate on nutritional health and oral-motor development. *Dent Clin North Am.* 2003;47(2):305–317.
13. Muntz HR. An overview of middle ear disease in cleft palate children. *Facial Plast Surg.* 1993;9:177.
14. Tannure NP, Oliveira CA, Maia LC, et al. Prevalence of dental anomalies in non-syndromic individuals with cleft lip and palate: a systematic review and meta-analysis. *Cleft Palate Craniofac J.* 2012;49(2):194–200.
15. Suzuki A, Nakano M, Yoshizaki K, et al. A longitudinal study of the presence of dental anomalies in the primary and permanent dentitions of cleft lip and/or palate patients. *Cleft Palate Craniofac J.* 2017;54(3):309–320.
16. Bokhout B, Hofman FX, van Limbeek J, et al. Incidence of dental caries in the primary dentition in children with a cleft lip and/or palate. *Caries Res.* 1997;31(1):8–12.
17. Ahluwalia M, Brasilsford SR, Tarelli E, et al. Dental caries, oral hygiene, and oral clearance in children with craniofacial disorders. *J Dent Res.* 2004;83(2):175–179.
18. Lucas VS, Gupta R, Ololade O, et al. Dental health indices and caries associated microflora in children with unilateral cleft lip and palate. *Cleft Palate Craniofacial J.* 2000;37(5):447–452.
19. Vichi M, Franchi L. Abnormalities of the maxillary incisors in children with cleft lip and palate. *ASDC J Dent Child.* 1995;62(6):412–417.
20. Hotz M, Perko M, Gnoinski W. Early orthopaedic stabilization of the praemaxilla in complete bilateral cleft lip and palate in combination with the Celesnik lip repair. *Scand J Plast Reconstr Surg Hand Surg.* 1987;21:45–51.
21. McNeil C. Orthodontic procedures in the treatment of congenital cleft palate. *Dent Rec.* 1950;70:126–132.
22. Hoffman JP. *De labiis leoporinvis/von Hasen-Scharten.* Heidelberg: Bergmann; 1686.
23. Smith KS, Henry BT, Scott MA. Presurgical dentofacial orthopedic management of the cleft patient. *Dent Clin North Am.* 2016;28(2):169–176.
24. Latham RA, Kusy RP, Georgiade NG. An extraorally activated expansion appliance for cleft palate infants. *Cleft Palate J.* 1976;13:253–261.
25. Grayson BH, Maull D. Nasoalveolar molding for infants born with clefts of the lip, alveolus, and palate. *Clin Plastic Surg.* 2004;31:149–158.

26. Garfinkle JS, King TW, Grayson BH, et al. A 12-year anthropometric evaluation of the nose in bilateral cleft lip-cleft palate patients following nasoalveolar molding and cutting bilateral cleft lip and nose reconstruction. *Plast Reconstr Surg*. 2011;127:1659–1667.

27. Santiago PE, Schuster LA, Levy-Bercowski D. Management of the alveolar cleft. *Clin Plast Surg*. 2014;41(2):219–232.

28. Attiguppe PR, Karuna YM, Yavagal C, et al. Presurgical nasoalveolar molding: a boon to facilitate the surgical repair in infants with cleft lip and palate. *Contemp Clin Dent*. 2016;7(4):569–573.

29. Sasaki H, Togashi S, Karube R, et al. Presurgical nasoalveolar molding orthopedic treatment improves the outcome of primary cheiloplasty of unilateral complete cleft lip and palate, as assessed by naris morphology and cleft gap. *J Craniofac Surg*. 2012;23(6): 1596–1601.

30. Ahmed MM, Brecht LE, Cutting CB, et al. 2012 American Board of Pediatric Dentistry College of Diplomates annual meeting: the role of pediatric dentists in the presurgical treatment of infants with cleft lip/cleft palate utilizing nasoalveolar molding. *Pediatr Dent*. 2012;34(7):e209–e214.

31. Vander Woude DL, Mulliken JB. Effect of lip adhesion on labial height in two-stage repair of unilateral complete cleft lip. *Plast Reconstr Surg*. 1997;100(3):567–572, discussion 573–574.

32. Chow I, Purnell CA, Hanwright PJ, et al. Evaluating the rule of 10s in cleft lip repair: do data support dogma? *Plast Reconstr Surg*. 2016;138:670.

33. Willadsen E. Influence of timing of hard palate repair in a two-state procedure on early speech development in Danish children with cleft palate. *Cleft Palate Craniofac J*. 2012;49(5):574–595.

34. Vig KW, Mercado AM. Overview of orthodontic care for children with cleft lip and palate, 1915-2015. *Am J Orthod Dentofacial Orthop*. 2015;148(4):543–556.

35. Coots BK. Alveolar bone grafting: past, present, and new horizons. *Semin Plast Surg*. 2012;26(4):178–183.

36. Ochs MW. Alveolar cleft bone grafting (Part II): secondary bone grafting. *J Oral Maxillofac Surg*. 1996;54:83–88.

37. Eppley BL. Alveolar cleft bone grafting (Part I): primary bone grafting. *J Oral Maxillofac Surg*. 1996;54:74–82.

38. Rosenstein SW. Early bone grafting of alveolar cleft deformities. *J Oral Maxillofac Surg*. 2003;61:1078–1081.

39. Kazemi A, Stearns JW, Fonseca RJ. Secondary grafting in the alveolar cleft patient. *Oral Maxillofac Surg Clin North Am*. 2002;14:477–490.

40. Bajaj AK, Wongworawat A, Punjabi A. Management of alveolar clefts. *J Craniofac Surg*. 2003;26(4):840–846.

41. Yu J, Glover A, Levy-Bercowski D, et al. Cleft orthognathic surgery. In: Guyton B, Eriksson E, Persing J, eds. *Plastic surgery indications and practice*. Philadelphia: Saunders; 2008:563–575.

42. Kloukos D, Fudalej P, Sequeira-Byron P, et al. Maxillary distraction osteogenesis versus orthognathic surgery for cleft lip and palate patients. *Cochrane Database Syst Rev*. 2016;(9):CD010403.

43. Kim J, Uhm KI, Shin D, et al. Maxillary distraction osteogenesis using a rigid external distractor: which clinical factors are related with relapse? *J Craniofac Surg*. 2015;26(4):1178–1181.

44. Silveira AD, Moura PM, Harshbarger RJ 3rd. Orthodontic considerations for maxillary distraction osteogenesis in growing patients with cleft lip and palate using internal distractors. *Semin Plast Surg*. 2014;28(4):207–212.

6
Fundamental Principles of Pediatric Physiology and Anatomy

JEFFREY N. BROWNSTEIN

CHAPTER OUTLINE

The treatment of children presents particular challenges to the health care professional. The body of the pediatric patient is not simply a miniaturized version of his or her adult counterpart; child physiology and anatomy significantly differ from those of an adult. A basic understanding of these physiologic and anatomic differences is necessary to ensure patient safety and provide effective care. Dentists who treat children must consider such differences when they are considering therapeutic alternatives for young patients, particularly pharmacologic therapies. Route and rate of drug administration, dosage, onset, duration of action, and likelihood of toxicity all may be influenced by the unique physiology and anatomy of the child.

This chapter will review the fundamental principles of pediatric physiology and anatomy as it relates to the practice of pediatric dentistry, placing particular emphasis on the use of sedatives, local anesthetics, and other pertinent pharmacologic agents. For the sake of simplicity, this material will be presented by organ system. Because a comprehensive review of these subjects is beyond the scope of this chapter, the text emphasizes only the principles that differ significantly from those of the adult patient. Wherever possible, clinical applications to pediatric dentistry are made.

Respiratory System (Fig. 6.1)

Anatomy

During the treatment planning phase, the dentist must complete an airway evaluation when considering the use of pharmacologic behavior guidance. This focused exam is considered a basic element in the preoperative examination and is aimed at identifying a potential disease or disorder that may increase morbidity and mortality. If warranted, the practitioner may then formulate alternative options for delivery of care to mitigate acknowledged risks.[1] An appreciation for anatomic variances is paramount when treatment plans include the use of minimal, moderate, or deep sedation or general anesthesia. A lack of consideration can ultimately result in ineffective or delayed management of a compromised airway secondary to the depressive effects of anxiolytic and sedative medications, especially in infants and young children with reduced oxygen reserves. Several anatomic features of the pediatric respiratory system predispose patients to obstruction and collapse of both large and small airways. A child's upper respiratory tract is prone to obstruction at multiple sites. Narrow nasal passages and obligate nasal breathing, tongue/oral cavity disproportion, hypertrophy of tonsillar tissues (Fig. 6.2), and decreased overall airway diameter in infants and young children predispose these patients to partial or complete upper airway obstruction (Fig. 6.3).[2,3] Additional risk may be generated by routine office procedures: a tightly sealed rubber dam covering the mouth and nares, gauze or cotton rolls elevating the resting tongue position, or a mouth prop posteriorly displacing the tongue all may increase the likelihood of upper airway obstruction. Surgical hemorrhage, salivary secretions, and edema associated with upper respiratory infections and seasonal allergies also can further compromise the pediatric airway and should be considered when a symptomatic child reports for an elective dental procedure. The airway of patients undergoing general anesthesia with endotracheal intubation poses an additional set of concerns. Bronchospasm, laryngospasm, acute subglottic edema with stridor, perioperative hypoxia, atelectasis, breath holding, and postextubation croup are among the complications most frequently encountered following dental surgery with general anesthesia. In the past, most clinicians recommended postponement of an elective sedation/general anesthesia procedure until the child had been free of upper respiratory symptoms for at least 1 week. Although there is no consensus on indications for canceling an elective procedure without endotracheal intubation, the literature suggests that signs and symptoms of lower tract involvement, such as fever of 38°C (100.4°F) or higher, lethargy, productive cough, wheezing, or tachypnea, in addition to a history of asthma are more commonly associated with general anesthesia-related morbidity. Similarly, if a bacterial infection is suspected, patients should be placed on a therapeutic regimen of antibiotics and the general anesthesia procedure postponed for at least 4 weeks.[4-6] Children with airway abnormalities secondary to craniofacial, neuromuscular, or central nervous system disorders should also be approached with particular caution (Table 6.1). In addition, extremely obese children (body

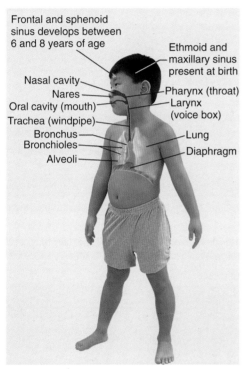

• **Figure 6.1** Respiratory system of a pediatric patient. (Modified from Leifer G. *Introduction to Maternity & Pediatric Nursing.* 6th ed. St Louis: Saunders; 2011.)

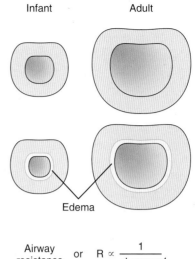

$$R \propto \frac{1}{\left(\dfrac{Lumen}{radius}\right)^4}$$

	Infant	Adult
Airway diameter	4 mm	8 mm
Airway diameter with edema	3 mm	7 mm
Airway resistance	↑ 16 x	↑ 3 x
Cross-sectional area	↓ 75%	↓ 44%

• **Figure 6.3** Effects of airway narrowing. Resistance to gas flow is inversely proportional to the fourth power of the radius of the airway lumen, meaning that small decreases in luminal diameter result in large increases in airway resistance. Because infants and children have smaller airways than adults at comparable levels, the same amount of airway narrowing (e.g., 1 mm) results in a disproportionate increase in resistance for these patients. This problem is compounded by the fact that the immature respiratory musculature of a pediatric patient is less efficient and therefore more prone to fatigue than that of an adult. (Redrawn from King C, Rappaport LD. Emergent endotracheal intubation. In: King C, Henretig FM, eds. *Textbook of Pediatric Emergency Procedures.* 2nd ed. Philadelphia: Lippincott Williams & Wilkins; 2008. Modified from Coté CJ, Todres ID. The pediatric airway. In: Cote CJ, Ryan JF, Todres ID, et al, eds. *A Practice of Anesthesia for Infants and Children.* 2nd ed. Philadelphia: WB Saunders; 1993.)

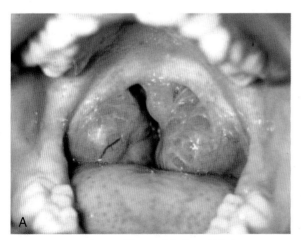
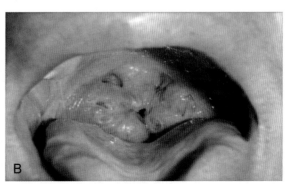

• **Figure 6.2** (A and B) Hypertrophic tonsils. (Courtesy Mark Saxen, DDS, PhD.)

TABLE 6.1	Congenital Conditions and Associated Clinical Features Pertaining to the Airway
Condition	**Clinical Feature**
Pierre Robin sequence	Micrognathia, macroglossia, glossoptosis, cleft lip and palate
Treacher Collins syndrome (mandibulofacial dysostosis)	Auricular and ocular defects, zygomatic and mandibular hypoplasia or aplasia, microstomia, choanal atresia, palatopharyngeal incompetence, cleft palate
Crouzon syndrome	Craniofacial synostosis, towering skull with proptosis, maxillary hypoplasia, beaked nose, high arched palate and malocclusion, cleft lip and/or palate, cervical vertebral fusions
Apert syndrome (acrocephalosyndactyly)	Craniofacial synostosis, maxillary hypoplasia, prognathism, cleft palate, tracheobronchial cartilaginous anomalies, cervical vertebral fusions
Goldenhar syndrome (hemifacial microsomia)	Auricular and ocular defects, zygomatic and mandibular hypoplasia, occipitalization of atlas, cleft lip and/or palate, velopharyngeal insufficiency and narrowed pharyngeal airway, cervical vertebral fusions
Down syndrome (trisomy 21)	Narrow nasopharynx, large tonsils and adenoids, macroglossia, poorly developed or absent bridge of the nose, small subglottic area, microcephaly, cervical spine abnormalities, atlantoaxial subluxation, broad short neck, obesity
Klippel-Feil syndrome	Congenital fusion of a variable number of cervical vertebrae, restriction of neck movement, cleft palate
Beckwith-Wiedemann syndrome (infantile gigantism)	Macroglossia, predisposition for development of various neoplasms involving the head and neck
Cherubism (familial fibrous dysplasia)	Tumorous lesions in the mandible and maxilla with intraoral masses, limited jaw closure and tongue displacement
Cretinism (congenital hypothyroidism)	Macroglossia, compression of the trachea, deviation of larynx/trachea, laryngeal nerve palsies, paradoxical vocal cord motion
Cri-du-chat syndrome (deletion 5p syndrome)	Microcephaly, micrognathia, laryngomalacia, stridor, cleft lip and/or palate, short neck, hemivertebrae
Von Recklinghausen disease (neurofibromatosis)	Tumors may occur in the larynx and right ventricle outflow tract, cervical spine abnormality, tongue lesions, and macroglossia
Hurler syndrome (mucopolysaccharidosis I)	Gargoyle facies, enlarged tongue, small mouth, profuse and thick secretions, upper airway obstruction due to infiltration of lymphoid tissue, abnormal tracheobronchial cartilages, stiff joints, kyphoscoliosis
Hunter syndrome (mucopolysaccharidosis II)	Similar but less severe than effects seen with Hurler syndrome
Pompe disease (glycogen storage disease II)	Macroglossia, muscle deposits, respiratory muscle weakness
Prader-Willi syndrome	Severe obesity, hypotonia
Osteogenesis imperfecta	Long bone and spine deformities, short neck, joint hyperextensibility, hypoplastic maxilla, occipitalization of upper cervical vertebrae
Moebius syndrome (congenital facial diplegia)	Hypoplasia of tongue and mandible, upper midfacial protrusion, high or cleft palate, microstomia, and hypotonia creating swallowing difficulty, lack of facial expression, drooling, aspiration risk
Saethre-Chotzen syndrome	Craniosynostosis, facial asymmetry, maxillary hypoplasia, narrow highly arched palate, cleft palate, cervical vertebral fusions
Rubenstein-Taybi syndrome	Facial deformation, highly arched palate, micrognathia, bifid uvula, palatal clefting, macroglossia, joint hyperflexibility, high potential for collapse of laryngeal walls
de Lange syndrome (Brachmann–de Lange syndrome)	Severe growth deficiency, recurrent respiratory infections, depressed nasal bridge, highly arched palate, short muscular neck, micrognathia, cleft palate, prone to regurgitation and aspiration

From Waage NS, Baker S, Sedano HO. Pediatric conditions associated with compromised airway: part I—congenital. *Pediatr Dent.* 2009;31(3):236–248.

mass index >40) may have airway difficulties related to excessive pharyngeal and neck tissues.[7,8]

The infant larynx (C3 to C4) resides superior to that of an adult (C4 to C5), and the epiglottis is proportionally larger, making vocal cord visualization potentially more problematic during intubation. Mandibular retrognathia or craniofacial changes, shortened thyromental distance, limitations on cervical mobility, and proclined maxillary incisors further complicate matters and may hamper emergent access to the airway as well. The infant vocal cords attach at a lower point anteriorly than posteriorly, altering its position slightly. This distorted angle occasionally results in difficulties during intubation, especially via a nasal approach. Beneath the vocal cords resides the narrowest part of an infant's larynx at the level of the only complete ring, the cricoid cartilage. This acute reduction in noncompliant cartilaginous circumference is a common site of edema resulting from traumatic intubation.

Acquired subglottic stenosis may also develop following prolonged airway intubation, as in premature patients with insufficient lung development who are supported by continuous mechanical ventilation or in rare cases as a consequence of gastroesophageal reflux disease (GERD).

Anatomic differences in the child's chest cage can also contribute to respiratory problems. The child's chest wall is more elastic than that of an adult, requiring lower ventilation pressures to expand the lungs. The sternum is less rigid, which means that ribs and intercostal muscles have less support. In the supine position, the child's ribs are more horizontally placed than those of the adult; this positional difference makes intercostal muscle retraction inefficient. Thus the diaphragm and abdominal musculature fatigue relatively quickly in children. Abdominal trauma or distention can further impede the movement of these muscles; crying and/or bag-valve-mask ventilation can lead to stomach insufflation and an increased risk of aspiration. Ventilation is primarily diaphragmatic. Anything that limits diaphragmatic excursions should be avoided, including the supine or Trendelenburg position, which promotes gastric organ pressure on the diaphragm. Instead, a 20- to 30-degree head-up position is recommended by many authors to prevent such pressure and thereby minimize risk of gastrointestinal regurgitation.

Lung infrastructure is different in the pediatric population as well. The majority of alveoli are formed after birth, with the adult number generally present between the sixth and eighth years of life. Although ratios of lung volume to body size are similar throughout the life span, children have a greater proportion of alveolar surface area in relation to lung size.[8–10]

Physiology

Because of this relative difference in alveolar surface area, children have a greater rate of *alveolar ventilation* (AV) per unit of area (a proportionally greater exchange of gas across the alveoli). However, the total volume of gas exchanged is less than that in adults, as is the *functional residual capacity* (FRC). FRC is defined as the volume of gas remaining in the lungs at the end of a normal expiration.

Drug Considerations

The AV/FRC ratio helps to determine the rate at which changes in inspired gas concentration affect a clinical response. AV supports transport of inhaled gas through the bloodstream and to the brain, whereas FRC determines how much gas remains in the lungs during normal breathing. Thus the increased AV/FRC ratio found in children results in a more rapid response to inhalation anesthetics and at lower concentrations. For this reason and also because of some unique aspects of the pediatric heart, discussed later in this chapter, children are at higher risk of overdose effects from inhalants, including hypotension, bradycardia, and hypoventilation. Careful monitoring of vital signs is therefore essential in children undergoing inhalation anesthesia for dental procedures.

Once in the blood, local anesthetic agents distribute to all tissues, with notably elevated levels in areas of increased perfusion, including the lungs. Therapeutic levels of local anesthetics have been shown to have a direct relaxant effect on bronchial smooth muscles. However, at elevated serum levels, profound respiratory depression parallels the toxic effects on the central nervous system.

With the exception of ketamine and nitrous oxide, the pronounced depressive effects associated with sedatives and general anesthetics on the respiratory system are well documented (Table 6.2).[11,12] Prolonged airway compromise deteriorating into complete respiratory arrest should be considered the most probable adverse consequence during sedation/anesthesia. Sedationists should pay particular attention when selecting and dosing pharmacologic agents in the pediatric population while also identifying individuals with

TABLE 6.2 Cardiopulmonary Effects of Common Procedural Sedative/Anesthetic Medications in Dentistry

Drug	Cardiac Effects	Pulmonary Effects
Meperidine *(Demerol)*	↓ BP, ↓ PVR, myocardial depression, ↑ HR	Respiratory depressant, possible chest wall rigidity
Morphine	↓ HR, ↓ BP	Respiratory depressant, ↑ airway resistance, apnea
Ketamine *(Ketalar)*	↑ BP, ↑ HR, ↑ CO (unless depleted catecholamine stores), ↑ myocardial O_2 consumption, possible arrhythmias	↑ airway secretions, slight ↓ RR, bronchodilation
Nitrous oxide	↑ LV filling pressure, ↓ PAP, ↓ PVR, ↓ CVP	Pulmonary vasodilation, rebound hypoxemia
Chloral hydrate	↓ BP, ↓ HR, possible arrhythmias	Respiratory depressant
Midazolam *(Versed)*	↓ BP, ↓ SVR, ↓ CO, ↑ HR	↑ RR *(at low doses)*, ↓ RR *(at high doses)*, ↑ upper airway obstruction, ↓ V_T, hypoxic respiratory drive
Diazepam *(Valium)*	↓ HR, ↓ BP, ↓ SVR	↓ V_T, ↓ minute volume, ↓ $PaCO_2$, hypoxic respiratory drive
Triazolam *(Halcion)*	Minimal effects on HR and BP	Slight ↓ RR, ↓ V_T
Hydroxyzine *(Vistaril)*	Minimal effects on BP and HR, arrhythmias	Minimal effects on RR
Diphenhydramine (Benadryl)	↓ BP, possible palpitations	Bronchodilation, nasal congestion, thickened secretions
Propofol *(Diprivan)*	↓ CO, ↓ BP, ↓ HR, myocardial depressant	↓ RR, ↑ $etCO_2$, $PaCO_2$, transient apnea

BP, Blood pressure; *CO,* cardiac output; *CVP,* central venous pressure; *etCO₂,* end-tidal carbon dioxide; *HR,* heart rate; *LV,* left ventricular; *O₂,* oxygen; *PaCO₂,* partial pressure of carbon dioxide; *PAP,* pulmonary artery pressure; *PVR,* peripheral vascular resistance; *RR,* respiratory rate; *SVR,* systemic vascular resistance; *Vₜ,* tidal volume.
Data from Tobias JD, Leder M. Procedural sedation: a review of agents, monitoring, and management of complications. *Saudi J Anaesth.* 2011;5(4):395–410; White P. *Perioperative Drug Manual.* 2nd ed. Philadelphia: Saunders; 2005.

an increased potential for airway obstruction. Physiologic monitoring is essential and should be based on the target level of sedation/anesthesia.

Cardiovascular System (Fig. 6.4)

Anatomy

Immediately after birth, the infant's cardiovascular system begins a series of complex changes that will continue for the next decade. After umbilical cord clamping and the first extrauterine breaths, pulmonary vascular resistance falls and the heart itself undergoes several changes, including closure of the ductus arteriosus and foramen ovale.

Physiology

Other physiologic changes continue throughout infancy and childhood. The heart rate, which averages about 120 beats per minute in the newborn, decreases throughout childhood, with a mean rate falling below 100 beats per minute by 4 years of age. Adult heart rates are generally realized by 10 to 12 years of age (Table 6.3).[13]

Cardiac output, defined as the product of heart rate and *stroke volume* (the amount of blood pumped by one contraction of the left ventricle), is influenced by several variables in the child. The infant heart is relatively inelastic and cannot make rapid changes in stroke volume. Thus the heart's rate of contraction is a much more important determinant of cardiac output in infants and young children than it is in adults. A significant drop in heart rate can result in decreased cardiac output and subsequent hypotension. At the same time, parasympathetic tone is more marked in the immature nervous system, resulting in a predisposition to significant bradycardias with vagal stimulation in younger children. Examples of stimuli provoking a vagal response include defecation, bladder distention, pressure on the eyeballs, placement of a throat pack, and tracheal intubation. Because of the potential for vagally induced bradycardia during intubation, children undergoing manipulation of the airway are frequently premedicated with atropine or a similar parasympathetic blocking agent.

Blood pressure, in contrast to heart rate, tends to increase throughout childhood. Mean systolic blood pressure in newborns ranges from 75 to 85 mm Hg, with an increase of 5 to 10 mm Hg over the first several weeks of life. Adult blood pressure values are generally achieved by early adolescence. Table 6.3 displays average blood pressures for children.[14]

Cardiac output also changes with age. Cardiac output per kilogram of body weight is highest in the newborn and gradually declines during the first several weeks of life. The relatively non-compliant infant myocardium adapts poorly to sudden changes in afterload; fluid overload and systemic hypertension produce cardiac failure more quickly in young children.[15,16]

Drug Considerations

Changes in cardiac output can have a dramatic impact on the uptake of inhaled anesthetic agents. A sudden decrease in heart rate results in decreased cardiac output, which in turn increases the rate of inhaled anesthetic uptake. Because 40% of a child's cardiac output perfuses the brain, increases in inhaled anesthetic uptake associated with decreased cardiac output can significantly depress the central nervous system. These depressant effects can include central reduction in vasomotor tone and peripheral

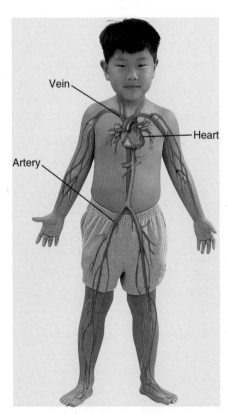

• **Figure 6.4** Cardiovascular system of a pediatric patient. (Modified from Leifer G. *Introduction to Maternity & Pediatric Nursing.* 6th ed. St Louis: Saunders; 2011.)

TABLE 6.3	**Vital Signs by Age**			
Age	Heart Rate[a] (Beats/Min)	Respiratory Rate[a] (Breaths/Min)	BLOOD PRESSURE[b] (mm Hg) (90TH PERCENTILE BP FOR 50TH PERCENTILE HEIGHT) Boys	Girls
Newborn	120–170	30–80	87/68	76/68
1 year	80–160	20–40	98/53	100/58
3 years	80–120	20–30	105/61	103/62
6 years	75–115	16–22	110/70	107/69
10 years	70–110	16–20	115/75	115/74
17 years	60–110	12–20	133/83	125/80

[a]Data from Seidel H, et al. *Mosby's Guide to Physical Examination.* 6th ed. St Louis: Mosby; 2006.
[b]"Normal" blood pressure is less than 90th percentile.
Modified from Johns Hopkins Hospital, Arcara K, Tschudy M. *The Harriet Lane Handbook.* 19th ed. St Louis: Mosby; 2012.

vasodilation, which can worsen the hypotension associated with significant bradycardia.

Because of these potential adverse effects, inhaled anesthetics should be used carefully in the pediatric population. These agents act more rapidly in children than in adults, and children are adequately sedated by gas concentrations lower than those required for adults.[9]

To minimize the hypotensive response associated with a potential drop in heart rate, pediatric patients should be well hydrated before elective procedures requiring inhaled or intravenous sedation. Recurrent vomiting, diarrhea, or poor oral intake in the days before the procedure are appropriate indications to reschedule.

The cardiovascular effect of local anesthetics is greatly dependent on the presence of vasoconstricting agents, which are regularly added to prolong the analgesic effect but subsequently stimulate the sympathetic nervous system. At recommended local anesthetic doses, this results in an increase in all physiologic cardiovascular functions. However, without its presence, commonly used dental local anesthetic agents have a suppressive effect on the cardiovascular system.

Although a multitude of hemodynamic effects associated with sedative/anesthetic agents have been demonstrated, dose-dependent adverse consequences are most common (see Table 6.2). Dentists providing office-based procedural sedation to children should have a full appreciation of the pharmacologic effects of each individual agent on the cardiovascular system and realize the potential for synergy, especially in the *nil per os* (NPO) hypovolemic pediatric patient.

Gastrointestinal and Hepatic Systems (Fig. 6.5)

There are several important physiologic differences in the child's gastrointestinal and hepatic activities as compared with those in the adult. Such variances alter drug pharmacokinetics and thus bioavailability. They include the following:

- *Gastric pH.* In infants and young children, the immature gastric mucosa secretes low levels of acid; adult levels of gastric acidity are generally not reached until 2 to 3 years of age. Before this time, the low acidity of the infant gut favors absorption of weakly acidic drugs such as penicillins and cephalosporins, whereas the absorption of weakly basic drugs such as the benzodiazepines is delayed.
- *Intestinal motility.* Due to decreased motility, gastric transit times are significantly longer during the neonatal period. Average emptying times in the young infant may approach 8 hours, and only achieve adult levels—2 to 3 hours—between 6 and 8 months of age. Extended emptying times combined with the irregular peristalsis of infancy generally result in decreased gastric absorption rates. Older infants, in contrast, demonstrate a reduction in enteral drug absorption as a result of amplified motility.
- *Excretory function.* As a result of immature excretory function and enzymatic activity, the secretion of bile and pancreatic fluid into the gastrointestinal tract is reduced and alters absorption, especially of lipophilic compounds.
- *Altered hepatic metabolism.* Many drugs are metabolized by the liver. Hepatic enzymes may act to detoxify a drug or alter it to a more potent or exploitable form. Because infants and young children are relatively deficient in these enzymes, medications are generally metabolized more slowly, and there is an increased risk of toxicity if they are not dosed correctly. Low levels of cytochrome P-450 enzymes in the first 2 months of life are associated with sluggish oxidation of benzodiazepines in the neonate, thus causing a prolonged clinical effect in this population. Liver function matures to adult capacities between ages 2 and 4 years.

Glucuronyltransferase, which conjugates drugs into an excretable form, is also deficient in the neonate but reaches adult levels after the first month of life. Morphine, acetaminophen, steroids, and sulfa antibiotics all are conjugated by glucuronyltransferase and thus should be used with caution in the neonate.

The infant liver is also deficient in pseudocholinesterase; enzyme levels are at 60% of adult levels for the first several months of life. Even when calculated on an adjusted body weight scale, succinylcholine doses do not reach adult levels until after 2 years of age. The effects of succinylcholine are therefore exaggerated in the infant. Deaths have been reported in association with succinylcholine administration to children with undiagnosed myopathies, and its routine use is no longer recommended. Succinylcholine is therefore administered with caution to infant patients, who may respond with prolonged apnea.

Renal System (Fig. 6.6)

Although drugs can be excreted by a number of physiologic routes, such as sweat, bile, and feces, the vast majority undergoes renal excretion. Renal blood flow and glomerular filtration are low in the first 2 years of life due to increased renal vascular resistance. Because of its immature state, the young kidney has a diminished capacity for the excretion of drugs or large sodium loads. Most renally excreted drugs are cleared by glomerular filtration, tubular transport, or a combination of both processes.

The glomerular filtration rate (GFR)—the volume of fluid filtered by the kidney per unit of time—doubles its newborn value by 2 months of age; adult levels are roughly five times the newborn

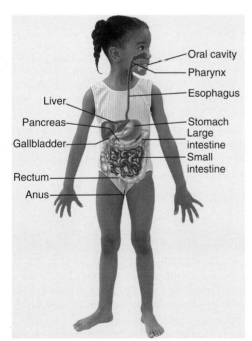

• **Figure 6.5** Gastrointestinal system of a pediatric patient. (Modified from Leifer G. *Introduction to Maternity & Pediatric Nursing.* 6th ed. St Louis: Saunders; 2011.)

Oral cavity
Pharynx
Esophagus
Liver
Pancreas
Gallbladder
Stomach
Large intestine
Small intestine
Rectum
Anus

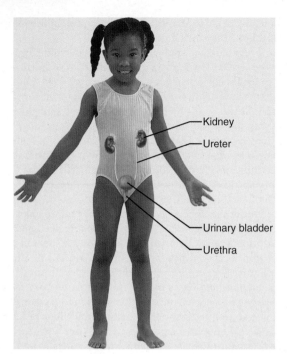

• **Figure 6.6** Renal system of a pediatric patient. (Modified from Leifer G. *Introduction to Maternity & Pediatric Nursing.* 6th ed. St Louis: Saunders; 2011.)

TABLE 6.4	American Society of Anesthesiologists Preoperative Fasting Guidelines	
Ingested Material	**Minimum Fasting Period (h)**	
Clear fluids (water, clear juices, or sports drinks)	2	
Breast milk	4	
Infant formula	6	
Nonhuman milk (bovine, soy, almond, coconut, etc.)	6	
Light meal (cereal, toast, crackers, or coffee with milk)	6	
Heavy meal (animal protein, or fried foods)	8	

Data from American Society of Anesthesiologists Committee. Practice guidelines for preoperative fasting and the use of pharmacologic agents to reduce the risk of pulmonary aspiration: application to healthy patients undergoing elective procedures: an updated report by the American Society of Anesthesiologists Committee on Standards and Practice Parameters. *Anesthesiology.* 2011;114(3):495–511.

level and are approached at 8 to 12 months of age. GFR participates in the excretion of such commonly used pediatric drugs as the penicillins, short-acting barbiturates, and phenobarbital; recommended dosages of these agents for infants and toddlers are calculated to consider the low infant GFR.

The term *tubular transport* describes a group of mechanisms that transfer drug and drug metabolites across the renal tubular epithelium. Drugs in which tubular transport plays an excretory role include morphine, atropine, and sulfa antibiotics. Many such drugs have decreased tubular transport rates in young infants and thus have much narrower margins of toxicity in this patient population. Tubular transport mechanisms generally mature by 7 months of age.[17,18]

Common side effects associated with sedation and anesthesia may include postoperative nausea and vomiting and diarrhea. Prolonged periods may result in depletion of a child's essential fluids and electrolytes, resulting in dehydration. This diminished physiologic state is poorly tolerated in young children, and management of perioperative fluids by clinicians and parents should be essential. In an effort to minimize the chance of gastric regurgitation, strict NPO instructions are essential prior to the onset of these procedures; however, prolonged adherence to such recommendations increases the probability of such occurrences. With this, it is suggested that practitioners closely adhere to the American Society of Anesthesiologists (ASA) guidelines for perioperative fasting (Table 6.4).[18]

Blood and Body Fluids

Terminology

Drug metabolism and excretion are profoundly affected by the size of various body fluid compartments. Fluid distribution among these compartments is significantly different in infancy and childhood, which in turn alters the action of certain drugs in this age group.

A brief review of body fluid nomenclature may be helpful at this point. The total body water space consists of the intracellular fluid (ICF) and extracellular fluid (ECF) compartments. The volume of distribution (V_d) is that volume into which a drug distributes in the body at equilibrium. Although V_d is usually measured in plasma (the volume of plasma at a given drug concentration that is required to account for all drug in the body), many drugs distribute into body tissues as well. Thus V_d may be estimated at many times the total plasma volume.

Physiology

Alterations in Body Fluids

As the child grows, changes in body mass are accompanied by changes in body fluid compartments. Although total body water equals 80% of the infant's weight, it makes up only 50% to 60% of normal adult body weight. Much of this volume loss comes from the ECF compartment. Because so much of the infant's weight is water, any water-soluble drug must be administered at higher levels per unit of body weight to attain therapeutic concentration in this age group.

Plasma Protein Differences

A number of plasma proteins function to bind drug in the bloodstream. Plasma proteins both transport a drug and render it less physiologically active while bound. Several of these proteins, including serum albumin and plasma globulin, are deficient in the newborn and young infant. Certain drugs that are highly protein-bound (e.g., clindamycin, ibuprofen, or naproxen) must be given at relatively low levels per unit of body weight in these patients. Because amide local anesthetics—such as lidocaine, mepivacaine, or bupivacaine—bind to serum proteins and albumin, free fractions may also become elevated. This, in turn, warrants extreme caution during administration to very young patients, as toxic effects may be more prevalent.

Body Habitus and Integument

Children are obviously smaller than adults. It makes intuitive sense that they need smaller drug doses to maintain therapeutic drug concentrations and that smaller doses are needed to produce toxicity. The "maximal safe dose" listed in standard drug reference manuals is potentially enough to overdose an undersized pediatric patient. Because of this, practitioners have recognized several formulas, including Young's and Fried's rules, to adjust an established adult dose to a safe dose for a pediatric patient based on the child's age:

Young's rule: Pediatric dosage

$$= \frac{\text{Age of child in years} \times \text{Adult dosage}}{\text{Age of child in years} + 12}$$

Fried's rule: Pediatric dosage

$$= \frac{\text{Age in months} \times \text{Adult dosage}}{150}$$

Since a wide degree of size variability exists among similarly aged children, a weight-based dosing formula, such as Clark's rule, became very popular[19]:

Clark's rule: Pediatric dosage

$$= \frac{\text{Child's weight in pounds} \times \text{Adult dosage}}{150}$$

Unfortunately, however, these calculations are not always precise. Not only are the pediatric patients smaller, but their proportions also differ from those of the adult. Because a child's height triples from birth to adulthood but the weight increases 20-fold over the same period, many professionals feel that body surface area (BSA) is the most accurate parameter on which to base drug dosage.[3,11,20] Measured in square meters, BSA is estimated by plotting the child's height and weight on a nomogram[21]:

Mostellar's formula: $\text{BSA (m}^2) = \dfrac{\sqrt{\text{height (cm)} \times \text{weight (kg)}}}{3600}$

The BSA method, however, should not be used in patients weighing less than 10 kg. The ratio of BSA to body weight is highest in the neonate and falls to about one-sixth of this level when adult proportions are reached, just before puberty. Although BSA is rarely used in the clinical setting—it is inconvenient to calculate and unwieldy to use—it has been shown to be proportional to multiple physiologic variables such as fluid requirements, oxygen consumption, metabolic rate, and cardiac output. Ultimately, contemporary clinicians now rely on published recommended pediatric dosing schedules created by the individual drug makers.

The tissue composition of infants and children differs as well, depending on developmental stage. Fat makes up 10% to 15% of full-term newborn weight; it increases to 20% to 25% during the first several months of life and then declines during the toddler and preschool years as the child becomes more active. Some commonly used dental sedatives (benzodiazepines and barbiturates) are lipid-soluble and extensively bound by fatty tissue, thus decreasing serum drug levels. It follows that children with lower percentages of body fat may be more sensitive to these agents.

Temperature Control

With a large surface-to-weight ratio; minimal subcutaneous adipose tissues; and poorly developed shivering, sweating, and vasoconstricting mechanisms, infants have difficulty maintaining their ideal body temperature, especially under general anesthesia. Hypothermic effects result in respiratory depression, decreased cardiac output, acidosis, prolonged duration of action of drugs, depleted platelet function, and an elevated risk for postoperative infection. In an effort to maintain a homeostatic physiologic state, thermoregulation precautions should be exercised during all sedative and general anesthetic procedures.

Summary

Child physiology and anatomy differ significantly from that of adults. A working knowledge of those differences is essential for the pediatric dental care provider who assesses and treats children at every developmental stage. Careful consideration of the unique needs in this variable patient population, along with assessing a patient's physical state using the ASA Physical Status Classification (Table 6.5),[22] will help practitioners to promote safe and effective care.

TABLE 6.5   ASA Physical Status Classification System for Dental Patient Care 2017

Classification	Definition	Examples (Including, But Not Limited To)
ASA I	A normal healthy patient and no risk during dental treatment	Healthy, nonsmoking, no or minimal alcohol use
ASA II	A patient with mild to moderate systemic disease and minimal risk during dental treatment	Mild to moderate systemic diseases without substantive functional limitations or healthy with extreme anxiety and fear toward dentistry. Example: current smoker, social alcohol drinker, pregnancy, obesity (30 < BMI < 40), well-controlled DM/HTN, mild lung disease
ASA III	A patient with moderate to severe systemic disease and increased risk during dental treatment.	One or more moderate to severe diseases with functional limitations. Example: poorly controlled DM or HTN, COPD, morbid obesity (BMI ≥40), active hepatitis, alcohol dependence or abuse, implanted pacemaker, moderate reduction of ejection fraction, ESRD undergoing regularly scheduled dialysis, history (>3 months) of MI, CVA, TIA, or CAD/stents

TABLE 6.5
ASA Physical Status Classification System for Dental Patient Care 2017—cont'd

Classification	Definition	Examples (Including, But Not Limited To)
ASA IV	A patient with severe systemic disease that is a constant threat to life and significantly increased risk during dental treatment	Recent (<3 months) MI, CVA, TIA, or CAD/stents, ongoing cardiac ischemia or severe valve dysfunction, severe reduction of ejection fraction, sepsis, DIC, ARD, or ESRD not undergoing regularly scheduled dialysis
ASA V	A moribund patient who is not expected to survive without the operation	Ruptured abdominal/thoracic aneurysm, massive trauma, intracranial bleed with mass effect, ischemic bowel in the face of significant cardiac pathology or multiple organ/system dysfunction
ASA VI	Patient declared brain-dead whose organs are being harvested for donor purpose	

The addition of "E" denotes emergency surgery: An emergency is defined as existing when delay in treatment of the patient would lead to a significant increase in the threat to life or body part. The addition of "P" denotes a pregnant patient.

ARD, Acute respiratory disease; *ASA,* American Society of Anesthesiologists; *BMI,* body mass index; *CAD,* coronary artery disease; *COPD,* chronic obstructive pulmonary disease; *CVA,* cerebrovascular accident; *DIC,* disseminated intravascular coagulation; *DM,* diabetes mellitus; *ESRD,* end-stage renal disease; *HTN,* hypertension; *MI,* myocardial infarction; *TIA,* transient ischemic attack.

From Fehrenbach M. ASA physical status classification system for dental patient care; 2017. http://www.dhed.net/ASA_Physical_Status_Classification_SYSTEM.html. Accessed September 11, 2017.
Modified from American Society of Anesthesiologists. ASA physical status classification system; 2014. https://www.asahq.org/resources/clinical-information/asa-physical-status-classification-system.

References

1. Committee on Standards and Practice Parameters, Apfelbaum JL, Connis RT, et al. Practice advisory for preanesthesia evaluation: an updated report by the American Society of Anesthesiologists Task Force on Preanesthesia Evaluation. *Anesthesiology.* 2012;116(3):522–538.
2. Chidananda Swamy MN, Mallikarjun D. Applied aspects of anatomy and physiology of relevance to paediatric anesthesia. *Indian J Anaesth.* 2004;48:333–339.
3. Amieva-Wang NE. Airway, breathing, and ventilation. In: Amieva-Wang NE, Shandro J, Sohoni A, et al, eds. *A Practical Guide to Pediatric Emergency Medicine: Caring for Children in the Emergency Department.* Cambridge, UK: Cambridge University Press; 2011:3–5.
4. Flick RP, Wilder RT, Pieper SF, et al. Risk factors for laryngospasm in children during general anesthesia. *Paediatr Anaesth.* 2008;18:1–7.
5. Tait AR, Maviya S. Anesthesia for the child with an upper respiratory tract infection: still a dilemma? *Anesth Analg.* 2005;100:59–65.
6. Singh P, Whyte S. Anaesthesia for elective ear nose and throat surgery in children. *Anaesth Intensive Care Med.* 2004;10(4):186–190.
7. Baker S, Paricio L. Pathologic pediatric conditions associated with a compromised airway. *Int J Paediatr Dent.* 2010;20:3–4.
8. Setzer M, Saade E. Childhood obesity and anesthetic morbidity. *Paediatr Anaesth.* 2007;17(4):321–326.
9. Hillier SC, Krishna G, Brasoveanu E. Neonatal anesthesia. *Semin Pediatr Surg.* 2004;13(3):142–151.
10. Seidel H, et al. *Mosby's Guide to Physical Examination.* 6th ed. St Louis: Mosby; 2006:395, 444.
11. White P. *Perioperative Drug Manual.* 2nd ed. Philadelphia: Saunders; 2005.
12. Mosteller RD. Simplified calculation of body surface area. *N Engl J Med.* 1987;317(17):1098.
13. Fleming S, Thompson M, Stevens R, et al. Normal ranges of heart rate and respiratory rate in children from birth to 18 years of age: a systemic review of observational studies. *Lancet.* 2011;377:1–17.
14. Sinaiko AR. Hypertension in children. *N Engl J Med.* 1996;335(26):1968–1973.
15. Kaelber DC, Pickett F. Simple table to identify children and adolescents needing further evaluation of blood pressure. *Pediatrics.* 2009;123(6):e972–e974.
16. Fernandez E, Perez R, Hernandez A, et al. Factors and mechanisms for pharmacokinetic differences between pediatric population and adults. *Pharmaceutics.* 2011;3:53–72.
17. Kearns GL, Adcock KG, Wilson JT. Drug therapy in pediatric patients. In: van Boxtel CJ, Santoso B, Edwards IR, eds. *Drug Benefits and Risks: International Textbook of Clinical Pharmacology.* New York: John Wiley & Sons; 2001:159–164.
18. Practice guidelines for preoperative fasting and the use of pharmacologic agents to reduce the risk of pulmonary aspiration: application to healthy patients undergoing elective procedures. *Anesthesiology.* 2011;114:495–511.
19. Shirkey HC. Drug dosage for infants and children. *JAMA.* 1965;193:443–446.
20. Tobias JD, Leder M. Procedural sedation: A review of agents, monitoring, and management of complications. *Saudi J Anaesth.* 2011;5(4):395–410.
21. Mosteller RD. Simplified calculation of body surface area. *N Engl J Med.* 1987;317(17):1098.
22. Fehrenbach M. ASA physical status classification system for dental patient care; 2017. http://www.dhed.net/ASA_Physical_Status_Classification_SYSTEM.html. Accessed September 11, 2017.

7

Assessment and Management of Pain in the Pediatric Patient

ELIZABETH S. GOSNELL AND S. THIKKURISSY

CHAPTER OUTLINE

The Impact and Management of Pain

Pain has often been referred to and labeled as the "fifth vital sign."[1] The English word *pain* is derived from an ancient Greek word meaning "penalty" and a Latin word meaning "punishment" as well as "penalty." When the term *pain* is used in clinical dentistry or medicine, it is synonymous with strong discomfort. It is important to realize that despite the distress experienced by the person in pain, pain has a necessary function. Pain signals real or apparent tissue damage that thereby energizes the organism to take action in relieving or alleviating its presence. In this sense, it is a desirable experience for maintaining and guiding a person's activities in life.

It is important to understand that pain is more than just a sensation and a consequential response. It is a highly complex, multifaceted interaction of physical, chemical, humoral, affective (emotional), cognitive, psychological, behavioral, and social elements. Certainly the determinants of how an individual interprets and reacts to pain are not clearly understood. However, the body of knowledge surrounding the understanding of pain has begun to evolve and is accelerating rapidly into a scientific and useful discipline. The onset and persistence of pain may be associated with comorbid symptoms, including increased suffering, reduced quality of life, and delayed recovery from the initial insult.[2]

An interesting and clinically relevant parallel experience to pain is the presence of anticipatory responses secondarily acquired from the pain experience. These are conceptualized and broadly referred to as "stress" and "fear." The perception of fear can profoundly influence the behavior and emotional responses of children. For example, the 4-year-old child who presents with painful, abscessed maxillary anterior teeth due to caries and poorly endures the injection of local anesthesia and extractions while immobilized may develop strong disruptive and avoidance behaviors. Such behaviors may include crying with or without tears, placing hands over the mouth, refusing to open, kicking, screaming, shaking the head, spitting, and biting. These may manifest during subsequent dental appointments.

The overwhelming majority of pharmacologic agents used in dentistry are administered to manage anxiety and pain. Generally the elimination of pain sensation in the dental setting requires blocking of pain perception either peripherally using local anesthesia or centrally with general anesthesia. Anxiety is managed in part or completely by pharmacologic and/or nonpharmacologic techniques. Anxiety and pain and their management in actual clinical practice overlap to a significant degree.

There is no single *best* technique to manage anxiety and pain. A practitioner may have a preferred technique, but one technique is not useful for all dental patients in all situations. The prudent and wise dentist has a working knowledge of several techniques and selects, on an individual basis, the one that appears to be most appropriate for a particular patient. In some cases, this may necessitate referral.

Definition of Pain

Pain is a highly personalized state often preceding tissue damage that is either real (e.g., skin laceration) or apparent (e.g., excess bowel distension) as a result of an adequate stimulus. Under normal circumstances, the state of pain implies that there is a simultaneous activation of cognitive, emotional, and behavioral consequences that provide both motivation and a direction for action.

Physiologically, pain involves neural signals that are transmitted over a multitude of pathways involving neurons that are specialized in space, biochemistry, size, and shape. These signals induce a host of secondary responses that may become organized in a hierarchy of systems involving portions of the central nervous system (CNS). At the physiologic level, some of these responses involve further transmission of neural signals and the release of neurochemicals and humorally active chemicals (e.g., γ-aminobutyric acid and endogenous opioids). Other systems within this response hierarchy include those that activate motor activities for purposeful escape.

Research has demonstrated that emotional and cognitive elements in the pain process play critical roles in the degree of pain awareness and, possibly more importantly, in the individual's ability to induce self-control while enduring pain.[3] For instance, cognitive mechanisms (e.g., cognitive dissociation) that reduce the *perceived* quality and quantity of discomfort can be effectively taught to a patient before the experience of pain. Children, through the process of suggestion, can be taught (to varying degrees) to ignore or to inhibit responsiveness to painful stimuli during cancer therapies.[4,5]

Theories of Pain Perception: Why and How Pain Is Experienced

Specificity

Historically it was believed that the pain experience occurred when a particular set of neurons was activated.[6,7] The neural receptors (i.e., free nerve endings) and their pathways were considered to be specialized for the perception of pain, just as other elements and pathways were rigidly designed as passages for other sensory information (e.g., the sensation of pressure).

Portions of this theory are reasonably accurate and remain prominent in our understanding of the pain mechanism, but the theory is inadequate to explain the multifaceted nature of the pain experience (e.g., the phantom pain in the missing limb experienced by an amputee).

Pattern

With the technologic ability to record stimulus-induced activity within neural pathways, a more sophisticated model of pain mechanisms arose. Neural activity recorded and amplified on an oscilloscope allowed some appreciation of the changes in timing and grouping of nerve action potentials as a consequence of modification in stimulus parameters. A light stroking across a patch of skin may provoke one or two isolated action potentials in large-diameter neurons servicing the area, whereas a hot iron may cause an initial burst followed by a steady discharge of action potentials in smaller neurons.

It was theorized that the recognition of painful stimuli by the individual was based primarily on the pattern of nervous activity that entered the CNS. Again, this theory was inadequate to explain the complexity of the pain experience, but it contributed significantly to the advancement of knowledge about pain mechanisms.[6,7]

Gate Control Theory

The gate control theory of pain (Fig. 7.1) was developed by Melzack and Wall in 1965 and is the most influential, comprehensive, and adaptive conceptualization of pain and its consequences to date. The theory proposes that various "gates" controlling the level of noxious input via small-fiber neurons to the spinal cord can be modulated by other sensory, large-fiber neurons, higher CNS input, or both. Postulated mechanisms for the gates include presynaptic inhibitory effects on secondary transmission cells in the spinal cord. This implies that large C fibers (e.g., those for touch) can cause partial depolarization of the nerve terminals of small α-δ fibers (e.g., for pain) resulting in the release of fewer "packets" of neurotransmitter molecules and a decreased likelihood that presynaptic cells will summate and fire.

A simplistic example would be the ameliorative inhibitory effect of the parent rubbing a "bumped" area of the knee immediately following a toddler's fall. The light rubbing disproportionately activates greater numbers of large fibers that inhibit previously activated small fibers. In dentistry, shaking of the lip during delivery of local anesthesia is commonly believed to distract or lessen the associated discomfort.

Transcutaneous electrical nerve stimulation (TENS), or the use of low-intensity electrical stimulation at peripheral sites, has been shown to relieve pain.[8] Although the mechanism for TENS-mediated pain relief is not known, it has been suggested that its segmental effects may be due to activation of large-diameter, primary afferent fibers that in turn inhibit small-fiber transmission as predicted by the gate theory. A similar mechanism may account for the effects of acupuncture. TENS has been shown to produce partial analgesia due to the electrical stimulation of tooth pulp in school-aged children.[9]

Proportionately more emphasis has been placed on the role and influence of higher CNS modulation of pain perception and reactivity.[3,10,11] This reorientation is partially the result of more sophisticated studies suggesting the need for a more comprehensive explanation of cognitive, behavioral, and emotional influences in

pain perception and control.[12] Discoveries of endogenous opioids, widespread locations of opioid receptors throughout the CNS, and unnatural (i.e., electrical) stimulation of CNS sites resulting in pain threshold elevations also have sparked renewed interest in pain research.

Neuromatrix

In more recent years the components of the CNS we generally refer to as higher levels of CNS functioning (i.e., above the midbrain) have become a popular focus of pain research. In one theory, a highly complex neuronal network or matrix purportedly exists and is referred to as the neuromatrix (Fig. 7.2). It is thought to have some genetic basis but can be influenced by the internal and external environment.[13] The uniqueness of the genetic makeup of the neuromatrix and its ultimate functional identity may aid in distinguishing each individual's "body self." It is through this neuromatrix that the cyclic processing and synthesis of neuronal activity may result in a characteristic pattern known as a neuro-signature. It has been theorized that neurosignatures can help explain complicated states like pain in individuals who experience a specified set of symptoms that have environmental, situational, or other influential mediators (e.g., emotions). This abstract model undoubtedly will stimulate a focus on future research to aid in diagnosing, understanding, and explaining many clinical conditions.

Central Nervous System Effects on Pain Perception and Control

An endogenous opioid system that is both complex in function and widespread throughout the mammalian CNS has been partially characterized and described.[14] Endogenous opioids are peptides that are naturally synthesized in the body and cause effects similar to those of opiates (e.g., morphine). β-Endorphin is one of the most potent peptides and has an N terminal identical to that of met-enkephalin, which was one of the first opioid peptides isolated.

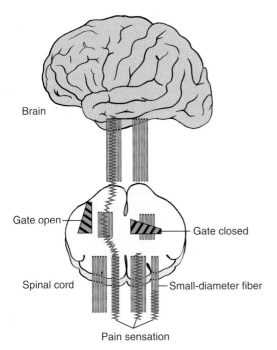

• **Figure 7.1** The gate control theory of pain. (From deWit SC. *Medical-Surgical Nursing: Concepts and Practice*. St Louis: Saunders; 2009.)

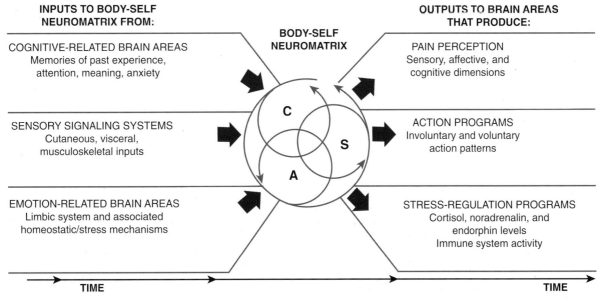

• **Figure 7.2** The neuromatrix. (Redrawn from Melzack R. Pain and the neuromatrix in the brain. *J Dent Educ*. 2001;65[12]:1378–1382.)

The active opioid peptides are cleaved from larger precursors and act at various CNS opioid receptor sites, including the spinal cord. The peptides are not equally potent but all are inactivated by naloxone, a narcotic antagonist, and each may contribute to selective and specialized mechanisms underlying the pain perception process.

Correspondingly, at least four opiate receptors have been characterized (μ, δ, κ, and nociceptin) throughout the CNS. However, the contribution of each in producing analgesia is not clear. Opioid ligands that bind to μ receptors produce potent analgesia when injected into the periaqueductal gray (PAG) area of the medulla. Other sites, extending from the hypothalamus to the rostral ventromedial medulla including the PAG, produce analgesia when properly stimulated electrically or by opiates. Curiously, the analgesic effects of nitrous oxide are believed to be partially mediated by endogenous opioid ligands, or it may be able to directly activate opiate receptors.[15]

There is evidence to suggest that this system develops early in CNS development and thus should be functional in younger children. The extent of its influence and the conditions necessary for its activation are not understood. Future studies will probably underscore the means and usefulness of activating this system in addressing clinical pain states.

Cognitive Elements of Pain Perception

Cognition is a complex process resulting in an appreciation and often subsequent recognition of potential consequences as a function of "knowing." Knowing involves a multitude of processes including but not limited to perceiving, organizing, judging, meaning, reasoning, and responding.

Cognition implies an awareness of internal and external environmental influences on oneself. It also insinuates that steps can be taken for one to gain control over those influences and use the control to alter one's response (e.g., coping). For instance, one may be experiencing some discomfort but can possibly diminish the degree of discomfort by practicing mental processes (e.g., imagining pleasant events or counting holes in a ceiling tile).

A person can cope with a variety of conditions, including stressful environments, depending on his or her perception of the situation. Factors such as consequences and repercussions of the situation, its timing, and individual resources are important to the outcome of coping strategies. Coping strategies may include hypnosis and relaxation techniques, imagery, modeling, distraction, and reconceptualization. Typically, therapeutic coping strategies of pain management have a number of common elements, including (1) an assessment of the problem, (2) reconceptualization of the patient's viewpoint, (3) development of appropriate skills (e.g., breathing and relaxation), (4) generalization and maintenance of those skills in preventing relapse, and (5) measurement of therapeutic success.[16]

Evidence supports the notion that coping skills in the context of pain and anxiety can be taught even to children, and the effectiveness of cognitive training can be evaluated through self-report or physiologic/behavioral measures. In one study, children who were undergoing restorative procedures were taught distraction and self-support techniques before undergoing dental procedures; they were subsequently compared with a group of children who were read stories. Self-report of anxiety for specific procedures (e.g., the injection) was less in those who received the cognitive training than in those who did not.[17] School-aged children who have had opportunities to exercise self-control in anxiety-provoking circumstances may be able to invoke their own personalized coping skills in preparation for an anticipated event during a dental appointment.

However, knowing ahead of time about impending discomfort can have a detrimental effect under certain conditions. For instance, the less time between informing a young child, who cognitively is incapable of significant coping strategies (i.e., 3 years or less), of a procedurally related painful stimulus (e.g., injection) and doing it allows correspondingly less time for interference behaviors to occur. It is even possible that the length of emotional outburst before and following the procedure may be reduced under these circumstances.

Some studies indicate that adults who are led to believe that they have some control over impending discomfort exhibit more tolerance of painful stimuli.[3] However, a strong *belief* in their ability to gain self-control is apparently an important factor in modulating the degree of discomfort. Those who lack this ability may place more trust in others (e.g., physician) and "suffer less" under their care.

Cognitive development and maturation are keys to the success of cognitive strategies. Anxiety reduction can be attained in the medical and dental environment as a function of age in school-aged cohorts. The extent to which these strategies can be successfully applied to preschoolers is yet to be determined. However, younger children are capable of significant pain modulation through processes resembling cognitive strategies. In one study, play therapy with needles and dolls before venipuncture resulted in a significantly more rapid return of heart rate and less body movement within 5 minutes of blood drawing compared with controls. This finding was interpreted as evidence of reduced anxiety in the children.[18]

Emotional Elements of Pain Perception

Although pain and the anticipation of painful stimuli (i.e., anxiety) invoke a personalized emotional experience, most humans have a common understanding of the attendant emotions of such experiences. Certainly we are adept at recognizing another's suffering and possibly even better attuned to appreciating another person's anticipation of discomfort.

The expression of emotional content during or preceding painful experiences is most likely a complex combination of a partially inherited yet learning-tempered phenomenon that occurs early in life. An infant's expression of discomfort resulting from inoculations changes with aging from a more diffuse, crying, and reflexive response to one of anticipation, attentiveness toward the noxious object, and sometimes expression of anger.[19,20]

The social response to pain can be a commanding and attention-gathering entity.[21] For example, the toddler who skins a knee during a fall initially may not react as if in pain until the parent secondarily reacts to the injury. Depending on the parental response, the child may burst into tears if the parent looks upset or not respond at all, based on the support of the parent's verbal encouragement.

Although one might conceive of the emotional elements of pain as being secondary to the pain itself, the emotional overtones may act in concert to modulate painful experiences. Indirect and anecdotal evidence suggests that certain pharmacologic agents (e.g., nitrous oxide and benzodiazepines) act on areas of the CNS responsible for emotional influence. A person feels the pain but is not particularly annoyed by it.

In contrast, emotional distress in anticipation of discomfort is known to lower pain thresholds and increase reactivity. Cognitive strategies designed to elicit positive emotional states can be effective in reducing anxiety and the degree of responsiveness to painful stimuli. (See Chapter 24 for a discussion of coping.)

Pediatric Pain Assessment

Appropriate pediatric pain assessment and management are highlighted in current clinical algorithms and research studies. Even so, pediatric pain continues to be underestimated and inadequately treated.[22] Pediatric pain is associated with increased risk for physical and psychological symptoms. In addition, there are coincident enormous health care expenditures associated with pediatric pain.[23,24] The assessment of children's pain can be challenging, especially for younger children or those with developmental delays.

Studies suggest that the developmental changes in response to painful stimuli occur early in infancy. In fact, anticipatory fears of sharp objects can be seen in children around 1 year of age.[25] A child's ability to communicate feelings becomes increasingly sophisticated as he or she matures, develops a broader vocabulary, and witnesses a variety of environments. Paralleling and reflecting the child's cognitive development are signs manifesting the evolution of coping skills.[26] The pain threshold tends to decline and the self-management of pain becomes more effective with increasing age in typically developing children.[27] Similar self-management trends are noteworthy in the young dental patient.[28] This phenomenon results from the interactions of multiple factors, including the maturation of coping skills, appreciation of self-control, and social influences.

The pain associated with dental or other medically imposed procedures might be instrumental in invoking the opportunity for the development and testing of certain self-control and coping mechanisms.[29] Many children are efficient with their coping skills and tolerate mild discomfort with little overt expression. A few lack good coping skills and display hysterical behaviors (e.g., extreme panic, screaming, and struggling) in anticipation of or during minor discomforts. Consequently, any assessment of a child's behavioral and cognitive responses to the dental environment should be considered in light of age-appropriate expressions, specific procedures, and the use of cognitive probes.

Studies have shown that health care providers tend to underestimate the pain experienced by children. A pain assessment tool, or pain scale, should be utilized to provide the practitioner a more objective method to assess and adequately manage pain in pediatric patients.

There are three types of pain assessment tools: self-report, observational/behavioral, and physiologic measurement. An *observational/behavioral assessment tool* is used for those patients who are very young or cognitively impaired; for example, preverbal children or those who are unable to understand the self-report scale. The *self-report assessment tool* is ideal but requires the child to be able to understand instructions and point to or verbalize his or her response. Certain *physiologic measurements*, especially heart rate, in conjunction with self-report of discomfort are thought to add another important dimension to the characterization of response specificity to painful stimuli.[30,31] Many assessment tools are available; those presented here have been shown to be most reliable and valid for the intended target population. It is important to note that the appropriate scale should be chosen depending on developmental age of the child. The chronologic age listed is only a guide.[23,32]

It may appear difficult to measure the degree of pain or discomfort experienced by young children, especially preschool children, because of their level of cognitive and language development. Several tools have been developed for this purpose, including nonverbal self-report techniques like the number of poker chips selected (Poker Chip Tool), the rating along a "pain thermometer" scale, and color selections.[33] Self-report measures of pain intensity are not sufficiently valid for children below 3 years of age. In addition, many children 3 to 4 years of age may not be able to accurately self-report their pain. As a result, an observational measurement tool may be used to assess pain intensity.[32] The FLACC (Face, Legs, Activity, Cry, Consolability) is a valid and reliable tool for children age 1 and above. This is a five-item scale in which raters score each of five categories from 0 to 2 with a total score range of 0 to 10 (Table 7.1).[34,35]

For children 4 to 12 years of age, the *Faces Pain Scale–Revised* (FPS-R) is a valid pain measurement tool. This self-report scale consists of six gender and ethnicity-neutral line drawings of faces

TABLE 7.1 **The Face, Legs, Activity, Cry, Consolability Behavioral Pain Assessment Scale**

	SCORING		
Categories	0	1	2
Face	No particular expression or smile	Occasional grimace or frown; withdrawn, disinterested	Frequent to constant frown, clenched jaw, quivering chin
Legs	Normal position or relaxed	Uneasy, restless, tense	Kicking or legs drawn up
Activity	Lying quietly, normal position, moves easily	Squirming, shifting back and forth, tense	Arched, rigid, or jerking
Cry	No cry (awake or asleep)	Moans or whimpers, occasional complaint	Crying steadily, screams or sobs; frequent complaints
Consolability	Content, relaxed	Reassured by occasional touching, hugging, or being talked to; distractible	Difficult to console or comfort

This is a five-item scale in which raters score each of five categories from 0 to 2 with a total score range of 0 to 10.
From Merkel SI, Voepel-Lewis T, Shayevitz JR, Malviya S. The FLACC: a behavioral scale for scoring postoperative pain in young children. *Pediatr Nurs.* 1997;23(3):293–297. The FLACC scale was developed by Sandra Merkel, MS, RN, Terri Voepel-Lewis, MS, RN, and ShobhaMalviya, MD, at C.S. Mott Children's Hospital, University of Michigan Health System, Ann Arbor, Michigan.

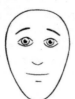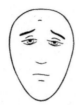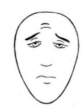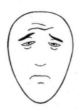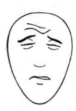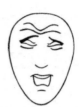

• **Figure 7.3** Faces Pain Scale–Revised. This is a self-report scale consisting of six line drawings of faces, scored 0 to 10 in pain intensity. (From International Association for the Study of Pain © 2001; Hicks CL, von Baeyer CL, Spafford P, et al. The Faces Pain Scale—Revised: toward a common metric in pediatric pain measurement. *Pain*. 2001;93[2]:173–183.)

• **Figure 7.4** Visual Analog Scale. This is a self-report scale. The patient marks a line signifying the intensity of pain experienced. (From Heller GZ, Manuguerra M, Chow R. How to analyze the Visual Analogue Scale: myths, truths, and clinical relevance. *Scand J Pain*. 2016;13:67–75.)

• **BOX 7.1** **Factors Exacerbating Children's Pain**

Intrinsic Factors

Child's cognitive development, anxiety, depression, and fear
Previous experience with inadequately managed pain (child's lack of control)
Experience of other aversive symptoms (nausea, fatigue, and dyspnea)
Child's negative interpretation of the situation

Extrinsic Factors

Anxiety and fears of parents and siblings
Poor prognosis
Invasiveness of treatment regimen
Parental reinforcement of extreme underreaction (stoicism) or overreaction to pain
Inadequate pain management practices of health care staff
Boring or age-inappropriate environment

that are scored 0 to 10 (Fig. 7.3); it has been translated into over 40 languages. The faces in this revised scale do not show a smile or tears at the extremes in order to avoid evoking the emotions or fear that may coincide with pain, but do not directly correlate with pain experienced. It is important for the person implementing the scale to use appropriate language, such as, "These faces show how much something can hurt. This face [point to face on far left] shows no pain. The faces show more and more pain [point to each from left to right] up to this one [point to face on far right]—it shows very much pain. Point to the face that shows how much you hurt [right now]." It is imperative to avoid using the words *happy* and *sad*. In addition, this scale is intended to measure how the child feels; this will not necessarily correlate with his or her facial expression.[36,37]

The *Visual Analog Scale* (VAS) is one of the most reliable and valid measurement tools for self-report of pain in children aged 8 and above. A VAS is a line approximately 100 mm in length, with each end anchored by extreme descriptors (e.g., *no pain* versus *severe pain*). The patient indicates the degree of perceived pain by making a mark on the line. The length of the line from the left-hand margin to the mark determines the magnitude of pain for that individual (Fig. 7.4). Certain physiologic measurements, especially heart rate, in conjunction with self-report of discomfort are thought to add another important dimension to the characterization of response specificity to painful stimuli.[30,31]

For children and adolescents with cognitive impairment (CI), the self-report measurement tools may not be applicable. Health care providers must be able to observe and assess the presence and intensity of pain in order to effectively manage pain for children with CI. For this population, the revised FLACC has been shown to be valid and reliable for postoperative pain assessment (Table 7.2). This observational scale takes into account the various facial expressions or bodily movements that may be exhibited. It incorporates additional behavioral descriptors including tremors, increased spasticity, jerking movements, changes in respiratory pattern, and verbal outbursts. Parents also have the ability to input their individual responses with open-ended descriptors in each category.[38]

Family and cultural elements are apparent in the mediation of pain-related expressions and their effects. An infant's cry may elicit protective and indulging types of behavior or, sadly, abusive behaviors in adult caretakers. Family members may respond

differentially to a child's painful expressions, with females being more supportive and soothing and males more coarse and distracting. Some societies are highly sensitive to infant distress whereas others are less sensitive. In addition, behavioral manifestations of pain as well as self-report measures are subject to effects of minimization, exaggeration, and the influence of social and contextual variables. There are strengths and flaws in any assessment method. For example, patients tend to choose the extreme facial expressions in the FPS-R. When appropriate, a combination of behavioral observation and self-report methods can be used in conjunction with physiologic measures.[23]

In summary, many factors may contribute to a child's perception of pain. McGrath and colleagues have listed factors that tend to exacerbate the pain in children with cancer and suggest developmental considerations for quantification of pain (Box 7.1 and Table 7.3).[39]

Pain Control With Analgesics

Pharmacologic relief of pain may occasionally be deemed necessary for the pediatric patient. The agents used for pain relief are termed *analgesics*. Ideally, analgesic drugs should relieve pain without significantly altering consciousness. Analgesics act either in the peripheral tissues, centrally in the brain and spinal cord, or both. Narcotic analgesics are thought to act primarily in the CNS. Nonnarcotic analgesics (e.g., nonsteroidal antiinflammatory drugs [NSAIDs] like ibuprofen) act to reduce inflammation in both the peripheral and CNS in order to decrease pain transmission. The great majority of dental pain in pediatric patients can and should be managed using nonnarcotic agents; however, children of all ages are capable of experiencing pain, and recently

TABLE 7.2	Revised Face, Legs, Activity, Cry, Consolability Scale

	Individual Behavior
Face 0. No particular expression or smile 1. Occasional grimace/frown; withdrawn or disinterested; appears sad or worried 2. Consistent grimace or frown; frequent/constant quivering chin, clenched jaw; distressed-looking face; expression of fright or panic Individualized behavior:_____	"Pouty" lip; clenched and grinding teeth; eyebrows furrowed; stressed looking; stern face; eyes wide open—looks surprised; blank expression; nonexpressive
Legs 0. Normal position or relaxed; usual tone and motion of limbs 1. Uneasy, restless, tense; occasional tremors 2. Kicking, or legs drawn up; marked increase in spasticity, constant tremors or jerking Individualized behavior:_____	Legs and arms drawn to center of body; clonus in left leg with pain; very tense and still; legs tremble
Activity 0. Lying quietly, normal position, moves easily; regular, rhythmic respirations 1. Squirming, shifting back and forth, tense or guarded movements; mildly agitated (e.g., head back and forth, aggression); shallow, splinting respirations, intermittent sighs 2. Arched, rigid, or jerking; severe agitation; head banging; shivering (not rigors); breath holding, gasping or sharp intake of breaths, severe splinting Individualized behavior:_____	Grabs at site of pain; nods head; clenches fists, draws up arms; arches neck; arms startle; turns side to side; head shaking; points to where it hurts; clenches fist to face, hits self, slapping; tense, guarded, posturing; thrashes arms; bites palm of hand; holds breath
Cry 0. No cry/verbalization 1. Moans or whimpers; occasional complaint; occasional verbal outburst or grunt 2. Crying steadily, screams or sobs, frequent complaints; repeated outbursts, constant grunting Individualized behavior:_____	States, "I'm okay" or "All done"; mouth wide open and screaming; states "Owie" or "No"; gasping, screaming; grunts or short responses; whining, whimpering, wailing, shouting; asks for medicine; crying is rare
Consolability 0. Content and relaxed 1. Reassured by occasional touching, hugging or being talked to; distractible 2. Difficult to console or comfort; pushing away caregiver, resisting care or comfort measures Individualized behavior:_____	Responds to cuddling, holding, parent, stroking, kissing; distant and unresponsive when in pain

This revised scale is useful for patients with cognitive impairment. The additional descriptors include facial expressions, bodily movements, and vocalizations that may signify behavioral changes. There are also open-ended descriptors for the parent to input information.
From Malviya S, Voepel-Lewis T, Burke C, et al. The revised FLACC observational pain tool: improved reliability and validity for pain assessment in children with cognitive impairment. *Paediatr Anaesth.* 2006;16(3):258–265.

TABLE 7.3	Age and Measures of Pain Intensity

Age	Self-Report Measures	Behavior Measures	Physiologic Measures
Birth to 3 years	Not available	Of primary importance	Of secondary importance
3–6 years	Specialized, developmentally appropriate scales available	Primary if self-report not available	Of secondary importance
>6 years	Of primary importance	Of secondary importance	Of secondary importance

From McGrath PJ, Beyer J, Cleeland C, et al. Report of the Subcommittee on Assessment and Methodologic Issues in the Management of Pain in Childhood Cancer. *Pediatrics.* 1990;86:814–817.

investigators have expressed concern that younger children and infants may be undertreated for pain following certain clinical procedures. Refer to Table 7.4 for an overview of analgesics used in children.

Nonnarcotic Analgesics

Generally the nonnarcotic analgesics are useful for mild to moderate pain, which includes the vast majority of dental procedural pain. The nonnarcotic analgesics differ from the narcotics in their site and mechanism of action, their adverse effect profile, and their analgesic ceiling effect, which is the dose at which maximum pain relief can be achieved. These drugs exert their antiinflammatory effects primarily at the peripheral nerve endings. The standard prototype drugs in this class are acetaminophen and NSAIDs. It should be noted that in most cases of dental procedural pain in children, the nonnarcotic analgesics should be considered first-line therapeutic agents.

TABLE 7.4	Commonly Used Analgesics for Children				
	Drug	Class	Generic Name	Trade Name	Dose
Mild to moderate pain	Acetylsalicylic acid	Salicylate, NSAID	Aspirin	Bayer Aspirin	10–15 mg/kg/dose q4–6h; maximum dose: 60–80 mg/kg/day up to 4 g/day
	Acetaminophen	Nonnarcotic analgesic	Acetaminophen	Tylenol; Tempra	10–15 mg/kg/dose q4–6h as needed; do **not** exceed 5 doses in 24 h
	Ibuprofen	NSAID	Ibuprofen	Advil; Children's Motrin	4–10 mg/kg/dose q6–8h; maximum daily dose: 40 mg/kg/day
	Acetaminophen and codeine	Nonnarcotic analgesic and narcotic analgesic	Acetaminophen and codeine	Tylenol with codeine; Tylenol 3	Codeine: 0.5–1 mg codeine/kg/dose q4–6h; maximum dose: 60 mg/dose Acetaminophen: 10–15 mg/kg/dose q4–6h; do **not** exceed 5 doses in 24 h Oral solution: 120 mg acetaminophen and 12 mg codeine/5 mL
Moderate to severe pain	Acetaminophen and hydrocodone	Nonnarcotic analgesic and Narcotic analgesic	Acetaminophen and hydrocodone	Lortab, Norco	Hydrocodone: 0.1–0.2 mg/kg/dose q4–6h as needed; maximum dose: 6 doses of hydrocodone/day Acetaminophen: 10–15 mg/kg/dose q4–6h; do **not** exceed five doses in 24 h Oral solution: 300 mg acetaminophen and 10 mg hydrocodone/15 mL 325 mg acetaminophen and 7.5 mg hydrocodone/15 mL 325 mg acetaminophen and 10 mg hydrocodone/15 mL

NSAID, Nonsteroidal antiinflammatory drug.

Acetaminophen

Acetaminophen (e.g., Tylenol, Tempra, and Datril) is the most common analgesic used in pediatrics in the United States today. It is an effective analgesic and antipyretic that is as potent as aspirin for the management of mild to moderate pain. Unlike aspirin, acetaminophen does not inhibit platelet function.[40] It also causes less gastric upset and has not been implicated in Reye syndrome. The primary disadvantage of acetaminophen is that it has no clinically significant antiinflammatory properties.

Toxicity as a result of overdose may result in acute liver failure with serious or fatal hepatic necrosis. The pathophysiology is related to transient elevations in serum aminotransferase levels in a proportion of subjects with hepatocellular injury. It is estimated that 15 g of acetaminophen is required in an adult to produce liver damage, or more than 3 g in a child under 2 years of age.[41] Allergic reactions are very rare. Acetaminophen is a good alternative analgesic in patients who do not require an antiinflammatory effect. See Table 7.4 for dosing information.

Nonsteroidal Antiinflammatory Drugs

The NSAIDs, principally derivatives of phenylalkanoic acid, exert their analgesic effects by inhibiting prostaglandin synthetase in the periphery and CNS. These agents possess analgesic and antiinflammatory properties that are superior to those of aspirin, especially for arthritis, and are effective for the management of acute pain following minor surgery or trauma. The NSAIDs produce fewer bleeding problems than aspirin because their inhibition of platelet aggregation is reversible after elimination by the body. Other side effects reported include gastrointestinal upset, rash, headache, dizziness, eye problems, hepatic dysfunction, and renal dysfunction. There are relatively few clinical drug trials evaluating NSAIDs in children, but common agents approved by the US Food and Drug Administration (FDA) for children are ibuprofen, naproxen, and tolmetin. Both ibuprofen and naproxen are available in oral suspension form.

Aspirin

Since its introduction in 1899, aspirin, a salicylate (acetylsalicylic acid), has found widespread use for its analgesic, antipyretic, antiplatelet, and antiinflammatory properties. Despite the advent of many newer drugs, aspirin remains a standard drug for comparison to other analgesics.

The most significant side effects of aspirin include alterations of coagulation by irreversible inhibition of platelet aggregation, gastric distress and dyspepsia, occult blood loss, and, very rarely, sensitivity reactions such as urticaria, angioneurotic edema, asthma, or anaphylaxis. The anticoagulant properties of aspirin are rarely a problem in children; however, aspirin should be avoided in patients with bleeding or platelet disorders and in those taking warfarin (Coumadin) or similar drugs.

The gastrointestinal effects of aspirin are the most common problems and may be modulated by administering the drug with food or by using a buffered or enteric-coated preparation, although absorption may be affected. The more severe allergic types of reactions have been shown to occur more often in patients with preexisting asthma, atopy, or nasal polyps, and aspirin should probably be avoided in patients with such a history. The possible association of aspirin with certain viral illnesses and the development of Reye syndrome (a poorly understood disease entity characterized by vomiting, prolonged lethargy and ultimately seizures and coma) has resulted in many practitioners opting for aspirin substitutes, particularly in children.[42] See Table 7.4 for dosing information.

Opioid Analgesics

The opioid analgesics, frequently referred to as narcotics, have been shown to interact with opioid receptors in the CNS.[43] These interactions result in the pharmacologic effects characteristic of the narcotics, including analgesia, sedation, and cough suppression. Narcotics are significantly more effective against severe and acute pain than the nonnarcotic analgesics, and they exhibit no ceiling effect for analgesia. However, they can produce serious adverse effects such as sedation, respiratory depression, and, with prolonged use, dependence and the possibility of addiction. Constipation can also be a problem, even with short-term use. Practitioners should know their state mandates when prescribing an opioid to a minor. Many states require specific consent to be obtained with the legal guardian as well as verification to ensure the patient has no open opioid prescriptions.[43]

There are many narcotic analgesics available, including morphine, meperidine (Demerol), fentanyl, codeine, hydrocodone (e.g., Norco, Vicodin, Lortab), oxycodone (e.g., Percocet), and hydromorphone (Dilaudid). Many of these drugs are available only in parenteral preparations. Codeine, hydrocodone, and oxycodone are available for oral use.

Narcotic Analgesics

Codeine is the standard of comparison for oral opioids. It is absorbed well when given orally and is a prodrug that must be converted to its active form, morphine, in the liver. It may be used for more significant pain that is not responsive to acetaminophen or NSAIDs. Codeine is much less potent than its relative, morphine. Side effects include nausea, sedation, dizziness, constipation, and cramps. Codeine may produce more serious side effects of respiratory depression and dependence. *For this reason, all other nonopioids should be considered as first-line analgesics.* According to the literature, "anoxic brain injuries and death have occurred in children with weight-appropriate dosing for codeine. There is a reported variance in pharmacogenetics based on cytochrome P450 family 2 subfamily D type 6 (CYP2D6), which may alter action of the drug."[44] According to the FDA, codeine has risks including slowed or difficult breathing and death, which appear to be a greater risk in children below age 12. Strongly consider recommending over-the-counter or other FDA-approved prescription medicines for pain management in children younger than 12 years and in adolescents younger than 18 years, especially those with certain genetic factors, obesity, or obstructive sleep apnea and other breathing problems.[45]

Hydrocodone and oxycodone have a better affinity for opioid receptors than codeine. Hydrocodone and oxycodone metabolism are both modulated by the same enzyme as codeine. However, the pharmacogenetics of these drugs is still unclear. Hydrocodone in combination with acetaminophen has been shown to provide safe and effective pain relief after tonsillectomy, and the World Health Organization, in its stepwise management of pain, recommends strong opioids such as oxycodone for moderate to severe pain in children.[46,47] These drugs are not first-line agents for pain management and should be reserved for moderate to severe "breakthrough" pain that is not relieved with a nonnarcotic analgesic agent alone.

Codeine, when in combination with another analgesic, usually acetaminophen (e.g., Tylenol with Codeine No. 3), is a Drug Enforcement Administration (DEA) Schedule III drug while hydrocodone and oxycodone are Schedule II drugs.

It is recommended that narcotics be given in combination with acetaminophen when administered orally for pediatric analgesia. See Table 7.4 for dosing information. The maximum allowable dose of acetaminophen with a narcotic is, however, *not* based on the codeine or hydrocodone component but rather the acetaminophen component. For children, do *not* exceed five doses in 24 hours.

It has been reported that children undergoing invasive restorative treatment require postoperative analgesia.[48,49] Since most cases of postoperative pain include an inflammatory component, NSAIDs are considered first-line agents in the treatment of mild to moderate postoperative pain.[50] When one agent is ineffective in controlling postoperative pain, an alternation between acetaminophen and ibuprofen may be used. Acetaminophen alternated every 3 hours with ibuprofen is known as multimodal analgesia and is based on the principle that these agents target different receptor sites.[51] It is rare that the recommended doses of acetaminophen or NSAIDs will not manage dental pain. In the uncommon situation where dental pain is refractory to these modalities, a more potent agent such as hydrocodone or oxycodone may be used. Practitioners should be careful to distinguish physiologic pain from a behavioral response. The duration of such drug usage should generally be brief, and a prolonged perceived need for analgesics should prompt reevaluation or further consultation to determine the etiology of persistent reported pain.

Regulations and guidelines are changing in regard to the use of narcotic agents in the pediatric population. It is the practitioner's responsibility to review these recommendations.

Dosing Schedule

Analgesics should be administered on a regular time schedule if moderate to severe pain is expected. This is called *around-the-clock dosing* and has been consistently shown to be the most effective way to decrease breakthrough pain because it keeps the plasma levels of analgesic stable. Advising parents to give a pain medicine "as needed" sometimes means that the child will not receive any medicine unless he or she is vocal in his or her complaints.[47] For dental pain, using an analgesic as prescribed (e.g., every 4 to 6 hours) for the first 36 to 48 hours is recommended.[50]

Pain Control With Local Anesthesia

Profound local anesthesia facilitates the successful treatment of patients, especially pediatric patients, by allaying their anxiety and discomfort during restorative and surgical procedures.

Good operator technique in obtaining local anesthesia in pediatric patients is essential and requires mastery of the following areas: (1) child growth and development (physical and mental), (2) behavior management, (3) sound technique, and (4) pharmacology of local anesthetics. As with any anesthetic administration, a thorough preoperative medical evaluation must be conducted before selection of technique and agent. This should include but not be limited to review of medical history, evaluation of the patients' weight and body mass index, potential for adverse drug interactions, and completion of medical consults as needed.[52]

Mechanisms of Action

Local anesthesia is used to alter pain perception at the peripheral level by blocking the propagation of nerve impulses. The initial process of pain perception involves the production of nerve impulses by a noxious stimulus that activates specialized nerve fibers—termed *nociceptors* and classified as A-delta and C fibers—that transmit pain information to the CNS. The nerve impulses travel along the nerve fibers via a process involving ion transport across the neuronal membrane.[53,54]

The primary effect of local anesthetic agents is to penetrate the nerve cell membrane and block receptor sites that control the influx of sodium ions associated with membrane depolarization.[54] The sequence of events involved in a local anesthetic block consists of (1) intraneuronal penetration of the local anesthetic and subsequent binding to a receptor site that exists on the inside of the cell membrane, (2) blockade of the sodium channels through which the sodium ions would normally enter during depolarization, (3) a decrease in sodium conductance, (4) depression of the rate of electrical depolarization, (5) failure to achieve threshold potential, and (6) lack of development of a propagated action potential and thus blockade of conduction of the nerve impulse.[54] Fig. 7.5

illustrates the local anesthetic mechanism. The net result is inhibition of neuronal excitability, which reduces the likelihood of action potential transmission. Therefore local anesthetics alter the reactivity of neural membranes to propagated action potentials that may be generated in tissues distal to the anesthetic block. Action potentials that enter an area of adequately anesthetized nervous tissue are blocked and fail to transmit information to the CNS.[54] In general, small nerve fibers are more susceptible to the onset of action of local anesthetics than large fibers. Accordingly, the sensation of pain is one of the first modalities blocked, followed by cold, warmth, touch, and at times, pressure.[52]

Local anesthetic agents are weak chemical bases and are supplied generally as salts, such as lidocaine hydrochloride. The salts may exist in one of two forms, either the uncharged free base or a cation whose charge is determined by its dissociation constant (pKa). The free-base form, which is lipid soluble, is capable of penetrating the nerve cell membrane. Penetration of the tissue and cell membrane is necessary for the local anesthetic to have an effect because the receptor sites are located on the inside of the cell membrane. Once the free base has penetrated the cell, it reequilibrates, and the cation is thought to be the form that then interacts with the receptors to prevent sodium conductance.[54] Local infection and inflammation can modify the normal local physiology of tissue by causing the release of neuroactive substances (e.g., histamine, leukotrienes, kinins, and prostaglandins) and by lowering the pH. These changes reduce the lipid solubility of the anesthetic and interfere with its ability to penetrate the nervous tissue. Blocking the nerve at a more proximal site distant from the infected area may be a viable alternative. Antibiotic administration may reduce the extent of infection and permit definitive treatment under local anesthesia that would otherwise be impossible.[54]

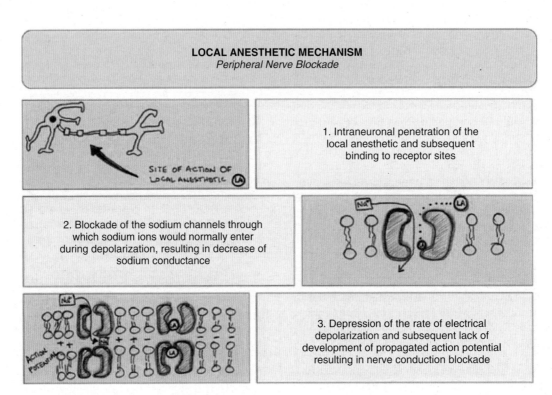

• **Figure 7.5** Mechanism of action of local anesthetic.

Local Anesthetic Agents

Esters

There is one commonly used ester anesthetic, benzocaine, a topical anesthetic. The major problem with the ester class of local anesthetics is their propensity to produce allergic reactions. Ester local anesthetics are hydrolyzed in the plasma by the enzyme pseudocholinesterase. Ester local anesthetics are metabolized to para-amino benzoic acid (PABA), which has been associated with allergic sensitization.[52,54,55]

Amides

The amides were introduced with the synthesis of lidocaine in 1943. These compounds are amide derivatives of diethylaminoacetic acid. They are relatively free from sensitizing reactions. Since lidocaine was synthesized, several other local anesthetics have been introduced for dental use. Amides are used more frequently because of their reduced allergenic characteristics and greater potency at lower concentrations. Amide local anesthetics are metabolized primarily in the liver. Therefore liver function may significantly affect the rate of metabolism. Significant liver dysfunction may result in slower metabolism and increased risk of local anesthetic toxicity. The amides commonly used include lidocaine, mepivacaine, prilocaine, bupivacaine, and articaine.[52,54,55]

Excretion of Local Anesthetics

For both ester and amide local anesthetics and their metabolites, the kidneys are the primary organ for excretion. Significant renal impairment may result in an inability to eliminate the local anesthetic, thus resulting in increased risk for toxicity.[52,54]

Local Anesthetic Properties

Individual local anesthetic agents differ from one another in their pharmacologic profiles (Table 7.5).[56] The reader may refer to additional readings for more in-depth information on local anesthetics that are rarely used in children. They vary in their potency, toxicity, onset time, and duration of action. All these characteristics may be clinically important, and all vary as a function of the intrinsic properties of the anesthetic agent itself and the regional anesthetic procedure employed. Furthermore, these characteristics may be modified by the addition of vasoconstrictors.

Potency

The intrinsic potency of a local anesthetic is the concentration required to achieve the desired nerve blockade and is best predicted by its lipid solubility. Greater lipid solubility allows the anesthetic to penetrate the nerve membrane more readily, which is 90% lipid.[54] Lidocaine, prilocaine, mepivacaine, and articaine have intermediate potency, and bupivacaine has the highest potency.[52] The efficacy of local anesthesia depends on the concentration of the anesthetic on a segment of the nerve. Beyond a fixed amount of local anesthetic necessary for blockage of neuronal impulses, any excess is wasteful and potentially dangerous. Failure to obtain anesthesia is most likely due either to operator error in depositing the solution sufficiently close to the nerve or to anatomic aberrations (e.g., accessory innervation).

Local anesthetics do not necessarily come in the same concentration; hence caution is needed to prevent exceeding toxic doses of local anesthesia, especially when used in combination with other agents affecting the cardiovascular system and the CNS (e.g., sedatives). As an example, two full cartridges (carpules) of 2% lidocaine without vasoconstrictor may be easily tolerated by an adult, but the same amount may exceed the maximal allowable dosage for a child. Great care must be taken when a 4% concentration of a local anesthetic (e.g., articaine) is used with children because the amount of local anesthetic is twice that of a 2% solution.

Onset Time

Onset time is the time required for the local anesthetic solution to penetrate the nerve fiber and cause complete conduction blockade. The pKa is the most important factor in determining onset time. The pKa, or dissociation constant, is a measure of the affinity of

TABLE 7.5 Common Local Anesthetics Used in Dentistry for Children

Anesthetic	Maxillary Block Pulp	Maxillary Block Soft Tissue	Mandibular Block Pulp	Mandibular Block Soft Tissue	Max Dosage mg/kg	mg/lb	Max Total Dose (mg)
Lidocaine					4.4	2.0	300
2% + 1:100,000 epinephrine	60	170	85	190			
Mepivacaine					4.4	2.0	300
3% plain	25	90	40	165			
2% + 1:100,000 epinephrine	60	170	85	190			
Articaine					7.0	3.2	500
4% + 1:100,000 epinephrine	60	190	90	230			
Prilocaine					6.0	2.7	400
4% plain	20	105	55	190			

a molecule for hydrogen ions. In order for the local anesthetic solution to diffuse through the nerve sheath, it must be in the free base form. For example, local anesthetics with a high pKa value will have fewer molecules available in the free base form, thus it is slow to diffuse through the membrane and has a slower onset of action. While both molecular forms (free base and cationic) of the local anesthetic are important in neural blockade, drugs with a lower pKa have a more rapid onset of action than those with a higher pKa.[54] The rates of onset time for local anesthetics are as follows: mepivicaine is fastest, articaine, lidocaine, and prilocaine have moderate onset time, and bupivicaine has the longest onset time.[52,54] The clinician must understand that conduction blockade requires time to become effective; otherwise, unnecessary pain may result from beginning a procedure too soon.

Duration

Duration of anesthesia is one of the most important clinical properties considered in choosing an appropriate local anesthetic agent for a given procedure and is best predicted by protein-binding characteristics. After the local anesthetic penetrates the nerve sheath, the molecule reequilibrates between the base and cationic forms. The cationic form binds to the sodium channel receptor sites. Local anesthetics have varying vasodilatory properties, which also affects the duration of action. The addition of a vasoconstrictor to the local anesthetic will slow absorption and uptake into the bloodstream, away from the injection site. Thus, a local anesthetic with increased protein-binding capacity and a vasoconstrictor will have a longer duration than an agent with decreased protein-binding capacity and no vasoconstrictor. See Table 7.5 for commonly accepted anesthetic durations.[54,56]

Regional Technique

A major factor that determines drug characteristics is the type of regional (local) anesthetic procedure employed. Depending on whether topical, infiltration, or a major or minor nerve block is employed, onset and duration of the various agents will vary. Potency is not affected.

Onset

Local anesthesia of the soft tissues by the infiltration technique occurs almost immediately with all of the local anesthetics. As more tissue penetration becomes necessary, the intrinsic latency of onset previously discussed plays a greater role. Generally, in dentistry, for any given drug the onset time required is shortest with an infiltration and longer for a peripheral nerve block.[52,54]

Duration

Duration of anesthesia varies greatly with the regional technique performed. For dental infiltration in the maxilla or inferior alveolar nerve (IAN) block in the mandible, 2% lidocaine with 1:100,000 epinephrine has an average soft tissue anesthetic duration of 180 to 300 minutes and pulpal anesthesia time of 40 to 60 minutes. Use of 3% mepivacaine plain (without epinephrine) provides approximately 20 minutes of pulpal anesthesia time with maxillary infiltration, but it provides 40 minutes for IAN block. Soft tissue anesthesia time with either technique is 120 to 180 minutes.[54]

Local anesthetic duration is significant when considering possible postoperative adverse reactions, mainly trauma. Young children are more likely to experience soft tissue injury as a result of prolonged numbness. This should be considered in choosing the local anesthetic and procedure.[57]

Other Factors

Dose

For consistently effective local anesthetic blocks, an adequate concentration and volume must be administered. However, increases in dosage must be limited by anesthetic toxicity concerns. To calculate the maximum dosage of an anesthetic, the child should be weighed in kilograms. The maximum recommended dosage of local anesthetics is listed in Table 7.5.[56] See Box 7.2 for an example of local anesthetic calculation.

Vasoconstrictors

Onset time, duration, and quality of block are also affected by the addition of vasoconstrictor agents such as epinephrine. Vasoconstrictor agents decrease the rate of systemic drug absorption by constricting the blood vessels and thus decreasing local blood flow, counteracting the vasodilatory effects of the local anesthetic and maintaining a higher anesthetic concentration at the injection site. This generally prolongs the duration of local anesthesia produced and increases the frequency with which adequate anesthesia is attained. Toxic effects of local anesthetics are reduced because absorption into the systemic circulation is delayed. Onset time of anesthesia may be shortened as well.

In pediatric dental patients, a vasoconstrictor is generally indicated because of the potential for increased systemic uptake in the pediatric physiology. This will produce a shorter duration of action and a more rapid accumulation of toxic levels in the blood. Finally, vasoconstrictors produce local hemostasis following local anesthetic infiltration into the operative field. This assists in postoperative hemorrhage control—an advantage in the management of young children undergoing dental extractions.

Vasoconstrictors are all sympathomimetic agents that carry their own intrinsic toxic effects. These include tachycardia, hypertension, headache, anxiety, tremor, and arrhythmias. It has been shown that 2% lidocaine containing a concentration of 1:200,000 epinephrine is as effective in increasing the depth and duration of local anesthesia block as higher concentrations of epinephrine, such as 1:100,000 or 1:50,000.[54,58] To prevent vasoconstriction toxicity in children, a concentration of 1:100,000 epinephrine

• BOX 7.2	Calculating Maximum Allowable Local Anesthetic
	Example of 2% Lidocaine With 1:100,000 Epinephrine

STEP 1	• Weight of child in kilograms (kg) • Weight (for example) = **20 kg**
STEP 2	• Multiple weight by maximum allowable dose of anesthetic • 20 kg × 4.4 mg/kg = **88 mg maximum allowable lidocaine**
STEP 3	• Divide maximum mg allowable of local anesthetic by mg of local anesthetic per carpule of local anesthetic • Result is maximum allowable number of carpules • 88 mg × 1 carpule/34 mg per carpule = **2.5 maximum allowable carpules**

should not be exceeded. For healthy patients, the maximum recommended dosage is limited by the dosage of the local anesthetic drug. In patients with cardiovascular disease, a medical consultation prior to local anesthetic with vasoconstrictor administration is warranted. In general, for patients with cardiovascular disease, the maximum recommended epinephrine dose of 0.04 mg should not be exceeded.[54,58] In addition, caution should be taken in patients taking medications with drug interactions; for example, β-adrenergic blockers and tricyclic antidepressants.[52,54,59] The reader is referred to textbooks of local anesthesia for a comprehensive discussion of vasoconstrictors in patients with cardiac disease.

Toxicity

The use of local anesthetics is so common in dentistry that the potential for toxicity with these agents can easily be overlooked. Toxic reactions to local anesthetics may be due to overdose, accidental intravascular injection, idiosyncratic response, allergic reaction, or interactive effects with other agents (e.g., sedatives).[54,60]

The dental practitioner should be familiar with the maximal recommended dose for all local anesthetic agents given as the dose per body weight (e.g., milligrams per kilogram). Simply knowing the total milligram dosage for an average adult is not adequate and may lead to overdose in pediatric patients.

One must be ever mindful of the pharmacokinetics of the local anesthetics used with children. Because of the higher cardiac output, higher basal metabolic rate, and higher degree of tissue perfusion in children, these agents tend to be absorbed more rapidly from the tissues. The less mature liver enzyme systems in very young children may detoxify these chemicals at a slower rate than in older children and adults. Additionally, altered glomerular filtration rates in the kidneys and the immature central nervous and cardiovascular systems likely are more susceptible to toxicity at lower drug levels than in adults. For these reasons, a precise local anesthetic technique, with aspiration, should be used. A vasoconstrictor is generally indicated, and a thorough knowledge of the intrinsic properties of local anesthetic agents is essential.

Above all, the recommended maximal safe dose of local anesthetic should be calculated precisely for each patient and must never be exceeded. Maximal safe doses for local anesthetics are listed in Table 7.5.[56]

Central Nervous System Reactions

At safe, therapeutic dosages of local anesthetic, no CNS effects of clinical significance have been noted.[54] At higher, toxic doses, adverse reactions may occur. The initial signs of overdose are seen in the CNS. Local anesthetic agents cause a biphasic reaction in the CNS as blood levels increase (excitation followed by depression). Although local anesthetics have depressant effects in general, they are thought to selectively depress inhibitory neurons initially, producing a net effect of CNS excitation. Subjective signs and symptoms of early anesthetic toxicity include circumoral numbness or tingling, dizziness, tinnitus (often described as a buzzing or humming sound), cycloplegia (difficulty in focusing the eyes), and disorientation. Depressant effects may be evident immediately. These include drowsiness, sedation, or even transient loss of consciousness. Objective signs may include muscle twitching, tremors, slurred speech, and shivering, followed by overt seizure activity. Generalized CNS depression characterizes the second phase of local anesthetic toxicity, sometimes accompanied by respiratory depression.[52,54,60]

Cardiovascular System Reactions

The cardiovascular response to local anesthetic toxicity is also biphasic. During the period of CNS stimulation, the heart rate and blood pressure may increase as a result of increased sympathetic activity. When plasma levels of the anesthetic increase, vasodilatation followed by myocardial depression occurs, with a subsequent fall in blood pressure. Bradycardia, cardiovascular collapse, and cardiac arrest may occur at higher levels of the agents. The depressant effect on the myocardium is essentially proportional to the inherent potency of the local anesthetic.[54]

Operator Technique

Local anesthesia may be obtained anatomically by one of three means:
1. *The nerve block,* which is the placement of anesthetic on or near a main nerve trunk. This results in a wide area of tissue anesthesia.
2. *The field block,* which is the placement of anesthetic on secondary branches of a main nerve.
3. *Local infiltration,* which is the deposition of the anesthetic on terminal branches of a nerve. Adequate diffusion of local anesthetic from local infiltration readily occurs in children because their bones are less dense than those of adults.[54]

Topical Anesthesia

Topical anesthesia is used to obtund the discomfort associated with the insertion of the needle into the mucosal membrane. The usefulness of topical anesthesia has been debated, although several studies have shown it to be more effective than placebo.[61] Several factors may be considered disadvantages in the application of a topical anesthetic, including the taste of the anesthetic, the period during which the patient anticipates the needle, and the establishment of a conditioned patient response from the needle immediately following the application of topical anesthetic.[62] However, the operator's effectiveness in interacting with children to distract them and aiding them to cope with their anxieties may supersede the disadvantages of topical anesthesia. Therefore the use of a benzocaine topical anesthetic that is available in an easy-to-control gel is recommended. The best results behaviorally and physiologically occur when the gel is used sparingly and applied to a very dry mucosal surface for at least 2 minutes.

A small amount of topical anesthetic should be applied with a cotton-tipped applicator to a mucosa that has been adequately dried and isolated with a 2- by 2-inch cotton gauze pad (Fig. 7.6). The topical anesthetic should be applied to the tissue for 2 minutes. When applied appropriately, topical anesthetics are effective for surface tissues up to 3 mm in depth.[54] This allows for atraumatic needle penetration of the mucous membrane. Although a toxic response to topical anesthesia is rare, as it is poorly absorbed into the cardiovascular system, application of an excessive amount should be avoided.[54]

Complications of Topical Anesthesia

An allergic reaction to benzocaine, as ester anesthetic, can potentially occur and should be addressed prior to use. It has been estimated that 1 in 7000 exposures to benzocaine may result in methemoglobinemia,[63,64] a condition whereby the typically ferrous (Fe^{+2}) state of iron, which is functional for oxygen transport, is oxidized to the ferric (Fe^{+3}) state. This results in a nonfunctional hemoglobin

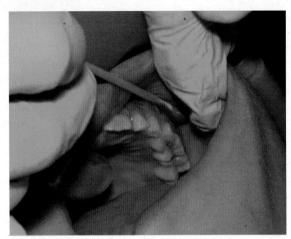

• **Figure 7.6** Application of topical anesthetic to maxillary vestibule for buccal infiltration. Note a minimum amount of anesthetic on the cotton-tip applicator. Technique: (1) Reflect tissue to expose injection site. (2) Dry soft tissue with 2 × 2 gauze. (3) Apply topical anesthetic gel with cotton-tipped applicator, slowly burnishing into tissues for 30 seconds (see manufacturer's recommendations). Remove applicator and proceed with injection.

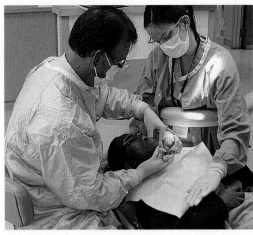

• **Figure 7.7** Preparing for the injection. Note the hand positions of the dentist and assistant in stabilizing the child's head and body during the injection.

that is incapable of binding to oxygen and may cause hypoxemia.[65] Overdosage (physiologic concentrations typically near or above 8% vs. the recommended 1%) of benzocaine may result in methemoglobinemia and tissue hypoxia, which in its initial stages is not detectable by pulse oximetry. It is imperative that clinicians use the minimal clinically effective required dose of benzocaine.[66] In addition, clinicians should discuss these risks with parents, who may purchase over-the-counter benzocaine to apply at home for teething discomfort.

Alternative Topical Anesthetics

Several studies report a significant decrease in pain perception from local anesthetic administration that is preceded by cooling of the injection site in lieu of a topical anesthetic gel. The cooling reported is varied, from a refrigerant spray to an ice-filled glove finger. The precoolant ice application time reported varied from 1 to 2 minutes and application time for the refrigerant spray was 5 seconds. This is a potential alternative to topical anesthetic gel and is an easy, reliable technique.[67–69]

Needle Selection

The needle gauge should be determined by the injection required. A short (20-mm) or long (32-mm) 27- or 30-gauge needle may be used for most intraoral injections in children, including mandibular blocks. Very little difference in discomfort level has been noted between the 25-gauge, 27-gauge, and 30-gauge needles for inferior alveolar injections; thus the 27-gauge needle would seem less likely to break or bend during injections and is preferred.[54] An extra-short (10-mm) 30-gauge needle is appropriate for maxillary anterior injections.

Because of the concern for inadvertent needle sticks, alternative needle delivery systems are now available, including retractable covers and self-sheathing needles. Injection delivery systems now have needles covered by a needle sheath and a retractable cover preventing needlesticks associated with resheathing needles after injection. If retractable needles are

not used, a needle holder should be in place to avoid two-hand resheathing.[54]

Injection Technique

Communicating at a level appropriate to the child's development is necessary in a pediatric dentistry practice. The dentist may have to modify his or her wording to accommodate the level of the child's understanding when discussing the injection. For instance, the child may be told that the tooth will be "going to sleep" after a "little pinch" is felt near his tooth. The dentist should not deny that the injection might hurt, because this denial may cause the child to lose trust in the dentist and confidence about the procedure. The dentist should minimize but not reinforce the child's anxieties and fears about the "pinch."

The discomfort of the injection may be lessened by counter-stimulation, distraction, and a slow rate of administration. Counterstimulation is the application of vibratory stimuli (e.g., shaking the cheek) or of moderate pressure (e.g., with a cotton-tipped applicator) to the area adjacent to the site of injection. These stimuli have a physical and psychological basis for modifying noxious input. Distraction can be accomplished by maintaining a constant monologue with the child and keeping his or her attention away from the syringe. The operator should always aspirate (i.e., gently pull back on the plunger of the dental syringe to cause negative pressure; aspiration of blood into the carpule occurs if the needle is in the blood vessel) and alter the depth of the needle if necessary and reaspirate before slowly injecting the anesthetic. This greatly decreases the likelihood of an intravascular injection. The recommended rate of injection is 1 mL per minute. Rapid injections tend to be more painful because of rapid tissue expansion. They also potentiate the possibility of a toxic reaction if the solution is inadvertently deposited in a blood vessel.[54]

The role of the dental assistant is important during transfer of the syringe and in anticipation of patient movement. During the transfer of the syringe from the assistant to the dentist, the child's eyes tend to follow the dentist. The eyes of the dentist should be focused on the patient's face (Fig. 7.7). The hand that is to receive the syringe is extended close to the head or body of the child. The body of the syringe is placed between the index and middle fingers, with the ring of the plunger slipped over the dentist's thumb by the assistant. The plastic sheath protecting the needle is then removed by the assistant. The dentist's peripheral vision guides the syringe to the patient's mouth in a slow, smooth movement.

Reflexive movements of the child's head and body should be anticipated.[54] The head can be stabilized by being held firmly but gently between the body and arm or hand of the dentist. The assistant passively extends his or her arm across the child's chest so that potential arm and body movements can be intercepted. The area of soft tissue that is to receive the injection is reflected by the free hand of the dentist and held taut, allowing the needle tip to easily penetrate the mucosa.[54] This hand can also be used to block the child's vision as the syringe approaches the mouth. Once tissue penetration by the needle has occurred, the needle should not be retracted in response to the child's reactions. Otherwise, if the child anticipates reinjection, his or her behavior may deteriorate significantly. Use of finger rests is strongly advocated. After administering local anesthetic, the syringe is carefully withdrawn and the needle is recapped by using a needle holder. After administration, the patient should never be left unattended.

Maxillary Primary and Permanent Molar Anesthesia

The innervation of maxillary primary and permanent molars arises from the posterosuperior alveolar nerve (permanent molars) and middle superior alveolar nerve (mesiobuccal root of the first permanent molar, primary molars, and premolars).

In anesthetizing the maxillary primary molars or permanent premolars, a supraperiosteal injection is indicated. The needle should penetrate the mucobuccal fold and be inserted to a depth that approximates that of the apices of the buccal roots of the teeth (Fig. 7.8). The solution should be deposited adjacent to the bone. The maxillary permanent molars may be anesthetized with a posterosuperior alveolar nerve block or by local infiltration.

Maxillary Primary and Permanent Incisor and Canine Anesthesia

The innervation of maxillary primary and permanent incisors and canines is by the anterosuperior alveolar branch of the maxillary nerve. Labial infiltration, or supraperiosteal injection, is commonly used to anesthetize the primary anterior teeth. The needle is inserted in the mucobuccal fold to a depth that approximates that of the apices of the buccal roots of the teeth (Fig. 7.9). Rapid deposition of the solution in this area is contraindicated because it produces discomfort during rapid expansion of the tissue. The innervation of the anterior teeth may arise from the opposite side of the midline. Thus it may be necessary to deposit some solution adjacent to the apex of the contralateral central incisor.

Palatal Tissue Anesthesia

The tissues of the hard palate are innervated by the anterior palatine and nasal palatine nerves. Surgical procedures involving palatal tissues usually require a nasal palatine nerve block or anterior palatine anesthesia. These nerve blocks are painful, and care should be taken to prepare the child adequately. These injections are not usually required for normal restorative procedures unless the procedure involves palatal tissue. However, if it is anticipated that the rubber dam clamp will impinge on the palatal tissue, a small amount of anesthetic solution should be deposited into the marginal tissue adjacent to the lingual aspect of the tooth. Adequate topical anesthesia at the injection site should be applied. Pressure anesthesia can be produced by applying pressure with a cotton applicator stick. It should be held firmly adjacent to the injection site and should produce blanching of the tissue. This should be maintained throughout administration. The palatal tissue is tightly bound to bone, so a slow deposition will limit the discomfort for the patient felt during tissue expansion. Blanching of the tissue will be observed (Fig. 7.10).

Mandibular Tooth Anesthesia

The IAN innervates the mandibular primary and permanent teeth. This nerve enters the mandibular foramen on the lingual aspect of the mandible. The position of the foramen changes by remodeling more superiorly from the occlusal plane as the child matures into adulthood. The foramen is at or slightly above the occlusal plane during the period of the primary dentition.[70] In adults it averages 7 mm above the occlusal plane. The foramen is approximately

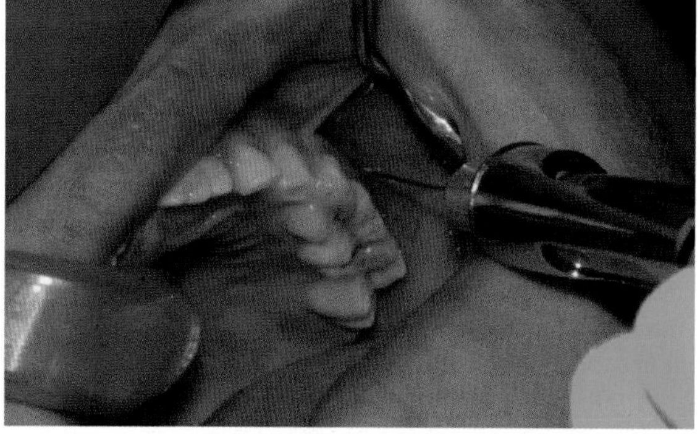

• **Figure 7.8** Buccal infiltration for anesthetizing maxillary primary molars. Technique: (1) Reflect tissue to expose injection site. (2) Orient bevel of needle parallel to the bone. (3) Insert needle in mucobuccal fold. (4) Proceed to depth that approximates the apices of the buccal roots of the molars. (5) The bevel of the needle should be adjacent to the periosteum of the bone. Aspirate. (6) Deposit the bolus of anesthetic slowly. (7) Remove needle and apply pressure with 2- × 2-inch gauze for 1 minute to obtain hemostasis.

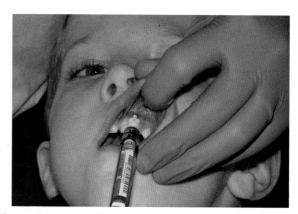

• **Figure 7.9** Labial infiltration of maxillary incisor area. Technique for maxillary primary and permanent incisors and canines: (1) Reflect tissue to expose injection site. (2) Orient bevel of needle parallel to the bone. (3) Insert needle in mucobuccal fold. (4) Proceed to depth approximating that of root apices. This depth is less in the primary dentition than in the permanent dentition. (5) The bevel of the needle should be adjacent to the periosteum of the bone. Aspirate. (6) Inject the bolus of anesthetic very slowly. (7) Remove needle and apply pressure to area with 2- × 2-inch gauze for hemostasis.

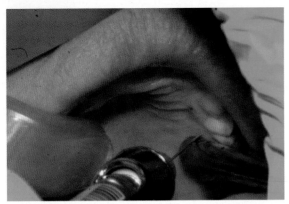

• **Figure 7.10** Palatal infiltration of primary molars anesthetizing the anterior palatine nerve. The cotton-tipped applicator is held firmly against the palatal tissue. The needle is inserted in the area between the applicator and tooth. The applicator may provide a masking or distracting effect. Technique: (1) Apply pressure with cotton-tipped applicator to site that is to receive the needle. (2) Insert needle with bevel oriented parallel to the bone immediately adjacent to the applicator. (3) Proceed to depth at which the bevel of the needle is adjacent to the periosteum and aspirate. (4) Inject the bolus of anesthetic very slowly. (5) Remove needle and apply pressure to area with 2- × 2-inch gauze for hemostasis.

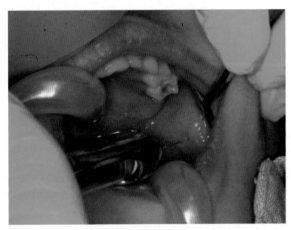

• **Figure 7.11** Inferior alveolar block. Technique: (1) With patient's mouth opened as wide as possible, place the ball of the thumb on the coronoid notch on the anterior border of the mandible. (2) Position the index and middle fingers on the external posterior border of the mandible. (3) Insert the needle with the bevel oriented parallel to the bone and at the level of the occlusal plane between the internal oblique ridge and the pterygomandibular raphe. The barrel of the syringe will be exiting the mouth adjacent to the lip commissure contralateral to the side that is to be anesthetized. (4) Insert the needle to a depth that is adjacent to the bone. Aspirate. (5) Slowly inject the bolus of anesthetic. (6) Remove the needle and apply pressure to area with 2- × 2-inch gauze for hemostasis.

midway between the anterior and posterior borders of the ramus of the mandible.

For the IAN block, the child is asked to open his or her mouth as wide as possible. Mouth props may aid in maintaining this position for the child. The ball of the thumb is positioned on the coronoid notch of the anterior border of the ramus and the fingers are placed on its posterior border. The needle is inserted between the internal oblique ridge and the pterygomandibular raphe (Fig. 7.11). The barrel of the syringe overlies the two primary mandibular molars on the opposite side of the arch and parallels the occlusal

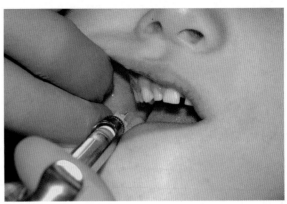

• **Figure 7.12** Long buccal nerve block. Technique: (1) Reflect tissue to expose site of injection. (2) Insert needle in the mucobuccal fold at a point distal and buccal to the most posterior molar. The bevel of the needle should be oriented parallel to the bone. (3) Insert needle to a depth that is adjacent to the bone. Aspirate. (4) Slowly inject the bolus of anesthetic. (5) Remove the needle and apply pressure to the area with 2- × 2-inch gauze for hemostasis.

plane. The needle is advanced until it contacts bone, aspiration is completed, and the solution is slowly deposited.[54,55]

Occasionally the IAN block is not successful. A second try may be attempted; however, the needle should be inserted at a level higher than that of the first injection. Care must be taken to prevent an overdose of anesthetic (see Table 7.5).

Local infiltration in the mandibular buccal vestibule adjacent to teeth has been advocated in an effort to diminish soft tissue anesthesia and possible soft tissue injury (i.e., lip biting) associated with an IAN block. However, using the mandibular infiltration technique versus a block is not of great value in prevention of soft tissue injuries since the lip still becomes anesthetized and the duration of soft tissue anesthesia may not be reduced significantly.[54,56]

Also, supplemental infiltration following an inferior alveolar block has been suggested. The effectiveness of these procedures is controversial, especially for conditions such as irreversible pulpitis.[71–73]

The long buccal nerve supplies sensory innervation to the molar buccal gingivae. It should only be anesthetized if manipulation of these tissues is anticipated. This may be done along with the IAN block after confirming the success of the block. A small quantity of solution is deposited in the mucobuccal fold at a point distal and buccal to the most posterior molar (Fig. 7.12).[54]

Some operators advocate the use of a periodontal ligament injection for anesthetizing singular teeth.[74] An advantage of this method is that limited soft tissue is anesthetized, which may prevent inadvertent tissue damage resulting from chewing after dental procedures. However, there is some evidence that this type of injection may produce areas of hypoplasia or decalcification on succedaneous teeth.[75]

Complications of Local Anesthesia

The complications of local anesthesia may include local and systemic effects.[54] Local complications may include masticatory trauma (Fig. 7.13), hematomas, infections, nerve damage by the needle, trismus, and, rarely, needle breakage in the soft tissue. These types of complications may be minimized by aspirating, decreasing needle deflection, and warning the parent and child that the soft tissue

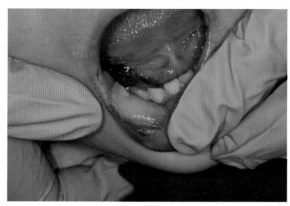

• **Figure 7.13** Masticatory trauma to lower lip that has been anesthetized with an inferior alveolar block.

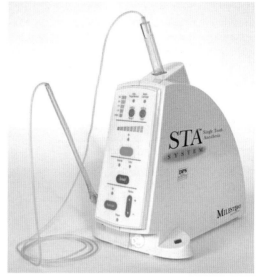

• **Figure 7.14** Single Tooth Anesthesia (STA) System, a computer-controlled local anesthetic delivery system including the wand hand piece. (Courtesy Milestone Scientific, Livingston, New Jersey, © 2010.)

will be anesthetized for a period of up to 1 to 2 hours after the restorative procedure. Paresthesia is persistent anesthesia beyond the expected duration. Potential etiologies may include trauma to the nerve, hemorrhage in or around the nerve, or trauma by the needle. The risk of permanent paresthesia has been estimated to be 1 : 1,200,000 for 0.5%, 2%, and 4% local anesthetics.[54] Paresthesia has been reported more often than is expected from the frequency of use with articaine and prilocaine.[57,76]

Phentolamine mesylate (PM) is a nonselective competitive α-adrenergic antagonist and also a vasodilator. When PM (OraVerse; Septodont, Lancaster, PA) is injected in the same area as a previous injection of local anesthetic, it is thought to facilitate the clearance of local anesthetic from the area via vasodilation, thus reducing the time of soft tissue anesthesia. Research has indicated a reduction in the duration of soft tissue anesthesia by approximately 45 minutes in children as young as 4 years of age.[77,78] However, the manufacturer recommends that PM not be used in children younger than 6 years of age or weighing less than 15 kg. One also must note that PM is not a true local anesthetic antagonist (as naloxone is to opioids), which means that it cannot be used to treat local anesthetic toxicity.

Systemic complications of local anesthetics include allergic reactions and cardiovascular and CNS dysfunction. Local anesthetic cartridges contain preservatives, organic salts, and vasoconstrictors. The preservative sodium bisulfite may be a source of allergic reaction and should be considered in the medical evaluation of the patient prior to its use. Concern about rubber products in local anesthetic cartridges as a source of allergic reactions has not been supported by any studies or case reports.[54] An allergic reaction can manifest in various ways, including urticaria, dermatitis, angioedema, fever, or anaphylaxis.[60] The practitioner should be prepared to manage emergencies as they arise (see Chapter 10).

As discussed earlier, the CNS responses to local anesthetics are complex and depend on plasma concentrations. Significant adverse events can occur when dose limits of local anesthetics are exceeded in the presence of sedatives, especially opioids. Management of overdoses may require oxygen supplementation, ventilatory support, and possible hospitalization. As discussed in Chapter 10, the dentist should be skillful in the management of emergency events.

Alternative Anesthesia Systems

In general, the conventional technique of local anesthesia delivery, in conjunction with behavioral guidance techniques, can successfully

be employed for children in the dental office. However, this experience can be overwhelming and disruptive to some children. In recent years, alternative delivery systems of dental anesthesia have been made available. These include buffered local anesthetic, computer-controlled local anesthetic delivery (C-CLAD) and vibratory devices.

The pH of an amide anesthetic with vasopressor is very low, approximately 3.5, which results in a burning sensation during administration. Increasing the pH of the cartridge of lidocaine HCl with epinephrine raises the pH to 7.4 and results in (1) increased patient comfort, (2) more rapid onset of anesthetic, and (3) decreased potential for postinjection injury. In order to buffer the local anesthetic, sodium bicarbonate ($NaHCO_3$) solution is mixed with the local immediately prior to administration. A system is available in which the local anesthetic cartridge is inserted into a mixing pen to consistently buffer the local solution. A prospective randomized double-blind crossover trial comparing traditional local administration with buffered local showed patients reported significant decreased pain when the buffered solution was administered.[79] However, in a similarly designed study with 6- to 12-year-old children, there were no significant differences in pain perception or onset time between the traditional local or buffered local anesthetic.[80]

Several C-CLAD systems are available. An example is the STA Single Tooth Anesthesia System, which utilizes the wand hand piece (Milestone Scientific, Livingston, NJ; Fig. 7.14). One of the advantages of the system is the thin, wand-like syringe that appears similar to a pen and is held like one. A foot control delivers the anesthetic at constant pressure and a relatively slow rate by a microprocessor-controlled regulator. Evidence suggests that these systems may appear less threatening to a young child. However, evidence is inconclusive in studies comparing the traditional local anesthetic administration with syringe to computerized local anesthetic administration and does not support a definitive recommendation.[81–85]

Vibratory devices that attach to dental syringes or are adjacent to the dental syringe are available. Examples include the VibraJect (Newport Coast, CA) and DentalVibe (BING Innovations LLC,

Boca Raton, FL). Their purported effectiveness is based on the gate control theory of pain and possibly auditory distraction. The VibraJect is an attachment to a traditional syringe that is intended to, as discussed earlier, activate large C fibers consistent with the gate theory of pain. Studies have been limited in the pediatric population, and there is inconclusive evidence to support a vibratory device over a conventional technique.[86,87]

Conclusion: Local Anesthetics

Profound local anesthesia is an essential and critical part of providing safe and effective dental care for any patient. The pediatric patient presents the additional challenges of an immature physiology, age-dependent communication skills, and an overlap between behaviors associated with age and those associated with pain. The dental team must ensure that local anesthetic is delivered appropriately and in a manner providing restorative or surgical care in a relatively comfortable environment.

References

1. Sollami A, Marino L, Fontechiari S, et al. Strategies for pain management: a review. *Acta Biomed*. 2015;86(suppl 2):150–157.
2. Liossi C, Howard RF. Pediatric chronic pain: biopsychosocial assessment. *Pediatrics*. 2016;138(5).
3. Weisenberg M. Cognitive aspects of pain. In: Wall PD, Melack R, eds. *Textbook of Pain*. New York: Churchill Livingstone; 1989.
4. Weisenberg M. Pain and pain control. *Psychol Bull*. 1977;84:1008–1041.
5. Zeltzer L, LeBaron S. Hypnosis and nonhypnotic techniques for reduction of pain and anxiety during painful procedures in children and adolescents with cancer. *J Pediatr*. 1982;101:1032–1035.
6. Melzack R, Wall PD. Pain mechanisms: a new theory. *Science*. 1965;150:971–979.
7. Sternbach R. *Pain: A Psychophysiological Analysis*. New York: Academic Press; 1968.
8. Woolf C. Segmental afferent fibre-induced analgesia: transcutaneous electrical nerve stimulation (TENS) and vibration. In: Wall PD, Melzack R, eds. *Textbook of Pain*. New York: Churchill Livingstone; 1989.
9. Abdulhameed SM, Feigal RJ, Rudney JD, et al. Effect of peripheral electrical stimulation on measures of tooth pain threshold and oral soft tissue comfort in children. *Anesth Progr*. 1989;36:52–57.
10. Lavigne JV, Schulein MJ, Hahn YS. Psychological aspects of painful medical conditions in children. I. Developmental aspects and assessment. *Pain*. 1986;27:133–146.
11. Lavigne JV, Schulein MJ, Hahn YS. Psychological aspects of painful medical conditions in children. II. Personality factors, family characteristics and treatment. *Pain*. 1986;27:147–169.
12. Rasnake LK, Linscheid TR. Anxiety reduction in children receiving medical care: developmental considerations. *J Dev Behav Pediatr*. 1989;10:169–175.
13. Melzack R. Pain—an overview. *Acta Anaesthesiol Scand*. 1999;43(9):880–884.
14. Fields HL, Basbaum AI. Endogenous pain control mechanisms. In: Wall PD, Melzack R, eds. *Textbook of Pain*. New York: Churchill Livingstone; 1989.
15. Eger E. *Nitrous Oxide*. New York: Elsevier; 1985.
16. Turk DC, Meichenbaum D. A cognitive-behavioural approach to pain management. In: Wall PD, Melzack R, eds. *Textbook of Pain*. New York: Churchill Livingstone; 1989.
17. Siegel LJ, Peterson L. Stress reduction in young dental patients through coping skills and sensory information. *J Consult Clin Psychol*. 1980;48:785–787.
18. Young MR, Fu VR. Influence of plan and temperament on the young child's response to pain. *Child Health Care*. 1988;18:209–215.
19. Craig KD, McMahon RJ, Morison JD, et al. Developmental changes in infant pain expressions during immunization injections. *Soc Sci Med*. 1984;19:1331–1337.
20. Izard CE, Hembree EA, Heubner RR. Infants' emotion expressions to acute pain: developmental change and stability to individual differences. *Dev Psychol*. 1987;23:105–113.
21. Frodi AM, Lamb ME. Sex differences in responsiveness to infants: a developmental study of psychophysiological and behavioral responses. *Child Dev*. 1978;49:1182–1188.
22. Perquin CW, Hazebroek-Kampschreur AA, Hunfeld JA, et al. Pain in children and adolescents: A common experience. *Pain*. 2000;87:51–58.
23. Cohen L, Lemanek K, Blound R, et al. Evidence-based assessment of pediatric pain. *J Pediatr Psychol*. 2008;33(9):939–955.
24. Groenewald C, Wright D, Palermo T. Health care expenditures associated with pediatric pain-related conditions in the United States. *Pain*. 2015;156(5):951–957.
25. Barr R. Pain in children. In: Wall PD, Melzack R, eds. *Textbook of Pain*. New York: Churchill Livingstone; 1989.
26. Brown JM, O'Keeffe J, Sanders SH, et al. Developmental changes in children's cognition of stressful and painful situations. *J Pediatr Psychol*. 1986;11:343–357.
27. Katz ER, Kellerman J, Siegel SE. Behavioral distress in children with cancer undergoing medical procedures: developmental considerations. *J Consult Clin Psychol*. 1980;48:356–365.
28. Zachary RA, Friedlander S, Huang LN, et al. Effects of stress-relevant and -irrelevant filmed modeling on children's responses to dental treatment. *J PediatrPsychol*. 1985;10:383–401.
29. Corah NL. Effect of perceived control on stress reduction in pedodontic patients. *J Dent Res*. 1973;52(6):1261–1264.
30. Winer GA. A review and analysis of children's fearful behavior in dental settings. *Child Dev*. 1982;53:1111–1133.
31. Scott P, Ansell B, Huskisson E. Measurement of pain in juvenile chronic polyarthritis. *Ann Rheum Dis*. 1977;36:186–187.
32. McGrath P, Walco G, Turk D, et al. Core outcome domains and measures for pediatric acute and chronic/recurrent pain clinical trials: PedIMMPACT recommendations. *J Pain*. 2008;9(9):771–783.
33. Hester N, Foster R, Kristensen K. Measurement of pain in children: generalizability and validity of the pain ladder and poker chip tool. *Adv Pain Res Ther*. 1990;15:79–84.
34. Merkel SI, Voepel-Lewis T, Shayevitz JR, et al. The FLACC: a behavioral scale for scoring postoperative pain in young children. *Pediatr Nurs*. 1997;23:293–297.
35. Merkel S, Voepel-Lewis T, Malviya S. Pain assessment in infants and young children: the FLACC scale. *Am J Nurs*. 2002;102(10):55–58.
36. Hicks CL, von Baeyer CL, Spafford PA, et al. The Faces Pain Scale-Revised: toward a common metric in pediatric pain measurement. *Pain*. 2001;93:173–183.
37. International Association for the Study of Pain. Faces pain scale-revised. http://www.iasp-pain.org/Education/Content.aspx?ItemNumber=1823. Accessed March 2, 2017.
38. Malviya S, Voepel-Lewis T, Burke C, et al. The revised FLACC observational pain tool: improved reliability and validity for pain assessment in children with cognitive impairment. *Pediatr Anaesth*. 2006;16:258–265.
39. McGrath PJ, Beyer J, Cleeland C, et al. American Academy of Pediatrics Report of the Subcommittee on Assessment and Methodologic Issues in the Management of Pain in Childhood Cancer. *Pediatrics*. 1990;86:814–817.
40. Shannon M, Berde CB. Pharmacologic management of pain in children and adolescents. *Pediatr Clin North Am*. 1989;36(4):855–871.
41. National Library of Medicine, National Institute of Diabetes and Digestive and Kidney Diseases. Liver disease. niddk.nih.gov. Accessed April 12, 2017.
42. American Academy of Pediatrics. Reye syndrome from caring for your baby and young child: birth to age 5. www.healthychildren.org. Accessed January 18, 2017.

43. Tyler DC. Pharmacology of pain management. *Pediatr Clin North Am.* 1994;41(1):59–71.
44. Chidambaran V, Sadhasivam S, Mahmoud M. Codeine and opioid metabolism: implications and alternatives for pediatric pain management. *Curr Opin Anaesthesiol.* 2017;30(3):349–356.
45. US Food and Drug Administration. FDA Drug Safety Communication: FDA restricts use of prescription codeine pain and cough medicines and tramadol pain medicines in children; recommends against use in breastfeeding women. https://www.fda.gov/Drugs/DrugSafety/ucm549679.htm. Accessed June 2017.
46. Sutters KA, Holdridge-Zeuner D, Waite S, et al. A descriptive feasibility study to evaluate scheduled oral analgesic dosing at home for the management of postoperative pain in preschool children following tonsillectomy. *Pain Med.* 2012;13(3):472–483.
47. Sutters KA, Miaskowski C, Holdridge-Zeuner D, et al. A randomized clinical trial of the efficacy of scheduled dosing of acetaminophen and hydrocodone for the management of postoperative pain in children after tonsillectomy. *Clin J Pain.* 2010;26(2):95–103.
48. Acs G, Drazner E. The incidence of postoperative pain and analgesic usage in children. *ASDC J Dent Child.* 1992;59(1):48–52.
49. Ashkenazi M, Blumer S, Eli I. Post-operative pain and use of analgesic agents in children following intrasulcular anaesthesia and various operative procedures. *Br Dent J.* 2007;202(5):E13, discussion 276-277.
50. American Academy of Pediatric Dentistry Council on Clinical Affairs. Policy on Pediatric Pain Management. Adopted 2012. aapd.org/media/policies_guidelines/P_painmangement. Accessed June 2017.
51. Lazo OL, White PF. The role of multimodal analgesia in pain management after ambulatory surgery. *Curr Opin Anesthesiol.* 2010;23:697–703.
52. Giovannatti JA Jr, Rosenberg MB, Phero JC. Pharmacology of local anesthetics used in oral surgery. *Oral Maxillofac Surg Clin North Am.* 2013;25:453–465.
53. Haas D. An update on local anesthetics in dentistry. *J Can Dent Assoc.* 2002;68(9):546–551.
54. Malamed S. *Handbook of Local Anesthesia.* 6th ed. Philadelphia: Elsevier; 2013.
55. Ogle O, Mahjoubi G. Local anesthesia: agents, techniques, and complications. *Dent Clin North Am.* 2012;56:133–148.
56. American Academy of Pediatric dentistry. Guideline on use of local anesthesia for pediatric dental patients. *Pediatr Dent.* 2016;38(6):204–210.
57. Adewumi A, Hall M, Guelmann M, et al. The incidence of adverse reactions following 4% Septocaine (Articaine) in children. *Pediatr Dent.* 2008;30(5):424–428.
58. Pallasch T. Vasoconstrictors and the heart. *J Calif Dent Assoc.* 1998;26(9):668–674.
59. Waits J, Cretton-Scott E, Childers N, et al. Pediatric psychopharmacology and local anesthesia: potential adverse drug reactions with vasoconstrictor use in dental practice. *Pediatr Dent.* 2014;36(1):18–23.
60. Chen A. Toxicity and allergy to local anesthesia. *J Calif Dent Assoc.* 1998;26(9):668–674.
61. Meechan JG. Effective topical anesthetic agents and techniques. *Dent Clin North Am.* 2002;46(4):759–766.
62. Kohli K, Ngan P, Crout R, et al. A survey of local andtopical anesthesia use by pediatric dentists in the United States. *Pediatr Dent.* 2001;23(3):265–269.
63. Kreshak A, Ly B, Edwards W, et al. A 3-year-old boy with fever and oral lesions. *Pediatr Ann.* 2009;38:613–616.
64. Bayat A, Kosinski R. Methemoglobinemia in a newborn: a case report. *Pediatr Dent.* 2011;33(3):252–254.
65. Cash C, Arnold D. Extreme methemoglobinemia after topical benzocaine: recognition by pulse oximetry. *J Pediatr.* 2017;181:319.
66. Lehr J, Masters A, Pollack B. Benzocaine-induced methemoglobinemia in the pediatric population. *J Pediatr Nurs.* 2012;27(5):583–588.
67. Kosaraju A, Vandewalle KS. A comparison of a refrigerant and a topical anesthetic gel as preinjection anesthetics: a clinical evaluation. *J Am Dent Assoc.* 2009;140(1):68–72.
68. Ghaderi F, Banakar S, Rostami S. Effect of pre-cooling injection site on pain perception in pediatric dentistry: a randomized clinical trial. *Dent Res J (Isfahan).* 2013;10(6):790–794.
69. Aminabadi NA, Farahani RM. The effect of pre-cooling the injection site on pediatric pain perception during the administration of local anesthesia. *J Contemp Dent Pract.* 2009;10(3):43–50.
70. Benham NR. The cephalometric position of the mandibular foramen with age. *ASDC J Dent Child.* 1976;43:233–237.
71. Aggarwal V, Jain A, Kabi D. Anesthetic efficacy of supplemental buccal and lingual infiltrations of articaine and lidocaine after an inferior alveolar nerve block in patients with irreversible pulpitis. *J Endod.* 2009;35(7):925–929.
72. Brandt RG, Anderson PF, McDonald NJ, et al. The pulpal anesthetic efficacy of articaine versus lidocaine in dentistry: a meta-analysis. *J Am Dent Assoc.* 2011;142(5):493–504.
73. Matthews R, Drum M, Reader A, et al. Articaine for supplemental buccal mandibular infiltration anesthesia in patients with irreversible pulpitis when the inferior alveolar nerve block fails. *J Endod.* 2009;35(3):343–346.
74. Malamed SF. The periodontal ligament (PDL) injection: an alternative to inferior alveolar nerve block. *Oral Surg Oral Med Oral Pathol.* 1982;53(2):117–121.
75. Brannstrom M, Lindskog S, Nordenvall KJ. Enamel hypoplasia in permanent teeth induced by periodontal ligament anesthesia of primary teeth. *J Am Dent Assoc.* 1984;109:735–736.
76. Haas D. Localized complications from local anesthesia. *J Calif Dent Assoc.* 1998;26(9):677–682.
77. Tavares M, Goodson JM, Studen-Pavlovich D, et al. Reversal of soft-tissue local anesthesia with phentolamine mesylate in pediatric patients. *J Am Dent Assoc.* 2008;139(8):1095–1104.
78. Hersh E, Lindemeyer R, Berg J, et al. Phase four, randomized, double-blind, controlled trial of phentolamine mesylate in two- to five-year-old dental patients. *Pediatr Dent.* 2017;39(1):39–45.
79. Malamed SF, Hersh E, Poorsattar S, et al. Reduction of local anesthetic injection pain using an automated dental anesthetic cartridge buffering system: a randomized, double-blind, crossover study. *J Amer Dent Assoc.* 2011;October.
80. Chopra R, Jindal G, Sachdev V, et al. Double-blind crossover study to compare pain experience during inferior alveolar nerve block administration using buffered two percent lidocaine in children. *Pediatr Dent.* 2016;38(1):25–29.
81. Allen KD, Kotil D, Larselere RE, et al. Comparison of a computerized anesthesia device with a traditional syringe in preschool children. *Pediatr Dent.* 2002;24(4):315–320.
82. Palm AM, Kirkegaard U, Poulsen S. The Wand versus traditional injection for mandibular nerve block in children and adolescents: perceived pain and time of onset. *Pediatr Dent.* 2004;26(6):481–484.
83. Klein U, Hunzeker C, Hutfless S, et al. Quality of anesthesia for the maxillary primary anterior segment in pediatric patients: comparison of the P-ASA nerve block using CompuMed delivery system vs traditional supraperiosteal injections. *J Dent Child.* 2005;72(3):119–125.
84. Dam D, Peretz B. The assessment of pain sensation during local anesthesia using a computerized local anesthesia (Wand) and a conventional syringe. *J Dent Child.* 2003;70(2):130–133.
85. Gibson RS, Allen K, Hutfless S, et al. The Wand vs. traditional injection: a comparison of pain related behaviors. *Pediatr Dent.* 2000;22:458–462.
86. Ching D, Finkelman M, Loo C. Effect of the DentalVibe injection system on pain during local anesthesia injections in adolescent patients. *Pediatr Dent.* 2014;36(1):51–55.
87. Roeber B, Wallace D, Rothe V, et al. Evaluation of the effects of the VibraJect attachment on pain in children receiving local anesthesia. *Pediatr Dent.* 2011;33(1):46–50.

8

Pain Reaction Control: Sedation

S. THIKKURISSY AND ELIZABETH S. GOSNELL

CHAPTER OUTLINE

The majority of pediatric dental patients can be treated in the conventional dental environment. By establishing good rapport with the patient and parent and by relying on sound behavior guidance techniques (see Chapter 24), the anxiety and pain of many pediatric dental patients can be managed effectively using only local anesthesia. In those children who are unable to tolerate dental procedures comfortably despite gentle encouragement and adequate local anesthesia, anxiety and pain control will have to go beyond communicative behavioral modification and physiochemical blockade of the anatomic pathways. Pharmacologic management is indicated for children who cannot be managed with traditional behavioral guidance techniques and local anesthesia.

The primary purpose of pharmacologic management of young patients is to minimize or eliminate anxiety. General anesthesia totally eliminates anxiety and elevates the pain reaction threshold. Sedation, depending on its depth, produces a relative reduction in anxiety, facilitating (1) an increased opportunity for the patient to use learned coping skills, and (2) a reduction in the reactions to painful stimuli. However, sedation and general anesthesia are not without risks against which the benefits of these techniques must be weighed. The degree of sedation depends on a host of factors related to both the drug(s) administered and certain characteristics of the patient (Fig. 8.1). Prominent drug factors include dose, route, and rate of administration, and important patient factors are age, general health, size, and metabolic rate. Importantly, sedation represents a continuum whose effects vary from minimal sedation (previously termed "anxiolysis") to moderate sedation (previously termed "conscious sedation") to deep sedation and general anesthesia. For the purposes of this textbook, the new terminology of minimal and moderate sedation will be adopted and replace conscious sedation, which was used in previous editions. Many dental schools teach some form of minimal sedation to the competence level, usually nitrous oxide/oxygen inhalation sedation and possibly oral minimal sedation. When moderate sedation is taught to competence in dental schools, it is usually an elective for select senior dental students and almost always focuses on techniques for adult patients. Specialized pediatric training is highly desirable for those planning on using moderate sedation for pediatric patients, particularly those 12 years and younger. Residency training beyond dental school that is formally accredited by the Commission of Dental Accreditation (CODA) is required for those providing deep sedation and general anesthesia.

In 1985 the American Academy of Pediatrics (AAP) and the American Academy of Pediatric Dentistry (AAPD) jointly endorsed "Guidelines for the Elective Use of Conscious Sedation, Deep Sedation, and General Anesthesia in Pediatric Patients."[1] These guidelines set the current standard of care for those who practice these sedation techniques for pediatric patients. The most recent cosponsored guidelines using the definitions of minimal, moderate, and deep sedation appeared in 2016 and can be broadly summarized (Table 8.1).[2]

The guidelines emphasize that the goals of sedation are to (1) guard the patient's safety and welfare; (2) minimize physical discomfort and pain; (3) control anxiety, minimize psychological trauma, and maximize the potential for amnesia; (4) control behavior and/or movement, which allows the safe completion of the procedure; and (5) return the patient to a state in which safe discharge from medical supervision, as determined by recognized criteria, is possible.

The purpose of this chapter is to focus on minimal and moderate sedation and its use, as an adjunct, in the management of anxiety

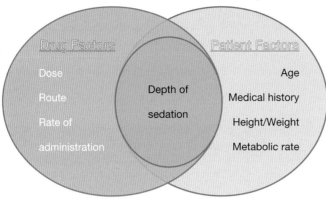

• **Figure 8.1** Depth of sedation based on drug and patient factors.

and pain control in pediatric patients. Because of the potential overlap of minimal sedation with moderate sedation and moderate sedation with deep sedation and general anesthesia, these modalities must be defined and delineated in the context of outlining what minimal and moderate sedation are and, more importantly, what they are not.

Minimal and Moderate Sedation

Minimal sedation is a drug-induced state during which patients respond normally to verbal commands. Although cognitive function and coordination may be impaired, ventilatory and cardiovascular functions are unaffected.

Moderate sedation is a drug-induced depression of consciousness during which patients respond purposefully to verbal commands (e.g., "open your eyes," either alone or accompanied by light tactile stimulation—a light tap on the shoulder or face, not a sternal rub). The caveat that loss of consciousness should be unlikely is

TABLE 8.1 **Definitions and Characteristics for Levels of Sedation**

	Minimal Sedation	Moderate Sedation	Deep Sedation
Definition	Drug-induced state during which patients respond normally to verbal commands	Drug-induced depression of consciousness during which patients respond purposefully to verbal commands or light tactile stimulation The caveat that loss of consciousness should be unlikely is a particularly important aspect of the definition of moderate sedation The drugs and techniques used should carry a margin of safety wide enough to render unintended loss of consciousness highly unlikely	Drug-induced depression of consciousness during which patients cannot be easily aroused but respond purposefully after repeated verbal or painful stimulation
Cognitive and physiologic functions	Although cognitive function and coordination may be impaired, ventilatory and cardiovascular functions are unaffected	No interventions are required to maintain a patent airway (i.e., patients should be able to maintain their airway without assistance), and spontaneous ventilation is adequate Cardiovascular function is usually maintained	The state and risks of deep sedation may be indistinguishable from those of general anesthesia
Personnel needed	2	2	3
Monitoring	Children who have received minimal sedation generally will not require more than observation and intermittent assessment of their level of sedation	There should be *continuous* monitoring of oxygen saturation and heart rate and *intermittent* recording of respiratory rate and blood pressure; these should be recorded in a time-based record	In addition to the equipment previously cited for moderate sedation, an ECG monitor and a defibrillator for use in pediatric patients should be readily available These vital signs must be documented every 5 minutes in a time-based record
Other considerations	Some children will become moderately sedated despite the intended level of minimal sedation; should this occur, the guidelines for moderate sedation will apply	Restraining devices should be checked to prevent airway obstruction or chest restriction If a restraint device is used, a hand or foot should be kept exposed The child's head position should be checked frequently to ensure airway patency A functioning suction apparatus must be present	One person must be available; his or her only responsibility is to constantly observe the patient's vital signs, airway patency, and adequacy of ventilation and to either administer drugs or direct their administration Patients receiving deep sedation should have an intravenous line placed at the start of the procedure or have a person skilled in establishing vascular access in pediatric patients immediately available

ECG, Echocardiogram.

a particularly important aspect of the definition of moderate sedation. The drugs and techniques used should carry a margin of safety wide enough to render unintended loss of consciousness highly unlikely.

For the very young patient or those patients with intellectual or physical impairments who are incapable of giving the usually expected verbal responses, a minimally depressed level of consciousness for that individual should be maintained. Unfortunately, this is usually contrasted with the need to overcome more primal and emotional responses often associated with such patients, necessitating deeper levels of sedation or general anesthesia. Note that moderate sedation suggests that a child may be in a state wherein eyes are temporarily closed; however, the child is arousable following a verbal prompt (i.e., opens his or her eyes) or responds to the degree that withdrawal *and* crying occur following mildly painful stimulus, such as an injection of local anesthetic. Withdrawal from painful stimuli and crying are prominent at this level of sedation, whereas deeper levels of sedation may result only in reflex withdrawal or reflex withdrawal and moaning. If arousal, as described previously,

does not occur, especially following a repeated moderately painful stimulus (e.g., trapezius muscle pinch), then the child is in a state of deep sedation and must be managed and monitored accordingly.

Currently, the minimal monitoring requirements for moderate sedation are:
- Pulse oximeter for monitoring oxygenation and pulse rate (Fig. 8.2A)
- Blood pressure cuff for monitoring circulation (see Fig. 8.2B)
- Precordial stethoscope or capnography to monitor ventilation (see Fig. 8.2C and D). Observation of chest movements and continuous verbal communication are acceptable for moderate sedation, but because continuous verbal communication may be undesirable for the child patient, a precordial stethoscope or capnography is usually required for moderate sedation and is always required for deep sedation.

If the patient enters a deeper level of sedation than the dentist is qualified to provide, the dentist must stop the dental procedure until the patient returns to the intended level of sedation.

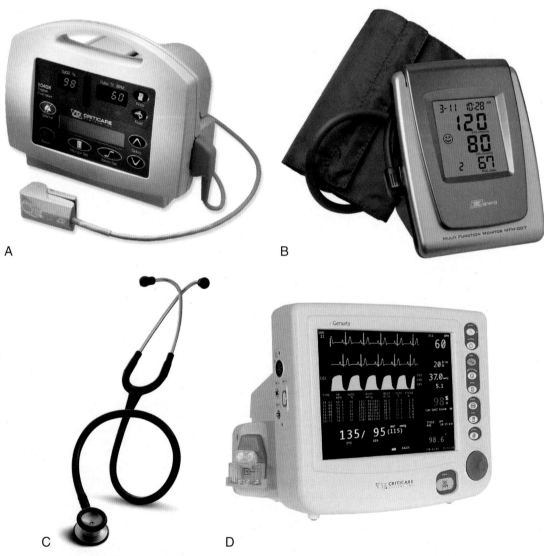

A

B

C

D

• **Figure 8.2** (A) Pulse oximeter. (B) Automatic blood pressure monitor. (C) Pediatric stethoscope. (D) Capnograph. ([A] and [D] Courtesy Criticare Systems, Inc., Waukesha, WI; [B] Courtesy Zewa Inc., Fort Myers, FL; [C] Courtesy 3M Littman Stethoscopes, St Paul, MN.)

Deep Sedation

Deep sedation is a controlled state of depressed consciousness or unconsciousness from which the patient is not easily aroused. Deep sedation may be accompanied by a partial or complete loss of protective reflexes, including the ability to maintain a patent airway independently and to respond purposefully to physical stimulation or verbal command. Young patients who are in deep sedation may respond with only a reflex withdrawal to an intensely painful stimulus, if at all. Monitoring requirements for deep sedation require a minimum of a pulse oximeter, capnography or precordial stethoscope, electrocardiography, and blood pressure cuff.

General Anesthesia

General anesthesia is a controlled state of unconsciousness accompanied by a loss of protective reflexes, including the inability to maintain an airway independently and respond purposefully to physical stimulation or verbal command.

Minimal and Moderate Versus Deep Sedation: A Critical Question

The difference between minimal and moderate versus deep sedation is a concept that must be comprehended thoroughly by those who sedate pediatric dental patients. Practitioners must realize that the goal of minimal and moderate sedation is a level of sedation that does not render the patient unconscious or unresponsive to verbal prompting or, at the most, to minimally painful stimuli. A reflex withdrawal response alone to repeated minimal or moderately painful stimuli is not appropriate for minimal and moderate sedation and is indicative of deeper levels of sedation. The patient under minimal and moderate sedation can respond appropriately to verbal commands or minimally noxious stimuli and is able to maintain a patent airway at all times. If sedation techniques are practiced in this manner, the patient's cardiovascular and respiratory functions should always be well maintained and acceptable for the age of the child.

Why is it a problem for the practitioner to move from the threshold of minimal and moderate sedation to deep sedation? The answer is simple: The patient has a much more frequent and serious risk of respiratory or cardiovascular complications during deeper levels of sedation. When the patient has a partial or complete loss of protective reflexes and cannot maintain an airway independently, hypoxemia, laryngospasm, pulmonary aspiration, and apnea may be serious or life-threatening outcomes.[3] Because the separation between moderate and deep sedation can sometimes be difficult to discern, it is the wise practitioner who obtains proper training in monitoring techniques and managing sedation before using pharmacologic management for children. Furthermore, the current guidelines indicate that the practitioner should be sufficiently trained to "rescue" the child should he or she enter a deeper level of sedation than that intended or otherwise become compromised. Although it is appropriate to activate Emergency Medical Services (EMS; call 911) in an emergency, the practitioner must not rely solely on the arrival and intervention of the EMS personnel. In other words, active intervention using basic or advanced life support must be accomplished by the practitioner and his or her staff while awaiting arrival of the EMS team. Management of the airway and ventilation is usually the most critical task to accomplish and master while awaiting the EMS team. Because the depth of sedation level is not always predictable, especially with oral routes of administration, the practitioner needs to be trained and able to rescue a child who enters a deeper level of sedation than originally intended or planned for the procedure.

For those practitioners who choose to practice deep sedation for pediatric patients, the guidelines are specific about requirements for a higher level of personnel training, as well as a higher level of vigilance in monitoring the patient's vital signs and level of sedation. They spell out requirements for personnel, the operating facility, intravenous access, monitoring procedures, and recovery care that carry a higher level of expectation and training than is the case with the use of minimal or moderate sedation.[2] In short, for practitioners who choose to use deep sedation, the standard of care specified in the guidelines is nothing less than stringent, and it is doubtful that many general practitioners or pediatric dentists currently have the training or facilities to undertake deep sedation in an office setting.

Reliance on the Guidelines as the Standard of Care for Minimal and Moderate Sedation

The AAP/AAPD guidelines establish a standard of care for minimal and moderate sedation of pediatric patients. In considering presedation events the guidelines focus on parental instructions, dietary precautions, and a preoperative health and physical evaluation. Essentially, the guidelines intensify the presedation activities, with a keen eye toward eliminating the possibility of sedation complications. They call also for documentation and recording of events during treatment (i.e., vital signs, medications given, and patient response).

The three standards in the guidelines that have most dramatically changed the manner in which pediatric sedation is practiced in the office setting relate to (1) personnel, (2) patient monitoring, and (3) preprocedural prescriptions. Relative to personnel, the guidelines specify that an assistant other than the dental operator must participate in the sedation procedure and that this assistant must be trained to monitor appropriate physiologic parameters and assist in any support or resuscitation measures required. Relative to intraoperative monitoring procedures during sedation, the guidelines specify continuous monitoring by a trained individual. A precordial stethoscope, blood pressure cuff, and pulse oximeter are considered the minimal equipment needed for obtaining continuous information on heart rate and respiratory rate.[4,5]

Preprocedural prescriptions refer to the practitioner giving a written prescription to the parent to obtain and administer the sedative agent(s) outside of the treatment facility. Preprocedural prescriptions to relieve anxiety (e.g., diazepam [Valium]) for older children who are extremely anxious may be helpful, although no strong evidence is available to support this notion. For younger children (i.e., preschool age), use of prescriptions outside of the treatment facility and without professional supervision is not appropriate. Drugs intended for sedation, particularly in a dose that has even a slight potential to make the child difficult to arouse or potentially lose consciousness, should never be administered at home by parents or guardians on the night before or during the day of sedation before transporting a child to a facility where a procedure will be performed (e.g., chloral hydrate, meperidine [Demerol], or high-dose benzodiazepines). Again, chloral hydrate and meperidine are not considered minor tranquilizers or antianxiety agents and thus should not be administered to a child outside of the dental office.

In summary, the guidelines have had a major impact on how the practitioner must approach the sedation of children. There are no systematic evaluations of the impact of the guidelines on safety in pediatric sedation; however, it is our opinion that these guidelines are having a dramatic impact in improving the safety of sedation in the dental office environment. Unfortunately, significant morbidity and mortality have occurred[6–9]; however, no deaths have occurred, to our knowledge, when the guidelines have been faithfully followed by the practitioner.

Routes of Administration

The primary routes of administration for minimal and moderate sedation are (1) inhalational; (2) enteral (e.g., oral or rectal); and (3) parenteral (e.g., intramuscular, subcutaneous, submucosal, intranasal, or intravenous). In reviewing these techniques, only the primary advantages and disadvantages will be discussed.

Inhalational Route (Nitrous Oxide)

Advantages

Nitrous oxide and oxygen administered with fail-safe dental delivery systems produce minimal sedation or light moderate sedation. Loss of consciousness and/or the inability to maintain a patent airway are almost impossible to achieve. The primary advantages of nitrous oxide for sedation in pediatric dentistry are discussed in the following sections.

Rapid Onset and Recovery Time

Because nitrous oxide has very low blood:gas solubility, it reaches a therapeutic level in the blood rapidly; conversely, blood levels decrease rapidly when nitrous oxide is discontinued.

Ease of Dose Control (Titration)

There are two ways to initially administer nitrous oxide to children. One is the standard titration technique used on adults, and the other is the rapid "induction" technique. For the standard titration technique, nitrous oxide should be started at 10% concentration and increased in increments ranging from 5% to 10%, until the patient becomes comfortable and clinical signs of optimal sedation are noted. The signs of optimal sedation that may be observed include slight relaxation of the limbs and jaw muscles, ptosis of the eyelids, a blank stare as if looking up at a star-filled evening sky, palms open, warm, and slightly moist, slight change in the pitch of the patient's voice, a lowered heart rate, and patient reports of being comfortable and relaxed. Each time the clinician increases the concentration, he or she should wait at least 30 to 60 seconds while talking with the child and watching for these signs of optimal sedation before deciding to increase the concentration again. The end point in terms of maximal concentration of nitrous oxide usually should not exceed 50% for children. Most children seem comfortable and demonstrate optimal signs of sedation in the concentration range of 35% to 50% nitrous oxide (Fig. 8.3A). The standard titration technique is primarily used for mildly to moderately anxious but cooperative children.

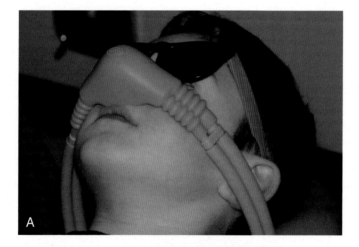

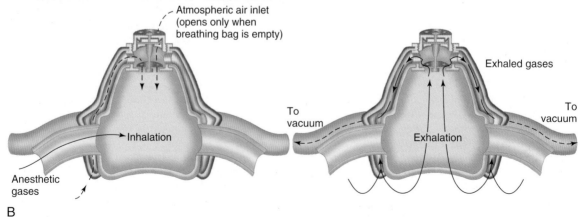

• **Figure 8.3** (A) Patient receiving inhalation sedation. (B) Scavenging nasal hood system. ([B] From Malamed SF. *Sedation: A Guide to Patient Management.* 5th ed. St Louis: Mosby; 2010.)

A second option to the standard titration technique of nitrous oxide administration is the rapid "induction" technique.[a] This technique is usually indicated for the mild to moderately anxious, potentially cooperative child who may be on the edge of losing coping abilities and needs to be controlled quickly by the clinician. The technique involves administering 50% nitrous oxide immediately to the patient without any titration steps.

In either technique, nitrous oxide should be discontinued if the child becomes disruptive or no longer breathes through the nitrous oxide hood. Gas flow should also be terminated if the child becomes nauseated or vomits, or both. In addition, good nitrous oxide hygiene is always indicated and includes the use of a scavenging system (see Fig. 8.3B), large operatories, rapid room air exchanges, supplemental movement of air (i.e., fans), and a nasal hood that adapts closely to the nose area of the face.

Lack of Serious Adverse Effects

Nitrous oxide is considered to be physiologically safe for the patient when administered with adequate oxygen. The most commonly encountered adverse effect is nausea, which should be very rare unless high concentrations of nitrous oxide are used. Poor technique with high concentrations may also result in an "excitement phase" in which the patient may become uncomfortable, uncooperative, and delirious, resembling a transitional stage to general anesthesia.

Disadvantages

The use of nitrous oxide in pediatric dentistry also has several disadvantages.

Weak Agent

Attempts to increase the concentration of nitrous oxide to control *moderately or severely* anxious patients will be fraught with failure and will not be pleasant for the operator or the patient.

Lack of Patient Acceptance

There are some patients (adults and children) who do not find the effects of nitrous oxide pleasant. These patients may become overtly noncompliant, removing the nasal mask or becoming otherwise uncooperative.

Inconvenience

In some areas, such as the maxillary anterior teeth, the use of a nitrous oxide nasal mask may hinder exposure of the area. This may be a problem, especially in small children.

Contraindications

Acute otitis media (middle ear infection) is a primary contraindication to nitrous oxide/oxygen use in children because it may enter the closed tympanic space and rupture the eardrum. Children with active pulmonary infection are not good candidates for nitrous oxide but also are generally not seen in the dental office. A history of asthma is not a contraindication to nitrous oxide. Older children with serious mental health concerns may respond inappropriately to the psychogenic effects of nitrous oxide, just as they may to other sedatives.

---

[a]The term "induction" is commonly used to describe entrance into general anesthesia, which is almost impossible with fail-safe dental nitrous oxide delivery systems and is not meant to imply entrance into a state of general anesthesia as used in this chapter.

Potential Chronic Toxicity

Retrospective survey studies of dental office personnel who were exposed to trace levels of nitrous oxide suggest a possible association with an increased incidence of spontaneous abortions, congenital malformations, certain cancers, liver disease, kidney disease, and neurologic disease.[10,11] These results underscore the necessity of scavenging (removing) waste gases adequately from the dental operatory, which, when properly provided for, significantly minimizes or eliminates these risks. It should be noted that it can be difficult to scavenge nitrous oxide adequately in the uncooperative child because gases that are exhaled through the mouth cannot be scavenged effectively.

Potentiation

Although nitrous oxide is a weak and very safe agent when used with oxygen as a sole sedative agent, deep sedation or general anesthesia may be easily produced if nitrous oxide is added to the effects of other sedative drugs given by another route, such as orally or intravenously. The combination of nitrous oxide with other sedation agents must be undertaken with extreme care and by an individual who has the proper training and experience.

Equipment

Equipment must be purchased, installed, tested for proper function, and maintained.

Practical Use of Inhalation Sedation Techniques

Nitrous oxide analgesia is relatively safe and effective for the treatment of children in the dental office. It is useful for decreasing minimal levels of anxiety and is indicated for patients who have the capacity to be compliant and follow instructions during nitrous oxide administration. Children who have nasal obstructions or are uncooperative when directed to breathe through the nose are poor candidates for nitrous oxide administration. The analgesic properties of nitrous oxide help to raise the pain threshold and may be used to lessen the discomfort during a local anesthetic injection. However, nitrous oxide will not eliminate the need for local anesthetic pain control in most children, except for very minor dental procedures (e.g., small class V preparations).

Nitrous oxide changes the patient's perception of the environment and the passage of time and is therefore helpful in managing children with short attention spans. This minimal dissociation may be perceived by some children as unpleasant, in which case the level of nitrous oxide concentration should be decreased or the administration discontinued.

A total liter flow rate per minute of gases should be established first with 100% oxygen. An adult will require 5 to 7 L/min, whereas a 3- to 4-year-old will require 3 to 5 L/min. While adjusting the controls, the dentist should use the "tell-show-do" technique with terminology appropriate for the age level of the child (e.g., "smell the happy air"). The nosepiece should be introduced with instructions to breathe nasally. Minimal finger pressure under the lower lip to produce an oral seal and gentle tapping of the nosepiece can be helpful to encourage nasal breathing in the young child.

After stabilization of the nosepiece and delivery of 100% oxygen for 3 to 5 minutes, the nitrous oxide level should be increased to 30% to 35% and administered for 3 to 5 minutes for the induction period. While administering the nitrous oxide, the dentist should talk gently to the child to promote relaxation and reinforce cooperative behavior. Although asking older children and adults if they feel tingling sensations in the fingers and toes is appropriate for verification of early signs of central nervous system (CNS) effects from the nitrous oxide, these suggestive questions to the young child may lead to undesirable body movements. An indication of such CNS effects would be minimal or continual movements of the fingers and toes in the young child.

Most dentists prefer to increase the level of nitrous oxide to 50% for 3 to 5 minutes to provide maximum analgesia for the local anesthetic injection; however, concentrations of nitrous oxide in excess of 50% are usually not indicated for dental office sedation. When the dental injection is completed, the nitrous oxide level should be reduced to 30% to 35% for a maintenance dose during the dental treatment; alternatively, 100% oxygen may be administered when the nitrous oxide is needed only for behavior management related to the dental injection.

Upon termination of nitrous oxide administration, inhalation of 100% oxygen for not less than 3 to 5 minutes is recommended to prevent diffusion hypoxia. This allows rapid diffusion of nitrous oxide from the venous blood into the alveolus while maintaining oxygenation, enabling the patient to return without incident to pretreatment activities. Inadequate oxygenation may produce such postoperative side effects as nausea, light-headedness, or dizziness, all of which can be reversed with continued oxygen administration.

It is important for the dentist to recognize that nitrous oxide analgesia should not be used as a substitute for the traditional behavioral approach to child management problems in the dental office. Nitrous oxide should be considered an adjunct to aid in management of minimal anxiety in the child who is capable of cooperating in the dental chair.

Oral Route

A route of administration used commonly for minimal and moderate sedation in pediatric dentistry is oral premedication.

Required Permit

Many states now require a special sedation permit for oral sedation of children 12 years or younger. It is prudent to review your state's rules regarding oral sedation of children.

Advantages
Convenience
Oral drug administration is generally easy and convenient, especially if the medication tastes good and can be delivered in low volume. Usually it is best to administer oral sedative medications in a separate, quiet room in the office where initiation of sedation can be facilitated by the parent in a conducive environment.

Economy
To administer oral sedative medications, no special office equipment needs to be purchased or maintained. However, special equipment is needed to monitor patients' vital signs and level of sedation, as specified in the guidelines.

Lack of Toxicity
If therapeutic doses are calculated for each patient (keeping the previous discussion on pharmacokinetics in mind) and single drugs are used in single doses, the oral route of sedation is extremely safe. However, if drug combinations are used or if two routes are combined (e.g., oral premedication followed by intravenous or inhalational medications), the chance of adverse side effects significantly increases.

Disadvantages
Variability of Effect
The biggest disadvantage of oral premedication is the fact that a standard dose must be used for all patients based generally on weight (or preferably, but unfortunately impractically, based on a body surface area). However, individuals of the same weight may respond quite differently to the same dose of drug, depending on many variables. Absorption of the drug from the gastrointestinal tract can be altered by several factors, such as the presence of food, autonomic tone, fear and anxiety, emotional makeup, fatigue, medications, and gastric emptying time. The patient may not cooperate in ingesting the medication or may vomit, making it impossible to estimate the true dose received. In some cases a paradoxical response may be seen, which may be due to a direct effect or loss of emotional inhibitions. In this case the patient may become agitated and more uncooperative rather than sedated and cooperative. These factors make the oral route of administration least dependable as far as certainty of effect is concerned. A second dose of oral medication to offset a presumably inadequate dose should never be given. Titration is not possible or safe with oral medication. If absorption of the initial dose has been delayed for any reason and a second dose is subsequently given on the assumption that the first dose was ineffective, both doses will eventually be absorbed, possibly resulting in a high serum level of the CNS depressant drug, leading to possible serious consequences such as respiratory arrest, cardiovascular collapse, and death.

Onset Time
Oral drug administration has the longest time of onset of any administration route used for sedation. The lag time varies from 15 to 90 minutes, depending on the drug, and the appropriate time should be allowed from the time of administration until treatment is attempted.

Oral premedication is very useful in pediatric dentistry, but its limitations must be clearly understood. An adequate dose must be given, and enough time must be allowed to elapse for absorption to take place before the desired effect can be expected.

Intranasal Route

The intranasal route is occasionally used in pediatric dentistry, especially for young children who may have difficulty drinking unpleasant tasting medication. In this situation the medication is sprayed or dripped into the nostrils.

Advantages
Technical Advantages
Similar to the intramuscular route, the intranasal route of administration requires little to no cooperation from child, and the full calculated dose is given with a high degree of certainty. A mucosal atomizer device (Fig. 8.4) is soft and improves patient comfort while also creating a "mist" of the drug that is more easily administered.

Absorption and Onset
The intranasal route bypasses the gastrointestinal tract and forgoes hepatic metabolism. Intranasally delivered drugs pass to the blood-brain barrier through the cribriform plate, allowing onset of the medication faster than the oral route.

Disadvantages
Discomfort
The drug may cause a burning sensation after delivery which can upset a pediatric patient. Although using a topical anesthetic spray

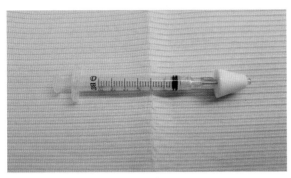

• **Figure 8.4** Mucosal atomizer device for intranasal sedation.

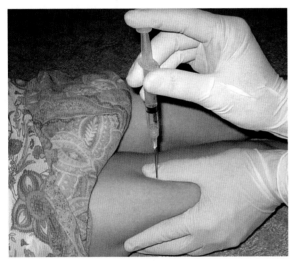

• **Figure 8.5** Intramuscular injection site: vastus lateralis. (From Malamed SF. *Medical Emergencies in the Dental Office.* 6th ed. St Louis: Mosby; 2007.)

prior to drug administration may minimize this disadvantage, this technique requires a young child to endure two drugs delivered intranasally, as well as issues as toxicity of topical/local anesthetics.

Effect

As with the oral and intramuscular routes, the drug effect cannot be titrated with intranasal delivery.

Liability Costs

Administration of parenteral medications increases the costs of malpractice coverage and may be subject to state dental laws that require permits for the use of parenteral sedation.

Intramuscular Route

The intramuscular route of drug administration (Fig. 8.5) involves injection of the sedative agent into a skeletal muscle mass. It also involves certain advantages and disadvantages when used in pediatric dentistry.

Advantages

Absorption

Absorption from an injection deep into a large muscle is much faster and more dependable than absorption from the oral route.

Technical Advantages

Technically, the intramuscular route of administration might be considered the easiest of all routes. It requires no special equipment except a syringe and needle. Patient cooperation is required for the oral route of administration, sometimes making it very difficult to give a full dose of a bitter-tasting medication to an uncooperative child. When intramuscular medications are administered, little or no patient cooperation is required, and the full calculated dose is given with a high degree of certainty. Even when a child requires restraint, intramuscular injections are easier to accomplish technically than placement of an intravenous cannula. Children and parents are familiar with this route of administration, even if it may be momentarily unpleasant.

Disadvantages

Onset

Absorption of the injected drug can be decreased or delayed by several factors. A patient who is cold or very anxious may experience peripheral vasoconstriction in the area of the injection, significantly decreasing the rate of absorption. Perhaps the biggest variable in onset is related to where the drug is actually deposited. If the drug is deposited deep into a large muscle mass, the high degree of vascularity there will allow quite rapid uptake. However, if some or the entire drug is deposited in fat or between muscle layers (all distinct possibilities in small, struggling children), absorption may be quite unpredictable.

Effect

A standardized dose is calculated based on the patient's weight, as with the oral route of administration. Drug effect cannot be titrated safely by administering additional doses for much the same reason as that described for the oral route (i.e., the possibility of cumulative overdose). A standard dose may have little or no effect in some children, whereas it may sedate others heavily.

Trauma

Injection sites that are devoid of large nerves and vessels are used for intramuscular injections, such as the middeltoid region, the vastus lateralis muscle of the thigh, and the gluteus medius muscle. Proper selection of the injection site and proper technique should minimize the possibility of tissue trauma. A hematoma may occur at any injection site.

Lack of Intravenous Access

The potential for more rapid side effects and toxicity is higher with the intramuscular route than with the inhalational or oral route. Compared with the intravenous route, a major disadvantage of the intramuscular route is the lack of a patent intravascular access (an intravenous catheter) in the event of a medical emergency.

Liability Costs

Malpractice insurance carriers generally charge a higher premium for dentists who administer parenteral sedatives in the dental office. In addition, most state dental practice acts have established requirements for permits for dentists who administer parenteral medications.

Subcutaneous Route

Occasionally, the subcutaneous route of administration is used in pediatric dentistry for sedation. In this situation the drug is most commonly injected into an intraoral submucosal space, not into a true subcutaneous space, as would be used for a tuberculin skin test, for example. In general, similar advantages and disadvantages apply to this route as to the intramuscular route, with the following exceptions.

Advantages
Site
For dental procedures, some drugs may be injected submucosally within the oral cavity, usually into the buccal vestibule. This may be less objectionable to some patients and parents than classical intramuscular or subcutaneous injection sites, and the dentist may find it more comfortable and convenient to perform.

Disadvantages
Technical Disadvantages
The rate of absorption is slower with the subcutaneous route than with the other parenteral routes. Blood supply to the subcutaneous tissue often is sparse compared with muscle. However, submucosal injections in the oral cavity have a relatively rapid effect because the vascularity is abundant.

Tissue Slough
Because the drug is deposited close to the surface of the skin or mucosa, the possibility of tissue sloughing is present. For this reason, only nonirritating substances should be given subcutaneously, and large volumes of solution should not be injected.

Liability Costs
Administration of parenteral medications increases the costs of malpractice coverage and may be subject to state dental laws that require permits for the use of parenteral sedation.

Intravenous Route

The intravenous route is the optimal and ideal route for administration of sedative agents.

Advantages
Titration
Among the parenteral routes, only the intravenous route allows exact titration to a desired drug effect. Because the drug is injected directly into the bloodstream, absorption is not a factor and the time to peak drug effect is consistent. Within a few circulation times, the intravenous drug will exert its maximal effect. Small, incremental doses may be given over a relatively short period until the desired level of sedation is achieved, thus avoiding underdosing or overdosing with a standardized, weight-based single bolus dose, as is necessary with oral, intramuscular, or subcutaneous injections.

Test Dose
With the intravenous route, a very small initial test dose can be administered, and a short time is allowed to pass to observe for an allergic reaction or extreme patient sensitivity to the agent.

Intravenous Access
In the event of a medical emergency, administration of emergency drugs is always best accomplished through the intravenous route. Establishing intravenous access after an emergency has occurred can be difficult and can consume precious time.

Disadvantages
The intravenous route would be used for all patients requiring sedation if it did not involve some disadvantages.

Technical Disadvantages
Establishment of intravenous access (venipuncture) is technically the most difficult skill that must be mastered in the practice of minimal and moderate sedation and requires some level of patient cooperation. Placing and maintaining an intravenous catheter in children can be difficult even for a seasoned clinician. The procedure requires both training and extensive practice. This is particularly true of younger children who rarely cooperate for placement of intravenous catheters.

Potential Complications
Because potent drugs are injected directly into the bloodstream, the intravenous route carries an increased potential for complications. Extravasation of drug into the tissues, hematoma formation, and inadvertent intraarterial injections are possible complications of a misplaced intravenous catheter. If the medication is injected too rapidly, exaggerated effects may be produced. An immediate anaphylactic allergic reaction may become life threatening more rapidly if it is due to an intravenous bolus of a drug than if it is due to an oral or intramuscular dose. All of these complications should be avoidable by using a test dose and a proper, careful technique. Thrombophlebitis is a rare complication that is attributable directly to the intravenous cannula or irritating intravenous medications.

Patient Monitoring
Because of the previously discussed increased potential of developing complications rapidly, the patient receiving intravenous sedation requires higher levels of monitoring.

Liability Costs
Again, because the intravenous route is a parenteral route, the liability costs are considerably higher than for oral administration. With the additional monitoring and the armamentarium required, intravenous sedation can be costly, but these costs have decreased as the use of monitors and intravenous equipment has become more common.

Pharmacologic Agents for Sedation

A large number of drugs are available for use in sedation and anesthesia. In this text, individual drugs or techniques will be put into perspective rather than discussed in detail. Three primary groups of drugs are used for sedation in pediatric dentistry in addition to nitrous oxide: the sedative-hypnotics, the antianxiety agents, and the narcotic analgesics (Table 8.2). Each group acts primarily in a different area of the brain and should be expected to produce a distinctive primary effect. The wise practitioner will understand which specific effect to expect from a given drug and will use the drug principally to achieve that effect.

Sedative-Hypnotics

The sedative-hypnotics are drugs whose principal effect is sedation or sleepiness. As the dose of a sedative-hypnotic drug is increased, the patient will become increasingly drowsy until sleep (hypnosis) is produced. Further increasing the dose can produce general anesthesia, coma, and even death. It is important to note that the primary effect of these drugs is not to decrease anxiety or to raise

TABLE 8.2	Minimal and Moderate Sedation: Pharmacologic Agents	
Group	Site of Primary Effect	Effect
Sedative-hypnotics	Reticular activating system	Sedation/sleep
Antianxiety agents	Limbic system	Decrease in anxiety
Narcotics	Opioid receptors	Analgesia

the pain threshold (analgesia). In fact, a sedative-hypnotic used alone may lower the pain reaction threshold in some cases by removing inhibitions. However, at inadequate dosages it may simply produce a patient who is more responsive to pain stimulation. The principal action of the sedative-hypnotics results from the initial primary effect of these drugs on the reticular activating system, an area of the brain involved in maintaining consciousness. Further increases in dose will affect other brain areas, especially the cortex.

The sedative-hypnotic drugs fall into three categories: barbiturates, such as pentobarbital, secobarbital, and methohexital; benzodiazepines, which will be discussed in the antianxiety section; and nonbarbiturates, such as chloral hydrate and paraldehyde.

Oral chloral hydrate, alone or in combination with other drugs, is a common sedative agent used in pediatric dentistry. When used in low doses (15 to 25 mg/kg; maximum 1000 mg), chloral hydrate can produce minimal and moderate sedation or it can have the opposite effect, producing a resistive and agitated patient, as occurs also with barbiturate sedation in children. Higher doses (30 to 50 mg/kg), especially in combination with other medications such as hydroxyzine (Atarax or Vistaril) or meperidine, can produce deeper levels of sedation. Therefore, due to the increased risk of respiratory depression and loss of consciousness, patients' vital signs and level of consciousness must be monitored closely.[12] Chloral hydrate is bitter tasting, which can produce management problems during administration. A final disadvantage is that chloral hydrate can induce nausea and vomiting secondary to gastric irritability.

The most commonly used oral barbiturate for pediatric sedation is pentobarbital. This is commonly used by pediatric medical radiologists but has not found much favor with pediatric dentists.

Antianxiety Agents

These drugs have the primary effect of removing or decreasing anxiety. The primary site of action of these agents is the limbic system, which is the "seat of the emotions." Theoretically, a dose exists for each antianxiety agent at which anxiety will be decreased without producing significant sedation. However, as doses are increased, the reticular activating system and then the cortex are affected, producing sedation as well as sleep. Thus some benzodiazepines are also classified as sedative-hypnotics. Because anxiety is often the primary problem in people with dental phobias, a primary effect against anxiety appears to be desirable, especially in reasonably cooperative adults. Antianxiety drugs possess a flatter dose-response curve, pharmacologically, than many of the sedative-hypnotics (especially barbiturates), allowing for a safer therapeutic index. This means that for most antianxiety drugs (e.g., diazepam), a larger difference exists between the dose that will produce loss of consciousness than is the case with a rapidly acting sedative-hypnotic (e.g., methohexital [Brevital]), which has a steep

dose-response curve (i.e., the difference between a minimally sedating dose and a general anesthetic dose is smaller). Drugs such as methohexital should not be used for sedation for this reason. The antianxiety agents produce no analgesia.

The antianxiety agents consist primarily of the benzodiazepines, such as diazepam, midazolam (Versed), and triazolam (Halcion). This group of agents is the one principally used for minimal and moderate sedation in adults. Midazolam is the only agent that has been extensively studied in children and is the most frequently used agent for pediatric oral sedation in medicine and dentistry. Midazolam possesses some positive characteristics, such as rapid onset and decreased likelihood of inducing loss of consciousness. However, midazolam has some characteristics that are not always beneficial to the practitioner for some operative procedures, such as short duration of action and the potential increased patient irritability primarily after dental local anesthetic administration. Flumazenil is a benzodiazepine antagonist and can reverse the effects of benzodiazepine-related sedation and overdose. As with many reversal agents, the practitioner must be aware that the duration of action of a reversal agent may not last as long as the effects mediated by the drug being reversed. Consequently, the reversal agent may have to be given parenterally in repeated doses.

Some of the antihistamines, such as hydroxyzine and diphenhydramine (Benadryl), possess both antianxiety and sedative-hypnotic properties. They are often classified with the antianxiety agents. These drugs are not very useful for sedation when used alone but are useful in combination with other drugs, such as chloral hydrate or meperidine (discussed later), as potentiating agents and also for their antiemetic properties.

Opioids

Opioids, commonly referred to as narcotics, were discussed previously in Chapter 7. These drugs are also used in sedation for their primary action of analgesia. The site of action of the narcotics is the opioid receptors of the CNS. These drugs modify the interpretation of the pain stimulus in the CNS and therefore raise the pain threshold. As the dose of the narcotic is increased, other effects such as sedation will occur. It should be recognized that sedation per se is not the principal end point sought from a narcotic. If narcotic dosage is increased to achieve sedation, serious adverse effects will be encountered, the most common of which are respiratory depression and apnea, which can lead to hypoxia and death. If sedation is desired, the narcotic should be considered an adjunct to a drug that produces sedation as its primary effect.

Narcotics may produce nausea and vomiting, especially when used alone. In high doses, narcotics may also induce cardiovascular depression. Narcotics strongly potentiate other CNS depressant drugs. Therefore the principal use of narcotics in minimal and moderate sedation should be to augment the effects of the sedative-hypnotic or antianxiety agents and to contribute some degree of analgesia that other agents do not provide. However, it should be noted that the analgesia obtained with narcotics cannot be used as a substitute for adequate local anesthesia. It should be appreciated that narcotics cause supraadditive respiratory depression when combined with sedative-hypnotics or antianxiety agents. This means that the respiratory depressant effect of the combination of agents is much greater than the additive respiratory depressant effects that would be expected.

The narcotic most commonly used in pediatric sedation techniques is meperidine. When considering the use of narcotics in pediatric dentistry, it is wise to remember the definition of minimal and moderate sedation as spelled out in the guidelines. To reiterate, the caveats that loss of consciousness should never occur in moderate sedation or be unlikely in moderate sedation are particularly important parts of the definitions of these sedative levels. Furthermore, for moderate sedation, the drugs and techniques used should carry a margin of safety wide enough to render unintentional loss of consciousness unlikely. Narcotics have steep dose-response curves. They must be used with extreme caution for minimal and moderate sedation because they carry a high risk of producing respiratory depression and loss of consciousness, especially if they are combined with other agents such as nitrous oxide. Naloxone is an opioid antagonist and can be administered parenterally to reverse the adverse effects of opioid-related sedation (e.g., respiratory depression).

Ketamine

The dissociative agent ketamine has had periods of popularity in pediatric dental practice. It produces a cataleptic state with profound analgesia and varying amnesia depending on dose. Because ketamine acts primarily on the thalamus and cortex, not on the reticular activating system, the patient does not appear to be asleep but rather dissociated from the environment. Respirations usually are not depressed with proper dosages. Stimulatory cardiovascular changes usually are produced, so tachycardia and increased blood pressure can be expected. Nystagmus and increased salivation are also common.

Ketamine is mentioned primarily to point out that it is classified as a general anesthetic because the patient under its influence is incapable of making appropriate responses to verbal commands or stimulation. It may cause respiratory depression and arrest in some patients, as well as delirium and hallucinations. Ketamine should be used only by practitioners qualified to administer general anesthesia.

Monitors

There are a host of monitors used during sedation and general anesthesia.[5] The most common are pulse oximeters, capnography, automated blood pressure cuffs, precordial stethoscopes, electrocardiography, and temperature probes. The mix of monitors required for any sedation will depend on the final depth of sedation. The most common monitors for minimal and moderate sedation are pulse oximeters, precordial stethoscopes, and automated blood pressure cuffs. These will be briefly outlined.

Pulse Oximeter

A pulse oximeter is a self-contained instrument that noninvasively monitors the degree of oxygen saturation of the patient's hemoglobin and the patient's pulse rate. Oxygen sensors placed across perfused tissue beds in which a pulse can be detected (e.g., the fingertip) determine oxygen saturation by measuring differences in the absorption of red and infrared light that is emitted by the sensors. Normally, the hemoglobin in arteries of healthy children and adults is 97% to 99% saturated (but is frequently read as 100% by pulse oximeters). The pulse oximeter is generally quite accurate, but some factors, such as patient movement artifacts, cold tissue beds, poor perfusion of tissue beds, and crying, may cause "false alarms" that incorrectly indicate low oxygen levels.

Precordial Stethoscope

A precordial stethoscope is essentially a stethoscope whose bell is temporarily attached to the chest wall and is used for monitoring ventilation (Fig. 8.6A and B). By listening through the stethoscope, the clinician can determine the respiratory rate and quality of air movement during breathing, as well as the heart sounds. The closer the bell of the stethoscope is placed to the precordial notch (i.e.,

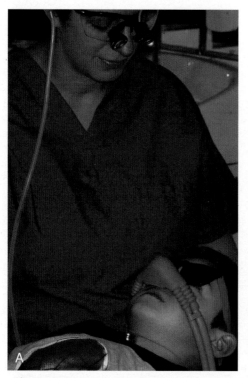
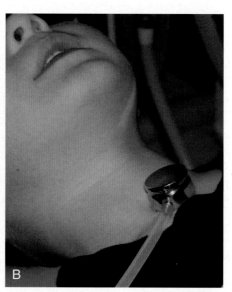

• **Figure 8.6** (A and B) Placement of precordial stethoscope for monitoring heart and respiratory sounds.

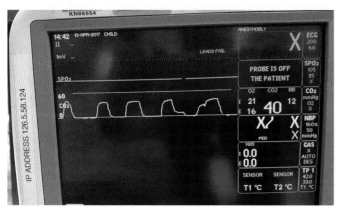

• **Figure 8.7** Capnograph monitor measuring concentration of carbon dioxide in respiratory gases.

in the soft tissue area immediately above the manubrium of the chest), the louder are the breathing sounds in comparison with the heart sounds. Partially occluded airways or restrictive airways have different sound qualities, including wheezing, stridor, and crowing. The precordial stethoscope is especially sensitive to competing operatory sounds (e.g., the pitch of the high-speed handpiece), and the operator must rely frequently on other clinical signs (e.g., chest excursions) or physiologic monitors (e.g., capnographs) (Fig. 8.7) to determine the stability and condition of the patient.

The Future

The level of training required for a dentist to administer sedation or anesthesia safely is currently under debate and is changing throughout the United States. In virtually all states, special permits are required to practice parenteral sedative techniques. Many states have instituted permits for adult and/or pediatric oral sedation as well.

Deep sedation and general anesthesia are grouped together for training requirements, medicolegal reasons, and purposes of malpractice insurance. *The clinician should remember that a sedation technique from which a patient is not easily aroused and may not respond purposefully to verbal commands at all times is, by definition, deep sedation.* The suggested educational requirement for administration of deep sedation or general anesthesia is completion of a CODA-accredited residency training program that provides comprehensive training in general anesthesia. All states have adopted

requirements for the administration of deep sedation and general anesthesia by dentists.

Summary

A pharmacologic approach to managing the behavior of uncooperative children in the dental office with sedation is very complex and requires additional training beyond the scope of this textbook. An undersedated child may continue to pose a management problem, whereas oversedation of a child may quickly become a life-threatening emergency in the dental office.

References

1. Consensus development conference statement on anesthesia and sedation in the dental office. National Institutes of Health. *J Am Dent Assoc.* 1985;111(1):90–93.
2. Cote CJ, Wilson S. Guidelines for monitoring and management of pediatric patients during and after sedation for diagnostic and therapeutic procedures: an update. *Pediatrics.* 2006;118(6):2587–2602.
3. Anderson JA, Vann WF Jr. Respiratory monitoring during pediatric sedation: pulse oximetry and capnography. *Pediatr Dent.* 1988;10(2):94–101.
4. Wilson S. Conscious sedation and pulse oximetry: false alarms? *Pediatr Dent.* 1990;12(4):228–232.
5. Wilson S. Review of monitors and monitoring during sedation with emphasis on clinical applications. *Pediatr Dent.* 1995;17(7):413–418.
6. Coté CJ, Karl HW, Notterman DA, et al. Adverse sedation events in pediatrics: analysis of medications used for sedation. *Pediatrics.* 2000;106(4):633–644.
7. Coté CJ, Notterman DA, Karl HW, et al. Adverse sedation events in pediatrics: a critical incident analysis of contributing factors. *Pediatrics.* 2000;105(4 Pt 1):805–814.
8. Jastak JT, Peskin RM. Major morbidity or mortality from office anesthetic procedures: a closed-claim analysis of 13 cases. *Anesth Progr.* 1991;38(2):39–44.
9. Krippaehne JA, Montgomery MT. Morbidity and mortality from pharmacosedation and general anesthesia in the dental office. *J Oral Maxillofac Surg.* 1992;50(7):691–698, discussion 98–99.
10. Cohen EN, Gift HC, Brown BW, et al. Occupational disease in dentistry and chronic exposure to trace anesthetic gases. *J Am Dent Assoc.* 1980;101(1):21–31.
11. Rowland AS, Baird DD, Weinberg CR, et al. Reduced fertility among women employed as dental assistants exposed to high levels of nitrous oxide. *N Engl J Med.* 1992;327(14):993–997.
12. Nathan JE, West MS. Comparison of chloral hydrate-hydroxyzine with and without meperidine for management of the difficult pediatric patient. *ASDC J Dent Child.* 1987;54(6):437–444.

9

Antimicrobials in Pediatric Dentistry

CINDY L. MAREK AND SHERRY R. TIMMONS

CHAPTER OUTLINE

The necessity for antimicrobial drug use in pediatric dentistry arises from a variety of circumstances, including odontogenic infections, oral wounds, periodontal disease, candidosis, and primary herpetic gingivostomatitis. Successful management of infections relies on the practitioner's knowledge of the microbiology of odontogenic and intraoral infections and the spectrum of activity, pharmacology, and adverse effects of the antimicrobial agents being prescribed. In addition, patient-specific factors such as overall health, concomitant medications, and the ability to afford or comply with the prescribed drug regimen must be considered. In the case of pediatric patients, compliance with unpalatable liquid medications can be especially problematic.

Antimicrobials (or antiinfectives) are substances that kill or suppress the growth or multiplication of microorganisms, either bacteria, viruses, fungi, or parasites. These agents exert selective toxicity, meaning dilute concentrations cause damage to microorganisms without causing harm to the host cells, thus allowing for safe and effective use. Selective toxicity occurs because the cells of microorganisms differ from human cells in their biochemistry, anatomy, and affinity for these substances.[1]

Antimicrobial Classification and Use

Microbiology

Antibiotics are defined as substances naturally produced by microorganisms (yeast or fungi) and used to inhibit bacteria and sometimes protozoa. Semisynthetic agents such as sulfonamides and fluoroquinolones also fall into this category.

Maximally effective antimicrobial therapy occurs after a definitive identification of the pathogen is made via culture or serologic testing, which is followed by susceptibility testing to determine which therapeutic agent is most effective against the pathogen. In outpatient dentistry the recognition of common causative pathogens, along with the most efficacious antimicrobial agents against those pathogens, is well established and microbiologic testing is rarely used.[2] However, culture and sensitivity testing can be useful in the treatment of recalcitrant infections, recurrent infections, postoperative infections, or suspected osteomyelitis or when the patient is significantly immunocompromised.[3]

The susceptibility of a microorganism to an antibiotic is based on the minimum inhibitory concentration (MIC), which is the lowest concentration of the drug which prevents growth of the microorganism. The organisms may still be viable, but they are no longer actively dividing.

The process of culture and sensitivity testing may take hours or days to complete. A rapid, preliminary identification of bacteria can often be obtained through a Gram stain (crystal violet) and microscopic evaluation. Bacteria that remain stained from crystal violet have a thick outer layer of peptidoglycan and are called gram-positive bacteria. Gram-negative bacteria have an outermost lipopolysaccharide membrane that does not retain the stain. Microscopic evaluation reveals morphology. Medically significant gram-positive pathogens are frequently cocci (spheres) rather than bacilli (rods).[1] Streptococci tend to appear in pairs or chains, whereas staphylococci form clusters.

Other common microbiologic tests include:

- Rapid catalase test—differentiates between staphylococci and streptococci.
- Blood agar plates (BAPs)—patterns of hemolysis (clearing around colonies) are used to differentiate streptococci. β-Hemolytic activity reveals lysis and complete digestion of red blood cell (RBC) contents. α-Hemolysis (*Streptococcus viridans*) causes partial lysis of RBCs and results in green/brown appearance on the plate. γ-Hemolysis refers to no hemolytic activity and the plate remains the original red color.
- Coagulase test—differentiates *Staphylococcus aureus*, a virulent coagulase positive microorganism, from *Staphylococcus epidermidis* (coagulase negative), which is a common blood culture contaminant.[1]

Chemotherapeutic Spectrum of Activity

An antibiotic's *spectrum of activity* refers to the species of microorganisms affected by the drug. Narrow-spectrum antibiotics are active against a single or limited group of microorganisms (e.g., some gram-positive organisms). Extended-spectrum antibiotics are effective against gram-positive organisms and a significant number of gram-negative organisms.

Broad-spectrum antibiotics act against a wide variety of species. These agents are often initially prescribed to neutropenic or critically ill patients while awaiting the results of culture and sensitivity testing. Administering broad-spectrum agents can significantly alter the normal flora and precipitate superinfection of a commensal organism to a pathogen (*Candida albicans*).[1] Practitioners should choose the narrowest spectrum antibiotic that will target the identified pathogen(s).

Bacteriostatic Versus Bacteriocidal Agents

Antimicrobial agents are classified as either bacteriostatic or bactericidal (Box 9.1). Bacteriostatic drugs limit the spread of the infection by halting bacterial growth and replication. This allows the body's immune system to attack, immobilize, and kill the pathogens. To eradicate the infection, the patient's host defense mechanisms must be intact. Host defense mechanisms can be compromised by a variety of conditions, including alcoholism, diabetes, malnutrition, advanced age, infection with human immunodeficiency virus, and immunosuppressant drugs. The effects of bacteriostatic antibiotics on microorganisms are reversible. If

Bactericidal	Bacteriostatic
Aminoglycosides	Clindamycin[a]
Carbapenems	Macrolides[a]
Cephalosporins	Sulfonamides
Fluoroquinolones	Trimethoprim
Metronidazole	Tetracyclines
Penicillins	
Vancomycin	

• **BOX 9.1 Bactericidal and Bacteriostatic Antibiotics**

[a]May be bactericidal against some organisms or at higher concentrations.
Data from Flynn TR. Principles of management of odontogenic infections. In: Miloro M, Ghali GE, Larsen PE, Waite PD, eds. Peterson's Principles of Oral and Maxillofacial Surgery. 2nd ed. Hamilton, Ontario: BC Decker, Inc.; 2004. Used with permission of PMPH USA, Ltd., Raleigh, North Carolina.

patient compliance is poor or the drug is discontinued before the organisms have been scavenged, a second cycle of the infection may occur because remaining viable bacteria will be able to grow and replicate.

Bactericidal drugs act independently of host immune defenses to cause cell death. These effects are irreversible—the microorganism will ultimately die following adequate drug exposure. Bactericidal drugs are preferred for most infections, including intraoral infections, due to the fact that they act largely independent of host factors, which is an important consideration for rapidly progressing infections or when the patient is immunocompromised. It should be noted that some antibiotics may be cidal to certain microorganisms and have a static effect on others or the effect may be concentration dependent.[4]

Many bactericidal drugs, including β-lactam antibiotics and vancomycin, act when the cell is actively growing or dividing. Concomitant administration of a bacteriostatic drug with a β-lactam antibiotic or similarly acting drug can interfere with the effectiveness of the bactericidal antibiotic.[4]

Categories of Antibiotic Use

The clinical use of antibiotics falls into one of three categories: prophylactic, empiric, or definitive. Prophylaxis is the use of antimicrobial chemotherapy to prevent an infection. Prophylactic therapy is intended for patients at high risk for developing an infection. Common reasons include disease states (previous bacterial endocarditis, uncontrolled diabetes), immunosuppressive drug therapy, and high-risk surgery.[1] Due to emerging resistance patterns and risk of superinfection, prophylactic administration of antibiotics should occur only when the benefit outweighs the risk. The duration of the prophylaxis regimen is dictated by the duration of risk.[1]

In medical and dental practice, most antibiotics are prescribed empirically. This approach works particularly well in dentistry, due to the extensive information available on both the causative organisms seen in dental infections and the best agents to eradicate them. Unless the infection is severe or rapidly spreading, a penicillin is generally the drug of choice assuming the patient does not have an allergy. If the infection fails to improve or worsens, then a broader-spectrum drug with good anaerobic activity is chosen.

Definitive antimicrobial therapy occurs following culture and susceptibility tests. Empiric therapy in medical practice often initially uses a broad-spectrum antibiotic, especially if the patient is seriously ill. After the organism is identified, the clinician should then choose an agent that is narrower in spectrum to target the specific pathogen.

The failure to transition to definitive therapy and the widespread use of empiric antibiotics in medicine are major factors contributing to the global burden of drug resistance.[1]

Antimicrobial Mechanisms of Action

Antimicrobial agents exert their effects on microorganisms through various mechanisms including: the inhibition of cell wall synthesis, inhibition of ribosomal protein synthesis, suppression of deoxyribonucleic acid (DNA) synthesis, disruption of cell membrane integrity, and alteration of cell membrane permeability.[5] Selected antimicrobial agents and their mechanisms of action are listed in Box 9.2.

In general, antimicrobials that suppress DNA synthesis or affect the cell wall or cell membrane tend to be bactericidal, whereas those that inhibit protein or folic acid synthesis result in a bacteriostatic effect. Understanding the mechanisms of action of antibiotics frequently used in dental practice is an important component of rational prescribing.

Inhibition of Cell Wall Synthesis

The β-lactam antibiotics classified according to their ring structure include penicillins (penams), cephalosporins (cephams), carbapenems, and monobactam, among others. These groups share the four-sided β-lactam ring structure, which imparts similar features of chemistry, mechanism of action, pharmacology, and immunologic characteristics.[6] Most β-lactams are fused to five- or six-membered rings; the exception is monobactam, which contains only the β-lactam ring. These agents selectively act on bacteria because they have cell walls versus mammalian cells that are encased by outer membranes.

β-Lactam antibiotics exert their bactericidal effects by disrupting bacterial cell wall synthesis. Bacterial cell walls consist of peptidoglycan, a cross-linked polymer of polysaccharides and polypeptides. Cross-linkage of peptides is necessary for the formation of a rigid cell wall that can withstand the osmotic pressure of the cytopasm.[6] Penicillin is a structural analogue of D-alanine and acts by competitively inhibiting the final transpeptidation reaction (removal of a terminal D-alanine) necessary to complete cross-linkage. Inhibiting transpeptidase (also known as penicillin-binding protein) halts peptidoglycan synthesis and ultimately results in cell death.

In some organisms the presence of β-lactam antibiotics causes the derepression of an endogenous autolysin. Autolysins are enzymes that selectively break down the rigid peptidoglycan matrix to allow for cell growth and division. Excessive amounts of autolysin will weaken the peptidoglycan and result in cell lysis.[6]

Vancomycin is a tricyclic glycopeptide antibiotic which disrupts cell wall synthesis by binding to the terminal D-alanine–D-alanine chains on the peptidoglycan cell wall, preventing elongation of the peptidoglycan chains (one step ahead of β-lactams).[1,6] Vancomycin requires active cell growth to exert bactericidal effects.[6] The large molecular size of the vancomycin molecule prevents the drug from entering gram-negative bacteria, limiting its spectrum of activity to aerobic and anaerobic gram-positive bacteria.[7] Vancomycin is effective against multiple drug-resistant organisms, including methicillin-resistant staphylococci and most enterococci and *Clostridium difficile*.[1]

Both β-lactam antibiotics and vancomycin exhibit time-dependent bactericidal effects. This means that the bactericidal activity continues as long as the serum concentrations are greater than the minimum bactericidal concentration (MBC) of the antimicrobial agent against the pathogens.

Inhibition of Protein Synthesis

Antimicrobials that inhibit protein synthesis target the bacterial ribosome which is structurally different from the human ribosome (70S vs. 80S in mammals).[5] The bacterial ribosome functions to translate messenger RNA, adding the correct amino acid to make the protein. The bacterial ribosome is composed of a 50S and 30S subunit. Macrolides and clindamycin both bind irreversibly to the same site on the 50S subunit, inhibiting translocation steps of protein synthesis.[7] Tetracycline antibiotics bind to the 30S subunit, blocking amino acyl-tRNA from adding amino acids to the protein, thus halting protein growth.[5,8]

Aminoglycosides (gentamycin, tobramycin, amikacin) irreversibly bind to the separated 30S ribosomal subunit and interfere with the microbial genetic code, producing a bactericidal effect.[7,9] Susceptible organisms have an oxygen-dependent transport system that allows the drug to enter the cell wall; therefore the agents are effective only against aerobic organisms.[9] A high degree of toxicity (nephrotoxicity and ototoxicity) limits their use. Aminoglycosides (usually gentamycin) are combined with β-lactam antibiotics to produce a synergistic effect. Cell wall inhibition by β-lactam enhances the entry of the aminoglycoside into the cell.[8]

Many agents that inhibit protein or DNA synthesis (aminoglycosides, quinolones) exhibit concentration-dependent killing

---

• BOX 9.2   Antimicrobial Mechanisms of Action

Inhibition of Cell Wall Synthesis
β-Lactam antibiotics
    Penicillins (penams)
    Cephalosporins (cephems)
    Monobactams
    Carbapenems
Vancomycin

Inhibition of Protein Synthesis
Bind 50S ribosome
    Clindamycin
    Macrolides

Bind 30S ribosome
    Aminoglycosides
    Tetracyclines

Suppression of DNA Synthesis
Fluoroquinolones

Alteration of Cell Membrane Permeability
Polyene antifungals
Azole antifungals

Data from Carroll KC, Morse A, Mietzner T, Miller S, et al., eds. Antimicrobial chemotherapy. In: Jawetz, Melnick, & Adelberg's Medical Microbiology. 27th ed. New York: McGraw-Hill; 2016:363–396.

of bacteria where the rate and extent of killing increases as the peak drug concentration increases.[9] These drugs also exhibit a "postantibiotic effect" where the inhibition of bacterial growth persists, even after a short exposure to the drug. Proposed mechanisms for this effect include slow recovery of bacteria after nonlethal drug exposure, the need to synthesize new proteins, and antibiotic occupation of the binding site.[4] The clinical advantage of drugs with long postantibiotic effects (aminoglycosides, azithromycin, fluoroquinolones) is longer dosing intervals. Fewer doses per day result in increased compliance.

Suppression of DNA Synthesis

Fluoroquinolones enter cells through passive diffusion and interfere with the action of DNA gyrase (topoisomerase II) and topoisomerase IV by complexing with the topoisomerase-DNA during bacterial growth. Topoisomerase enzymes change the topography of DNA by causing transient breaks in the helix which are necessary for relaxation of the supercoiled DNA and successful bacterial cell division. They are "involved in the crucial processes of DNA replication, transcription, and recombination."[7] Fluoroquinolone-mediated cell death occurs through a variety of mechanisms that destabilize and inactivate the bacterial DNA.

Alteration of Cell Membrane Permeability

Ergosterol is a sterol that resides on the cell membranes of fungi and acts to maintain cell membrane integrity, similar to mammalian cholesterol. Polyene antimycotic agents (amphotericin B, nystatin) are a subset of macrolide antibiotics that bind to ergosterol on the cell membranes of fungi. The bound drug molecules form a pore in the ergosterol which allows electrolytes and small molecules to leak out of the cell.[10]

Azole antifungals (fluconazole, itraconazole, ketoconazole) act to prevent the conversion of lanosterol to ergosterol by inhibiting fungal cytochrome P450. Without the protective layer of ergosterol, the cell membrane becomes permeable, leaking intracellular contents.[10] Interestingly, the azoles have an antagonistic effect on the polyene antimycotics—they can only bind to ergosterol.[11]

Adverse Effects of Antimicrobials

Allergic Reactions

Antimicrobials and other drugs trigger immunologic reactions through activation of the adaptive immune system. Patients may experience an allergic reaction to a medication upon first exposure due to cross-reactivity between the current medication and one previously taken.[12] Associated reactions may be immediate (anaphylaxis or hives) or delayed (drug fever, skin rashes).[1]

The true incidence of allergic reactions to medications is far lower than reported by patients or caregivers. Reactions to medications such as gastrointestinal (GI) intolerance, nausea, hypotension, or dizziness are often considered allergies to the drug, when they are adverse events (side effects). The clinician should follow up any report of a drug allergy with questions to determine the likelihood of a true allergic event.

Patients will report an allergy to penicillin, for example, when the reaction occurred in a parent or sibling because they believe the response is hereditary in nature. When the reaction to the medication is unknown, the patient should be considered allergic to the drug until proven otherwise through a drug history report or sensitivity testing. When it has been determined the patient experienced intolerance to a drug as opposed to an allergy, it should be noted as such and discussed with the patient or caregiver.

Photosensitivity Reactions

Drug photosensitivity reactions have been associated with antimicrobials, nonsteroidal antiinflammatory drugs (NSAIDs), thiazide diuretics, and other classes of topical and systemic medications. Photosensitivity reactions can be either phototoxic or, rarely, photoallergic in nature.

Phototoxic reactions to medications occurs when the drug becomes activated through exposure to sunlight or ultraviolet A (UV-A) light. The reaction can occur quickly, within minutes to hours of exposure, and causes an acute inflammatory response in the areas exposed to light. The resulting erythema resembles an exaggerated sunburn. Symptoms include rapid onset of burning sensation, edema, erythema, and occasional blisters. Lighter-skinned patients tend to be more prone to this problem.[13]

Medications such as nonsteroidal antiinflammatory agents, fluoroquinolone antibiotics, and tetracyclines exhibit this reaction, primarily interacting with UV-A light. The occurrence of photosensitivity with doxycycline is estimated to be up to 35% and is a dose-dependent reaction.[13] In addition, acyclovir, azithromycin, and itraconazole have been associated with photosensitivity, although the incidence is less frequent. Counseling patients to avoid direct sunlight and the use of tanning facilities during antimicrobial treatment and administering the medications in the evening when possible will help to minimize this adverse effect.[13]

Photoallergic reactions are immune-mediated and occur less often than phototoxic reactions. These reactions are usually due to longer UV-A wavelengths (>315 nm) and will develop in patients who are already sensitized. Similar to allergic dermatitis, "the reaction can appear as solar urticaria or as eczematous or as lichenoid dermatitis on predominantly light-exposed areas."[13]

Long QT Interval Syndrome

The QT interval on the electrocardiogram (ECG) represents the time it takes to fire an impulse through the ventricles and then repolarize—in other words, how long it takes for the heart to recover after contraction. Long QT syndrome (LQTS) is due to a defect in the heart's ion channels and increases the risk for torsades de pointes, a potentially life-threatening ventricular tachycardia.

LQTS can be congenital or acquired. Congenital LQTS risk factors include congenital deafness and children with sudden death, known LQTS, or syncope in family members.[14] Acquired LQTS can be caused by medications, especially if the patient has an underlying genetic predisposition. Although macrolide antibiotics account for a majority of the cases, fluoroquinolones and clindamycin are also known to cause this disorder.[7]

Drug-Drug Interactions

The number of recognized interactions between antimicrobial agents and other medications is ever increasing as metabolic enzymes and drug transporters continue to be identified.[15]

Therefore it is impossible for clinicians to be aware of all the possible drug-drug interactions for medications they prescribe. Comprehensive online drug information resources often contain a "drug interaction checker" that will analyze a list of medications to determine the likelihood and severity of drug-drug interactions.

Obtaining a thorough history of current prescription medications, over-the-counter agents, along with herbal and dietary supplements is a prerequisite to prescribing any medication.

Antibacterial Agents

Penicillins

All penicillins (penams) share the general structure of a thiazolidine ring attached to a β-lactam ring that carries a free amino group, thus forming the 6-aminopenicillanic acid core (Fig. 9.1). Substituents to the core structure at the site of the amino group give rise to the individual drugs in this class, each possessing unique antibacterial and pharmacologic properties. These characteristics place the individual drugs within one of three general classes (Table 9.1).

Absorption of orally administered penicillins varies from 15% to 80%, due in part to their chemical degradation by stomach acids, degree of binding to foods, and buffering.[5] Oral absorption of most penicillins is impaired by food, and they should be given 1 hour before or 2 hours after a meal. Exceptions are penicillin VK and amoxicillin, which can be given without regard to meals. Penicillins have short half-lives and need to be dosed three to four times daily. Penicillin concentrations in most tissues equal serum concentrations.

Most penicillins are minimally metabolized and are primarily excreted by the kidneys. The elimination half-life of these agents will increase as renal function declines, thus dosage adjustments are necessary for patients with significant renal impairment. Antistaphylococcal penicillins (oxacillin, nafcillin) are partially eliminated by the liver and require dosage adjustment in patients with hepatic disease.

Penicillins exhibit time-dependent killing of bacteria, in part because they do not enter the cell cytoplasm. Without postantibiotic effect, therapeutic success relies on the drug concentration remaining greater than the MBC throughout the entire dosing interval because only bacterial cells actively growing will be affected by the drug.[6] Patients must adhere to the dosing regimen as closely as possible, and the dosage interval should be given in hours as opposed to "three times daily."

Penicillin G and V

Penicillin G, discovered by Alexander Fleming in 1928, was first available commercially in 1942, ushering in the antibiotic era. The activity of penicillin G was originally defined in units, with 1600 units equal to 1 mg. Newer, semisynthetic penicillins are dosed on a milligram (mg) basis.

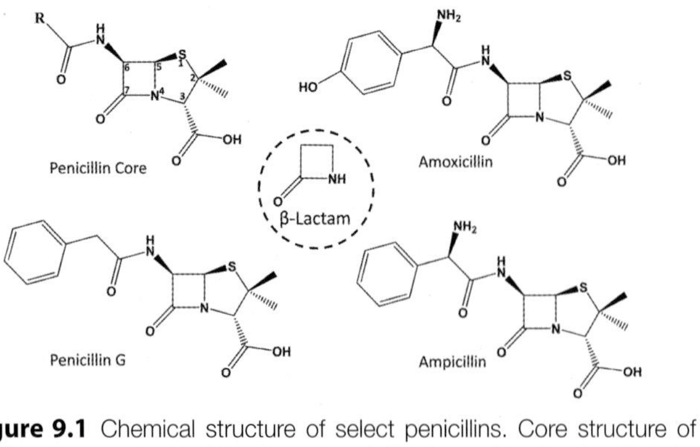

Penicillin G and penicillin V (phenoxymethylpenicillin) are "natural" penicillins, with a narrow-spectrum of activity due to the development of penicillinases (β-lactamases active against penicillins). Staphylococci, initially sensitive to penicillin G, are now considered highly resistant. Natural penicillins still maintain activity against other gram-positive cocci and bacilli and gram-negative cocci.

Benzathine and procaine salts of penicillin G are designed for depot intramuscular injections which are used to provide prolonged blood and tissue levels. Penicillin G benzathine intramuscular injections are primarily used to treat *Treponema* infections and to eradicate colonization of group A β-hemolytic streptococci in chronic carriers. Benzathine is the least soluble salt form of penicillin G, thus providing the longest duration of action (up to 3 weeks).[1,5,6]

Penicillin G procaine is usually given once daily and injected into the midlateral thigh or upper outer quadrant of the gluteus maximus. In infants and small children, injection into the midlateral muscles of the thigh is preferred to avoid injury to the sciatic nerve (from a gluteal injection). Blood levels obtained from an injection of penicillin G procaine are prolonged, but low compared with intravenous (IV) administration of penicillin G potassium.[1,5,6]

IV administration of penicillin G is preferred to the intramuscular route, due to the discomfort associated with the administration

• **Figure 9.1** Chemical structure of select penicillins. Core structure of the β-lactam ring along with selected penicillin drugs showing the diversity of the R side chain. (From Pichichero ME, Zagursky R. Penicillin and cephalosporin allergy. *Ann Allergy Asthma Immunol.* 2014;112[5]: 404–412.)

TABLE 9.1 Penicillins

Drug Class and Name	Route	Acid Stable	Penicillinase Resistant
Penicillins			
Penicillin G benzathine	IM	No	No
Penicillin G potassium	IV, (IM)	No	No
Penicillin G procaine	IM	No	No
Penicillin V	PO	Yes	No
Antistaphylococcal Penicillins			
Cloxacillin	PO[a]	Yes	
Dicloxacillin	PO	Yes	
Oxacillin	PO,[a] IM, IV	Yes	Yes
Nafcillin	IM, IV	No	Yes
Extended-Spectrum Penicillins			
Aminopenicillins			
Amoxicillin	PO	Yes	No
Ampicillin	PO, IM, IV	Yes	No
Amoxicillin/clavulanic acid	PO	Yes	Yes
Piperacillin/tazobactam	IM, IV	No	Yes
Ticarcillin/clavulanic acid	IM, IV	No	Yes

[a]No oral formulations are currently on the US market.
IM, Intramuscular; *IV*, intravenous; *PO*, oral.

of large doses. Oral penicillin G is no longer used because it is subject to degradation in the presence of stomach acid.

Penicillin V and amoxicillin have chemical structures that enhance their stability in acidic environments and result in improved oral absorption (bioavailability). Penicillin V is administered orally as the potassium salt and is dosed at 6-hour intervals. Penicillin VK can be taken without regard to meals. Historically, penicillin VK has been the drug of choice to treat mild to moderate dental infections in nonallergic patients.

Amoxicillin and Ampicillin

Ampicillin and amoxicillin are the two aminopenicillins remaining on the US market. These agents have an extended spectrum over penicillin V, but resistance has emerged with gram-negative bacilli and other microorganisms due to widespread use.

The aminopenicillins have similar spectrums of activity, but amoxicillin is the preferred agent over ampicillin for a variety of reasons. Amoxicillin may be taken without regard to meals and is dosed every 8 hours. Ampicillin must be dosed every 6 hours. Food decreases both the rate of oral absorption and the peak plasma concentrations of ampicillin; therefore it must be given on an empty stomach. In addition, amoxicillin is more bioavailable than ampicillin; improved oral absorption reduces the incidence of diarrhea.

Amoxicillin has replaced penicillin VK as the drug of choice for the prevention of infective endocarditis by the American Heart Association because amoxicillin produces higher and longer sustained blood levels than penicillin VK. Ampicillin is still used in IV prophylaxis regimens because amoxicillin is not available in an IV dosage form in the United States.

Amoxicillin/Clavulanate

Clavulanate potassium (the potassium salt of clavulanic acid) is a β-lactamase inhibitor which is added to amoxicillin to prevent inactivation by bacterial enzymes. β-Lactamase inhibitors (clavulanate, sulbactam, tazobactam) irreversibly bind to β-lactamase.[1] These agents are not active against all β-lactamase enzymes. It is important to note that β-lactamase inhibitors do not enhance the intrinsic activity of the antibiotic or extend the drug's spectrum of activity. The inhibitors simply bind up the β-lactamase enzymes, allowing the drug to kill the bacteria.

The manufacturer recommends taking amoxicillin/clavulanate at the beginning of a meal to enhance the absorption of clavulanate and to decrease GI irritation. Clavulanate can cause severe diarrhea if given in excess. It is especially important for practitioners to understand that not all dosage forms of amoxicillin/clavulanate are appropriate for children.

Amoxicillin/clavulanate products contain different ratios of amoxicillin to clavulanate, ranging from 2 mg amoxicillin:1 mg clavulanate for the 250/125-mg oral tablet to 16 mg amoxicillin:1 mg clavulanate in the 1000/62.5-mg extended release tablet. Therefore these products are not interchangeable. Because both the 250- and 500-mg oral tablets of amoxicillin/clavulanate contain 125 mg of clavulanate, two of the 250-mg tablets cannot be substituted for one of the 500-mg tablets.

Likewise, 250-mg chewable tablets (62.5 mg clavulanate) are not equivalent to 250-mg oral tablets (125 mg clavulanate). The 250-mg oral tablet should not be used until the pediatric patient weighs at least 40 kg or more. Even though children may be able to swallow an oral tablet, they should be given either the chewable tablet or the suspension until they weigh at least 40 kg. Dosages listed for this product are based on the amoxicillin component.

The appropriate dosage form listed with the dosage recommendation should always be used to avoid overdosing clavulanate in children (Box 9.3).[16-19]

Cephalosporins (Cephams)

Cephalosporins are closely related in structure and function to penicillins, with a six-membered dihydrothiazine ring replacing the five-membered thiazolidine ring. In general, their spectrum of activity is broader than that of penicillins, due to a greater stability in the presence of β-lactamases. Currently there are five generations of cephalosporins, with successive generations becoming broader in spectrum adding antianaerobic activity, antipseudomonal activity, and enhanced stability to β-lactamases.

The first-generation cephalosporins available for oral use are cephalexin and cefadroxil. The second-generation cephalosporins are more stable against gram-negative β-lactamases but have weaker gram-positive activity.[1] Oral second-generation agents include cefaclor, cefprozil, cefuroxime, and loracarbef. The cephamycins have good intrinsic activity against anaerobes, but the *Bacteroides fragilis* group is becoming increasingly resistant.[1]

The third-generation agents exhibit greater gram-negative activity, good streptococcal activity, but less staphylococcal activity than earlier generations.[1] These agents are associated with a high incidence of *C. difficile*–induced diarrhea, and resistance in gram-negative rods is widespread. Cefepine is the only fourth-generation agent and has the broadest activity of all cephalosporins.

Cephalosporins have traditionally played a small role in dental pharmacotherapeutics. Some first- and second-generation orally available agents may be of use in select patients with a history of penicillin allergy (non-type I).

Clindamycin

Clindamycin is a lincosamide antibiotic, chemically unrelated to erythromycins. There is no cross-allergenicity between macrolides and clindamycin. Clindamycin has significant activity against nonenterococcal gram-positive organisms and numerous anaerobes, including *B. fragilis*. It is both bacteriostatic and bactericidal. Clindamycin is nearly 100% bioavailable via the oral route, but oral doses are lower than IV doses due to gastric intolerance. It has good distribution in all fluids (except the cerebrospinal fluid [CSF]) and penetrates bone and abscesses. Clindamycin is taken up by phagocytic cells and fibroblasts, which deliver the antibiotic to areas of inflammation and infection.[8]

Clindamycin's activity against oral pathogens makes it the drug of choice for significant oral infections. It is available in a pediatric powder for solution that contains 75 mg clindamycin/5 mL (100-mL bottle) in addition to the 150-mg and 300-mg capsules. The solution is not very palatable.

Clindamycin is associated with an increased risk of *C. difficile* infection (CDI). *C. difficile* is a spore-forming anaerobic bacillus that produces a toxin that can cause a variety of serious GI symptoms.[20,21] A large study by Adams et al. found "recent exposure to fluoroquinolones, clindamycin, and third-generation cephalosporins, and to multiple classes of antibiotics"[20] are associated with the subsequent diagnosis of community-acquired CDI in children. The study identified exposure to proton pump inhibitors, outpatient medical clinics, and family members with CDI as additional risk factors. Surprisingly, 40% of children diagnosed with CDI in this study had no preceding antibiotic

---

• BOX 9.3   Adverse Reactions of Penicillins and Cephalosporins

An estimated 10% of the population report having a penicillin allergy, yet more than 90% of these patients do not demonstrate immunoglobulin E (IgE) antibodies upon skin testing.[17] An estimated 97% of patients with a confirmed IgE-mediated allergy will tolerate cephalosporins and 99% will tolerate carbapenems.[17] However, β-lactams remain the leading cause of drug-induced anaphylaxis and anaphylactic deaths in the United States.[7,17]

The chemical structure of β-lactam antibiotics provides multiple antigenic determinates (β-lactam ring, attached ring structure, R-group side chains) that can react with antibodies in patients with IgE-mediated allergic reactions. Patterns of sensitization vary in populations. Cross-allergenicity exists for all penicillins. The scientific literature differs on the issue of cross-sensitivity between penicillin groups and cephalosporins.

There is evidence that the R1 side chain off the β-lactam ring can determine the rate of cross-reactivity between penicillins and cephalosporins.[16,18] The aminopenicillins, amoxicillin, and ampicillin have the same R-group side chains as several first- and second-generation cephalosporins. These cephalosporins should be avoided in patients with known penicillin allergies (Table 9.2).[16,18]

Risk factors for penicillin allergy include a history of allergic reactions to multiple drugs (especially antibiotics), atopic disease (asthma, nasal polyps, allergic rhinitis),[7] and multiple exposures to the drug. Penicillin skin testing is a valuable aid in determining if a patient can safely use penicillins.

Penicillins can cause multiple types of allergic reactions, but the immediate IgE reactions pose the most acute threat. These reactions can begin within seconds to an hour after drug exposure. Symptoms may include urticaria, bronchospasm, wheezing, hypotension, skin erythema, and angioedema. Nearly all fatal anaphylactic reactions occur within the first 60 minutes after penicillin exposure.[7]

Less than 5% of patients receiving an aminopenicillin may experience a mild, pruritic rash that may occur at any time during the course of therapy and rarely occurs up to 2 weeks after the cessation of the antibiotic.[19] The cause of the reaction is unknown but does not increase the risk of penicillin allergy. This rash will occur in nearly all patients with mononucleosis or cytomegalovirus.[7]

TABLE 9.2   Aminopenicillins That Cross-React With Cephalosporins

Penicillin	Cephalosporins That Cross React	Common R1 Side Chain
Amoxicillin	Cefaclor[a]	
Ampicillin	Cefadroxil[b]	
	Cefatrizine[b]	
	Cefprozil[a]	
	Cephalexin[b]	
	Cephradine[b]	

[a]Second generation.
[b]First generation.
Penicillin and cephalosporins known to have a risk of allergic cross-reaction. These cephalosporins should be avoided in patients who are allergic to penicillin.
Patients who are selectively allergic to amoxicillin or ampicillin should avoid the cephalosporins listed, because they have similar R1-group chains.
From Campagna JD, Bond MC, Schabelman E, Hayes BD. The use of cephalosporins in penicillin-allergic patients: a literature review. *J Emerg Med.* 2012;42(5):612–612.

---

exposure, highlighting the importance of recognizing other factors that lead to community-acquired CDI in both children and adults.[20]

Macrolides

The macrolides are a group of antibiotics with a macrocyclic lactone structure. Erythromycin was the first drug available in this class, but it is rarely used nowadays due to GI intolerance, frequent dosing, and multiple drug interactions. The newer macrolides, azithromycin and clarithromycin, are among the most frequently prescribed antibiotics in the outpatient setting, due to their activity against a broad range of respiratory pathogens. Not surprisingly, resistance is increasing to these newer agents, especially in *Streptococcus pneumoniae*.[1]

Macrolides should not be prescribed to patients who have a known hypersensitivity to any other macrolide as these drugs show cross-sensitivity. All macrolides are eliminated through the liver. The macrolides have numerous drug interactions and can prolong the QT interval. These agents should be used with caution in patients with preexisting heart conditions, especially arrhythmias.

Macrolides have moderate coverage over many streptococci but poor coverage of anaerobes and other oral pathogens, limiting their usefulness in dentistry. Due to the ever-increasing list of drug-drug and drug-disease interactions with these agents, it is important to always check for interactions before prescribing macrolides.

Azithromycin

Azithromycin exhibits significant intracellular penetration and concentrates within phagocytes and fibroblasts, thus the levels in tissues are much greater than in plasma. This drug has a long half-life in children (32 to 64 hours). Through selective uptake by fibroblasts and phagocytic cells, tissue concentrations may be 100 to 1000 times that of blood.[7] Azithromycin is available in 250-, 500-, and 600-mg oral tablets and as a 100-mg/5 mL and 200-mg/5 mL powder for suspension. IV azithromycin is sometimes combined with an IV β-lactam when atypical pathogens are suspected for inpatients with community-acquired pneumonia.[8]

The most common adverse effects in pediatric patients receiving azithromycin are GI effects which are dose-related. Azithromycin is not appreciably metabolized.

Clarithromycin

GI adverse effects are the most commonly reported adverse reactions associated with the use of clarithromycin and include diarrhea, nausea, vomiting, and up to a 19% rate of dysgeusia (metallic taste). All pediatric dosing recommendations are based on the immediate-release product formulations (tablet and oral suspension).[22] Immediate-release products can be taken without regard to meals and should be given every 12 hours, as opposed to twice daily, to avoid peak and trough variations. The manufacturer recommends giving the product with food if GI irritation occurs. Clarithromycin is available as 250- and 500-mg oral tablets, 500-mg extended-release tablets, and 125-mg/5 mL and 250-mg/5 mL powder for suspension.

Clarithromycin should be avoided in patients with hepatic disease because production of the active metabolite is reduced. It is partially eliminated by the kidneys; therefore patients with renal impairment may require dosage adjustment.

Metronidazole

Metronidazole belongs to the nitroimidazole class of antibiotics and is active against protozoa in addition to anaerobic bacteria. It is bactericidal to anaerobic organisms through formation of free radicals that inhibit DNA synthesis and cause DNA degradation.[23] This agent is equally effective against dividing and nondividing cells. Metronidazole is metabolized in the liver and should be used with caution in patients with hepatic dysfunction, due to decreased clearance and possible accumulation of metronidazole and its metabolites. Adverse effects include GI effects (nausea, epigastric distress, GI discomfort) and dysgeusia (metallic taste).

Oral metronidazole is the drug of choice for the treatment of mild to moderate *C. difficile* colitis. Metronidazole can be combined with amoxicillin or a cephalosporin for the treatment of periodontal disease or to enhance anaerobic coverage when a patient has risk factors for *C. difficile* colitis. The gram-negative anaerobes seen in acute orofacial infections and periodontal disease are very sensitive to metronidazole.

Because metronidazole does not affect aerobic organisms, it should not be used as single-agent therapy for dental infections. There is less resistance to metronidazole by *B. fragilis* than seen with clindamycin.[1]

Metronidazole inhibits alcohol-metabolizing enzymes, leading to an accumulation of acetaldehyde and the development of disulfiram-like adverse effects. Patients should not consume alcohol during metronidazole therapy and for at least 3 days after discontinuation.

Commonly available commercial dosage forms include 250- and 500-mg oral tablets. Metronidazole is a very bitter medication. Compounding pharmacists can grind up the tablets and make a pediatric suspension, but the taste cannot be masked and children will refuse the medication. FIRST-Metronidazole 100 and FIRST-Metronidazole 50 are commercially available compounding kits that use the benzoate salt of metronidazole to make a grape-flavored oral suspension.[24] The benzoate salt is nearly tasteless and the product should be more readily accepted by children. Both the 100-mg/mL and 50-mg/mL kits make 150 mL of suspension. The suspension must be shaken well before each use to ensure the correct dose. Although most pharmacies will not have these products in stock, they can usually be ordered and arrive the next day. Unfortunately, most insurance companies will not pay for these products and the cost of the 100-mg/mL suspension will be at least $130.

Fluoroquinolones

Fluoroquinolones (ciprofloxacin, levofloxacin, ofloxacin, etc.) are bactericidal antibiotics with broad-spectrum activity for a variety of gram-positive, gram-negative, and atypical organisms.[1] The overuse of these agents has led to increasing levels of resistance. The American Academy of Pediatrics Committee on Infectious diseases recommends reserving the use of these agents for infections caused by multidrug-resistant pathogens for which there is no safe and effective alternative.[25]

Adverse effects of these agents include photosensitivity, prolongation of the QT interval, and peripheral neuropathy. Historically, there has been a hesitancy to use this class of drugs in the pediatric population because arthropathy and osteochondrosis were seen in testing of juvenile animals. Unless indicated as an agent of choice after culture and sensitivity testing, there is no indication for the use of these agents in dentistry.

Antifungal Agents

Polyenes

Nystatin and amphotericin B bind to the ergosterol in the fungal cell membrane and form pores in the fungal cell membrane which allows leakage of the cell contents and eventual cell death.[1] Nystatin is considered a poor antifungal in activity. Amphotericin B has a broad spectrum of action, is fungicidal, and was the mainstay for IV treatment of systemic fungal infections prior to the development of the echinocandins and broad-spectrum azoles. Called "ampho terrible," the drug was noted for nephrotoxicity and infusion-related reactions. All patients have adverse reactions to systemic amphotericin B. Topical amphotericin B suspension was available on the US market for a few years but was discontinued by the manufacturer. This leaves nystatin, a poor antifungal, as the only topical polyene for the treatment of oral candidiasis.

Systemic toxicity of antifungal agents is due to their lack of selectivity for fungal versus human cells. Fungi, like us, are eukaryotic organisms which evolved with the animal kingdom. Common cellular and molecular processes and constituents make it more difficult to find a "target" to selectively affect fungi.

Nystatin

Nystatin is a topical polyene antifungal with a similar structure to amphotericin B. Nystatin binds to sterols in human and fungal cells. Though it is more selective for ergosterol than cholesterol, this lack of target specificity renders nystatin too toxic to administer IV. Nystatin is usually considered fungistatic, but can be cidal with high concentrations or highly susceptible organisms.[26] Nystatin is not absorbed orally.

Commercially available nystatin suspensions contain 100,000 µ/mL and are usually formulated with 33% to 50% sucrose to enhance stability. For mild oropharyngeal candidiasis, the suggested regimen by the Infectious Disease Society of America (ISDA) is 4 to 6 mL given four times daily for 7 to 14 days.[27] According to the ISDA guidelines, patients should swish the suspension in the mouth for several minutes before swallowing. Although the suspension can be swallowed, it can cause nausea and diarrhea. Many patients object to the taste of the oral suspension.

There is disagreement as to how long therapy should continue in immunocompetent patients. Some sources say therapy should continue for at least 10 days or for 48 hours after remission.[1] Shorter courses of therapy for oral candidiasis often result in recurrence of the infection. For this reason the ISDA and some drug references recommend a 14-day course of therapy.[28]

Azole Antifungals

The azoles inhibit fungal cytochrome P450, which results in decreased ergosterol production and a fungistatic effect. Fungal cytochrome P450s are 100 to 1000 times more sensitive to the azoles than are mammalian cells.[29] Azole effects on cytochrome P450 result in numerous, often serious, interactions with other drugs. Azoles are structurally divided into two groups: imidazoles and triazoles. The imidazoles consist of ketoconazole, miconazole, and clotrimazole.

Ketoconazole, approved by the US Food and Drug Administration (FDA) in 1981, was the first azole on the US market. Currently the FDA limits the use of oral ketoconazole to certain life-threatening systemic fungal infections, due to the risk of fatal liver damage, life-threatening drug interactions, and decreased sex hormone production in patients taking systemic ketoconazole. The two other members of the class are too toxic for systemic use and only available topically. The triazole class of antifungals has expanded to include broader-spectrum agents.

Newer azoles are available in both oral and IV dosage forms and are primarily indicated for serious systemic infections. These include voriconazole, a derivative of fluconazole, which has better antifungal specificity and improved efficacy than the parent compound. Voriconazole can be used in children as young as 3 years of age and is especially valuable in the treatment of mold infections. Posaconazole, an itraconazole analogue, is more active against a broader range of fungi and approved for adolescents. Isavuconazonium is the newest azole antifungal with an expanded spectrum of activity for invasive aspergillosis and mucormycosis in adults.[1]

Clotrimazole

Clotrimazole is available for topical use only. When used intraorally as a troche, only small amounts are absorbed and then metabolized in the liver. Usual administration is via 10-mg lozenges (troches), which are to be dissolved slowly in the mouth five times daily for 7 to 14 days.[30] The troches are FDA approved for children 3 years of age and older.[31]

Miconazole

Miconazole is also an imidazole antifungal available only for topical use. When used intraorally, the drug appears to be poorly absorbed.[32] For the treatment of oral candidiasis, a 50-mg adhesive buccal tablet is placed on the canine fossa once daily for 14 days. The buccal tablet is FDA indicated for patients aged 16 years and older. In clinical trials, patients using the buccal tablet experienced GI adverse events that included diarrhea, nausea, vomiting, and taste disturbances.[32] Average adherence of the buccal tablet is 15 hours.[33] One course of therapy costs approximately $1000, and insurance companies have been reluctant to pay for this product.

Fluconazole

The introduction of fluconazole in 1990 was hailed as a great advance in antifungal pharmacotherapy. Fluconazole has high oral bioavailability and good GI tolerance and is more selective for fungal cells than ketoconazole.[11,29] It is highly active against many species of candida. Fluconazole is FDA approved for children 6 months of age and older, although it is used in neonates to treat fungal meningitis.[34]

Fluconazole has been associated with QT prolongation and affects several cytochrome P450 enzymes (CYP2C9, CYP3A4), leading to multiple drug interactions. A search of the online database Clinical Pharmacology listed 70 drug products that had the potential for severe interactions with fluconazole and several hundred others that had lower levels of drug-drug interactions.[34]

A loading dose of fluconazole equal to two times the usual daily dose is given on the first day of therapy. With a loading dose, steady state plasma levels are achieved within 2 days of initiating therapy. Without a loading dose, it may take 5 to 10 days to achieve steady state.[34] The renal clearance of fluconazole is higher in children compared with adults, accounting for the higher doses given to children. The elimination half-life is approximately 15 to 20 hours in children compared with 30 hours for adults. Fluconazole is available for IV use and in a 50-, 100-, 150-, and 200-mg oral tablet and a 10-mg/mL and 40-mg/mL powder for suspension.

Itraconazole

Itraconazole is broader in spectrum than fluconazole, but its usefulness is limited for several reasons. Itraconazole has a daunting adverse effect profile which includes hepatotoxicity. It is a stronger inhibitor of cytochrome P450 enzymes meaning drug-drug interactions would be more severe. Itraconazole is a negative inotrope, which weakens the strength of myocardial contractility, and as such should not be used in patients with heart failure. It has extensive black box warnings for congestive heart failure, cardiac effects, and drug interactions. Itraconazole can cause prolonged QT interval.[35]

Oral itraconazole absorption is erratic, and so the manufacturer has come up with multiple complexed formulations that are not interchangeable. The oral capsules have lower bioavailability than the solution and therefore should not be used for systemic fungal infections. The solution must be taken on an empty stomach, whereas the capsules should be taken with a full meal. Like ketoconazole, absorption is improved by gastric acidity, so having patients take their dose with a carbonated beverage will improve absorption. Because of the poor bioavailability of itraconazole, extemporaneous compounds with this product will not be effective.

Antiherpetic Agents

Anti–herpes simplex virus (HSV) and varicella-zoster agents are nucleoside analogues that get phosphorylated intracellularly to become activated. Activated agents insert into the viral DNA strand and halt replication via several mechanisms. These agents are effective against HSV and varicella-zoster virus (VZV). In addition, they are effective only against actively replicating viruses, so they do not affect the latent herpes virus genome. These agents are thought to show cross-sensitivity.

Acyclovir

Acyclovir is 10 times more potent against herpes viruses (HSV-1, HSV-2) than against VZV and is approved for neonates.[36] Acyclovir is renally eliminated, and dose and dosing intervals must be adjusted to avoid neurotoxicity. The drug can also precipitate out in the urine and damage the kidneys, so patients should be well hydrated while on high-dose therapy. Dosage of acyclovir should be based on ideal body weight. Obese patients are at risk of drug-induced nephrotoxicity or neurotoxicity secondary to overdosage based on actual weight.[36] In addition to IV preparations, acyclovir is available in a 200-mg capsule, 400- and 800-mg tablets, and a 200-mg/5 mL suspension.

A 50-mg buccal adhesive acyclovir tablet is FDA approved for herpes labialis in adults. The package inserts state that one tablet should be applied within 1 hour of prodromal symptoms and prior to appearance of lesions. Two tablets cost more than $300, and most insurance companies will not pay for the product. Acyclovir is also available in a topical cream ($175 per gram) or ointment ($30 per gram) for extraoral use in patients with herpes labialis. Efficacy and insurance coverage are both doubtful.

Valacyclovir

Valacyclovir is a prodrug which is converted to acyclovir in vivo. The prodrug has greater bioavailability than acyclovir, allowing for less frequent dosing. Valacyclovir is FDA approved for children 12 years of age and older for herpes labialis and 2 years of age and older with chickenpox.[37] Valacyclovir is available in 500-mg and 1-g caplets. The prescribing package insert for Valtrex provides instructions for pharmacists on making an extemporaneous suspension from the caplets which makes 100 mL of either a 25- or 50-mg/mL suspension.[37]

Special Considerations in the Pediatric Patient

Barriers to Compliance

Patient adherence to prescribed drug regimens decreases as the number of doses per day increase. In antimicrobial chemotherapy, dose omissions allow plasma concentrations to fall below the MIC, where the drug is no longer clinically effective. At subtherapeutic doses, antimicrobials exert selective pressure resulting in the emergence of drug-resistant organisms. The consequences of nonadherence result in a poor therapeutic outcome for the patient and add to the community burden of drug resistance.[38]

Practitioners must consult the patient/caregiver when prescribing an antibiotic regimen to both assess and address possible barriers to compliance with the prescribed dosing regimen. This is especially important in the dental setting for two reasons: we primarily prescribe antimicrobials with short half-lives which need to be dosed three to four times daily, and the agents most commonly used are β-lactam antibiotics, which have little to no postantibiotic effect. In many situations, it may not be feasible to prescribe a medication that needs to be dosed every 6 hours. Late doses frequently turn into missed doses.

Children experience many barriers regarding drug therapy. Institutions such as schools and daycare facilities may have policies that prohibit students from bringing medications to school. Institutions often require that all medications be kept in a central location and in the original labeled container for liability issues. In schools, it is generally the student's responsibility to go to the office to obtain the medication.

If it is determined that the medication will need to be dosed outside the home, the parent should be instructed to ask the pharmacy for an additional labeled container and extra oral syringes with caps for liquid medications. If the parent is stressed or inexperienced, the practitioner can write "additional labeled container and syringes for school" on the face of the prescription. This solves half the problem. The other half is to get the child to the medication. Parents should discuss the issue with the teacher who can release/remind the student to obtain his/her medication. In addition, the parent can text the child or teacher as a reminder.

When children are old enough to understand and cooperate with their medication regimens, they should be given some responsibility for taking their medications. Dentists should discuss this in appropriate terms with both the parents and child. Eliciting cooperation and involvement may enhance compliance.

Unfortunately, for some children, the parent/caregiver may pose the biggest barrier to compliance by not filling the prescription or failing to comply with the dosing regimen. When there is any index of suspicion regarding the child's caregiver, the prescription can be called into the pharmacy. The dentist can later telephone the pharmacy to ascertain that the prescription has been dispensed. Setting up return appointments to closely follow the patient can be helpful. If it is determined that the child will not receive adequate care at home, hospitalization may be in the best interest of the patient.

Accurate Dosing

Pediatric patients are more susceptible to drug dosing errors than adults. The most common harmful pediatric medication error is improper dose/quantity of medication which can be a result of improper dose calculation by the prescriber or improper measurement of a liquid medication at home.[39]

Most pediatric medications are dosed by the child's weight. One study showed that 83% of parents were able to report the child's current weight within 10 lb. However, 60% of the parents who were in error reported the child weighing more than 100 lb, which would place them in the adult dosing range for many medications.[40]

Adverse effects of antimicrobials are frequently dose related (GI upset, diarrhea, etc.) and will result in noncompliance and increase the risk of treatment failure. The consequences of underdosing antimicrobial agents may have the same result—a poor outcome for the patient. To avoid dosage errors, practitioners should weigh the child in the office before prescribing medications and record the weight in kilograms because pediatric dosing recommendations are generally given as mg/kg/day or mg/kg/dose.

Numerous studies have shown that parents often measure liquid medications incorrectly. When administering liquid medications to children, adults tend to use dosing cups, teaspoons, and droppers.[40] These devices are not as accurate as using an oral syringe, which is the recommended measuring device for pediatric liquids by The Joint Commision.[39] However, oral syringes are used in a minority (perhaps less than 20%) of households.[40] Parents may have the belief that oral syringes are only for babies, and older children may resist taking a medication via oral syringe for the same reason.

Medicine cups are the most frequently reported device used by parents to measure liquid medications. Parents usually dispense an excessive dose when using marked plastic medicine cups to measure a liquid medication.[41] Parents should be educated on the importance of accurate dosing of liquid medications to children. The dose should always be measured via oral syringe to ensure accuracy.[39] Once measured, the liquid can then be placed in a medicine cup for administration if the patient objects to an oral syringe.

Unpalatable Medications

Many children resist taking liquid antimicrobials due to their disagreeable taste or smell or because of previous experiences with other medications. Refusal to take medications can result in battles of will between parents and children that escalate during the course of therapy. This almost inevitably leads to nonadherence with the dosage regimen and early discontinuation of the medication.

Clindamycin pediatric solution has the deserved reputation of being the worst tasting antibiotic liquid. The product smells horrible and tastes even worse. However, there are ways to overcome a child's reluctance to take liquid medications, even clindamycin solution. Administering bad-tasting medications with an oral syringe will limit the surface area that comes into contact with the medication. It also masks the medication odor better than a medicine cup. Liquids that do not taste good often have an objectionable smell, and this is especially true with some antimicrobial agents.

A common error is to warn the parent regarding a "distasteful" liquid medication in front of or within hearing distance of the child or any siblings. An even more common mistake is to not give the parent an action plan regarding drug administration if the child has a history of medication refusal or if the product is known to be problematic.

Leaving a bad-tasting medication on a child's palate will lead to increased reluctance as the duration of therapy continues. A successful countermeasure for bad-tasting medications is to have a small cup of cold grape soda ready as a "chaser" as soon as the child swallows the medication. Grape is one of the best flavors available to mask foul-tasting and bitter medications. Grape soda is much better than grape juice because the carbonation helps to lift the taste off the palate. Milk, orange juice, and even other flavors of soda do not work nearly as well. Fortunately, grape is a favorite flavor in the pediatric population. It is worth a parent's trip to the store to start this routine.

Another method that can be used in difficult situations is a sugar syringe. This is useful if the correct dose of medication is available in capsule form or a tablet that can be split to achieve the desired dose. Parents should be instructed to remove the plunger from an oral syringe and then cap it. Fill the syringe to the 2-mL mark with sugar, then add the finely crushed tablet or capsule contents to the top of the sugar. Layer another 2-mL of sugar on top of the medication. Slowly drip water into the syringe until the sugar at the bottom becomes a slurry. Then add the plunger and immediately administer the contents of the syringe. The bad-tasting medication is surrounded by sugar and often goes down without being noticed by the child.

Clinical Use of Antimicrobials in Pediatric Dentistry

Bacterial Infections

Necrotizing Ulcerative Gingivitis, Necrotizing Ulcerative Periodontitis, Necrotizing Ulcerative Stomatitis

Necrotizing ulcerative gingivitis (NUG), necrotizing ulcerative periodontitis (NUP), and necrotizing ulcerative stomatitis (NUS) are a group of diseases that can affect specific intraoral structures such as gingiva, periodontal tissues, and mucosa. Various microorganisms have been isolated from affected tissues and include *Fusobacterium nucleatum, Borrelia vincentii, Prevotella intermedia, Porphyromonas gingivalis, Selenomonas sputigena,* and other anaerobic organisms.[42] Additional theories for etiology include a role for viruses, such the human herpesviruses (HHVs). Several factors have been identified as potential triggers for these conditions, and these include stress, altered immune status, trauma, illness, smoking, malnutrition, and lack of sleep.[43,44] NUG presents as necrotic, craterlike ulcerations that initially affect the interdental papilla with progression to free gingival margins and extension to adjacent tissues (NUP, NUS). Spontaneous hemorrhage, halitosis, as well as fever, lymphadenopathy, and malaise have also been reported. Management of these conditions includes the débridement of local factors, topical antiseptics, and oral hygiene instructions, as well as antibiotics such as penicillin and metronidazole, which may be indicated in patients with fever and/or lymphadenopathy.

Periapical Abscess

This acute inflammatory condition is associated with pulpal necrosis resulting in purulence within the alveolus at the apex of a nonvital tooth. Both aerobic and anaerobic bacteria have been isolated from these lesions. Periapical abscesses can present with pain to percussion, extrusion of the tooth within the socket, and soft tissue swelling in the periradicular region. If the infection spreads into intraosseous medullary spaces, osteomyelitis can develop.[45] Extension through the cortical plate into adjacent soft tissues can result in sinus track formation. This condition can be accompanied by fever and lymphadenopathy. Management may include incision and drainage, appropriate therapy for the nonvital tooth (root canal therapy or extraction), and pain control with analgesics. A localized lesion with appropriate drainage does not require antibiotic therapy. Antibiotic therapy would be indicated for the patient who is immunocompromised or who develops cellulitis.

Periodontal Abscess

A periodontal abscess is an acute infection that presents with purulence in a periodontal pocket. Both aerobic and anaerobic bacteria have been isolated from these lesions. Frequently, foreign material implantation is identified. This condition presents as a localized swelling with redness of the gingiva. There may be pain, tooth mobility, and tenderness to percussion, but the associated tooth responds to vitality testing. If a sinus track develops, purulent exudate may be noted. The amount of bone loss and attachment loss can be variable. Management includes drainage through the periodontal pocket to avoid fenestration, as well as débridement and curettage. Systemic antibiotics may be indicated if fever and/or lymphadenopathy is identified.

Pericoronitis

Pericoronitis is an acute or subacute gingival inflammatory reaction around a partially erupted, impacted, or erupting tooth. When food, debris, and/or microorganisms accumulate underneath the overlying soft tissue, an inflammatory reaction can develop.[42] Pericoronitis has a predilection for mandibular first and second molars in adolescents and mandibular third molars in young adults. Patients may present with severe, painful inflammation of gingiva, soft tissue edema, taste alterations, foul taste or odor, trismus, and abscess formation. Fever, lymphadenopathy, and malaise may also be present. Management includes irrigation below the soft tissue flap, antiseptic rinses, and alleviation of the condition through surgical removal of the overlying soft tissue or tooth extraction. Systemic antibiotics may be indicated if fever and/or lymphadenopathy is identified.

Cervicofacial Cellulitis/Facial Space Infections

Cervicofacial cellulitis develops when an abscess cannot develop a path of drainage. There is extension of acute edema and infection via the spread of the exudate into the adjacent facial soft tissues.[45] Various microorganisms such as *S. aureus*, alpha-hemolytic streptococci, and gram-negative and anaerobic bacteria have been isolated from these lesions. In addition, *Haemophilus influenzae* type B has been identified in cases of buccal cellulitis in infants. These patients present with diffuse swelling of buccal and/or submandibular facial areas. The swelling is firm, ill-defined, red, and warm to the touch. Pain, fever, lymphadenopathy, and malaise have been reported. Depending on the areas of involvement, patients may also present with trismus or dysphagia. The condition is usually diagnosed using blood cultures, fine-needle aspiration, or biopsy. Management includes hospitalization, maintaining a secure airway, as well as bacterial culture and sensitivity testing. Incision and drainage and systemic antibiotics are indicated.

Acute Suppurative Sialadenitis

Acute suppurative sialadenitis develops when ductal obstruction causes backflow of saliva and retrograde infection of salivary ducts and/or glands. The condition can affect the major or minor salivary glands and can present as unilateral or bilateral involvement. *S. aureus, Streptococcus pyogenes, Streptococcus pneumococci*, and other microorganisms have been identified with this condition.[46] There will be painful, indurated swelling of the affected gland. The area may feel warm to palpation, the ductal orifice may appear inflamed, and purulent drainage may be identified. A sialolith may or may not be present. Malaise, fever, and tender lymphadenopathy can be present, and trismus may be noted. The condition is diagnosed through cultures, magnetic resonance imaging (MRI), or computed tomography (CT) imaging and/or a sialogram. Management includes bacterial culture and antibiotic sensitivity testing with appropriate antibiotic therapy. If present, the sialolith should be removed.

Actinomycosis

Actinomycosis is a chronic, suppurative granulomatous infection that can be seen in the clinical context of a grossly carious tooth or a tooth with previous root canal therapy. It can also be associated with an impacted tooth, periodontitis, or periimplantitis. The majority of cases are asymptomatic. Anaerobic gram-positive bacteria such as *Actinomyces israelii, Actinomyces odontolyticus, Actinomyces naeslundii, Actinomyces gerencseriae*, and *Actinomyces viscosus* have been isolated. This condition is often localized to the mandible and mandibular angle regions. There is often a cervicofacial asymptomatic, slow-growing, hard swelling. Trismus may be present. Abscesses and draining sinus track or gingival parulis can develop, and a yellow purulent exudate (sulfur granules) is pathognomonic for this condition. The condition is diagnosed via culturing the exudate and isolation of the microorganism or by biopsy. Management includes prolonged antibiotic regimens (penicillin, doxycycline, clindamycin, erythromycin, and tetracycline), as well as surgical débridement and management of the original source of infection.

Viral Infections

Primary Herpetic Gingivostomatitis

Primary herpetic gingivostomatitis is the most common acute viral infection affecting the oral mucosa. The condition is caused by infection with HHV-1 or HHV-2, and transmission occurs through direct contact. The condition peaks between 2 and 4 years of age, and lesions are widely distributed on keratinizing and nonkeratinizing tissues. The most frequent sites of involvement include gingiva, tongue, palate, labial mucosa, buccal mucosa, tonsils, and posterior pharynx.[46] The condition presents as an abrupt onset of fever and malaise. Typically there will be intraoral discomfort and red, swollen mucosa with small vesicles. These vesicles rupture within 24 hours, resulting in shallow, painful, small ulcerations with a pseudomembrane and red halo. The ulcers can progressively coalesce. Lesions continue to develop for 3 to 5 days, and the condition heals within 7 to 10 days without scarring. Bilateral tender lymphadenopathy, fever, malaise, and perioral lesions may be present. Diagnosis can be made using culture, cytology, serology for antibody titers, and/or biopsy. Management includes palliative care and may include systemic antiviral therapy when indicated.[47] Although eating is

often painful, fluid intake should be encouraged with the young child to prevent dehydration. Parents should be advised not to use products that contain benzocaine in infants or young children with primary herpetic gingivostomatitis, due to reports of benzocaine gel–related cases of methemoglobinemia.

Secondary Herpetic Infections

Secondary herpetic infections occur through reactivation in a patient previously infected with HHV-1 or HHV-2. After the primary infection the virus remains latent in neural ganglion until reactivated. Predisposing factors that have been identified include illness, trauma, stress, UV light, and immunosuppression. The most common sites of involvement include the lips (herpes labialis) and intraoral keratinized tissues such as hard palate, dorsal tongue, and attached gingiva. This condition may present with a prodrome described as burning, tingling, itching, or paresthesia. There will be discrete small vesicles arranged in clusters which rupture within 2 to 3 days, leaving 1- to 3-mm areas of ulceration that heal within 6 to 10 days.[46] Lesions of herpes labialis can also be secondarily infected by skin flora. Recurrent herpes in an immunocompromised patient can present on any mucosal site. Diagnosis can be made using culture, cytology, serology for antibody titers, and/or biopsy. Management includes palliative care and appropriate systemic antiviral therapy ideally given at the time of prodrome.[47]

Varicella

VZV/HHV-3 causes the primary infection of chickenpox and presents as a recurrent infection in the form of herpes zoster (shingles). Patients most at risk for the recurrent infection include elderly, medically complex, and immunocompromised patients. Recurrent infection usually presents in a unilateral distribution along a trigeminal nerve and extends to the midline. Chickenpox presents as a cutaneous rash that initially appears on the face and trunk with extension to others sites. It starts as erythematous skin lesions that progress to vesicles and pustules that rupture into a hardened crust. The vesicles are surrounded by a rim of erythema. The condition can present in successive crops of lesions every 2 to 3 days which remain contagious prior to the exanthema until all lesions crust. Oral involvement can proceed skin involvement and frequent oral sites of involvement include the palate, vermilion border, and buccal mucosa, as well as the gingiva. The intraoral vesicles will rupture and form small round shallow erosions with a red halo. Chickenpox is often accompanied by tender lymphadenopathy, fever, and malaise. Diagnosis is made through cytology, serology, biopsy, or polymerase chain reaction (PCR) testing of vesicular fluid. Management includes palliative care with antiviral medications reserved for individuals at risk for severe disease. Systemic antivirals are also considered for secondary household members.

Fungal Infections

Candidiasis/Candidosis

Candidiasis is the most common intraoral superficial mycosis. It most often involves *C. albicans*, but *C. tropicalis, C. krusei*, and *C. glabrata* have also been identified. Predisposing factors for infection include xerostomia, anemia, uncontrolled diabetes mellitus, malignancies, immunodeficiency, and medications such as antibiotics. The infant with cleft lip and/or palate is particularly susceptible to candida infections because of the pooling of breast milk or formula in the areas of clefting which serve as a reservoir for the organism. Parents and caregivers should be encouraged to cleanse the oral cavity of the cleft lip/palate infant with a clean, moist washcloth after each feeding.

The most frequent sites of involvement for candida infections include the soft palate, buccal mucosa, and tongue. Pseudomembranous candidosis (thrush) presents as white removable papules or plaques with erythematous underlying tissue.[48] Patients with thrush may report a burning sensation or pain. Angular cheilitis presents as red, fissuring, and crusting in the commissure region, while erythematous candidosis (which includes denture stomatitis) presents as red patches accompanied by a burning sensation primarily affecting the dorsal tongue and palate. Diagnosis can be made using cytologic smears, culture, and histopathologic examination. Management of most forms of candidiasis includes topical or systemic antifungals, whereas angular cheilitis may have concomitant *S. aureus* infection requiring both antifungal and antibacterial medications.[49]

Antimicrobial Prophylaxis

Per the American Heart Association, antibiotic prophylaxis should be considered for individuals with artificial heart valves, a history of infective endocarditis, heart transplant patients with a history of valvular problems, and some patients with congenital cardiac conditions. Congenital conditions needing prophylaxis may include unrepaired cyanotic congenital heart disease, palliative shunts and conduits, defects repaired with prosthetic material or a device during the first 6 months after repair, and repaired defects with a residual defect remaining at the site or adjacent to the site of the prosthetic patch or prosthetic device.

References

1. Gallagher JC, MacDougall C. *Antibiotics Simplified*. 4th ed. Burlington, MA: Jones & Bartlett Learning; 2017.
2. Becker DE. Antimicrobial drugs. *Anesth Prog*. 2013;60(3):111–123.
3. Flynn TR. Principles of management of odontogenic infections. In: Miloro M, Ghali GE, Larsen PE, et al, eds. *Peterson's Principles of Oral and Maxillofacial Surgery*. 2nd ed. Hamilton, Ontario, Canada: BC Decker Inc; 2004.
4. Lampiris HW, Maddix DS. Clinical use of antimicrobial agents. In: Katsung BG, Trevor AG, eds. *Basic and Clinical Pharmacology*. 13th ed. New York: McGraw-Hill; 2015:873–885.
5. Carroll KC, Morse A, Mietzner T, et al, eds. Antimicrobial chemotherapy. In: *Jawetz, Melnick, & Adelberg's Medical Microbiology*. 27th ed. New York: McGraw-Hill; 2016:363–396.
6. Deck DH, Winston LG. Beta-lactam and other cell wall & membrane-active antibiotics. In: Katsung BG, Trevor AG, eds. *Basic and Clinical Pharmacology*. 13th ed. New York: McGraw-Hill; 2015:769–787.
7. Kumar P. Pharmacology of specific drug groups: antibiotic therapy. In: Dowd FJ, Johnson BS, Mariotti AJ, eds. *Pharmacology and Therapeutics for Dentistry*. 7th ed. St Louis: Elsevier; 2017:457–487.
8. Deck DH, Winston LG. Tetracyclines, macrolides, clindamycin, chloramphenicaol, streptogramins & oxazolidones. In: Katsung BG, Trevor AG, eds. *Basic and Clinical Pharmacology*. 13th ed. New York: McGraw-Hill; 2015:788–798.
9. Deck DH, Winston LG. Aminoglycosides & spectinomycin. In: Katsung BG, Trevor AG, eds. *Basic and Clinical Pharmacology*. 13th ed. New York: McGraw-Hill; 2015:799–806.
10. Sheppard D, Lampiris HW. Antifungal agents. In: Katsung BG, Trevor AG, eds. *Basic and Clinical Pharmacology*. 13th ed. New York: McGraw-Hill; 2015:825–834.
11. Park N, Shin K, Kang MK. Antifungal and antiviral agents. In: Dowd FJ, Johnson BS, Mariotti AJ, eds. *Pharmacology and Therapeutics for Dentistry*. 7th ed. St Louis: Elsevier; 2017:488–503.
12. Schnyder B, Pichler WJ. Mechanisms of drug-induced allergy. *Mayo Clin Proc*. 2009;84(3):268–272.
13. Vassileva SG, Mateev G, Parish LC. Antimicrobial photosensitive reactions. *Arch Intern Med*. 1998;158(18):1993–2000.
14. Paulussen ADC, Aerssens J. Risk factors for drug-induced long-QT syndrome. *Neth Heart J*. 2005;13(2):47–56.
15. Pai MP, Momary KM, Rodvold KA. Antibiotic drug interactions. *Med Clin North Am*. 2006;90(6):1223–1255.
16. Campagna JD, Bond MC, Schabelman E, et al. The use of cephalosporins in penicillin-allergic patients: a literature review. *J Emerg Med*. 2012;42(5):612–620.
17. Blumenthal KG, Solensky R. Allergy evaluation for immediate penicillin allergy: kin test-based diagnostic strategies and cross-reactivity with other beta-lactam antibiotics. In: Feldweg AM, ed. Waltham, MA: UpToDate Inc. http://www.uptodate.com. Accessed June 1, 2017.
18. Pichichero ME, Zagursky R. Penicillin and cephalosporin allergy. *Ann Allergy Asthma Immunol*. 2014;112(5):404–412.
19. Solensky R. Penicillin allergy: delayed hypersensitivity reactions. In: Atkinson NF, ed. Waltham, MA: UpToDate Inc. http://www.uptodate.com. Accessed June 1, 2017.
20. Adams DJ, Eberly MD, Rajnik M, et al. Risk factors for community-associated *Clostridium difficile* infection in children. *J Pediatr*. 2017;186:105–109.
21. Elsevier/Gold Standard, Inc. Azithromycin monograph, Clinical Pharmacology [database online]; 2017. http://www.clinicalpharmacology.com. Accessed May 30, 2017.
22. Lexicomp Online, Clarithromycin monograph, Pediatric and Neonatal Lexi-Drugs Online, Hudson, Ohio: Wolters Kluwer Clinical Drug Information, Inc.; 2017. Accessed May 30, 2017.
23. Deck DH, Winston LG. Miscellaneous antimicrobial agents; disinfectants, antiseptics & sterilants. In: Katsung BG, Trevor AG, eds. *Basic and Clinical Pharmacology*. 13th ed. New York: McGraw-Hill; 2015:865–872.
24. FIRST®-Metronidazole 100 package insert, CutisPharma, Wilmington, MA. September 2016.
25. Jackson MA, Schutze GE, American Academy of Pediatrics Committee on Infectious Diseases. The use of systemic and topical fluoroquinolones. *Pediatrics*. 2016;138(5):e20162706.
26. Elsevier/Gold Standard, Inc. Nystatin monograph. Clinical Pharmacology [database online]; 2017. http://www.clinicalpharmacology.com. Accessed May 30, 2017.
27. Pappas PG, Kauffman CA, Andes DR, et al. Clinical practice guideline for the management of candidiasis: 2016 update by the Infectious Disease Society of America. *Clin Infect Dis*. 2016;62(4):e1–e50.
28. Lexicomp Online® Nystatin (Topical) (AHFS DI [Adult and Pediatric] Monograph) [database online]. Hudson, Ohio: Lexi-Comp, Inc. Accessed June 23, 2017.
29. Carroll KC, Morse SA, Mietzner TA, et al, eds. Medical mycology. In: *Jawetz, Melnick, & Adelberg's Medical Microbiology*. 27th ed. New York: McGraw-Hill; 2016:657–704.
30. Mycelex® (clotrimazole) troche product package insert. Bayer Corporation. West Haven, CT, April 2001.
31. Elsevier/Gold Standard, Inc. Clotrimazole monograph, Clinical Pharmacology [database online]; 2017. http://www.clinicalpharmacology.com. Accessed May 30, 2017.
32. Elsevier/Gold Standard, Inc. Miconazole monograph, Clinical Pharmacology [database online]; 2017. http://www.clinicalpharmacology.com. Accessed May 30, 2017.
33. Oravig® (miconazole adhesive buccal tablet) product package insert, DARA BioSciences, Inc, Raleigh NC, April 2015.
34. Elsevier/Gold Standard, Inc. Fluconazole monograph (pediatric), Clinical Pharmacology [database online]; 2017. http://www.clinicalpharmacology.com. Accessed June 2, 2017.
35. Elsevier/Gold Standard, Inc. Itraconazole monograph, Clinical Pharmacology [database online]; 2017. http://www.clinicalpharmacology.com. Accessed June 2, 2017.

36. Elsevier/Gold Standard, Inc. Acyclovir monograph (pediatric), Clinical Pharmacology [database online]; 2017. http://www.clinicalpharmacology.com. Accessed June 2, 2017.

37. Elsevier/Gold Standard, Inc. Valacyclovir monograph (pediatric), Clinical Pharmacology [database online]; 2017. http://www.clinicalpharmacology.com. Accessed June 2, 2017.

38. Vrijens B, Urquhart J. Patient adherence to prescribed antimicrobial drug dosing regimens. *J Antimicrob Chemother.* 2005;55(5):616–627.

39. The Joint Commission. Sentinel Event Alert, Issue 39: Preventing pediatric medication errors; April 11, 2008. https://www.jointcommission.org/sentinel_event_alert_issue_39_preventing_pediatric_medication_errors/. Accessed May 20, 2017.

40. Tanner S, Wells D, Scarbecz M, et al. Parent's understanding of and accuracy in using measuring devices to administer liquid oral pain medication. *J Am Dent Assoc.* 2014;145(2):141–149.

41. Yin HS, Mendelsohn AL, Wolf MS, et al. Parents' mediation administration errors: role of dosing instruments and health literacy. *Arch Pediatr Adolesc Med.* 2010;164(3):181–186.

42. Cawson RA, Odell EW, eds. Gingivitis and periodontitis. In: *Cawson's Essentials of Oral Pathology and Medicine.* 8th ed. Philedelphia: Churchill Livingstone; 2008:77–98.

43. Neville BW, Damm DD, Allen CM, et al, eds. Periodontal diseases. In: *Oral and Maxillofacial Pathology.* 4th ed. Canada: Elsevier; 2016:140–163.

44. Marty M, Palmieri J, Noirrit-Esclassan E, et al. Necrotizing periodontal diseases in children: a literature review and adjustment of treatment. *J Trop Pediatr.* 2016;62(4):331–337.

45. Neville BW, Damm DD, Allen CM, et al, eds. Pulpal and periodontal diseases. In: *Oral and Maxillofacial Pathology.* 4th ed. Canada: Elsevier; 2016:111–139.

46. Laskaris G, ed. Viral infections. In: *Color Atlas of Oral Diseases in Children and Adolescents.* New York: Georg Thieme Verlag; 2000.

47. Goldman RD. Acyclovir for herpetic gingivostomatitis in children. *Can Fam Physician.* 2016;62(5):403–404.

48. Green L, Dolen WK. Chronic candidiasis in children. *Curr Allergy Asthma Rep.* 2017;17(5):31.

49. Reddy RCJ, Jeelani S, Duraiselvi P, et al. Assessment of effectiveness of fluconazole and clotrimazole in treating oral candidiasis patients: a comparative study. *J Int Soc Prev Community Dent.* 2017;7(2):90–94.

10
Medical Emergencies

MATTHEW COOKE AND R. JOHN BREWER

Medical Emergencies in the Pediatric Dental Office

Medical emergencies occur within the practice of pediatric dentistry.[1] A medical emergency is defined as a sudden, unexpected deviation from the normally expected pattern (normal physiology). Emergencies can occur with anyone: the patient, parent/guardian, or other individuals who accompany the patient, the dentist, or the staff.[1]

Morbidity

All types of medical emergencies occur. Some are seen more frequently (allergic reactions, asthma, cardiac arrest, diabetes mellitus, hyperventilation, seizures, and syncope) and will be discussed later in the chapter. Acute events result in morbidity, a diseased state, disability, or poor health due to any cause.[2]

Mortality

Emergencies in the pediatric dental office may threaten the patient's life. However, only on rare occasions is death the outcome. Objectives in medical emergency training include management of morbidity to prevent mortality.[1]

"Swiss Cheese Model" of Accident Causation

Medical emergencies are the result of system failure.[3] Every step in a process has the potential for failure. The ideal system is similar to sliced Swiss cheese. This model is often referred to as the "Swiss cheese model" of accident causation.[3] The holes represent opportunities for failure, and each slice serves as a "defensive layer" in the process. An error may allow a problem to pass through a hole in one layer, but in the next layer the holes are in different places, allowing the issue to be identified. Each layer serves as a defense against additional errors which impact the total outcome (Fig. 10.1A).[3] Catastrophic errors occur when the holes align for each step in the process, allowing all defenses to be defeated (see Fig. 10.1B).[3]

The Swiss cheese model includes both active and latent failures or "sins of commission and sins of omission." Active failures are the unsafe acts which can directly cause an accident. Latent failures refer to not acting when indicated to prevent or manage a situation. Both types of failure contribute to catastrophic outcomes. The Swiss cheese model is respected and considered useful, but it may not explain all medical emergencies in the pediatric dental office.[4]

Fear, anxiety, and pain are often associated with the surgical specialty of pediatric dentistry. Acute stress reactions result in surges of endogenous catecholamines.[1] The physiologic response may be conducive to the development of a medical emergency.[5] Add highly vasoactive drugs—local anesthetics and vasoconstrictors—used for almost all pediatric dental procedures, and the probability for a medical emergency increases.[1] Other drugs, such as antibiotics, sedatives, and analgesics, also carry the potential for producing acute, life-threatening reactions from toxicity or allergy.[1]

Recognition and action are key steps. Because pediatric dentists are not routinely managing medical emergencies, there may be uneasiness when expected to handle a crisis in the dental office.

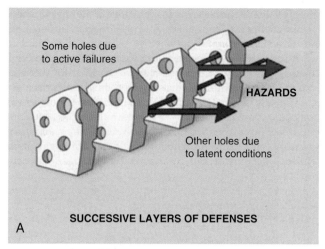
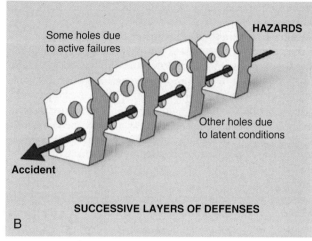

• **Figure 10.1** (A–B) Swiss cheese illustration. (From Reason J. *Human Error.* Cambridge: Cambridge University Press; 1990.)

However, what may be an emergency to one provider may be a normal occurrence to another.[6] Responsibilities of the pediatric dentist include prevention, preparation, basic life support (BLS), basic emergency medicine procedures, and procurement of help.[7] Patients may require transfer by Emergency Medical Services (EMS) personnel to an appropriate medical facility for definitive diagnosis and treatment. Upon recognition of a medical emergency, the pediatric dentist should attempt to stabilize the patient.

Prevention of Medical Emergencies

Undoubtedly, preventing the occurrence of medical emergencies is most desired.[1] Studies show that a complete system evaluation of all dental patients can prevent approximately 90% of life-threatening situations.[8–10] The remaining 10% will occur despite the best preventive efforts.[9] Knowledge of acute and chronic conditions allows for medical optimization and risk reduction, thus decreasing the probability of a medical emergency.[1,9] Completing a pretreatment assessment or evaluation is essential and is accomplished with a complete medical history and physical examination. A medical consultation should be considered, when indicated.[1]

History and Physical Examination

Knowledge of existing medical conditions, which predispose the patient, will prevent the vast majority of emergency situations.[1,8,9] Assessment of the patient's psychological outlook to dental treatment should also be included. The medical history is generally obtained via a written questionnaire, which is completed by the patient or parent.[11,12] Many standardized forms are available, but they may require modification for pediatric dental practice. These forms should include questions pertaining to any present or past medical conditions, allergies or adverse drug reactions, hospitalizations, surgeries, and medications (Fig. 10.2). Questions regarding dental concerns as well as past dental treatment are frequently included (see Chapter 14). The dentist should review this form, note positive findings, and conduct a brief interview with the patient to clarify and expand on the questionnaire. Clarifications and further explanations of positive findings should also be written by the dentist in the record, documenting that these questions were thoroughly addressed.[12] An example of this would be if a parent notes "asthma"

on the medical history form. Asthma is the second most prevalent chronic condition in pediatric patients and it has multiple forms (mild, intermittent through severe, persistent). It is the responsibility of the pediatric dentist to obtain more information than the mere fact that the patient currently has or has had asthma in the past. The dentist should further document the frequency and severity of the asthma attacks, what causes them, how they are managed, and whether or not past episodes were ever so severe that treatment was emergently needed in the hospital or emergency room. Also, it is prudent to determine when the last attack occurred, and finally whether the patient is breathing easily today. Based on the assessment of these documented clarifications, the dentist may feel comfortable providing the needed dental treatment at that appointment or may decide to postpone treatment until the patient is medically optimized by his or her physician.[12]

The physical examination should include baseline vital signs (blood pressure, pulse rate and rhythm, respiratory rate and character), a thorough head and neck examination, and observation of general appearance (gait, mental status, skin tone and color, etc.).[12] Further physical evaluation should be dictated by the dentist's training, expertise, and plan.[12,13]

A complete history and physical examination will give the pediatric dentist insight into preexisting conditions that potentially may lead to a medical emergency.[1,12] Conditions involving the cardiac, pulmonary, and endocrine systems are of greatest concern. Patients with a history of seizures also warrant special consideration. Knowledge allows the development of treatment protocols that decrease the likelihood of a serious medical event. These protocols may involve prophylaxis for infective endocarditis, proper timing of appointments, or the use of sedation/anesthesia for stress-induced conditions.[1,13–15]

Medical Consultation

Consultation with the physician of a medically compromised patient is highly advised prior to treatment.[1,12] The outdated concept of obtaining "medical clearance" from a medical consultant before initiation of a dental procedure has now been superseded by requesting the consultant's statement that "the patient is in optimal condition for the planned procedure."[1,12] The information obtained should help the dentist develop the safest treatment plan for the mutual patient.

Patient Monitoring

Monitoring is continuous observation of physiologic parameters over time.[13] The dentist and/or trained staff member should always be monitoring/observing the patient.[12–24] The level of monitoring necessary to safely treat a pediatric dental patient depends on the procedure to be provided, the patient's underlying medical condition, and the management technique used.[1,13,23,24]

When changes are detected, an intervention can be implemented, preventing potentially dangerous situations.

Monitor/observe the general appearance of the patient, including the level of consciousness, level of comfort, muscle tone, color of the skin and mucosa, and respiratory pattern. For the majority of healthy patients being treated with local anesthesia alone or with minimal sedation as defined by the American Dental Association, this is all the monitoring that is necessary.[23] The patient should never be left alone once drugs (local anesthetics or sedative agents) are administered.[21,22,24,25]

Moderate sedation requires a time-based record including blood pressure, pulse, and pulse oximetry. Waveform capnography is strongly recommended.[13] A precordial stethoscope should also be

---

MEDICAL HISTORY

Child's Full Name _____ Date of Birth _____/_____/_____

Child's Physician/Pediatrician _____ Child's Pediatrician's Telephone:_____

Pediatrician's Address: _____

Medications or Treatments

1. Is your child up to date on immunizations? ☐ No ☐ Yes
2. Is your child currently taking any medication (prescription, over-the-counter medicines, or inhalers)? ☐ No ☐ Yes
3. Has your child ever received radiation or chemotherapy or is it planned? ☐ No ☐ Yes

If yes to any of the above, please explain: _____

Allergies

1. Is your child allergic to any medication? ☐ No ☐ Yes
2. Is your child allergic to latex? ☐ No ☐ Yes
3. Any other allergies such as skin, food, etc.? ☐ No ☐ Yes

If yes to any of the above, please explain: _____

Please indicate if your child has or has a history of any of the following:

Growth and Development:

☐ Birth complications/premature   ☐ Physical growth   ☐ Delayed growth   ☐ Intellectual disabilities
☐ Behavioral problems/disorders   ☐ Learning disabilities   ☐ Communication difficulties   ☐ None of these

If yes to any of the above, please explain: _____

Central Nervous System:

☐ Cerebral palsy   ☐ Epilepsy (seizures)/convulsions   ☐ Fainting   ☐ Autism spectrum disorder
☐ Speech, hearing, vision problems   ☐ Hydrocephaly   ☐ None of these

If yes to any of the above, please explain: _____

Heart Problems:

☐ Congenital heart disease   ☐ Heart murmur   ☐ Heart damage from rheumatic fever
☐ High blood pressure   ☐ Any other heart problems   ☐ None of these

If yes to any of the above, please explain: _____

Blood:

☐ Blood transfusion   ☐ Anemia   ☐ Sickle cell disease/trait   ☐ Cancer
☐ Bruise easily   ☐ Frequent nosebleeds   ☐ Bleed excessively from small cuts   ☐ None of these
☐ Other blood disorder

If yes to any of the above, please explain: _____

Breathing:

☐ Asthma   ☐ Shortness of breath   ☐ Difficulty in breathing
☐ Pneumonia   ☐ Cystic fibrosis   ☐ Any other breathing problem   ☐ None of these
☐ Snoring   ☐ Obstructive sleep disorder

If yes to any of the above, please explain: _____

• **Figure 10.2** Sample medical history questionnaire.

Digestive system:

☐ Stomach/intestinal problems   ☐ Hepatitis   ☐ Jaundice or liver problems   ☐ Other

☐ Eating disorders/problems   ☐ Unexplained weight loss   ☐ Reflux/GERD   ☐ None of these

If yes to any of the above, please explain: _____

Reproductive/Urinary system:

☐ Bladder/kidney problem   ☐ Is the patient pregnant or possibly pregnant?   ☐ None of these

If yes to any of the above, please explain: _____

Glands:

☐ Diabetes   ☐ Thyroid disorders   ☐ Gland problems   ☐ None of these

If yes to any of the above, please explain: _____

Skin:

☐ Skin problems   ☐ Rash/hives, eczema   ☐ Cold sores or canker sores   ☐ None of these

If yes to any of the above, please explain: _____

Arms/Legs:

☐ Limitations of arms or legs   ☐ Arthritis   ☐ Joint bleeding   ☐ None of these

☐ Joint replacement   ☐ Muscular dystrophy   ☐ Muscle weakness

If yes to any of the above, please explain: _____

Hospitalizations

Has your child been hospitalized?   ☐ No   ☐ Yes

If yes, please list hospital, date, and reason: _____

Please check any of the illnesses that your child has now, has recently been exposed to, or has had in the past:

☐ HIV/AIDS   ☐ Tuberculosis (TB)

☐ Scarlet fever   ☐ Methicillin resistant staphylococcus aureus (MRSA)

☐ Substance abuse, alcoholism, drug addiction

☐ Upper respiratory infection, common cold, sinus infection, or tonsillitis

☐ Sexually Transmitted disease (genital herpes, gonorrhea, syphilis, other)

Is your child presently being seen by a physician?   ☐ No   ☐ Yes

If yes, for what reason:

_____

Is there any other significant medical history pertaining to this child or his/her family that the dentist should be told?

☐ No   ☐ Yes

If yes, describe: _____

_____

| _____ | _____ | _____ |
| Signature (Parent or guardian) | Relationship to child | Date |

• **Figure 10.2, cont'd**

used (Fig. 10.3).[13] Electrocardiography monitoring should be considered, though at this time it is not a requirement for moderate sedation in children under 12 years of age.[13] These measures are particularly important for patients with whom continual verbal contact is difficult or undesirable.[13] (See Chapter 8 for a detailed discussion of monitoring during sedation.) Deep sedation and general anesthesia require advanced monitoring, as the patient is unconscious.[21,22] (Note: These services should only be provided by practitioners who are properly trained.) Presedation and discharge vital signs, including pulse rate, respiratory rate, and blood pressure, should always be obtained unless prevented by the lack of patient cooperation.[13] Patients should return to baseline prior to discharge.[13,21,22]

Preparing for Office Emergencies

It is imperative that all dentists and staff members master BLS at the health care provider (HCP) level of training.[1,26] It is

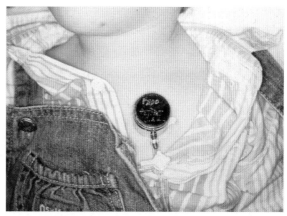

• **Figure 10.3** Use of a precordial stethoscope.

recommended that dentists and staff also receive additional medical emergency training which includes simulated medical emergency scenarios. Advanced Cardiac Life Support (ACLS) and Pediatric Advanced Life Support (PALS) are required if providing office-based sedation.[13,21,27,28] The reader is referred to the American Heart Association's publications on emergency cardiovascular care.

Personal Preparation

While it cannot be expected that the practicing dentist will be able to diagnose and manage every possible medical emergency, it is possible to anticipate which emergency situations are most likely to arise in the dental office, as well as those that have the greatest potential to cause patient morbidity or mortality.[1,29] Emergency situations that might logically occur as a direct result of medications or techniques used must not only be anticipated but well understood.[1] Examples include local anesthetic toxicity reactions and respiratory depression secondary to sedation.[29] The dentist must also be prepared to quickly carry out an action plan to manage the situation.[29,30] Personal preparation for the dentist should include, at a minimum, a working knowledge of the signs, symptoms, course, and therapy for common treatable conditions.[29,30]

Staff Preparation

The office should have an emergency plan in place. Each team member should know what is expected in an emergency.[1,30–35] Responsibilities of the team include dentist and staff providing patient care, staff to phone 911, staff for documentation, staff for assisting other patients and family members, and staff to direct EMS to the patient.

A team approach to medical emergencies will provide for organized management of emergency situations.[1,30] Regularly scheduled mock medical emergency drills will keep the team protocol running smoothly and reduce panic in an actual emergency.[30,31]

Backup Medical Assistance

The dentist and staff should be expected to manage a medical emergency until EMS arrives. There are cases where response times have been 20 to 40 minutes for emergencies in the dental office, including cardiac arrests.[1,25,27] Dentists and staff should not rely on other physicians in close proximity to help manage emergencies. It is the dentist's responsibility to be prepared to handle the emergency until EMS arrives on the scene.[1,30,31,34] Paramedics should be requested over basic emergency medical technicians when feasible.[1]

Office Preparation: Emergency Equipment

Table 10.1 details recommended emergency equipment for the pediatric dental office. Emergency equipment for pediatric patients must be appropriately sized (infant through adolescent) and available (Fig. 10.4).[1,13,29,31]

Oxygen is the primary emergency drug in the dental office.[31] It requires specialized equipment for administration. An oxygen source capable of delivering greater than 90% oxygen at flows of 10 L/min for a minimum of 1 hour is ideal. This means that an "E" cylinder is the minimum size required. Pediatric dental patients rarely suffer myocardial infarction or cardiac arrest as the initiating medical event.[28] Drug-induced respiratory depression and loss of a patent airway during unconsciousness are much more likely to

TABLE 10.1	Emergency Equipment	
Equipment	**Description**	**Quantity**
Suction and suction tips	High-volume suction system	Office suction
	Large-diameter round-ended suction tip (Yankauer suction)	Minimum of 2
Oxygen delivery system	Positive pressure via bag valve mask device (AMBU bag)	Minimum 1 infant, 1 child, 1 small adult, 1 large adult
	Nasal cannulas basic oxygen mask	
	Nonrebreather oxygen masks	
Airways	Oral and nasal (with appropriate sizes)	1 of each size
Patient monitor	Stethoscope, pulse oximeter, glucometer	1 of each
	Blood pressure cuffs (pediatric and adult)	
Automatic external defibrillator	Pediatric and adult pads available	1 of each
Syringes for drug administration	Disposable syringes and 18-g needle	4 3-mL syringes

If performing office-based sedation it is advised to have the following emergency equipment:
Advanced airways
    i-gels/LMA adult and pediatric (with hands-on medical emergency training)
Cardiac monitor
Capnography
IV/IO equipment
Mucosal atomization devices
Nebulizer masks

IO, Intraosseous; *IV,* intravenous; *LMA,* laryngeal mask airway.

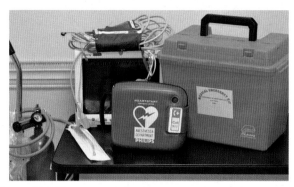

• **Figure 10.4** Recommended emergency equipment for the pediatric dental office.

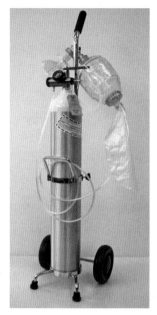

• **Figure 10.5** Bag-valve-mask apparatus to deliver positive pressure ventilation to a nonbreathing patient.

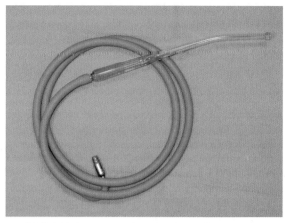

• **Figure 10.6** A Yankauer type of suction tip enables effective suctioning without damaging surrounding tissue.

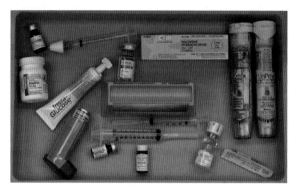

• **Figure 10.7** Emergency drugs.

occur.[13,36,37] Hypoxemia (low oxygen content in the arterial blood) will be the final common pathway to morbidity and mortality in the majority of severe pediatric medical emergency situations.[28,36,37] Therefore, establishment and maintenance of a proper airway and respiratory function is paramount.[13,31]

Adequate oxygenation is easily ensured by the administration of supplemental oxygen.[28] If the patient is adequately breathing spontaneously, oxygen may be delivered by way of a facemask, nasal mask, or nasal cannula prongs.[28] A nonrebreather facemask should be available, as this delivers the highest concentration of oxygen to the spontaneously breathing patient for the most serious medical emergencies.[28] However, should the patient cease breathing during an emergency situation, positive pressure ventilation will be necessary.[28] Although mouth-to-mouth ventilation, or preferably mouth-to-mask ventilation, is possible, this delivers only about 17% oxygen from the rescuer's lungs and is not ideal, but certainly better than no ventilation in a patient who is not breathing.[31] A positive-pressure oxygen delivery system (bag-valve-mask device) that can be connected to a high-flow oxygen source is considered essential equipment to deliver oxygen to the apneic patient (Fig. 10.5).[13,28,31] The bag-valve-mask device, face masks, and oxygen cylinder should all be together in one central location in the office.[1,13,31]

A high-volume suction device is another piece of equipment that is considered essential for the management of medical emergencies.[1,13,28] Emergency situations, especially those involving an obtunded patient, often induce vomiting.[38,39] The aspiration of vomitus can be disastrous, leading to pneumonia and death.[38–42] This can usually be minimized or prevented by proper patient positioning and suctioning.[39] Most dental offices contain high-volume suction equipment for restorative dentistry purposes. A Yankauer type of suction configured and connected to the high-volume evacuation dental suction unit is recommended for suctioning the mouth and pharynx (Fig. 10.6).

Other emergency items that may be needed include syringes and needles for drug administration, oropharyngeal and nasopharyngeal airways, basic monitoring devices which are appropriately sized, and automated external defibrillators (AEDs) capable of electrical therapy delivery for both children and adults.[1,31] For pediatric dentists who provide office-based sedation, the armamentarium for establishing intravenous (IV) access and advanced airway equipment (i-gels/laryngeal mask airways [LMA], endotracheal tubes) should be available.[13,21]

Emergency Drugs

Medical emergencies do not always require rescue drugs.[1,29] Emergency drugs should be administered when there is a clear indication that the agent is needed.[31] There are 10 basic drugs (Table 10.2) that a pediatric dentist should have in their emergency kit (Fig. 10.7).[1,23,27–31] Pediatric dentists who provide office-based sedation are required to have additional drugs available.[13,20,21]

TABLE 10.2   **Emergency Drugs**

Albuterol

Indications:	Treatment of bronchospasm in either asthma attack or allergic reaction
Action:	B$_2$ adrenergic receptor agonist, which causes bronchodilation
How Supplied:	Metered dose inhaler and premixed 2.5 mg/3 mL nebulized solution
Amount to Keep in Office:	1 inhaler and 3 premixed albuterol for nebulized treatments
Dosage:	2 puffs; ideally should have a spacer; may repeat as needed 2.5 mg/3 mL premixed via O$_2$ powered nebulizer; may repeat as needed
Side Effects:	Tachycardia, anxiety, shakiness in arms, hands, legs, feet

Aspirin

Indications:	Suspected acute coronary syndrome or myocardial infarction
Action:	Antiplatelet agent; inhibits thromboxane synthesis
How Supplied:	Chewable tablet (81 mg preferable)
Amount to Keep in Office:	1 bottle baby aspirin (81 mg)
Dosage:	(4) 81 mg chewable
Side Effects:	Dyspepsia (initially)

Diphenhydramine

Indications:	Allergic reactions of slower onset, or less severity than anaphylaxis; adjunct drug with epinephrine in severe allergic reactions
Action:	Histamine (H$_1$) receptor antagonist that blocks the response of the H$_1$ receptor to histamine
How Supplied:	50 mg/mL vial and oral tabs 25 mg/tab
Amount to Keep in Office:	(3) 50 mg vials and (1) box of 25 mg tablets
Dosage:	1 mg/kg IM/IV; max 50 mg
Side Effects:	Dry mouth, sedation

Epinephrine

Indications:	Anaphylaxis, severe persistent asthma, bronchospasm
Action:	Sympathomimetic that stimulates both α- and β-adrenergic receptors, increasing heart rate and blood pressure, relaxing bronchial smooth muscle, and inhibiting histamine's action (antagonism of the physiologic effects of histamine)
How Supplied:	1:1000 (1 mg/mL) ampule, auto injector 0.3 mg/mL (EpiPen) and 0.15 mg auto injector (EpiPen Jr)
Amount to Keep in Office:	(1) EpiPen Adult, (1) EpiPen Jr, and (2) 1:1000 ampules (>30 kg) (15–30 kg)
Dosage:	Adult: 0.3 mL (0.3 mg) Pediatric: IM pediatric dose 0.01 mg/kg up to a maximum of 0.3 mg/dose
Side Effects:	Sinus tachycardia, supraventricular tachycardia and ventricular tachycardia, hypertension, chest pain, anxiety, and headache

Glucose (Oral)

Indications:	Treatment of very low blood sugar (hypoglycemia), most often in people with diabetes mellitus
Action:	Will raise blood sugar if patient is able to swallow
How Supplied:	37.5 g tube
Amount to Keep in Office:	(4) 37.5 g tubes
Dosage:	Swallow 37.5 g; may repeat as necessary
Side Effects:	N/A

Midazolam (Versed)

Indications:	Anticonvulsant for management of status epilepticus (recurrent of sustained seizures >2 min) or seizures from local anesthetic overdose
Action:	Anticonvulsant; enhances GABA-A receptor activity

TABLE 10.2   Emergency Drugs—cont'd

How Supplied:	5 mg/mL in 1-, 2-, 5-, 10-mL vials
Amount to Keep in Office:	1 mg/mL and 5 mg/mL in 10-mL vial; (1) vial each is suggested
Dosage:	IV/IM/IN: Adult 2 mg (max dose 10 mg); pediatric dose 0.2 mg/mg; supplemental doses may be considered if seizures have not resolved within 5–10 min
Side Effects:	Sedation; respiratory depression or arrest

Naloxone

Indications:	Blocks or reverses the effects of opioid medication, including depressed respiratory effort or loss of consciousness. Naloxone is used to treat a narcotic overdose in an emergency situation.
Action:	Opioid antagonist
How Supplied:	0.4-mg/mL vials; 0.4-mg/mL multi-dose vials; 2-mg prefilled syringe
Amount to Keep in Office:	(5) 0.4 mg/mL vials or (1) 0.4 mg/mL multi-dose vial
Dosage:	Adult dose 0.4 mg–2 mg every 3–5 min; max dose: 10 mg
	IV/IM/IN: Pediatric dose 0.01–0.1 mg/kg every 3–5 min as needed based on response; max dose: 10 mg
Side Effects:	Abrupt reversal of opioid effects in persons who are physically dependent on opioids may precipitate an acute withdrawal syndrome, which may include aches, fever, sweating, runny nose, sneezing, weakness, shivering or trembling, nervousness, restlessness or irritability, diarrhea, nausea or vomiting, abdominal cramps, increased blood pressure, and tachycardia; flash pulmonary edema potential for resedation

Nitroglycerin

Indications:	Chest pain as a result of angina or myocardial infarction
Action:	Nitrates cause reduction in left and right ventricular preload through peripheral arterial and venous dilation (predominantly venous)
How Supplied:	Tablets 0.4 mg or spray 0.4 mg metered dose
Amount to Keep in Office:	1 bottle
Dosage:	0.4 mg sublingual every 3–5 min until pain is resolved Administer only if the blood pressure is above 100 systolic and the heart rate is between 60–100 beats per minute
Side Effects:	Headache, facial flushing, hypotension

Oxygen

Indications:	Any medical emergency where the patient is having respiratory distress and hypoxemia
Action:	Increased concentrations of oxygen will increase the amount of oxygen dissolved in the blood, relieving the symptoms caused by low oxygen levels in tissues
How Supplied:	Cylinders
Amount to Keep in Office:	Minimum (1) E cylinder with adjustable regulator 0–15 L
Dosage:	If pulse oximetry is <94%, medium to high concentration, 8–15 L/min via basic or rebreather mask. If pulse oximetry is >94%, low concentration is all that is necessary, 2–4 L via nasal cannula.
Side Effects:	Increased myocardial ischemia/damage when given in high concentrations, when pulse oximetry is >94%

Flumazenil (Romazicon)

Indications:	Indicated to reverse oversedation and respiratory depression Required if sedating with benzodiazepines
Action:	Benzodiazepine antagonist
How Supplied:	0.1 mg/mL, 5 mL, and 10 mL multi-dose vials[a]
Amount to Keep in Office:	(1) 0.1 mg/5 mL multi-dose vial
Dosage:	Adult dose: 0.2 mg IN/IM repeat every minute; max dose is 1 mg
	Pediatric dose: 0.01 mg/kg IN/IM with a maximum dose of 0.2 mg as initial dose; may repeat up to max dose of 1 mg
Side Effects:	May induce seizure activity; potential for resedation

[a]Not FDA approved.

FDA, US Food and Drug Administration; *GABA*, γ-aminobutyric acid; *IM*, intramuscular; *IN*, intranasal; *IV*, intravenous.

It is recommended that the pediatric dentist assemble his or her own drug kit as opposed to purchasing a commercial kit (Fig. 10.8).[31,43-45] Most commercially available emergency kits are not only expensive, but frequently not optimal or tailored to an individual practitioner's needs.[1,31] One of the biggest dangers of owning a commercially available emergency kit is gaining a false sense of security simply by purchasing it. Emergency drugs, along with emergency equipment, should be stored in one location, where they are easily accessible and known to the entire dental team.[1,30,31]

The pediatric dentist is responsible for knowing what drugs are available, along with indications, contraindications, dosages, and side effects.[28,31,43-45] When an emergency occurs, this may be difficult to remember; therefore, it is advised to have a set of emergency drug cards as a reference.[28,45,46] It is also important to know the expiration date of rescue drugs and keep them current.[1,30,31]

Various state regulations may require specific drugs not listed in Table 10.2. The list contains only superficial information and must be expanded upon as needed.

Aspirin

Although this drug is unlikely to be needed by the pediatric patient, he or she is brought to the dental office by adults who may require emergency medical management.

Epinephrine

Epinephrine is the treatment of choice for life-threatening emergencies including anaphylactic reactions and severe asthmatic attacks unresponsive to albuterol.[1,31,47] It is also an early ACLS drug for cardiac arrest.[27] If a pediatric dentist is administering drugs to patients, including local anesthetics, epinephrine must be available in case of allergy.[1,31]

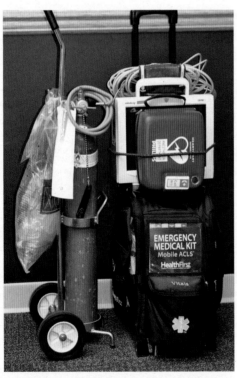

• **Figure 10.8** Emergency equipment kit.

Glucose

Simple sugar, as opposed to complex carbohydrates, should be available for ingestion in cases of suspected hypoglycemic shock.[31] Examples of simple sugar include sugar packets emptied into coffee, nondiet soda, or dissolving candies such as Life Savers.[31] IV dextrose can be given by those competent in establishing IV access.

Other Optional Medications

The pediatric dentist may consider having available a respiratory stimulant, such as ammonia inhalant crushable capsules.[29,45] Commonly, these drugs are found in dental offices taped to cabinets in the operatory to help arouse a patient with unconsciousness secondary to suspected syncope.[1] Other medications to consider in the emergency kit include a corticosteroid, such as methylprednisolone (Solu-Medrol) or hydrocortisone (Solu-Cortef) for acute adrenal insufficiency.[1,48,49] These may also serve as an adjunct to allergy management.[47]

Other agents for cardiovascular urgencies or emergencies could be included. Drugs used in the treatment of hypotension, hypertension, tachycardia, and bradycardia should be available for use by pediatric dentists with advanced training (ACLS and PALS) and are well versed in their use.[25,27]

Management of Medical Emergencies in the Dental Office

Medical emergencies should be approached systematically.[29,31] Certain basic action principles should be applied (Box 10.1).[1,29,31] Management should proceed in a similar fashion for every situation, understanding that a definitive diagnosis may not always be obvious. This will improve efficacy and efficiency while reducing anxiety and confusion for the dental team.[29-31]

Position

For patients who are unconscious or have a decreased level of consciousness, they should be placed supine.[30] This will minimize the work of the heart, increase return of pooled blood from the extremities, and increase vital blood flow to the brain. If the patient is awake, the patient can be placed in a position of comfort (sitting position or semireclined).[30]

> **• BOX 10.1 Steps for Management of Medical Emergencies**
>
> The five basic steps include (the C, A, B's):
> (P)—Position
> (C)—Circulation
> (A)—Airway
> (B)—Breathing
> (D)—Definitive Treatment
>   For all emergencies:
> 1. Discontinue dental treatment.
> 2. Call for assistance/someone to bring oxygen and emergency kit.
> 3. Position patient to ensure open and unobstructed airway.
> 4. Monitor vital signs.
> 5. Be prepared to support respiration, support circulation, provide cardiopulmonary resuscitation, and call for emergency medical services.

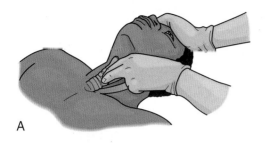 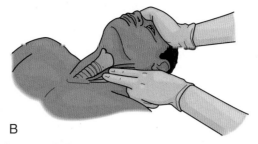

• **Figure 10.9** (A–B) Palpation of the carotid artery. (From Sorrentino S, Remmert L. *Mosby's Textbook for Nursing Assistants.* 9th ed. St Louis: Elsevier; 2017.)

• **BOX 10.2** Compressions

The compression rate is 100–120 per minute. Compressions are done in the lower half of the sternum, mid-nipple line. The compression depth is as follows:

Adult (puberty and above): 2″–2.4″ in depth
Child (age 1 to prepuberty): 2″ in depth
Infant (discharge from hospital to age 1): 1½″ in depth
    The compression to ventilation ratio is:
30:2 single rescuer
30:2 two rescuer adult
15:2 two rescuer, infant and pediatric cardiopulmonary resuscitation

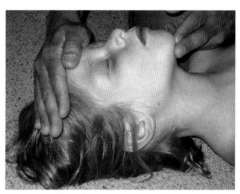

• **Figure 10.10** Head-tilt-chin-lift maneuver. (From Malamed SF. *Medical Emergencies in the Dental Office.* 7th ed. St Louis: Elsevier; 2015.)

Circulation ("C")

The first assessment step is to determine if the patient has a pulse.[27,28,46] The carotid pulse is the easiest and most accurate in the adult and child patient (Fig. 10.9).[30] The carotid artery lies just under the sternocleidomastoid muscle in the neck. Do not palpate both carotid arteries simultaneously as pressure on the baroreceptors of the carotid sinuses may precipitate reflex brady-cardia.[27] When assessing the infant, the brachial pulse should be palpated.[28,46]

While assessing pulse, evaluate chest movement.[28,46] If there is good rise and fall of the chest and a pulse, the patient likely has circulation. If the patient has no chest movement or a very slow, gasping type of breathing (agonal breathing), then assume there is no circulation.[27,28,46] Begin chest compressions immediately (Box 10.2).[46] EMS should simultaneously be activated. Allow full recoil of the chest after each compression; do not lean on the chest after each compression.[46] Compressions should be fast and deep.[46]

Airway ("A")

If the supply of oxygen to the lungs is interrupted, rapid deterioration will occur, resulting in brain cell damage, cardiac arrest, and death.[1,28,30] After determining the patient has a pulse, assess for an adequate airway.[27,28,46] The upper airway may be obstructed by progressive swelling, trauma, a foreign body, or other factors.[50,51]

The most common cause of airway obstruction is the tongue.[52] When a patient becomes obtunded or unconscious, the musculature supporting the mandible and tongue will become relaxed. This allows the base of the tongue to fall against the posterior pharyngeal tissues creating an obstruction. Children with enlarged tonsils are particularly vulnerable to this type of airway obstruction.[53] Tilting the head back (head-tilt maneuver or cervical extension, Fig. 10.10) and thrusting the jaw forward (chin-lift or jaw-thrust maneuver)

will help open the obstructed airway.[30] Oral or nasal airway devices are also useful in keeping the tongue forward in the unconscious or deeply obtunded patient.[27,28] These devices should not be used in conscious patients, as they tend to induce gagging and vomiting.[28]

If the airway is obstructed by a foreign body, such as a cotton roll or dental device, management depends on the patient's condition.[26,30] If the patient is conscious and can cough or vocalize, allow him or her to expel the object with his or her own efforts.[26] If after a short period of time this is clearly ineffective, or if the patient uses the universal choking sign of placing the hands around the neck, the initial step should be to deliver abdominal thrusts (Heimlich maneuver).[26,54–57] Sitting or standing behind the patient, place one fist below the xiphoid process over the mid- to upper abdomen; clench it with the other hand and pull up and back forcefully.[26,54] This maneuver pushes the diaphragm up and produces a sustained forceful increase in intrathoracic pressure, expelling air through the larynx and hopefully dislodging the obstruction.[26,54] Abdominal thrusts should be performed in rapid succession until successful or loss of consciousness.

The abdominal thrust may be modified for the patient who is lying down (as in the dental chair). The rescuer delivers the thrust with the heel of the hand from the side or front of the patient. The abdominal thrust should not be performed in infants less than 1 year old because of their relatively large abdominal organs (especially the liver), which could be damaged.[26] In these cases, a chest thrust maneuver should be delivered. Use the heel of the hand positioned over the mid-sternum, similar to the position of chest compressions during cardiopulmonary resuscitation (CPR).[26]

If the object is not expelled, consciousness will be lost. EMS should be activated as soon as possible. Begin CPR or BLS, chest compressions, and head-tilt-chin-lift maneuver.[26,28] If a foreign body is visible, remove it, but do not perform blind finger sweeps because they may push obstructing objects farther into the pharynx and may damage the oropharynx.[26] Attempt to give two breaths and continue with cycles of chest compressions and ventilations.[26,28] There should be only very brief intermittent evaluations of the upper airway to determine if the foreign body has been dislodged or could be seen and removed. If ventilations are difficult because of the obstruction, reattempt head-tilt/jaw-thrust and consider an oral or nasal airway.[26,28] Caution should be used when placing an airway so as not to distalize the foreign object, worsening the obstruction.[58] Dentists with training may perform laryngoscopy, endotracheal intubation, transtracheal jet ventilation, or cricothyroidotomy, if skilled in these techniques.[31]

Breathing ("B")

Once the airway is managed, rise and fall of the chest should be observed.[1] If there is no rise and fall of the chest, or breathing appears to be inadequate, then ventilating the patient is necessary.[26] In the office setting, ventilation is best achieved by using an appropriately sized bag valve mask.[26,58,59] A bag-valve-mask system, such as an AMBU bag (Ballerup, Denmark), is considered essential emergency equipment for every dental office.[31] The bag valve mask may require two people to operate correctly.[28] One rescuer seals the mask, making the letter "C" and "E" with their fingers and the other squeezes the bag to ventilate (Fig. 10.11). The bag valve mask should be connected to an oxygen source (E tank at minimum) at 15 L/min to ensure 100% oxygen delivery.[28] Bag-mask ventilation is the most critical emergency management skill to master.[59,60]

If there is a palpable pulse (≥60 beats per minute) but there is inadequate breathing, give rescue breaths at a rate of 12 to 20 breaths per minute (1 breath every 3 to 5 seconds) until spontaneous breathing resumes.[26] Reassess the pulse every 2 minutes.[26]

Ventilate with 100% oxygen. Do not hyperventilate, as outcomes are worse when patients are hyperventilated.[27,28,61,62] If unable to properly ventilate using a bag valve mask, an oral or nasal airway should be inserted.[28] Consider an advanced technique when unsuccessful with the oral or nasal airway.[28,31] For the novice intubator, an effective advanced technique may be the i-gel LMA (Intersurgical Ltd, Wokingham, Berkshire, UK) (Fig. 10.12).[31,63,64]

Definitive Therapy ("D")

The "D" represents definitive therapy.[1,30] Once the patient is positioned and circulation, airway, and breathing are managed, then various treatment options, including drug administration, should be considered.[30,65] The decision to administer definitive drug therapy should be based on risk versus benefit.[1] If the cause is clear or was precipitated by a treatment or drug administration, definitive therapy may be indicated and essential.[28,30,65]

Common Medical Emergencies

Allergic Reactions

The primary agents employed in pediatric dentistry that provoke allergic reactions are the penicillins and latex.[65,66] Sulfite antioxidants in local anesthetics containing vasoconstrictors and ester-type local anesthetics used in topical products are also known triggers.[67,68] Common pediatric oral sedative agents and amide local anesthetics rarely cause allergic reactions.[1,68]

Allergy is a hypersensitivity response by the immune system to antigens that are recognized as foreign.[69] Several types of allergic reactions may occur.[70] They range from mild to severe and treatment varies depending on the type of reaction.[70–72] The type I, immediate, or anaphylaxis reaction is of most concern.[1,71,72]

A mild reaction would be an isolated skin rash or small number of hives.[71] For this patient, administering 25 to 50 mg of oral diphenhydramine or 1 mg/kg for pediatric patients is appropriate. The patient should be monitored to make sure symptoms do not worsen.[1,29] These patients may be discharged from the office with a prescription for diphenhydramine 1 mg/kg for children or 25 to 50 mg for adults every 6 hours for 24 hours.[1] A methylprednisolone dose pack may also be considered.[73] The patient and parent should also be instructed to seek immediate medical attention if symptoms worsen (increased redness, rash, or difficulty breathing).[1]

Rapid-onset allergic skin reactions manifest as systemic redness, urticaria (itching, hives), erythema (rash), or angioedema (localized swelling measuring several centimeters in diameter).[1,71] In this case as long as there is no airway involvement, diphenhydramine 1 mg/kg up to 50 mg should be administered intramuscularly (IM).[65] Activate EMS if recovery is not immediate.[1] Recognize that this

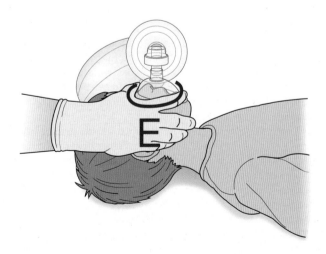

• **Figure 10.11** Hand position ("C and E") for bag valve mask for ventilation.

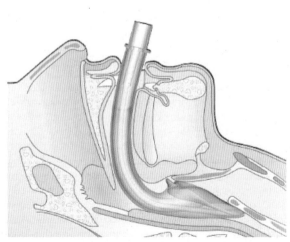

• **Figure 10.12** The i-gel single use supraglottic airway device. (Courtesy Intersurgical Inc., East Syracuse, NY.)

A severe reaction most likely will occur suddenly and manifest in all systems:
Skin: flushing, urticarial, and angioedema
Respiratory: wheezing, laryngeal edema, respiratory distress
Cardiovascular: hypotension, tachycardia, dizziness, loss of consciousness, cardiovascular collapse
Gastrointestinal: abdominal cramps, nausea, vomiting, diarrhea

moderate reaction may rapidly progress to a severe/anaphylactic reaction, which a true life-threatening emergency (Box 10.3).[74]

As a general rule, the more rapid the onset and the more intense the symptoms, the more severe the generalized reaction will become.[1,74] Edema that involves the face and neck may rapidly progress to airway obstruction and death.[74] Respiratory symptoms follow skin reactions in generalized anaphylaxis.[1,74] Constriction of bronchial smooth muscle causes respiratory distress. The principal recognizable sign is wheezing, a distinctive breathing sound associated with bronchoconstriction and similar to an asthmatic attack.[74] As the obstruction worsens, the patient has increasing difficulty exchanging adequate volumes of air.[74]

Cardiovascular involvement, which could lead to life-threatening hypotension, occurs in 45% of patients.[47,74] Hypotension is produced by the vasodilating effects of histamine and other mediators of the response. Reflex tachycardia, arrhythmias, and eventually cardiac arrest may follow. The management of a severe, immediate reaction is discussed below.[47,74]

Management

Terminate the suspected agent, begin basic life support protocol (CABs), activate EMS, and administer 0.3 mg of epinephrine IM for an adult or 0.15 mg for the pediatric patient (EpiPen and EpiPen Jr, respectively)[1,47,76] (Fig. 10.13). Epinephrine at the dose of 0.01 mg/kg to a maximum initial dose of 0.3 mg must be administered to reverse the deleterious effects of histamine (bronchoconstriction and vasodilation).[1,47,76] Administration may need to be repeated every 5 to 15 minutes if symptoms reoccur and EMS is not yet on the scene.[47] Oxygen therapy, two puffs of the albuterol inhaler, and diphenhydramine may also be administered. The patient who suffers from severe anaphylaxis must be transported to the hospital for additional treatment with antihistamines and corticosteroids.[47]

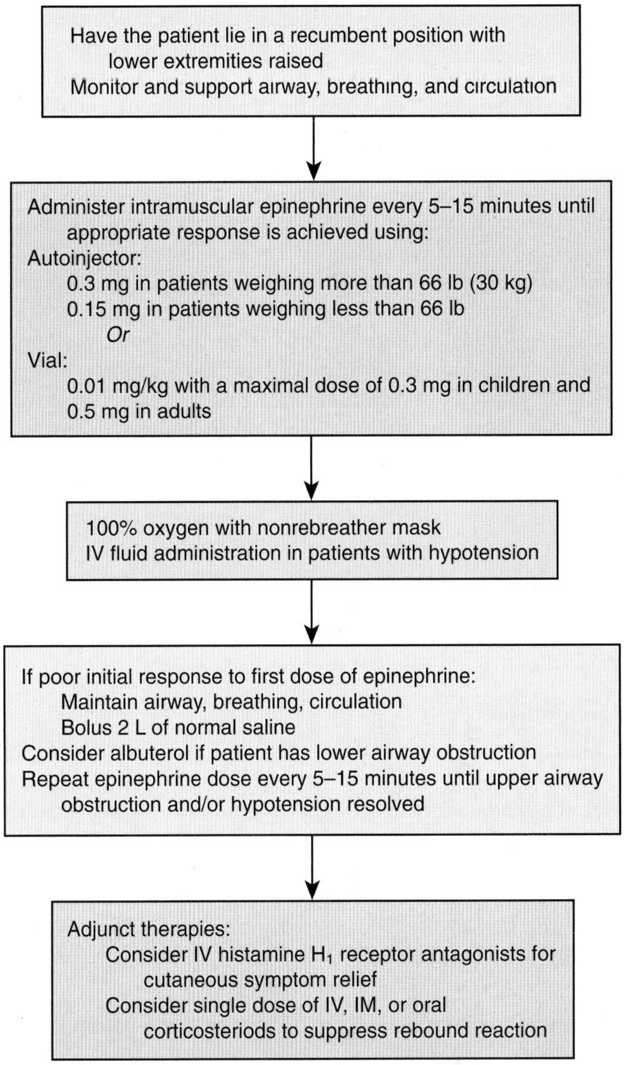

Asthma (Acute Bronchospasm)

Asthma is a common medical emergency that may occur in the dental office.[1,29,65] It is estimated that approximately 17 million Americans suffer from asthma.[76] This results in approximately 2 million visits to the emergency department each year and approximately 5000 to 6000 deaths per year.[1,76]

Asthma is an inflammatory disorder of the airway that results in intermittent airflow obstruction.[77,78] The pathophysiology of asthma is complex. Asthmatic patients have extreme sensitivity of the airway, with an increased contractile response and excessive tenacious secretions. Sudden constriction of hyperreactive smooth muscle in the bronchial wall causes bronchospasm and the characteristic wheezing.[1,79] Thick, tenacious secretions and bronchial wall edema plug small airways, each leading to airway compromise.

• **Figure 10.13** Management of anaphylaxis in the outpatient setting. *IM,* Intramuscular; *IV,* intravenous. (Data from Lieberman P, Kemp SF, Oppenheimer J, et al. The diagnosis and management of anaphylaxis: an updated practice parameter. *J Allergy Clin Immunol.* 2005;115(3 suppl 2):S483–S523.)

The signs and symptoms of an acute asthma attack include chest congestion, cough, wheezing, dyspnea, use of accessory muscles, anxiety, restlessness, apprehension, tachypnea, tachycardia, increase in blood pressure, diaphoresis, confusion, nasal flaring, and cyanosis.[1]

The primary type of asthma in children is allergic or extrinsic asthma, which is mediated by immunoglobulin (IgE) antibodies.[1,79] This asthma attack is triggered by specific allergens such as pollens, dust, and molds.[79,80] The process may produce various signs and symptoms from mild wheezing and coughing to severe dyspnea, cyanosis, and even death.[78–80]

Acute attacks of extrinsic asthma usually occur with diminishing frequency as the child ages and may disappear in later life.[1] In adults, the primary type of asthma is intrinsic asthma. With intrinsic asthma, attacks may be precipitated by infections, cold weather, exercise, and stress.[81,82] Some overlap may occur in the types of asthma.

A thorough history should be documented in the record including how often attacks occur, how severe they have become (if emergency department visits or hospitalization have been required), what triggers attacks, and what medications are being taken. All attempts should be made to avoid precipitating factors. If the patient is taking medications, he or she should be instructed to continue taking them before the dental appointment.[1] The patient should be instructed to bring his or her albuterol inhaler to the dental appointment, should it be needed. The patient may be using other inhalers, such as corticosteroid inhalers, but albuterol is the important rescue inhaler that is needed.[29,65] If patients with asthma begin to wheeze and develop respiratory distress in the dental office, they should be allowed to sit upright where they are usually more comfortable.[1] The patient should take two puffs from the albuterol inhaler. If the inhaler is not available, the dentist should give the patient the inhaler from the office emergency kit. In the vast majority of cases, albuterol inhalation will be sufficient to abort an asthmatic attack.[1] If this fails to reverse the bronchospasm, oxygen should be administered. This may likely be Status Asthmaticus, a true medical emergency.[29,78,83] If the dentist believes the attack may be life-threatening, 0.01 mg/kg (maximal initial dose, 0.3 mg) of epinephrine (1 : 1000) should be injected IM and EMS activated.[29] Epinephrine should be beneficial within a few minutes in most cases. Early administration of a corticosteroid IM may also be helpful in severe attacks, although the onset is rather slow.[73]

Management

Terminate the dental procedure. Reassure the patient and place him/her in a position of comfort. Assess CABs and administer two puffs of albuterol inhaler or 2.5 mg Albuterol/3 mL nebulized solution via an oxygen-powered nebulizer mask at 6 L/min. If the patient is unresponsive to treatment, activate EMS. Reassess CABs; deliver oxygen in high concentration; and consider administering epinephrine 0.3 mg (1 : 1000) IM for an adult or 0.15 mg (1 : 1000) for a child (EpiPen and EpiPen Jr).[1,29,84]

Cardiac Symptoms (Acute Coronary Syndrome)

Pediatric dentists will not see many patients with acute coronary syndrome (ACS). However, parents and grandparents who accompany the patient may develop these symptoms.[1] The chief complaint is usually chest pain. This pain is typically described as tightness or pressure in the chest. The severity can range from minimal to a severe crushing-type of discomfort. Pain may radiate to the neck, back, jaw, and/or down one or both arms. Associated symptoms include dyspnea, nausea, vomiting, and diaphoresis.[27,85] The patient may also experience profound weakness.[27]

Management

Place the patient in a position of comfort and perform physical assessment with vital signs. Activate EMS and administer aspirin (81 mg × 4 chewable) and nitroglycerin 0.4 mg (if the heart rate is between 60 and 100 and BP is >100 systolic). Administer oxygen at 4 L/min if the pulse oximeter is less than 90%. Repeat nitroglycerin as needed every 5 minutes (up to three times) as long as heart rate and blood pressure remain stable.[85]

Cardiac Arrest

According to the American Heart Association, the annual incidence rate for out-of-hospital nontraumatic sudden acute cardiac arrest is 326,200 cases and 9 out of 10 victims die.[86,87] This event can happen anywhere including the dental office and affects people of all ages including infants.[1]

The most common causes of sudden cardiac arrest are thrombosis, cardiomyopathy, and prolonged Q-T interval.[1,87] Predisposing cardiac conditions may go undetected, and drugs, such as attention deficit hyperactivity disorder medications, antidepressants, and antibiotics, could contribute.[88] Some of the warning signs that may indicate impending cardiac arrest include dizziness or feeling light-headed during or after exertion, brief loss of consciousness for no apparent reason, or a family member who dies suddenly under the age of 50.[88–93] If cardiac arrest occurs, recognizing the problem is vital, because timely management is critical.[1,27,28]

Management[27,28]

Assess the circulation by checking for a pulse while simultaneously looking for adequate chest rise and fall. Activate EMS and obtain the AED with the emergency kit and oxygen. Begin chest compressions at a rate of 100 to 120 a minute, with good recoil at the appropriate depth, as described earlier in this chapter, until the AED arrives. Once the AED arrives, turn it on, and follow the voice prompts. If a shock is advised and delivered and the patient does not recover, immediately resume chest compressions and ventilations at the appropriate intervals. If an advanced airway is placed (LMA, i-gel), compressions become continuous and the ventilations are given at a rate of 1 breath every 6 seconds. The AED will analyze every 2 minutes. Continue BLS until EMS arrives or the patient has a return of spontaneous circulation. The AED is indicated for everyone including infants. Pediatric electrodes should be used for children under 55 lb (25 kg).[28]

Diabetic Emergencies

Diabetes mellitus is a disease involving insulin production and/or resistance.[94] Decreased insulin or insulin insensitivity leads to impairments in carbohydrate, fat, and protein metabolism. This disorder is characterized by hyperglycemia when left untreated.[95] Chronic hyperglycemia predisposes to vascular compromise with subsequent dysfunction of the cardiovascular system, peripheral nervous system, kidneys, and other body systems.[1,94]

Type 1 or insulin-dependent diabetes mellitus occurs most commonly in children.[96] It results from loss of pancreatic β cell function, which produces endogenous insulin.[1,95] Therefore, exogenous insulin is required by daily parenteral administration to control blood glucose levels.[1,95]

Emergencies in children may be the result of hypoglycemia or hyperglycemia.[1] If plasma insulin levels remain low or at zero for a prolonged period, blood glucose levels will become extremely elevated. This glucose, however, cannot be used by certain tissues because of the lack of insulin, causing cells to metabolize fat and proteins to produce needed energy. The breakdown of fat and protein produces ketones and other metabolic acids, which may result in a condition known as diabetic ketoacidosis (DKA).[95] This condition could lead to coma and death.[1] Ketoacidosis requires several days to develop, during which time the patient appears ill. It does not occur suddenly in a previously alert and well patient. Therefore, this disorder will generally not lead to an acute emergency in the dental office. Regardless, if the diabetic patient does not look well, and particularly if the breath has an acetone-like odor, he or she should be instructed to seek medical attention immediately.[1,95]

If a diabetic patient, who appears well, has a sudden deterioration in cognition or loss of consciousness in the dental office, the condition is more likely to be due to acute hypoglycemia or insulin shock.[1,65,95] The usual scenario involves a patient who has taken his or her morning insulin and has forgotten to eat a meal or has ingested inadequate carbohydrates.[1]

Exercise and stress may also increase carbohydrate utilization and lower blood glucose concentrations.[97,98]

Glucose and oxygen are the primary metabolic sources for brain cells.[95] As serum glucose levels decrease, symptoms appear.[98] The sympathetic nervous system will attempt to raise blood glucose levels, resulting in tachycardia, hypertension, anxiety, and sweating.[94,95] If not corrected, the patient will develop slurred speech, ataxia, and eventually loss of consciousness.[1] Seizures may also occur.

Most diabetic patients are well attuned to this phenomenon and carry a carbohydrate source to be ingested in this event.[98,99] However, if carbohydrate is not ingested and the blood glucose concentration continues to decrease, cerebral function will deteriorate. Alterations in mood, strange activity, and inappropriate responses to questions may be early clinical indicators.[94,95] Patients in this condition may be confused with those having excessive alcohol ingestion.[1]

Recommend patients continue with their daily regimen and eat their normal diet.[1] This should prevent hypoglycemia (<80 mg/dL blood glucose). The exception to this rule is when patients are instructed to have nothing by mouth (NPO) before sedation or general anesthesia.[99,100]

Management[1,101]

Place the patient in a position of comfort and assess (CABs) the patient. Obtain a blood glucose (if possible) and provide definitive care.[1] Management of hypoglycemia involves the administration of glucose.[98,99] The oral route is used if the patient is conscious and is experiencing early symptoms. Oral glucose tabs 37.5 g can be administered and repeated as necessary. Sugar dissolved in juice or a sugar-containing soft drink may also be used. Simple sugars are more rapidly absorbed than complex carbohydrates. Should the patient become unconscious, BLS should be initiated. Definitive care requires IV access and 50% dextrose IV. This will rapidly bring a return to consciousness. Administering glucose orally is unadvisable if the patient is significantly obtunded or unconscious, as aspiration or airway obstruction may occur. Glucagon may also be considered.

Hyperventilation Syndrome

Hyperventilation syndrome is a maladaptive anxiety reaction that primarily occurs in apprehensive patients who attempt to hide their anxiety.[102] The syndrome is often triggered by an anxiety-provoking event such as local anesthetic adminstration.[1] The patient is usually unaware of the fact that he or she is breathing rapidly. Respiratory rates increase (25 to 30 breaths/min) with an increase in tidal volume. Increased ventilation causes a marked reduction in the blood carbon dioxide.[102,103] The decrease in the arterial partial pressure of carbon dioxide ($PaCO_2$), referred to as hypocarbia, causes a physiologic vasoconstriction of the arteries supplying the brain. The result of the decreased blood flow leaves the patient feeling dizzy and light-headed, which further enhances the anxiety, worsening the condition in a vicious cycle.[1] Other symptoms that may occur include numbness and tingling of the extremities and perioral area, muscle twitching and cramping, seizures, and loss of consciousness.[102–104]

Management

Management of hyperventilation involves early recognition.[1] Reassurance, patient rapport, and calmly coaching the patient to

breathe slowly may be sufficient to stop the process.[1] Oxygen administration will worsen the syndrome.[103] If the cycle cannot be broken, steps should be taken to increase the $PaCO_2$.[1] This can be accomplished simply by having the patient rebreathe exhaled CO_2-containing air. Raising $PaCO_2$ should reverse the process. Extended periods of rebreathing are not recommended, as hypoxia should be avoided.[1] Sedation or general anesthesia for future treatment may be appropriate.

Seizures

Seizures are clinical manifestations of paroxysmal excessive neuronal brain activity.[1] Uncontrolled electrical discharge within the central nervous system (CNS) results in sensory or motor activity, altered visceral function, abnormal motor movements, changes in mental acuity, and unconsciousness.[1]

There are various types of seizures. Generalized (tonic-clonic) seizures may be life-threatening.[1] Generalized seizures are manifested in four phases: the prodromal phase, the aura, the convulsive (ictal) phase, and the postictal phase. The prodromal phase consists of subtle changes that occur over minutes to hours. It is usually not clinically evident to the practitioner or the patient. The aura is a neurologic experience that the patient goes through immediately before the seizure. It is specifically related to the trigger areas of the brain in which the seizure activity begins. It may consist of a taste, a smell, a hallucination, motor activity, or other symptoms. A given patient's aura is often the same for all seizures. As the CNS discharge becomes generalized, the ictal phase begins.[105]

Consciousness is lost, the patient falls to the floor, and tonic, rigid skeletal muscle contraction occurs. Clonic movements begin, producing rapid jerking of the extremities and trunk. Breathing may be labored during this period, and patients may injure themselves. This tonic-clonic phase usually lasts 1 to 3 minutes.[105–107] As the clonic phase ends, the muscles relax and movement stops. A significant degree of CNS depression is usually present during this postictal phase.[105] Caution must be exercised in the postictal phase as there may be respiratory depression. Often, the patient has amnesia from the prodromal phase throughout the entire seizure.[1]

Management[1,29]

Management of a seizure consists of clearing the area, gentle immobilization (stabilization), and positioning of the patient to prevent self-injury.[1,108,109] Postictal management is critical as this is when the patient is likely to become obtunded or hypoglycemic.[108] Ensure adequate ventilation (airway management) and provide supportive care, as indicated. Consider a blood glucose level to rule out hypoglycemia if the patient is unarousable.[1,108]

Single seizures do not require drug therapy because they usually are self-limiting. Should the ictal phase last longer than 5 minutes or if seizures continue to develop with little time between them, a condition called *status epilepticus* has developed.[105,106] This may be a life-threatening medical emergency, since the uncontrolled muscle activity can result in hyperthermia, hypoglycemia, increased oxygen consumption, tachycardia, hypertension, impaired ventilation, and cardiac arrhythmias.[106,107] IV administration of an benzodiazepine anticonvulsant (diazepam, lorazepam, or midazolam) should be administered.[110] In the pediatric dental office, where IV access may not be available, the condition may be managed with IM midazolam, 0.2 mg/kg to a maximum of 10 mg or intranasal midazolam 0.2 mg/kg up to 1 to 2 mg.[111–113] Airway management postadministration is essential as benzodiazepines can cause respiratory depression. EMS should be activated for transport to the hospital.[111]

Syncope

Syncope is the most common medical emergency in the dental office.[114,115] Less common in young children, it is very prevalent among teenagers and young adults.[1] Factors that predispose patients to syncope include, but are not limited to, anxiety, pain, and stress.[1,116]

Vasodepressor syncope, or the simple faint, is the most common type of syncope and cause for loss of consciousness in the dental office.[1] This maladaptive stress reaction activates the fight-or-flight response of the sympathetic nervous system. Endogenous epinephrine and norepinephrine are released into the circulation, resulting in a large increase in blood flow to the muscles of the body. If the muscles are contracting, as would be the case if the individual were running, normal blood flow is maintained. However, in the dental chair, little or no muscle contraction is occurring, thus the blood pools in the muscles, effectively decreasing the relative blood volume available to the central circulation and therefore the brain. The heart rate initially increases in an attempt to maintain the blood pressure, but as ventricular filling decreases because of poor venous return, reflex mechanisms slow the heart rate to improve filling of the ventricles. Thus, a patient who is anxious with initial hypertension and tachycardia develops hypotension and bradycardia. Cerebral perfusion is then compromised, causing loss of consciousness or fainting. Early in the process, as blood flow to the brain decreases, the patient feels dizzy or light-headed. This phase of the condition is called *presyncope,* and the patient may lose normal skin color in the face and lips. Presyncope usually begins rapidly.[1]

If presyncope is recognized in a susceptible patient and managed quickly, loss of consciousness may be prevented. Management consists of positioning the patient supine, lowering the head, and raising the legs above the heart to augment blood flow to the brain by gravity. Cardiac output will be increased and adequate cerebral perfusion will be restored. Administration of oxygen is appropriate in any emergency involving a decrease in brain perfusion.

If the process of syncope continues, the sympathetic nervous system will fatigue, and the parasympathetic nervous system will suddenly become dominant. This vagal response results in a sudden, severe decrease in heart rate and blood pressure. Blood flow to the brain is compromised, and consciousness is lost. However, if the patient is quickly placed in the supine position with legs elevated, loss of consciousness from syncope will likely resolve. Although consciousness may be regained fairly quickly, recovery of heart rate and blood pressure may be quite slow. If loss of consciousness does not return in less than 1 minute, it is not syncope. All syncope cannot be assumed to be vasovagal; however, treatment is essentially the same.[1,116]

Management[1,29,65]

Position the patient supine, with legs slightly elevated, and administer oxygen. Airway, breathing, and circulation should be monitored and supported as needed. Tight and constrictive clothing should be loosened and vital signs monitored. Ammonia inhalants may stimulate and be beneficial.[29]

If recovery of consciousness is delayed beyond 5 minutes or is incomplete after 15 to 20 minutes, medical assistance should be sought.[1] Drug therapy is usually not indicated with syncope unless the heart rate or blood pressure remains dangerously depressed

after positioning. In such a case, epinephrine could increase heart rate and improve cardiac output.[27]

Following a syncopal episode, the patient may be discharged after a period of watchful waiting and return of vital signs to acceptable levels. The risk of repeat syncope is, however, greater for some time after the episode.[116] The patient should not operate a vehicle and should arrange for alternative transportation if needed.[1]

Recommendations

Dentists treating pediatric patients should:
- Be prepared by further expanding on this material.
- Become familiar with other potential medical emergency situations that may occur in the dental office.
- Understand drug-related emergencies that may result from pharmacologic agents being utilized in daily practice.

References

1. Malamed SF. *Medical Emergencies in the Dental Office.* 7th ed. St Louis: Elsevier; 2015.
2. Morbidity. In: *Dorland's Illustrated Medical Dictionary.* 32nd ed. Philadelphia: Elsevier; 2012.
3. Reason J. *Human Error.* New York: Cambridge University Press; 1990.
4. Reasons J. Human error: models and management. *BMJ.* 2000;320(7237):768–770.
5. Dionne RA, Phero JC, Becker DE, eds. *Management of Pain & Anxiety in the Dental Office.* Philadelphia: Saunders; 2002.
6. Malamed SF. *Sedation: A Guide to Patient Management.* 4th ed. St Louis: Mosby; 2003.
7. Goldberger E. *Treatment of Cardiac Emergencies.* 5th ed. St Louis: Mosby; 1990.
8. McCarthy FM. *Essentials of Safe Dentistry for the Medically Compromised Patient.* Philadelphia: WB Saunders; 1989.
9. McCarthy FM. Sudden, unexpected death in the dental office. *J Am Dent Assoc.* 1971;83(5):1091–1092.
10. Mastuura H. Analysis of systemic complications and deaths during dental treatment in Japan. *Anesth Prog.* 1990;36:219–228.
11. McCarthy FM. A new patient-administered medical history developed for dentistry. *J Am Dent Assoc.* 1985;111:595.
12. Malamed SF. Knowing your patients. *J Am Dent Assoc.* 2010;141 (suppl):3s–7s.
13. American Academy of Pediatrics, American Academy of Pediatric Dentistry. Guideline for monitoring and management of pediatric patients during and after sedation for diagnostic and therapeutic procedures: update 2016. *Pediatr Dent.* 2016;38(special issue):216–245.
14. American Dental Association. Guidelines for the Use of Sedation and General Anesthesia by Dentists, as adopted by the October 2007 ADA House of Delegates. Chicago: American Dental Association; 2007.
15. American Society of Anesthesiologists Task Force on Sedation and Analgesia by Non-Anesthesiologists. Practice guidelines for sedation and analgesia by non-anesthesiologists. *Anesthesiology.* 2002;96(4):1004–1017.
16. Haas DA. An update on local anesthetics in dentistry. *J Can Dent Assoc.* 2002;68(9):546–551.
17. American Academy of Pediatric Dentistry. Policy on medically necessary care. *Pediatr Dent.* 2016;38(special issue):18–22.
18. American Academy of Pediatric Dentistry. Proceedings of the Consensus Conference: Behavior Management for the Pediatric Dental Patient. American Academy of Pediatric Dentistry. Chicago; 1988.

19. American Academy of Pediatric Dentistry. Special issue: proceedings of the conference on behavior management for the pediatric dental patient. *Pediatr Dent.* 2004;26(2):110–183.
20. American Academy of Pediatric Dentistry. Guideline on use of nitrous oxide for pediatric dental patients. *Pediatr Dent.* 2016;38(special issue):211–215.
21. American Academy of Pediatric Dentistry. Guideline on use of anesthesia personnel in the administration of office-based deep sedation/general anesthesia to the pediatric dental patient. *Pediatr Dent.* 2016;38(special issue):246–250.
22. Excerpted from Continuum of Depth of Sedation: Definition of General Anesthesia and Levels of Sedation/Analgesia; 2014, of the American Society of Anesthesiologists (ASA).
23. American Dental Association Guidelines for the Use of Sedation and General Anesthesia by Dentists. Adopted by the ADA House of Delegates, October 2016.
24. American Academy of Pediatric Dentistry. Guideline on use of local anesthesia for pediatric dental patients. *Pediatr Dent.* 2016;38(special issue):204–210.
25. Boynes SG, Moore PA, Lewis CL, et al. Complications associated with anesthesia administration for dental treatment in a special needs clinic. *Spec Care Dentist.* 2010;30(1):3–7.
26. Atkins DL, Berger S, Duff JP, et al. Web-based integrated guidelines for cardiopulmonary resuscitation and emergency cardiovascular care—part 11: pediatric basic life support and cardiopulmonary resuscitation quality. American Heart Association. ECCguidelines.heart.org.
27. Link MS, Berkow LC, Kudenchuk PJ, et al. Part 7: adult advanced cardiovascular life support. *Circulation.* 2015;132:S444–S464.
28. de Caen AR, Berg MD, Chameides L, et al. Part 12: pediatric advanced life support: 2015 guidelines update. *Circulation.* 2015;132:S526–S542.
29. Guideline for managing medical emergencies. *Pediatr Dent.* 2016;38(special issue):451–452.
30. Haas DA. Preparing dental office staff members for emergencies: developing a basic action plan. *J Am Dent Assoc.* 2010;141(suppl):8s–13s.
31. Rosenburg M. Preparing for medical emergencies. The essential drugs and equipment for the dental office. *J Am Dent Assoc.* 2010;141(suppl):14s–19s.
32. Weaver WD, Cobb LA, Hallstrom AP, et al. Factors influencing survival after out-of-hospital cardiac arrest. *J Am Coll Cardiol.* 1986;7(4):752–757.
33. Eisenber MS, Bergner L, Hallstrom A. Cardiac resuscitation in the community; importance of rapid provision and implications for program planning. *JAMA.* 1979;241(18):1905–1907.
34. Malamed SF. Managing medical emergencies. *J Am Dent Assoc.* 1993;124:40–45.
35. Academy of General Dentistry. Medical Emergencies: Video Journal of Dentistry. 3:3, Chicago, 1994.
36. Coté CJ, Karl HW, Notterman DA, et al. Adverse sedation events in pediatrics: analysis of medications used for sedation. *Pediatrics.* 2000;106(4):633–644.
37. Coté CJ, Notterman DA, Karl HW, et al. Adverse sedation events in pediatrics: a critical incident analysis of contributing factors. *Pediatrics.* 2000;105(4 Pt 1):805–814.
38. Duncan GH, Moore P. Nitrous oxide and the dental patient: a review of adverse reactions. *J Am Dent Assoc.* 1984;108:213–219.
39. Cote CJ, Goudsouzian NG, Liu LMP, et al. Assessment of risk factors related to the acid aspiration syndrome in pediatric patients—gastric pH and residual volume. *Anesthesiology.* 1982;56:70–72.
40. Campbell RL, Paulette SW. Pulmonary aspiration during general anesthesia. *Anesth Prog.* 1986;33(2):98–101.
41. Hupp JR, Peterson LJ. Aspiration pneumonitis etiology, therapy, and prevention. *J Oral Surg.* 1981;39(6):430–435.
42. Warner MA, Warner ME, Warner DO, et al. Perioperative pulmonary aspiration in infants and children. *Anesthesiology.* 1999;90:66–71.
43. Pallasch TJ. This emergency kit belongs in your office. *Dent Manage.* 1976;16(9):43–45.
44. American Dental Association (ADA). *ADA Guide to Dental Therapeutics.* Chicago: ADA; 2015.
45. Hegenbarth MA, American Academy of Pediatrics Committee on Drugs. Preparing for pediatric emergencies: drugs to consider. *Pediatrics.* 2008;121(2):433–443.
46. 2015 American Heart Association Guidelines for CPR and ECC. Dallas, American Heart Association, 2015.
47. Joint Task Force on Practice Parameters; American Academy of Allergy, Asthma and Immunology; American College of Allergy, Asthma and Immunology; Joint Council of Allergy, Asthma and Immunology. The diagnosis and management of anaphylaxis: an updated practice parameter. *J Allergy Clin Immunol.* 2005;115(3 suppl 2):S483–S523. (Published correction appears in *J Allergy Clin Immunol.* 2008;122[1]:68.)
48. Leshin M. Acute adrenal insufficiency; recognition management and prevention. *Urol Clin North Am.* 1982;9(2):229–235.
49. Wogan JM. Endocrine disorders. In: Marx J, ed. *Rosen's Emergency Medicine Concepts and Clinical Practice.* 5th ed. St Louis: Mosby; 2002:1770–1785.
50. Safar P, Excarraga L, Change F. A study of upper airway obstruction in the unconscious patient. *J Appl Physiol.* 1961;14:760.
51. Boidin MP. Airway patency in the unconscious patient. *Br J Anaesth.* 1985;57(3):306–310.
52. Linscott MS, Horton WC. Management of upper airway obstruction. *Otolaryngol Clin North Am.* 1979;12(2):351–373.
53. Harless J, Ramaiah R, Bhananker S. Pediatric airway management. *Int J Crit Illn Inj Sci.* 2014;4(1):65–70.
54. Heimlich HJ. A life-saving maneuver to prevent food-choking. *JAMA.* 1975;234(4):398–401.
55. Langhelle A, Sunde K, Wik L, et al. Airway pressure with chest compressions versus Heimlich manoeuvre in recently dead adults with complete airway obstruction. *Resuscitation.* 2000;44:105–108.
56. Sternbach G, Kiskaddon RT. Henry Heimlich: a life-saving maneuver for food choking. *J Emerg Med.* 1985;3:143–148.
57. Redding JS. The choking controversy: critique of evidence on the Heimlich maneuver. *Crit Care Med.* 1979;7:475–479.
58. Hartrey R, Bingham RM. Pharyngeal trauma as a result of blind finger sweeps in the choking child. *J Accid Emerg Med.* 1995;12:52–54.
59. Stockinger ZT, McSwain NE Jr. Prehospital endotracheal intubation for trauma does not improve survival over bag-valve-mask ventilation. *J Trauma.* 2004;56:531–536.
60. Pitetti R, Glustein JZ, Bhende MS. Prehospital care and outcome of pediatric out-of-hospital cardiac arrest. *Prehosp Emerg Care.* 2002;6:283–290.
61. Aufderheide TP, Sigurdsson G, Pirrallo RG, et al. Hyperventilation-induced hypotension during cardiopulmonary resuscitation. *Circulation.* 2004;109:1960–1965.
62. Wik L, Kramer, Johansen J, et al. Quality of cardiopulmonary resuscitation during out-of-hospital cardiac arrest. *JAMA.* 2005;293:299–304.
63. Samarkandi AH, Seraj MA, el Dawlatly A, et al. The role of laryngeal mask airway in cardiopulmonary resuscitation. *Resuscitation.* 1994;28(2):103–106.
64. Kim YY, Kang GH, Kim WH, et al. Comparison of blind intubation through supraglottic devices and direct laryngoscopy by novices: a simulation manikin study. *Clin Exp Emerg Med.* 2016;3(2):75–80.
65. Reed K. Basic management of medical emergencies: recognizing a patient's distress. *J Am Dent Assoc.* 2010;141 suppl:20s–24s.
66. Anderson JA, Adkinson NF Jr. Allergic reactions to drugs and biologic agents. *JAMA.* 1987;258(20):2891–2899.
67. Aldrete JA, Johnson DA. Allergy to local anethetics. *JAMA.* 1969;207:356–357.
68. Lang ML, Lubken WC, Goering A. Insights for specialties: oral surgery, periodontics, and endodontics. In: Basset KB, DiMarco AC, Naughton DK, eds. *Local Anesthesia for the Dental Professional.* Upper Saddle River, NJ: Pearson Education; 2010:397.

69. *Mosby's Dictionary of Medicine, Nursing, & Health Professionals.* 7th ed. St Louis: Mosby; 2006.
70. Lachmann PH, ed. *Clinical Aspects of Immunology.* 5th ed. Boston: Blackwell Scientific; 1993.
71. Lindzon RD, Silvers WS. Anaphylaxis. In: Marx JA, Hockberger RS, Walls RM, eds. *Rosen's Emergency Medicine Concepts and Clinical Practice.* 5th ed. St Louis: Mosby; 2002.
72. Sicherer SH, Leung DY. Advances in allergic skin disease, anaphylaxis, and hypersensitivity reactions to food, drugs, and insect stings. *J Allergy Clin Immunol.* 2004;114:118–124.
73. Methylprednisolone (Medrol, Medrol Dosepak) package insert, Pharmacia & Upjohn Co, Division of Pfizer Inc, New York.
74. Arnold JJ, Williams PM. Anaphylaxis: recognition and management. *Am Fam Physician.* 2011;84(10):1111–1118.
75. Deleted in review.
76. National Center for Health Statistics. Health, United States, 2016: with chartbook on long-term trends in health. Hyattsville, MD: 2017. https://www.cdc.gov/nchs/data/hus/hus16.pdf. Accessed December 22, 2017.
77. Sveuem RJ. Childhood asthma. Balancing efficacy and adherence for optimum treatment. *Postgrad Med.* 2005;118:43–50.
78. Yang KD. Asthma management issues in infancy and childhood. *Treat Respir Med.* 2005;4(1):9–20.
79. Daniele RP. Pathophysiology of asthma. In: Fishman AP, ed. *Pulmonary Diseases and Disorders.* 2nd ed. New York: McGraw-Hill; 1988.
80. Morwood K, Gills D, Smith W, et al. Aspirin-sensitive asthma. *Intern Med J.* 2005;35:240–246.
81. Lucas SR, Platts-Mills TA. Physical activity and exercise in asthma: relavence to etiology and treatment. *J Allergy Clin Immunol.* 2005;115:928–934.
82. Hudgel DW, Langston L, Sclner JC. Viral and bacterial infections in adults with chronic asthma. *Am Rev Respir Dis.* 1979;120:393–397.
83. Lencher KI, Saltoun C. Status asthmaticus. *Allergy Asthma Proc.* 2004;25(4 suppl 1):S31–S33.
84. Pollart SM, Compton RM, Elward KS. Management of acute asthma exacerbations. *Am Fam Physician.* 2011;84(1):40–47.
85. American Heart Association. Web-based integrated guidelines for cardiopulmonary resuscitation and emergency cardiovascular care—part 9: acute coronary syndromes. ECCguidelines.heart.org.
86. Writing Group Members, Mozaffarian D, Benjamin EJ, et al. Executive summary: heart disease and stroke statistics—2016 update: a report from the American Heart Association. *Circulation.* 2016;133(4):447–454.
87. Go AS, Mozaffarian D, Roger VL, et al. Heart disease and stroke statistics—2014 update. A report from the American Heart Association. *Circulation.* 2014;129(3):e28–e292.
88. Lopshire JC, Zipes DP. Sudden cardiac death: better understanding of risks, mechanisms, and treatment. *Circulation.* 2006;114:1134–1136.
89. Mäkikallio TH, Barthel P, Schneider R, et al. Frequency of sudden cardiac death among acute myocardial infarction survivors with optimized medical and revascularization therapy. *Am J Cardiol.* 2006;97(4):480–484.
90. Goldenberg I, Jonas M, Tenenbaum A, et al. Current smoking, smoking cessation, and the risk of sudden cardiac death in patients with coronary artery disease. *Arch Intern Med.* 2003;163(19):2301–2305.
91. Chugh SS, Reinier K. Predicting sudden death in the general population: another step, N terminal B-type natriuretic factor levels. *Circulation.* 2009;119:2863–2864.
92. Das MK, Zipes DP. Fragmented QRS: a predictor of mortality and sudden cardiac death. *Heart Rhythm.* 2009;6(3 suppl):S8–S14.
93. Chugh SS, Reinier K, Singh T, et al. Determinants of prolonged QT interval and their contribution to sudden death risk in coronary artery disease: the Oregon Sudden Unexpected Death Study. *Circulation.* 2009;119(5):663–670.
94. Cydulka RK, Stiff J. Diabetes mellitus and disorders of glucose homeostasis. In: Marx JA, Hockberger RS, Walls RM, eds. *Rosen's Emergency Medicine: Concepts and Clinical Practice.* 5th ed. St Louis: Mosby; 2002:1635–1664.
95. Sherwin RS. Diabetes mellitus. In: Golman I, Ausiello D, eds. *Cecil Textbook of Medicine.* 22nd ed. Philidelphia: WB Saunders; 2003.
96. Centers for Disease Control and Prevention. National Diabetes Fact Sheet: general Information and National Estimates on Diabetes in the United States, 2005. Atlanta, US Department of Health and Human Services, Centers for Disease Control and Prevention, 2005.
97. Arogyasami J, Conlee RK, Booth CL. Effects of exercise on insulin-induced hypoglycemia. *J Appl Physiol.* 1990;69:686–693.
98. Cooke DW, Plotnick L. Type 1 diabetes mellitus in pediatrics. *Pediatr Rev.* 2008;29:374–385.
99. American Diabetes Association. Management of dyslipidemia in children and adolescents with diabetes. *Diabetes Care.* 2003;26:2194–2197.
100. Marks JB. Perioperative management of diabetes. *Am Fam Physician.* 2003;67(1):93–100.
101. Hazinski MF, Shuster M, Donnino MW, et al. Highlights of 2015 American Heart Association Guidelines Update for CPR and ECC. Dallas: American Heart Association; 2015.
102. Masoka Y, Jack S, Warburton CH, et al. Breathing patterns associated with trait anxiety and breathlessness in humans. *J Physiol.* 2004;54:465–470.
103. Folgering H. The pathophysiology of hyperventilation syndrome. *Monaldi Arch Chest Dis.* 1999;54:365–372.
104. Foster GT, Vaziri ND, Seasoon CS. Respiratory alkalosis. *Respir Care.* 2001;46:384–391.
105. Pollack CV, Pollack ES. Seizures. In: Marx JA, Hockberger RS, Walls RM, eds. *Rosen's Emergency Medicine: Concepts and Clinical Practice.* 5th ed. St Louis: Mosby; 2002:1445–1455.
106. Sirven JL, Waterhouse E. Management of status epilepticus. *Am Fam Physician.* 2003;68:469–476.
107. Chen JW, Wasterlain CG. Status epilepticus: pathophysiology and management in adults. *Lancet Neurol.* 2006;5:246–256.
108. Scheur ML, Pedley TA. The evaluation and treatment of seizures. *N Engl J Med.* 1990;323:1468–1474.
109. Giovanntti JA Jr. Aspiration of a partial denture during an epileptic seizure. *J Am Dent Assoc.* 1981;103:895.
110. Mahmoudian T, Zadeh MM. Comparison of intranasal midazolam with intravenous diazepam for treating acute seizures in children. *Epilepsy Behav.* 2004;5:253–255.
111. Brophy GM, Bell R, Claassen J, et al. Guidelines for the evaluation and management of status epilepticus. *Neurocrit Care.* 2012;17(1):3–23.
112. Wolfe TR, McFarlane TC. Intranasal midazolam therapy for pediatric status epilepticus. *Am J Emerg Med.* 2006;24(3):343–346.
113. Midazolam Injection USP (package insert). Akorn Inc., Lake-Forest, IL.
114. Fast TB, Martin MD, Ellis TM. Emergency preparedness: a survey of dental practitioners. *J Am Dent Assoc.* 1986;112:499–501.
115. Malamed SF. Beyond the basics: emergency medicine in dentistry. *J Am Dent Assoc.* 1997;128:843–854.
116. Feinberg AN. Syncope in the adolescent. *Adolesc Med.* 2002;13:553–567.

11

Dental Public Health Issues in Pediatric Dentistry

HOMA AMINI, JONATHAN D. SHENKIN, AND DONALD L. CHI

CHAPTER OUTLINE

Of the primary challenges facing the dental profession is ensuring that all children and adults enjoy the benefits of good oral health. Though treatment of children in an office setting is the cornerstone of pediatric dental practice, it cannot address all the needs of all children because of limited access to dental care and limited capacity. Thus, to optimize the oral health of all children, community-based, public health approaches are necessary. This chapter provides an overview of dental public health and outlines ways in which the oral health of children is enhanced by various public health activities.

Definition of Dental Public Health

Dental public health is defined as "the science and art of preventing and controlling dental diseases and promoting dental health through organized community efforts."[1] A common misconception about dental public health is that its primary objective is the delivery of dental care to low-income persons. Although this is important, the actual delivery of dental care is only one aspect of dental public health. The three major core functions of public health, as identified by the 1988 Institute of Medicine study, are assessment, policy development, and assurance.[2] The major activities of dental public health can be divided into these same categories. Examples of core dental public health activities that affect the oral health of children are given in Box 11.1.

Role of the Individual Practitioner

Dental professionals are in a unique position to improve the oral health of their patients and their community. They not only provide direct dental care for individual patients, they are also the primary advocates for the oral health of children. Engaging in advocacy efforts to promote better oral health is a responsibility of all dental professionals, and it can occur at multiple levels including individual, community, and policy/legislative levels.

It is important for the individual practitioner to understand that the oral health status and needs of children receiving care in a private practice setting may not represent the status and needs of *all* children in the community. Children with unmet dental needs frequently do not utilize dental care regularly. The challenge for dentists, therefore, is to look beyond the individual dental office and make a broad assessment of their community's needs while assessing their own role in enhancing the oral health of the entire community.

The Association of State and Territorial Dental Directors (ASTDD) developed and disseminated a needs assessment model last revised in 2003, designed to help communities identify and address their oral health needs.[3,4] This model is known as the ASTDD Seven-Step Model (Fig. 11.1). It provides a straightforward approach for identifying the oral health needs of a community and for designing a program to meet these needs based on available resources. A community-based needs assessment will also provide an excellent opportunity to educate a community about the importance of oral health.[4]

In addition to participating in needs assessment activities, practitioners are often called on to participate in other public health activities, including advocating fluoridation of community water supplies, participating in school and community health promotion activities, advocating for physicians to be reimbursed for the application of fluoride varnish for at-risk children, and advising policy makers regarding dental care programs including Medicaid. Support and guidance for the individual practitioner becoming involved in dental public health activities can be sought from a variety of sources, including the oral health components of state public health agencies, county boards of health, dental/medical societies, and various community boards and organizations.

One important issue practitioners often find themselves involved with is enhancing access to dental care for members of their communities. This topic is discussed in the following sections.

Assessment

1. Documenting the oral health status of children through epidemiologic surveys
2. Assessing the supply and availability of dentists to meet the needs of children
3. Assessing the status of water fluoridation in communities
4. Assessing the need for dental care for children with special health care needs
5. Identifying barriers to dental access
6. Screening children before entering school

Policy Development

1. Developing policies and advocating for legislative action to ensure access to oral health services for low-income, underserved, hard-to-reach, and vulnerable children
2. Developing programs that focus on primary and secondary prevention
3. Developing programs to provide dental care to children with special health needs or without access to adequate dental care
4. Adopting state rules mandating oral health screening for children entering school for the first time

Assurance

1. Encouraging and coordinating efforts to provide oral health education and promotion in schools, clinics, community settings, and other settings
2. Expanding or establishing new dental clinical sites (e.g., Community Health Center expansions)
3. Developing promotional activities by the State Health Agency to meet the oral health needs of a specific target group or community
4. Targeting topical and systemic fluoride programs to areas with nonfluoridated water supplies and high-risk populations
5. Including an oral health component in all school health initiatives
6. Establishing school-based prevention programs and school-based or school-linked dental clinics as components of comprehensive school health
7. Establishing programs to train medical professionals and other health-related workers to recognize oral health problems, including early childhood caries
8. Integrating oral health services into appropriate health, education, and social service programs (e.g., Maternal and Child Health; nutrition; Women, Infants, and Children; health promotion; school health)

Modified from Association of State and Territorial Dental Directors. Guidelines for State and Territorial Oral Health Programs. June 2010.

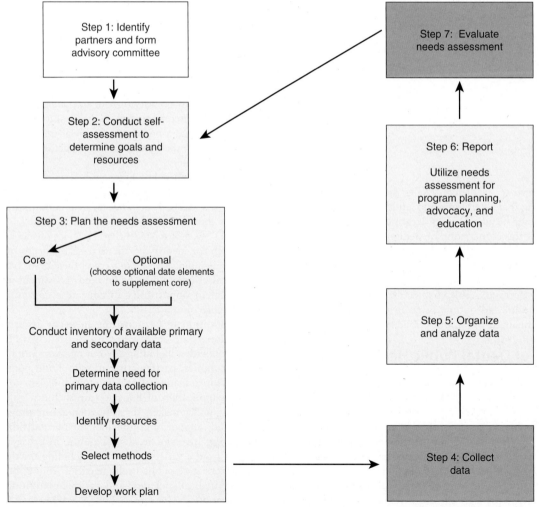

• **Figure 11.1** Association of State and Territorial Dental Directors Seven-Step Needs Assessment Model. (Redrawn from *Association of State and Territorial Dental Directors.* Assessing oral health needs: ASTDD Seven-Step Model. www.astdd.org/oral-health-assessment-7-step-model/. Accessed August 24, 2017.)

Access to Care

Although regular dental care contributes substantially to good oral health for millions of children, a significant number of children and adults have serious problems receiving the care they need. These children are most often from low-income or minority families, and unfortunately these groups tend to experience more oral disease than other children.[5-7] Some of the factors that can limit access to dental care for these children are (1) lack of finances (including lack of third-party coverage), (2) lack of transportation and geographic isolation, (3) language and cultural barriers, and (4) availability of dental providers who accept Medicaid.

Another major factor that limits use of dental services is lack of perceived need for care and low oral health literacy. Although financial, cultural, behavioral, social, and biological factors are among the major determinants of oral health, literacy skills are hypothesized to contribute to oral health outcomes. Oral health literacy is defined as "the degree to which individuals have the capacity to obtain, process, and understand basic oral health information and services needed to make appropriate health decisions."[8] Individual patient skills, the provider's ability to communicate effectively and accurately, and the informational demands placed on patients by health care systems impact health literacy. Low health literacy has been linked to poor health outcomes, lower use of preventive services, increased use of hospital emergency rooms, and higher health care costs.

Dental Participation in Medicaid

Historically, financial limitations have been among the most formidable barriers for low-income children in receiving health care. In 1965, the federal government attempted to reduce these financial barriers by creating the Medicaid program (Title 19), which pays for medical and dental care for eligible low-income children. Adult dental coverage under Medicaid is optional, and covered services vary widely from state to state. However, coverage for child dental services is mandatory because of a 1968 amendment to the Medicaid program creating the Early and Periodic Screening, Diagnostic and Treatment (EPSDT) program.[9] The purpose of the EPSDT program is to identify the health problems of children as early as possible and to provide comprehensive preventive and remedial care.

Since 1965, the Medicaid program has been the primary public insurance program for the financing of dental services for low-income children in the United States. Most children below the poverty level who receive dental care do so through the Medicaid (Title 19) program.[10] In 1997, the State Children's Health Insurance Program (SCHIP) was started to expand public insurance to children in families with incomes too high to qualify for Medicaid but not adequate to purchase private insurance; the program is now simply known as the CHIP program.[11] In January 2015, the Affordable Care Act (ACA) required that all children who were up to 133% of the federal poverty level be transitioned from CHIP programs to Medicaid. As of 2015, states covered children in their CHIP program either through an expansion of their existing Medicaid program (9 states), a separate child health program (13 states), or a combination of the two (29 states).[12]

Although Medicaid and CHIP have been successful in improving access to dental services for some, in 1996 a report from the Inspector General of the US Department of Health and Human Services (DHHS) indicated that only one in five Medicaid-eligible children receive any dental services annually.[13] However, the number of children receiving dental services under Medicaid has grown continuously since 2000. By 2012, almost half of all children under age 20 were reported to receive dental services, compared with 29.3% in 2000. The percentage of children under age 20 receiving preventive dental services increased from 23.2% to 42.4%, and for dental treatment services the rate increased from 15.3% to 22.9%.[14]

One of the biggest barriers to dental care is the lack of dentists willing to accept Medicaid-enrolled children. Rates of participation vary by state and by the definition of participation.[15] The most common reason cited by dentists for their lack of participation in Medicaid was the low reimbursement rates.[16] Other nonfinancial issues, however, were important as well. For example, in a study from Iowa, although dentists were more likely to rank low fees as the most important problem, more dentists said that broken appointments were a more important problem in their practice than low fees.[17] Dentists who were less busy and those who believed that dentists have an ethical obligation to treat Medicaid enrollees were most likely to be accepting all new Medicaid patients in their practice. A number of states have increased reimbursement rates to try and improve dentists' acceptance of Medicaid enrollees. Several other states have been forced to raise Medicaid reimbursement rates after being successfully sued because of poor access to dental care. Michigan chose a different approach and improved dentist participation in Medicaid by "carving out" the dental portion of their Medicaid program in 39 counties to Delta Dental of Michigan to remove the stigma that Medicaid has among dentists and increase reimbursement rates. By 2007, there had been 27 lawsuits in 21 jurisdictions aimed at improving reimbursement rates for dental services in Medicaid.[18]

As of 2016, in the 50 states and the District of Columbia, 4 Medicaid programs offer no dental services for adults, 13 offer emergency dental care only, 19 offer limited coverage, and the remaining 15 offer comprehensive services, a vast improvement over recent years.[19] Reducing or eliminating dental services for adults may result in an increase in modeling of poor behavior for children, and evidence clearly shows parental oral health status impacts that of their children.[20]

The Pediatric Dental Benefit Within the Affordable Care Act

One of the largest changes in health care coverage in the history of the United States involved implementation of the ACA by President Barack Obama in 2010. While private dental benefits for adults were completely absent from the law, a pediatric dental benefit was included.

For adults, states were given the option under the ACA of expanding Medicaid, which included dental benefits of some kind in most scenarios. Between 2013 and 2016, there was an increase of 15.5 million people enrolled in Medicaid or CHIP.[21]

Despite the best of intentions, the ACA lacked an effective pathway to provide comprehensive dental coverage for children due to several loopholes. The law allowed several variations that either eliminated mandated dental coverage for children or provided for a large deductible that made dental coverage available only when large health expenditures had been met by the family.[22]

In addition, in 2011 the Obama administration sided with states in opposing lawsuits against cuts in Medicaid rates that could result in further reductions in access for children and their parents/guardians.[23]

There is no telling the future of Medicaid under the new Donald Trump administration, though predictions are generally quite negative for the future of the program.[24] Both houses of Congress took initial steps to repeal the ACA by January 2017. It is unknown what it will be replaced with, nor how dentistry will fit into any new health care scheme.[25]

Federally Qualified Health Centers

As part of his "Great Society" plan to eliminate poverty, President Lyndon Johnson funded eight neighborhood health centers in 1965. This neighborhood health center concept has continued to develop and expand through the years and has evolved into a nationwide network of roughly 1200 federally qualified health centers (FQHCs), which includes Community Health Centers, Migrant Health Centers, Health Care for the Homeless programs, and public housing primary care programs. The mission of these centers is to increase access to affordable health care services for low-income families. FQHCs are located throughout the country in areas where barriers limit access to primary health care for a significant portion of the population. These barriers can be economic, geographic, and/or cultural. FQHCs provide primary and preventive health care services including dental care in many centers.

Fiscal year (FY) 2015 collections for FQHCs were $20 billion. Program statistics from the 2015 Uniform Data System (UDS) for that same year were as follows[26,27]:

- Total users: 24.3 million
- Total patients who received a dental service: 5.2 million
- Total physicians: 11,867
- Total nurse practitioners/physician assistants: 9664
- Total dentists: 4108
- Total hygienists: 1920

The role of FQHCs in the provision of oral health care for individuals who would otherwise not be able to access or afford care will likely increase in years to come.

Children and Dental Public Health

This textbook is organized by children's developmental stages. It works well to discuss dental public health issues within this same developmental context. The remainder of this chapter is devoted to introducing some dental public health issues as they relate to children of different age groups.

Barriers to Care for Infants and Toddlers From Low-Income Families

Dental care for infants and toddlers from low-income families presents a dilemma for several reasons. These children often (1) lack financial access to care, (2) have caregivers who fail to recognize the importance of early dental visits, (3) have difficulty finding a dentist who accepts Medicaid, (4) have difficulty finding a dentist who will treat children younger than 3 years, and (5) are not advised by the patient's primary care physician to seek dental care at an appropriate age.

Dental care for children should begin in infancy. This is especially true for low-income children who are at higher risk for disease. Although it is true that many children never experience decay in their primary dentition, others experience severe decay. For young children, particularly those under age 3 years, such treatment often requires hospitalization and general anesthesia. Thus, for low-income children with severe decay, the costs of treatment can

be very high and present a major barrier to patients, parents, and practitioners.

Despite EPSDT program requirements that eligible children visit a dentist by age 3 years (or younger in some states), the use of dental services by low-income children ages 0 to 3 years remains extremely low.[28] Continuing efforts are needed to convey the importance of early dental visits for this group of children. Primary care medical care providers play an important role in screening infants during medical well-baby visits and referring to dentists, but most young infants in Medicaid who see medical providers multiple times fail to see a dentist by age 1.[29] In addition, oral health screening and counseling should be a part of existing public health programs where young children appear for other services. Successful integration of oral health activities, including prevention, education, and screening, has already occurred in many public health programs, including Maternal Child Health Clinics and Women, Infants, and Children (WIC) Clinics.

Project Head Start

Head Start is the largest preschool program in the country and serves children from low-income families and children with disabilities. It was established in 1965 and is administered by the DHHS. Head Start is a comprehensive child development program that serves children from birth to age 5 years, pregnant women, and their families. They are child-focused programs and their overall goal is to increase the school readiness of young children in low-income families.

In 1994, Congress approved the development of Early Head Start, serving pregnant women, infants, and toddlers. Whereas the preschool program serves children in a classroom setting, Early Head Start mostly serves pregnant women, infants, and toddlers through weekly home visits of 90 minutes each for the entire family.

Also in 1994, Head Start and Early Head Start began providing services through community child care centers (Fig. 11.2). Many grantees now have formal partnership agreements that extend Head Start program performance standards to these community organizations.

Head Start operates in all 50 states, the District of Columbia, Puerto Rico, Virgin Islands, and Outer Pacific Islands. In addition, Head Start provides child development services to migrant children and families and Indian tribal nations. Head Start is organized by "grantees"; in 2015, federal funding for Head Start programs was just over $8 billion and served just under a million children. By year end in 2015, 91% of Head Start enrolled children had a dental home.[30]

Head Start has historically maintained a strong commitment to the health of children and their families enrolled in its programs. This commitment reflects the documented connection between school readiness and good health, including good oral health. Head Start and Early Head Start have a mandatory dental component requiring all enrolled children to receive a dental examination complete with prophylaxis as well as follow-up care for necessary restorative treatment. Head Start programs establish and maintain dental records for children enrolled in their program, but the necessary dental treatment is usually provided by dental professionals in the community or with public health clinics. Head Start programs are the payer of last resort for necessary dental treatment for children enrolled in their program who are not eligible for funding from Medicaid or other sources. This unique public-private partnership has been instrumental in helping ensure access to care for

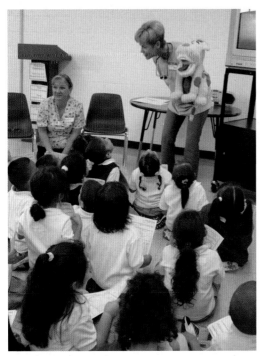

• **Figure 11.2** Dental hygienists provide education to Head Start children. (From Geurink KV. *Community Oral Health for the Dental Hygienist.* 3rd ed. St Louis: Saunders; 2012.)

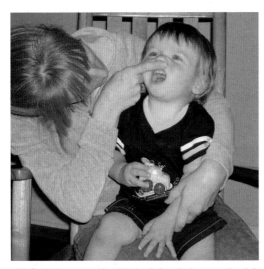

• **Figure 11.3** Mother uses the "lift the lip" technique to check her child's mouth for decay. (From Bird DL, Robinson DS. *Modern Dental Assisting.* 10th ed. St Louis: Saunders; 2012.)

low-income preschool children nationwide. One of the stated goals of Head Start is to attempt to link families to an ongoing health care system to ensure that the child continues to receive comprehensive health care even after leaving the Head Start program.[31]

All Head Start grantees have a health services manager, who must ensure that families, staff, and community resources are coordinated for the delivery of quality health services to children. This work includes training families and staff to conduct ongoing observations to spot signs of health problems, including "lift the lip" techniques (Fig. 11.3). The health services manager and staff recruit and build professional relationships with community health

and dental professionals to work toward good health for all children.

Special Medicaid Dental Programs

A number of state Medicaid program have implemented special programs to improve the oral health of young enrollees. One example is the Access to Baby and Children Dentistry (ABCD) program in Washington State. ABCD is a public-private partnership in which care coordinators help to connect families and dental offices, where children under age 6 years can receive additional preventive care, and dentists receive advanced training in pediatric dentistry behavior management techniques and enhanced reimbursements.[32] Preliminary studies have shown that ABCD improves dental care utilization and leads to less dental disease.[33,34] Similar programs exist in North Carolina (focusing on medical care providers) and Iowa.[35–37]

School-Based Dental Care

The attainment of school age presents another unique opportunity for enhancing the oral health of children. Schools are a logical site for promoting oral health through educational and prevention programs and delivering dental services to school-aged children because they provide a high concentration of children at the same location.[38] The United States has enjoyed a long tradition of successfully implementing oral health activities in school settings. The Centers for Disease Control and Prevention has established guidelines for school-based dental services through Coordinated School Health programs, which were set up to improve basic health outcomes in school-based settings.[39] Examples of services that can be provided in these settings include oral health education, fluoride mouth rinsing (FMR), sealant placement, oral health screenings and referrals, and comprehensive restorative care.

Health education, including oral health education, has long been considered an important part of school curricula in the United States. Dentists and other dental health professionals often have the opportunity to contribute to these activities by visiting classrooms and participating in health fairs or other special events. Oral health information presented in these forums can generate interest and stimulate changes in knowledge and attitudes. However, it is important for the oral health professional to understand that these changes are commonly short-lived and that desired behavioral changes require regular, long-term follow-up.[40]

School-based FMR programs in the United States had been a common public health prevention strategy for 30 years. A recent Cochrane review estimated that FMR resulted in a 27% reduction in decayed, missing, and filled tooth surfaces in permanent teeth.[41] In 1988, an estimated 3.25 million children were participating in FMR programs in 11,683 schools.[42] However, between 2003 and 2011, the number of FMR programs had decreased 15%.[43] The number of children participating in FMR programs was down to about 800,000.[42,43] Historically, school-based FMR programs have been most commonly targeted toward schools where the majority of children do not have access to fluoridated drinking water, regardless of the socioeconomic level of the students. The general decline in the caries rate among children has caused researchers to question the cost-effectiveness of these programs, which has resulted in the large decline in its use today.[44] These programs are most likely to be cost-effective when targeted at schools with additional risk factors besides a lack of water fluoridation (e.g., low-income status, high caries rate, lack of access to primary care). Typically, children participating in school-based FMR programs rinse once a week with 10 mL of a 0.2% sodium fluoride solution. Mouth rinsing activities are generally supervised by a classroom teacher, a school nurse, or other persons with appropriate training.

School-based sealant programs have become increasingly popular as a means of increasing the prevalence of sealants among low-income children.[45–48] Although pit and fissure sealants have been known to be effective in preventing dental decay for more than 30 years,[49] in 1989 only 11% of US school children had dental sealants on their teeth. More than a decade later some improvements had been attained in the most recent National Health and Nutrition Examination Survey (NHANES) (2011–2014), with 43.6% of children having a dental sealant. Of note is the nearly doubling in percentage of children living in poverty with a dental sealant present during this time frame, from 22.5% to 38.7%.[50–52] In 2009, school-based/school-linked dental sealant programs were identified in 33 states and reached about 500,000 children.[50] These programs usually target schools with a high percentage of low-income children (based on eligibility for free and reduced cost meal programs). Certain grades are usually chosen to participate, based on the eruption patterns of the permanent molars. Because of the timing of eruption for first permanent molars, second grade is a common age to initiate sealant programs. The majority of sealant programs use a four-handed approach, with each team generally providing sealants to 10 to 15 children a day (Fig. 11.4).

Silver diamine fluoride is an inexpensive topical medicament applied to carious lesions that helps with caries control and management. Studies conducted in school settings show that it is effective and safe.[53,54] The US Food and Drug Administration recently approved silver diamine fluoride as a tooth desensitizer. Silver diamine fluoride is commercially available in the United States and is being used off-label to arrest caries.

Oral health screenings are carried out in schools under a number of different circumstances. Often, oral health screenings are provided as part of health fairs or in combination with other educational/promotional activities. The purpose of these screenings is generally to identify gross problems and to refer children for dental care. A minimum of equipment is needed for this level of screening: a penlight and tongue blade are often sufficient. When screenings are performed in conjunction with school-based sealant programs or as part of surveys gathering data on the oral health status of children, the mirror and explorer examination is often more complete.

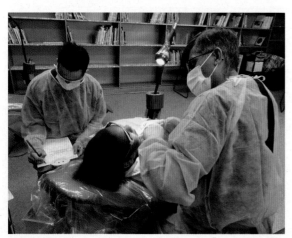

• **Figure 11.4** Dentists place dental sealants as part of a school-based sealant program. Commonly, through one of these programs, exams and sealants are provided to children in second through sixth grades.

Following school-based oral health screenings, referrals for follow-up care are generally made to area dentists, FAHCs, or school-based clinics. Only rarely are school-based screenings or examinations intended to take the place of complete dental examinations by dentists outside the school. This information should be communicated to parents and guardians of children who are screened in school-based settings so that they understand the intent of the school-based screening and the limitations of the procedures provided (e.g., no radiographs).

Comprehensive school-based dental care is not common in the United States, although some school-based programs providing a wide range of services have existed for more than 80 years. In Virginia, comprehensive school-based dental programs were first introduced in 1921, with ongoing programs functioning ever since.[55] Although examples of school-based programs offering comprehensive care can be found in the United States, perhaps the best known model for comprehensive school-based dentistry is the School Dental Service of New Zealand, which has been in existence for more than 60 years.[56] However, New Zealand continues to have large oral health disparities from childhood throughout adulthood. The likely explanation is that their dental care system relies on the belief that treating disease will mitigate the dental disease process, instead of focusing on the early prevention of dental diseases.[57]

School-based dental care can increase both access and use of dental services for children who do not or cannot receive care in the private sector. School-based dental programs, regardless of scope, should be planned carefully to optimize chances for success. The most fundamental aspect of planning involves a careful assessment of the need for school-based dental services and ongoing evaluation of such programs. School-based programs should not attempt to replace services provided in the private sector, nor should they compete for patients who are adequately served by existing resources. A profound piece missing from school-based dental clinics is that parents are not part of the educational component of the visit; in the long term, this is one of the most significant services of a preventive dental visit. Experimental intense education efforts fail to improve oral health outcomes in school-based settings when compared with outcomes attributable to education through traditional dental services, because parental modeling is the most significant determinant of patient behavior.[58]

The Challenge of Adolescence

Providing oral health care to adolescents can be a rewarding experience for the practitioner. This is generally a very teachable age, with most adolescents acutely interested in their appearance and their health. For some adolescents, however, daily life challenges may make dental care a very low priority. Adolescence is a period of life typically associated with increased risks in the areas of health and education[59]; however, over the past two decades the overall health of teenagers has greatly improved[60]:

- In 1991, 26% of teenagers did not wear a seat belt, whereas in 2015 only 6% did not.
- In 1991, 28% of teenagers had smoked a cigarette at least once in the past 30 days, whereas in 2009, only 10.8% had.
- In 1991, 51% of teenagers had at least one drink of alcohol in the past 30 days, but in 2009 32.8% had.
- In 1991, 19% of teenagers had sexual intercourse with four or more persons, whereas in 2009, less than 11.5% had.

Two new indicators that are relevant today in studies of adolescent behavior are related to texting and driving in the past 30 days (41.5%) and use of vapor or e-cigarettes.

One area where we have witnessed a decline in health among adolescents has been the surge in obesity rates. Between 1980 and 2008, the percentage of adolescents aged 12 to 19 years who were obese increased from 5% to 18%, and in 2014 it rose to 20.5%.[61,62]

Needless to say, the oral health needs of adolescents are often overshadowed by other pressing concerns.

The term "at risk" has become a general term used to describe people in trouble[63] and is often used to categorize adolescents who are not likely to succeed in school or in life because of one or more factors.[64] Factors that can place an adolescent at risk may include, but are not limited to, chemical dependency, teenage pregnancy, poverty, disaffection with school and society, emotional and physical abuse, physical and emotional disabilities, and learning disabilities.[65]

Many of these same factors can affect an adolescent's oral health and ability or willingness to seek dental care. Low-income adolescents experience more decay than other adolescents,[66] and adolescents with risk factors of poverty, teenage pregnancy, low grades, or disaffection with school are less likely to use or receive dental care than other adolescents.[67]

As with other age groups, lack of finances is a significant barrier to oral health care for at-risk adolescents. It is estimated that between 2008 and 2014, the percentage of adolescents living in poor or low-income families increased from 51% to 59%.[68] Nonfinancial barriers to care also exist and may include (1) low priority given to oral health, (2) no perceived need for dental care, (3) a dislike for going to the dentist, (4) lack of dentist office hours that do not interfere with school and other activities, and (5) lack of transportation. These barriers can make it especially difficult for adolescents with special health care needs to transition to adult-centered care.[69,70]

Addressing the oral health needs of at-risk teens is a relatively newly recognized problem, and strategies for dealing with this problem have not been as well developed as for other age groups. Possible strategies that may offer solutions include integrating oral health services into comprehensive school-based health centers, offering screening and referral programs in community settings frequented by teens, and maximizing the participation of adolescents in the EPSDT program.[71]

CHILD ABUSE AND NEGLECT

Suzanne Fournier

Child abuse and neglect are unfortunate and emotionally charged aspects of the more general problem of family dysfunction in our society. Since the 1960s these themes have received increased attention from the legal and health professions. By 1966, each of the 50 states had drafted legislation describing the responsibilities of professionals to report suspected abuse of children.

The same laws that mandate dentists to report suspected abuse often also protect them from legal litigation brought by angry and vengeful parents. These laws also delineate the legal implications for the dentist who knowingly and willfully fails to report suspected child abuse. In general, the dentist who fails to report such cases is considered guilty of charges ranging from a simple misdemeanor to a felony depending on the law of the state. Penalties may include fines or jail sentences.[1] Typically, under the law the dentist is civilly liable for any damages to the child caused by a failure to report abuse.

The technical aspects of identifying and documenting abuse are well established, and a dental office should include a policy describing procedures related to its identification. The American Academy of Pediatric Dentistry (AAPD) offers dentists educational material about management of child abuse if encountered in the course of dental treatment.[2] While examining a child, the dentist may encounter a suspicious lesion. The dentist should attempt in a nonthreatening manner to discern separately from both the patient and parent the etiology of the injury. If discrepancies arise between the two accounts of the injury or the reported etiology does not match the injury, the suspicion of abuse is present and appropriate authorities should be informed. Dentists are not obligated to investigate or prove child mistreatment, only suspicion of abuse. The investigation, especially the child interview, should be left to trained professionals.

Reports can be made in one of three ways. If the provider is afraid for the child's immediate safety, the local police should be notified immediately before the child is allowed to leave the office. If neglect is suspected, the provider can either call in a report to their state's Department of Children and Families Services (DCFS) or most DCFS websites have a form that can be completed and faxed. Regardless of the manner in which a report is made, the provider is required by law to make the report immediately after being made aware of the case. According to the American Academy of Pediatrics, the rate of abuse and neglect resulting in fatalities is correlated with poverty.[3] However, abuse and neglect can occur at any socioeconomic level.

Normal areas for children to be bruised are typically boney protuberances, such as chins, elbows, shins, and knees. Bruising circumferential to upper arms, neck, ears, and other such soft tissues should induce suspicion of abuse. Physical abuse can be caused by burning, slapping, hitting, choking, twisting, pulling, and pinching; broken teeth, burns in unlikely places or in patterns, and lacerations and bruises in patterns and various stages of healing should alert the dentist.[2] Tears to the lingual frenum are extremely rare accidental injuries and may be due to forced feeding. The adage "children who don't cruise rarely bruise" reminds us that injury is rare for children younger than 6 months. Fig. 11.5 depicts some examples of physical abuse possibly noticeable during a dental examination. Children who are victims of physical abuse may exhibit behaviors ranging from those similar to attention deficit with hyperactivity disorder,[5] to not making eye-contact with a provider and appearing withdrawn. Additionally, wearing clothing that is inappropriate for the weather (such as sweatshirts in 80°F heat) may indicate hiding of bruises.

Sexual abuse is far more difficult to identify and may be beyond the purview of the dentist. Areas affected by sexual abuse would not be readily seen by the dentist; however, the sexually abused child may demonstrate inappropriate behaviors with the dentist, be suggestive in speech, exhibit language delays,[6] or alternatively flinch at benign touch. Sexually transmitted diseases found in a prepubescent child would indicate sexual abuse and would require a referral to an appropriate medical professional for examination, testing, and treatment.[7,8] Bruising of the palate may be associated with forced oral sex.

Neglect may be less easily identifiable. Often, poor oral health is the trigger that prompts a dentist to investigate further the possibility of neglect. The dentist should look at the child's overall hygiene and clothing as well as dental hygiene. Suspicion of poor nutrition may arise from dry and unkempt hair, dirty clothing, and apparent lack of medical care as evidenced by skin lesions such as impetigo. The dentist is responsible for taking the same approach to neglect as to abuse; reporting of such cases is mandatory.[9] By recognizing dental neglect in child patients, child abuse may be curtailed. Abused children have higher levels of untreated dental disease (i.e., neglect) than their non-abused peers. The AAPD defines dental neglect as "the willful failure of parent or guardian to seek and follow through with treatment necessary to ensure a level of oral health for adequate function and freedom

Continued

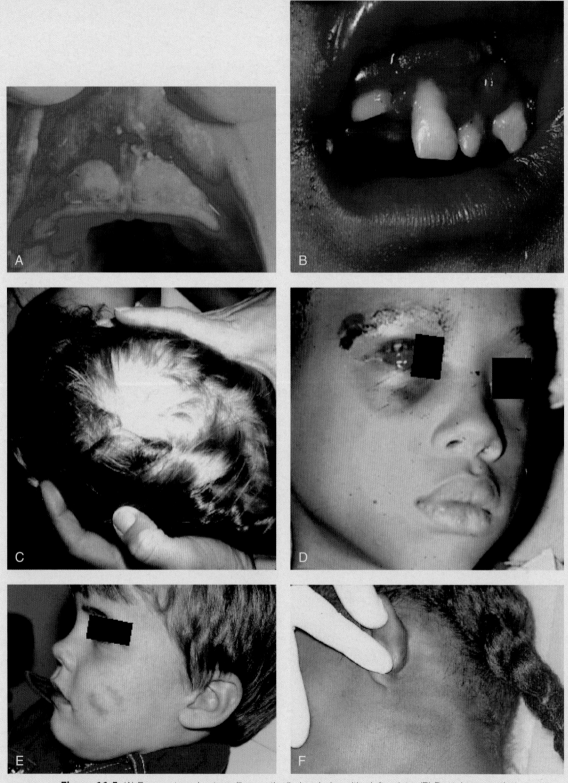

• **Figure 11.5** (A) Frenum tear due to pulling on the lip in a baby with cleft palate. (B) Dental trauma that has gone untreated in the primary dentition. (C) Loss of hair on scalp due to pulling by abuser. (D) Eye injuries from beating, which should also involve the bridge of the nose if received from an accidental fall (such as from a bicycle), but does not. (E) Bite mark on the cheek showing imprints of maxillary and mandibular teeth in a characteristic pattern. (F) Bruises from a slap showing finger pattern, paying attention to the handedness of the parent (i.e., right-handed people tend to hit the left side of the child whereas left-handed people tend to strike the right side of their victims).

CHILD ABUSE AND NEGLECT—cont'd

from pain and infection."[2] Additionally, failure of the parent or guardian to follow through with treatment once he or she is informed that the aforementioned conditions exist would also constitute neglect.[2] Social service agencies may become involved to assist families or to move the child from both an abusive and neglectful situation into a safer environment. While reporting is both an ethical and legal mandate, the dentist may find that dental neglect is but one problem area for that child and should not become frustrated with the inability of social services to effect dental care immediately when more serious issues are yet to be resolved.

References

1. Price S OLR research report: penalties for failing to report suspected child abuse; January 23, 2012 (cited April 27, 2017). Hartford, CT: Connecticut General Assembly, Office of Legislative Research. Report No. 2012-R-0058. https://www.cga.ct.gov/2012/rpt/2012-R-0058.htm. Accessed August 24, 2017.
2. American Academy of Pediatric Dentistry. Guideline on oral and dental aspects of child abuse and neglect. *Pediatr Dent.* 2016;38(special issue):177–180.
3. Block RW. No surprise: the rate of fatal child abuse and neglect fatalities is related to poverty. *Podiatrics.* 2017;130(5).
4. Weissenberger S, Ptacek R, Klicperova-Baker M, et al. ADHD, lifestyles and comorbidities: a call for an holistic perspective—from medical to societal intervening factors. *Front Psychol.* 2017;8:454.
5. Brownlie EB, Graham E, Bao L, et al. Language disorder and retrospectively reported sexual abuse of girls: severity and disclosure. *J Child Psychol Psychiatry.* 2017;58(10):1114–1121.
6. McNeese MC, Hebeler JR. The abused child: a clinical approach to identification and management. *Clin Symp.* 1977;29:1–36.
7. Levin AV. Otorhinolaryngologic manifestations. In: Levin AV, Sheridan MS, eds. *Munchausen Syndrome by Proxy: Issues in Diagnosis and Treatment.* New York: Lexington Books; 1995:219–230.
8. Katner D, Brown C, Fournier S. Considerations in identifying pediatric dental neglect and the legal obligation to report. *J Am Dent Assoc.* 2016;147(10):812–816.
9. Harris JC, Balmer RC, Sidebotham PD. British Society of Paediatric Dentistry: a policy document on dental neglect in children. *Int J Paediatr Dent.* 2009 May 14. [Epub ahead of print].

References

1. American Board of Dental Public Health. *Informational Brochure.* Gainesville, FL: The Board; 2009.
2. National Academy of Sciences, Institute of Medicine. *The Future of Public Health.* Washington, DC: National Academy Press; 1988.
3. Association of State and Territorial Dental Directors' Guidelines for State and Territorial Dental/Oral Health Programs. Essential Public Health Services to Promote Oral Health in the United States; January 3, 1997.
4. Kuthy RA, Siegal MD. Assessing oral health needs: ASTDD seven-step model. www.astdd.org/oral-health-assessment-7-step-model/. Accessed August 24, 2017.
5. Blackwell DL. Family structure and children's health in the United States: findings from the National Health Interview Survey, 2001-2007. *Vital Health Stat 10.* 2010;246:1–166.
6. Dye BA, Arevalo O, Vargas CM. Trends in pediatric dental caries by poverty status in the United States, 1988-1994 and 1999-2004. *Int J Paediatr Dent.* 2010;20(2):132–143.
7. Rizk SP, Christen AG. Falling between the cracks: oral health survey of school children ages five to thirteen having limited access to dental services. *J Dent Child.* 1994;61(5–6):356–360.
8. Amini H, Casamassimo PS, Lin HL, et al. Readability of the American Academy of Pediatric Dentistry education materials. *Pediatr Dent.* 2007;29(5):431–435.
9. US Congress, House of Representatives. An Act to Amend the Social Security Act; January 2, 1968. Public Law 90-248, HR 12080.
10. US Congress, Office of Technology Assessment. *Children's Dental Services Under the Medicaid Program: Background Paper.* Washington, DC: US Government Printing Office; 1990.
11. Centers for Medicare & Medicaid Services. The Children's Health Insurance Program. https://www.medicaid.gov/chip/index.html. Accessed August 24, 2017.
12. Kaiser Family Foundation. CHIP program name and type as of May 2015. http://kff.org. Accessed August 24, 2017.
13. US Office of the Inspector General. *Children's Dental Services Under Medicaid: Access and Utilization.* DHHS Publication No. OEI-0993-00240, Washington, DC: Department of Health and Human Services, Office of the Inspector General, 1996.
14. Steinmetz A, Bruen B, Ku L. Children's use of dental care in Medicaid: federal fiscal years 2000-2012; 2014. https://www.medicaid.gov/medicaid/benefits/downloads/dental-trends-2000-to-2012.pdf. Accessed August 24, 2017.
15. Ku L, Sharac J, Bruen B, et al. Increased use of dental services by children covered by Medicaid: 2000-2010. *Medicare Medicaid Res Rev.* 2013;3(3):E1–E13.
16. Borchgrevink A, Snyder A, Gehshan S. *The Effects of Medicaid Reimbursement Rates on Access to Dental Care.* Washington, DC: National Academy for State Health Policy; March 2008.
17. Damiano PC, Kanellis MJ, Willard JC, et al. *A Report on the Iowa Title XIX Dental Program: Final Report to the Iowa Department of Human Services.* Iowa City: University of Iowa Public Policy Center and College of Dentistry; 1996.
18. Perkins J. National health law program: docket of Medicaid cases to improve dental access; 2007. http://www.healthlaw.org/component/jsfsubmit/showAttachment?tmpl=raw&id=00Pd00000077hKuEAI. Accessed January 8, 2018.
19. Hinton E, Paradise J. Access to dental care in Medicaid: spotlight on nonelderly adults; 2016. http://kff.org/medicaid/issue-brief/access-to-dental-care-in-medicaid-spotlight-on-nonelderly-adults/. Accessed August 24, 2017.
20. Dye BA, Vargas CM, Lee JJ, et al. Assessing the relationship between children's oral health status and that of their mothers. *J Am Dent Assoc.* 2011;142(2):173–183.
21. Gates A, Rudowitz R, Artiga S, et al. Issue brief: two year trends in Medicaid and CHIP enrollment data: findings from the CMS Performance Indicator Project; 2016. http://www.kff.org/medicaid/issue-brief/two-year-trends-in-medicaid-and-chip-enrollment-data-findings-from-the-cms-performance-indicator-project/. Accessed August 24, 2017.
22. Reusch C. FAQ: pediatric oral health services in the Affordable Care Act; 2014. https://www.cdhp.org/resources/165-faq-pediatric-oral-health-services-in-the-affordable-care-act. Accessed August 24, 2017.
23. Pear R. Administration opposes challenges to Medicaid cuts. *New York Times;* May 28, 2011:A23.
24. Sperling G. The quiet war on Medicaid. *New York Times;* December 25, 2016:A19.
25. Cowan R, Cornwell S. US House votes to begin repealing Obamacare; 2017. http://www.reuters.com/article/us-usa-obamacare-idUSKBN14X1SK. Accessed August 24, 2017.
26. Health Resources & Services Administration (HRSA). 2016 health center program grantee data. https://bphc.hrsa.gov/uds/datacenter.aspx. Accessed August 24, 2017.
27. Health Resources and Services Administration (HRSA). Table 5: staffing and utilization; 2015. https://bphc.hrsa.gov/uds/datacenter.aspx?q=t5&year=2015&state=. Accessed August 24, 2017.

28. Brickhouse TH, Rozier RG, Slade GD. The effect of two publicly funded insurance programs on use of dental services for young children. *Health Serv Res.* 2006;41(6):2033–2053.

29. Chi DL, Momany ET, Jones MP, et al. Relationship between medical well baby visits and first dental examinations for young children in Medicaid. *Am J Public Health.* 2013;103(2):347–354.

30. US Department of Health & Human Services; Administration for Children & Families. Head Start program fact sheets; 2015. https://eclkc.ohs.acf.hhs.gov/hslc/data/factsheets/2015-hs-program-factsheet.html. Accessed August 24, 2017.

31. US Government Printing Office. *Head Start Program Performance Standards for Operation of Head Start Programs by Grantees and Delegate Agencies, Chapter XIII.* Washington, DC: Office of Human Development Services, Department of Health and Human Services; 1995:231.

32. Donahue GJ, Waddell N, Plough AL, et al. The ABCDs of treating the most prevalent childhood disease. *Am J Public Health.* 2005;95(8):1322–1324.

33. Lewis C, Teeple E, Robertson A, et al. Preventive dental care for young, Medicaid-insured children in Washington state. *Pediatrics.* 2009;124(1):e120–e127.

34. Kobayashi M, Chi D, Coldwell SE, et al. The effectiveness and estimated costs of the access to baby and child dentistry program in Washington State. *J Am Dent Assoc.* 2005;136(9):1257–1263.

35. Stearns SC, Rozier RG, Kranz AM, et al. Cost-effectiveness of preventive oral health care in medical offices for young Medicaid enrollees. *Arch Pediatr Adolesc Med.* 2012;166(10):945–951.

36. Zilversmit L, Kane DJ, Rochat R, et al. Factors associated with receiving treatment for dental decay among Medicaid-enrolled children younger than 12 years of age in Iowa, 2010. *J Public Health Dent.* 2015;75(1):17–23.

37. Chi DL, Momany ET, Mancl LA, et al. Dental homes for children with autism: a longitudinal analysis of Iowa Medicaid's I-Smile program. *Am J Prev Med.* 2016;50(5):609–615.

38. Marx E, Wooley SF. *Health Is Academic: A Guide to Coordinated School Health Programs.* New York: Teachers College Press; 1998.

39. Association of State and Territorial Dental Directors (ASTDD) Best Practices Committee. Best practice approach: improving children's oral health through coordinated school health programs; 2011. www.astdd.org/docs/BPASchoolCSHP.pdf. Accessed August 24, 2017.

40. Burt BA, Eklund SA. *Dentistry, Dental Practice, and the Community.* 6th ed. St Louis: Saunders; 2005.

41. Marinho VCC, Chong LY, Worthington HV, et al. Fluoride mouth rinses for preventing dental caries in children and adolescents. *Cochrane Database Syst Rev.* 2016;(7):CD002284.

42. Burt BA, Eklund SA. *Dentistry, Dental Practice, and the Community.* 6th ed. St Louis: Elsevier Saunders; 2005.

43. Association of State and Territorial Dental Directors. School-based fluoride mouthrinse programs policy statement; 2011. https://www.astdd.org/docs/school-based-fluoride-mouthrinse-programs-policy-statement-march-1-2011.pdf. Accessed January 3, 2018.

44. Marinho VC, Higgins JP, Logan S, et al. Fluoride mouthrinses for preventing dental caries in children and adolescents. *Cochrane Database Syst Rev.* 2003;(3):CD002284.

45. Gooch BF, Griffin SO, Gray SK, et al. Preventing dental caries through school based sealant programs: updated recommendations and review of evidence. *J Am Dent Assoc.* 2009;140(10):1356–1365.

46. Griffin SO, Jones KA, Lockwood S, et al. Impact of increasing Medicaid dental reimbursement and implementing school sealant programs on sealant prevalence. *J Public Health Manag Pract.* 2007;13(2):202–206.

47. Klein SP, Bohannan HM, Bell RM, et al. The cost and effectiveness of school-based preventive dental care. *Am J Public Health.* 1985;75(4):382–390.

48. Siegal MD, Detty AM. Do school-based sealant programs reach higher risk children? *J Public Health Dent.* 2010;70(3):181–187.

49. Simonsen RJ. Retention and effectiveness of dental sealant after 15 years. *J Am Dent Assoc.* 1991;122(10):34–42.

50. Griffin SO, Wei L, Gooch BF, et al. Vital signs: dental sealant use and untreated tooth decay among U.S. school-aged children. *MMWR Morb Mortal Wkly Rep.* 2016;65:1141–1145.

51. National Institute of Dental and Craniofacial Research. Dental sealants in children (age 6-11). www.nidcr.nih.gov/DataStatistics/FindDataByTopic/DentalSealants/Children.htm. Accessed August 24, 2017.

52. US Public Health Service, National Center for Health Statistics. *Dental Services and Oral Health: United States, 1989.* PHS Publ No 93-1511, Series 10, No 183. Washington, DC; Government Printing Office; 1992.

53. Chu CH, Lo EC, Lin HC. Effectiveness of silver diamine fluoride and sodium fluoride varnish in arresting dentin caries in Chinese pre-school children. *J Dent Res.* 2002;81(11):767–770.

54. Llodra JC, Rodriguez A, Ferrer B, et al. Efficacy of silver diamine fluoride for caries reduction in primary teeth and first permanent molars of schoolchildren: 36-month clinical trial. *J Dent Res.* 2005;84(8):721–724.

55. Day KC, Doherty J. Celebrating 75 years of dental public health in Virginia. *Va Dent J.* 1996;73(3):8–11.

56. Nash DA. Developing a pediatric oral health therapist to help address oral health disparities among children. *J Dent Educ.* 2004;68(1):8–20.

57. New Zealand Health Ministry, National Health Committee. *Improving Child Oral Health and Reducing Child Oral Health Inequalities.* Wellington, NZ: National Health Committee; May 2003.

58. Hietasalo P, Seppa L, Lahti S, et al. Cost-effectiveness of an experimental caries-control regimen in a 3.4-yr randomized clinical trial among 11-12-yr-old Finnish schoolchildren. *Eur J Oral Sci.* 2009;117:728–733.

59. National Academy of Sciences, Institute of Medicine. *Adolescent Health Services: Missing Opportunities.* Washington, DC: National Academies Press; 2009.

60. Eaton DK, Kann L, Kinchen S, et al. Youth risk behavior surveillance—United States, 2009. *MMWR Surveill Summ.* 2010;59(5):1–142.

61. Ogden CL, Carroll MD, Curtin LR, et al. Prevalence of high body mass index in US children and adolescents, 2007–2008. *JAMA.* 2010;303(3):242–249.

62. Ogden CL, Carroll MD, Fryar CD, et al. *Prevalance of Obesity Among Adults and Youth: United States, 2011-2014.* NCHS Data Brief, No 219. Hyattsville, MD: National Center for Health Statistics; 2015.

63. Tidwell R, Garrett SC. Youth at risk: in search of a definition. *J Counsel Dev.* 1994;72:444–446.

64. Capuzzi D, Gross D. *Youth at Risk.* Alexandria, VA: American Association for Counseling and Development; 1989.

65. Oral Health Coordinating Committee, Public Health Service. Toward improving the oral health of Americans: an overview of oral health status, resources, and care delivery. *Public Health Rep.* 1993;108(6):657–672.

66. Dye BA, Thornton-Evans G. Trends in oral health by poverty status as measured by Healthy People 2010 objectives. *Public Health Rep.* 2010;125(6):817–830.

67. Harvey HL. Factors Affecting the Utilization of Dental Services by Adolescents [*thesis*]; 1996. Iowa City: University of Iowa.

68. Jiang Y, Ekono M, Skinner C. *Basic Facts About Low-Income Children: Children 12 through 17 Years, 2014.* New York: National Center for Children in Poverty, Mailman School of Public Health, Columbia University; 2016.

69. Nowak AJ, Casamassimo PS, Slayton RL. Facilitating the transition of patients with special health care needs from pediatric to adult oral health care. *J Am Dent Assoc.* 2010;141(11):1351–1356.

70. Cruz S, Neff J, Chi DL. Transitioning from pediatric to adult dental care for adolescents with special health care needs: adolescent and parent perspectives—part one. *Pediatr Dent.* 2015;37(5):442–446.

71. English A. Early and periodic screening, diagnosis, and treatment program (EPSDT): a model for improving adolescents' access to healthcare. *J Adolesc Health.* 1993;14(7):524–526.

12

Dental Caries

NORMAN TINANOFF

Dental caries is perhaps the most prevalent chronic disease. The outcome of the disease is dental decay. The disease is the result of a complex interaction between acid-producing tooth-adherent bacteria and fermentable carbohydrates. Over time, the acids in the dental plaque may demineralize enamel and dentin in the fissures and the smooth surfaces of the tooth. The earliest visual sign of dental caries is the so-called white spot lesion. If demineralization continues, the surfaces of the white spot will cavitate resulting in a cavity. However, if the demineralization environment is reduced or eliminated, white spot lesions may remineralize and not progress. Risk for caries includes factors such as high numbers of cariogenic bacteria, high-frequency sugar consumption, inadequate salivary flow, insufficient fluoride exposure, poor oral hygiene, and poverty. The approach to caries prevention should be based on patient-centered and evidence-based practices

regarding the reduction of risk factors and increase in preventive factors. Caries management, if overt disease is present, should be focused on assessment of patient compliance and whether the disease will continue to progress, as well as tissue-preserving approaches.

Consequences of Dental Caries

The seriousness and societal costs of dental caries in children are enormous. Dental caries is still a major public health problem in high-income countries and is increasing in many low- and middle-income countries. The consequences of dental caries often include high treatment costs, loss of school days, pain causing diminished ability to learn, hospitalizations and emergency room visits, disabilities and even death, reduced oral health-related quality of life, and other problems such as being ashamed to smile and problems eating.

Although practitioners deal with children in dental pain periodically, there are few studies of the epidemiology of children's dental pain. One study of Head Start children in Maryland reported that 16.6% of children with caries complained of a toothache and 8.9% cried because of a toothache.[1] With regard to objective data for hospital visits due to dental problems in children, the Texas Children's Hospital in Houston reported 636 emergency room dental visits for children less than 5 years of age between 1997 and 2001, of which 73% were for nontraumatic dental problems.[2] A California study of emergency department visits showed that the rate for preventable visits for children under 6 years of age was 189 per 100,000 in 2005, and 203 per 100,000 in 2007.[3] With regard to the cost of dental care, a national study of children under age 18 found that dental care was $539 per year in 2005.[4] That cost now is considerably higher due to medical inflation. By any estimate, dental caries has a major effect on children's quality of life, physical health, and family and societal costs.

Epidemiology of Dental Caries

Primary Teeth

Information from the National Health and Nutrition Examination Survey (NHANES) has been used to follow changes in dental caries prevalence in US children. This national study is more reliable than other surveys because of its large sample size, national representativeness, and careful standardization of examiners. Furthermore, because these surveys include socioeconomic factors, insights can be derived regarding the prevalence of dental caries and its treatment in US children at various income levels. Studies conducted between 1988 and 2004 have shown a consistent relationship of dental caries prevalence with poverty levels in the United States, with those that are near poor or poor often having twice the caries prevalence found in nonpoor children. Also of interest was that there was found a consistent increase in caries prevalence in children in all socioeconomic levels in the 10 years between surveys (Table 12.1).[5] Therefore one can conclude that, in general, poverty has a major impact of caries prevalence in children, but the reasons for the effect has not been determined and may be related to preventive behaviors and diet.

Another important finding from examining NHANES data in 2- to 5-year-old children over quarter of a century is the remarkable shifts in decay and filled teeth over time. This national data show that mean number of decayed tooth surfaces was constant over the years, except for the 2001–2002 and 2011–2012 surveys. Remarkably, the 2011–2012 survey reported an approximately 75% reduction from the previous survey. Also of great interest is that even though the 2011–2012 survey showed a large reduction in mean decayed teeth, the number of filled teeth proportionally increased (Fig. 12.1).[6] The large reduction in dental caries and the large increase in filled surfaces may indicate greater access to care for 2- to 5-year-old children.

In the United States many studies of caries prevalence in preschool populations often are derived from convenience samples of Head Start and Women, Infant, and Children (WIC) populations that may be greatly different from national data. Fig. 12.2 is an overview of US epidemiologic studies of caries prevalence between 1988 and 2012 that shows higher caries prevalence from selected state populations than from the three national studies (NHANES, 1988–1994, 1999–2004, and 2011–2012). The greater caries prevalence from state surveys is probably due to lower socioeconomic status of the state samples (e.g., Head Start, WIC children) compared with national samples that are generalizable to the whole US population. The greater variability of prevalence in these state studies also is probably due to the many local factors that may have influence on caries prevalence in the different locations, such as water fluoridation, access to care, and socioeconomic levels. One should recognize that national surveillance survey data might not reflect the caries prevalence of specific population of interest.

Permanent Teeth

From the 2011–2012 NHANES survey, it is apparent that caries prevalence also remains high in permanent teeth of US children. This most current survey found that children aged 6 to 8 had a caries prevalence of 14% in their permanent teeth, and children aged 9 to 11 had a prevalence of 29%. Approximately 6% of children aged 6 to 11 had untreated dental caries in the permanent teeth. The high caries prevalence at age 6 to 8 years old is remarkable, since the permanent teeth generally start erupting around age 6. With regard to the association of race/ethnicity and dental caries in permanent teeth, the 2011–2012 survey found that caries was highest in Hispanic 6- to 11-year-old children (27%), compared to 19% for non-Hispanic white children and 18% for non-Hispanic Asian children (18%).[7]

The dental caries prevalence also was found to be high in adolescents, with 50% of the 12- to 15-year-olds, and 57% in 16- to 19-year-olds having experienced dental caries in their permanent teeth. With regard to untreated dental caries, 12% of children aged 12 to 15 had untreated caries, and 19% of children aged 16 to 19 had untreated caries.[7] As these epidemiologic studies of both primary and permanent teeth show, dental caries experience is still highly prevalent in children of all ages, with a large percentage of teeth with caries not having treatment.

Dental Caries Factors

Enamel

The earliest macroscopic evidence of a dental carious lesion is known as a white spot lesion. Such lesions are best seen after the tooth surface is cleaned and air-dried. These lesions form

TABLE 12.1	US Prevalence of Dental Caries in the Primary Dentition of Children, 2 to 8 Years Old by Poverty Status and Survey Years		
		NHANES 1988–1994	NHANES 1999–2004
2–5 years	Poor	35.5	41.8
	Near-poor	29.1	30.4
	Nonpoor	14.0	17.8
6–8 years	Poor	60.6	65.7
	Near-poor	54.0	61.1
	Nonpoor	38.4	39.4

Poor = 0% to 99% of federal poverty level.
Near poor = 100% to 199% of federal poverty level.
Nonpoor = >200% of poverty level.
NHANES, National Health and Nutrition Examination Survey.
Data from Dye BA, Tan S, Smith V, et al. Trends on oral health status: United States, 1988–1994 and 1999–2004. National Center for Health Statistics. *Vital Health Stat.* 2007;11(248):1–92.

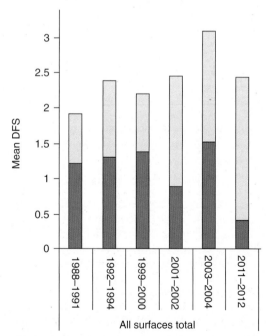

• **Figure 12.1** Decayed and filled primary tooth surfaces *(DFS)* for children ages 2 to 5 in the United States between 1988 and 2012. Dark bars represent mean decayed tooth surfaces; light bars represent mean filled tooth surfaces. (Modified from Dye BA, Hsu K-L, Afful J. Prevalence and measurement of dental caries in young children. *Pediatr Dent.* 2015;37: 200–216.)

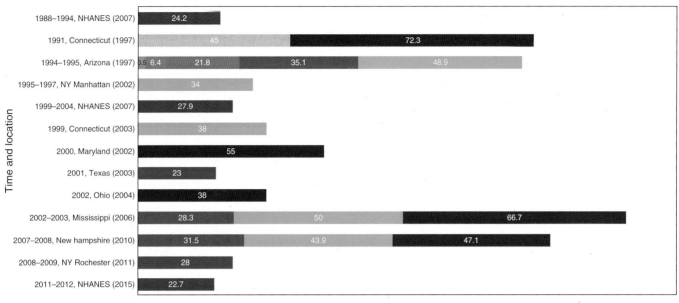

Caries prevalence %

• **Figure 12.2.** Caries prevalence of US studies of children under age 6, listed chronically between 1988 and 2012. Left-hand column shows dates that study was conducted, location, and publication date. *NHANES,* National Health and Nutrition Examination Survey. (Unpublished data from Alkuhl H, Tsai YJ, Tinanoff N, 2017.)

in areas of plaque accumulation, such as in occlusal fissures, on interproximal surfaces, and the gingival thirds of teeth. The enamel at the white spot stage is hard, and the surface may or may not be rougher than surrounding areas not affected by demineralization (Fig. 12.3).

A white spot lesion indicates that there already has been considerable loss of enamel in the affected area due to demineralization from acids derived from bacterial metabolism. If demineralization of the white spot continues, the surface will cavitate, resulting in a cavity. However, if the demineralization environment is reduced or eliminated, white spot lesions may remineralize. Evidence of remineralized white spot lesions is indicated by the lesions not enlarging, as well as lesions no longer on the gingival margin as the tooth erupts (Fig. 12.4).

Thin ground sections of teeth visualized by polarized light microscopy illustrate the process of demineralization and remineralization often associated with white spot lesions (Fig. 12.5). The outermost 30 microns of the white spot lesion often is called the surface zone. This area on ground section appears relatively intact but may be more porous that sound enamel. The surface zone remains relatively intact due to remineralization from calcium, phosphate, and fluoride in saliva. Subjacent to the surface zone is the "body of the lesion" which is the most demineralized part of the lesion. It has a pore volume of 5% to 25%[8] and is visualized as dark brown with polarizing microscopy due to this loss of enamel. If the lesion continues to progress, the surface zone will develop small defects allowing acids to more rapidly diffuse below the surface. If a demineralizing environment continues, the surface enamel will be undermined and a cavitation will occur. Once cavitation occurs, bacteria can readily invade the underlying dentin and are less likely to be affected by preventive treatments.

There is a certain amount of uncertainty regarding treatment of white spot lesions because, as mentioned before, these lesions may be progressing, arrested, or remineralizing. Besides clinical

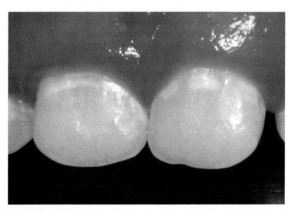

• **Figure 12.3** White spot lesions on the gingival third of primary incisors.

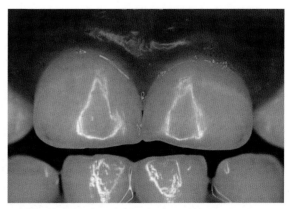

• **Figure 12.4** Arrested white spot lesions on primary central incisors, suggested by lesions at a distance from the gingival margin.

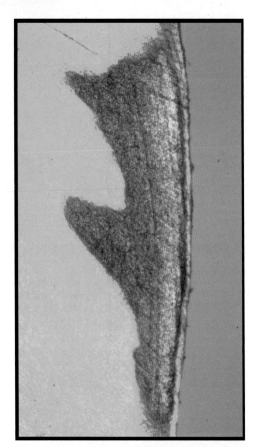

• **Figure 12.5** Thin ground section of a white spot lesion visualized with polarized light microscopy. The body of the lesion is dark due to the larger pore volume produced by demineralization. The surface is intact and perhaps more dense due to remineralization. (Courtesy Dr. J. Wefel.)

findings to help determine activity of these initial lesions, there has been a movement to use caries risk assessment tools to assess potential progression of caries for individual teeth and for individuals (details later in this chapter). If a lesion is considered active, then the management goal should be an individualized patient approach to reduce the cariogenic environment by affecting the patient's diet and acid-forming bacteria, as well as evidence-based preventive measures, such as fluoride and sealants.

Caries Microbiology

The understanding of the microbiology of dental caries has progressed with the general field of microbiology. The specific plaque hypothesis, proposed by Loesche, considered that only certain bacterial species were responsible for disease.[9] With the development of microbial media specifically for oral streptococci species (such as mitis salivarius bacitracin, kanamycin agar), investigators conducted numerous studies that showed strong association of the so-called *Streptococcus mutans (S. mutans)* with dental caries prevalence and incidence. *S. mutans* was believed to contribute to caries because of their ability to adhere to tooth surfaces, produce copious amounts of acid, and survive and continue metabolism at low pH conditions. With the advent of DNA techniques, the bacteria that was previously described as *S. mutans* was actually a group of several species (mutans streptococci [MS]) that included the species *S. mutans, S. sobrinus, S. cricetus,* and *S. rattus.*[10] Importantly, the species *S. mutans* is the most common in man with over 98% of

adults harboring this bacterium, followed by *S. sobrinus* that is found in 5% to 35% of individuals.[11] Since most clinical studies and evaluations used in dental practice identify and quantitate these streptococci by semi-selective media that cannot distinguish between *S. mutans* and *S. sobrinus*, it is most appropriate to refer to the findings from cultural techniques as the group of bacteria (i.e., MS).

The ecological plaque hypothesis proposed in 2004 advanced the understanding of bacterial cariogenicity by identifying how MS relate to other bacteria in the plaque biofilm. It was shown that low pH values in dental plaque because of frequent sugar consumption leads to alterations in tooth adherent biofilm, favoring bacteria that can survive and thrive in acidic conditions.[12] Thus, the acid production by bacteria not only is a key factor to tooth demineralization, but it also affects the microbial composition of plaque. Because MS are resistant to acid conditions and can continue to metabolize in low pH environments, they have a competitive advantage over other plaque bacteria, and consequently will numerically become a more dominant species in low pH dental plaque environments.

Recent advances in molecular biology allow further understanding of the factors involved in the cariogenicity of dental plaque. Techniques such as 16S rRNA gene sequencing reveal a complex host-bacterial community interaction that does not fit the single microbial pathogenicity model developed from culturing bacteria with selective media. Molecular methods still support the concept that MS is a key pathogen in dental caries, and that frequent carbohydrate consumption selects bacteria that are more acidogenic and aciduric. However, molecular biology reveals the complexity of the biofilm by identifying other bacteria that may be associated with caries (e.g., *Lactobacillus* species, *Veillonella, Actinomyces, Bifidobacterium, Scardovia, Fusobacterium, Prevetella, Candida,* etc.) and gives further understanding of the contribution and interaction of bacterial community members in disease and in health.[13]

Molecular genetics techniques such as DNA fingerprinting and ribotyping also have increased the understanding of early colonization of children with MS. These studies show strong evidence that mothers are the primary source of MS colonization of their children.[14] The exact method of transmission is not known, but it is suspected to be due to close maternal-child contact and sharing of food and utensils. Colonization with MS at an early age is an important risk factor for early caries initiation. Studies have shown that the earlier MS is detected in children, the higher the caries experience.[15]

Addressing the management of dental caries as a microbial disease assists in individualizing patient care based on a patient's level of cariogenic microorganisms. Furthermore, knowledge of the microbiology allows understanding of the caries mechanisms, including frequent sugar consumption, that results in low plaque pHs that foster demineralization as well as allowing MS to have a competitive advantage over less cariogenic microorganisms.

Preventing Dental Caries

Education and Changing Oral Health Behaviors

Educational programs to prevent or reduce the incidence of dental caries may involve written material or conversations with parents or child to reduce high frequency sugar consumption, brushing teeth twice daily with fluoridated toothpaste, or participate in frequent professional visits. However, outcomes suggest that educational programs improve knowledge, yet only have a temporary effect on plaque levels, and have no discernible effect on caries incidence.[16] Despite these limitations, oral health education continues to be an important component of preventive dental programs.

The technique of motivational interviewing (MI) to change health behaviors has shown effectiveness in improving uptake of educational messages, altering oral health behaviors (brushing, visiting the dentist, diet management), and decreasing dental caries.[17] The MI approach attempts to understand patient's expectations, beliefs, perspectives, and concerns about changing their health behaviors; and the counseling is calibrated to the patient's level of readiness to change. Counseling is nonjudgmental, without coercion or premature suggestions of change options. Patients are given the autonomy to make their own decisions about change.

Diet

Due to the high prevalence of dental caries, as well as childhood obesity, more attention is now being devoted to the amount of sugar-sweetened foods and beverages children consume daily. With regard to dental caries, simple sugars (e.g., sucrose, glucose, and fructose) readily facilitate growth and metabolism of MS and other acidogenic and acid-tolerating bacteria species. With frequent sugar consumption, the bacteria that are attached to the teeth produce acid that will reduce the pH of the environment and produce tooth demineralization. Fruit juices, fruit flavored drinks, and soft drinks have a substantial cariogenic potential because of their high sugar content and their frequent consumption between meals.

Since 2015, national and international organizations have developed recommendations for daily sugar consumption that address obesity and dental caries risk in children. Their recommendation for children ages 4 to 8 is that added sugar should be less than 10% of daily calorie consumption, or approximately 32.5 g sugar.[18,19] To put the recommendations on sugar consumption into perspective, one must understand that the amount of sugar in products commonly consumed often exceeds the daily recommendation. Table 12.2 lists the sugar content of several foods and

beverages commonly consumed by children at recommended serving sizes.[20]

From Table 12.2 it is apparent that certain foods and beverages, particularly beverages that children consume often, have substantial quantities of sugar. In many cases, consuming just one 8-ounce drink is close to the daily sugar consumption recommendation for children. To reduce the risk of dental caries and obesity in children, health professionals and parents should be aware of the sugar content of processed foods and beverages, as well as current daily sugar-consumption recommendations. Additionally, dental professionals need to become more engaged in identifying children who have high sugar consumption and provide dietary information or referral for dietary counseling.

Tooth Brushing

The role of tooth brushing in the prevention of tooth decay has long been considered self-evident. Yet there is little evidence to support the notion that tooth brushing per se reduces caries. The relationship between individual oral hygiene status and caries experience is weak, and instructional programs designed to reduce caries incidence by promoting oral hygiene have failed.[21] However, there is convincing evidence for the decay-preventing benefit of tooth brushing when used with a fluoride-containing toothpaste.[22] To prevent fluorosis from excessive swallowing of toothpaste, children under age 3 should brush with a "smear" of fluoridated toothpaste and children over 3 years should brush with a pea-sized amount.[23] To maximize the beneficial effect of fluoride in the toothpaste, teeth should be brushed twice daily, and rinsing after brushing should be kept to a minimum or eliminated altogether.[24]

Optimally Fluoridated Water

Community water fluoridation is the most equitable and cost-effective method of delivering fluoride to all members of most communities. Water fluoridation at the level of 0.7 to 1.2 mg fluoride ion/L (ppm F) was introduced in the United States in the 1940s. Since fluoride from water supplies is now one of several sources of fluoride, the Department of Health and Human Services in 2015 recommended not to have a fluoride range in community water supplies, but rather recommended the lower limit of 0.7 ppm F.[25] In some countries, such as the United States, where the majority of food and drink processing is done in cities with optimally fluoridated water supplies, children living in low-fluoride areas also receive some of the benefits of fluoridated water from consumption of processed foods. This has been termed the "halo effect" and is believed to be a major factor in caries reduction in children residing in nonfluoridated areas.

Fluoride Supplements

Fluoride supplements were introduced in the late 1950s to give anticaries benefits to populations that resided in areas where optimally fluoridated water was not available. Fluoride supplementation programs were based on the premise that the cariostatic effect of fluoride was predominately systemic rather than topical, and that systemic doses of fluoride should be equivalent to those ingested from optimally fluoridated water. Summaries of trials of the effect of systemic fluoride supplements on dental caries showed a 50% to 80% caries reduction in primary teeth where the age of initiation was 2 years or younger (21 trials), and a 39% to 80% reduction in permanent teeth (34 trials).[26] However, one must be cautious

TABLE 12.2	Examples of Sugar Content in Foods and Beverages Commonly Consumed by Children
Foods and Beverages[a]	Grams of Sugar
Sports drink (20 oz)	34
Soda (8 oz)	26
100% orange juice (8 oz)	24
Chocolate milk 8 oz)	24
Yogurt with fruit (170 g)	24
Juice drink (8 oz)	21
Ice cream (62 g)	13
Children's cereal (29 g)	10
Cookies (25 g)	8

[a]Suggested serving size on package.
Note: 24 g of sugar equals 6 teaspoons of sugar, or 96 calories.
From Tinanoff N, Holt K. Children's sugar consumption: obesity and dental caries. *Pediatr Dent.* 2017;39(1):12–13.

of the conclusions of these investigations since they were reported at a time of much greater caries incidence than the present, and methods and analysis of some studies weaken confidence in the findings.

The dose of fluoride supplements has varied over the years and generally has been adjusted downward to reduce the risk of fluorosis. The Centers for Disease Control and Prevention in 2001 further recommended that fluoride supplements be administered only to children at high risk for dental caries, and stated that, for children under age 6, practitioners and parents should weigh the risks for caries with and without fluoride supplements versus the potential for enamel fluorosis.[27] Thus, current recommendations for fluoride supplementation are based on fluoride content of the water, the child's age, and the child's caries risk (Table 12.3).[28]

Irrespective of efficacy, there are issues associated with administration of fluoride supplements that make supplementation not the first-line approach for caries prevention in preschool children. Concerns with fluoride supplementation include: children, whether living in a fluoridated or nonfluoridated area, ingest sufficient quantities of fluoride from toothpaste, beverages, and foods; parents of high-risk children often do not comply with a fluoride supplement regimen; and many practitioners prescribe fluoride supplements without testing the child's water supply for fluoride content and without considering the caries-risk status of a child.

Professionally Applied Topical Fluorides

Until recently, the agents for professionally applied fluoride treatments were 5% sodium fluoride varnish (NaF; 22,500 ppm F), and 1.23% acidulated phosphate fluoride (APF; 12,300 ppm F) gel. These products have been shown to be effective in numerous clinical trials in children and adults, although some of the evidence is from studies conducted 20 to 30 years ago. Fluoride varnish has superseded the traditional fluoride gel treatments because of ease of use and its safety due to single-dose dispensers. The efficacy of fluoride varnish in primary teeth when used at least twice a year has been reported in at least four randomized controlled trials.[29] Products now come in dispensers of either 0.25, 0.4, or 0.6 mL of varnish, corresponding to 5.5, 8.8, or 13.2 mg fluoride, respectively. Other topical fluoride products, such as 0.2% sodium fluoride mouthrinse (900 ppm F) and brush-on gels/pastes (e.g., 1.1% NaF; 5000 ppm F), also have been shown to be effective in reducing dental caries in permanent teeth.[29]

TABLE 12.3   Current Fluoride Supplement Schedule[a]

| Age | FLUORIDE CONCENTRATION IN COMMUNITY DRINKING WATER | | |
	<0.3 Ppm	0.3–0.6 Ppm	>0.6 Ppm
0–6 months	None	None	None
6 months–3 years	0.25 mg/day	None	None
3–6 years	0.5 mg/day	0.25 mg/day	None
6–16 years	1.0 mg/day	0.50 mg/day	None

[a]Only for children at high caries risk.[27]
Modified from American Academy of Pediatric Dentistry, Council on Clinical Affairs. Guideline on fluoride therapy; 2014. http://www.aapd.org/media/Policies_Guidelines/G_FluorideTherapy1.pdf. Accessed August 25, 2017.

Silver diamine fluoride (SDF) is a topical fluoride that contains 5% (weight/volume [w/v]) fluoride and 24% to 27% (w/v) silver. The reaction of SDF with exposed dentin structure reportedly results in calcium fluoride deposits on the tooth surface and a deposition of silver phosphate layer. Silver, like other heavy metals, has an antimicrobial effect with substantivity.[30] As a result, the caries disease process may arrest soon after application. The black-stained dentin after treatment with SDF has been associated with arrested caries. Proponents of SDF suggest that it be applied twice yearly to be an effective interim therapy in reducing caries risk in primary teeth.[31] As of 2017, there are only five studies with control groups examining the efficacy of SDF, limiting the evidence that clinicians have for using SDF in managing caries.[32]

Antimicrobials

Some antimicrobial agents, such as chlorhexidine, iodine, probiotics, and xylitol, have been proposed to reduce dental caries by suppressing acidogenic and acid-tolerating bacteria species adherent to teeth. One comprehensive systematic review found that most antimicrobials produced a moderate reduction in cariogenic bacterial levels following their topical use, but bacterial regrowth occurs and new carious lesions developed once the treatment has ceased, particularly in high-risk children.[33] There also is evidence of a suppression of MS in new mothers and perhaps reducing MS acquisition in their children; however, the long-term effect of caries reduction in the children is lacking.[33] Another systematic review examined the effect of xylitol in reducing dental caries; it found that xylitol had a small effect on reducing dental caries, and studies were of low quality, making the preventive action of xylitol uncertain.[34]

Sealants

Numerous reports have shown that dental sealants are safe and highly effective in preventing pit and fissure caries in primary and permanent teeth, reducing dental caries by over 70% after 2- to 3-year follow-up.[35] With regard to evidence of effectiveness, a Cochrane review found that sealants placed on the occlusal surfaces of permanent molars in children and adolescents reduces dental caries up to 48 months when compared to no sealant.[36] Studies incorporating recall and maintenance have reported sealant success levels of 80% to 90% after 10 or more years.[37] After placement, sealants greatly reduce the number of viable bacteria in the covered fissures, including S. mutans and lactobacilli. Thus, sealants may effectively seal a sound fissure, as well as minimize the progression of noncavitated fissure carious lesions.[36,37]

There are reviews and clinical trials that have evaluated techniques for placement of sealants. One review has shown that teeth cleaned prior to sealant application with a toothbrush prophylaxis exhibited a similar or higher success rate compared to those sealed after handpiece prophylaxis.[38] In addition, there is limited and conflicting evidence to support mechanical preparation with a bur prior to sealant placement and is not recommended.[39]

Caries Risk Factors

Caries risk assessment has the goal of estimating the incidence of caries (i.e., the number of new cavitated or incipient lesions) during a certain time period, or the likelihood that there will be a change in the size or activity of lesions already present. Even though caries risk data in dentistry still are not sufficient to quantitate the models, the process of determining risk should be a necessary component in the clinical decision-making process.

The process of determining risk gives the provider and the patient an understanding of the disease factors, anticipates if there will be caries progression or stabilization, and aids in determining the intensity of preventive procedures and recall intervals. Caries risk assessment models currently involve a combination of factors including previous caries experience, diet, microflora, maternal factors, plaque, and enamel defects, as well as social, cultural, and behavioral factors (Tables 12.4 and 12.5).

Previous Carious Experience

One of the best predictors of future caries is previous caries experience.[40] Children under the age of 5 with a history of dental caries should automatically be classified as being at high risk for future decay. However, the absence of caries is not a useful caries risk predictor for infants and toddlers because, even if these children are at high risk, there may not have been enough time for carious lesion development. Since white spot lesions are the precursors to cavitated lesions, they will be apparent before cavitations. These white spot lesions are most often found on enamel smooth surfaces close to the gingiva.

Dietary Factors

There is abundant epidemiologic evidence that dietary sugars, especially sucrose, are a factor affecting dental caries prevalence and progression.[41] The intensity of caries in children may be due to frequency of sugar consumption. High frequency sugar consumption enables repetitive acid production by cariogenic bacteria that are adherent to teeth. Daily consumption of sugar-containing drinks, especially during the night, and daily sugar intake have been shown as independent risk factors in the development of caries.[42]

Microbiologic Factors

MS are most associated with the dental caries process and key to the understanding of caries in preschool children. MS contribute to caries formation with their increased ability to adhere to tooth surfaces, produce copious amounts of acid, and survive and continue metabolism at low pH conditions. Preschool children with high colonization levels of MS have greater caries prevalence, as well as a much greater risk for new lesions than those children with low levels of MS.[43,44] Additionally, colonization with MS at an early age is an important factor for early caries initiation.[45]

Maternal Factors

Colonization of the oral cavity with MS in children is generally regarded as a result of transmission of these organisms from the child's primary caregiver.[46] No definitive modes have been confirmed, but the burden of MS in the mother from dental caries, the economic level of the family, as well as the feeding practices and health habits that allowed salivary transfer from mother to infants have been suggested.[46] Also parents' history of abscessed teeth has been found to be a predictor of their child's urgent need for restorative treatment.[47]

TABLE 12.4   Caries Risk Assessment for 0- to 5-Year-Olds

Factors	High Risk	Moderate Risk	Low Risk
Biological			
Mother/primary caregiver has active caries	Yes	—	—
Parent/caregiver has low socioeconomic status	Yes	—	—
Child has >3 between-meal sugar-containing snacks or beverages per day	Yes	—	—
Child is put to bed with a bottle containing natural or added sugar	Yes	—	—
Child has special health care needs	—	Yes	—
Child is a recent immigrant	—	Yes	—
Protective			
Child receives optimally fluoridated drinking water or fluoride supplements	—	—	Yes
Child has teeth brushed daily with fluoridated toothpaste	—	—	Yes
Child receives topical fluoride from health professional	—	—	Yes
Child has dental home/regular dental care	—	—	Yes
Clinical Findings			
Child has >1 decayed/missing/filled surfaces	Yes	—	—
Child has active white spot lesions or enamel defects	Yes	—	—
Child has elevated mutans streptococci levels	Yes	—	—
Child has plaque on teeth	—	Yes	

Modified from American Academy of Pediatric Dentistry, Council on Clinical Affairs. Guideline for caries-risk assessment and management of infants, children and adolescents; 2014. http://www.aapd .org/media/Policies_Guidelines/G_CariesRiskAssessment7.pdf. Accessed August 25, 2017. Copyright © 2016–2017 by the American Academy of Pediatric Dentistry, reproduced with permission.

TABLE 12.5	Caries Risk Assessment for Children Over Age 6 Years			
Factors		High Risk	Moderate Risk	Low Risk
Biological				
Patient is of low socioeconomic status		Yes	—	—
Patient has >3 between-meal sugar-containing snacks or beverages per day		Yes	—	—
Patient has special health care needs		—	Yes	—
Patient is recent immigrant		—	Yes	—
Protective				
Patient receives optimally fluoridated drinking water		—	—	Yes
Patient brushes teeth daily with fluoridated toothpaste		—	—	Yes
Patient receives topical fluoride from health professional		—	—	Yes
Additional home measures (e.g., xylitol, MI paste, antimicrobial)		—	—	Yes
Patient has dental home/regular dental care		—	—	Yes
Clinical Findings				
Patient has ≥1 interproximal lesions		Yes	—	—
Patient has active white spot lesions or enamel defects		Yes	—	—
Patient has low salivary flow		Yes	—	—
Patient has defective restorations		—	Yes	—
Patient wearing an intraoral appliance		—	Yes	—

Modified from American Academy of Pediatric Dentistry, Council on Clinical Affairs. Guideline for caries-risk assessment and management of infants, children and adolescents; 2014. http://www.aapd .org/media/Policies_Guidelines/G_CariesRiskAssessment7.pdf. Accessed August 25, 2017. Copyright © 2016–2017 by the American Academy of Pediatric Dentistry, reproduced with permission.

Visible Plaque

Studies demonstrate a correlation between visible plaque on primary teeth and caries risk.[48] One study found that 91% of the children are correctly classified as to caries risk solely based on the presence or absence of visible plaque.[49] Most interesting is a study of 39 children, aged 12 to 36 months, that found a positive correlation between the baseline MS and plaque regrowth, suggesting that the presence of plaque on the anterior teeth of young children is related to MS colonization.[50] The potential for visible plaque to be an accurate predictor of caries risk and MS colonization in young children is encouraging since this screening method is relatively easy.

Enamel Developmental Defects

Lack of enamel maturation or the presence of developmental structural defects in enamel may increase the caries risk in preschool children. Such defects enhance plaque retention, increase MS colonization, and in severe cases, the loss of enamel enables greater susceptibility to tooth demineralization. A strong correlation is found between the presence of enamel hypoplasia and high counts of MS.[51] Enamel defects in the primary dentition are most associated with pre-, peri-, or postnatal conditions such as low birth weight and the child's or mother's malnutrition or illness.[52]

Socioeconomic Status

Despite the consistent evidence demonstrating the importance of socioeconomic status on caries risk, there is limited understanding of the underlying mechanisms that account for these disparities. Nevertheless, there is consistent evidence to support a strong association between socioeconomic status, as represented by income, and caries prevalence. Preschool children from low-income families are more likely to have caries.[53] In addition, children with immigrant backgrounds have three times higher caries rates than nonimmigrants.[54]

Care Pathways for Caries Management

Care pathways (also called clinical pathways, protocols, care paths, and evidence-based care) are tools used to guide management of complex health care decisions in medicine since the 1980s.[55] Care pathways assist in clinical decision making by providing criteria regarding diagnosis and treatment that lead to recommended courses of action. They are based on evidence from current peer-reviewed literature and the considered judgment of expert panels. These pathways are updated frequently with new technologies and emerging evidence. In dentistry, care pathways can individualize and standardize decisions concerning the management of caries based on a patient's risk levels, age, and compliance with preventive strategies. Such protocols should yield greater probability of success and better cost-effectiveness of treatment than less standardized treatment.

Current dental caries care pathways are based on results of clinical trials, systematic reviews, national guidelines, and expert panel recommendations. The care pathways shown in Tables 12.6 and 12.7 are from the Guidelines of the American Academy of Pediatric Dentistry (AAPD)[56] and reflect radiographic protocols from the American Dental Association (ADA),[57] and fluoride

TABLE 12.6 Example of a Care Pathway for Caries Management for a 3- to 5-Year-Old Child

| Risk Category | Diagnostics | INTERVENTIONS | | | |
		Fluoride	Diet	Sealants[f]	Restorative
Low risk	• Recall every 6–12 months • Radiographs every 12–24 months • Baseline MS	• Twice daily brushing with fluoridated toothpaste[e]	No	Yes	• Surveillance[b]
Moderate risk Parent engaged	• Recall every 6 months • Radiographs every 6–12 months • Baseline MS[a]	• Twice daily brushing with fluoridated toothpaste[e] • Fluoride supplements[c] • Professional topical treatment every 6 months	Counseling	Yes	• Active surveillance[d] of incipient lesions • Restoration of cavitated or enlarging lesions
Moderate risk Parent not engaged	• Recall every 6 months • Radiographs every 6–12 months • Baseline MS[a]	• Twice daily brushing with fluoridated toothpaste[e] • Professional topical treatment every 6 months	Counseling, with limited expectations	Yes	• Active surveillance[d] of incipient lesions • Restoration of cavitated or enlarging lesions
High risk Parent engaged	• Recall every 3 months • Radiographs every 6 months • Baseline and follow up MS[a]	• Brushing with 0.5% fluoride (with caution) • Fluoride supplements[c] • Professional topical treatment every 3 months	Counseling	Yes	• Active surveillance[d] of incipient lesions • Restoration of cavitated or enlarging lesions
High risk Parent not engaged	• Recall every 3 months • Radiographs every 6 months • Baseline and follow up MS[a]	• Brushing with 0.5% fluoride (with caution) • Professional topical treatment every 3 months	Counseling, with limited expectations	Yes	• Restore incipient, cavitated, or enlarging lesions

[a]Salivary mutans streptococci bacterial levels.
[b]Periodic monitoring for signs of caries progression.
[c]Need to consider fluoride levels in drinking water.
[d]Careful monitoring of caries progression and prevention program.
[e]Parental supervision of a "pea-sized" amount of toothpaste.
[f]Indicated for teeth with deep fissure anatomy or developmental defects.
MS, Mutans streptococci.
Modified from American Academy of Pediatric Dentistry, Council on Clinical Affairs. Guideline for caries-risk assessment and management of infants, children and adolescents; 2014. http://www.aapd.org/media/Policies_Guidelines/G_CariesRiskAssessment7.pdf. Accessed August 25, 2017. Copyright © 2016–2017 by the American Academy of Pediatric Dentistry, reproduced with permission.

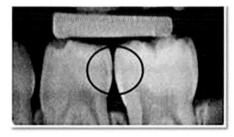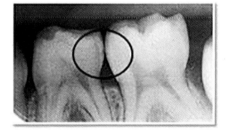

• **Figure 12.6** Active surveillance: Serial radiographs, 13 months apart, showing no caries progression on the proximal surfaces of mandibular molars. Parents complied by brushing the child's teeth twice daily with fluoridated toothpaste.

protocols based on the Centers for Disease Control and Prevention,[27] American Dental Association,[29] and the Scottish Intercollegiate Guideline Network.[58] Protocols for pit-and-fissure sealants are based on the ADA's and AAPD's recommendations for the use of pit-and-fissure sealants.[35] Active surveillance (prevention therapies and close monitoring) of enamel lesions is based on the concept that treatment of disease may only be necessary if there is disease progression,[59] that caries progression has diminished over recent decades,[60] and that the majority of interproximal radiographic enamel lesions are not cavitated.[61]

It is known that traditional surgical intervention of dental caries restores the tooth structure but does not stop the disease process. Additionally, many lesions do not progress, or with preventive treatment, lesions may arrest. Therefore, the principle of "active surveillance" (i.e., preventive measures along with monitoring signs of arrestment or progression) may be indicated for the management of some lesions in patients that will be compliant with preventive procedures. Active surveillance, as part of decisions in care pathways, will promote patient-centered decisions based on an individual's risk and success of preventive interventions (Fig. 12.6).

TABLE 12.7	Example of a Care Pathway for Caries Management for a Child Over 6 Years Old				
		INTERVENTIONS			
Risk Category	Diagnostics	Fluoride	Diet	Sealants[d]	Restorative
Low risk	• Recall every 6–12 months • Radiographs every 12–24 months	• Twice daily brushing with fluoridated toothpaste[e]	No	Yes	• Surveillance[a]
Moderate risk Patient/parent engaged	• Recall every 6 months • Radiographs every 6–12 months	• Twice daily brushing with fluoridated toothpaste[e] • Fluoride supplements[b] • Professional topical treatment every 6 months	Counseling	Yes	• Active surveillance[c] of incipient lesions • Restoration of cavitated or enlarging lesions
Moderate risk Patient/parent not engaged	• Recall every 6 months • Radiographs every 6–12 months	• Twice daily brushing with fluoridated toothpaste[e] • Professional topical treatment every 6 months	Counseling, with limited expectations	Yes	• Active surveillance[c] of incipient lesions • Restoration of cavitated or enlarging lesions
High risk Patient/parent engaged	• Recall every 3 months • Radiographs every 6 months	• Brushing with 0.5% fluoride • Fluoride supplements[b] • Professional topical treatment every 3 months	• Counseling • Xylitol	Yes	• Active surveillance[c] of incipient lesions • Restoration of cavitated or enlarging lesions
High risk Patient/parent not engaged	• Recall every 3 months • Radiographs every 6 months	• Brushing with 0.5% fluoride • Professional topical treatment every 3 months	• Counseling, with limited expectations • Xylitol	Yes	• Restore incipient, cavitated, or enlarging lesions

[a]Periodic monitoring for signs of caries progression.
[b]Need to consider fluoride levels in drinking water.
[c]Careful monitoring of caries progression and prevention program.
[d]Indicated for teeth with deep fissure anatomy or developmental defects.
[e]Less concern about the quantity of toothpaste.
Modified from American Academy of Pediatric Dentistry, Council on Clinical Affairs. Guideline for caries-risk assessment and management of infants, children and adolescents; 2014. http://www.aapd.org/media/Policies_Guidelines/G_CariesRiskAssessment7.pdf. Accessed August 25, 2017. Copyright © 2016–2017 by the American Academy of Pediatric Dentistry, reproduced with permission.

References

1. Vargas CM, Monajemy N, Khurana P, et al. Oral health status of preschool children attending Head Start in Maryland 2000. *Pediatr Dent.* 2002;24(3):257–263.
2. Ladrillo TE, Hobdell MH, Caviness C. Increasing prevalence of emergency department visits for pediatric dental care 1997-2001. *J Am Dent Assoc.* 2006;137(3):379–385.
3. California Health Care Foundation. Emergency department visits for preventable dental conditions in California; 2009. http://www.chcf.org/~/media/MEDIA%20LIBRARY%20Files/PDF/PDF%20E/PDF%20EDUseDentalConditions.pdf. Accessed March 26, 2017.
4. Iida H, Lewis C, Zhou C, et al. Dental care needs, use and expenditures among U.S. children with and without special health care needs. *J Am Dent Assoc.* 2010;141:79–88.
5. Dye BA, Tan S, Smith V, et al. Trends on oral health status: United States, 1988-1994 and 1999-2004. National Center for Health Statistics. *Vital Health Stat.* 2007;11(248):1–92.
6. Dye BA, Hsu K-L, Afful J. Prevalence and measurement of dental caries in young children. *Pediatr Dent.* 2015;37:200–216.
7. Dye BA, Thornton-Evans G, Li X, et al. *Dental Caries and Sealant Prevalence in Children and Adolescents in the United States, 2011-2012.* NCHS Data Brief, no 191. Hyattsville, MD: National Center for Health Statistics; 2015.
8. Darling AL. Studies of the early lesion of enamel caries with transmitted light, polarized light and radiography. *Braz Dent J.* 1956;101:289–297.
9. Loesche WJ. Clinical and microbiological aspects of chemotherapeutic agents used according to the specific plaque hypothesis. *J Dent Res.* 1979;58:2404–2412.
10. Coykendall AL. Proposal to elevate the subspecies of *Streptococcus mutans* to species status, based on their molecular composition. *Int J Syst Bact.* 1997;27:26–30.
11. Russell RR. Changing concepts in caries microbiology. *Am J Dent.* 2009;22:304–310.
12. Marsh PD. Dental plaque as a microbial biofilm. *Caries Res.* 2003;38:204–211.
13. Gross EL, Beall CJ, Kutsch SR, et al. Beyond *Streptococcus mutans*: dental caries onset linked to multiple species by 16S rRNA community analysis. *PLoS ONE.* 2012;7(10):e47722.
14. Douglass JM, Li Y, Tinanoff N. Association of mutans streptococci between caregivers and their children. *Pediatr Dent.* 2008;30:375–387.
15. Berkowitz RJ. Mutans streptococci: acquisition and transmission. *Pediatr Dent.* 2006;28:106–109.
16. Kay EJ, Locker D. Is dental health education effective? A systemic review of current evidence. *Community Dent Oral Epidemiol.* 1996;24:231–235.
17. Borelli B, Tooley EM, Scott-Sheldon LAJ. Motivational interviewing for parent-child health interventions: a systematic review and meta-analysis. *Pediatr Dent.* 2015;37:254–265.
18. US Department of Health and Human Services. *U.S. Department of Agriculture. 2015-2020 dietary guidelines for Americans.* 8th ed. Washington, DC: USDHHS and USDA; 2015. https://health.gov/dietaryguidelines/2015/guidelines/. Accessed August 25, 2017.

19. World Health Organization. *Guideline: Sugars Intake for Adults and Children*. Geneva, Switzerland: World Health Organization; 2015.

20. Tinanoff N, Holt K. Children's sugar consumption, obesity and dental caries. *Pediatr Dent*. 2017;39(1):12–13.

21. Andlaw RJ. Oral hygiene and dental caries: A review. *Int Dent J*. 1978;28:1–6.

22. Santos AP, Oliveira BH, Nadanovsky P. Effects of low and standard fluoride toothpastes on caries and fluorosis: systematic review and meta-analysis. *Caries Res*. 2013;47(5):382–390.

23. Wright JT, Hanson N, Ristic H, et al. Fluoride toothpaste efficacy and safety in children younger than 6 years. *J Am Dent Assoc*. 2014;145(2):182–189.

24. Sjögren K, Birkhed D. Factors related to fluoride retention after toothbrushing and possible connection to caries activity. *Caries Res*. 1993;27(6):474–477.

25. US Public Health Service. Recommendation for fluoride concentration in drinking water for the prevention of dental caries. *Public Health Rep*. 2015;130(4):318–331.

26. Murray JJ, Naylor MN. Fluorides and dental caries. In: Murray JJ, ed. *Prevention of Oral Disease*. Oxford: Oxford University Press; 1996.

27. Centers for Disease Control and Prevention. Recommendations for using fluoride to prevent and control dental caries in the United States. *MMWR Recomm Rep*. 2001;50(RR–14):1–42.

28. American Academy of Pediatric Dentistry, Council on Clinical Affairs. Guideline on fluoride therapy; 2014. http://www.aapd.org/media/Policies_Guidelines/G_FluorideTherapy1.pdf. Accessed August 25, 2017.

29. Weyant RJ, Anselmo T, Beltrán-Aguilar ED, et al. Topical fluoride for caries prevention: clinical recommendations with a systematic review. *J Am Dent Assoc*. 2013;144:1279–1291.

30. Rosenblatt A, Stamford TC, Niederman R. Silver diamine fluoride: a caries "silver-fluoride bullet." *J Dent Res*. 2009;88(2):116–125.

31. Crystal YO, Niederman R. Silver diamine fluoride treatment considerations in children's caries management. *Pediatr Dent*. 2016;38(7):446–471.

32. Cheng LL. Limited evidence suggesting silver diamine fluoride may arrest dental caries in children. *J Am Dent Assoc*. 2017;148(2): 120–122.

33. Li Y, Tanner A. Effect of antimicrobial interventions on the oral microbiota associated with early childhood caries. *Pediatr Dent*. 2015;37:226–244.

34. Marghalani A, Guinto E, Minhthu P, et al. Xylitol and dental caries in children: a systematic review. *Pediatr Dent*. 2017;39:217–224.

35. Wright JT, Crall JJ, Fontana M, et al. Evidence-based clinical practice guideline for the use of pit-and-fissure sealant. *J Am Dent Assoc*. 2016;147(8):672–682.

36. Oong EM, Griffin SO, Kohn W, et al. The effect of dental sealants on bacteria levels in caries lesions: a review of the evidence. *J Am Dent Assoc*. 2008;139:271–278.

37. Simonsen RJ. Retention and effectiveness of dental sealants after 15 years. *J Am Dent Assoc*. 1991;122:34–42.

38. Gray SK, Griffin SO, Malvitz DM, et al. A comparison of the effects of toothbrushing and hand piece prophylaxis on retention of sealants. *J Am Dent Assoc*. 2009;140:38–46.

39. Dhar V, Chen H. Evaluation of resin based and glass ionomer based sealants placed with or without tooth preparation—a two year clinical trial. *Pediatr Dent*. 2012;34:46–50.

40. Fontana M, Zero DT. Assessing patient's caries risk. *J Am Dent Assoc*. 2006;17:1231–1239.

41. Sheiham A, James WPT. Diet and dental caries: the pivotal role of free sugars reemphasized. *J Dent Res*. 2015;94(10):1341–1347.

42. Rodrigues CS, Sheiham A. The relationship between dietary guidelines, sugar intake and caries in primary teeth in low-income Brazilian 3-year-olds: a longitudinal study. *Int J Paediatr Dent*. 2000;10:47–55.

43. Thibodeau EA, O'Sullivan DM. Salivary mutans streptococci and dental caries patterns in pre-school children. *Community Dent Oral Epidemiol*. 1996;24:164–168.

44. Edelstein BL, Ureles SD, Smaldone A. Very high salivary *Streptococcus mutans* predicts caries progression in young children. *Pediatr Dent*. 2016;38(4):325–330.

45. Alaluusua S, Renkonen OV. *Streptococcus mutans* establishment and dental caries experience in children from 2 to 4 years old. *Scand J Dent Res*. 1983;91:453–457.

46. Douglass JM, Li Y, Tinanoff N. Literature review of the relationship between mutans streptococci in adult caregivers and mutans streptococci and dental caries in their children. *Pediatr Dent*. 2008;30:375–387.

47. Southward LH, Robertson A, Edelstein BL, et al. Oral health of young children in Mississippi Delta child care centers: a second look at early childhood caries risk assessment. *J Public Health Dent*. 2008;68:188–195.

48. Alaluusua S, Malmivirta R. Early plaque accumulation—a sign for caries risk in young children. *Community Dent Oral Epidemiol*. 1994;22:273–276.

49. Alanen P, Hurskainen K, Isokangas P, et al. Clinician's ability to identify caries risk subjects. *Community Dent Oral Epidemiol*. 1994;22:86–89.

50. Lee CL, Tinanoff N, Minah G, et al. Effect of mutans streptococci colonization on plaque formation and regrowth. *J Public Health Dent*. 2008;68:57–60.

51. Li Y, Navia JM, Caufield PW. Colonization by mutans streptococci in the mouths of 3- and 4-year-old Chinese children with or without enamel hypoplasia. *Arch Oral Biol*. 1994;39:1057–1062.

52. Seow WK. Enamel hypoplasia in the primary dentition: a review. *J Dent Child*. 1991;58:441–452.

53. Vargas CM, Crall JJ, Schneider DA. Sociodemographic distribution of pediatric dental caries: NHANES III, 1998-1994. *J Am Dent Assoc*. 1998;129:1229–1241.

54. Nunn ME, Dietrich T, Singh HK, et al. Prevalence of early childhood caries among very young urban Boston children compared with US children. *J Public Health Dent*. 2009;69:156–162.

55. Kinsman L, Rotter T, James E, et al. What is a clinical pathway? Development of a definition to inform the debate. *BMC Med*. 2010;8:31.

56. American Academy of Pediatric Dentistry, Council on Clinical Affairs. Guideline for caries-risk assessment and management of infants, children and adolescents; 2014. http://www.aapd.org/media/Policies_Guidelines/G_CariesRiskAssessment7.pdf. Accessed August 25, 2017.

57. ADA Council on Scientific Affairs. The use of dental radiographs. Update and recommendations. *J Am Dent Assoc*. 2006;137:1304–1312.

58. Scottish Intercollegiate Guidelines Network (SIGN). *Dental Interventions to Prevent Caries in Children: A National Clinical Guideline*. SIGN publication no. 138. Edinburgh: SIGN; 2014. http://www.sign.ac.uk/assets/sign138.pdf. Accessed August 25, 2017.

59. Parker C. Active surveillance: toward a new paradigm in the management of early prostate cancer. *Lancet Oncol*. 2004;5:101–106.

60. Warren JJ, Levy SM, Broffitt B, et al. Longitudinal study of non-cavitated carious lesion progression in the primary dentition. *J Public Health Dent*. 2006;66:83–87.

61. Anusavice KJ. Present and future approaches for the control of caries. *J Dent Educ*. 2005;69:538–554.

PART **2**

Conception to Age Three

Without question, the development of a child from conception to age 3 years is the most dramatic in terms of growth and development. Dentally, the predentate neonate will have grown into a toddler with a complete primary dentition consisting of 20 teeth. Ideally, the foundation for a lifetime of good oral health is established during this timeframe. Never will there be a time when the impact of others will influence the oral health as much as it will during these years. The importance of getting stakeholders, consisting of parents and guardians as well as dental professionals, to buy in to the concept of infant and toddler dental care cannot be overemphasized. This is a challenging age group for all those involved. Precooperative behavior is the norm. Children of this age can be a challenge to work on by both dental professionals and parents/guardians. Why is it so critical for the dental professional to see patients at such a young age? How does one go about developing an effective infant/toddler oral health program? How do we recruit parents to buy in to the concept of good home care for these young patients? Why is good home care even more important for the child with special health care needs? The answers to these questions are addressed in this section.

13

The Dynamics of Change

ERIN L. GROSS AND ARTHUR J. NOWAK

Physical Changes

Body

The gestation of a human being lasts approximately 9 months and begins at the moment the ovum is fertilized by the sperm cell. At the moment of penetration of the ovum wall, the sperm releases 23 chromosomes into the ovum, which also releases from a dissolving nucleus 23 chromosomes of its own. The human infant begins life with these 46 chromosomes. The fertilized cell begins to expand by the process of mitosis. The first division of the fertilized ovum into two cells usually takes place in 24 to 36 hours.

The time from conception to birth is often described in three phases. The first phase, the period of the ovum, is measured from fertilization to implantation. This period lasts until the dividing ovum, or blastocyst, becomes attached to the wall of the uterus. This period lasts for approximately 10 to 14 days. The next period lasts 2 to 8 weeks and is called the period of the embryo. This period is most important because of the cell differentiation that occurs during this time. It is during this period that all the major organs appear. The third and last period, which starts at 8 weeks and lasts until delivery at approximately 40 weeks, is called the period of the fetus. This period is characterized by maturation of the newly formed organs.

Fig. 13.1 shows the difference in body proportions as a child matures from the fetal stage through newborn, toddler, adolescent, and early adult stages of life. No year is more dramatic in terms of growth than the first year of life, during which most children undergo a 50% increase in length and almost a 200% increase in weight. Toward the end of the first year of life, the growth rate slows. After the first birthday, the growth rate stabilizes and the height and weight increments of the child remain relatively predictable all the way to adolescence.

There are no accurate predictors of the child's final height before age 3 years. However, at age 3, correlations between the child's height and weight at maturity are fairly strong. The process of a newborn changing into an adult is one of elongation. The legs, at first shorter than the trunk, become longer. In addition, the length of the child's trunk, compared with his or her breadth, becomes considerably greater.

As the body changes and matures, the infant is afforded increasingly sophisticated postural and locomotive actions. Table 13.1 shows some of the physical and cognitive developmental hallmarks of a child during his or her first 18 months of life. (Piagetian psychology, as well as object permanency and causality, is discussed in this chapter's section on cognitive development.)

By age 2 years, a child has the gross motor skills to run, climb, walk up and down steps, and kick a ball. His fine motor skills allow him to stack blocks (up to six), make parallel crayon strokes, and turn the pages of a book one page at a time. Table 13.2 shows a variety of motor skills and the mean age at which they are acquired.

The nervous system of the child grows dramatically from birth until age 3 years. By the end of the second year the child's brain has already attained 75% of its adult weight.[1]

Craniofacial Changes

Intrauterine Growth and Development

The organization and complexity of growth and development are nowhere more evident than in the changes that take place in the head and face (Table 13.3). The human face begins its first observable growth during the fourth week of intrauterine life with the development of the branchial apparatus. The branchial apparatus is first seen as a series of ridges on the lateral aspect of the cephalic end of the embryo at approximately the third week of intrauterine life. A 1-month-old embryo has no real face, but the key primordia have already begun to gather. These slight swellings, depressions, and thickenings then rapidly undergo a series of mergers, rearrangements, and enlargements that transform them from a cluster of separate masses into a face (Fig. 13.2).[2]

Sperber[3] described the presomite stage of development (21 to 31 days), during which the 3-mm embryo develops at its cranial end five mesenchymal elevations or processes. The five mesenchymal elevations constitute the initial features of the face. These include the frontonasal process, two maxillary processes, and two mandibular arches. These processes grow differentially, and by obliterating the

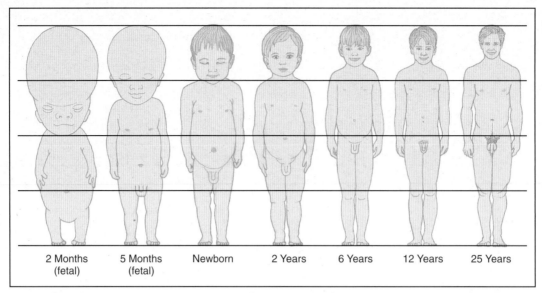

| 2 Months (fetal) | 5 Months (fetal) | Newborn | 2 Years | 6 Years | 12 Years | 25 Years |

• **Figure 13.1** The changing proportions of the human body from 2 months in utero to adulthood. (From James SR, Nelson K, Ashwill J. *Nursing Care Of Children: Principles and Practice*. 4th ed. St Louis: Saunders; 2013.)

TABLE 13.1 **Cognition, Play, and Language**

Piagetian Stage	Age	Object Permanence	Causality	Play	Receptive Language	Expressive Language
I	Birth to 1 month	Shifting images	Generalization of reflexes		Turns to voice	Range of cries (hunger, pain)
II	1–4 months	Stares at spot where object disappeared (looks at hand after yarn drops)	Primary circular reactions (thumb sucking)		Searches for speaker with eyes	Cooing Vocal contagion
III	4–8 months	Visually follows dropped object through vertical trajectory (tracks dropped yarn to floor)	Secondary circular reactions (re-creates accidentally discovered environmental effects, e.g., kicks mattress to shake mobile)	Same behavioral repertoire for all objects (bangs, shakes, puts in mouth, drops)	Responds to own name and to tones of voice	Babbling Four distinct syllables
IV	9–12 months	Finds an object after watching it hidden	Coordination of secondary circular reactions	Visual motor inspection of objects Peek-a-boo	Listens selectively to familiar words Responds to "no" and other verbal requests	First real word Jargoning Symbolic gestures (shakes head no)
V	12–18 months	Recovers hidden object after multiple visible changes of position	Tertiary circular reactions (deliberately varies behavior to create novel effects)	Awareness of social function of objects Symbolic play centered on own body (drinks from toy cup)	Can bring familiar object from another room Points to parts of body	Many single words—uses words to express needs Acquires 10 words by 18 months
VI	18 months to 2 years	Recovers hidden object after invisible changes in position	Spontaneously uses nondirect causal mechanisms (uses key to move wind-up toy)	Symbolic play directed toward doll (gives doll a drink)	Follows series of two or three commands Points to pictures when named	Telegraphic two-word sentences

From Zuckerman BS, Frank DA. Infancy. In: Levine MD, Carey WB, Crocker AT, et al., eds. *Developmental-Behavioral Pediatrics*. Philadelphia: Saunders; 1983:91.

TABLE 13.2	Median Age and Range in Acquisition of Motor Skills		
		AGE IN MONTHS	
Motor Skill		Median	Range[a]
Transfers objects hand to hand		5.5	4–8
Sits alone 30 s or more		6.0	5–8
Rolls from back to stomach		6.4	4–10
Has neat pincer grasp		8.9	7–12
Stands alone		11.0	9–16
Holds crayon adaptively		11.2	8–15
Walks alone		11.7	9–17
Walks up stairs with help		16.1	12–23
Walks up stairs both feet on each step		25.8	19–30

[a]5th to 95th percentile.
Modified from Bayley N. *Manual for the Bayley Scales of Infant Development*. New York: Psychological Corporation; 1969. From Zuckerman BS, Frank DA. Infancy. In: Levine MD, Carey WB, Crocker AT, et al., eds. *Developmental-Behavioral Pediatrics*. Philadelphia: Saunders; 1983.

TABLE 13.3	Developing Structures of the Head and Face
Developing Structures	Initiation (Weeks in Utero)
Neural plate	2
Buccopharyngeal membrane	2
Mandibular arch initiation	3
Hypoglossal muscles (tongue)	5
Medial and lateral nasal processes	5
Lens of the eye	5
Retina	5
External carotid artery	6
Eustachian tube	6
Larynx	6
Maxillary process	6
External auditory meatus	7
Nasal septum	8
Two palatal shelves fuse together	8
Palatal shelves fuse with nasal septum	10
Ossification of craniofacial skeleton	10
Eyelids completely formed and closed	10
Eyelids open	28

the midline and joins with the lateral nasal fold of the frontonasal process. As this is happening, a shelflike process (the palatal process) develops on the medial side of each maxillary process. These two palatal processes move toward the midline, where they fuse. This palatal fusion is normally completed by the eighth intrauterine week. The mandibular processes fuse at the midline somewhat before the maxillary and nasal processes (Fig. 13.4). The palate grows more rapidly in width than in length during the fetal period as a result of midpalatal sutural growth and appositional growth of the lateral alveolar margins. A failure in the fusion of the processes gives rise to oral or facial clefts or both. In the mandible, the cartilaginous skeleton of the first branchial arch, known as Meckel cartilage, provides a form for the development of the mandible.

The muscles of mastication, which include the temporalis, the masseter, and both the medial and lateral pterygoids, and the trigeminal nerve are all derived from the first branchial arch. At approximately 60 days of gestation, the embryo has acquired all of its basic morphologic characteristics and enters the fetal period, which is marked by osseous development.

Rapid orofacial development is characteristic of the advanced development of the cranial portion of the embryo compared with its caudal portion. The different rates of growth result in a pear-shaped embryonic disk, with the head region forming the expanded portion of the pear. Because of this early development at the cranial end of the embryo, the head constitutes nearly half of the total body size during the postsomite embryonic period (fourth to eighth weeks).

The dominance of head growth and development in the embryonic period is not maintained in the fetal period. Accordingly, the proportions of the head are reduced from approximately one-half of the entire body length at the end of the embryonic period to approximately one-third at the fifth month.

During the fetal period, the eyeballs, following the neural pattern of growth, initially grow rapidly. This contributes to the widening of the face. Interestingly, the nasal cavity and the nasal septum are believed to have a considerable influence in determining facial form, by acting either as a matrix for development or as a biomechanical template.

The growth of the nasoseptal region contributes to frontomaxillary, frontonasal, frontozygomatic, and zygomaticomaxillary sutural changes. The expansion of the eyeballs, the brain, and the sphenooccipital synchondrosal cartilage also acts in separating the facial sutures. The overall effect of these diverse forces of expansion is osseous buildup on the posterior surface of the facial bones.[4]

During the fetal period the relative sizes of the maxilla and mandible vary widely when compared with each other. Throughout the preceding embryonic stage, the mandible is considerably larger than the maxilla. However, in the fetal stage the maxilla becomes more developed than the mandible. Subsequently, the mandible grows at a greater pace and equals the size of the maxilla by the 11th week in utero. Then, between the 13th and 20th weeks in utero, mandibular growth again lags relative to the maxilla. At birth, the mandible tends to be retrognathic to the maxilla.[5] During the remainder of its intrauterine existence the fetus undergoes a process of growth and maturation and a reorganization of the spatial relationships among various structures.[6]

Rapid and extensive growth characterizes the ensuing 7 months of fetal life. An expansion of the cranium occurs during this fetal period as the result of a combination of growth processes, including interstitial, endochondral, and sutural or translational growth. The cartilage remnants of the chondral cranium that persist between the bones are known as synchondroses.

ectodermal grooves between them, they eventually contour the features of the face.

The oral cavity of the embryo is bounded by the frontonasal process and by the maxillary and mandibular processes of the first branchial arch (Fig. 13.3). Each maxillary process moves toward

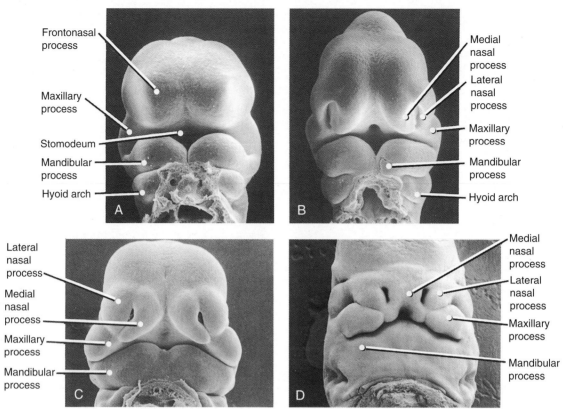

• **Figure 13.2** Scanning electron micrographs of mouse embryos (except D, which is a human specimen), resemble human embryos at comparable stages of development. (A) This stage is approximately 24 days after conception in the human and shows the division of the first brachial arch into the maxilla and mandible and the hyoid arch. (B) At approximately 31 days in the human, the medial and lateral nasal processes are recognizable alongside the nasal pit. (C) Fusion of the median nasal, lateral nasal, and the maxillary processes forms the upper lip. Fusion of the maxillary and mandibular processes establishes the width of the mouth (approximately 36 days in the human). (D) At 42 days gestation in humans, more definitive fusion has taken place, and the mouth and nose are readily evident. Still, this stage portrays a map of the potential cleft sites most commonly observed in facial development. (Courtesy Dr. K. Sulik. [A to C] From Proffit WR, Fields HW. *Contemporary Orthodontics*. 4th ed. St Louis: Mosby; 2007.)

In addition, the cranial base undergoes selective appositional remodeling by resorption and apposition. This process is mediated by activity on the part of the bone-forming cells (osteoblasts) and by bone-destroying cells (osteoclasts).

The major remodeling of the early facial skeleton that occurs throughout the remainder of the fetal period begins in the fetus at approximately 14 weeks. Before this time, the bones enlarge in all directions from their respective ossification centers. Remodeling, a process that accompanies growth, starts when the definitive form of each of the individual bones of the face and cranium is attained (Fig. 13.5).[6]

Growth and Development After Birth

At birth, the bony face and skull show little differentiation among individuals. Newborns have tiny mouths and virtually no chins. Their faces are small, although their eyes, in comparison with the small face, are exceedingly large. The forehead and top of the head are relatively large. It is difficult to imagine the diversity of individual looks that will develop over the course of childhood and adolescence from such similar infant faces (Fig. 13.6).

The maxilla of the newborn is very low frontally and relatively small. By the age of 9 months, the jaw has become considerably wider and higher. There is also a remarkable increase in size of the maxillary sinus. At birth, the bones that compose the cranium are not fused and are separated by six membrane-filled gaps called fontanels (Fig. 13.7). These gaps completely close by ossification within 2 years of birth.

The face of the newborn appears broad and flat. The lower jaw appears underdeveloped and receded. The overall broadness of the face results from the lack of vertical growth, which is yet to commence. The horizontal dimensions are more nearly adultlike. According to Ranly,[7] the upper face height of the newborn is only 43% of adult height. Similarly, the total face height of the newborn is only 40% of adult face height. This demonstrates that the most striking and complex growth of the head is associated with the face. After an initial spurt during the first 3 years, the rate of increase of these dimensions slows. It remains steady until the adult size is reached. The cranium of the infant, as represented by cranial width and length, is closer to adult size than any other part of the head. This can be explained by the development of the brain, which by the eighth month of intrauterine life has all of the nerve cells it will ever have. The growth of the cranial vault is complete before that of the maxilla, and maxillary growth is complete before mandibular growth. This is an example of the cephalocaudal growth gradient, which indicates that the cranial structures are closer to their adult size during infancy and childhood

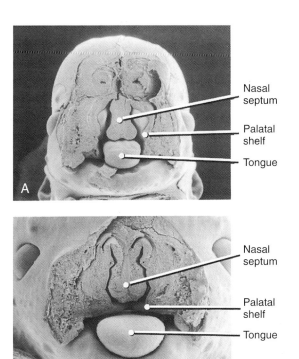

• **Figure 13.3** Scanning electron micrographs of mouse embryos sectioned in the frontal plane. (A) Before elevation of the palatal shelves showing their margins extending to the level of the lateral borders of the tongue. (B) Following elevation of the palatal shelves. (Courtesy Dr. K. Sulik. From Proffit WR, Fields HW. *Contemporary Orthodontics*. 4th ed. St Louis: Mosby; 2007.)

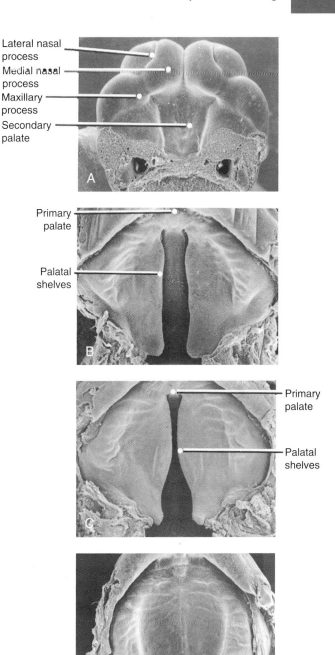

• **Figure 13.4** These scanning electron micrographs of human specimens (except A, which is a mouse specimen) show several stages of palate closure from 53 to 59 days after conception. (A) At the completion of primary palate closure. (B) Palatal shelves during elevation. (C) Just before fusion of the shelves. (D) The secondary palate following fusion. (Courtesy Dr. K. Sulik. From Proffit WR, Fields HW. *Contemporary Orthodontics*. 4th ed. St Louis: Mosby; 2007.)

than other body parts.[8] Symphyseal growth increases the width of the mandible. By the second year, the symphysis is closed and growth becomes localized in the mandible, as well as in the nasomaxillary complex. An enormous metamorphosis has taken place, but many more changes need to occur before the child's adult appearance is realized.

Dental Changes

This section addresses the growth, development, and eruption of each tooth unit from initiation to complete eruption. By definition, *growth* signifies an increase, expansion, or extension of any given tissue. For example, a tooth *grows* as more enamel is deposited by ameloblasts. *Development* addresses the progressive evolution of a tissue. A tooth *develops* as the ameloblasts develop from less specific ectodermal tissue and as the dentinoblasts develop from unspecialized mesoderm.

Teeth are formed by tissues originating from both ectoderm and mesoderm. At approximately 6 weeks in utero, the basal layer of the oral epithelium of the fetus shows increased activity and enlargement in the areas of the future dental arches. This increase and expansion give rise to the dental lamina of the future tooth germ. As the tooth bud develops, it reaches a point at which it is recognized as the cap stage. At this time, it begins to incorporate mesoderm into its structure. Therefore the tooth-forming organ is initially formed from ectoderm but shortly thereafter includes mesoderm.

The expansion of tissue on the epithelial borders represents the beginning of the life cycle of the tooth. The ectoderm will become responsible for the future enamel, and the mesoderm will become primarily responsible for pulp and dentin. The tooth germ is accountable for the development of the following three formative tissues:

1. Dental organ (epithelial)
2. Dental papilla
3. Dental sac

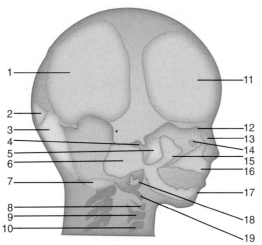

• **Figure 13.5** Human skull at approximately 3 months. Intramembranous bones are shown in a *tannish-yellow* color. Cartilage is represented by a *light orange* color, and bones developing by endochondral ossification are indicated by a *light gray* color. Approximate time of appearance for each bone is indicated in parentheses. *1,* Parietal bone (10 weeks). *2,* Interparietal bone (8 weeks). *3,* Supraoccipital (8 weeks). *4,* Dorsum sellae (still cartilaginous). *5,* Temporal wing of sphenoid (2 to 3 months; the basisphenoid appears at 12 to 13 weeks, orbitosphenoid at 12 weeks, and presphenoid at 5 months). *6,* Squamous part of temporal bone (2 to 3 months). *7,* Basioccipital (2 to 3 months). *8,* Hyoid (still cartilaginous). *9,* Thyroid (still cartilaginous). *10,* Cricoid (still cartilaginous). *11,* Frontal bone (7½ weeks). *12,* Crista galli (still cartilaginous; inferiorly, the middle concha begins ossification at 16 weeks, the superior and inferior conchae at 18 weeks; the perpendicular plate of ethmoid begins ossification during the first postnatal year, the cribriform plate during the second postnatal year, the vomer at 8 fetal weeks). *13,* Nasal bone (8 weeks). *14,* Lacrimal bone (8½ weeks). *15,* Malar (8 weeks). *16,* Maxilla (end of sixth week; premaxilla, 7 weeks). *17,* Mandible (6 to 8 weeks). *18,* Tympanic ring (begins at 9 weeks, with complete ring at 12 weeks; petrous bone, 5 to 6 months). *19,* Styloid process, still cartilaginous. (Redrawn from Enlow DH. *Handbook of Facial Growth.* Philadelphia: Saunders; 1982; Modified from Patten BM. *Human Embryology.* 3rd ed. New York: McGraw-Hill; 1968.)

The 6-week-old fetus demonstrates 10 sites of epithelial activity on the occlusal (soft tissue) border of both the developing maxilla and the mandible.[9] These sites are lined up next to each other and ultimately predict the position of the 10 primary teeth in both the maxilla and the mandible (Fig. 13.8).

In addition to developing 20 primary teeth, each unit also develops a dental lamina that is responsible for the development of the future *permanent* tooth.[9] The primary centrals, laterals, and canines produce a dental lamina for the future permanent centrals, laterals, and canines. The primary first and second molars produce a dental lamina for the future permanent first and second premolars. The permanent molars develop from and on three successive locations on one dental lamina, extending distally from each of the primary second molars (Fig. 13.9).[9]

An analysis of the successive periods of growth of the tooth germ can be organized by the following stages of the life cycle of the tooth[9]:

Growth
    Initiation
    Proliferation
    Histodifferentiation
    Morphodifferentiation
    Apposition
Calcification
Eruption
Attrition

Growth

Initiation

The initiation stage is first noticed in the 6-week-old fetus (Fig. 13.10). As the word *initiation* suggests, this stage is recognized by the initial formation of an expansion of the basal layer of the oral cavity immediately above the basement membrane. The basal layer is a row of organized cells lined up on the basement membrane, which is a tissue division line between the ectoderm (epithelium)

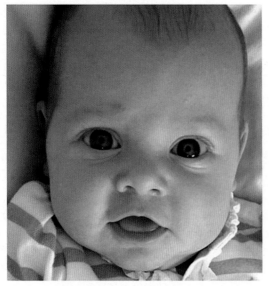
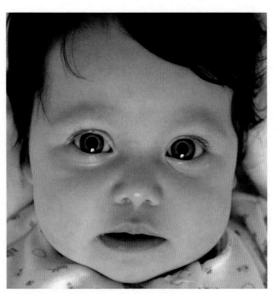

• **Figure 13.6** The small nose, lips, jaws, ears, and chin are shared among young babies. Babies have a uniformity of appearance. With growth, of course, the subtle differences among young babies' faces become explicit and easily recognized.

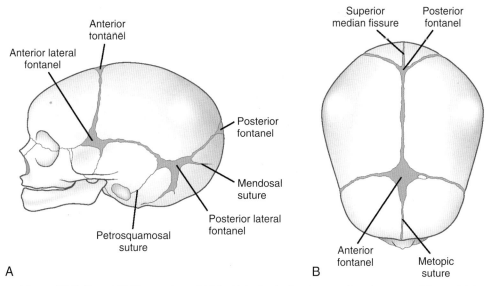

• **Figure 13.7** (A and B) The cranium at birth. Note the fontanels, one at each corner of the parietal bones. (From Slovis TL. *Caffey's Pediatric Diagnostic Imaging.* 11th ed. St Louis: Mosby; 2008.)

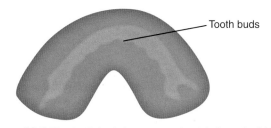

• **Figure 13.8** The tooth buds in an approximately 8-week-old fetus.

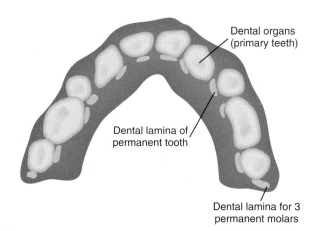

• **Figure 13.9** The dental organs and dental lamina in an approximately 4-month-old fetus.

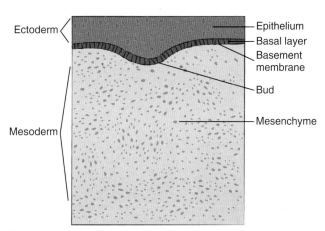

• **Figure 13.10** The initiation stage of the life cycle of the tooth in an approximately 5- to 6-week-old fetus.

and the mesoderm (Fig. 13.11). The cells of the basal layer are the innermost cells of the oral epithelium (ectoderm) adjacent to the basement membrane.

At 10 specific intermittent locations along the basement membrane, the cells of the basal layer multiply at a much faster rate than the surrounding cells.[10] This development occurs at that point on the oral epithelium that is the tooth bud and is responsible for the initial growth of that tooth (Fig. 13.12).

It can be noted that the times of initiation of the various teeth differ.[11] This period of tooth development is also recognized as the

bud stage. Such a description assists in visually understanding the developmental process of the immature tooth.

Proliferation

Proliferation is a multiplication of the cells of the initiation stage and an expansion of the tooth bud, resulting in the formation of the tooth germ (Fig. 13.13). The tooth germ is a result of the prolific epithelial cells forming a caplike appearance with the subsequent incorporation of the mesoderm. This incorporation of mesodermal tissue below and within the cap gives rise to the dental papilla.

The mesenchyme (mesoderm) surrounding the dental organ and dental papilla is the tissue that will form the dental sac. The dental sac ultimately gives rise to the supporting structures of the tooth. These structures are the cementum and periodontal ligament.

As the tooth germ continues to proliferate in an irregular fashion, it produces a caplike appearance. This stage is called the cap stage (Fig. 13.14). Like the bud stage, it is so referenced for visual identification. As the cap begins to form, the mesenchyme changes

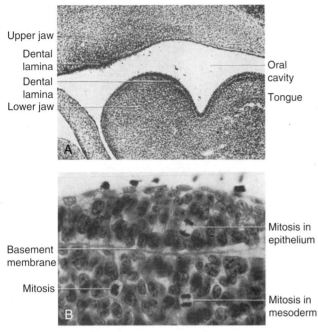

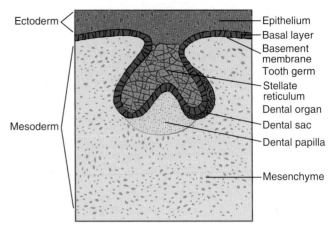

• **Figure 13.13** The proliferation stage of the life cycle of the tooth in an approximately 9- to 11-week-old fetus.

• **Figure 13.11** Initiation of tooth development. Human embryo 13.5 mm long, fifth week. (A) Sagittal section through upper and lower jaws. (B) High magnification of thickened oral epithelium. (From Orban B. *Dental Histology and Embryology*. 2nd ed. New York: McGraw-Hill; 1929.)

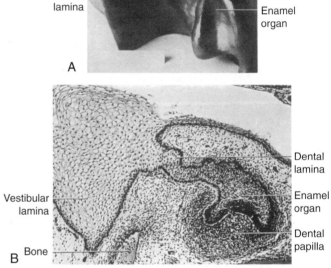

• **Figure 13.14** Cap stage of tooth development. Human embryo 60 mm long, 11th week. (A) Wax reconstruction of the dental organ of the lower lateral incisor. (B) Labiolingual section through the same tooth. (From Orban B. *Dental Histology and Embryology*. 2nd ed. New York: McGraw-Hill; 1929.)

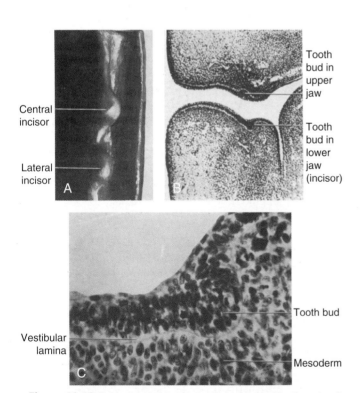

• **Figure 13.12** Bud stage of tooth development (proliferation stage). Human embryo 16 mm long, sixth week. (A) Wax reconstruction of the germs of the central and lateral lower incisors. (B) Sagittal section through upper and lower jaws. (C) High-magnification view of the tooth germ of the lower incisor in bud stage. (From Orban B. *Dental Histology and Embryology*. 2nd ed. New York: McGraw-Hill; 1929.)

within the cap, which initiates the development of the dental papilla.

The dental papilla evolves from the mesenchyme invaginating the inner dental epithelium and generates the pulp and dentin. The dental sac also comes into being by a marginal condensation in the mesenchyme surrounding the dental organ and dental papilla. The stellate (starlike) reticulum (network) is an organization of cells within the descending portion of the dental organ that is enamel-forming tissue referred to as the enamel pulp. During this stage the tooth germ has all the necessary formative tissues to embrace the development of a tooth and its periodontal ligament.[9]

In summary, the tooth germ consists of all the necessary elements for the development of the complete tooth. The germ is composed of the following three distinct parts: (1) dental organ, (2) dental papilla, and (3) dental sac. The dental organ produces the enamel.

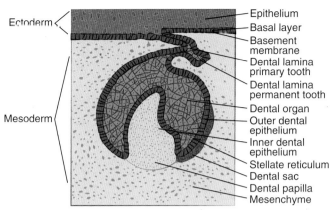

• **Figure 13.15** The histodifferentiation stage of the life cycle of the tooth. Approximately 14-week-old fetus.

The dental papilla generates the dentin and pulp. The dental sac gives rise to the cementum and periodontal ligament.[9]

Histodifferentiation

The histodifferentiation stage is marked by the histologic difference in the appearance of the cells of the tooth germ because they are now beginning to specialize (Fig. 13.15). The cap continues to grow and begins to look more like a bell. The image of a bell is registered because the extensions of the cap grow deeper into the mesoderm. This part of development is appropriately called the bell stage, and the tissue within the bell gives rise to the dental papilla.

The dental organ is now completely surrounded by the basement membrane and is divided into an inner and outer dental epithelium. The dental organ ultimately becomes enamel.

The condensation of the tissue (mesoderm) adjacent to the outside of the bell is responsible for the dental sac. The dental sac ultimately gives rise to the cementum, which covers the tooth's root, and to the periodontal ligament, which attaches the tooth to the bone adjacent to the tooth roots.

The dental lamina continues to shrink, with the result that it looks more like a cord. The dental lamina for the permanent successor becomes obvious as an extension of the dental lamina of the primary tooth. The basal layer continues to exist and is now divided into an inner and an outer dental epithelium. The stellate reticulum expands and organizes to incorporate more intercellular fluid in preparation for the formation of enamel (Figs. 13.16 to 13.18).

Morphodifferentiation

The morphodifferentiation stage, as the name implies, is the stage at which the cells find an arrangement that ultimately dictates the final size and shape of the tooth (Fig. 13.19).[11] This stage is called the advanced bell stage (see Fig. 13.19). The cells of the inner dental epithelium become the ameloblasts, which produce the enamel matrix. As the ameloblasts begin their formation, the tissue of the dental papilla immediately adjacent to the basement membrane begins to differentiate into odontoblasts (Figs. 13.20 and 13.21). The odontoblasts and the ameloblasts are responsible for the formation of dentin and enamel, respectively.

Although the development of dentin is not clearly understood, structures have been identified that show progressive changes. The first change in dentin formation to be seen is a thickening of the basement membrane of the inner dental epithelium and the pulp

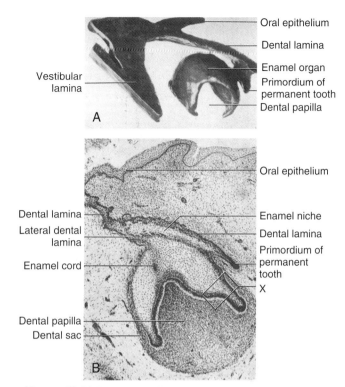

• **Figure 13.16** Bell stage of tooth development. Human embryo 105 mm long, 14th week. (A) Wax reconstruction of lower central incisor. (B) Labiolingual section of the same tooth. X designates inset (see Fig. 13.17). (From Orban B. *Dental Histology and Embryology*. 2nd ed. New York: McGraw-Hill; 1929.)

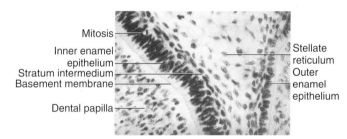

• **Figure 13.17** The four layers of the epithelial dental organ in high magnification (inset X of Fig. 13.16). (From Orban B. *Dental Histology and Embryology*. 2nd ed. New York: McGraw-Hill; 1929.)

developed by the dental papilla. The membrane from the mesenchyme of the pulp consists of fine reticular fibrils. A continuation of growth is noted by a formation of irregular spiraling fibers from deep in the pulp that entangle with the reticular fibrils from the mesenchyme of the pulp. These long spiraling fibers are known as Korff fibers and assist in the structural support of the developing dentin (Fig. 13.22).[9]

The specialized cells of the previous stage now arrange themselves in a manner that gives each tooth its prescribed size and shape. There is a disappearance of the dental lamina, except for the dental lamina proper immediately adjacent to the developing primary tooth.

The dental lamina proper continues to proliferate to the lingual of the primary tooth which initiates the development of the permanent tooth. The primary tooth germ now becomes a free

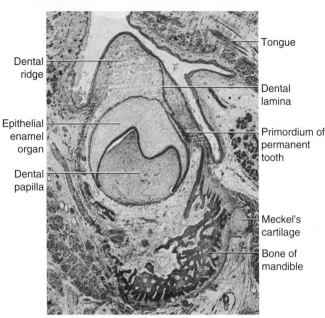

• **Figure 13.18** Advanced bell stage of tooth development. Human embryo 200 mm long, age approximately 18 weeks. Labiolingual section through the first primary lower molar. (From Bhaskar S. *Synopsis of Oral Histology*. St Louis: Mosby; 1962:44.)

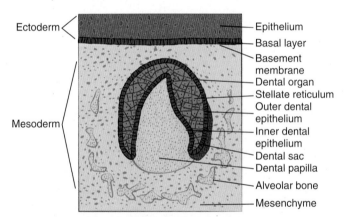

• **Figure 13.19** The morphodifferentiation stage of the life cycle of the tooth in an approximately 18-week-old fetus.

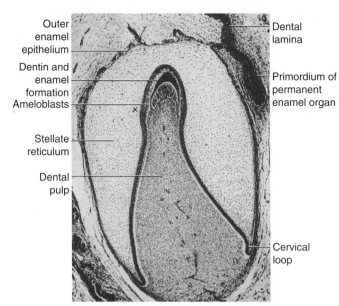

• **Figure 13.20** Tooth germ (lower incisor) of a human fetus (fifth month). Beginning of dentin and enamel formation. The stellate reticulum at the tip of the crown reduced in thickness. *X* designates inset (see Fig. 13.21). (From Diamond M, Applebaum E. The epithelial sheath: histogenesis and function. *J Dent Res.* 1942;21:403.)

internal organ.[11] The specialized cells found during the histodifferentiation stage and the organization of these specialized cells during the morphodifferentiation stage prepare the tooth for the development of various tissues of enamel, dentin, pulp, cementum, and periodontal ligament.

Apposition

Whereas the morphodifferentiation stage dictates the size and shape of the tooth, the appositional stage occurs when the network or tissue matrix of the tooth is formed (Fig. 13.23). Cells that have the potential for the deposition of extracellular matrix fulfill the plan of the tooth germ established by previous stages. The growth is appositional, additive, and regular. This accounts for the layered appearance of enamel and dentin.[9] The organized special tissues now deposit incremental layers of enamel and dentin matrix. The matrices layered by ameloblasts and odontoblasts begin from a growth center along the dentinoenamel and dentinocemental junctions (Figs. 13.24 and 13.25).

Calcification

Calcification occurs with an influx of mineral salts within the previously developed tissue matrix (Fig. 13.26). The chemical structure of enamel consists of approximately 96% inorganic material and approximately 4% organic material and water. The inorganic portion is composed primarily of calcium and phosphorus, with a small portion of several other compounds and elements, such as carbon dioxide, magnesium, and sodium, to mention a few (Table 13.4).

Calcification begins with the precipitation of enamel in the cusp tips and incisal edges of the teeth and continues with the production of more layers on these small points of origin. This results in older, more mature enamel at the cusp tips and incisal edges, and newer enamel at the cervical region (see Figs. 13.24 and 13.25).

The calcification of enamel and dentin is a very sensitive process that takes place over a long period. Therefore calcification irregularities noted in any fully developed tooth can often be equated with a specific systemic disturbance.[11] In the cross-section of the clinical crown of a tooth that has been prepared for histologic view, there are apparent lines or bands, which are called the incremental lines of Retzius (Fig. 13.27). Depending on how the section is prepared (either longitudinally or horizontally), the incremental lines of Retzius may appear as lines or circles (Fig. 13.28). These lines or circles represent the developmental pattern of the developing tooth.

The degree of variation of any line usually reflects a reaction to a change in the physiologic processes of growth and development of the tooth. For instance, in primary teeth there is an incremental line of Retzius called the neonatal line or neonatal ring (Fig. 13.29). This neonatal line is attributable to the abrupt change in certain body processes of the fetus when it is born. At birth, there is enough of a change or insult to the newborn's systems to cause a growth change that is reflected dentally as a neonatal ring.[9] This ring is actually the result of disturbances in the growth and calcification of the tooth.

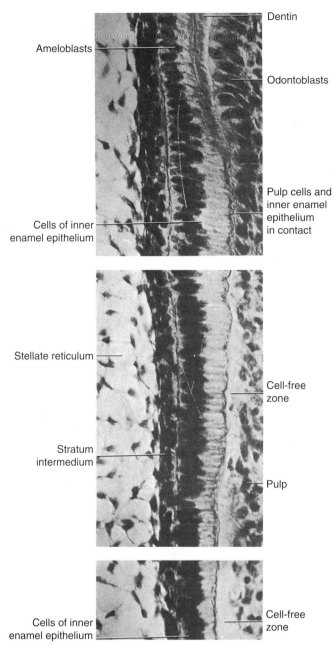

• **Figure 13.21** High-magnification view of the inner dental epithelium from inset *X* in Fig. 13.20. In the cervical region the cells are short, and the outermost layer of the pulp is cell free. Occlusally the cells are long and the cell-free zone of the pulp has disappeared. The ameloblasts are again shorter where dentin formation has set in, and enamel formation is imminent. (From Diamond M, Applebaum E. The epithelial sheath: histogenesis and function. *J Dent Res*. 1942;21:403.)

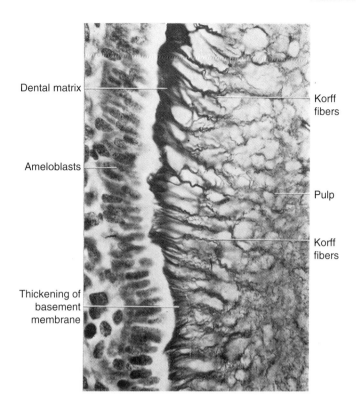

• **Figure 13.22** Thickening of the basement membrane between pulp and inner dental epithelium, leading to the development of Korff fibers. (From Bhasker SN, ed. *Orban's Oral Histology and Embryology*. 11th ed. St Louis: Mosby; 1990.)

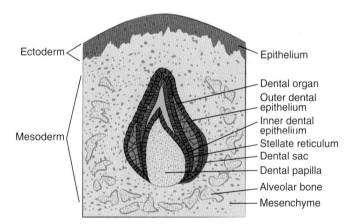

• **Figure 13.23** The apposition stage of the life cycle of the tooth.

In summary, the aspect of enamel maturation called calcification involves the hardening of the previously formed matrix by the precipitation of mineral salts (inorganic calcium salts). This calcification is a slow, gradual process beginning at the cusp tips or incisal edge of the tooth (see Fig. 13.25).

Eruption

It is necessary to mention root development before addressing eruption (Fig. 13.30). The developmental process of the crown of the tooth involves many overlying processes occurring at the same time. The same is true for the root. Root development has correlations with eruption. When formation of the clinical crown of the tooth has been completed, the inner and outer epithelia appear to fold over at the cementoenamel junction and continue their growth without any tissue between them. Previously, stellate reticulum occupied this space. The inner and outer dental epithelia without the stellate reticulum is referred to as Hertwig epithelial root sheath, which is responsible for the size and shape of the root and eruption of the tooth (Fig. 13.31).[9]

Eruption can be categorized into three different phases: (1) preeruptive phase, (2) eruptive phase (prefunctional), and (3) eruptive phase (functional). The preeruptive phase is that period

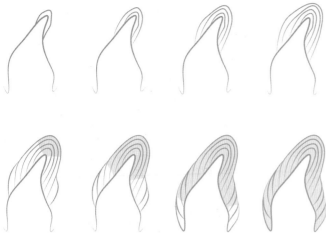

• **Figure 13.24** Enamel matrix formation and maturation. Formation follows an incremental pattern; maturation begins at the tip of the crown and proceeds cervically in cross-relation to the incremental pattern. (Redrawn from Bhasker SN, ed. *Orban's Oral Histology and Embryology*. 11th ed. St Louis: Mosby; 1990.)

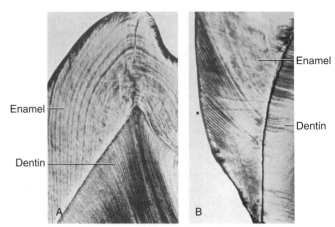

• **Figure 13.27** Incremental lines of Retzius in longitudinal ground sections. (A) Cuspal region. (B) Cervical region *(x)*. (From Bhasker SN, ed. *Orban's Oral Histology and Embryology*. 11th ed. St Louis: Mosby; 1990.)

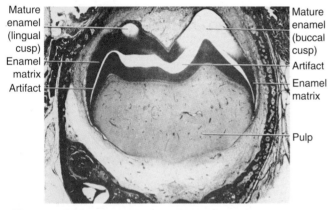

• **Figure 13.25** Buccolingual section through a deciduous molar. Maturation of the enamel has started in the lingual cusp; it has fairly well progressed in the buccal cusp. Note the gradual transition between the enamel matrix and the fully matured enamel. (From Bhasker SN, ed. *Orban's Oral Histology and Embryology*. 11th ed. St Louis: Mosby; 1990.)

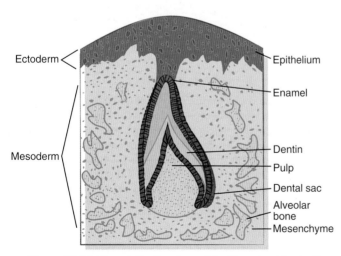

• **Figure 13.26** The calcification stage of the life cycle of the tooth.

TABLE 13.4 Chemical Contents of Enamel, Dentin, Cementum, and Bone

	Enamel	Dentin	Cementum, Compact Bone
Water (%)	2.3	13.2	32
Organic Matter (%)	1.7	17.5	22
Ash (%)	96.0	69.3	46
In 100 g of Ash:			
Calcium (g)	36.1	35.3	35.5
Phosphorus (g)	17.3	17.1	17.1
Carbon Dioxide (g)	3.0	4.0	4.4
Magnesium (g)	0.5	1.2	0.9
Sodium (g)	0.2	0.2	1.1
Potassium (g)	0.3	0.07	0.1
Chloride (g)	0.3	0.03	0.1
Fluorine (g)	0.016	0.017	0.015
Sulfur (g)	0.1	0.2	0.6
Copper (g)	0.01		
Silicon (g)	0.003		0.04
Iron (g)	0.0025		0.09
Zinc (g)	0.016	0.018	
Lead (g)	**Whole Teeth** 0.0071–0.037	**Bone** 0.002–0.02	

Small amounts of: Ce, La, Pr, Ne, Ag, Sr, Ba, Cr, Sn, Mn, Ti, Ni, V, Al, B, Cu, Li, Se

Data from Sicher H. *Orban's Oral Histology and Embryology*. 5th ed. St Louis: Mosby; 1962. Compiled by Dr. Harold C. Hodge.

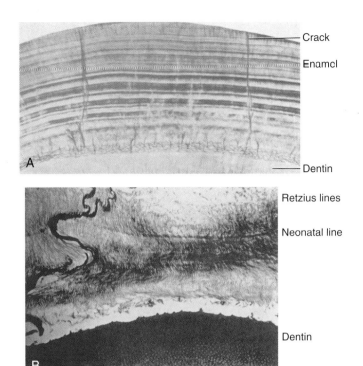

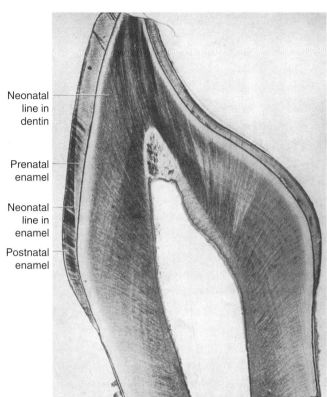

• **Figure 13.28** (A) Incremental lines of Retzius in transverse ground section, arranged concentrically. (B) Decalcified paraffin section of exfoliated primary molar (×20). Heavy dark lamella runs from darkly stained dentin to surface in an irregular course independent of developmental pattern. Approximately parallel to dentin surface, a number of incremental lines are visible, one of which, the neonatal line, is accentuated. (From Bhasker SN, ed. *Orban's Oral Histology and Embryology*. 11th ed. St Louis: Mosby; 1990.)

• **Figure 13.29** Neonatal line in the enamel. Longitudinal ground section of a primary canine. (From Schour I. The neonatal line in the enamel and dentin of the human deciduous teeth and first permanent molar. *J Am Dent Assoc*. 1936;23:1946. Copyright by the American Dental Association. Reprinted with permission.)

during which the tooth root initiates its formation and begins to move toward the surface of the oral cavity from its bony vault. The prefunctional eruptive phase consists of that period of development of the tooth root through gingival emergence. Most eruption tables report the time that the tooth can first be seen in the mouth (Figs. 13.32 and 13.33). The tooth root is usually approximately one-half to two-thirds of its final length at the time of gingival emergence.

After the tooth has erupted into the oral cavity and contacts its antagonist (opposing tooth in the opposite arch), it is considered to be in the functional eruptive phase. Teeth remain a dynamic unit in that some type of movement, no matter how slight, is always taking place. Teeth continue to move and erupt as necessary as the body continues to change throughout life.[11]

There has been considerable speculation about the causes of tooth eruption. Some examples of causes of tooth eruption frequently cited are (1) root formation, (2) proliferation of Hertwig epithelial root sheath, (3) proliferation of the connective tissue of the dental papillae, (4) growth of the jaw, (5) pressures from muscular action, (6) pressure at the apical part of the tooth, and (7) apposition and resorption of bone. Because myriad events are occurring at the time of eruption, it is difficult to single out any one process as the primary cause of tooth eruption.

The process of exfoliation of primary teeth is caused by the eruptive pressure of the permanent successor at the apex of the primary tooth and its surroundings. The eruptive pressure stimulates the development of osteoclasts. A progressive resorption of the

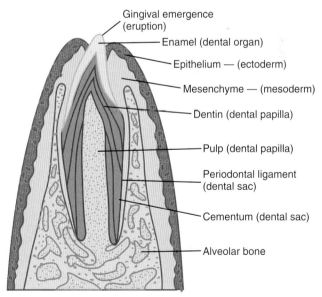

• **Figure 13.30** The eruption stage of the life cycle of the tooth.

tooth root, dentin, and cementum, as well as adjacent bone, is completed by the action of the osteoclasts.

Attrition

Attrition is the wearing of teeth during function (Fig. 13.34). It is a normal physiologic process that occurs as teeth occlude with

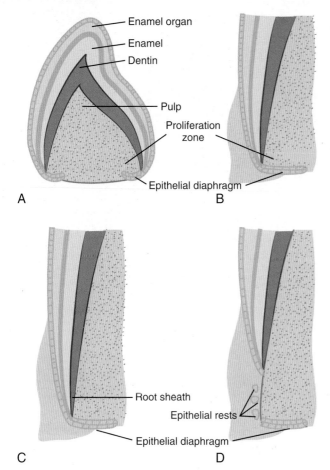

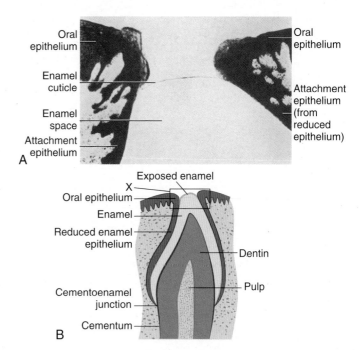

• **Figure 13.32** (A and B) Tooth emerges through a perforation in the fused epithelia. *X* in B indicates area from which the photomicrograph was taken. ([B] Redrawn from Bhasker SN, ed. *Orban's Oral Histology and Embryology*. 11th ed. St Louis: Mosby; 1990.)

• **Figure 13.31** Three stages in root development. (A) Section through a tooth germ showing the epithelial diaphragm and proliferation zone of the pulp. (B) Higher magnification view of the cervical region of A. (C) Imaginary stage showing the elongation of Hertwig epithelial sheath between the diaphragm and future cementoenamel junction. Differentiation of odontoblasts in the elongated pulp. (D) In the cervical part of the root, dentin has been formed. The root sheath is broken up into epithelial rests and is separated from the dentinal surface by connective tissue. Differentiation of cementoblasts. (Redrawn from Bhasker SN, ed. *Orban's Oral Histology and Embryology*. 11th ed. St Louis: Mosby; 1990.)

those in the opposing dental arch. Certain types of foods and associated habits may contribute to more or less wear for individuals.[11] The effects of attrition on occlusion are compensated for by further functional eruption.

Fig. 13.35 summarizes the life cycle of the tooth from initiation through attrition.

Primary Dentition Development Up to Age 3 Years

Table 13.5 demonstrates the various stages of development of the teeth from conception to adolescence.[12] The primary teeth begin to form at 6 weeks in utero, and the enamel of all of the primary teeth is usually completed by the first year of age (Figs. 13.36 and 13.37). The first primary teeth to erupt are the primary mandibular central incisors at 6 months of age, and all of the primary teeth generally erupt by age 2.

Permanent Dentition Development Up to Age 3 Years

The first permanent molar is the first tooth to show germ formation, which occurs at age 3½ to 4 months in utero. It is followed by

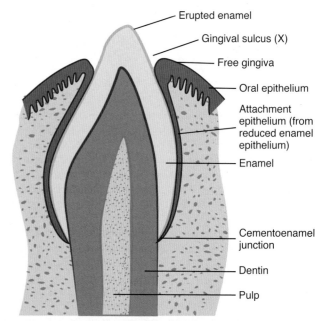

• **Figure 13.33** The attached epithelial cuff and gingival sulcus at an early stage of tooth eruption. Bottom of sulcus is at *X*. (Redrawn from Bhasker SN, ed. *Orban's Oral Histology and Embryology*. 11th ed. St Louis: Mosby; 1990.)

the central and lateral incisors, which demonstrate formation at 5 to 5½ months in utero. The canines are the only other permanent teeth that begin formation before birth, at 5½ to 6 months in utero. The first and second premolars and the second and third molars demonstrate germ formation after birth.

At birth, the only permanent teeth that show a trace of hard tissue formation are the first permanent molars.[9] With the exception of the third molars, all permanent teeth demonstrate hard tissue formation by 3 years of age (see Table 13.5).[12]

See Box 13.1 for a glossary of terms from this section.

Cognitive Changes

The human infant has long been regarded as a cognitively incompetent creature because of his or her helplessness. Many psychologists now recognize that there is cognitive ability in the newborn. There is evidence that newborns experience sensations of pain, touch,

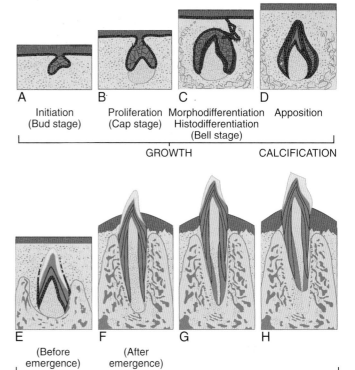

• **Figure 13.35** (A–H) The life cycle of the tooth. (Redrawn from Schour I, Massler M. Studies in tooth development: the growth pattern of human teeth. *J Am Dent Assoc*. 1940;27:1785. Copyright by the American Dental Association. Reprinted with permission.)

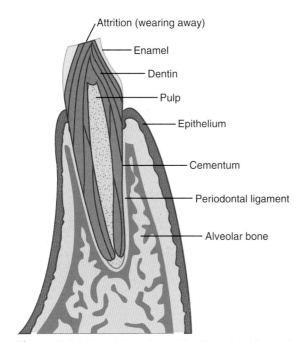

• **Figure 13.34** The attrition stage of the life cycle of the tooth.

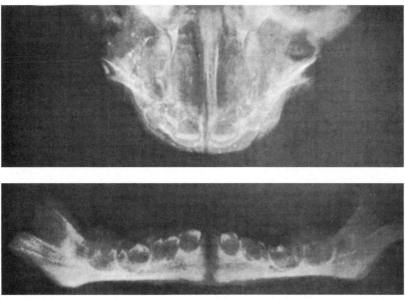

• **Figure 13.36** Wet specimen from 8-month-old fetus. Note areas of dental calcification in the mandibular incisors, canines, and primary first molars, as well as in the maxillary central and lateral incisors and first primary molars. There is only slight calcification in the maxillary canines and cusp tips of the second primary molars. (From McCall JO, Wald SS. *Clinical Dental Roentgenology*. 4th ed. Philadelphia: Saunders; 1957.)

TABLE 13.5   Chronology of the Human Dentition

Tooth	Hard Tissue Formation Begins	Amount of Enamel Formed at Birth	Enamel Completed	Eruption	Root Completed
Primary Dentition					
Maxillary					
Central incisor	4 months in utero	Five-sixths	1½ months	7½ months	1½ years
Lateral incisor	4½ months in utero	Two-thirds	2½ months	9 months	2 years
Canine	5 months in utero	One-third	9 months	18 months	3¼ years
First molar	5 months in utero	Cusps united	6 months	14 months	2½ years
Second molar	6 months in utero	Cusp tips still isolated	11 months	24 months	3 years
Mandibular					
Central incisor	4½ months in utero	Three-fifths	2½ months	6 months	1½ years
Lateral incisor	4½ months in utero	Three-fifths	3 months	7 months	1½ years
Canine	5 months in utero	One-third	9 months	16 months	3¼ years
First molar	5 months in utero	Cusps united	5½ months	12 months	2¼ years
Second molar	6 months in utero	Cusp tips still isolated	10 months	20 months	3 years
Permanent Dentition					
Maxillary					
Central incisor	3–4 months	—	4–5 years	7–8 years	10 years
Lateral incisor	10–12 months	—	4–5 years	8–9 years	11 years
Canine	4–5 months	—	6–7 years	11–12 years	13–15 years
First premolar	1½–1¾ years	—	5–6 years	10–11 years	12–13 years
Second premolar	2–2¼ years	—	6–7 years	10–12 years	12–14 years
First molar	At birth	Sometimes a trace	2½–3 years	6–7 years	9–10 years
Second molar	2½–3 years	—	7–8 years	12–13 years	14–16 years
Mandibular					
Central incisor	3–4 months	—	4–5 years	6–7 years	9 years
Lateral incisor	3–4 months	—	4–5 years	7–8 years	10 years
Canine	4–5 months	—	6–7 years	9–10 years	12–14 years
First premolar	1¾–2 years	—	5–6 years	10–12 years	12–13 years
Second premolar	2¼–2½ years	—	6–7 years	11–12 years	13–14 years
First molar	At birth	Sometimes a trace	2½–3 years	6–7 years	9–10 years
Second molar	2½–3 years	—	7–8 years	11–13 years	14–15 years

After Logan WHG, Kronfeld R. Development of the human jaws and surrounding structures from birth to the age of fifteen years. *J Am Dent Assoc.* 1933;20:379–427 (slightly modified by McCall and Schour). Copyright by the American Dental Association.

and changes in bodily position. In addition, it is known that infants can smell, see, and hear from the first day of life. Cognitive competence explains how and why an infant explores a nursing mother's fingers and studies her face.

In 1984 Mussen and coworkers[13] noted that there are four major areas of cognitive development which occur during the first year of a child's life. The first is the area of perception. Even very young infants have the ability to perceive movement, facial relationships, and color (see Table 13.1).

The second prominent cognitive area is the recognition of information. Infants recognize certain stimuli such as a face when viewed from various and different observational angles. In such a case, it is contended that children have developed mental schemes or representations of things encountered in their consciousness and that these schemes contain some but not all of the crucial elements of the object or event. This allows them to recognize the similarity of new objects compared with old ones because of their ability to generalize these crucial elements.

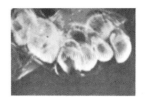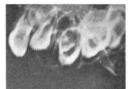

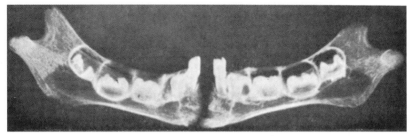

• **Figure 13.37** Wet specimen from infant at birth. Note areas of dental calcification similar to those shown in Fig. 13.36. Maxillary calcification is slightly less advanced. (From McCall JO, Wald SS. *Clinical Dental Roentgenology*. 4th ed. Philadelphia: Saunders; 1957.)

The third important cognitive area is the ability to categorize. Children group things together by way of shape, color, and use as early as 1 year of age.

Enhancement of memory is the fourth area of cognitive development noted in the first year of life. Even very young infants have been shown to have some memory. At age 6 months and older, the ability to recall past experiences appears obvious. At this age, most children have the ability to recall events and to use the information gained from that event to help them form a reaction to new situations. Two theories are of interest in the study of cognition in infants. The first is learning theory. The concept of conditioning is derived from that body of thought. Essentially there are two types of conditioning: classical and operant. *Classical conditioning* occurs when two stimuli are paired together. For instance, sucking the nipple, if paired often enough with hearing a lullaby, eventually leads the infant to initiate sucking when he hears the lullaby. *Instrumental* or *operant conditioning* occurs when a child's actions are reinforced or rewarded; rewarded behavior is behavior that is likely to occur again. When parents smile in response to their baby's smile, the baby will smile again to get the same response.

The cognitive development theory of Jean Piaget is the other theory of interest in the attempt to understand infant cognition. According to Piaget,[14] much of the intellectual development of the child from birth to the age of 2 years results from the interactions of the child with objects in the his or her environment. Although Piagetian theory is not without some controversy regarding its accuracy, it is extremely useful to researchers, clinicians, parents, and other observers of infants because Piaget based his conclusions on observations of his own children's behavior. The behaviors he witnessed are common to all children.

In 1954 Piaget described the first 2 years of life as a period of sensorimotor development, which he divided into six discrete stages.[15] Piaget contended that during this time the child must develop knowledge in the following three areas:

1. *Object permanence:* Objects continue to exist even when they are not perceivable by the child.
2. *Causality:* Objects have uses, and events have causes. Piaget used the term *circular reaction* (primary, secondary, and tertiary) to describe the changes that occur in this area. A primary circular reaction describes re-creating an already known satisfying action,

such as thumb sucking. A secondary circular reaction is the re-creating of an accidentally discovered cause and effect. Tertiary circular reactions involve experimentation, and, as one might guess, such behaviors often exasperate the child's parents.

3. *Symbolic play:* One object can represent another.

The language development of the infant is, at first, very slow. The mean expressive vocabulary (words used) of an 18-month-old is 10 words. At this time, the receptive vocabulary (the words they understand) of the child is considerably higher than the expressive vocabulary. Toward the end of the second year, the expressive vocabulary of children develops extraordinarily quickly. In 1983 Levine and colleagues[15] noted that the mean vocabulary of a 3-year-old child is 1000 words.

Table 13.1 coordinates the six stages of the sensorimotor stage of development with cognition, play, and language development.

Emotional Changes

There are many human emotions, such as shame, guilt, anger, joy, fear, and sadness. Emotions can be discerned by observing behavioral reactions (crying), measuring physiologic responses (increased heart rate), or ascertaining a person's thoughts and reactions ("I'm depressed").

In assessing the emotional state of young children, the latter two methods of discernment are of little or no value. As a general rule, in the first year of a child's life, adults assign whatever emotion they believe that the child should feel in a particular situation. Thus a wide range of interpretation exists. When an 18-month-old child spills milk, one parent may interpret the child's crying as frustration over his or her awkwardness, another as guilt for the mistake, and yet another as fear of or sadness about having nothing else to drink.

It is also evident that in older children and adults, the true description of an emotion is strongly influenced by how a person reacts to, analyzes, and studies his or her own feelings. Thus, for the same stimulus, one person may laugh and another may cry. In very young children, ascertaining such subtleties as these is not possible. The excited babbling of a 3-month-old, which parents label as joy, may more appropriately be called excitement.

There appears to be an awakening of emotional states within the child between 4 months and 10 months of age. In 1984 Mussen

• BOX 13.1 Glossary

Ameloblast: One of a group of cells originating from the ectoderm from which the dental enamel is developed; an enamel cell. The ameloblasts cover the papilla of the enamel organ

Apposition: Appositional growth is that stage of the life cycle of the developing tooth during which a layerlike deposition of a nonvital extracellular secretion is laid down in the form of tissue matrix

Attrition: Due to rubbing and friction. In dentistry, the term refers to the natural wearing away of the substance of a tooth under the stress of mastication

Basal layer: Basal is an adjective meaning pertaining to or situated near a base. In the developing tooth, the basal layer is that tissue at the junction of the ectoderm and mesoderm

Basement membrane: The delicate, transparent, membranous layer of cells underlying the epithelium of mucous membranes and secreting glands at the junction of the ectoderm and mesoderm

Bud stage: The initial expansion of cells of the ectoderm in the developmental life cycle of the tooth

Calcification: The process by which organic tissue becomes hardened by a deposit of calcium salts within its substance

Cap stage: The stage of tooth development after the bud stage and before the bell stage, which is caused by unequal growth of the cells of the basal layer descending into the mesoderm, resulting in the appearance of a cap

Cementoblast: One of the cells arising from the mesoderm from which the cementum of the tooth is developed

Cementum: The layer of bony tissue covering the root of a tooth. It differs in structure from ordinary bone by containing a greater number of Sharpey fibers (see "Sharpey fibers")

Dental lamina: *Dental*—pertaining to a tooth or teeth; *lamina*—a thin leaf or plate of something, such as bone; *dental lamina*—dental ridge; a band of thickening of the epithelium along the margin of the gum, in the embryo, from which the enamel organ is ultimately developed

Dental organ (enamel organ): A process of epithelium forming a cap over the dental papilla from which the enamel is developed

Dental papilla: A process of condensed mesenchyme within the dental organ and cap from which the dentin and dental pulp are formed

Dental sac: A process of condensed mesenchyme surrounding the dental organ and dental papilla from which the cementum and periodontal ligament are formed

Dentinoblast: A cell found on the pulpal side of the dentinoenamel junction differentiated from an odontoblast to form dentin

Ectoderm: The outer layer of the primitive (two-layered) embryo from which the epidermis and the neural tube are developed

Enamel pulp: The soft material from which the dental enamel is developed

Eruption: The act of breaking out, appearing, or becoming visible. For a tooth, it is the process of moving through alveolar bone into the oral cavity

Hertwig epithelial root sheath: An investment of epithelial cells around the unerupted tooth and inside of the dental follicle, which are derived from the enamel organ

Histodifferentiation: A stage of the life cycle of the tooth identified by the cells of the embryonic tissue becoming specialized. The proliferating cells of ectoderm and mesoderm take on a definite change in this stage to be able to produce enamel, dentin, and cementum

Initiation: A stage of the life cycle of the tooth identified as the first point of its development

Mesenchyme: The embryonic connective tissue; that part of the mesoderm whence are formed the connective tissues of the body as well as the blood vessels and lymphatic vessels

Mesoderm: The middle of three layers of the primitive embryo

Morphodifferentiation: A stage of the life cycle of the tooth identified as that period producing form or shape

Odontoblast: One of the cylindrical connective tissue cells that form the outer surface of the dental pulp adjacent to the dentin. They are connected by protoplasmic processes. Each odontoblast has a long, threadlike process, the dental fibril (or fiber of Tomes), which extends through the dentinal tubule to the dentoenamel junction

Odontoclast: One of the cells that help to absorb the roots of the primary teeth. They occur between the primary teeth and the erupting permanent teeth

Periodontal ligament: *Periodontal*—situated or occurring around a tooth; pertaining to the periodontal membrane that attaches the tooth to alveolar bone

Periodontal membrane: The connective tissue occupying the space between the root of a tooth and the alveolar bone and furnishing a firm connection between the root of the tooth and the bone

Proliferation: The reproduction or multiplication of similar forms; a stage in the life cycle of the tooth bud just after the initiation stage

Sharpey fibers: Cementum is the covering of the tooth root surface. There is also a cementoid tissue covering the cementum, and it is lined with cementoblasts to maintain a dynamic state. There are connective tissue fibers passing through these cementoblasts from the periodontal ligament into the cementum. The embedded portion of the fiber in the cementum is the Sharpey fiber

Stellate reticulum: *Stellate*—shaped like a star or stars; *reticulum*—a network, especially a protoplasmic network in cells; *stellate reticulum*—the reticular connective tissue–like epithelium forming the enamel pulp of the developing tooth

Tooth bud: The initial identification of the developing tooth by the expansion of certain cells in the basal layer of the oral epithelium (ectoderm only)

Tooth germ: The rudiment of a tooth, consisting of a dental sac and including the dental papilla and dental organ (enamel organ)

---

and colleagues[16] noted that infants were capable of displaying fearful behavior, as well as anger or frustration. As a child approaches his or her first birthday, sadness on separation from a parent, joy on reunion, and jealousy of peers or siblings become reliable findings.

Infant and childhood fears are interesting to clinicians who treat children and must be taken into account when formulating a strategy for dealing with the child. Uncertainty and certainty are a pair of elements that emerge early in infancy and can lead to fear or lack of fear. For instance, if the first time the jack in a jack-in-the-box jumps up it startles the child, the child may avoid the toy until later, when he recognizes at what part of the tune the jack will jump out. Avoiding startling situations is important in helping children react in new environmental situations.

Fear of strangers is almost a universal finding after 7 to 12 months of age, although its intensity varies from child to child.

Another very common fear in this age group is fear of separation from the parents. This fear starts around 6 months of age, peaks between 13 and 18 months of life, and then declines. The basis for the onset of this fear is probably the result of developing a remembrance of the parent even when the parent is not present (i.e., object permanence). Because of this mental process, separation becomes distressful. In 1974 Goin-DeCarie[17] suggested that infants with a dysfunctional relationship with their mothers develop permanency much later than those whose mothers have been consistent and affectionate.

The onsets and peaks of separation anxiety appear to be the same in children from a variety of cultures, although the rate of diminishment of the fear varies greatly.[18] It should be noted that the problem of separation anxiety is fairly well controlled by most children by 36 to 40 months of age and by many children by 32 to 36 months of age. In 1967 Ainsworth[19] concluded that children who have strong relationships with their primary caregivers could use that relationship as a place from which to venture into wider social circles by exploration. Conversely, children with poorly developed relationships with their caregivers are not able to undertake such exploration because they lack a sense of security.

Social Changes

The First Year

In the first year of life, the child is utterly and completely dependent on the parents. Mothering is extremely important to the child at this time. In the first several months, the child does not show a clear differentiation among people. The baby may coo or smile at parents as well as strangers.

Nonreflexive smiling occurs at 2 to 3 months, and this represents the first major social behavior of the infant other than crying. With this smile, the child begins to understand what a behavior other than crying can do to expand his or her influence in the home.

The most important social interaction to occur during the first year of life is the development of strong and secure attachments to nurturing and caring adults. Research has shown that children who are started in high-quality daycare environments early in life do not suffer developmental social consequences compared with children raised solely by their mothers at home.

The Second Year

The 1-year-old child is capable of great social progress during the second year of development. The advent of language skills allows the child to learn and to relate to the family. Socially, children seek to exert their will. A need to test independence starts to surface. Effective and consistent parenting strategies become very important.

Role model observation becomes important at this age and remains so for years to come. Role models who display a consistent behavior are the most effective. Children who observe nonaggressive ways of handling frustration are likely to acquire a similar approach. Unfortunately, children who witness violent or aggressive behavior consistently are just as likely to adopt that particular approach.

The maintenance of affection between parent and child and increasing verbal approval and disapproval are important at this age. Discipline should be educational, not punitive. Parents should be reminded that 1- and 2-year-old children have not acquired internal controls and that often temper tantrums are normal and are best left unnoticed. Physical punishment, beyond an attention-getting technique by a parent (e.g., one painless thump on the buttocks), is usually contraindicated and can actually make a misbehaving child behave worse.

The Third Year

Typically it is late in the second year or early in the third year when children start to feed themselves without assistance from their parents. The third year is also when potty training generally starts. This training process should not be started too soon and should never become a source of conflict between the child and the parent. Parents are well advised to wait until the child is physically, mentally, and socially ready to begin this arduous task.

The third year can be a demanding one for parents. The period for children between the second and third birthdays has been labeled the "terrible twos." Children in the third year may use the word "no!" anytime they want to display resistance. Children of this age can be an embarrassment to their parents because they do not hesitate to state their observations in front of everyone ("Aunt Jane is fat!"). Genital manipulation is not an uncommon practice at this age, and this may be trying for parents as well.

By the end of the third year, the child is asking "how" and "why" questions. The child's unique identity is beginning to surface, and he or she can integrate the standards of others into his or her own life. Because of this and because of increased communication skills, the 3-year-old child is capable of a variety of social interchanges with other people. Historically, this ability to communicate at a child's third birthday marked the entry date for many children into a program of dental care. It is now well understood and one of the premises of this textbook that, from a prevention standpoint, age 3 years is much too late for a child's first dental appointment.

References

1. Hurlock EB. *Child Development*. New York: McGraw-Hill; 1950.
2. Stewart RE, Barber TK, Troutman KC, et al. *Pediatric Dentistry: Scientific Foundations and Clinical Practice*. St Louis: Mosby; 1982.
3. Sperber GH. *Craniofacial Embryology*. Bristol, United Kingdom: John Wright and Sons; 1978.
4. Proffit WR. *Contemporary Orthodontics*. St Louis: Mosby; 1982.
5. Fields HW. Craniofacial growth from infancy through adulthood. *Pediatr Clin North Am*. 1991;38:1053–1088.
6. Caffey J. *Pediatric X-Ray Diagnosis*. Chicago: Year Book; 1950.
7. Ranly DM. *A Synopsis of Craniofacial Growth*. New York: Appleton-Century-Crofts; 1980.
8. Enlow DH. *Handbook of Facial Growth*. Philadelphia: Saunders; 1982.
9. Orban BJ. *Oral Histology and Embryology*. St Louis: Mosby; 1957.
10. Schour I, Massler M. Studies in tooth development: the growth pattern of human teeth. Part II. *J Am Dent Assoc*. 1940;27:1918–1931.
11. Brauer JC, Demeritt WW, Higley LB, et al. *Dentistry for Children*. New York: McGraw-Hill; 1959.
12. Finn SB. *Clinical Pedodontics*. Philadelphia: Saunders; 1973.
13. Mussen PH, Conger JJ, Kagan J, et al. *Child Development and Personality*. 6th ed. New York: Harper & Row; 1984.
14. Piaget J. *The Construction of Reality in the Child*. New York: Basic Books; 1954.
15. Levine MD, Carey WB, Crocker AC, et al. *Developmental Behavioral Pediatrics*. Philadelphia: Saunders; 1983.
16. Mussen PH, Conger JJ, Kagan J, et al. *Child Development and Personality*. 6th ed. New York: Harper & Row; 1984.
17. Goin-DeCarie T. *The Infant's Reaction to Strangers*. New York: International Universities Press; 1974.
18. Kagan J, Kearsley R, Zelaso P. *Infancy: Its Place in Human Development*. Cambridge, MA: Harvard University Press; 1978.
19. Ainsworth MDS. *Infancy in Uganda: Infant Care and the Growth of Love*. Baltimore: Johns Hopkins University Press; 1967.

14

Examination, Diagnosis, and Treatment Planning of the Infant and Toddler

KARIN WEBER-GASPARONI

Infant Oral Health

In 1986 the American Academy of Pediatric Dentistry (AAPD) adopted a position on infant oral health, recommending that the first visit occur within 6 months of the eruption of the first primary tooth.[1] This bold recommendation was based on the recognition that many 3-year-old children had already experienced dental caries and, more troubling, that those who had experienced caries remained susceptible to future decay, even with subsequent preventive intervention.[2] Prior to the adoption of this policy, physicians claimed responsibility for the oral health of the child younger than 36 months of age.[3] The rationale, although somewhat circuitous, assumed that children visited a physician at regular intervals soon after birth but did not see a dentist until later in life. Unfortunately, physicians' knowledge and inclination to practice preventive dentistry have been shown to be lacking. Dental caries in pediatric patients continues to be a serious health problem, even though the prevalence has been reduced since 1960. National data on dental caries in children and adolescents in the United States for 2011–2012 showed that nearly 37% of children aged 2–8 years had experienced dental caries in their primary teeth, whereas 21% of children aged 6–11 and 58% of adolescents aged 12–19 had experienced dental caries in their permanent teeth.[4] Therefore it remains to be seen whether the medical community involvement and interventions can effect a change in that pattern.

Implementing a major shift in health philosophy, such as instituting infant oral health visits to dentists, is not without problems. Some dentists are reluctant to see these children because of expectations of negative behavior, complex dental needs, a lack of understanding of preventive opportunities, and concern about reimbursement for procedures.[5] Rightfully, physicians question whether a shift in practice that places infants in dental offices will work, given the reluctance of dentists and the scarcity of pediatric dentists who might see these children.

The purpose of this chapter is to describe the objectives, procedures, and rationale for infant oral health. The goal would be that dentists would gain a better knowledge of these practices and become more comfortable in treating patients in this age group.

Goals of Infant Oral Health

Initiating oral health care during infancy is ideal for a variety of reasons: dental caries have not had time to develop, habits have not become detrimental, and the entire dental preventive armamentarium is available.[6] Infant oral health affords the unique opportunity to start with a clean slate with the goal of maintaining good oral health throughout life. At no other point in life will the dentist have the same level of parental concern, attention, and compliance. The goals can be summarized by the following six tenets.

Break the Cycle of Early Childhood Caries

Although early childhood caries is relatively inexpensive to prevent, it is a pandemic disease among select populations, including very young children of low-income, racial, and ethnic minority groups. The prevalence of early childhood caries in disadvantaged groups can be as high as 70%.[7] Untreated cases of early childhood caries can lead to potentially life-threatening infection, pain, failure to thrive, learning difficulties, hospitalizations, and emergency room visits.[1,8] Early childhood caries progresses rapidly and by the time treatment is sought, the disease can be extensive enough to warrant the use of sedation or general anesthesia. Consequently, the overall costs to treat early childhood caries are quite high.[9] Of concern is the cyclic nature of early childhood caries, in which children afflicted remain at risk throughout childhood, even when preventive services are available.[2]

Disrupt the Acquisition of Harmful Microflora

Research suggests that children are inoculated with caries-initiating bacteria by vertical transmission from caretakers, primarily mothers. The relationship between maternal salivary levels of mutans streptococci (MS) and the risk of infant infection seems to be relatively strong because mothers with high levels of MS tend to have children with high levels, whereas those with low levels tend to have children with low levels.[10] If a child's caretaker harbors virulent organisms, then transmission via kissing, sharing food and eating utensils, or other contact can occur and initiate the caries process.[11] This process is described in detail in Chapter 12. On the plus side of this acquisition model is the potential to prevent transmission by reducing the caretaker's bacterial inoculum through dental treatment, increased oral health literacy, improved oral health dietary and hygiene habits,[12] and to a lesser extent through the use of antibacterial chemotherapeutic agents.[13] Recent preventive strategies emphasize the importance of maintaining a child's favorable oral health environment and healthy biofilm by establishing a low-sugar diet, adequate fluoride exposure, and effective oral hygiene practices.[14] Prenatal counseling coupled with maternal oral health and infant oral health forms the chain for prevention of bacterial acquisition.

Manage the Risk/Benefit of Habits

Infancy gives rise to many habits, and those affecting the oral cavity are described later in this chapter in the section under "Nonnutritive Sucking Habits." Traditionally, dentists were usually called on only to deal with lingering habits in older children that were causing deleterious dental problems. The opportunity to provide counseling to parents during infant oral health visits allows the dentist to enter the habit continuum and work with the family to mitigate deleterious effects and transition the child out of the habit. The goal would be a gentle waning of the habit, which would negate the need to correct habit-related malocclusions.

Establish a Dental Home for Health or Harm

The concept of a dental home is defined by the AAPD as "the ongoing relationship between the dentist and the patient, inclusive of all aspects of oral health care delivered in a comprehensive, continuously accessible, coordinated, and family-centered way. The dental home should be established no later than 12 months of age and includes referral to dental specialists when appropriate."[15] This concept is derived from the American Academy of Pediatrics (AAP) definition of a medical home.[16] Our physician colleagues understand the benefits of establishing a doctor-family relationship. Care is initiated with nonthreatening preventive services and if an emergency occurs, parents know where to turn. If questions arise, reliable and trusted information is available, and if treatment is needed, a firm foundation of trust has been built. As with the medical home, the early establishment of a dental home has the

potential to provide more effective and less costly dental care when compared with dental care provided in emergency care facilities or hospitals.[17,18] The US Surgeon General's report notes quite clearly that those children who have a dentist are more likely to receive preventive services.[19] Research has shown that early preventive oral health care targeted to high-risk populations can lower overall dental costs and yield better oral health outcomes.[20] Reports of preschool-aged, Medicaid-enrolled children have shown that the earlier a preventive dental visit occurred, the more likely these children were to use subsequent preventive services and experience lower dentally related costs.[21] In addition, the number and cost of dental procedures among high-risk children have been reported to be less for children seen at an earlier age versus later, confirming the fact that the sooner a child is seen by a dentist, the less treatment needs they are likely to have in the future.[22]

Impart Optimal Fluoride Protection

Fluoride remains dentistry's best preventive tool, and optimal fluoride exposure is the foundation of early intervention. Recent systematic reviews support the efficacy of fluoride toothpaste and in-office fluoride varnish applications as effective measures for early childhood caries prevention.[23,24] Twetman and Dhar[24] regard the daily use of fluoride toothpaste initiated immediately after the eruption of the first tooth as the best clinical preventive practice for early childhood caries. One concern is that children of this age are at greatest risk of developing fluorosis due to excessive amounts of fluoride being ingested. For this reason, the current AAPD guideline on fluoride therapy recommends the use of no more than a smear or rice-sized amount of fluoridated toothpaste for children 3 years of age and younger.[25] Chapter 15 details the safety and toxicity concerns of fluoride in this age group.

Arming the Parents Through Anticipatory Guidance

Parental involvement has become a cornerstone of child health care. Because infant oral health is so heavily dependent on protective factors at home, the parent becomes a cotherapist. The dentist must empower the parent to provide good preventive measures at home but, even more, to anticipate the oral health changes in the rapidly growing child. This is accomplished through the concept of anticipatory guidance, as described later in this chapter.

Concepts of Infant Oral Health

Risk Assessment

The predentate infant presents with a clean slate in terms of acquired dental conditions and diseases, but as the child grows and expands his or her world, this changes. Considering risks that go beyond infectious disease and encompass trauma and injury, orthodontic problems, and compliance with oral hygiene and dietary practices helps to maximize a child's opportunity to achieve good oral health. Risk assessment is defined as identification of factors known or believed to be associated with a condition or disease for purposes of further diagnosis, prevention, or treatment. According to the AAPD guidelines, *"risk assessment: 1. fosters the treatment of the disease process instead of treating the outcome of the disease; 2. gives an understanding of the disease factors for a specific patient and aids in individualizing preventive discussions; 3. individualizes, selects, and determines frequency of preventive and restorative treatment for a patient; and 4. anticipates caries progression or stabilization.*"[2] An essential part of the infant oral health visit is an individualized review of risk factors. By eliminating the risk factors before disease occurs, the disease process can be prevented in the immediate as well as distant future. An example would be the infant who sleeps with a bottle or sippy cup of a sugar-sweetened beverage but who presents with no overt dental caries. Intervention would focus on eliminating the habit and diminishing the risk of developing early childhood caries. Taking into consideration that the etiology of early childhood caries is multifactorial and complex, current caries risk assessment models entail a combination of factors including diet, fluoride exposure, host susceptibility, and microflora analysis and consideration of how these factors interact with social, cultural, and behavioral factors. More comprehensive models that include social, political, psychological, and environmental determinants of health are also available.[26–28] An excellent example is the conceptual model on children's oral health proposed by Fisher-Owens and colleagues.[26] This multilevel conceptual model recognizes the complex interplay of causal factors and describes the influences on oral health outcomes at the individual, family, and community levels over the classic Keyes biologic model (Fig. 14.1). It incorporates five key domains of determinants of health: genetic and biologic factors, the social environment, the physical environment, health behaviors, and dental and medical care. Lastly, this model incorporates the aspect of time, recognizing the evolution of oral health diseases (e.g., caries) and influences on the child-host over time. Table 12.4 in Chapter 12 depicts a caries risk assessment form developed by the AAPD, which can be used by dental providers to identify risk factors for dental caries development in children from birth to 5 years of age.[2] The AAPD has also developed caries management protocols, with the objective to assist providers in

the decisions regarding individualized treatments. These protocols are based on the patients' caries risk level, age, and parental compliance with recommended preventive strategies. This aids practitioners in determining the types and frequency of diagnostic, preventive, and restorative care for dental caries management. Such protocols increase the probability of successful and cost-effective treatments. An example of a caries management protocol for children 1 to 2 years of age is shown in Table 14.1.[2]

Anticipatory Guidance

Anticipatory guidance is defined as proactive counseling that addresses the significant physical, emotional, psychological, and developmental changes that will occur in children during the interval between health supervision visits. Anticipatory guidance is the complement to a risk assessment. It addresses protective factors aimed at preventing oral health problems. An example of anticipatory guidance would be a discussion on ambulation of an infant with a warning about possible tooth trauma that often occurs as the infant learns to stand and walk. Topics to address in this age group include oral development, fluoride adequacy, nonnutritive habits, diet and nutrition, oral hygiene, and injury prevention.[29] These six areas capture the major concerns related to the oral conditions of dental caries, periodontal disease, trauma, and malocclusion.

Health Supervision

Health supervision is defined as the longitudinal partnership between the dentist and family that is individualized to maximize healthy outcomes for that particular child. This is a departure from the

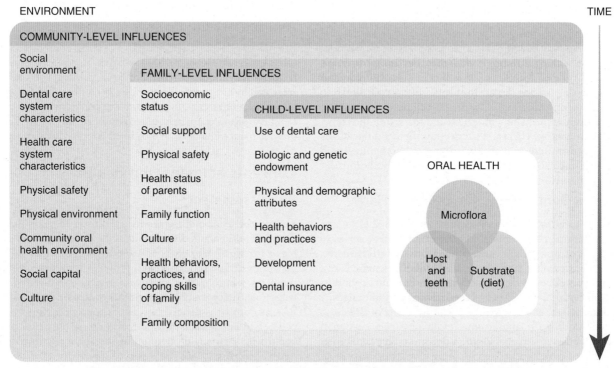

• **Figure 14.1** A multifactorial model of early childhood caries depicting possible roles for the child, the family, and the community beyond the classical biologic infectious disease model. (Redrawn from Fisher-Owens SA, Gansky SA, Platt LJ, et al. Influences on children's oral health: a conceptual model. *Pediatrics.* 2007;120[3]:e510–e520.)

TABLE 14.1	Example of a Caries Management Protocol for 1- to 2-Year-Olds			
		INTERVENTIONS		
Risk Category	**Diagnostics**	**Fluoride**	**Diet**	**Restorative**
Low risk	Recall every 6–12 months Baseline MS[a]	Twice daily brushing with fluoridated toothpaste[b]	Counseling	Surveillance[c]
Moderate risk Parent engaged	Recall every 6 months Baseline MS[a]	Twice daily brushing with fluoridated toothpaste[b] Fluoride supplements[d] Professional topical treatment every 6 months	Counseling	Active surveillance[e] of incipient lesions
Moderate risk Parent not engaged	Recall every 6 months Baseline MS[a]	Twice daily brushing with fluoridated toothpaste[b] Professional topical treatment every 6 months	Counseling, with limited expectations	Active surveillance[e] of incipient lesions
High risk Parent engaged	Recall every 3 months Baseline and follow up MS[a]	Twice daily brushing with fluoridated toothpaste[b] Fluoride supplements[d] Professional topical treatment every 3 months	Counseling	Active surveillance[e] of incipient lesions Restore cavitated lesions with ITR or definitive restorations
High risk Parent not engaged	Recall every 3 months Baseline and follow up MS[a]	Twice daily brushing with fluoridated toothpaste[b] Professional topical treatment every 3 months	Counseling, with limited expectations	Active surveillance[e] of incipient lesions Restore cavitated lesions with ITR or definitive restorations

[a]Salivary MS bacterial levels.
[b]Parental supervision of a "smear" amount of toothpaste.
[c]Periodic monitoring for signs of caries progression.
[d]Need to consider fluoride levels in drinking water.
[e]Careful monitoring of caries progression and prevention program.
ITR, Interim therapeutic restoration; *MS,* mutans streptococci.
From American Academy of Pediatric Dentistry. Clinical guideline on caries-risk assessment and management for infants, children, and adolescents. *Pediatr Dent.* 2016;38(special issue):142–149.

"every 6-month recall" approach that is all too common to dental practices and has no strong evidence-based support. Some children require more frequent visits and others less. In infant oral health, the dentist assesses risk at the initial exam, offers preventive advice using anticipatory guidance, and administers necessary treatment and prevention services. Outcomes are the measures that indicate success. These can be physical (reduction in gingival inflammation), cognitive (understanding of the caries process), or behavioral (elimination of nighttime feeding habits). For example, the presence of plaque on primary teeth in infants is a strong predictor of future dental caries, so after oral hygiene instruction, parents can monitor success by looking for the presence of plaque.[30] A desired outcome would be absence of plaque. Another example would be instructing parents to check their child's teeth for initial signs of early childhood caries by lifting the child's lip to look for white spot lesions. This lift-the-lip protocol is recommended periodically based on the child's risk. A desired outcome would be a parent who arranges an earlier dental visit because they have noted the presence of white spot lesions. The goal is to educate parents with tools (anticipatory guidance) to affect outcomes in addition to measures (outcomes) they can monitor. It is worth noting that individuals with special health care needs may require the dental team to develop individualized preventive and treatment strategies that take into consideration the unique needs and disabilities of the patient.

Infant Oral Health as a Diagnostic Process

The best way to envision the infant oral health visit is to compare it with the traditional medical model used for the diagnosis of disease. The medical model uses a stepwise approach beginning with a chief complaint, history, physical examination, differential diagnosis, and treatment plan. Infant oral health intervention assumes that the child has no oral disease but may be prone to disease due to risk behaviors such as high consumption of sugar-sweetened beverages or lack of fluoride. Conceptually, these risk factors will eventually lead to disease if not addressed. Conversely, if the risk factors are eliminated, the child will be free of disease.

In infant oral health the chief complaint may be a generic interest in prevention. The infant oral examination is equivalent to the well-baby visit for oral health. The health history is replaced with a focused risk-based history aimed at predisposing factors for dental conditions. The patient examination looks for existing disease in addition to physical factors that predispose the child to oral disease. The differential diagnosis is replaced with a risk profile that is individualized to the child. Instead of a treatment plan, the family receives anticipatory guidance with directives to eliminate risk and impart protective factors. They are given measurable outcomes to determine progress toward wellness. Both of these factors make the parents a part of the therapeutic alliance. The recall interval is designed to give parents time to address risk and for the dentist to reassess progress, institute preventive measures if needed, and ensure that disease has not manifested.

Elements of the Infant Oral Health Visit

Risk Assessment

The parent or guardian is the historian for the child. In Chapter 19 the general health history is discussed in depth. The focus of this section is on historical elements related to oral disease risk. Box 14.1 depicts a risk assessment form for infant oral health.[31] Historical risk elements can be divided into perinatal factors, diet and nutrition, fluoride adequacy, oral hygiene, bacteria transmission, oral habits, injury prevention, and oral development. The clinician should combine the general health history responses with those

focused on the risk of oral disease. When used in combination, this will form an individualized historical risk profile for the child, which helps in determining preventive and treatment strategies. Perinatal factors are important because of the attendant oral effects associated with premature birth. Although experts have concluded that prematurity does not predispose a child to an increased risk of dental caries,[32] some low birth weight children receive special diets, have hypoplastic dentitions,[33] and have developmental disabilities that place them at higher risk. Diet and nutrition questions should focus on breastfeeding, bottle and sippy-cup use and the transition to an open cup, frequency of sugar-sweetened beverages and snacks, and special diets.

The AAP recommends "exclusive breastfeeding for about 6 months, followed by continued breastfeeding as complementary foods are introduced, with continuation of breastfeeding for 1

• BOX 14.1   Risk Assessment Form for Infant Oral Health

Health History
Did birth mother have problems during pregnancy?
Was your child premature?
Was your child's birth weight low?
Were there any complications at birth?
Does your child have any health problems?
Current and/or previous medication(s)?
Any history of allergies and/or allergic reactions?
Any history of hospitalization?
Notes _____

Dental History
Has your child been to the dentist before?
Current or previous history of dental pain?
Is pain preventing your child to eat, drink, sleep, and or perform daily activities?

Diet and Nutrition
Is/was your child breastfed/bottle-fed? Duration, timing, and frequency?
Does your child sleep with a bottle/spill-proof cup? Content?
Does your child drink from a spill-proof cup during the day?
Content, amount, and frequency?
What does your child like to snack on and how frequently?
Does your child consume sugared snacks and beverages on a regular basis?
Is your child on a special diet?
Notes _____

Fluoride Adequacy
What is the main water source from which your child is drinking: city water (unfiltered, Brita/Pur filter), city water (filtered, reverse osmosis), well water, or bottled water?
Do you know the fluoride level of your child's drinking water?
Does your child take fluoride supplements?
If yes, dosage and frequency?
Do you use fluoridated toothpaste for your child?
If yes, frequency and amount placed on toothbrush?
Notes _____

Oral Hygiene
Do you clean your child's teeth/gums?
Do you use a toothbrush to clean your child's teeth? Timing and frequency?
Any problems with positioning and/or child's cooperation during the toothbrushing?
Notes _____

Bacteria Transmission
Does the child's mother (intimate caregiver) have any untreated decay?
Do you and your child share the same eating utensils and/or cups?
Do you kiss your child on the mouth?
Notes _____

Oral Habits
Does your child use a pacifier?
Does your child suck a thumb or finger(s)?
Does your child grind teeth day or night?
Frequency, duration, and intensity of oral habits?
Notes _____

Injury Prevention/Trauma
Is your child walking?
Is your home childproofed?
Do you use a car seat for your child?
Has your child had an oral/facial injury?
Notes _____

Oral Development
Does your child have any teeth?
Child's age (in months) when first tooth erupted: _____
Has your child experienced teething problems?
Have you noticed any oral problems in your child?
Notes _____

Clinician's Assessment
Demographic Information:
Is the child from a low socioeconomic status family?
Is the child from a minority group?
Is the child from a family with low oral health literacy skills?

Clinical Findings
Presence of visible plaque on teeth, cavitated and/or noncavitated lesions (white spot lesions), enamel hypoplasia, enamel defects, retentive or stained pits/fissures?

Iatrogenic Factors
Does the child use any oral appliance?
Notes _____

Modified from American Academy of Pediatric Dentistry (AAPD). Risk assessment. In: ABCs of Infant Oral Health. Chicago: AAPD; 2000.

year or longer as mutually desired by mother and infant."[34] Because of the developmental, economic, health, nutritional, immunologic, psychological, and social advantages that breastfeeding provides to mothers and their children, clinicians should promote and encourage optimal breastfeeding habits.[35] In a systematic review,[36] higher frequency of breastfeeding up to 12 months was associated with reduced caries risk. However, with the introduction of other dietary carbohydrates and inadequate oral hygiene, breastfeeding beyond 12 months of age increased a child's risk for developing caries. Although human milk alone cannot cause caries, in vitro studies have found breastfeeding in combination with other carbohydrates to be highly cariogenic.[37] Therefore the best recommendation for caries prevention clinicians can provide to mothers who are willing to breastfeed, including at nighttime, is to establish a diet low in simple carbohydrates and sugars when other foods and beverages are introduced in addition to breastfeeding, brush the child's teeth at least twice a day, especially at bedtime, and consider a smear amount of fluoride toothpaste.

Another component of the infant risk assessment is a determination of fluoride adequacy and current oral hygiene practices. Fluoride adequacy refers to a consideration whether the drinking water (community vs. bottled) provides optimal fluoride. It also addresses the effectiveness of fluoride dentifrice in reducing dental caries and the appropriate amount to decrease the risk of fluorosis. Oral hygiene practices are assessed by asking the parents how involved they currently are with cleansing of the oral structures. Such questioning should lead to a discussion of tooth-cleaning implements, timing, and frequency, as well as positioning of the child for oral care and the amount of fluoride toothpaste used. The means of bacteria transmission from mother/caregiver to the infant and ways to avoid such transmission should be thoroughly discussed. The discussion of habits establishes a baseline for families and enables the dentist to counsel parents on the risks and benefits of behavioral habits throughout early childhood. Historical information on injury prevention moves beyond purely dental trauma to general health issues like play objects, electrical cords, home childproofing, and car seat use. Oral development is covered to assess the presence of teeth, eruptive disorders, and teething problems. Finally, the clinician evaluates the family's oral health literacy, educational/socioeconomic background, and assesses the presence of clinical factors (e.g., plaque, white spot lesions, enamel defects) known to place a child at a higher risk for developing early childhood caries.

Oral Examination and Assessment of Clinical Risk Factors

The oral examination of the infant is a quick process but differs from the typical child examination in several ways:
- Use of a dental chair is unnecessary and the least preferred approach.
- The parent participates as a learner and immobilizer.
- Teaching about the oral cavity occurs during the examination process.
- The child may cry, which is useful.

The preferred approach to the infant examination is the knee-to-knee position (Fig. 14.2) in which a parent and a dental provider sit facing each other. Their knees should touch and ideally, mesh slightly, creating a flat surface on which the child can rest. The infant initially is held facing the parent and then reclined onto the lap of the dentist. The parent has the infant's legs straddling their torso and uses their elbows to hold the child's feet in place. The parent is responsible for holding the child's hands and the

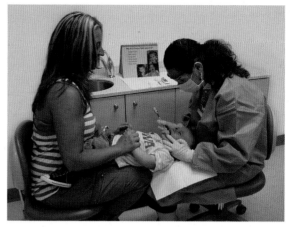

• **Figure 14.2** Knee-to-knee clinical examination position for dentist, child, and parent. Parent and dentist face each other with knees touching while parent holds child on lap with child facing parent. Parent carefully lays child in dentist's lap while holding child's hands.

dentist stabilizes the child's head. The examination can occur wherever a suitable light source can be found. The closeness of the parent and provider may concern some parents and should be explained before the procedure begins.

During the examination, which may take only seconds, the dentist has the opportunity to demonstrate oral hygiene and point out oral structures of importance. Most infants will cry briefly during the examination, affording a wide-open mouth! Parents may need to be assured that crying is a normal response and is to be expected. At the completion of the examination, the child is returned to the parent, who can cuddle and console the child as needed.

Children of this age are far more likely to have seen a physician for regular visits, so delays in cognitive, physical, emotional, and gross motor development are usually known by the parents prior to the first dental visit. However, dentists should be familiar with developmental milestones for children from birth to age 3 years (Table 14.2) and advise families of the need for a medical evaluation when problems are noted or suspicion of developmental problems exists. Furthermore, by knowing these developmental milestones, child behaviors and abilities are easier to relate to when providing anticipatory guidance to the parent.

The dentist should expect to see a healthy oral cavity in most infants. Table 14.3 shows some common oral conditions of infants and their management. In addition, Chapter 2 addresses some uncommon pathologic conditions of infancy, including dental lamina cysts (Bohn nodules and Epstein pearls), congenital epulides, eruption cysts, and neuroectodermal tumors of infancy. The infant exam should assess the child's developmental status, as well as the condition of the dentition in terms of caries, hypoplasia, and plaque accumulation. Assessment and discussion of atypical frenum attachments that may be associated with breastfeeding difficulties should also occur during the oral examination of an infant. It is important for the dentist to understand the normal head, neck, and oral presentations of an infant so that they are more likely to recognize abnormal presentations. These normal findings are described in Table 14.4.

Risk Profiling

From the historical and clinical data obtained from the parent and child, the dentist can create a risk profile using the same six areas

TABLE 14.2	Selected Developmental Characteristics of the Child Aged 6 Months to 3 Years		
6–9 months		**12–13 months**	**24 months+**
Intellectual Development			
Opens for a spoon		Copies sounds and actions	3- to 4-word sentences
Imitates actions of adults		Understands simple commands	Puts toys in groups
Turns to locate sounds		Tries to accomplish simple acts	Name five body parts
Gross/Fine Motor Skills			
Rolls over		Stands with hand held	Scribbles; draws shapes
Becomes able to sit independently		Sits without support	Kicks/throws ball
Picks up objects with fingers		Feeds self raisins	Puts on/takes off clothes
Psychological Development			
Laughs and squeals with delight		Shows affection to adults	Changeable feelings
Screams if annoyed		Fear of strangers	Recognizes emotions
Dental implications		Fear of separation	Understands commands
Needs physical support		Sippy cup use	Prone to falls/trauma
Can hold bottle alone			
Physiologic Height (75th percentile)			
Boys = 69.7–74.0 cm		77.7 cm	89.9 cm
Girls = 67.8–72.4 cm		76.3 cm	88.7 cm
Weight (75th percentile)			
Boys = 8.49–9.88 kg		10.91 kg	13.44 kg
Girls = 7.83–9.24 kg		10.23 kg	12.74 kg
Pulse (90th percentile)			
120/min		120/min	110/min
Respiration (50th percentile)			
30/min		28/min	25/min
Blood Pressure			
105/67 mm Hg		105/69 mm Hg	106/68 mm Hg

of anticipatory guidance addressed earlier. The risk profile might be simple or complicated by obstacles that may be difficult to surmount, such as special diets or profound disabilities. Parents should be provided with explanations and a prognosis of how a particular risk factor may influence the oral health of their child.

Anticipatory Guidance

Anticipatory guidance, which improves oral health behaviors while decreasing the risk of early childhood caries, is of crucial importance. It presumes that developmental information should cover the period until the next health supervision visit. Box 14.2 shows a list of topic areas for anticipatory guidance and the knowledge base needed for each area. These should be considered when discussing anticipatory guidance for children younger than 36 months. An example of a basic checklist of recommendations for infants which can be added to for unique situations is provided in Table 14.5.[38]

Teething and caries prevention are common topics discussed during the anticipatory guidance process. Symptoms associated with tooth eruption continue to be controversial. Similar opinions regarding teething symptoms have been consistently reported by parents and health professionals for decades across numerous cultures. However, although some studies have reported fever, drooling, diarrhea, irritability, and sleep disturbances to be related to tooth eruption, others found no association of these symptoms with the eruption of teeth.[39] Gingival irritation, irritability, and drooling were the most frequent signs and symptoms of primary tooth eruption in a meta-analysis published between 1969 and 2012. In addition, an analysis of body temperature showed that tooth eruption could lead to a rise in temperature not characterized as fever.[40] The discrepancy observed among studies reflects the possible bias and subjectivity of caregivers' reports of teething symptoms. Moreover, teething might be the culprit for the common childhood diseases (i.e., diarrhea, respiratory, and ear infections) during the first 3 years of life. Tooth eruption overlaps with the timing when infants are in the oral stage exploring the environment. By introducing objects and fingers into their mouths, infants are at risk of exposure to viruses and bacteria that can cause illnesses.

TABLE 14.3	Infant Oral Pathology and Unusual Clinical Findings

Condition Description and Illustration	Clinical Findings and Management
Ankyloglossia (tongue-tie) 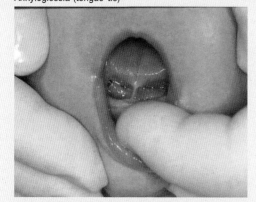	Prevalence ranges from 0.02%–10.7% Frenum may be short, thick, muscular of fibrotic May be associated with breastfeeding difficulties, failure to thrive, swallowing, articulation among other complications Coryllos classifications of tongue-tie: type 1, type 2, and type 3 Frenotomy is a treatment option
Natal and neonatal teeth 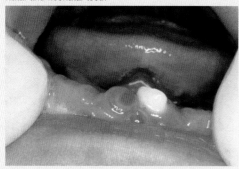	Natal teeth present at birth and neonatal present within 30 days of birth Incidence 1–2 per 6000 births 90% are primary; 10% supernumerary; 85% mandibular Extract supernumeraries; primary teeth left if not highly mobile Can be aspiration risk; nursing obstacle
Riga-Fede disease 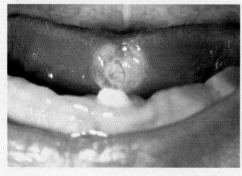	Actually traumatic ulcer of ventral surface of tongue from tooth May cause active bleeding and discomfort Treatment options are observation, cessation of breastfeeding, or smoothing/removal of the offending tooth

Health professionals should alert caregivers that if teething symptoms are present, they are expected to be mild. Parents should always consult with a physician if their child presents with robust and persistent symptoms. A discussion with parents of safe teething toys that are made of nontoxic materials should occur. Parents should be advised not to use teething products that contain benzocaine. Since the US Food and Drug Administration (FDA) first warned about potential dangers in 2006, the agency has received 29 reports of benzocaine gel–related cases of methemoglobinemia, a condition which reduces the amount of oxygen carried in the bloodstream and can result in death in the most severe cases. The agency repeated the warning in April 2011 and remains particularly concerned about the use of over-the-counter benzocaine products in infants for relief of pain from teething. For these reasons the FDA recommends that parents and caregivers not use benzocaine products for children younger than 2 years of age, except under the advice and supervision of a health care professional.[41] The FDA has released a warning regarding the potential dangers in connection with homeopathic teething tablets and gels. Consumers are advised of the lack of proven benefits of these products and recommended to stop their use. Difficulty breathing, seizures, excessive sleepiness, muscle weakness, and constipation are among the several adverse effects reported.[42]

Parental counseling geared toward primary prevention of dental disease must involve timely family education, instruction, and motivation. Because the etiology of early childhood caries is multifactorial and significantly influenced by health behaviors,[14] preventive messages for expectant parents and parents of very young children should target risk factors known to place children at a higher risk for developing caries (e.g., early MS contamination,

	Diagnostic	
Structure	Technique	Normal Characteristics
Head	Visualization	Disproportionately large
Hair	Visualization	Thin and fine
Scalp	Visualization/ palpation	Open fontanels
Temporomandibular joint	Palpation/ manipulation	Short condyles/flat fossae
Skin	Visualization	Soft, smooth
Neck	Palpation	Weak musculature Soft airway cartilage
Lips	Visualization	Full, cupid's bow
Oral Cavity		
Dental arches	Visualization	Edentulous/tooth bulges
Frenula	Visualization	High placement on alveolus
Palate	Visualization	Prominent median raphe/rugae
Gingivae	Visualization	Pink, hydrated, flaccid around teeth

TABLE 14.4 Elements of Head and Neck Examination of Infants

poor oral hygiene habits, high sugar consumption frequency). Motivational problems develop when parents are not interested in changing behaviors or feel that the changes require excessive effort. Two effective motivational approaches used for early childhood caries prevention that share similar psychological philosophies are motivational interviewing and self-determination theory.[43–46] Both psychological approaches are based on the concept that supporting a person's autonomy is a key element in changing human behavior.[47] Therefore, when motivating parents to adopt healthier behaviors for themselves and/or their children, it is important that health professionals satisfy the parent's psychological need for autonomy. This can be accomplished by promoting the parents' interest and curiosity in, appreciation for, and value of the message by relating the message to their own personal goals. Providing rationales for requested behaviors, especially those perceived to be uninteresting or particularly effortful, is helpful. In addition, using informational and noncontrolling language while avoiding pressuring directives such as "you should" or "you have to" improves parental compliance. Lastly, the provider should acknowledge the parents' perspective on the challenges of health care and be accepting of their expressions of negative affect and resistance to the health message being delivered. Health care professionals should be sensitive to how they can effectively communicate their recommendations so that parents can perceive these requests as behaviors worth pursuing.[45]

• BOX 14.2 Parent/Caregiver Information for Infant Oral Health

Child's name: _____
Child's next dental care visit: _____

Overall Health (Follow These Recommendations for a Healthier Child)
☐ Continue routine medical care with physician
☐ Child requires immediate care _____
_____

Diet and Nutrition (Follow These Recommendations to Provide the Child With a Diet That Reduces the Risk of Tooth Decay)
☐ Maintain healthy diet, OK as is
☐ Only water in bottles and/or spill-proof cups, except at meals or snacks
☐ Avoid nighttime feeding to sleep or in the middle of the night after 6 months of age or when teeth are present
☐ Transition from bottle/spill-proof cup to open cup as soon as child can drink adequate amount of fluids by open cup
☐ Encourage consumption of milk at meals and snacks
☐ Limit juice intake to no more than 4–6 ounces a day at meals or snacks
☐ Avoid sugar-sweetened beverages (e.g., juice drinks, soda pop, sports drinks) at all times
☐ Replace sugar-containing snacks with cheese, fruits, and other protein snacks
☐ Decrease frequency of snacks (particularly sweets) during the day
☐ Limit snacking to three structured snacks per day
☐ Change diet _____
_____

Oral Hygiene (Follow These Recommendations to Help Keep Child's Mouth Clean and Free of Plaque)
☐ Child's teeth should be brushed by an adult
☐ Brush the child's teeth twice a day, especially before bedtime
☐ Clean infant's mouth using a wet washcloth

☐ Use a soft toothbrush as soon as the first baby teeth appear (erupt)
☐ Special instructions _____
_____

Fluoride Adequacy (Follow These Recommendations to Provide the Child With the Right Amount of Fluoride That Both Reduces the Risk of Tooth Decay and Repairs Early Decayed Areas)
☐ Use a smear amount of fluoride toothpaste
☐ Use a pea-sized amount of fluoride toothpaste
☐ Do not use fluoride toothpaste

Oral Habits (Follow These Recommendations to Discourage the Child's Oral Habit That Can Lead to Poor Tooth Alignment or an Improper Bite)
☐ Thumb/finger sucking habit—discourage by age _____
☐ Pacifier use—discourage by age _____
☐ Use pacifier that conforms to lips and cheeks and supports lips
☐ Bruxism (grinding) or other habit _____
_____

Injury Prevention (Follow These Recommendations to Provide a Safe and Childproofed Home Environment)
☐ Childproof your home to prevent injuries such as choking, drowning, falls, poisoning, and electrical burns
☐ Use infant/child car seat
☐ Other protective device _____
_____

Oral Development (These Recommendations Will Increase Your Awareness of Oral Development Issues That Can Affect the Child)
☐ Current total primary teeth (baby teeth)
_____

• BOX 14.2   Parent/Caregiver Information for Infant Oral Health—cont'd

☐ Next tooth to erupt

☐ Special recommendations for teething symptoms

☐ Child requires further assessment

☐ Use antibacterial rinses _____

☐ Don't share a toothbrush with the child
☐ Don't lick or suck on the child's hands, pacifier, or bottle
☐ Don't share the same eating utensils with the child (cups, spoons, and forks)

Parent/Caregiver Special Recommendations (These Recommendations Will Help You Decrease the Transmission of Decay-Causing Bacteria to the Child and Their Risk of Developing Tooth Decay)

☐ Seek dental treatment and routine checkups to keep your mouth and teeth healthy

TABLE 14.5   Anticipatory Guidance Knowledge Base for Pre-3-Year-Old Care

Areas of Anticipatory Guidance	Knowledge Base for Area
Oral and Dental Development	
Eruption	Normal range, delay, acceleration and potential etiologies, sequence, occlusion, and exfoliation. Eruption problems including malposition, cyst formation, teething, Riga-Fede disease, and bruxism
Teeth	Color, shape, staining causes, role in speech, and chewing
Soft tissue	Mucosal color, ulceration, alveolar anatomy, and congenital abnormalities
Anatomy	Structures, integrity, and color
Fluorides	
Systemic	Water fluoridation procedures, supplementation, fluoride vehicles, timing, storage safety, fluorosis risk, bottled water, breast milk, formula, prenatal fluorides, and halo effect in diet
Topical	Role of dentifrice, storage safety, caries and fluorosis risks, swallowing amounts of dentifrice for age, and supplementation issues (if indicated)
Nonnutritive Habits	
Assessment	Frequency, duration, and intensity. Thumbs, fingers, pacifiers, toys, or blankets. Perceived emotional benefit to child. Effects on oral cavity. Interventions currently being used
Management	Interventions to discontinue the habit. Techniques, effectiveness, and safety of interventions. Life cycle of habits. Systemic effects of habits
Diet and Nutrition	
Feeding	Food in caries paradigm. Breastfeeding, weaning, and effect(s) on teeth and jaws. Formula feeding, frequency, and content of formulas. Development of feeding skills
Snacking	Snacking frequency and contents. Food choices. Safety and general health benefits
Diet	Infant food choices and evolution of pre-3-year-old diet
Problems and issues	Obesity concerns, picky eating, ethnic variations, and food aspiration
Oral Hygiene	
Science	Role of plaque (caries paradigm). Plaque removal goals. Developmental issues

Continued

TABLE 14.5	Anticipatory Guidance Knowledge Base for Pre-3-Year-Old Care—cont'd
Areas of Anticipatory Guidance	**Knowledge Base for Area**
Activity	Type of cleaning currently performed Parental involvement Frequency and duration Devices Dentifrice
Problems and issues	Positioning difficulties Child resistance and behavior Taste of dentifrice, choices Technical skills of parents Role of flossing, injury
Injury Prevention	
General issues	Accidental injury awareness Car safety Choking risks of toys and food Matching skills with activity Childproofing and poisoning safety
Oral health issues	Normal anatomy Trauma assessment and management Dental home access numbers for emergency management Snacking safety Fluoride safety Medication use for oral problems Signs of child abuse Helmet safety

From Casamassimo PS, Nowak AJ. Anticipatory guidance. In: Berg JH, Slayton RL, eds. *Early Childhood Oral Health*. 2nd ed. Hoboken, NJ: Wiley-Blackwell; 2016.

Growth and Development Treatment Planning

In rare instances, there may be an orthodontic or craniofacial component to the infant oral health visit, as would be the case with a child with a cleft lip or palate or a significant craniofacial abnormality. These patients should be referred to a craniofacial team for management and followed routinely by the primary care dentist for basic oral health needs.

Parents often express interest in occlusal development and may press the dentist to discuss future orthodontic needs. Growth is difficult to predict at this age, but the dentist should take the opportunity to discuss eruption, spacing, and occlusion with the parents as a part of anticipatory guidance. Chapter 28 discusses early orthodontic treatment planning at an age when treatment is far more realistic in terms of child cooperation.

Nonnutritive Sucking Habits

Parents often inquire about their child's habits, particularly thumb and pacifier habits. Such questions are common because oral habits are very prevalent in young children and negative effects of long-term habits on the dentition are well documented. Traditionally, dentists' involvement in nonnutritive sucking habits occurred only after prolonged habits produced clear damage to the dentition and raised parental concern. The dentist was consulted for advice on how to stop the nonnutritive sucking habit. This scenario still occurs with frequency, but early anticipatory guidance aimed at preventing the prolong engagement of oral habits is a more effective role that dentists can have in nonnutritive sucking habits. However,

before such guidance can be given, the dentist must have a thorough understanding of how and why nonnutritive sucking habits develop, how they affect oral structures, and what duration of habitual behavior may cause harm.

Origins of Nonnutritive Sucking Habits

Sucking behaviors are believed to arise from psychological needs, mainly from the physiologic need for nutrition. Normally developed infants have an inherent biologic drive for sucking. Psychoanalytic theorists and learning theorists differ in their explanation of why human infants possess a sucking drive and why it might persist beyond infancy, but they are in agreement that this drive is a normal developmental characteristic.[48] According to the psychoanalytic theory, nonnutritive sucking behaviors (such as pacifier, thumb, or finger sucking) arise out of erotic pleasure derived from oral stimulation. Persistence of substantial nonnutritive sucking beyond the so-called oral phase (approximately 3 years of age) reflects a psychological disturbance suggestive of an inability to manage stress or anxiety. Conversely, the learning theory suggests that nonnutritive sucking is an adaptive response that is often rewarded and that becomes a learned habit without psychological manifestations. Given the prevalence of nonnutritive sucking behaviors in normally developed children, the learning theory explanation is the most widely accepted. An alternative, yet complementary, theory proposed by Larsson and Dahlin[49] suggests that if an infant sucking need is not satisfied at the breast, the infant's fingers will be used as a substitute.

Prevalence of Nonnutritive Sucking Habits

It has been reported that well over 90% of children engaged in nonnutritive sucking at some time during their first year of life.[50]

Prolonged nonnutritive sucking habits may have negative consequences to the orofacial structures; therefore habits that continue beyond the toddler years are more concerning than those that terminate earlier. On average, children cease these habits by 24 to 36 months of age, and those who continue tend to be from better educated or higher income families.[51] Numerous studies document that thumb and finger sucking habits are more likely to persist longer than pacifier habits.[50,52] Pacifier habits rarely persist beyond the preschool years because of peer pressure that occurs when children enter kindergarten. This has led to the suggestion that when a digit habit develops, a pacifier should be encouraged as a substitute for the digit.[52,53]

The length of time of actual engagement (duration) of a habit is perhaps the single most important factor to consider when assessing the risk for habit-induced malocclusions. Other factors that also need to be considered include the amount of time a child engages in a particular habit per day (frequency) and the forcefulness (intensity) associated with the child's sucking pattern. For example, a child who sucks on a pacifier for only a few minutes before falling asleep at night would be expected to be at less risk for developing a malocclusion than a child who has a pacifier in the mouth several hours a day with a sucking intensity that results in audible sounds. Therefore parents should be instructed to limit the time a pacifier is in the infant's mouth and avoid ad lib use throughout the day.[54]

Effects and Mechanisms of Nonnutritive Sucking Habits on the Dentition

Numerous studies published before the mid-1960s found that finger sucking generally leads to reduced overbite, increased overjet, protrusion of the maxillary incisors, and a narrowing of the maxillary posterior arch width.[55]

Studies of the primary dentition have found sucking habits to be associated with a higher prevalence of malocclusion in the primary dentition, including class II canine and molar relationships, anterior open bite, increased overjet, decreased maxillary arch width, and increased mandibular arch width, resulting in an increased likelihood of posterior crossbite. Digit habits are more commonly associated with excessive overjet and anterior open bite, whereas pacifier habits are associated with posterior crossbites and class II canine relationships.[50,52,56–58] Pacifier habits, even if discontinued by 2 years of age, represent an increased risk for malocclusion. Open bites tend to resolve with the cessation of pacifier habits, whereas crossbites are more likely to persist after habits stop. Comparisons between conventional pacifiers and so-called orthodontic pacifiers have suggested that there is little if any difference in their effects on orofacial structures.[51]

The differences in digit and pacifier effects on the orofacial structures are likely due to the different forces applied. Pacifiers, presumably because they extend farther into the mouth, tend to force the tongue downward, applying lateral outward pressure against the lower arch. At the same time, the sucking action activates the muscles surrounding the mouth, which increases cheek pressure and results in greater medial force applied to the upper arch. Pacifiers tend to widen the mandibular arch and narrow the maxillary arch, resulting in posterior crossbites. Fingers or thumbs, because of the weight of the arm, tend to apply forward and slightly upward pressure on the maxillary incisor region, with accompanying backward and downward pressure on mandibular incisors; the net effect of digit habits is greater overjet and a tendency toward open bite.

The risk of acute otitis media (middle ear infection) may be higher among children using pacifiers. Some studies have linked pacifier use to early cessation of breastfeeding,[54] whereas others have concluded that pacifier use is a marker of breastfeeding difficulties, reduced motivation to breastfeed, and parental choice to bottle-feed rather than a true cause of early weaning.[59,60] Some studies have suggested that pacifier use may be beneficial in reducing sudden infant death syndrome, a benefit that potentially far outweighs the risks associated with acute otitis media or possible breastfeeding cessation.[61]

Recommendations

Traditional thinking has held that as long as oral habits cease by age 6 or 7 years, effects on the occlusion self-correct; therefore habits are of little consequence in the development of lasting malocclusions. This was based mostly on clinical observations, not longitudinal data. More recent studies have demonstrated that habits of longer duration are associated with higher prevalence of malocclusions, with some potential harm if habits continue between 24 and 36 months and greater risk for malocclusions if habits persist past 48 months of age.[56,58] Prolonged pacifier or digit habits past 48 months are associated with detrimental effects on the occlusion in the late deciduous dentition[52] and past 60 months in the mixed dentition.[58] Given the physiologic and psychological need for sucking in the first year of life, it is neither prudent nor realistic to recommend elimination of habits before 12 or 24 months of age.[56] Therefore anticipatory guidance to parents during infant oral health visits should advocate for cessation of nonnutritive habits no later than 36 months of age.[56,58] Because digit habits are likely to cause malocclusions of greater severity than those caused by pacifier habits and because digit habits are more difficult to overcome than pacifier habits, substitution of a pacifier habit for a digit habit may be advisable.

Office Readiness for Infant Oral Health

Infant care represents a deviation from routine office practice in several ways. A large component of it may be done by auxiliary personnel rather than by the dentist. It does not routinely require the same armamentarium that would be used for an older patient. The examination location can be in the operatory but can just as well be in a well-lit, comfortable conference room or play area. Radiographs would be considered an exception in most infant visits.

A dental record is still required but may be abbreviated. However, the essentials of a medical and dental history, examination record, treatment plan, and progress note remain. Patient education brochures and other instructional material should be available for this particular age group. The dental team can be enlisted in developing the time, place, and protocol for in-office infant oral health visits. This allows the team the opportunity to use their knowledge to provide parental education, as well as to work with small children, which is a joy for most pediatric dental personnel. Finally, in a busy office, the logistics of the infant dental appointment require some thought because it ties up auxiliaries and, if done outside the dental operatory area, necessitates a change in staff flow patterns.

Responsibility of Nondental Professionals Regarding Infant Oral Health

Lack of access to dental care is a major barrier for the establishment of a dental home at an appropriate and desirable young age. Health care professionals, such as pediatricians, physicians, and nurse practitioners, are more likely to serve children in their first 3 years of life than dental professionals. It has been reported that only 2% of Medicaid-enrolled children had a dental visit before age 1 when compared with 99% who had well-baby visits.[62] Therefore it is important that medical providers understand their crucial role in alleviating oral health disparities by including dental health as part of their practices for those children yet to establish a dental home. Medical professionals have an opportunity to implement primary prevention early in a child's life and establish lifelong positive oral health habits. Access to medical care is not as challenging as is the access to dental care. In addition, well-child care visits start early in life and occur very frequently. For this reason, it is critical that child health professionals become knowledgeable about oral health issues. They should be aware of the infectious and transmissible nature of bacteria that cause early childhood caries, caries risk factors, methods of oral health risk assessment, anticipatory guidance, and appropriate timing for effective intervention and referral. The AAP released a policy statement in 2003 regarding the role of pediatricians and other pediatric primary care providers on oral health. The recommendation was made that these professionals incorporate preventive oral health education into their practices and include oral health risk assessments for children by 6 months of age.[3] In 2008 this role was further reinforced with the AAP Policy Statement, *Preventive Oral Health Interventions for Pediatricians*.[63] In 2011 the AAP released a policy statement regarding the oral health of indigenous children of Canada and the United States due to the high caries rates observed among these populations.[64] A most recent AAP Policy Statement on "Maintaining and Improving the Oral Health of Young Children" was released in 2014.[65] In this comprehensive document, topics on the etiology and pathogenesis of dental caries, caries risk assessment, and anticipatory guidance (dietary counseling, oral hygiene, fluoride, oral habits, dental/orofacial injuries, and referral by age 1) are thoroughly discussed.[65]

Lack of knowledge on oral health issues has been reported as one of the most significant barriers for medical professionals to provide oral health–related services.[66,67] In an attempt to increase the oral health knowledge and skills of medical professionals and offer them the tools and support they need to provide early dental intervention, the AAP has developed numerous training programs, resources, and easy-to-use tools that are available through web-based modules and training videos, journal articles, and newsletters. Some examples of these resources include the AAP's *Children's Oral Health* website,[68] Bright Futures Guidelines on Promoting Oral Health,[69] Children's Dental Health Project,[70] and the National Maternal and Child Oral Health Resource Center.[71] Another resource with abundant information on oral health is the 2009 issue of the journal *Academic Pediatrics* that was devoted entirely to children's oral health. It compiled background papers from the 2008 AAP National Summit on Children's Oral Health.[72] In an attempt to incorporate available evidence into practical tools that can be used by medical practitioners and other nondental health care professionals to assess the caries risk levels of children 0 to 3 years of age, the AAPD created a caries risk assessment form to be used specifically by these health professionals. This caries risk assessment form is intended to help nondental health care providers and parents understand the factors that contribute to or protect young children from caries. An example of this form is shown in Table 14.6.[2]

It is crucially important that medical educators make an effort to include oral health as a required component in both pediatric and family medicine residency programs and offer continuing education programs for all child health professionals. Research has

TABLE 14.6   Caries Risk Assessment Form for 0- to 3-Year-Olds (for Physicians and Nondental Health Care Providers)

Factors	High Risk	Low Risk
Biologic		
Mother/primary caregiver has active caries	Yes	
Parent/caregiver has low socioeconomic status	Yes	
Child has >3 between-meal sugar-containing snacks or beverages per day	Yes	
Child is put to bed with a bottle containing natural or added sugar	Yes	
Child has special health care needs	Yes	
Child is a recent immigrant	Yes	
Protective		
Child receives optimally fluoridated drinking water or fluoride supplements		Yes
Child has teeth brushed daily with fluoridated toothpaste		Yes
Child receives topical fluoride from health professional		Yes
Child has dental home/regular dental care		Yes
Clinical Findings		
Child has white spot lesions or enamel defects	Yes	
Child has visible cavities and fillings	Yes	
Child has plaque on teeth	Yes	

Circling those conditions that apply to a specific patient helps the practitioner and parent to understand the factors that contribute to or protect from caries. Risk assessment categorization of low or high is based on preponderance of factors for the individual. However, clinical judgment may justify the use of one factor (e.g., frequent exposure to sugar-containing snacks or beverages, more than one decayed/missing/filled surface) in determining overall risk.

Overall assessment of the child's dental caries risk: High ☐   Moderate ☐   Low ☐

From American Academy of Pediatric Dentistry. Clinical guideline on caries-risk assessment and management for infants, children, and adolescents. *Pediatr Dent.* 2016;38(special issue):142–149.

shown that incorporation of infant oral health education in pediatric residency programs can improve oral health knowledge, confidence, and behavior of residents while delivering oral health care services.[73,74] The same has been observed in training programs for practicing medical providers.[75–77] Extensive programs in Washington,[76] North Carolina,[77] and California[78] focused on training medical professionals in providing preventive dental services such as counseling, oral screening, risk assessment, fluoride application, and referral. They also addressed issues regarding Medicaid reimbursement for these preventive services. Overall results of these training sessions were positive in terms of increased oral health knowledge, integration of preventive services in the medical offices, and improved accuracy among these professionals in identifying children needing referrals. Survey results from pediatricians who rotated through University of Iowa's Infant Oral Health Program (IOHP) during their residency are encouraging. These pediatricians, compared with those who graduated prior to the inclusion of this rotation in their training curriculum, were more knowledgeable about important early childhood caries preventive measures, such as parental brushing and use of smear amount of fluoride toothpaste, for the young child. In addition, these pediatricians were more likely to examine the teeth of children 3 years of age and younger.[79]

Collaborative efforts and effective communication between medical and dental homes is essential to prevent oral disease and promote oral and overall health, especially among young high-risk children. The historical separation between dentistry and medicine and a general conception that the mouth be treated separate from the rest of the body has greatly inhibited these collaborations. Medical professionals can play an important role in children's oral health by providing primary prevention and coordinated care. Equally, dentists can also improve the overall health of children not only by treating dental disease, but also by proactively recognizing child abuse, preventing traumatic injuries through anticipatory guidance, and preventing obesity by longitudinal dietary counseling and monitoring of weight status.[80] In addition, dentists can have an important role in assessing immunization status, developmental milestones (i.e., fine/gross motor skills, speech, language, social interactions) for potential delays, disabilities such as autism spectrum disorders, and appropriate referral to therapeutic services.[81] The unique opportunity dentists have to help address overall health issues strengthens as children get older, because compliance with annual well-child visits decreases whereas dental recall visits increase. Research shows that children aged 6 to 12 years are, on average, four times more likely to visit a dentist than a pediatrician.[82,83] Leadership and collaboration among the disciplines of dentistry, medicine, nursing, and other health organizations are also critical to overcome the obstacles that prevent a greater participation of primary care providers in oral health care delivery. On one hand, medical professionals face barriers such as time constraints, limited reimbursement for preventive oral health care services, and difficulties in finding dentists that will accept their referrals of children younger than 3 years of age.[84,85] On the other hand, despite the fact that pediatric dentistry is reported to be the most sought-after postdoctoral training program,[86] there are still not enough pediatric dentists in the United States to care for the dental needs of all children.[5] Consequently, general dentists must treat these children or at least alleviate the burden of their dental disease by providing measures for caries prevention early in life. However, national data indicate that very few general dentists treat children younger than 4 years of age.[5] Unfortunately, not all dental schools have made hands-on IOHPs a reality in their predoctoral programs. Consequently, it is not realistic to expect general dentists to provide early intervention if dental school programs do not adequately train and increase their students' learning experiences in treating infants and toddlers. In addition, poor Medicaid reimbursement fees and a limited dental workforce whose distribution does not match population needs also prevents young children from receiving professional primary preventive dental care. In their commentary paper, Casamassimo and Seale[87] discussed the ongoing debate of how prepared our graduating dentists are to treat low-income minority children younger than 5 years of age known to be at higher risk for caries. In their 2014 survey directed toward predoctoral pediatric dentistry program directors, it was reported that approximately half of the dental schools in the United States expose their students to infant oral health. However, an increase from 2004 to 2014 of approximately one-third of dental school predoctoral programs establishing external rotations in community-based programs was reported.[87] These programs, such as one established at the University of Iowa in 1998, have been successful in showing that community-based programs can be integrated into the dental school curricula as a means of increasing the training of future general dentists on infant oral health care, while providing important preventive dental care for young children with high caries risks.[88]

Although the medical profession has acted to increase participation of pediatric primary care providers in delivering oral health care services for young children, few medical practitioners in isolated areas of the country have assumed this responsibility. More action is required to increase education about preventive oral health care in medical schools and residency programs, to make continuing education programs available nationwide, to lobby policy makers about the importance of reimbursement for pediatric oral health care services, and to establish more effective collaboration between dentistry and medicine.

References

1. American Academy of Pediatric Dentistry. Guideline on perinatal and infant oral health care. *Pediatr Dent*. 2016;38(special issue):150–154.
2. American Academy of Pediatric Dentistry. Clinical guideline on caries-risk assessment and management for infants, children, and adolescents. *Pediatr Dent*. 2016;38(special issue):142–149.
3. American Academy of Pediatrics, Section on Pediatric Dentistry. Policy statement on oral health risk assessment timing and establishment of the dental home. *Pediatrics*. 2003;111:1113–1116.
4. Dye BA, Thornton-Evans G, Li X, et al. *Dental Caries and Sealant Prevalence in Children and Adolescents in the United States, 2011–2012. NCHS data brief, no 191*. Hyattsville, MD: National Center for Health Statistics; 2015.
5. Seale NS, Casamassimo PS. Access to dental care for children in the United States: a survey of general practitioners. *J Am Dent Assoc*. 2003;134(12):1630–1640.
6. Nowak AJ. Rationale for the timing of the first oral evaluation. *Pediatr Dent*. 1997;19:8–11.
7. Warren JJ, Kramer KWO, Dawson DV, et al. Factors associated with caries in very young American Indian children. *J Dent Res*. 2013;92(Special Issue A):Abstract #2876.
8. Acs G, Lodolini D, Kaminsky S, et al. Effect of nursing caries on body weight in a pediatric population. *J Pediatr Dent*. 1992;14:302–305.
9. Kanellis MJ, Damiano PC, Momany ET. Medicaid costs associated with the hospitalization of young children for restorative dental treatment under general anesthesia. *J Public Health Dent*. 2000;60(1): 28–32.
10. Caulfield PW. Dental caries—a transmissible and infectious disease revisited: a position paper. *Pediatr Dent*. 1997;19:491–498.
11. Wan AKL, Seow WK, Purdie DM, et al. A longitudinal study of *Streptococcus mutans* colonization in infants after tooth eruption. *J Dent Res*. 2003;82(7):504–508.
12. Dye BA, Vargas CM, Lee JJ, et al. Assessing the relationship between children's oral health status and that of their mothers. *J Am Dent Assoc*. 2011;142(2):173–183.
13. Rethman MP, Beltrán-Aguilar ED, Billings RJ, et al. American Dental Association Council on Scientific Affairs Expert Panel on nonfluoride caries-preventive agents. Nonfluoride caries-preventive agents: executive summary of evidence-based clinical recommendations. *J Am Dent Assoc*. 2011;142(9):1065–1071.
14. Albino J, Tiwari T. Preventing childhood caries: a review of recent behavioral research. *J Dent Res*. 2016;95(1):35–42.
15. American Academy of Pediatric Dentistry. Definition of dental home. *Pediatr Dent*. 2016;38(special issue):12.
16. American Academy of Pediatrics Ad Hoc Task Force on the Definition of the Medical Home. The medical home. *Pediatrics*. 1992;90(5):774.
17. Kempe A, Beaty B, Englund BP, et al. Quality of care and use of the medical home in a state-funded capitated primary care plan for low-income children. *Pediatrics*. 2000;105(5):1020–1028.

18. American Academy of Pediatrics Council on Children with Disabilities. Care coordination: integrating health and related systems of care for children with special health care needs. *Pediatrics*. 2005;116(5):1238–1244.

19. US Department of Health and Human Services. *Oral health in America: a report of the Surgeon General, Bethesda, MD, National Institute of Dental and Craniofacial Research*. National Institutes of Health; 2000.

20. Savage MF, Lee JY, Kotch JB, et al. Early preventive dental visits: effects on subsequent utilization and costs. *Pediatrics*. 2004;114(4):418–423.

21. Lee JY, Bouwens TJ, Savage MF, et al. Examining the cost-effectiveness of early dental visits. *Pediatr Dent*. 2006;28(2):102–105.

22. Nowak AJ, Casamassimo PS, Scott J, et al. Do early dental visits reduce treatment and treatment costs for children? *Pediatr Dent*. 2014;36(7):489–493.

23. Li Y, Tanner A. Effect of antimicrobial interventions on the oral microbiota associated with early childhood caries. *Pediatr Dent*. 2015;37(3):226–244.

24. Twetman S, Dhar V. Evidence of effectiveness of current therapies to prevent and treat early childhood caries. *Pediatr Dent*. 2015;37(3):246–253.

25. American Academy of Pediatric Dentistry. Guideline on fluoride therapy. *Pediatr Dent*. 2016;38(special issue):181–184.

26. Fisher-Owens SA, Gansky SA, Platt LJ, et al. Influences on children's oral health: a conceptual model. *Pediatrics*. 2007;120(3):e510–e520.

27. Seow KW. Environmental, maternal, and child factors which contribute to early childhood caries: a unifying conceptual model. *Int J Paediatr Dent*. 2012;22(3):157–168.

28. Lee JY, Divaris K. The ethical imperative of addressing oral health disparities: a unifying framework. *J Dent Res*. 2014;93(3):224–230.

29. Nowak AJ, Casamassimo PS. Using anticipatory guidance to provide early dental intervention. *J Am Dent Assoc*. 1995;126:1156–1164.

30. Alaluusua S, Malmivirta R. Early plaque accumulation—a sign for caries risk in young children. *Community Dent Oral Epidemiol*. 1994;22:273–276.

31. American Academy of Pediatric Dentistry (AAPD). Risk assessment. In: *ABCs of Infant Oral Health*. Chicago: AAPD; 2000.

32. Seow KW. Effects of premature birth on oral growth and development. *Aust Dent J*. 1997;42:85–90.

33. Burt BA, Pai S. Does low birthweight increase the risk of caries? A systematic review. *J Dent Educ*. 2001;65:1024–1027.

34. American Academy of Pediatrics. Section on breastfeeding: breastfeeding and the use of human milk. http://pediatrics.aappublications.org/content/pediatrics/early/2012/02/22/peds.2011-3552.full.pdf. Accessed June 17, 2017.

35. Salone LR, Vann WF Jr, Dee DL. Breastfeeding: an overview of oral and general health benefits. *J Am Dent Assoc*. 2013;144(2):143–151.

36. Tham R, Bowatte G, Dharmage SC, et al. Breastfeeding and the risk of dental caries: a systematic review and meta-analysis. *Acta Paediatr*. 2015;104(467):62–84.

37. Erickson PR, Mazhari E. Investigation of the role of human breast milk in caries development. *Pediatr Dent*. 1999;21(2):86–90.

38. Casamassimo PS, Nowak AJ. Anticipatory guidance. In: Berg JH, Slayton RL, eds. *Early Childhood Oral Health*. 2nd ed. Hoboken, NJ: Wiley-Blackwell; 2016:178–179.

39. Wake M, Hesketh K, Lucas J. Teething and tooth eruption in infants: a cohort study. *Pediatrics*. 2000;106(6):1374–1379.

40. Massignan C, Cardoso M, Porporatti AL, et al. Signs and symptoms of primary tooth eruption: a meta-analysis. *Pediatrics*. 2014;137(3):1–17.

41. US Food and Drug Administration. Benzocaine and babies: not a good mix. https://www.fda.gov/ForConsumers/ConsumerUpdates/ucm306062.htm. Accessed June 17, 2017.

42. Voelker MSJ. Safe relief for teething symptoms. *JAMA*. 2016;316(19):1957.

43. Weinstein P, Harrison R, Benton T. Motivating parents to prevent caries in their young children: one-year findings. *J Am Dent Assoc*. 2004;135(6):731–738.

44. Ismail AI, Ondersma S, Jedele JM, et al. Evaluation of a brief tailored motivational intervention to prevent early childhood caries. *Community Dent Oral Epidemiol*. 2011;39(5):433–448.

45. Weber-Gasparoni K, Reeve J, Ghosheh N, et al. An effective psychoeducational intervention for early childhood caries: part I. *Pediatr Dent*. 2013;35(3):241–246.

46. Weber-Gasparoni K, Warren JJ, Reeve J, et al. An effective psychoeducational intervention for early childhood caries: part II. *Pediatr Dent*. 2013;35(3):247–251.

47. Vansteenkiste M, Williams GC, Resnicow K. Toward systematic integration between self-determination theory and motivational interviewing as examples of top-down and bottom-up intervention development: autonomy or volition as a fundamental theoretical principle. *Int J Behav Nutr Phys Activ*. 2012;9(23):1–11.

48. Johnson ED, Larson BE. Thumb-sucking: literature review. *J Dent Child*. 1993;60:385–391.

49. Larsson FE, Dahlin GK. The prevalence and the etiology of the initial dummy- and finger-sucking habit. *Am J Orthod*. 1985;87(5):432–435.

50. Warren JJ, Levy SM, Nowak AJ, et al. Non-nutritive sucking behaviors in pre-school children: a longitudinal study. *Pediatr Dent*. 2000;22:187–190.

51. Adair SM, Milano M, Lorenzo I, et al. Effects of current and former pacifier use on the dentition of 24- to 59-month-old children. *Pediatr Dent*. 1995;17:437–444.

52. Bishara SE, Warren JJ, Broffitt B, et al. Changes in the prevalence of nonnutritive sucking patterns in the first 8 years of life. *Am J Orthod Dentofacial Orthop*. 2014;130(1):31–35.

53. Larsson E. Dummy- and finger-sucking habits with special attention to their significance for facial growth and occlusion. 1. Incidence study. *Sven Tandlak Tidskr*. 1971;64:667–672.

54. Adair SM. Pacifier use in children: a review of recent literature. *Pediatr Dent*. 2003;25(5):449–458.

55. Larsson E. Dummy- and finger-sucking habits with special attention to their significance for facial growth and occlusion. 4. Effect on facial growth and occlusion. *Sven Tandlak Tidskr*. 1972;65:605–634.

56. Warren JJ, Bishara SE, Steinbock KL, et al. Effects of oral habits' duration on dental characteristics in the primary dentition. *J Am Dent Assoc*. 2001;132(12):1685–1693.

57. Warren JJ, Bishara SE. Duration of nutritive and nonnutritive sucking behaviors and their effects on the dental arches in the primary dentition. *Am J Orthod Dentofacial Orthop*. 2012;121(4):347–356.

58. Warren JJ, Slayton RL, Bishara SE, et al. Effects of nonnutritive sucking habits on occlusal characteristics in the mixed dentition. *Pediatr Dent*. 2015;27(6):445–450.

59. Clements MS, Mitchell EA, Wright SP, et al. Influences on breastfeeding in Southeast England. *Acta Paediatr Scand*. 1997;86:51–56.

60. Kramer MS, Barr RG, Dagenais S, et al. Pacifier use, early weaning, and cry/fuss behavior. *JAMA*. 2001;2286:322–326.

61. Mitchell EA, Taylor BJ, Ford RPK, et al. Dummies and sudden infant death syndrome. *Arch Dis Child*. 1993;68:501–504.

62. Chi DL, Momany ET, Jones MP, et al. An explanatory model of factors related to well baby visits by age three years for Medicaid-enrolled infants: a retrospective cohort study. *BMC Pediatr*. 2013;13(158):1–9.

63. American Academy of Pediatrics, Section on Pediatric Dentistry and Oral Health. Policy statement on preventive oral health intervention for pediatricians. *Pediatrics*. 2008;122(6):1387–1394.

64. American Academy of Pediatrics, Committee on Native American Child Health, Canadian Paediatric Society, First Nations, Inuit and Métis Committee. Policy statement on early childhood caries in indigenous communities. *Pediatrics*. 2011;127(6):1190–1198.

65. American Academy of Pediatrics, Section on Oral Health. Maintaining and improving the oral health of young children (policy statement). *Pediatrics*. 2014;134(6):1224–1229.

66. Lewis CW, Boulter S, Keels MA, et al. Oral health and pediatricians: results of a national survey. *Acad Pediatr*. 2009;9:457–461.

67. Sanchez OM, Childers NK, Fox L, et al. Physicians' views on pediatric preventive dental care. *Pediatr Dent*. 1997;19:377–383.

68. American Academy of Pediatrics. Children's oral health. www.aap.org/oralhealth/. Accessed June 17, 2017.
69. Bright Futures. Guidelines for health supervision of infants, children and adolescents, promoting oral health. https://pediatriccare.solutions.aap.org/book.aspx?bookid=990. Accessed June 17, 2017.
70. Children's Dental Health Project. About children's dental health project. www.cdhp.org/about_cdhp/about_childrens_dental_health_project. Accessed June 17, 2017.
71. National Maternal and Child Oral Health Resource Center. Homepage. https://www.mchoralhealth.org. Accessed June 17, 2017.
72. Mouradian WE, Slayton RL, eds. Special issue on children's oral health: background papers from the American Academy of Pediatrics National Summit on Children's Oral Health, November 7-8, 2008. http://www.academicpedsjnl.net/article/S1876-2859(09)00309-X/pdf. Accessed June 17, 2017.
73. Douglass JM, Douglass AB, Silk HJ. Infant oral health education for pediatric and family practice residents. *Pediatr Dent.* 2005; 27:284–291.
74. Schaff-Blass E, Rozier RG, Chattopadhyay A, et al. Effectiveness of an educational intervention in oral health for pediatric residents. *Ambul Pediatr.* 2006;6(3):157–164.
75. Pierce KM, Rozier RG, Vann WF. Accuracy of pediatric primary care providers' screening and referral for early childhood caries. *Pediatrics.* 2002;109:82–94.
76. Mouradian WE, Schaad DC, Kim S, et al. Addressing disparities in children's oral health: a dental-medical partnership to train family practice residents. *J Dent Educ.* 2003;67:886–895.
77. Rozier RG, Sutton BK, Bawden JW, et al. Prevention of early childhood caries in North Carolina medical practices: implications for research and practice. *J Dent Educ.* 2003;67:876–885.
78. Dooley D, Moultrie NM, Heckman B, et al. Oral health prevention and toddler well-child care: routine integration in a safety net system. *Pediatrics.* 2016;137(1):1–8.
79. Kleinheksel B, Leary K, Qian F, et al: Pediatricians' behavior, comfort, and knowledge after infant oral health training (poster #278). *American Academy of Pediatric Dentistry 70th Annual Meeting Session,* Washington DC, May 27, 2017.
80. Tseng R, Vann WF Jr, Perrin EM. Addressing childhood overweight and obesity in the dental office: rationale and practical guidelines. *Pediatr Dent.* 2010;32(5):417–423.
81. Scharf RJ, Scharf G, Stroustrup A. Developmental milestones. *Pediatr Rev.* 2016;37(1):25–38.
82. Brown EJ. Quality AFHRA, ed. *Children's Dental Visits and Expenses, United States, 2003. Statistical brief no. 117.* Rockville, MD: Agency for Healthcare Research and Quality; 2006.
83. Selden TM. Compliance with well-child visit recommendations: evidence from the Medical Expenditure Panel Survey, 2000-2002. *Pediatrics.* 2016;118(6):e1766–e1778.
84. Casamassimo PS. Oral health in primary care medicine: practice and policy challenges. *Am Fam Physician.* 2004;70:2074–2076.
85. Krol DM. Educating pediatricians on children's oral health: past, present, and future. *Pediatrics.* 2004;113:487–492.
86. Stewart RE, Sanger RG. Pediatric dentistry for the general practitioner: satisfying the need for additional education and training opportunities. *J Calif Dent Assoc.* 2014;42(11):785–789.
87. Casamassimo P, Seale NS. Educating general dentists to care for U.S. children: how well are we doing and what can we do better? *J Calif Dent Assoc.* 2014;42(11):779–783.
88. Weber-Gasparoni K, Kanellis MJ, Qian F. Iowa's public health-based infant oral health program: a decade of experience. *J Dent Educ.* 2010;74(4):363–371.

15

Prevention of Dental Disease

KEVIN L. HANEY AND KAY S. BEAVERS

CHAPTER OUTLINE

Dental caries and periodontal diseases are among the most common bacterial diseases affecting humans. Even though substantial reductions in the levels and severity of these diseases and their sequelae have been documented in most Western nations, millions of children worldwide continue to experience caries, periodontal disease, tooth loss, and malocclusions. Much of dental disease could be prevented if patients or those responsible for providing oral health care to patients engaged in daily oral hygiene practices, had access to optimal systemic and topical fluorides, maintained sound dietary practices, and sought professional dental care on a regular basis. Dental diseases and their sequelae are largely preventable.

The goal of this chapter is to provide clinicians with guidelines that can help oral health care providers keep infants and toddlers free from preventable oral disease. The stakeholders involved in infant oral health extend beyond just dental personnel. They include the patients, their parents, pediatricians and medical specialists, as well as anyone else interested or responsible for a child's health and well-being. Planning for a lifetime of oral health should begin shortly after conception and should continue regularly to ensure that risk factors for oral disease are recognized early and dealt with effectively throughout pregnancy, infancy, childhood, and adolescence.

The mouth plays a major role in the life of a human being. All nutrients pass through it, it helps create the sounds and expressions through which we communicate with others, and it is a major component of our overall appearance. A healthy mouth with a full complement of teeth and a functional, aesthetic occlusion is a goal that dental professionals should promote and seek to achieve for the patients under their care.

Prenatal Counseling

For more than a century, the medical profession has recognized the importance of providing prenatal counseling and care to expectant mothers. Oral health care is important to the expectant mother as well. Whereas some studies report an association between the presence of maternal periodontitis and both preeclampsia and preterm births, the causal link has been difficult to demonstrate consistently.[1-5] Regardless, dental professionals can make an important contribution in this primary preventive effort by attending to women's oral health during pregnancy and providing prenatal counseling related to infant oral health and oral development.

Prenatal counseling is generally provided in conjunction with programs conducted in community hospitals, neighborhood health centers, and office-based settings. Regardless of where the program is conducted, close collaboration among members of the various health professions and community support groups (e.g., dentists, physicians, nurses, nutritionists, social workers) is important to ensure appropriate scheduling of educational presentations and reinforcement of concepts.

Although many oral health-counseling programs have been developed in recent years, the goals of the programs are similar (Box 15.1). Regardless of the setting, time allotted, and staff involved, the programs should be individualized to the greatest extent possible and should provide parents with information about the development of oral structures and functions, dental disease processes, and recommended preventive measures. Such programs should provide information on the importance of the mother's diet and health-related behaviors during pregnancy (including the effects of drugs, tobacco, and alcohol), the importance of maternal oral health care during pregnancy, and recommended scheduling of maternal dental treatment (Box 15.2).

Knowing that there is a strong relationship between the levels of *Streptococcus mutans* in expectant mothers and the caries experience of their offspring, prenatal counseling should include a discussion on interventions that can disrupt the transmission of these virulent organisms.[6] Interventions that can suppress maternal *S. mutans* reservoirs include dietary changes that reduce the frequency of simple carbohydrate consumption, chemotherapeutic applications such as topical fluorides and topical chlorhexidine, and the elimination of existing caries by either tooth restoration or extraction.[7,8] In addition, evidence suggests that xylitol-containing products can significantly reduce maternal levels of *S. mutans*.[9-11] Xylitol is a sugar alcohol that is used as a low-calorie sugar substitute. It is available in a variety of forms that include gums, mints, nasal sprays, toothpastes and gels, xylitol-containing beverages and snacks, and wipes (Fig. 15.1), which are promoted to cleanse the oral

• BOX 15.1 A Model of Prenatal Counseling

Purpose
To educate parents about dental development of the child
To educate parents about dental disease and prevention
To provide a suitable environment for the child
To strengthen and prepare the child and dentition for life

Methods
Education concerning development, prevention, and disease
Demonstration of oral hygiene procedures
Counseling to instill preventive attitudes and motivation
Evaluation of learning, acceptance, and needs

Content
External Component (Parents)
Parents' education concerning dental disease and oral hygiene
Parents' motivation for plaque removal program
Changes in mother's oral health
Intake of sweets
Pregnancy gingivitis
Myths and misconceptions about pregnancy and dentition
Parents' dental treatment

Internal Component (Parents and Child)
Parents' education/development of child
Effect of lifestyle on child
Habits (smoking, alcohol consumption)
Intake of sweets
Exposure to disease (e.g., rubella, syphilis)
Effect of drugs on child (e.g., tetracyclines)
Nutrition
    Calcium
    Vitamins
    Fluorides
Essential nutrients
Child's needs after birth
Breastfeeding versus bottle feeding
Fluoride supplementation
Teething
Hygiene
Nonnutritive sucking
First visit

• BOX 15.2 Dental Treatment for Women During Pregnancy

First Trimester
Consult with woman's physician.[a]
Emergency treatment only

Second Trimester
Elective and emergency treatment
Radiographs can be used with adequate protection.

Third Trimester
Emergency treatment only
Avoid supine position.
Radiographs can be used with adequate protection.

Throughout Pregnancy
Plaque control program for parents of child
Local anesthetic is anesthetic of choice.
Avoid the use of drugs if at all possible. If drugs are needed, use only those proved safe for use during pregnancy and use in consultation with a physician.
The use of a general anesthetic for dental treatment during pregnancy is contraindicated.

[a]The first trimester is most crucial; however, in these litigious times it would probably be wise to consult with the woman's physician during the last two trimesters, especially if there is a major problem.

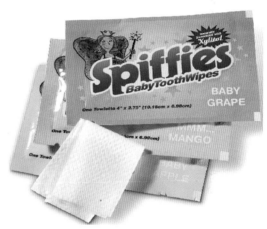

• **Figure 15.1** Premoistened wipes containing xylitol used for cleaning the oral cavity (Spiffies Baby ToothWipes). (Courtesy Practicon Dental, Greenville, NC.)

cavities of infants. Consumption of 6 to 10 g of xylitol per day at three different time intervals has been shown to reduce levels of *S. mutans* in adults.[12] Reducing levels in mothers can help delay the colonization of their offspring, which in turn has the potential to reduce the caries activity in these children.[10,13]

The timing and sequence of eruption of teeth should be discussed during prenatal counseling. Variations are common and a frequent source of parental anxiety. Teething should also be mentioned because it most likely will be the first postnatal oral issue that

parents confront. Teething is a natural phenomenon that usually occurs with little or no associated problems. Nevertheless, some infants exhibit signs of systemic distress including a slight rise in body temperature (typically lower than 101°F), diarrhea, dehydration, increased salivation, skin eruptions, and gastrointestinal disturbances.[14-16] Increased fluid consumption, a nonaspirin analgesic, and palliative care consisting of the use of teething rings to apply cold and pressure to the affected areas generally reduce the symptoms and result in a happier infant.[17] If symptoms persist for more than 24 hours or if body temperature exceeds 101°F, a physician should be consulted to rule out the possibility of other common diseases and conditions of infancy.

Prenatal counseling programs should also provide guidelines for parents about the timing of establishing a dental home. In the past, guidelines have recommended that children without symptoms of disease be scheduled for their first dental examination beginning at age 3 years. Today professional guidelines have incorporated the importance of earlier attention to oral health during infancy, particularly for children at elevated risk for the development of dental caries.[18–20] Programs designed to provide comprehensive preventive measures now stress the importance of initiating professional visits with a risk assessment within 6 months of the eruption of a child's first tooth or no later than age 12 months (Fig. 15.2).[21]

Several educational programs are available that provide comprehensive and practical information designed to assist health professionals and families to more effectively promote the health and well-being of children and adolescents. The American Academy of Pediatrics' *Bright Futures: Guidelines for Health Supervision of Infants, Children, and Adolescents* is one such program.[22] These programs not only stress the importance of the early initial exam to assess the infant's risk for dental disease but also provide anticipatory guidance and guidelines to help establish follow-up appointments based on the outcomes of the caries risk assessment.[23]

Caries Risk Assessment

Another innovation in designing preventive programs is based on the concept of the caries risk assessment as detailed in Chapter 14. The risk of developing dental disease varies among children and over time for each child. Assessing each child's risk for common dental diseases and identifying specific risk factors on a regular basis allow the practitioner to more effectively individualize oral health supervision and preventive measures.

Risk assessments for dental caries based on a single risk indicator are unlikely to reliably differentiate between those at high and low risk because caries is a complex disease process. Accordingly, various multifactorial models have been developed. The risk assessment protocol developed by the American Academy of Pediatric Dentistry, as detailed in Chapter 14 and presented in Table 14.1 and Box 14.1, is one such model. Based on the risk level, the clinician can personalize and initiate a comprehensive preventive program for the child. Risk status should be reassessed periodically to detect changes in the child's clinical, environmental, and general health conditions. The American Academy of Pediatrics also endorses the early risk assessment as well as the establishment of a dental home by 12 months of age.[18]

Establishing a Dental Home

All children should have a place where they can receive appropriate health care provided by physicians, dentists, and other allied health professionals. The health provider should know the child and parent and should establish a level of trust and responsibility with the family. Doing so allows for optimal cooperation and opens avenues of communication between the family and the provider. Most parents establish such an environment early with respect to medical care for their infants and toddlers. To complement the medical home, all infants and toddlers should have an established dental home as well. The concept of a dental home was introduced in 2002 as a means to address the epidemic of early childhood caries as well as other oral health issues that pertained to the pediatric patient.[24] The proposal that the first dental visit should take place earlier than 3 years of age, which had been customary, was a major change in philosophy. This recommendation was based on the fact that although dental caries had been declining in the permanent dentition for decades, the rates of early childhood caries had been static and had even begun to worsen in more recent years.[25] It was recognized that by 3 years of age, the damage from caries had already occurred and dental professionals were forced into surgical modes of treatment that included restorations and extractions as opposed to preventive measures of treatment. The benefits of early initial exams have been supported by studies showing that early enrollment of children into oral health care programs increases parental compliance with preventive measures,[26] reduces caries activity,[27–29] and results in lower expenses for dental care over time.[30]

The dental home should include accessible facilities and comprehensive oral health services geared toward the needs of children and their families. Whether this dental home is located in a private practice, a community health center, or at the neighborhood hospital, it should be supervised by dentists trained in primary pediatric care. By establishing a dental home early, parents will be appropriately counseled during the early infant years and have a facility to contact immediately in case of an orofacial traumatic injury. The dental home should provide all of the services listed in Box 15.3. Today's children should have established medical homes as well as established dental homes as part of their comprehensive health care programs.[24,31]

Fluoride Administration

Rationale

Significant reductions in the prevalence of dental caries have been documented in older children and adults in the United States and other countries over the past several decades.[25] Although the reason for this decline is unknown, most experts include increased availability of fluorides as one of the primary contributing factors. In

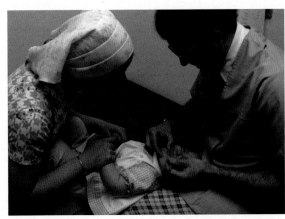

• **Figure 15.2** First dental visit for a 15-month-old child. The dentist is demonstrating how to brush the boy's teeth. (Courtesy John Warren, University of Iowa.)

• BOX 15.3   Services Provided by the Dental Home

1. Schedule early dental visits at approximately 12–18 months of age.
2. Assess the risk of the infant and toddler for future dental disease.
3. Evaluate the fluoride status of the infant and make appropriate recommendations.
4. Demonstrate to caretakers the appropriate method for cleaning teeth.
5. Discuss the advantages/disadvantages of nonnutritive sucking.
6. Be prepared to treat the infant/toddler if early childhood caries is diagnosed or to make the appropriate referral.
7. Be available 24 hours a day, 7 days a week to deal with any acute dental problems.
8. Recognize the need for specialty consultation and referrals.

spite of these advances, caries remains a relatively common yet largely preventable disease of childhood. Because of the importance of fluoride in this regard, the contemporary dental practitioner should understand the basis for using the many available forms of fluoride.

Mechanisms of Action

Although the precise mechanisms by which fluorides prevent dental caries are not fully understood, three general mechanisms are typically acknowledged: (1) increasing the resistance of the tooth structure to demineralization, (2) enhancing the process of remineralization, and (3) reducing the cariogenic potential of dental plaque.

The effects of fluoride are usually classified as either systemic or topical. Systemic effects can be obtained through the ingestion of foods that contain natural levels of fluoride, water that contains natural fluoride or to which fluoride has been added, and dietary fluoride supplements. Topical benefits are available from the previously mentioned sources as a result of their contact with the teeth as well as from fluoride toothpastes, fluoride mouth rinses, and other more concentrated forms of fluoride that are self-administered or applied professionally.

The decision to administer various forms of fluoride depends primarily on the age of the child and the results of their caries risk assessment. For children determined to be at moderate or high risk for developing caries, the optimal use of topical fluorides should be considered.

Systemic Fluorides

Water Fluoridation

Water fluoridation remains the cornerstone of any sound caries prevention program. It is not only the most effective means of reducing caries but also remains the most cost-effective, cost-saving, convenient, and reliable method of providing the benefits of fluoride to the general population because it does not depend on individual compliance.[33,34] Early studies documented caries reductions of 40% to 50% in the primary dentition and 50% to 65% in the permanent dentition of children and adolescents exposed to fluoridated water from birth.[35] More recent studies have reported that the mean decayed-missing-filled surfaces (dmfs) of children with continuous residence in fluoridated areas is approximately 18% lower than that of children with no exposure. When corrected to remove children who have been exposed to topical or supplemental fluorides, the mean dmfs was 25% lower in the group exposed continuously to water fluoridation.[36]

Many water supplies contain significant levels of natural fluoride, especially in the midwestern and southwestern sections of the country. Although it is relatively expensive to remove existing fluoride from a community water source, it is relatively inexpensive to add fluoride to a community water source. Numerous fluoride-deficient community water supplies have been artificially fluoridated at a cost of less than $0.50 per person, depending on the size of the community. In 2012, over 210 million US individuals (75% of the population served by public water systems) received optimally fluoridated water. This reflects an increase from 195 million (72.4%) reported in 2008.[37,38]

The issue of accurately determining an individual's fluoride water concentration is compounded by the increasing prevalence of home water filtration and purification units. These filtration units are often installed at either a point source such as a faucet

or refrigerator line or centrally installed to where they filter all the water that enters a household. The complexity of the issue is due to the fact that some filtration units, such as those that function by reverse osmosis, alter fluoride concentrations, while other units, such as charcoal filtration systems, do not alter fluoride concentration. The most accurate way of determining fluoride concentration in a household that uses a filtration unit is to collect and test a water sample that has been processed through the filtration system.

As part of their responsibility in promoting oral health, dentists have an obligation to educate the public about the effectiveness and safety of community water fluoridation. Involvement at the local level in support of this proven preventive measure can be one of the major contributions a dentist can make to enhance the oral health of all children in his or her community.

Dietary Fluoride Supplements

Fluoride supplements provide an alternative source of dietary fluoride for children who are at high risk of developing caries and whose primary source of drinking water is deficient in fluoride. In addition, those children who either reside in communities with fluoridated water but who do not rely on optimally fluoridated water as their primary water source or those who use filtration systems that remove fluoride from their water source could potentially benefit from fluoride supplements.

The use of bottled and processed waters for drinking and cooking has become increasingly popular in recent years. The total US consumption of bottled water was estimated at more than 9.1 billion gallons in 2012.[39,40] Consumers are turning to these water sources as alternatives to tap water, which they believe is contaminated with microorganisms, pesticides, herbicides, industrial waste, and heavy metals. The fluoride content of these bottled waters generally has been found to exhibit wide variability, usually below optimal concentrations.[41–45] Current regulations do not require manufacturers of bottled water to list the fluoride concentration on the label. Although optimally fluoridated bottled water is commercially available, it is infrequently used by consumers. Hence, dentists must be aware of the bottled water products readily available in their community and be prepared to obtain fluoride analyses when necessary. Furthermore, all parents, including those who reside in areas where water is fluoridated, should be questioned about the sources of fluid in their infants' diets and should realize that fluoride supplements are advisable for at-risk children who consume very little fluoridated water.

Fluoride supplements can be as effective as fluoridated water in preventing caries[46–48]; however, their effectiveness depends largely on the degree of parental compliance. Supplements are commercially available in liquid and tablet forms, both with and without vitamins. The fluoride-vitamin formulations are not inherently superior to supplements without vitamins in terms of reducing caries. Unfortunately the parents of children at high risk of developing caries often fail to comply with fluoride supplement regimens.[49] The combination of fluoride and vitamins may improve parental compliance, thereby providing greater benefits.[50] These fluoride-vitamin combinations should only be recommended for those children determined to be deficient in their fluoride consumption. Prescribing fluoride-vitamin combinations to the child already using an optimally fluoridated water source exposes that child to the risk of developing fluorosis.

Liquid preparations are recommended for younger patients who may have difficulty in chewing or swallowing tablets. Liquid supplements without vitamins are dispensed in preparations that

• **BOX 15.4** **Sample Supplemental Fluoride Prescription**

Eight-month-old whose drinking water contains less than 0.1 ppm fluoride:
Rx: Sodium fluoride solution 0.5 mg/mL (0.25 mg F⁻)
Disp: 50 mL
Sig: Dispense 1.0 mL of liquid in mouth before bedtime

Three-year-old whose drinking water contains 0.2 ppm fluoride:
Rx: Sodium fluoride tablets 0.25 mg fluoride/tablet (0.55 mg NaF/tablet)
Disp: 180 tablets
Sig: Chew one (1) tablet, swish, and swallow after brushing at bedtime. Nothing per os (NPO) for 30 min.

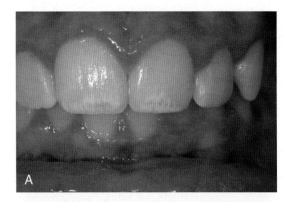

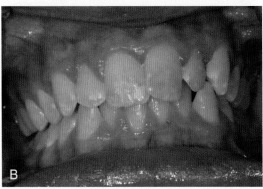

• **Figure 15.3** Examples of mild (A) and moderate (B) fluorosis. (Courtesy John Warren, University of Iowa.)

provide a fluoride dose of 0.125 mg/drop, 0.25 mg/drop, or 0.5 mg/mL; liquid supplements with vitamins are dispensed in preparations that provide 0.25 mg/mL and 0.5 mg/mL. Fluoride supplements in chewable tablet form for older patients are available without vitamins in doses of 0.25 mg, 0.5 mg, and 1.0 mg of fluoride, and fluoride-vitamin combinations are available in doses of 0.5 mg and 1.0 mg.

The fluoride in most dietary supplements is incorporated as sodium fluoride. One milligram of fluoride is equivalent to approximately 2.2 mg of sodium fluoride. When prescribing fluoride supplements, the practitioner should clearly specify the dose that is to be dispensed in terms of fluoride ion, sodium fluoride, or both. Examples of prescriptions for dietary fluoride supplements are given in Box 15.4.

In order to obtain both topical and systemic effects, fluoride supplements should be allowed to contact the teeth before being swallowed. With liquid preparations, this can be achieved by placing the drops directly on the child's teeth or by placing them in the child's food or drink, although the latter practice may reduce the bioavailability of the fluoride. Older children should be encouraged to "chew and swish" their tablets or allow the tablets to dissolve in the mouth before swallowing to prolong the contact of the fluoride with the outer surfaces of the teeth. Eating, drinking, and toothbrushing should be delayed for at least 30 minutes after taking a fluoride supplement. Administration at bedtime once toothbrushing is complete is ideal because it can eliminate the temptation that a child may have to eat or drink. In addition, salivary flow is diminished at night, which in turn can potentially increase the topical effects of bedtime administered fluoride by increasing the salivary concentration when compared with levels that might be obtained by daytime administration.

The dosage of fluoride that should be prescribed depends on the age of the child and the fluoride concentration of his or her drinking water. The fluoride concentration of a central community water supply can be determined by contacting the local or state department of health or the local water authority. *My Water's Fluoride* is a detailed website provided by the Centers for Disease Control and Prevention where consumers from participating states can access the fluoride status of their public water system.[51] For persons who do not obtain their drinking water from a central supply, water samples should be tested for fluoride content. This service usually is provided by state health departments, schools of dentistry, or commercial firms. Alternatively, in-office analyses of water fluoride concentrations can be performed by clinicians using a relatively inexpensive handheld colorimeter. Although less precise than more expensive fluoride electrodes, comparisons have shown that

colorimetric assays closely correlate with electrode findings and generally result in comparable supplementation recommendations.[52] When results of electrode findings and colorimetric assays differ, corresponding supplementation recommendations based on colorimetry tend to be lower, thereby minimizing the potential for adverse outcomes (e.g., fluorosis; Fig. 15.3). Because of the potential for considerable variations in fluoride levels in water obtained from different wells in the same area, it is important that each individual noncentral water source be sampled to accurately determine the appropriate level of fluoride supplementation for each patient. Table 15.1 shows the daily dosage schedule for fluoride supplementation that is currently recommended by the American Dental Association.[53]

Until recently, fluoride supplements were generally recommended for all children whose drinking water contained suboptimal levels of fluoride. However, consistent with the growing emphasis on risk assessment and risk-based preventive practices, recent recommendations call for fluoride supplements to be prescribed for children at high risk for dental caries whose primary drinking water has a low fluoride concentration.[33] These newer recommendations also call for dentists, physicians, and other health care providers to weigh the risk for caries without fluoride supplements, the caries prevention offered by supplements, and the potential for enamel fluorosis to develop in children younger than 6 years. In addition, parents and caregivers must be informed of both the benefits of fluoride protection and the possibility of developing enamel fluorosis.

Infants, whose primary and permanent teeth are undergoing maturation and calcification, are particularly vulnerable to the effects of excess fluoride. Since 1978, fluoridated water is no longer used in the manufacture of ready-to-use infant formulas.[54] A problem

TABLE 15.1	Supplemental Fluoride Dosage Schedule		
	CONCENTRATION OF FLUORIDE IN WATER		
Age	<0.3 ppm F⁻	0.3–0.6 ppm F⁻	>0.6 ppm F⁻
Birth–6 months	0	0	0
6 months to 3 years	0.25 mg	0	0
3–6 years	0.50 mg	0.25 mg	0
6 years up to at least 16 years	1.00 mg	0.50 mg	0

occurs when concentrated or powdered infant formulas, which can contain some fluoride, are reconstituted with an optimally fluoridated water. This poses the risk of overexposure to the infant. The American Dental Association recommends that when an infant formula needs to be reconstituted before use, it can be done with optimally fluoridated drinking water, although dental professionals should caution parents and caregivers of infants as to the risk of developing fluorosis.[55]

The fact that the prevalence of fluorosis has been significantly reduced in optimally fluoridated areas suggests that additional exposure to traditional sources of ingested fluoride may not be a major etiologic factor. That conclusion is further supported by studies suggesting that fluoride ingestion from dietary sources has remained relatively constant since the 1950s.[56] Notable exceptions in the pediatric population include a lowering of fluoride concentrations in infant formulas,[57] causing a reduction in fluoride exposure, and increased availability of fluoridated beverages in nonfluoridated areas (e.g., soft drinks prepared with fluoridated water) with the potential for additional fluoride intake.[58] This latter phenomenon has been called the "halo effect," reflecting the concept of extended water fluoridation effects beyond fluoridated communities.

Because it is common for infants and children to experience several contacts with a physician before their first dental visit, dentists providing treatment for children should become aware of the prescribing practices of local physicians and be prepared to offer advice about appropriate fluoride supplementation. In addition, dentists can provide input into local prenatal care programs so that expectant parents can be made aware of the benefits and appropriate use of fluorides.

Prescribing systemic fluorides during pregnancy to benefit the developing teeth was once a common practice in the United States. However, in 1966 the US Food and Drug Administration banned the promotion of prenatal fluoride supplements in the United States.[59] Safety was not the overriding issue in this decision. Rather, the decision was based on a lack of evidence about the effectiveness of prenatal fluoride supplements in preventing caries in offspring. Data from human studies suggest that the placenta is not an effective barrier to the passage of fluoride to the fetus and that there is a direct relationship between the serum fluoride concentrations of the mother and the fetus.[60,61] A study reported that 5-year-olds whose mothers were provided 1 mg of fluoride daily during prenatal months 4 through 9 had no statistically significant differences in their caries status than the control group. In addition, there was a risk, albeit low, for the development of mild fluorosis. Therefore there continues to be no support for prenatal fluoride supplementation.[62,63]

Topical Fluorides

Topical fluoride use for children up to age 3 years ordinarily consists of conscientious use of a moderate amount of fluoride-containing toothpaste applied by a parent or caregiver. Children whose teeth contain structural defects or who exhibit decalcified areas or other indicators that place them at moderate or high risk for developing caries, or toddlers who have previously experienced caries (i.e., early childhood caries), may receive additional topical applications in the form of professionally administered (e.g., fluoride varnish) or parentally applied concentrated preparations. Regardless of whether toothpaste or a more concentrated form of fluoride is applied, care should be taken to minimize the amount that is ingested. For the child who is either unable or unwilling to expectorate, either nonfluoridated toothpaste or only a smear of fluoridated toothpaste should be applied to the toothbrush. A parent or guardian should always be directly involved in the brushing process, as children in this age group have not yet developed the manual dexterity to adequately remove plaque from all surfaces of their teeth.

Fluoride Varnish

Fluoride varnish was first introduced in Europe in 1964. More than 48 years of clinical studies have since demonstrated that fluoride varnish is a safe and highly effective means of preventing decay. Based on these studies, the American Dental Association rates the quality of evidence as "high" for the efficiency of fluoride varnish to prevent and control dental caries in both primary and permanent teeth.[64] Although the preventive effects are strongest in infants, toddlers, and preschool children before caries has been detected, studies have shown that even for those children with a high risk of developing caries in the primary dentition, fluoride varnish is effective in reducing rates of decay.[65]

Fluoride varnish first became available in the United States in 1991, when the US Food and Drug Administration approved its use as a cavity varnish. Today there are a multitude of fluoride varnish products available to the dental professional. Although approved for use as a cavity varnish and for the management of hypersensitivity, the most common use of fluoride varnish is in the prevention of tooth decay. The therapeutic use of fluoride varnish for caries prevention in the United States is termed "off-label" use. This concept is sometimes confusing to those who may misinterpret it to mean that it is either illegal or unethical to use a product for an unapproved (as opposed to disapproved) use. However, the Federal Food, Drug, and Cosmetic Act does not limit the manner in which dentists may use approved drugs. It is often considered accepted medical or dental practice to use drugs for purposes other than that for which the drug originally received approval.[66]

Fluoride varnish is considered by many to be ideally suited for application to the teeth of pediatric dental patients. Its ease of application makes it attractive for use with young or precooperative patients needing topical fluoride treatments. Most fluoride varnishes consist of 5% sodium fluoride (2.26% fluoride ion) and are therefore more concentrated than most other professionally applied fluoride products. They are often sweetened with xylitol and contain a variety of flavoring agents, which has improved their acceptance among the pediatric population over that of earlier formulations. In addition, many of the varnishes available today are tooth-colored as opposed to the caramel color of the original products. When used clinically, only a small amount is needed. Less than 0.5 mL of varnish is typically required to coat the teeth of a young child. Other potential uses for fluoride varnish include application to identified areas of high risk—such as decalcified areas, deep pits, and fissures that cannot be sealed—and around orthodontic appliances in patients with poor oral hygiene.

Fluoride varnish is easy to apply by disposable brush. Varnish application may be preceded by professional prophylaxis but may also be applied after brushing with a toothbrush. The teeth should be dried before application with either compressed air or dry gauze. Fluoride varnish can be applied to all tooth surfaces or may be selectively applied to sites at higher risk for caries (i.e., decalcified sites or maxillary anterior teeth in children at risk for early childhood caries). It is not necessary to wait for the varnish to dry before releasing the patient because the varnish sets upon contact with the oral fluids. After varnish application, eating and drinking should be delayed for at least 30 minutes. Toothbrushing is not recommended until the following day so that the varnish will remain in contact with the teeth for as long as possible.

Fluoride varnish can be applied one to four times a year. Although one yearly application has been shown to have some benefit,[64] the American Dental Association recommends at least two applications a year, or every 6 months. Applications at 3-month intervals are recommended for those at high risk for caries.[65]

Safety and Toxicity

When used properly, fluoride in various forms can enhance the oral health status of infants and children. As is true of many other substances, however, when used improperly these same agents have the potential to produce objectionable side effects. Therefore each member of the dental profession has a responsibility to educate patients about the appropriate storage and use of these products.

Acute toxicity can result from the accidental ingestion of excessive amounts of fluoride. The manifestations of acute fluoride toxicity are usually limited to nausea and vomiting, but deaths have occasionally been reported as a result of excessive fluoride ingestion.[67] The amount of ingested fluoride necessary to produce acute symptoms is directly related to the weight of the individual. Precautions should be employed to prevent the accidental ingestion of concentrated forms of fluoride by all children, especially infants and very young children. The lethal dose of fluoride for a typical 3-year-old is approximately 500 mg, but the dose would be proportionately less for a younger and smaller child.

To avoid the possibility of ingestion of large amounts of fluoride, it is recommended that no more than 120 mg of supplemental fluoride be prescribed at any one time.[33] Likewise, prescriptions for concentrated topical fluoride preparations intended for home use (e.g., 0.5% fluoride gels that contain 5 mg of fluoride per milliliter) should be limited to 30 to 40 mL. Ingestion of moderate volumes of fluoride mouth rinses and toothpastes containing 1 mg or less of fluoride per milliliter would not be expected to cause severe symptoms, although nausea and vomiting could result.

Parents should be encouraged to store these and all potentially harmful substances out of the reach of small children. Chewable fluoride tablets are often sweetened with xylitol and artificial flavors and can be confused as a candy or treat by young children. If a child ingests excessive amounts of fluoride, the recommended approach is to call a local poison control center. The suspected amount of ingestion should be available, which will help to determine whether a child would need to report to an emergency department or if the child could be monitored at home. Milk, calcium carbonate, and aluminum/magnesium–based antacids are recommended to slow absorption. Vomiting should not be induced unless recommended by the poison control center. Syrup of ipecac and activated charcoal are not recommended.[69]

Repeated ingestion of lesser amounts of fluoride can result in manifestations of chronic fluoride toxicity, the most common of which is dental fluorosis. Infants and young children who cannot fully control their swallowing reflex or who do not understand that they should expectorate products intended only for topical application may regularly swallow significant amounts of fluoride toothpaste. This amount of fluoride may be significant in children who also receive fluoride from fluoridated water, fluoride supplements, or other dietary sources.[70,71] In light of concern about potential increases in the prevalence of dental fluorosis, parents should be cautioned to supervise their children closely and limit the amount of fluoride toothpaste used by young children. Use of toothpaste also may be limited for infants under 3 years of age who are considered to be at low risk for the development of dental caries.

Another potential source of excessive fluoride ingestion is the inappropriate prescribing of fluoride supplements. Health care providers may be unaware that some water supplies in their area may contain varying amounts of natural fluoride, or they may assume that the level of fluoride is relatively consistent among sources. Unless samples of drinking water are analyzed for each patient, fluoride supplements might inadvertently be prescribed when they are not indicated.[72,73]

Fluoride plays a critical role in the prevention of dental caries in children. Therefore dentists who assume responsibility for the oral health of children should be knowledgeable about the safe and appropriate use of the various forms of available fluoride.

Diet

Chapter 12 details the dental disease process and the relationships among host, bacteria, and substrate. Diet plays an important role in this disease process. It is important to establish dietary habits early in the child's life that promote physical growth and development and create an environment conducive to optimal oral health.

Although considerable research to determine the potential role of various foods in promoting dental disease continues, available evidence suggests that the solubility and adhesiveness of foods are important factors. Foods that stick to the teeth and tissues for long periods and dissolve slowly are more likely to promote the production of acids that lower the pH of the oral environment.

A pH below 5.5 provides an environment for bacterial growth and decalcification of enamel.[74]

Initially, the infant's diet consists primarily of milk, whether from the breast, the bottle, or both. Bovine milk has a higher calcium, phosphorus, and protein content than human milk and contains 4% lactose compared with 7% lactose in human milk.[75] The buffering capacity of human milk is very poor. Consequently, both human and bovine milk have the potential to promote development of caries and, when inappropriately provided to infants without daily oral hygiene care, can lead to early childhood caries. Infants should never be given a bottle containing milk or other sweetened beverages as a means to pacify them during the day, at naptime, or at bedtime. If a naptime or bedtime bottle is customary, the infant should be held by the parent while feeding from the bottle. Upon finishing, the infant should be placed in the bed without the bottle. If there is a need for additional sucking, a pacifier is preferable to the bottle. If parents continue to insist on prolonged use of a bottle, the contents should be limited to water.

Feeding infants by breast is popular in both the United States and Europe. Data suggest that the incidence if breastfeeding has steadily increased in recent years. The Centers for Disease Control and Prevention reported in 2014 that 79% of newborn infants were breastfeeding. By 6 months of age that rate had dropped to 49% and fell further to 29% by 12 months of age.[76] While current data does not appear to achieve the Healthy People 2020 goal of 60.6% of 6-month-olds who breastfeed,[77] the recent trend toward meeting the goal appears to be positive.

As noted earlier, because of its composition, breast milk may contribute to acid production and promote enamel demineralization. This generally only occurs when another carbohydrate source is available for bacterial fermentation and the buffering capacity is exceeded.[78] Infants who are breastfed "on demand" may suckle 10 to 40 times in a 24-hour period and are at risk for the consequences of prolonged acid production. Nevertheless, many feel that the benefits of breastfeeding outweigh any harmful effects. Dentists should advise mothers who breastfeed "on demand" to clean their infant's teeth frequently, verify that systemic fluoride intake is optimal, and monitor dietary habits carefully.[79]

Surveys report that most 2-month-old infants in the United States are fed foods other than milk or infant formulas, even though several organizations—including the American Academy of Pediatrics, American College of Obstetricians and Gynecologists, American Academy of Family Physicians, World Health Organization, and the United Nations Children's Fund—recommend exclusive breastfeeding for the first 6 months of life.[80] At 6 months, iron-fortified dry cereal is recommended, followed by one to two new commercially or home-prepared foods each week. Sound eating habits established during infancy assist in the continuation of sound habits later in life. Making an infant drain the last drop from the bottle or finish the last spoonful in the dish is not recommended. Forcing infants to eat when they indicate a desire to stop may contribute to overeating, frequent snacking, and obesity in later life.[81]

Usually by the time the posterior primary teeth have erupted and the infant is sitting in a high chair for meals, the child has been introduced to a variety of foods. Parents should be advised about appropriate snack foods that are not only nutritious but also "safe for teeth." Finger foods (e.g., soft fruits and vegetables, cereals without sugar coatings, gelatin cubes, salt-free crackers, and cheeses) are acceptable and should be introduced as the infant develops chewing patterns and swallowing reflexes to handle these new foods. Foods with a high percentage of carbohydrates should be avoided, as should foods that stick to the teeth and are slow to dissolve.

Natural fruit juices and artificially fortified fruit juices are frequently introduced to the infant. Pediatricians recommend that juices not be given to the infant in a bottle, in a covered cup, or at bedtime. Juices should not be introduced into the diet of infants before 6 months of age. Habitual and prolonged use of juices in the bottle can lead to early childhood caries.[82] Once fruit juices are introduced, they should be limited to 4 to 6 ounces per day through the preschool years.[82] Flavored milks such as chocolate and strawberry milk typically have a high sugar content; their intake should be limited.

Home Care

The initiation of a program to ensure an optimal environment for oral health should begin in infancy.[22] Parents should be informed that it is their responsibility to carry out this program, with information and guidance available from the dentist and staff.

Dental professionals have long provided direction to parents about their child's dental health, with the major emphasis being on caries prevention. The changing patterns of dental caries in children, increasing parental concerns about additional oral health issues, the increasing number of single-parent families, and dentistry's ability to deal with issues other than dental caries have broadened the counseling role in dental health care delivery for children.

Anticipatory guidance is the term used to describe a proactive, developmentally based counseling program that focuses on the needs of a child at a particular stage of life. The concept of a developmentally relevant, one-on-one intervention between dentist and parent offers a popular alternative to the traditional one-sided caries prevention message. Anticipatory guidance gives parents the chance to talk about their child, get age-appropriate information, and look ahead at how growth and the environment will affect their child's oral health in the future. It broadens dentistry's reach into related areas that have implications for the oral health of the child. Finally, it gives the dental professional a consistent staged format for counseling and record keeping and avoids the common routine repetition that often fails to provide effective motivation for children and parents alike.

A sound dental preventive program includes many facets: dietary management, optimal systemic fluorides, and ongoing plaque control. All are important, but plaque removal in the infant and young child is often neglected and misunderstood.

Studies have confirmed that bacteria responsible for the development of dental caries are present at the time of eruption of the primary teeth. The acquisition of these bacteria is usually vertically transmitted from caregiver to child. The timing of this acquisition is influenced by a multitude of factors including high maternal bacterial levels, low birth weight, early tooth emergence, and low salivary IgA antibody levels.[83] Growth of cariogenic bacteria and certain components of the infant's diet combine to promote the development of plaque and the subsequent production of acid. This acidic environment is conducive to demineralization of enamel and, eventually, cavitation. In addition, the gingiva is subjected to daily insult from the products of bacterial metabolism, which can lead to marginal gingivitis.

Daily removal of plaque promotes sound enamel and healthy gingiva. Early initiation of plaque removal helps to establish a lifelong habit of oral care. A disease-free mouth brings happiness and satisfaction not only to the parents and children but also to the dental team that provides the counseling and encouragement.

Once the parents have been informed of the dental disease process and have been charged with the responsibility of cleaning their child's teeth daily, counseling should be provided that addresses suitable locations for performing the procedure, devices for plaque removal, pros and cons of dentifrice use, positioning of the infant, and techniques for effective plaque removal. Initially, oral hygiene for the infant should probably be performed at routine intervals during the day, such as bath time, bedtime, or after meals. As the infant grows, the knee-to-knee position (see Fig. 14.1) becomes preferable. Bathrooms (the usual site for oral hygiene for older children and adults) are often crowded and not designed for infant safety.

Positioning the infant for visibility and control is important. Whether the parent uses the changing table, a bed top, countertop, or the knee-to-knee position, appropriate stabilization, visibility, and control of the lips, tongue, and cheeks are important for a thorough and pleasant hygienic experience.

A slightly moistened hand towel or introductory oral hygiene device may be used to gently clean the predentate mouth. These can be introduced as a daily routine as soon as the newborn arrives home from the hospital. Doing so at such an early age helps condition the newborn to the concept that at least once a day, mother or father or some caregiver is going to introduce an object into their mouth to cleanse their oral cavity. This will simplify the transition to a toothbrush, which should occur once teeth have erupted. A wet, soft-bristled brush with a small head size can be used for this. Toddlers who are introduced to oral hygiene practices for the first time are less accepting of the practice compared to those who have had a routine established since birth. The parents of the reluctant child should be advised to be persistent. With time, the tooth cleaning activity becomes an accepted part of the daily routine.

PLAQUE REMOVAL INNOVATIONS FOR INFANTS AND TODDLERS

M. Catherine Skotowski

There are several products in the oral health care market designed to assist parents in cleansing the mouth of an infant or toddler that do not resemble the traditional shape of a toothbrush. Small cotton finger cloths that fit over the finger of an adult (Fig. 15.4A) have been marketed as an introductory oral hygiene device for pre-dentate infants. They help remove plaque and food debris, stimulate the gingival tissues, and help when introducing oral cleansing at a very early age. They are not efficient at removing plaque in pits and fissures, and a transition to a soft bristled toothbrush should be made once primary molars erupt. Another popular oral cleansing device for a very young child resembles a small circular rubber ring with a few tufts of bristles at one end (Fig. 15.4B). The easy-to-grasp shape allows a child or an adult to stimulate the gums and cleanse the oral cavity without the risk of over insertion.

Historically, toothbrushes for infants and toddlers have been miniature replicas of adult toothbrushes, varying primarily by size and character designs added to appeal to young children. In recent years, considerable research and study have been invested in exploring better designed, more functional toothbrushes for this age group, focusing on the shape and design of the toothbrush itself. Recognizing that parents should be the primary plaque removers for young children, some manufacturers have produced toothbrushes with longer handles for easier parental brushing. Some manufacturers are designing brush heads to meet the specific needs of the developing dentition. Most still feature soft bristles, but efforts have been made to alternate the lengths of the bristles to accommodate different surfaces of the teeth. Some designs feature soft rubber padding around the brush head to make it gentle to the gums. Innovations in the shape of the handle have evolved to improve the grip as well as to promote angling of the bristles at the optimal 45 degrees.

Along with the attention focused in recent years on the shape and design of toothbrushes for young children, much research and study continue on the marketability of toothbrushes based on their color and character designs. Keeping current with the latest trends in this area is imperative because most often the consumer selects the product with the most eye appeal. The fact that the toothbrush has been designed to assist with better plaque removal is an added bonus.

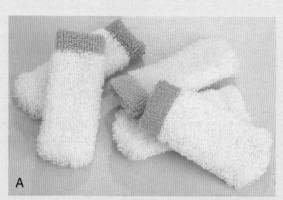
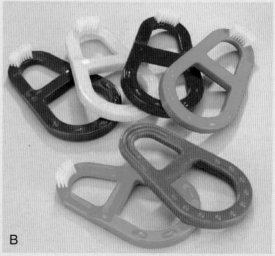

• **Figure 15.4** (A) Single-finger swabs used to clean the oral cavity before toothbrushing age (Tenders Pre-Toothbrushes). (B) Infant/toddler safety toothbrushes. (Courtesy Practicon Dental, Greenville, NC.)

References

1. Matevosyan NR. Periodontal disease and perinatal outcomes. *Arch Gynecol Obstet*. 2011;283(4):675–686.

2. Swati P, Thomas B, Vahab SA, et al. Simultaneous detection of periodontal pathogens in subgingival plaque and placenta of women with hypertension in pregnancy. *Arch Gynecol Obstet*. 2012;285(3): 613–619.

3. Politano GT, Passini R, Nomura ML, et al. Correlation between periodontal disease, inflammatory alterations and pre-eclampsia. *J Periodontal Res*. 2011;46(4):505–511.

4. Baccaglini L. A meta-analysis of randomized controlled trials shows no evidence that periodontal treatment during pregnancy prevents adverse pregnancy outcomes. *J Am Dent Assoc*. 2011;142(10):1192–1193.

5. Jeffcoat MK, Geurs NC, Reddy MS, et al. Current evidence regarding periodontal disease as a risk factor in preterm birth. *Ann Periodontol*. 2006;6:183–188.

6. American Academy of Pediatrics. Section on oral health. http://pediatrics.aappublications.org/content/134/6/1224l. Accessed May 31, 2017.

7. Livingston HM, Dellinger TM, Holden R. Considerations in the management of the pregnant patient. *Spec Care Dentist*. 1998; 18:183–188.

8. American Academy of Pediatric Dentistry. Guideline on perinatal oral health care. *Pediatr Dent*. 2011;33(special issue):118–123.

9. Isokangas P, Söderling E, Pienihäkkinen K. Occurence of dental decay in children after maternal consumption of xylitol chewing gum, a follow-up from 0 to 5 year of age. *J Dent Res*. 2000;79(11): 1885–1889.

10. Söderling E, Isokangas P, Pienihäkkinen K, et al. Influence of maternal xylitol consumption on acquisition of mutans streptococci by infants. *J Dent Res*. 2000;79(3):882–887.

11. Söderling E, Isokangas P, Pienihäkkinen K, et al. Influence of maternal xylitol consumption on mother-child transmission of mutans streptococci: 6-year follow-up. *Caries Res*. 2001;35(3):173–177.

12. Ly KA, Milgrom P, Rothen M. Xylitol, sweeteners, and dental caries. *Pediatr Dent*. 2006;28:154–163.

13. Kohler B, Andreen I, Jonsson B. The earlier the colonization by mutans streptococci, the higher the caries prevalence at 4 years of age. *Oral Microbiol Immunol*. 1988;3:14–17.

14. Barlow BS, Kanellis MJ, Slayton RL. Tooth eruption symptoms: a survey of parents and health professionals. *J Dent Child*. 2002;69:148–150.

15. Macknin ML, Piedmonte M, Jacobs J, et al. Symptoms associated with infant teething: a prospective study. *Pediatrics*. 2000;105:747–752.

16. Wake M, Hesketh K, Lucas J. Teething and tooth eruption in infants: a cohort study. *Pediatrics*. 2000;106:1374–1379.

17. King DL. Teething revisited. *Pediatr Dent*. 1994;16:179–182.

18. American Academy of Pediatrics. Oral health risk assessment timing and establishment of the dental home. *Pediatrics*. 2003;111:1113–1116.

19. American Academy of Pediatric Dentistry. Guideline on infant oral health care. *Pediatr Dent*. 2011;33(special issue):124–128.

20. American Academy of Pediatric Dentistry. Guideline on periodicity of examination, preventive dental services, anticipatory guidance/counseling, and treatment for infants, children, and adolescents. *Pediatr Dent*. 2016;38(6):133–140.

21. Nowak AJ. Rationale for the timing of the first oral evaluation. *Pediatr Dent*. 1997;19:8–11.

22. Hagan JF, Shaw JS, Duncan P. *Bright Futures: Guidelines for Health Supervision of Infants, Children, and Adolescents*. 4th ed. Elk Grove Village, IL: American Academy of Pediatrics; 2017.

23. Nowak AJ, Casamassimo PS. Using anticipatory guidance to provide early dental intervention. *J Am Dent Assoc*. 1995;126:1155–1163.

24. Nowak AJ, Casamassimo PS. The dental home: a primary care concept. *J Am Dent Assoc*. 2002;133:93–98.

25. Dye BA, Tan S, Smith V, et al. Trends in oral health status: United States 1988-1994 and 1999-2004. *Vital Health Stat 11*. 2007;(248):1–92.

26. Gagon F, Catellier P, Artieu-Gauthier I, et al. Compliance with fluoride supplements provided by a dental hygienist in homes of low-income parents of preschool children in Quebec. *J Public Health Dent*. 2007;67:60–63.

27. Nowak AJ, Casamassimo PS. The dental home. In: Berg JH, Slayton RL, eds. *Early Childhood Oral Health*. Singapore: Wiley-Blackwell; 2009:154–169.

28. Coulter C, Brill W. Benefits of establishing a dental home: a retrospective chart review. Poster presentation, American Academy of Pediatric Dentistry, 2007, San Antonio.

29. Lee G, Getzin A, Indurkhya A, et al. Changes in referrals and oral findings after implementation of an oral health program at the Children's Hospital Primary Care Clinic. Poster presentation, American Academy of Pediatric Dentistry, May 2007, San Antonio.

30. Savage M, Lee J, Kotch J, et al. Early preventive dental visits: effect on subsequent utilization and costs. *Pediatrics*. 2004;114:418–423.

31. American Academy of Pediatric Dentistry. Policy on the dental home. *Pediatr Dent*. 2011;33(special issue):24–25.

32. Deleted in review.

33. American Academy of Pediatric Dentistry. Guideline on fluoride therapy. *Pediatr Dent*. 2011;33(special issue):153–156.

34. Griffin SO, Jones K, Tomar SL. An economic evaluation of community water fluoridation. *J Public Health Dent*. 2001;61:78–86.

35. US Department of Health, Education, and Welfare. Evaluatory Surveys of Long-Term Fluoridation Show Improved Dental Health, USPHS Publication No. 84-22647. Atlanta, March 1979.

36. Brunelle JA, Carlos JP. Recent trends in dental caries in U.S. children and the effect of water fluoridation. *J Dent Res*. 1990;69(special issue):723–727.

37. Centers for Disease Control and Prevention. Populations receiving optimally fluoridated public drinking water–United States, 2000. *MMWR Morb Mortal Wkly Rep*. 2002;51:144–147.

38. Centers for Disease Control and Prevention. Community water fluoridation: statistics. www.cdc.gov/fluoridation/basics/index.htm. Accessed March 26, 2017.

39. ADA Division of Communication. For the dental patient. The facts about bottled water. *J Am Dent Assoc*. 2003;134:1287.

40. Hogan C. U.S. consumption of bottled water shows continued growth, increasing 6.2 percent in 2012; sales up 6.7 percent. www.bottledwater.org/us-consumption-bottled-water-shows-continued-growth-increasing-62-percent-2012-sales-67-percent. Accessed March 26, 2017.

41. Flaitz CM, Hill EM, Hicks MJ. A survey of bottled water usage by pediatric dental patients: implications for dental health. *Quintessence Int*. 1989;20:847–852.

42. Johnson SA, DeBiase C. Concentration levels of fluoride in bottled drinking water. *J Dent Hyg*. 2003;77:161–197.

43. Nowak AJ, Nowak MV. Fluoride concentration of bottled and processed waters. *Iowa Dent J*. 1989;75:28.

44. Stannard J, Rovero J, Tsamtsouris A, et al. Fluoride content of some bottled waters and recommendations for fluoride supplementation. *J Pedod*. 1990;14:103–107.

45. Tate WH, Snyder R, Montgomery EH, et al. Impact of source of drinking water on fluoride supplementation. *Pediatrics*. 1990;86:419–421.

46. Driscoll W. The use of fluoride tablets for the prevention of dental caries. In: Forrester D, Schultz E, eds. *International Workshop on Fluorides and Dental Caries Reductions*. Baltimore: University of Maryland; 1974:25–96.

47. Hargreaves JA. Water fluoridation and fluoride supplementation: considerations for the future. Proceedings of a Joint IADR/ORCA International Symposium on Fluorides: mechanisms of action and recommendations. *J Dent Res*. 1990;69(special issue): 765–770.

48. Thylstrup A. Clinical evidence of the role of pre-eruptive fluoride in caries prevention. *J Dent Res*. 1990;69(special issue):742–750.

49. Levy SM, Kiritsy MC, Slager SL, et al. Patterns of dietary fluoride supplement use during infancy. *J Public Health Dent*. 1998;58:228–233.

50. Hennon DK, Stookey GK, Muhler JC. The clinical anticariogenic effectiveness of supplementary fluoride-vitamin preparations. Results at the end of three years. *J Dent Child*. 1996;33:3–11.

51. Centers for Disease Control and Prevention. My water's fluoride. https://nccd.cdc.gov/DOH_MWF/Default/Default.aspx. Accessed March 26, 2017.

52. Edelstein BL, Cottrel D, O'Sullivan D, et al. Comparison of colorimeter and electrode analysis of water fluoride. *Pediatr Dent*. 1992;14:47–49.

53. American Dental Association. Evidence-based clinical recommendations on the prescription of dietary fluoride supplements for caries prevention. Council on Scientific Affairs. *J Am Dent Assoc*. 2010;141:1480–1489.

54. Tinanoff N. Use of fluoride. In: Berg JH, Slayton RL, eds. *Early Childhood Oral Health*. 1st ed. Singapore: Wiley-Blackwell; 2009:92–109.

55. American Dental Association. Evidence-based clinical recommendations regarding fluoride intake from reconstituted infant formula and enamel fluorosis. *J Am Dent Assoc*. 2011;142:79–87.

56. Pendrys DG, Stamm JW. Relationship of total fluoride intake to beneficial effects and enamel fluorosis. *J Dent Res*. 1990;69(special issue):529–538.

57. Johnson J Jr, Bawden JW. The fluoride content of infant formula available in 1985. *Pediatr Dent*. 1987;9:33–37.

58. Clovis J, Hargreaves JA. Fluoride intake from beverage consumption. *Community Dent Oral Epidemiol*. 1988;16:11–15.

59. Food and Drug Administration. Statements of general policy or interpretation, oral prenatal drugs containing fluoride for human use. *Fed Reg*. October 20 1966.

60. Ekstrand J, Whitford GM. Fluoride metabolism. In: Ekstrand J, Fejerskow O, Siluentone LM, eds. *Fluoride in Dentistry*. Copenhagen: Munksgaard; 1988:165–166.

61. Shen YW, Taves DR. Fluoride concentrations in the human placenta and maternal and cord blood. *Am J Obstet Gynecol*. 1974;19:205–207.

62. Leverett DH, Adair SM, Vaughan BW, et al. Randomized clinical trial of the effect of prenatal fluoride supplements in preventing caries. *Caries Res*. 1997;31:174–179.

63. American Academy of Pediatric Dentistry. Guideline on oral health care for the pregnant adolescent. *Pediatr Dent*. 2011;33(special issue):137–141.

64. Weintraub JA, Ramos-Gomez F, June B. Fluoride varnish efficacy in preventing early childhood caries. *J Dent Res*. 2006;85:172–176.

65. American Dental Association, Council on Scientific Affairs. Professionally applied topical fluoride. *J Am Dent Assoc*. 2006;137:1151–1159.

66. Food and Drug Administration. Use of approved drugs for unlabeled indications. *FDA Drug Bull*. 1982;12:4–5.

67. American Association of Poison Control Centers. 2010 Annual Report of the National Poison Data System (NPDS): 28th Annual Report. *Clin Toxicol*. 2011;49:910–941.

68. Deleted in review.

69. American Academy of Pediatrics. Poison treatment in the home. American Academy of Pediatrics Committee on Injury, Violence and Poison Prevention. *Pediatrics*. 2003;112:1182–1185.

70. Crall JJ. Biological implications and dietary supplementation. In: Pinkham JR, ed. *Pediatric Dental Care: An Update for the 90s*. Evansville, IN: Bristol-Myers Squibb; 1991:25–27.

71. Tinanoff N. Comment on urinary excretion of fluoride following ingestion of MFP toothpastes by infants ages two to six years. *Pediatr Dent*. 1985;7:345.

72. Kuthy RA, McTigue DJ. Fluoride prescription practices of Ohio physicians. *J Public Health Dent*. 1987;47:172–176.

73. Woolfolk NW, Faja BW, Bagramian RA. Relation of sources of systemic fluoride to prevalence of dental fluorosis. *J Public Health Dent*. 1989;49:78–82.

74. Stephan RM. Changes in the hydrogen ion concentration on tooth surfaces and in carious lesions. *J Am Dent Assoc*. 1940;27:718–723.

75. Rugg-Gunn AJ, Roberts GJ, Wright WG. Effect of human milk on plaque pH in situ and enamel dissolution in vitro compared with bovine milk, lactose and sucrose. *Caries Res*. 1985;19:327–334.

76. Centers for Disease Control and Prevention. Breastfeeding report card—United States; 2014. https://www.cdc.gov/breastfeeding/pdf/2014breastfeedingreportcard.pdf. Accessed March 26, 2017.

77. United States Breastfeeding Committee. Healthy people 2020: breastfeeding objectives. http://www.usbreastfeeding.org/p/cm/ld/fid=221. Accessed January 8, 2018.

78. Erickson P, Mazhari E. Investigation of the role of human breast milk in caries development. *Pediatr Dent*. 1999;21:86–90.

79. Hallonsten AL, Wendt LK, Mejere I, et al. Dental caries and prolonged breast feeding in 18-month-old Swedish children. *Int J Paediatr Dent*. 1995;5:149–155.

80. American Academy of Pediatrics. Breastfeeding and the use of human milk. *Pediatrics*. 2005;115(2):496–506.

81. Fomon S. *Nutrition of Normal Infants*. St Louis: Mosby; 1993.

82. American Academy of Pediatrics. The use and misuse of fruit juice in pediatrics. *Pediatrics*. 2000;107:1210–1213.

83. Li Y, Caufield PW, Dasanayake HW, et al. Mode of delivery and other maternal factors influence the acquisition of *Streptococcus mutans* in infants. *J Dent Res*. 2005;84(9):806–811.

16

Introduction to Dental Trauma: Managing Traumatic Injuries in the Primary Dentition

GIDEON HOLAN AND DENNIS J. MCTIGUE

CHAPTER OUTLINE

An injury to the teeth of a young child can have serious and long-term consequences, leading to their discoloration, malformation, or possible loss. The emotional impact of such an injury can be far-reaching. It is therefore important that the dentist treating children is:

1. Knowledgeable in the techniques for managing traumatic injuries
2. Readily available during and after office hours to provide treatment

If either of these conditions cannot be met, the child suffering a dental injury should immediately be referred to a specialist.

The purpose of this chapter is to provide a straightforward approach to managing dental injuries in the primary dentition. Techniques for diagnosis, treatment, and follow-up care are described. Fundamental issues covered in this chapter—such as the classification of injuries, history, examination, and pathologic sequelae of trauma—pertain to both the primary and permanent dentitions. Chapter 35 will focus on the management of injuries to young permanent teeth and will refer to this chapter for the information just noted. The principles gleaned from both chapters should enable the dentist to manage the great majority of dental injuries encountered in children.

Etiology and Epidemiology of Trauma in the Primary Dentition

The most frequently injured teeth in the primary dentition are the maxillary incisors. Primary molars are rarely injured, and when injury occurs, it is usually due to indirect trauma (e.g., blows to the underside of the chin, causing the mandible to close forcefully against the maxilla).[1] Primary incisors tend to be luxated more than permanent teeth. This is due to the spongy nature of the bone in young children and to the lower root/crown ratio in comparison with that of permanent teeth. It has been reported that injuries occurring while a child is using a pacifier tend to be tooth displacement rather than fractures.[2]

Although reports of injuries in preschool children presenting for dental treatment show that the majority of children suffer from luxation injuries,[3,4] epidemiologic studies in the community show that crown fractures (mainly enamel fractures) are the most common injuries to the primary teeth.[5–8] It has also been found that the incidence of an injury is higher among children who have already experienced a previous traumatic crown fracture.[9] These injuries, however, may result in only minor inconveniences that do not motivate parents to seek professional dental advice.

By the age of 5 years, up to 40% of boys and 30% of girls have experienced traumatic injuries to their teeth.[10] The peak age of injuries to the primary teeth is 2 to 4 years when children are developing mobility skills.[11] Children with protruding incisors, as in developing class II malocclusions, are two to three times more likely to suffer dental trauma than children with normal incisal overjets.[12–16]

Another major cause of dental injuries in young children is automobile accidents. Unrestrained children who are seated or standing often hit the dashboard or windshield when the car is stopped suddenly. All states now have laws mandating the use of child restraints in automobiles, and it is hoped that universal adoption of these laws will decrease the incidence of such trauma to children.[17]

Children with chronic seizure disorders experience an increased incidence of dental trauma. Frequently, these high-risk children wear protective headgear, and the fabrication of custom mouth guards for them is indicated as well (see Chapter 41).

Another serious cause of dental injuries to young children is child abuse. Often overlooked by the dental profession, up to 50% of abused children suffer injuries to the head and neck. Cardinal signs of abuse are injuries in various stages of healing, tears of labial frena, repeated injuries, and injuries whose clinical presentation is not consistent with the history reported by the parent.[5] Battered children frequently lie to protect their parents or out of fear of retaliation. Dentists are required by law to report cases of suspected child abuse (see Chapter 11 for more specific details).

Classification of Injuries to Teeth

Tooth fractures may involve the crown, root, or both (Figs. 16.1–16.3; see also Figs. 35.1–35.3). Fractures of the crown may be limited to the enamel, may involve the dentin, or may include the pulp. Injury to the pulp is the most complicated and demanding to manage.

As just mentioned, luxation (displacement) injuries are the most common types of injuries to primary teeth that are treated in the dental office. These injuries damage supporting structures of the teeth, which include the periodontal ligament (PDL) and the alveolar bone (see Fig. 16.1). The PDL is the physiologic "hammock" that supports the tooth in its socket. Maintaining its vitality is the primary objective in the management of all luxation injuries. Several types of luxation injury occur.[10]

1. Concussion: The tooth is not mobile and is not displaced. The PDL absorbs the injury and is inflamed, which leaves the tooth tender to biting pressure and percussion.
2. Subluxation: The tooth is loosened but is not displaced from its socket.
3. Intrusion: The tooth is driven into its socket. This compresses the PDL and commonly causes a crushing fracture of the alveolar socket (Fig. 16.4 and see Fig. 35.15).
4. Extrusion: This is a central dislocation of the tooth from its socket (Fig. 16.5 and see Fig. 35.16A). The PDL is usually torn in this injury.
5. Lateral luxation: The tooth is displaced in a labial, lingual, or lateral direction. The PDL is torn, and contusion or fracture of the supporting alveolar bone occurs (Fig. 16.6 and see Fig. 35.16B).
6. Avulsion: The tooth is completely displaced from the alveolus. The PDL is severed, and fractures of the alveolus may occur (Fig. 16.7 and see Fig. 35.17).

History

Obtaining an adequate medical and dental history is essential to proper diagnosis and treatment. The medical history should

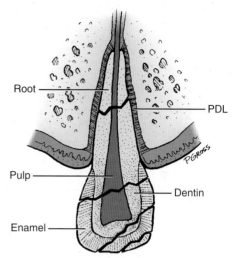

• **Figure 16.1** Classification of tooth injuries. Tooth fractures may involve enamel, dentin, or pulp and may occur in the crown or the root. *PDL*, Periodontal ligament.

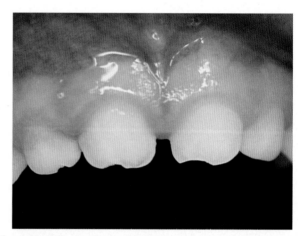

• **Figure 16.2** Fracture of enamel and dentin in both maxillary primary central incisors.

already be on record if the child suffering an injury is brought to his or her regular dentist. Frequently, however, a parent will take an injured child to the closest dentist or to one known to treat children. Thus, with the confusion of a young injured child entering the office for possibly the first time and disrupting the day's schedule, the potential to forget to gather important historical information is great. The use of a trauma assessment form to help record data and organize the management of care is highly recommended (Fig. 16.8).

Medical History

Routine data on the patient's general health should be obtained. Historical information particularly relevant to the dental injury includes the following:

1. Cardiac disease, which may necessitate prophylaxis against infectious endocarditis
2. Bleeding disorders
3. Allergies to medications
4. Seizure disorders
5. Medications
6. Status of tetanus prophylaxis

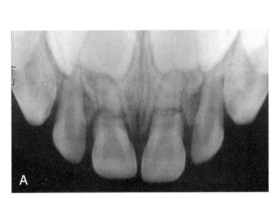
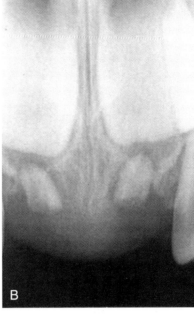

• **Figure 16.3** (A) Root fracture of both maxillary primary central incisors. (B) Apical fragments of the root fractured maxillary primary central incisors after extraction of the coronal fragments.

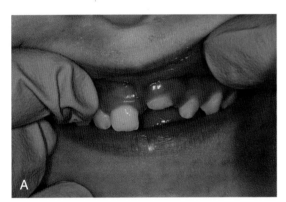
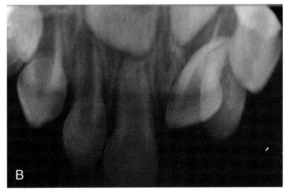

• **Figure 16.4** (A) Intruded maxillary left primary central incisor. (B) Periapical radiograph showing the left maxillary primary central incisor after intrusion. The shortened and more opaque image of the intruded tooth, as compared with that of the right central incisor, indicates that the root has been pushed labially and away from the underlying permanent tooth. (From McTigue DJ. Managing injuries to the primary dentition. *Dent Clin North Am.* 2009;53[4]:627–638.)

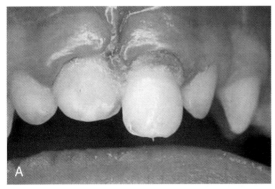
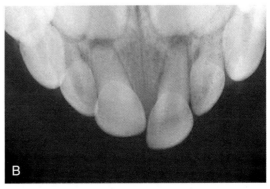

• **Figure 16.5** Extrusion of the left maxillary primary central incisor. (A) Clinical view. (B) Radiographic view. Notice the pulp canal obliteration in the right maxillary primary central incisor, which resulted from a previous injury.

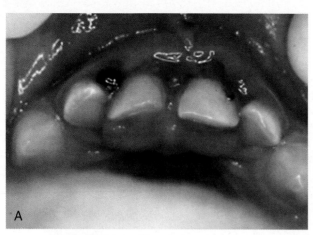 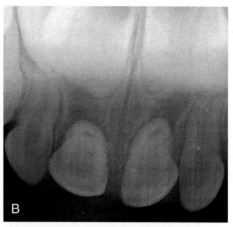

• **Figure 16.6** Lingual luxation of both maxillary primary central incisors. (A) Clinical view. (B) Radiographic view.

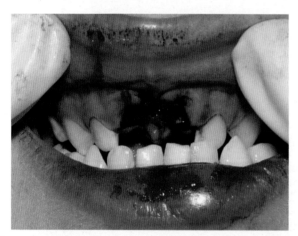

• **Figure 16.7** Avulsion of maxillary right and left primary central incisors.

The issue of tetanus protection is particularly important when a child has suffered a dirty wound (an avulsion), a deep laceration, or an intrusion injury in which soil is embedded in the tissues. Wounds containing necrotic tissue, dirt, and foreign material should be cleaned and debrided as an essential part of tetanus prophylaxis. Children acquire active immunity through a series of five injections of adsorbed tetanus toxoid, usually completed by the age of 4 to 6 years. These are normally administered as part of the diphtheria-tetanus-pertussis immunizations. Children should then receive a booster of tetanus toxoid at 11 to 12 years of age and again 5 years later.[18] An increasing number of reports have indicated that children in the United States are not receiving their childhood immunizations appropriately. If there is any question about the adequacy of a child's tetanus protection, the child's physician should immediately be consulted.

History of the Dental Injury

Three important questions are asked in gathering the dental history: *when, where,* and *how* did the accident occur? The time elapsed since the injury occurred is a major factor in determining the type of treatment to be provided. The dentist should also determine whether the tooth had been injured previously or whether the injury had first been treated elsewhere.

Where the injury occurred sheds light on its severity. Did the toddler slip and hit the coffee table in the living room, or did she fall off her parent's bicycle in the park? This information can help to determine the need for tetanus prophylaxis as well as signal a need to rule out more serious injury to the child.

How the accident occurred obviously provides the dentist with the most information regarding severity. Serious head injuries should be ruled out by asking if the child lost consciousness, has vomited, or is disoriented as a result of the accident. Positive findings indicate potential central nervous system injury, and medical consultation should be immediately obtained.[19] Significant head injuries can lead to symptoms many hours after the initial trauma in such cases parents are cautioned to watch for the signs noted previously for 24 hours, which includes waking the child every 2 to 3 hours through the night.[20–22]

As previously discussed, the possibility of child abuse can also be ruled out through a careful dental history. Any history of previous dental injuries should also be determined because their sequelae may complicate diagnosis of the current injury.

Directing attention to the specific teeth involved, the dentist should ask the child if there is spontaneous pain from any teeth. Positive findings here may indicate pulp inflammation that is due to a fractured crown or injuries to the supporting structures, such as the extravasation of blood into the PDL. Does the child experience a thermal change with sweet or sour foods? If so, dentin or pulp may be exposed. Are the teeth tender to the touch or tender while chewing? Does the child note a change in occlusion? These findings may indicate a luxation injury or an alveolar fracture.

Oral Health Quality of Life

"Does impaired dental esthetics following traumatic injuries to the primary dentition affect the child's quality of life"? This question was investigated, and contradictory findings were presented. One study found that 4- to 5-year-olds have negative social perceptions and self-perceptions regarding altered dental esthetics,[23] while other publications reported that the oral health-related quality of life of the children and their families was not influenced by traumatic dental injuries.[24,25]

Clinical Examination

Once the medical and dental histories are complete, the dentist is ready to begin the clinical examination. It is very tempting to focus immediately on a fractured or displaced tooth and thus miss other important injuries. A disciplined approach to a complete clinical examination should be followed in diagnosing every traumatic injury.

Extraoral Examination

A complete examination should rule out injuries to the child's facial bones. The facial skeleton should be palpated to determine discontinuities of facial bones.[26] Extraoral wounds and bruises should be recorded. The temporomandibular joints should be palpated, and any swelling, clicking, or crepitus should be noted. Mandibular function in all excursive movements should be checked. Any stiffness or pain in the child's neck necessitates immediate referral to a physician to rule out cervical spine injury.

Intraoral Examination

All soft tissues should be examined and any injuries recorded. The presence of foreign matter in lacerations of the lips and cheeks, such as tooth fragments or soil, should be identified. Removal at the initial appointment will eliminate chronic infection and disfiguring fibrosis.

The occlusion should be checked to identify possible occlusal disturbances that may result from oral luxation of the maxillary incisors.

Each tooth in the mouth should be examined for fracture, pulp exposure, and dislocation. In some crown fractures, only a very thin layer of dentin remains over the pulp, so that the pulp's outline can be seen as a pink tinge on the dentin. The dentist should be very careful not to perforate this dentin with an instrument.

SCHOOL of DENTISTRY
DEPARTMENT of PEDIATRIC DENTISTRY

Child's Name ____________ Student ____________
Age ______ Sex ______ Race ______ Faculty ____________
Place of Injury ____________ Chart No. ______ Date ______
Date of Injury ____________
Time of Injury ____________
Time Elapsed Since Injury ____________

HISTORY
Chief Complaint ____________ Previous Trauma ____________
Past Medical History ____________
Past Dental History ____________
How Injury Occurred ____________
Tetanus Protection: ☐ No Yes ☐ Date of Last Booster ____________

EXTRAORAL ASSESSMENT

CNS Status
☐ Unconsciousness ☐ Amnesia
☐ Unequal Pupil Size ☐ Headache
☐ Fixed Pupil ☐ Nausea
☐ CSF from Ears ☐ Disorientation
☐ CSF from Nose ☐ Loss of Smell
☐ Nystagmus ☐ Seizure
☐ Vertigo
Describe ____________

Hard Tissue
☐ Cranial Fracture ☐ Zygoma Fracture
☐ Mandibular Fracture ☐ Infection
☐ Maxillary Fracture
Describe ____________

Soft Tissue
☐ Laceration ☐ Abrasion
☐ Contusions ☐ Infection
☐ Swelling ☐ Embedded Material
Describe ____________

INTRAORAL ASSESSMENT

Hard Tissue
☐ Alveolar Fracture ☐ Palatal Fracture
Describe ____________

Soft Tissue
☐ Lips ☐ Frenum
☐ Buccal Mucosa ☐ Tongue
☐ Gingiva ☐ Palate
Describe ____________

Dental Occlussion
Molar ______ Cuspid ______
Overjet ______ mm Overbite ______ %
Open Bite ______ Crossbite ______
Classification Deviation Induced by Trauma ______
Describe ____________

RADIOGRAPHS
☐ Periapical ☐ Occlusal
☐ Lateral Anterior ☐ Panorex
Other ____________
Pathology ____________

• **Figure 16.8**

Continued

DENTAL FINDINGS

| Fracture | Class I | Class II | Class III | Class IV |

Draw Injury

41   42   31   32

12   11   21   22

Involved Teeth _____

Tooth Response — Pulp and PDL

Tooth No.			
Exposure			
Hemorrhage			
Heat			
Cold			
Contamination			
Percussion			
Mobility			
Vitalometer			

Displacement
□ Intrusion   □ Subluxation
□ Extrusion   □ Lateral Luxation
□ Avulsion

Color
□ Normal   □ Dark   □ Light

SUMMARY AND DIAGNOSIS

Crown _____

Pulp _____

Root _____

Periapical Tissue _____

Alveolar Process _____

Root Displacement _____

Restoration _____
Fragments _____

TREATMENT

Soft Tissues _____
Pulp _____
Restoration _____
Splinting _____
Medication _____

Recall Follow-up
□ 2 weeks   □ 3 weeks   □ 6 weeks
□ 3 months   □ 6 months
Other _____

• **Figure 16.8, cont'd** Trauma assessment form. *CNS,* Central nervous system; *CSF,* cerebrospinal fluid; *PDL,* periodontal ligament.

Displacement of teeth should be recorded, as well as horizontal and vertical tooth mobility. Increased mobility of an injured primary tooth is an indication of damage to the PDL unless the tooth is near natural exfoliation. Reaction to palpation and percussion of teeth is recorded. Percussion sensitivity is a good indicator of PDL inflammation.

Pulpal vitality testing is not routinely performed in the primary dentition. This is because the testing requires a relaxed and cooperative patient who can report reactions objectively, and some young children lack the ability to do so.

Radiographic Examination

Indications for Radiographs

Radiographs are an important part of the diagnosis and management of dental injuries. They allow the clinician to detect root fractures, extent of root development, size of pulp chambers, periapical radiolucencies, extent and type of root resorption, degree of tooth displacement, position of unerupted teeth, relationship between the injured primary teeth and their permanent successors, jaw fractures, and the presence of tooth fragments and other foreign bodies in soft tissues. Although some radiographs will show negative findings at the initial appointment, they are nonetheless important as baseline documentation. Subsequent radiographic evidence can thus be compared with the initial films.

Radiographic Techniques

There is no "standard series" of radiographs for dental injuries. All films taken should clearly show the apical areas of traumatized teeth (see Fig. 19.15E).

To determine the presence of foreign bodies such as tooth fragments in the lips or tongue, one-fourth of the normal exposure

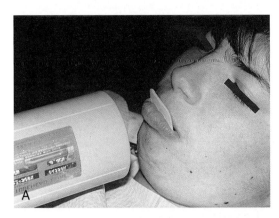

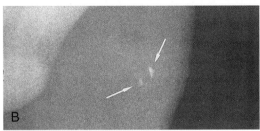

• **Figure 16.9** (A) Positioning film to detect the presence of tooth fragments in the lip. (B) Radiograph demonstrating tooth fragments in lip *(arrows)*.

time is used. The film is placed beneath the tissue to be examined, and the radiograph is exposed (Fig. 16.9).

Timing of Follow-up Radiographs

As noted previously, many pathologic changes are not immediately apparent in radiographs. After approximately 3 weeks, periapical radiolucencies that are due to pulpal necrosis can usually be detected. In addition, inflammatory root resorption may be evident at this time. After approximately 6 to 7 weeks, replacement resorption, or ankylosis, can be seen. Thus there is adequate rationale to obtain postoperative radiographs at 1 month following the injury. In the absence of any clinical signs or symptoms—such as the development of swelling, fistula, mobility, tooth discoloration, or pain—additional films are not indicated until 6 months after the injury. If changes are to appear radiographically, they usually do so by this time.

Emergency Care

Injuries to the Hard Dental Tissues

Cracks and Fractures of the Enamel and Dentin Without Pulp Exposure

Enamel cracks and small fractures are common findings in primary teeth (see Fig. 16.2). It is believed that even fractures exposing dentin in primary teeth have no deleterious effect on the pulp and need not be covered.[27] In the case of larger fractures, treatment is often indicated to restore esthetics. Various methods have been suggested to restore the fractured crown, including the use of strip crowns, preformed esthetic crowns, and open-faced steel crowns (see Chapter 22).

If it is decided to avoid crown restoration, possibly due to the child's age and/or behavior, sharp edges at the fracture line can be smoothened with abrasive disks to prevent irritation to the tongue

and lips. The exposed dentin should be carefully examined to ensure that there is no exposure of the pulp. If tooth fracture is associated with a wounded lip, then a radiograph of the lip should be obtained to rule out the presence of tooth fragments trapped in the soft tissue (see Fig. 16.9). Late complications, such as coronal discoloration (see later), usually are attributed not to the fractured crown but to overlooked minor displacement of the tooth and obstruction of blood supply to the pulp.

Fractures of the Enamel and Dentin With Pulp Exposure

Deep fracture of the crown may be associated with exposure of the pulp, usually at the pulp horn. If the pulp horn is exposed at its incisal edge, it may not bleed and therefore may go unnoticed. A red point of blood can be seen if the pulp is exposed at a deeper level. If not treated immediately, a widely exposed pulp may proliferate, resulting in a pulp polyp.[28]

Several treatment options are available for crown fracture with pulp exposure in primary teeth, including pulpotomy, root canal treatment, and extraction.[29] The vitality of the tissue and the time elapsed since the injury dictate the treatment of choice. If the pulp tissue is vital, a cervical pulpotomy can be performed (see Chapter 23). Ram and Holan suggest that a partial pulpotomy technique is indicated to preserve pulp vitality in a young primary tooth with a wide-open apex and thin root dentin walls.[30]

Pulp exposure is sometimes overlooked or neglected, and no treatment is rendered. The unavoidable outcome is a necrotic and infected pulp with consequent swelling or fistula. If massive external inflammatory root resorption is detected or if the follicle of the underlying permanent tooth bud is involved in the inflammatory process, the tooth must be extracted as soon as possible. Leaving such teeth untreated increases the risk of damage to the permanent incisor. If there is no evidence of inflammatory external root resorption, some clinicians attempt to save these teeth with complete pulpectomies. The principle of this treatment is complete removal of the necrotic pulp, filling the pulp canal with a resorbable paste, and providing esthetic restoration of the crown. (For further details, see Chapter 23.)

Permanent incisors succeeding infected and root-treated primary incisors show mild enamel defects that could be attributed to both the inflammatory process and overinstrumentation during the endodontic procedure.[31]

Crown-Root Fractures

Fractures involving both the crown and the root of primary teeth are rare. The teeth in this type of injury are split into two or more fragments, with one main fragment remaining firm and the other fragment becoming loose because of injury to its periodontal fibers (Fig. 16.10). The two fragments should be separated to determine whether the pulp has been exposed. The loose fragment should be removed, allowing inspection of the main fragment's exposed dentin. Pulpotomy is the suggested treatment for such exposures, with subsequent esthetic reconstruction of the crown. If the fracture goes deep into the alveolus, creating a periodontal pocket in the space previously occupied by the loose fragment, both fragments should be extracted.

Root Fractures

Root fractures are also rare in primary teeth.[32] Both fragments may remain close to each other, with the tooth presenting slight mobility and sensitivity to percussion (see Fig. 16.3). If the coronal fragment is pushed away from the apical part of the root, it frequently assumes a lingual inclination that may interfere with the occlusion unless the child has an open bite. In this case, the coronal fragment should be extracted. Attempts to remove the apical fragment should be avoided, as such action may harm the developing permanent successor. These apical fragments usually resorb as part of the physiologic process of tooth replacement.[32] If no disturbance to the child's occlusion exists, the tooth may be left untreated and the parents provided with instruction for thorough oral hygiene and soft diet for a limited time (see "Information and Instructions for Parents," later in this chapter). The PDL attached to the mobile coronal fragment may recover, with decrease in tooth mobility and sensitivity to percussion. Unlike permanent teeth, there is no intention to cause repair of the fracture with calcified tissue in root-fractured primary teeth; thus immobilization of the tooth, though reported in the literature as a treatment option,[33] is unnecessary. Splinting the tooth is recommended only to alleviate sensitivity during routine function.

Injuries to the Chin

An injury to the chin may produce a sudden forceful closure of the mandibular teeth with their maxillary opponents. As a result, a wide range of injuries may affect molar teeth.[34] These include minor enamel fractures, fractures with dentin exposure that may imitate a carious lesion on the radiograph, crown root fractures with or without pulp exposure,[35] and injuries to the

PDL.[36] In addition, fracture of the mandible may occur mainly in the symphysis, mental, and subcondylar areas (Fig. 16.11).[37] These injuries have also been correlated with cervical spine fractures.[38]

The exposed dentin in fractured posterior teeth increases the risk of pulp irritation and may become carious. It can therefore be covered by a composite resin if the area of exposure is small. If the fracture is large or extends below the gum line, a stainless steel crown is preferable. When the pulp is exposed and the crown restorable, pulpotomy and a stainless steel crown is the treatment of choice. Otherwise the tooth must be extracted and space maintenance considered.

Injuries to the Supporting Tissues

Concussion and Subluxation

Teeth suffering concussion injuries are sensitive to percussion without any additional sign. Subluxated teeth also present increased mobility and widening of the periodontal space. If the teeth are examined shortly after the injury, signs of bleeding from the gingival crevice can be seen (Fig. 16.12). Concussion and subluxation are mild injuries that often go unnoticed. Parents, if questioned, may recall the injury when a late complication develops, such as tooth discoloration (see "Coronal Discoloration").[39]

Usually no treatment is required except for a soft diet for a limited time and thorough oral hygiene to prevent contamination of the damaged PDL (see "Information and Instructions for Parents").

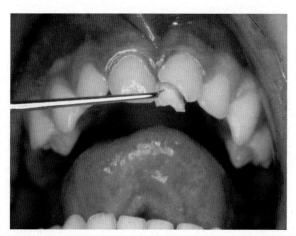

• **Figure 16.10** Clinical view of a left maxillary primary central incisor with crown-root fracture. The palatal fragment is mobile and attached by gingival fibers only.

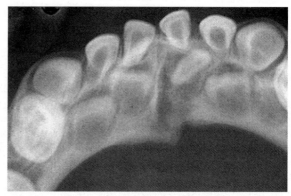

• **Figure 16.11** Fracture of the mandible in a baby as a result of trauma to the chin.

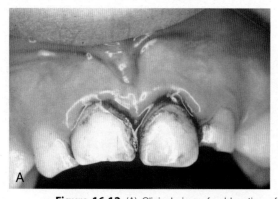

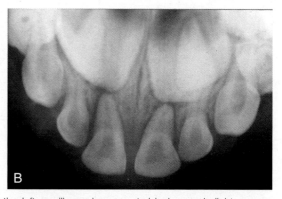

• **Figure 16.12** (A) Clinical view of subluxation of the left maxillary primary central incisor and slight extrusion of the adjacent central incisor. (B) Radiograph of both teeth showing widening of the periodontal ligament.

Intrusion

Intrusion is one of the most complicated injuries to the primary incisors. Clinically, the tooth may disappear completely into the surrounding tissues, or the incisal part may remain visible with its clinical crown shorter than that of an adjacent nontraumatized tooth. Following intrusion the PDL is compressed and the root surface is tightly pressed against the alveolar bone, resulting in reduced mobility. Percussion of an intruded tooth produces a metallic sound and does not provoke pain. Bleeding from the gingival sulcus is visible shortly after the injury. A swollen upper lip due to edema and/or hemorrhage can often be seen.

The root of the primary incisor is normally close to the labial surface of the permanent tooth. If the root of the primary tooth is pushed against the crown of the permanent incisor, it may severely damage the developing tooth bud. Immediate removal of the primary tooth may relieve the pressure and minimize the damage.[40] It is therefore extremely important to determine as soon as possible after the injury if the root of the primary tooth contacts the permanent tooth or has been pushed labially and away from the labial surface of the permanent successor. Fortunately, the root apex of maxillary primary incisors has a labial curvature, leading the root away from the permanent tooth in more than 80% of cases.[41]

Several clinical and radiographic signs support the diagnosis of labial alignment of the root:
- Palatal inclination of the crown
- Hemorrhage and hard swelling palpated in the vestibule due to fracture of the labial bone plate by the root of the primary tooth
- A shortened and more opaque image of an intruded incisor as compared with an adjacent nondisplaced tooth (see Fig. 16.4)
- Proper alignment of the permanent successor as seen on a periapical radiograph

Absence of such signs should alert the operator to suspect palatal displacement of the primary tooth root with subsequent displacement of the permanent tooth.

Some authors suggest the use of lateral extraoral radiographs, although a study has shown that this technique does not contribute to assessment of the relation between the root of the intruded tooth and the labial surface of the permanent tooth. In addition, it is only beneficial in children younger than 20 months.[42]

Intruded incisors that do not risk the permanent teeth can be left to spontaneously reerupt. Reeruption begins within 2 to 3 weeks but can be delayed for more than 6 months. In many cases the teeth do not erupt back to their original position but into a rotated alignment (see Fig. 16.23, later). An estimate of reeruption can be made by measuring the distance between the incisal edge of a partially intruded tooth and a tongue depressor placed between fully erupted teeth on either side of the intruded tooth (Fig. 16.13). Repeated measurements at recall visits allow estimation of the rate of reeruption. It should be emphasized that increase of the clinical crown (the distance between the incisal edge and the gingival margins) is not an indication of reeruption. Decrease in the size of edematous gums may erroneously be viewed as reeruption. Surgical reposition and splinting of the intruded primary incisor has also been suggested as a treatment option.[43–45]

Extrusion

An extruded tooth is clinically elongated relative to adjacent unaffected teeth. The tooth presents increased mobility and sensitivity to percussion. Bleeding from the gingival sulcus can be seen shortly

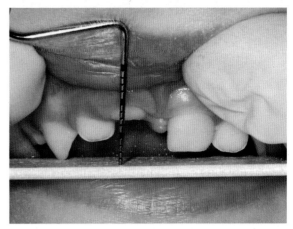

• **Figure 16.13** Measuring the positions of intruded maxillary right primary incisors relative to their antimeres using a tongue depressor.

after the injury. A periapical radiograph of an extruded tooth will show widening of the PDL, especially around the apex (see Fig. 16.5). The more the tooth moves out of the alveolar socket, the higher the chances of disruption of the blood supply and development of pulp necrosis. Extrusions resemble lingual luxation in many features; thus the approach to both types of injuries should be similar (see later).

Lingual Luxation

In the case of lingual luxations, the crown moves in a palatal direction while the apex is pushed labially. It is sometimes difficult to distinguish between lingual luxation and intrusion. The palatal inclination of the crown may interfere with the occlusion unless the child has an open bite. The tooth presents increased mobility and sensitivity to percussion. Signs of bleeding may be evident around the tooth (see Fig. 16.6A). The upper lip is often swollen, with signs of hemorrhage due to fracture of the labial bone plate by the tooth apex. A periapical radiograph will show a radiolucent gap between the apex and the alveolar bone (see Fig. 16.6B). The luxated tooth presents a shortened and more opaque image as compared with an adjacent unaffected tooth.

Many clinicians recommend extraction of severely luxated primary teeth because they may potentially damage the succeeding permanent incisor. Some parents insist that everything be done to save anterior primary teeth, and if the child is seen shortly after the injury and before the formation of a coagulum, the tooth can be repositioned. The tooth must then be splinted for 7 to 14 days, and root canal treatment is indicated because rupture of the blood supply to the pulp is expected in cases of severe luxation.[31] The cost-benefit ratio of retaining these teeth and the potential for injury to the succeeding permanent teeth must be explained to the parents.

In the case of open bite without occlusal interference, the functional forces of the tongue may push the crown into a labial position. Occlusal interferences can sometimes be eliminated by creating an intentional open bite by adding composite "buttons" to the occlusal surface of the maxillary or mandibular first molars. These are removed as soon as the functional forces push the lingually luxated tooth into its original position. This technique is indicated when the luxated teeth are seen after the formation of a blood clot in the alveolus several hours after the injury. Extraction of the luxated teeth is indicated in the case of severe fracture of the labial bone plate.

Parents should be provided with strict instructions for good oral hygiene to prevent migration of microorganisms between the root and the gums with subsequent infection of the PDL (see "Information and Instructions for Parents").

Avulsion

Avulsion of a primary incisor is a common outcome of dental trauma in young children (see Fig. 16.7). The high crown/root ratio of primary incisors and the resilience of the bone are contributing factors. In about 75% of cases involving avulsion of a primary incisor, the developing permanent successor is damaged.[46] Most articles, textbooks, and guidelines recommend that avulsed primary incisors should not be replanted because the permanent tooth may be damaged during insertion of the root back to its socket.[47,48] Case reports suggest shortening of the root by 2 to 3 mm before replantation to prevent such damage.[49] If a child arrives at the dental office with a tooth that has been avulsed and replanted by his or her parents, the parents should be apprised of the risks and costs versus benefits of keeping that tooth. A splint and root canal treatment with a resorbable paste will be required in the attempt to save the tooth until its natural exfoliation and to prevent inflammatory resorption of the root.

Avulsed primary teeth should be accounted for to rule out potential aspiration. If the tooth cannot be found, the child should be referred for further evaluation by a pediatrician.[50]

Information and Instructions for Parents

Emergency Telephone Call

Diagnosis of traumatic injuries to primary teeth should never be based solely on information provided by parents over the telephone or a text message. Occasionally, however, parents call stating that their child injured a primary tooth and asking how urgent it is to bring the child to the dental office. The dentist's main concerns are risk of damage to the permanent teeth in case of intrusion and risk of aspiration in case of avulsion. So if the injury sounds like a serious luxation, the child should be seen as soon as possible. The management of other conditions can be postponed until the next day without risking the prognosis.

Information and Instructions Provided at the Emergency Visit

Parents should be informed about possible complications of the injury, prognosis of the injury, and the likelihood of damage to the permanent successors. Instructions for parents are aimed at preventing late complications (e.g., infection of the PDL and pulp necrosis) following injuries to the primary teeth and detecting such complications as soon as possible. Early detection allows appropriate treatment that may prevent further damage to the injured primary tooth or to its permanent successor.

In cases of luxation injuries, parents should be given strict instructions for their child's oral hygiene. Thorough cleaning and plaque removal all around the injured teeth are imperative. Application of an antiseptic medicament, such as 0.2% chlorhexidine gluconate, to the injured gingivae can improve the chances for healing. Because preschool children may swallow the solution while rinsing, cotton-tipped applicators soaked with the solution should be used to gently apply the antiseptic to the gingival crevices of the injured teeth. This should be repeated several times a day, especially after meals, for 7 days. At this time the gingival fibers are expected to be healed.

The child should be placed on a soft diet for several days to prevent intense forces on the tooth and to allow its stabilization. Antibiotics are necessary only in cases of severe tooth luxation and heavy damage to the oral soft tissues.

The timing of follow-up examinations is based on the type of injury sustained. Pathologic sequelae such as pulpal necrosis and inflammatory root resorption can frequently be detected radiographically in 1 month. Parents should be instructed to bring the child in earlier if they suspect any deterioration in the condition of the injured teeth, such as redness, swelling, or the appearance of a fistula in the gums above the injured tooth and, in case of discoloration, increased mobility or sensitivity of the tooth.

Pathologic Sequelae of Trauma to the Teeth

Complications following traumatic injuries to primary teeth may appear shortly after the injury (e.g., infection of the PDL or dark discoloration of the crown) or after several months (e.g., yellow discoloration of the crown and external root resorption). It is currently not possible to accurately identify the histopathologic condition of a dental pulp based on clinical symptoms. The following terms describe a spectrum of clinical signs and symptoms that accompany inflammation and degeneration of the pulp and/or PDL.

Reversible Pulpitis

The pulp's initial response to trauma is pulpitis. Capillaries in the tooth become congested, a condition that can be clinically apparent upon transillumination of the crown with a bright light. Teeth with reversible pulpitis may be tender to percussion if the PDL is inflamed (e.g., following a luxation injury). Pulpitis may be totally reversible if the condition causing it is addressed, or it may progress to an irreversible state with necrosis of the pulp.

Infection of the Periodontal Ligament

Infection of the PDL becomes possible when detachment of the gingival fibers from the tooth in a luxation injury allows invasion of microorganisms from the oral cavity along the root to infect the PDL. Loss of alveolar bone support can be seen on a periapical radiograph (Fig. 16.14). This diminishes the healing potential of the supporting tissues. Subsequently, increased tooth mobility accompanied by exudation of pus from the gingival crevice will require extraction of the injured tooth. Parents should be informed about the risk of infection and provided with appropriate instructions to minimize such risk.

Irreversible Pulpitis

Irreversible pulpitis may be acute or chronic, and it may be partial or total. Acute, irreversible pulpitis following a dental injury can be painful if the exudate accompanying the pulpal inflammation cannot vent. Most frequently in children, however, inflammatory exudates are quickly vented and the pulpitis progresses to a chronic, painless condition.

Pulp Necrosis and Infection

Two main mechanisms can explain how the pulp of injured primary teeth becomes necrotic: (1) infection of the pulp in cases of untreated crown fracture with pulp exposure and (2) interrupted blood supply to the pulp through the apex in cases of luxation injury leading to ischemia. Not all luxation injuries result in a necrotic pulp. Surprisingly, intruded primary teeth, unlike permanent teeth, maintain the vitality of their pulp.[41] Though untreated teeth with exposed pulps are expected to develop swelling or fistulas, injured teeth with avascular necrosis may remain asymptomatic both clinically and radiographically.[51] Loss of pulp vitality due to a traumatic injury at an early stage of root development results in the arrest of dentin apposition and cessation of root development (Fig. 16.15).

Periapical radiolucencies indicative of a granuloma or cyst are frequently evident radiographically in necrotic anterior teeth (Fig. 16.16A). In addition, a parulis is often clinically evident at the level of the involved tooth's root apex (see Fig. 16.16B). Controversy exists regarding the most appropriate treatment of primary anterior teeth with necrotic pulps. Some clinicians treat them with a pulpectomy technique similar to that used in permanent teeth.[52] A resorbable paste is packed into the thoroughly cleansed canal (see Chapter 23). Other clinicians choose to extract these teeth because of the potential for damage to the developing permanent tooth buds. It is generally agreed that pulpectomy is contraindicated in primary teeth with gross loss of root structure, advanced internal or external resorption, or periapical infection involving the crypt of the succedaneous tooth.

Coronal Discoloration

As a result of trauma, the capillaries in the pulp occasionally hemorrhage, leaving blood pigments deposited in the dentinal tubules. In mild cases, the blood is resorbed and very little discoloration occurs, or that which is present becomes lighter in several weeks. In more severe cases, the discoloration persists for the life of the tooth (Fig. 16.17).

From a diagnostic standpoint, discoloration of primary teeth does not necessarily mean that the tooth is nonvital, particularly when the discoloration occurs 1 or 2 days after the injury. Dark discoloration that persists for weeks or months after the injury is more indicative of a necrotic pulp.[51,53] Nevertheless, in the primary dentition of a healthy child, color change alone does not indicate

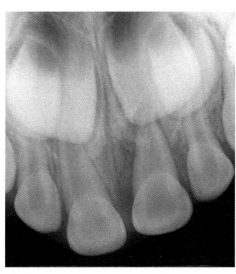

• **Figure 16.14** Infection of the periodontal ligament. This radiograph shows the left maxillary primary central incisor following injury to the supporting tissues. Infection of the attachment apparatus resulted in loss of alveolar bone at the medial aspect of the root.

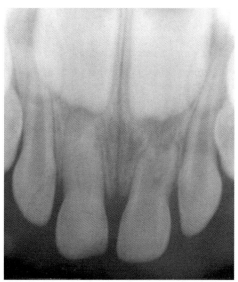

• **Figure 16.15** Periapical radiograph of the premaxilla of a 42-month-old child. Both maxillary primary central incisors were injured at 18 months. The left incisor presents arrest of dentin apposition due to pulp necrosis. The pulp of the fractured right incisor reacted by pulp canal obliteration. Notice the two radiopaque stripes in the root canal.

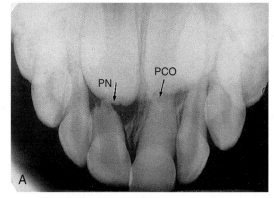

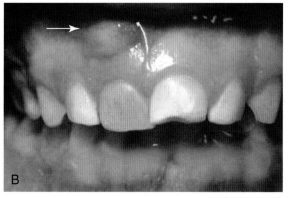

• **Figure 16.16** (A) Pulp canal obliteration *(PCO)* in the patient's left primary central incisor and pulp necrosis *(PN)* in the right primary central incisor. (B) In the same patient, a parulis is present at the apical level of the necrotic right central incisor *(arrow)*.

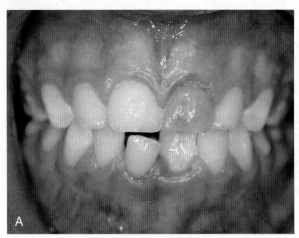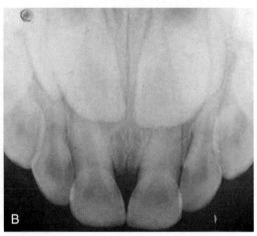

• **Figure 16.17** (A) Left maxillary primary central incisor 1 year after color change due to trauma. This clinical view shows no pathologic signs except dark discoloration. (B) Periapical radiograph showing no pathology associated with the injury.

a need for pulp therapy or extraction of the tooth. Additional signs and symptoms of infection—such as periapical radiographic radiolucency, mobility, swelling, fistula, or pain—must be evident before further treatment is indicated.

Crown discoloration is the external expression of changes in the pulp-dentin complex that become visible through the almost transparent enamel. Crown discoloration of primary incisors is a common posttraumatic finding and is often the only evidence of trauma to the tooth. Discoloration of a primary tooth can be noticed earlier and seen better if viewed from the palatal aspect by transillumination than by direct observation of its labial aspect. The variety of colors is traditionally divided into three main groups: pink-red, yellow, and dark (gray-brown-black).

Pink discoloration that is observed shortly after the injury may represent intrapulpal hemorrhage. Rupture of blood vessels in the pulp as a result of the injury allows extravasation of red blood cells into the surrounding pulpal tissue, resulting in a reddish hue of the crown that becomes visible shortly after the injury.

A reddish hue noticed long after the injury is usually due to internal resorption in the pulp chamber. In both cases follow-up is the only treatment option. Although the hemorrhage eventually dissolves and disappears, the resorption process continues and results in early loss of the crown. The apical part of the root can be left untouched, awaiting its spontaneous resorption. It can be removed if necessary, but care must be taken not to damage the permanent successor.

Yellow discoloration of primary incisors can be seen when the dentin is thick and the pulp chamber narrower than usual. This condition is termed pulp canal obliteration (PCO). It has been shown that PCO can be seen on radiographs without the corresponding yellow discoloration of the crown.[54] Although PCO is a pathologic process, it has no known deleterious effects and therefore does not necessitate any treatment except follow-up. (See further discussion later.)

Dark discoloration of primary teeth is the most controversial posttraumatic complication in terms of the significance of the change in tooth color. The term "dark" refers to a variety of shades, including black, gray, brown, and intermediate hues.

When the pulp becomes necrotic or when pulpal hemorrhage occurs, red blood cells lyse and release hemoglobin. Hemoglobin and its derivatives, such as hematin molecules that contain iron ions, invade the dentin tubules and stain the tooth dark.[55,56] If the pulp remains vital and eliminates the pigments, the dark discoloration may fade, with subsequent restoration of the original color.[57] If the pulp loses its vitality and cannot eliminate the iron-containing molecules, the tooth may remain discolored.

If dark discolored primary incisors present additional signs such as swelling, fistula, or a periapical radiolucent defect, the diagnosis of pulp necrosis is easy. Controversy exists when the dark coronal discoloration is the only evidence of trauma to the tooth (see Fig. 16.17A). It has been found that over 70% of untreated dark discolored primary incisors remained without radiographic or clinical pathology.[58] Furthermore, asymptomatic primary incisors with persistent dark discoloration of the crown following trauma contain a necrotic or partially necrotic pulp.[41] It is not yet clear why some teeth acquire different hues of dark discoloration. An attempt to investigate the variations in the dark colors failed to show a correlation between the various shades and the condition of the pulp.[59] A study evaluating the effect of root canal treatment compared with follow-up only of asymptomatic dark discolored primary incisors showed that there is no difference in the fate of the primary incisors and the eruption pattern and appearance of the permanent successors.[60] It is therefore important to note that in the primary dentition of a healthy child, color change alone does not indicate a need for pulp therapy or extraction of the tooth.

Rapidly Progressing Root Resorption

Rapidly progressing root resorption (previously referred to as "inflammatory" resorption) can occur either on the external root surface or internally in the pulp chamber or canal (see Fig. 35.13). It occurs subsequent to luxation injuries and is related to a necrotic pulp and an inflamed PDL.[61] It can progress very rapidly, destroying a tooth within months. Clinicians who choose to treat a patient with this condition when it occurs in the primary dentition use a resorbable paste of calcium hydroxide, iodoform or zinc oxide, and eugenol as an endodontic filling material. The operator should be aware of the possibility that the zinc oxide eugenol paste may not be completely resorbed with the root of the primary incisor and remain permanently in the surrounding tissue.[62]

Internal Resorption

The predentin, an unmineralized layer of organic material, covers the inner aspect of the dentin and protects it against access of odontoclasts. When the pulp becomes inflamed, as in cases of traumatic injury, the odontoblastic layer may lose its integrity and expose the dentin to odontoclastic activity, which is then seen on radiographs as radiolucent expansion of the pulp space. Eventually this process reaches the outer surface of the root, causing root perforation. If the coronal dentin is completely resorbed, the red color of the resorbing tissue becomes visible through the enamel.

External Resorption

The cementoblast layer and the precementum serve as a shield, protecting the root from involvement in the perpetual remodeling process of the surrounding bone. In nontraumatized primary teeth, external root resorption is part of the physiologic process of replacing the primary dentition with permanent teeth. In primary incisors sustaining traumatic injuries, external root resorption may appear as an accelerated unfavorable pathologic reaction. A variety of patterns of pathologic external root resorption can be seen in primary incisors following traumatic injury.

Rapidly progressing external root resorption, as in permanent teeth, is a rapid process characterized clinically by increased mobility of the tooth, sensitivity to percussion, a dull sound produced by percussion, and often a fistula or swelling in the gums above the tooth. Radiographically the PDL space is widened and the root surface is irregular (Fig. 16.18). This condition may develop within a few weeks of the injury. Removal of the necrotic and probably infected pulp may stop the rapid phase of the resorption process; however, because of the unfavorable preexisting conditions, the benefit of root canal filling in saving the tooth is questionable. Traumatized primary incisors with rapidly progressing external root resorption and evidence of infection should therefore be extracted. It has been shown that root canal treatment in traumatized and infected primary incisors is highly correlated with enamel defects in the permanent teeth.[63]

External surface root resorption is characterized by gradual elimination of the root dentin with preservation of the PDL. The resorption process affects the apex of the root only, which becomes rounded, and progresses until natural exfoliation or traumatic avulsion occurs (Fig. 16.19). As the resorption progresses, bone replaces the space previously occupied by the root and separates the primary tooth and its permanent successor. Sometimes an intermediate stage exists in which osteoclasts attack the root along its apical half, leaving the coronal half unaffected. This type of external root resorption has been termed "atypical external root resorption."[58,64,65] The apical half is finally completely resorbed,

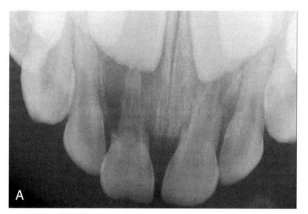 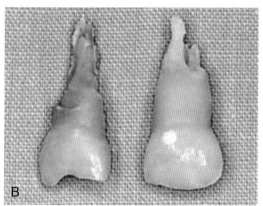

• **Figure 16.18** (A) Periapical radiograph of the maxillary primary central incisors showing external inflammatory root resorption as a result of traumatic injury several months earlier. (B) The affected teeth after extraction. Notice the irregularity of the resorbed root surface.

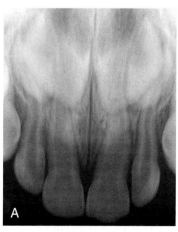 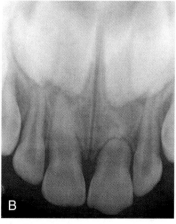 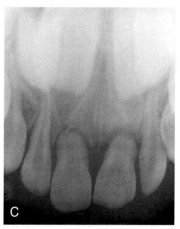

• **Figure 16.19** Periapical radiograph of maxillary primary central incisors with external surface root resorption. (A) Shortly after the injury. (B) Twelve months after the injury. (C) Twenty-seven months after the injury.

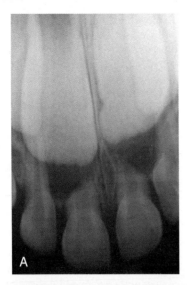

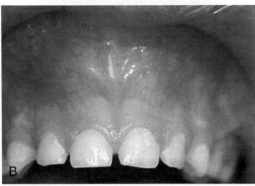

• **Figure 16.20** (A) External root resorption associated with expansion of the follicle of the developing permanent tooth. (B) Clinical view that shows no pathologic signs except a hard expansion of the bone in the vestibule above the tooth.

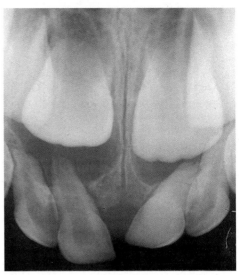

• **Figure 16.21** Radiograph showing an infected expansion of the follicle of the permanent incisors with deflection of the right maxillary permanent central incisor from its normal alignment.

leaving a shortened root with a rounded apex. The clinical appearance imitates that of natural but early exfoliation.

Root resorption associated with expansion of the permanent tooth follicle can be seen mainly, but not exclusively, in traumatized incisors with dark coronal discoloration (Fig. 16.20A). The follicle of the permanent tooth expands gradually and often does not become visible until close to the normal shedding age, even if the teeth were injured at an early age. Expansion of the follicle of the permanent tooth is rarely expressed clinically, and dark coronal discoloration is the only reason to suspect it.[66]

Occasionally, the hard expansion of the labial bone above the injured primary incisors can be observed or, better, palpated (see Fig. 16.20B). Usually, the primary tooth sheds normally and is followed by normal eruption of the permanent teeth.[58]

Occasionally, a dilated follicle becomes infected or the permanent tooth is deflected from its normal alignment (Fig. 16.21). Immediate extraction of the primary incisors is mandatory in these cases.

Replacement External Root Resorption

Replacement external root resorption, also known as ankylosis, results after irreversible injury to the PDL. Alveolar bone directly contacts and fuses with the root surface.[61] As the alveolar bone

undergoes normal physiologic osteoclastic and osteoblastic activity, the root is resorbed and replaced with bone. Ankylosis occurs more often in intruded primary teeth, and they eventually become infraoccluded (Fig. 16.22).[41] Ankylosed primary teeth should be extracted if they cause a delay in or an ectopic eruption of a developing permanent tooth.

Pulp Canal Obliteration

PCO is the result of intensified activity of the odontoblasts that results in accelerated dentin apposition. Gradually, the pulp space narrows to a state in which it cannot be seen on a radiograph (see Figs. 16.5B, 16.15, 16.16A, and 16.22). PCO is a common finding in primary incisors following traumatic injuries[67,68] and is often associated with yellow coronal discoloration. As yet, however, the exact mode by which the impact to the tooth affects the odontoblasts is obscure. Although scientifically defined as a pathologic process, clinically it is not regarded as having deleterious effects. Ninety percent of primary teeth that have undergone PCO resorb normally[69]; therefore treatment in the primary dentition is usually not indicated.

Complications Following Intrusion

Approximately two-thirds of intruded primary incisors reerupt and survive without any complications more than 3 years after the injury.[41] In most cases, however, the teeth do not return to their original position but reerupt into a rotated alignment (Fig. 16.23). If the child still uses a pacifier, it may occupy the space of the crown of the intruded tooth and prevent its reeruption back to the occlusal level. Intruded primary teeth may fail to reerupt if the root has been pushed out of the alveolar bone into the surrounding soft tissues (Fig. 16.24). These teeth should be extracted. Another reason for failure of intruded incisors to reerupt is damage to the PDL during the injury that results in ankylosis. It is not yet clear whether intervention is needed to remove the ankylosed tooth or if the root can be resorbed spontaneously with subsequent exfoliation of the tooth.

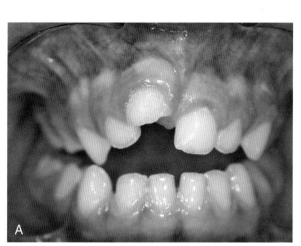
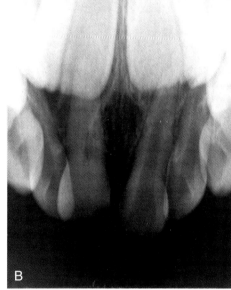

• **Figure 16.22** (A) Clinical view showing infraposition of the maxillary right primary central incisor following an intrusion injury many months previous. (B) Radiograph demonstrating ankylosis and pulp canal obliteration of the intruded primary incisor.

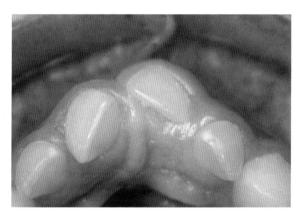

• **Figure 16.23** Clinical view of the maxillary primary incisors. Both central incisors were completely intruded and reerupted several weeks after the injury but into a rotated alignment. The teeth are clinically asymptomatic.

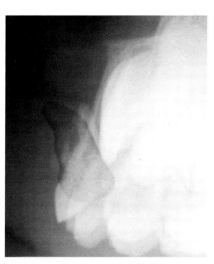

• **Figure 16.24** Lateral extraoral radiograph showing an intruded maxillary primary central incisor that has been pushed out of the labial alveolar bone plate.

Periodontal breakdown due to infection is the main reason for loss of primary incisors following intrusion.[41] This can be prevented by maintaining optimal oral hygiene (see "Information and Instructions for Parents"). Surprisingly, pulp necrosis following intrusion of primary incisors is not a common finding,[41] and unlike the recommendations for intruded permanent teeth, removal of the pulp is not recommended. Even if the apex of an intruded primary incisor avoids contact with its permanent successor, the permanent tooth may have still been damaged. It could have been affected during the sudden movement of the primary tooth from its original position to its final alignment. This explains the discrepancy found between the low percentage (10% to 20%) of primary incisors pushed toward the developing permanent teeth[41] and the high percentage (38% to 77%) of affected permanent teeth following intrusion of their primary predecessors.[46,70–72] The impact of intrusion of primary incisors on their permanent successors varies from discoloration and dysplasia of the enamel to eruption disturbances and crown dilacerations.[73]

Complications Following Avulsion

Several outcomes of early loss of primary incisors have been described in the dental literature.[74] Loss of space can be expected if the injury occurred before eruption of the primary canines and in children with a crowded dentition.[75] If primary incisors are lost before the child masters articulation, speech development may be affected.[76,77] However, articulation becomes normal after eruption of the permanent teeth.[78] The impact to the primary incisor pushes the tooth into the surrounding tissues before the tooth is completely detached from the PDL and damages the permanent successors in 38% to 85% of cases.[79,80] The younger the child is when injured, the higher the prevalence of damage to the permanent teeth.[46] Delayed and ectopic eruption of permanent incisors in cases of avulsion of their primary predecessors have been described and attributed to lack

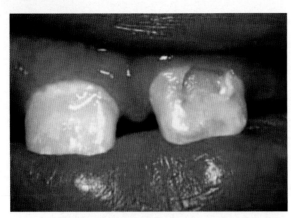

• **Figure 16.25** Hypoplasia of the patient's maxillary left permanent central incisor as a result of intrusion of a primary incisor.

of guidance, development of scar tissue, and deflection of the developing permanent tooth bud by the injured primary incisor.[10]

Injuries to Developing Permanent Teeth

The most damaging sequelae of injuries to primary teeth are their effects on the unerupted developing permanent teeth. Anatomically, the permanent anterior teeth develop close to the apices of primary incisors (see Fig. 16.24). Thus a periapical pathologic process that is due to necrotic pulps, intrusion injuries, or overinstrumentation of primary root canals can irreversibly damage the permanent teeth. If the injury occurs during the development of the permanent tooth crown, enamel hypoplasia or hypocalcification may occur (Fig. 16.25). These injuries can also alter the path of the developing permanent tooth crown, causing root dilaceration or ectopic eruption. For these reasons, the clinician should plan management of injuries to primary teeth with the ultimate objective of preventing or minimizing damage to the succeeding permanent teeth. Enamel calcification of permanent central incisor crowns is usually completed by age 4 years, so the risk of injury to them is greater in children younger than that.

References

1. Sasaki H, Ogawa T, Kawaguchi M, et al. Multiple fractures of primary molars caused by injuries to the chin: report of two cases. *Endod Dent Traumatol.* 2000;16(1):43–46.
2. Ostergaard BH, Andreasen JO, Ahrensburg SS, et al. An analysis of pattern of dental injuries after fall accidents in 0- to 2-year-old children—does the use of pacifier at the time of injury make a difference? *Int J Paediatr Dent.* 2011;21(5):397–400.
3. Kirzioglu Z, Karayilmaz H, Erturk MS, et al. Epidemiology of traumatised primary teeth in the west-Mediterranean region of Turkey. *Int Dent J.* 2005;55(5):329–333.
4. Sandalli N, Cildir S, Guler N. Clinical investigation of traumatic injuries in Yeditepe University, Turkey during the last 3 years. *Dent Traumatol.* 2005;21(4):188–194.
5. Granville-Garcia AF, de Menezes VA, de Lira PI. Dental trauma and associated factors in Brazilian preschoolers. *Dent Traumatol.* 2006;22(6):318–322.
6. Jorge KO, Moyses SJ, Ferreira e Ferreira E, et al. Prevalence and factors associated to dental trauma in infants 1-3 years of age. *Dent Traumatol.* 2009;25(2):185–189.
7. Viegas CM, Scarpelli AC, Carvalho AC, et al. Predisposing factors for traumatic dental injuries in Brazilian preschool children. *Eur J Paediatr Dent.* 2010;11(2):59–65.
8. Dutra FT, Marinho AM, Godoi PF, et al. Prevalence of dental trauma and associated factors among 1- to 4-year-old children. *J Dent Child.* 2010;77(3):146–151.
9. Correa-Faria P, Paiva SM, Ramos-Jorge ML, et al. Incidence of crown fracture and risk factors in the primary dentition: a prospective longitudinal study. *Dent Traumatol.* 2016;32(6):450–456.
10. Andreasen JO, Andreasen FM, Andersson L, eds. *Textbook and Color Atlas of Traumatic Injuries to the Teeth.* 4th ed. Copenhagen: Blackwell Munksgaard; 2007:891.
11. Veire A, Nichols W, Urquiola R, et al. Dental trauma: review of common dental injuries and their management in primary and permanent dentitions. *J Mich Dent Assoc.* 2012;94(1):41–45.
12. Feldens CA, Kramer PF, Ferreira SH, et al. Exploring factors associated with traumatic dental injuries in preschool children: a Poisson regression analysis. *Dent Traumatol.* 2010;26(2):143–148.
13. El Karmi RF, Hamdan MA, Rajab LD, et al. Prevalence of traumatic dental injuries and associated factors among preschool children in Amman, Jordan. *Dent Traumatol.* 2015;31(6):487–492.
14. Norton E, O'Connell AC. Traumatic dental injuries and their association with malocclusion in the primary dentition of Irish children. *Dental Traumatol.* 2012;28(1):81–86.
15. Bonini GC, Bonecker M, Braga MM, et al. Combined effect of anterior malocclusion and inadequate lip coverage on dental trauma in primary teeth. *Dent Traumatol.* 2012;28(6):437–440.
16. Feldens CA, Borges TS, Vargas-Ferreira F, et al. Risk factors for traumatic dental injuries in the primary dentition: concepts, interpretation, and evidence. *Dent Traumatol.* 2016;32(6):429–437.
17. Governors Highway Safety Association. Child passenger safety. www.ghsa.org/html/stateinfo/laws/childsafety_laws.html. Accessed August 28, 2017.
18. Centers for Disease Control and Prevention (CDC). Updated recommendations for use of tetanus toxoid, reduced diphtheria toxoid and acellular pertussis (Tdap) vaccine from the Advisory Committee on Immunization Practices, 2010. *MMWR Morb Mortal Wkly Rep.* 2011;60(1):13–15.
19. Davis MJ, Vogel L. Neurological assessment of the child with head trauma. *ASDC J Dent Child.* 1995;62(2):93–96.
20. Tecklenburg FW, Wright MS. Minor head trauma in the pediatric patient. *Pediatr Emerg Care.* 1991;7(1):40–47.
21. Palchak MJ, Holmes JF, Vance CW, et al. A decision rule for identifying children at low risk for brain injuries after blunt head trauma. *Ann Emerg Med.* 2003;42(4):492–506.
22. Pandor A, Goodacre S, Harnan S, et al. Diagnostic management strategies for adults and children with minor head injury: a systematic review and an economic evaluation. *Health Technol Assess.* 2011;15(27):1–202.
23. Soares FC, Cardoso M, Bolan M. Altered esthetics in primary central incisors: the child's perception. *Pediatr Dent.* 2015;37(5):29–34.
24. Feldens CA, Day P, Borges TS, et al. Enamel fracture in the primary dentition has no impact on children's quality of life: implications for clinicians and researchers. *Dent Traumatol.* 2016;32(2):103–109.
25. Viegas CM, Scarpelli AC, Carvalho AC, et al. Impact of traumatic dental injury on quality of life among Brazilian preschool children and their families. *Pediatr Dent.* 2012;34(4):300–306.
26. Kaban LB. Diagnosis and treatment of fractures of the facial bones in children 1943-1993. *J Oral Maxillofac Surg.* 1993;51(7):722–729.
27. Andreasen JO, Lauridsen E, Andreasen FM. Contradictions in the treatment of traumatic dental injuries and ways to proceed in dental trauma research. *Dent Traumatol.* 2010;26(1):16–22.
28. Abdel Jabbar NS, Aldrigui JM, Braga MM, et al. Pulp polyp in traumatized primary teeth—a case-control study. *Dent Traumatol.* 2013;29(5):360–364.
29. Kupietzky A, Holan G. Treatment of crown fractures with pulp exposure in primary incisors. *Pediatr Dent.* 2003;25(3):241–247.
30. Ram D, Holan G. Partial pulpotomy in a traumatized primary incisor with pulp exposure: case report. *Pediatr Dent.* 1994;16(1):44–48.
31. Holan G. Conservative treatment of severely luxated maxillary primary central incisors: case report. *Pediatr Dent.* 1999;21(7):459–462.

32. Majorana A, Pasini S, Bardellini E, et al. Clinical and epidemiological study of traumatic root fractures. *Dent Traumatol*. 2002;18(2):77–80.

33. Kim GT, Sohn M, Ahn HJ, et al. Intra-alveolar root fracture in primary teeth. *Pediatr Dent*. 2012;34(7):e215–e218.

34. Holan G. Traumatic injuries to the chin: a survey in a paediatric dental practice. *Int J Paediatr Dent*. 1998;8(2):143–148.

35. Hariharan VS, Rayen R. Case report: management of crown-root fracture in lower first primary molar caused by injury to the chin: report of an unusual case. *Eur Arch Paediatr Dent*. 2012;13(4):217–220.

36. Holan G. Periodontal breakdown and pathologic root resorption of primary molars following traumatic injuries to the chin: case report. *Pediatr Dent*. 1997;19(6):425–426.

37. Hurt TL, Fisher B, Peterson BM, et al. Mandibular fractures in association with chin trauma in pediatric patients. *Pediatr Emerg Care*. 1988;4(2):121–123.

38. Bertolami CN, Kaban LB. Chin trauma: a clue to associated mandibular and cervical spine injury. *Oral Surg Oral Med Oral Pathol*. 1982;53(2):122–126.

39. Sheinvald-Shusterman K, Holan G. Parents' ability to recall past injuries to maxillary primary incisors in their children. *Dent Traumatol*. 2012;28(4):273–276.

40. Andreasen JO. The influence of traumatic intrusion of primary teeth on their permanent successors. A radiographic and histologic study in monkeys. *Int J Oral Surg*. 1976;5(5):207–219.

41. Holan G, Ram D. Sequelae and prognosis of intruded primary incisors: a retrospective study. *Pediatr Dent*. 1999;21(4):242–247.

42. Holan G, Ram D, Fuks AB. The diagnostic value of lateral extraoral radiography for intruded maxillary primary incisors. *Pediatr Dent*. 2002;24(1):38–42.

43. Soporowski NJ, Allred EN, Needleman HL. Luxation injuries of primary anterior teeth—prognosis and related correlates. *Pediatr Dent*. 1994;16(2):96–101.

44. Shanmugam HV, Arangannal P, Vishnurekha C, et al. Management of intrusive luxation in the primary dentition by surgical repositioning: an alternative approach. *Aust Dent J*. 2011;56(2):207–211.

45. Hirata R, Kaihara Y, Suzuki J, et al. Management of intruded primary teeth after traumatic injuries. *Pediatr Dent J*. 2011;21:94–100.

46. Ravn JJ. Developmental disturbances in permanent teeth after intrusion of their primary predecessors. *Scand J Dent Res*. 1976;84(3):137–141.

47. Andreasen JO, Andreasen FM. Injuries to the primary dentition. In: *Essentials of Traumatic Injuries to the Teeth*. Copenhagen: Munksgaard; 1990.

48. Malmgren B, Andreasen JO, Flores MT, et al. International Association of Dental Traumatology guidelines for the management of traumatic dental injuries: 3. Injuries in the primary dentition. *Dent Traumatol*. 2012;28(3):174–182.

49. Holan G. Replantation of avulsed primary incisors: a critical review of a controversial treatment. *Dent Traumatol*. 2013;29(3):178–184.

50. Holan G, Ram D. Aspiration of an avulsed primary incisor. A case report. *International J Paediatr Dent*. 2000;10(2):150–152.

51. Holan G, Fuks AB. The diagnostic value of coronal dark-gray discoloration in primary teeth following traumatic injuries. *Pediatr Dent*. 1996;18(3):224–227.

52. Tannure PN, Fidalgo TK, Barcelos R, et al. Analysis of root canal treated primary incisor after trauma: two year outcomes. *J Clin Pediatr Dent*. 2012;36(3):257–262.

53. Cardoso M, de Carvalho Rocha MJ. Association of crown discoloration and pulp status in traumatized primary teeth. *Dent Traumatol*. 2010;26(5):413–416.

54. Borum MK, Andreasen JO. Sequelae of trauma to primary maxillary incisors. I. Complications in the primary dentition. *Endod Dent Traumatol*. 1998;14(1):31–44.

55. Pindborg JJ. *Pathology of the Dental Hard Tissues*. Copenhagen: Munksgaard; 1970.

56. Marin PD, Bartold PM, Heithersay GS. Tooth discoloration by blood: an in vitro histochemical study. *Endod Dent Traumatol*. 1997;13(3):132–138.

57. Heithersay GS, Hirsch RS. Tooth discoloration and resolution following a luxation injury: significance of blood pigment in dentin to laser Doppler flowmetry readings. *Quintessence Int*. 1993;24(9):669–676.

58. Holan G. Development of clinical and radiographic signs associated with dark discolored primary incisors following traumatic injuries: a prospective controlled study. *Dent Traumatol*. 2004;20(5):276–287.

59. Soxman JA, Nazif MM, Bouquot J. Pulpal pathology in relation to discoloration of primary anterior teeth. *ASDC J Dent Child*. 1984;51(4):282–284.

60. Holan G. Long-term effect of different treatment modalities for traumatized primary incisors presenting dark coronal discoloration with no other signs of injury. *Dent Traumatol*. 2006;22(1):14–17.

61. Tronstad L. Root resorption—etiology, terminology and clinical manifestations. *Endod Dent Traumatol*. 1988;4(6):241–252.

62. Nivoloni Tannure P, Barcelos R, Farinhas J, et al. Zinc oxide-Eugenol paste retained in gingival mucosa after primary teeth pulpectomy. *Eur J Paediatr Dent*. 2010;11:101–102.

63. Holan G, Topf J, Fuks AB. Effect of root canal infection and treatment of traumatized primary incisors on their permanent successors. *Endod Dent Traumatol*. 1992;8(1):12–15.

64. Holan G, Yodko E, Sheinvald-Shusterman K. The association between traumatic dental injuries and atypical external root resorption in maxillary primary incisors. *Dental Traumatol*. 2015;31(1):35–41.

65. Mortelliti GM, Needleman HL. Risk factors associated with atypical root resorption of the maxillary primary central incisors. *Pediatr Dent*. 1991;13(5):273–277.

66. Holan G, Yodko E. Radiographic evidence of traumatic injuries to primary incisors without accompanying clinical signs. *Dent Traumatol*. 2017;33(2):133–136.

67. Mello-Moura AC, Bonini GA, Zardetto CG, et al. Pulp calcification in traumatized primary teeth: prevalence and associated factors. *J Clin Pediatr Dent*. 2011;35(4):383–387.

68. Santos BZ, Cardoso M, Almeida IC. Pulp canal obliteration following trauma to primary incisors: a 9-year clinical study. *Pediatr Dent*. 2011;33(5):399–402.

69. Jacobsen I, Sangnes G. Traumatized primary anterior teeth. Prognosis related to calcific reactions in the pulp cavity. *Acta Odontol Scand*. 1978;36(4):199–204.

70. Altun C, Cehreli ZC, Guven G, et al. Traumatic intrusion of primary teeth and its effects on the permanent successors: a clinical follow-up study. *Oral Surg Oral Med Oral Pathol Oral Radiol Endod*. 2009;107(4):493–498.

71. de Amorim Lde F, Estrela C, da Costa LR. Effects of traumatic dental injuries to primary teeth on permanent teeth–a clinical follow-up study. *Dent Traumatol*. 2011;27(2):117–121.

72. Skaare AB, Aas AL, Wang NJ. Enamel defects on permanent successors following luxation injuries to primary teeth and carers' experiences. *Int J Paediatr Dent*. 2015;25(3):221–228.

73. Carvalho V, Jacomo DR, Campos V. Frequency of intrusive luxation in deciduous teeth and its effects. *Dent Traumatol*. 2010;26(4):304–307.

74. Holan G, Needleman HL. Premature loss of primary anterior teeth due to trauma–potential short- and long-term sequelae. *Dent Traumatol*. 2014;30(2):100–106.

75. Levine N. Injury to the primary dentition. *Dent Clin North Am*. 1982;26(3):461–480.

76. Riekman GA, el Badrawy HE. Effect of premature loss of primary maxillary incisors on speech. *Pediatr Dent*. 1985;7(2):119–122.

77. Adewumi AO, Horton C, Guelmann M, et al. Parental perception vs. professional assessment of speech changes following premature loss of maxillary primary incisors. *Pediatr Dent*. 2012;34(4):295–299.

78. Gable TO, Kummer AW, Lee L, et al. Premature loss of the maxillary primary incisors: effect on speech production. *ASDC J Dent Child*. 1995;62(3):173–179.

79. von Arx T. Developmental disturbances of permanent teeth following trauma to the primary dentition. *Aust Dent J*. 1993;38(1):1–10.

80. Ravn JJ. Sequelae of acute mechanical traumata in the primary dentition. A clinical study. *ASDC J Dent Child*. 1968;35(4):281–289.

17

Congenital Genetic Disorders and Syndromes

REBECCA L. SLAYTON AND PIRANIT NIK KANTAPUTRA

CHAPTER OUTLINE

As health care professionals, the information gained from the Human Genome Project has created many opportunities as well as challenges. This information provides clinicians with the ability to understand diseases at a molecular level. In addition, diseases that were once thought to be influenced primarily by environmental factors are now known to have genetic factors that modulate their severity. More recently, gene-environment interactions and epigenetic factors have been shown to contribute to disease susceptibility. Access to the sequence of the entire human genome will continue to facilitate the identification of additional disease genes and contribute to a better understanding of the complex interactions that occur between genes and regulatory proteins. The ability to identify single-nucleotide changes (referred to as polymorphisms) will lead to an understanding of individual risk factors for disease and how to tailor prevention and treatment strategies at an individual rather than a global level. These advances have guided recent efforts to develop precision medicine approaches to care.[1] The complete sequencing of microbial genomes will provide an understanding of what makes some strains of bacteria more virulent than others and will aid in the development of more effective therapeutic interventions.

There are also challenges involved in the management and use of information generated by the Human Genome Project. It will be important to anticipate how this information might be used in ways that are unethical or detrimental to individuals or groups of people. Information about genetics and genetic research is reported almost daily in newspapers and magazines and on the radio, television, and Internet. This often means that a patient may hear of a new discovery before it is published in a scientific journal. Health professionals must be prepared to answer patients' questions and must know how and where to refer them for additional information or counseling. Practicing dental clinicians provide the front line as diagnosticians and for the referral of patients and families for genetic testing and counseling involving many conditions with oral health consequences. This requires a basic understanding of the genetics of human disease, knowledge of the types of genetic testing that are available, and sensitivity to the family's concerns.

Practicing dentists are confronted daily with conditions that are either primarily genetic or have a significant genetic contribution in their etiologies. Common conditions such as tooth agenesis are now known in many cases to be caused by specific genetic mutations. Many syndromes involve craniofacial structures and have associated dental anomalies. Frequently other major malformations are present

The understanding of genetics and the genetic basis of disease has increased dramatically over the last 30 years. During this time, scientists have ascertained the sequence of the entire human genome (more than 3 billion nucleotides of DNA) and have discovered new ways in which diseases and disease susceptibility are inherited.

in addition to the craniofacial anomalies. Advances in the Human Genome Project have led to the discovery of the genetic basis of many of these disorders that include craniofacial and dental anomalies as part of the spectrum of the disease. Understanding the disease at this level permits the practitioner to provide a more precise diagnosis of the disease, a more appropriate treatment, and a more accurate prognosis of the outcomes of care.

Dental practitioners are aware of the environmental and behavioral risk factors that contribute to poor oral health. Patients and their parents are routinely counseled about the risks involved with cigarette smoking, smokeless tobacco, alcohol, poor oral hygiene, sweetened beverages, a diet high in carbohydrates, and traumatic injuries to the head and mouth. It is clear that the two most common dental diseases—dental caries and periodontal disease—are complex and have both environmental and genetic components. As information about the genetic makeup of individuals increases, there will be additional genetic susceptibility or resistance factors identified that will influence the severity of oral diseases. Once these factors are identified, there will be tests that can be performed well before the occurrence of disease. This will permit practitioners to educate patients about the importance of their behaviors and to tailor their preventive strategies more specifically for each patient. Some of these will be in-office tests, whereas others will require the use of an outside laboratory. The application of appropriate tests and ultimately the interpretation of the test results and the management of the oral disease will be the responsibility of the dentist. Therefore practicing dentists must understand the basis of the test, how it is performed, and how the results are interpreted. Understanding the basis for many of the genetic tests available today requires an understanding of basic genetic concepts as well as the current technologies that are available for testing.

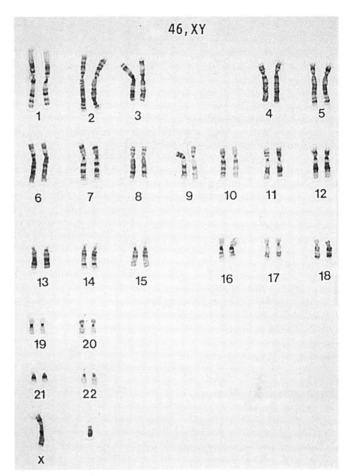

• **Figure 17.1** Karyotype of a normal male.

Basic Genetic Concepts

A person's genome is made up of the DNA in all 46 chromosomes in the nucleus of each cell of the body. Each cell has 23 pairs of chromosomes. One chromosome of each pair is inherited from each parent. Two of the chromosomes are called sex chromosomes (X and Y), whereas the remaining chromosomes (numbered 1 through 22) are called autosomes. Males have one X and one Y chromosome; females have two X chromosomes. In each cell of a female, one of the X chromosomes is randomly inactivated. This is an important determinant of the severity of X-linked genetic disorders, as discussed later. The technique used to look at all of the chromosomes in a cell and to determine the sex of a fetus from amniotic fluid is called karyotyping (Fig. 17.1). This technique also identifies major chromosomal anomalies such as trisomy (an extra chromosome), translocations of one part of a chromosome to another, or large chromosomal deletions.

Each chromosome is made up of a double-stranded DNA helix composed of a series of four nucleotides and a sugar-phosphate base. Each of the four nucleotides (adenine, thymine, cytosine, and guanine) is paired with a specific complementary nucleotide to form the double helix. Adenine always pairs with thymine, and cytosine always pairs with guanine. The ability of a single strand of DNA to bind to a complementary strand of DNA or RNA forms the basis of many of the diagnostic tests performed today.

Genes are sequences of DNA that are transcribed into messenger RNA and then translated into proteins. Each chromosome contains thousands of genes. The entire human genome is estimated to have approximately 30,000 genes. The exquisite control of gene expression is essential for the proper growth, development, and functioning of an organism.

Although each cell contains the same DNA and therefore the same genes, only a small percentage of those genes are active or expressed, depending on the time of development and the type of cell. Cells in the epidermis need different proteins than cells in the developing tooth or in the kidney, and each cell type has a complex regulatory process to ensure that the right genes are expressed and translated into the necessary proteins at the proper time.

Molecular Basis of Disease

Traditionally, genetic diseases have been thought of in terms of mendelian inheritance patterns. This means that a mutation present in a gene transmitted to a child from one or both parents results in the child's either having the disease or being a carrier of the disease. As we have learned more about genetics, additional mechanisms of inheritance have been identified that make it more challenging to predict both the occurrence and the severity of disease. It is not uncommon for a genetic disease to be the result of a new or fresh mutation. In this case, there would be no history of the disorder on either side of the family. Recently, it has been found that advanced paternal age is associated with craniosynostotic syndromes such as Apert and Crouzon syndromes.[2] Other types of nonmendelian inheritance patterns include imprinting, DNA triplet repeat expansion, mitochondrial DNA defects, and complex disorders in which multiple genes may be involved and in which sequence changes increase or decrease a person's susceptibility to disease.

Inheritance Patterns

Autosomal Dominant

In autosomal dominant inheritance, the transmission is vertical from parent to child. An affected parent has a 50% chance of passing along the defective gene to a child of either sex. Autosomal dominant inheritance may occur in the family initially as a new mutation or may have been present in the family for multiple generations. Dentinogenesis imperfecta is an example of an autosomal dominant disorder. The gene for type II dentinogenesis imperfecta has been identified (dentin sialophosphoprotein; *DSPP*) and is located on chromosome 4. Other autosomal dominant disorders include achondroplasia, some forms of amelogenesis imperfecta, and Marfan syndrome. Some individuals may carry the mutation without having the disease but being capable of transmitting the mutation to their children. This occurrence is called incomplete (reduced) penetrance.

Autosomal Recessive

An autosomal recessive disorder becomes manifest only when an individual has two copies of the mutant gene. Most frequently each parent has one copy of the defective gene and is a carrier, and there is a 25% chance that both mutant genes will be passed on to their offspring. Male and female offspring will be equally likely to be affected. Fifty percent of the time the offspring will get one copy of the mutant gene from one parent and will be carriers, and 25% of the time the offspring will get two normal copies of the gene. Although autosomal recessive disorders are relatively uncommon, the carrier status in certain populations can be significant. For example, 1 in 25 people of northern European descent are carriers of cystic fibrosis.[3] Genetic diseases more common among people of Asian and African descent are beta-thalassemia and sickle cell anemia, respectively.[4,5]

X-Linked

Mutations in genes located on the X chromosome result in X-linked genetic disorders. Since females have two X chromosomes and one is randomly inactivated in each cell, they are carriers and do not normally manifest the disorder. Males, on the other hand, have only one X chromosome, which is inherited from their mothers. A son has a 50% chance of inheriting the defective gene from his mother and manifesting the disease. A daughter also has a 50% chance of inheriting the defective gene from her mother but will then be a carrier. X-linked disorders often appear to skip a generation because an affected male will only pass the mutation in his X chromosome to his daughter, and she will serve as a carrier to the next generation. Disorders with X-linked inheritance include factor VIII deficiency (hemophilia), X-linked hypohydrotic ectodermal dysplasia, fragile X syndrome, and X-linked amelogenesis imperfecta. Occasionally, as a result of nonrandom X inactivation, females may have mild symptoms of an X-linked disorder.

Chromosomal Anomalies

In the previous examples, defects in one or both copies of a gene are responsible for the occurrence of a genetic disorder. Some disorders result from defects in chromosomes that result in extra copies of one or more genes, entire deletions of one or more genes, or translocation of one part of a chromosome with another. Generally chromosomal anomalies result in multiple physical defects as well as mental and developmental delay. Down syndrome is the result of a trisomy (three copies) of all or part of chromosome 21. The duplicated part of the chromosome leads to an extra copy of all the genes on that part of the chromosome. The dosage of gene products in each cell is highly regulated. Extra copies of genes lead to excess gene products that interfere with the necessary balance in the cell. Extra or missing chromosomal material frequently results in miscarriages and/or multiple birth defects.

Multifactorial Inheritance

Most common diseases of adulthood (such as diabetes, hypertension, and manic depression) as well as most congenital malformations (cleft lip/palate and neural tube defects) are the result of multiple genes and gene-environment interactions rather than a single gene defect. This is also true for the most common dental diseases (periodontal disease and dental caries). Multifactorial traits are thought to result from the interaction between multiple genes with multiple environmental factors. The most convincing evidence for this type of inheritance comes from twin studies. If a trait is multifactorial with a significant genetic component, monozygotic (identical) twins will both have the disease significantly more frequently than dizygotic (fraternal) twins. This has been demonstrated in multiple studies for dental caries among twins raised apart and provides strong evidence that there is a genetic component to dental caries susceptibility.[6,7] More recently, researchers have completed a genomewide association study designed to identify genetic loci associated with the susceptibility or resistance to dental caries.[8] These include *MMP10*, *MMP14*, and *MMP16*[9]; enamel matrix genes[10]; *MPPED2* and *ACTN2*[11]; and the region near the gene *PKD2*.[12]

Nontraditional Inheritance

Other types of inheritance patterns that do not fit the traditional mendelian patterns and have been identified fairly recently are imprinting and triplet repeat expansion. Imprinted genes are turned off by methylation of the gene. This process controls the level of expression of a particular gene in the offspring. Depending on whether the imprinted gene is inherited from the mother or father determines if the child has a particular disease. In some cases, if the imprinted gene is inherited from the father, the child has one disease, but if the same imprinted gene is inherited from the mother, the child has a different disease. Two disorders that exemplify this are Prader-Willi syndrome and Angelman syndrome. If the child inherits the imprinted gene region from their father, they have Prader-Willi syndrome and if inherited from their mother, it is manifested as Angelman syndrome.[13]

DNA triplet repeat expansion is a phenomenon where strings of repeated nucleotides increase in number. For example, within a particular gene, there may be 200 copies of the trinucleotide repeat "TAG." Smaller numbers of repeats are often referred to as a premutation, but when the repeats are expanded in an offspring, they may cause the gene to be inactivated (often by methylation). Diseases caused by this type of defect include Huntington chorea and fragile X syndrome.

Epigenetic mechanisms affect the expression of genes and can be caused by environmental chemicals, developmental processes, drugs, or aging. These changes are not the result of DNA sequence alterations but rather are caused by factors such as DNA methylation and histone acetylation. These modifications activate and deactivate parts of the genome at specific times and in specific cells. Epigenetic tags react to environmental stimuli such as diet, toxins, and physical activity. Since these tags can be maintained over multiple generations, offspring may be influenced by epigenetic changes that occurred in grandparents or great grandparents and may not have been manifested in the parents. Although the term *epigenetics* was coined in 1942, its relevance to inheritance of disease susceptibility has attracted substantial attention in recent years. There is evidence to suggest that epigenetics plays a part in autism,[14] suicidal ideation,[15] cancer,[16] and periodontal disease.[17] Future studies on the epigenome are likely to lead to new approaches to risk assessment and the treatment of complex disorders.

Dentist as Dysmorphologist

The word *dysmorphic* describes faulty development of the shape or form of an organism. Facial features in a child are frequently referred to as dysmorphic when they vary from what is considered normal. Features such as the spacing between the eyes, the position and shape of the ears, and the relative proportions of the maxilla and mandible are either within the range of normal or vary enough to be considered dysmorphic. Many genetic syndromes result in dysmorphic facial features that frequently help to diagnose the syndrome. For example, children with Down syndrome have inner epicanthal folds, upslanting palpebral fissures, and maxillary hypoplasia. This causes unrelated children with Down syndrome to have a similar appearance to each other.

There are four basic mechanisms that result in structural defects during development. The first is malformation, the second is deformation due to mechanical forces, the third is disruption where there is a breakdown of tissues that were previously normal, and the fourth is dysplasia. Dysplasia is caused by a failure of normal organization of cells into tissues. It is not uncommon for humans to have at least one "minor" malformation. This includes things such as hair whorls, inner epicanthal folds, aberrant positioning of oral frenula, or preauricular pits. Although the occurrence of single anomalies such as these is relatively common and often presents as a familial trait, there are a number of studies that have demonstrated that a child who has three minor anomalies has a much greater chance of having a major anomaly such as a defect in brain or heart development.[18–20] This illustrates why it is important for health care professionals to be careful observers of their patients and to be familiar with the facial features that are considered to be normal or aberrant.

In general, the children seen in a dental practice fit into one of three categories. They may be normally developed in every way, they may have been diagnosed with a developmental anomaly of some type (either physical or mental), or they may have a developmental anomaly that has not been diagnosed. Pediatric dentists and general dentists are in the unique position of seeing their patients regularly, even when the patient does not perceive

a dental problem. This is in contrast to the typical physician who may only see patients when they are ill. This frequent interaction between dentists and their patients gives the dentist the opportunity to observe a child's growth and development and to note changes that are not within the range of normal. As health care professionals, it is incumbent on all dentists to recognize disease in their patients and to make the appropriate referrals for definitive diagnosis and treatment.

Dentists are trained to observe and examine the mouth, face, and other craniofacial structures. Coincidentally, many inherited diseases in humans involve malformations of the craniofacial region. Accurate diagnosis of developmental anomalies and their related disorders relies on the ability of the clinician to recognize and differentiate between normal and dysmorphic physical characteristics. According to the text *Smith's Recognizable Patterns of Human Malformation*, 12 of the 26 categories of malformations used for diagnostic purposes involve features of the head or neck.[21] Several are limited to oral structures, such as hypodontia, microdontia, micrognathia, and cleft lip/palate. In addition, having an understanding of the full spectrum of malformations associated with certain syndromes is essential for the safe and effective treatment of patients with these disorders.

Because dentists concentrate their diagnostic expertise on the face and mouth, they may be more likely to observe anomalies that are suggestive of major developmental malformations. Dentists who can recognize potential genetic disorders can also provide a valuable service to their patients by offering appropriate referral to a medical geneticist or a genetic counselor.

Ocular Anomalies

Minor anomalies that affect the eyes and ocular region include widely spaced eyes (hypertelorism) (Fig. 17.2), inner epicanthal folds (Fig. 17.3), slanting of the palpebral fissures (upward or downward) (Figs. 17.4 and 17.5), a fused eyebrow (synophrys), blue sclera, and coloboma of the iris ("cat eye") (Fig. 17.6).

Auricular Anomalies

There are a number of minor anomalies that affect the outer ear (auricle) and the preauricular region. These include preauricular tags or pits (Fig. 17.7), low-set and malformed ears (Fig. 17.8), protruding ears, and slanted ears.

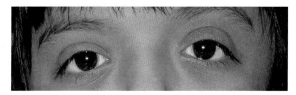

• **Figure 17.2** Hypertelorism.

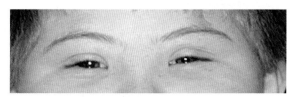

• **Figure 17.3** Inner epicanthal fold.

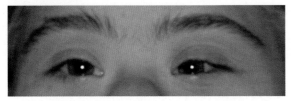

• **Figure 17.4** Upslanting palpebral fissures.

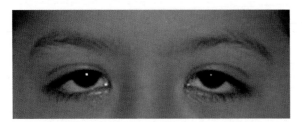

• **Figure 17.5** Downslanting palpebral fissures.

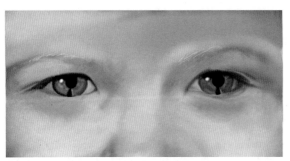

• **Figure 17.6** Coloboma of the iris. (From Kaban LB, Troulis MJ. *Pediatric Oral and Maxillofacial Surgery*. St Louis: Saunders; 2004.)

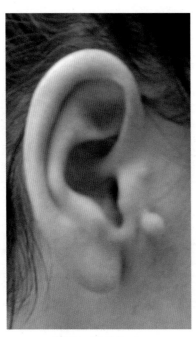

• **Figure 17.7** Ear tag.

Anomalies of the Mouth and Oral Region

Cleft lip alone or combined with a cleft palate, although not a minor anomaly, can occur independently from other malformations and is then considered nonsyndromic. Other anomalies in this region include lower lip pits (Fig. 17.9), bifid uvula, macroglossia, and prominent or full lips. Attached or short frenum, as seen with ankyloglossia ("tongue tie") (Fig. 17.10), or low attached maxillary labial frenum is also a fairly common anomaly in the oral region.

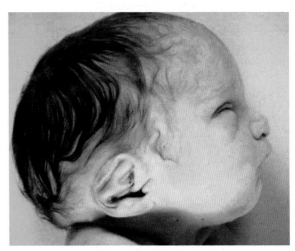

• **Figure 17.8** Low-set malformed ears. (From Gilbert-Barness E, Kapur RP, Oligny LL, et al. *Potter's Pathology of the Fetus, Infant and Child*. 2nd ed. St Louis: Mosby; 2007.)

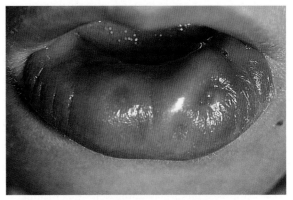

• **Figure 17.9** Lower lip pits.

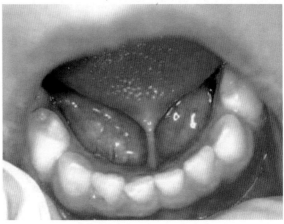

• **Figure 17.10** Ankyloglossia.

Dental Anomalies

Anomalies of tooth development are relatively common and may occur as an isolated finding or in association with other minor and major anomalies. Hypodontia is the developmental absence of one or more primary or permanent teeth. Although there are a number of syndromes in which hypodontia is a feature, the occurrence of one or more missing teeth (other than third molars) is estimated to be 6%, with reported ranges between 0.15% and 16.2%.[22] Anomalies of teeth follow patterns that reflect the time of development when the malformation occurs. For example, disruptions in tooth initiation result in hypodontia or supernumerary teeth, whereas disruptions during morphodifferentiation lead to anomalies of size and shape, such as macrodontia (Fig. 17.11), microdontia (Fig. 17.12), taurodontism (Fig. 17.13), dens invaginatus (Fig. 17.14), and dens evaginatus. Malformations that occur during histodifferentiation, apposition, and mineralization result in dentinogenesis imperfecta (Fig. 17.15), amelogenesis imperfecta (Fig. 17.16), denti n dysplasia, and enamel hypoplasia (Fig. 17.17).

Aside from managing the oral health of patients, a dentist's first responsibility is to recognize disease, whether it is in the mouth or in another part of the body. An additional responsibility is to know what to do when anomalies are identified in a patient. We are fortunate to be in an era where there is a wealth of information at our fingertips. With access to a computer and the Internet, both health care practitioners and the lay public can find information about a specific disorder in minutes. There are a number of extremely valuable and reliable resources on the Internet, including databases of published research articles, databases for inherited or rare diseases, and websites dedicated to information about specific syndromes (Box 17.1). For those without access to the Internet, there are a variety of valuable and frequently updated textbooks that provide information about syndromes that involve craniofacial anomalies.[21,23]

Why is it important for dentists to pay attention to potential developmental problems with their child patients, and what should dentists do if a developmental anomaly or syndrome is suspected? First, the dentist is responsible for the patient's overall health, not just the health of the mouth or teeth. Patients rely on health care providers to diagnose problems and inform them of those problems so that they can obtain appropriate and timely treatment. Second, there are many syndromes with features that influence how a dentist provides care for patients. For example, many children with Noonan

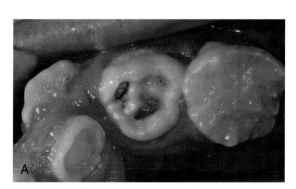
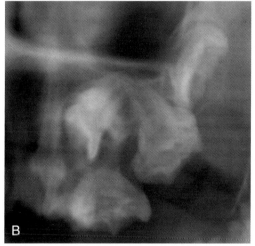

• **Figure 17.11** Clinical (A) and radiographic (B) images of primary molars with macrodontia.

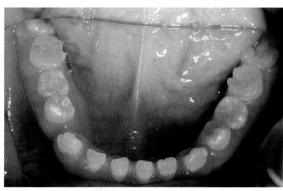

• **Figure 17.12** Permanent teeth with microdontia.

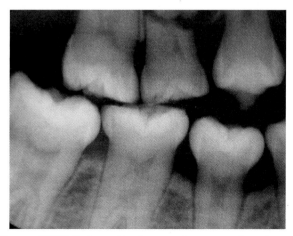

• **Figure 17.13** Radiographic image of permanent molars with taurodontism.

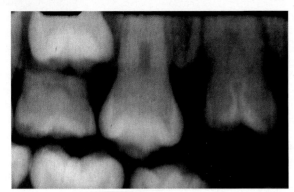

• **Figure 17.14** Radiographic image of permanent canine with dens invaginatus.

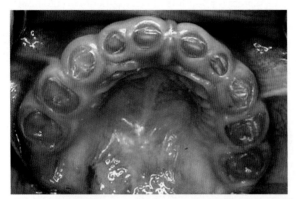

• **Figure 17.15** Dentinogenesis imperfecta in the primary dentition.

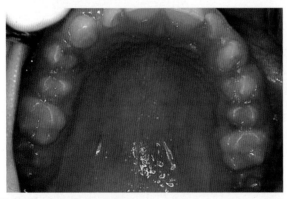

• **Figure 17.16** Amelogenesis imperfecta in the permanent dentition.

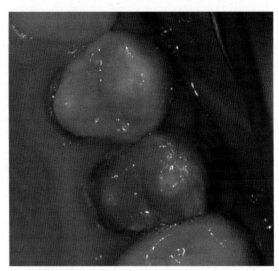

• **Figure 17.17** Enamel hypoplasia of a permanent second premolar. (Courtesy Dr. John Warren, University of Iowa, Iowa City, Iowa.)

> • BOX 17.1 **Sources of Genetic Information**
>
> National Center for Biotechnology Information: https://www.ncbi.nlm.nih.gov/
> Online Mendelian Inheritance in Man: https://www.omim.org/
> National Human Genome Research Institute: www.genome.gov/
> Genetic Education for Health Professionals: www.ashg.org/education/
>   Health_Professionals.shtml
> Genetic Alliance: geneticalliance.org/
> Gene Expression in Tooth: bite-it.helsinki.fi/
> National Organization for Rare Disorders: www.rarediseases.org/
> National Foundation for Ectodermal Dysplasias: www.nfed.org/
> National Society of Genetic Counselors: www.nsgc.org/
> American Society of Human Genetics: www.ashg.org/
> National Newborn Screening and Genetics Resource Center:
>   genes-r-us.uthscsa.edu/
> March of Dimes: www.marchofdimes.com/
> FACES: The National Craniofacial Association: www.faces-cranio.org/
> American Cleft Palate-Craniofacial Association: www.acpa-cpf.org/

syndrome have a congenital heart defect that may require the use of prophylactic antibiotics before dental treatment. Patients with Down syndrome frequently have congenital cardiac anomalies and, in addition, are at higher risk for periodontal disease as adults. Both of these characteristics require that a dentist modify the way he or she provides treatment to such patients.

When an anomaly is suspected but not diagnosed, the dentist should know how to gather the appropriate background information from the parent and, if necessary, refer the patient to a medical geneticist for further evaluation. Most teaching hospitals have a department of medical genetics that a child could be referred to for evaluation. In some areas, there are also outreach clinics where medical geneticists and genetic counselors travel to smaller towns to evaluate patients. Availability of genetic counselors in a particular area (in the United States) can be determined from the website of the National Society of Genetic Counselors (http://www.nsgc.org/page/find-a-gc-search). The database can be searched by entering a ZIP code and the number of miles a patient is able or willing to travel for care. Alternatively, practitioner name, practice type, or location can be used as search queries. As with any referral, it is important to send a letter or email to the physician or genetic counselor explaining why you are sending the patient for evaluation.

When discussing potential developmental anomalies with parents, it is important to be very sensitive to their concerns and to avoid causing undue alarm. Depending on the circumstances, it may be best to observe the child at multiple appointments (assuming that there are treatment needs) and to get to know the family better before broaching the subject. On the other hand, when there are obvious concerns and a timely diagnosis is indicated, an immediate referral should be made. One group of disorders that a dentist is likely to be the first to diagnose is the ectodermal dysplasia syndromes. Frequently parents become concerned when their 2- or 3-year-old child does not have any visible teeth or has conically shaped teeth. This should be recognizable to a dentist who sees children as a developmental anomaly that warrants further investigation. At this age, children frequently have sparse hair, but the combination of hypodontia, sparse hair, and dry skin should lead a dentist to refer this child to determine if he or she has a form of ectodermal dysplasia. Similarly, if a child who is 10 or 12 years old has not lost any primary teeth, a dentist should investigate further to determine the reason why the teeth have not exfoliated. In children with cleidocranial dysplasia, Gardner syndrome, and tricho-rhino-phalangeal syndrome, multiple supernumerary teeth may be present that block the eruption of the permanent teeth; but there is also a genetic defect that keeps teeth from erupting even after the supernumerary teeth are removed.

Because the genetic defects that cause many dominantly inherited syndromes can occur as new mutations, the child may be the first person in the family to experience the disorder. It is always important to ask about family history of disease, but absence of disease in the family does not preclude the occurrence of disease in the offspring.

When the child has been diagnosed with a particular disorder, frequently the disorder is rare enough that a dentist may not be familiar with it. In this case, it is important to gather as much information about the characteristics of the disorder before treating the child. Again, one of the most useful resources for this is the Internet. The database known as Online Mendelian Inheritance in Man (OMIM; www.ncbi.nlm.nih.gov/omim) is maintained and updated regularly by Johns Hopkins University. The database can be searched by entering the name of the syndrome or by entering clinical characteristics of the syndrome, such as hypodontia and sparse hair. After searching for a particular term, the database will give a list of disorders that include that term within the text of the description of the disorder. In addition, there are references that are linked to the National Library of Medicine database of published literature, PubMed (see Box 17.1), so that abstracts of articles about the disorder can be easily accessed or downloaded. This is a free database that is available to anyone with an Internet connection. Information about syndromes is also available via the National Organization for Rare Disorders (NORD; www.rarediseases.org/). This site also has a large database of rare diseases. To view full reports of a disease you must be registered. Two reports per day are available at no charge to registered users. There is currently no charge for registration.

Syndromes/Disorders With Craniofacial Anomalies

It is not possible in a single chapter to discuss every syndrome that includes malformations involving the face or mouth. The following section focuses on a subset of disorders that are either more commonly seen in the dental office or have such dramatic dental and oral manifestations that all dentists should be aware of them. It is recommended that every dental office has access to information about genetic disorders via both the Internet and one or more textbooks.

Down Syndrome

Inheritance pattern: Chromosomal; sporadic
Gene(s): Trisomy 21

General manifestations: Intellectual disability; hypotonia; cardiac anomaly in about 40% of cases; dry skin; increased risk for leukemia (ALL and AML); increased risk for atlantoaxial instability

Craniofacial/dental manifestations: Brachycephaly; inner epicanthal folds; upslanting palpebral fissures; small ears; microdontia; increased risk for periodontal disease, delayed exfoliation of primary teeth, and delayed eruption of permanent teeth[21]

Dental treatment considerations: When treating children with Down syndrome (Fig. 17.18), the primary concerns are to determine the need for subacute bacterial endocarditis prophylaxis and the child's ability to cooperate. If a child has had surgery to repair a congenital heart defect, he or she may or may not need subacute bacterial endocarditis prophylaxis, depending on when the surgery was performed and on the presence of any residual defect. This should be confirmed with the parent or the child's cardiologist. The behavior of children with Down syndrome varies from one child to another, just as it does for typically developed children. It is not fair to assume in advance that such a child will be uncooperative for dental treatment. On the other hand, some children and young adults with Down syndrome may be very uncooperative and difficult to examine in the traditional dental setting. When behavior is an issue, it may be necessary to use general anesthesia and/or to refer the child to a specialist in order to provide quality care. It is important to note that patients with Down syndrome are much more susceptible to periodontal disease. The dentist should make this clear to the parent and should stress early development of good oral hygiene habits including thorough, supervised daily tooth brushing with a fluoridated toothpaste; flossing; and, when necessary, the use of an antibacterial mouth rinse such as 0.12% chlorhexidine.

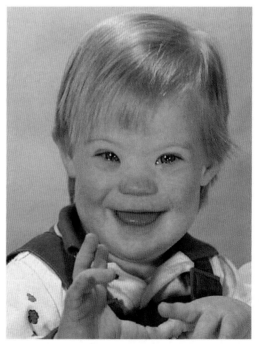

• **Figure 17.18** Typical facies of a child with Down syndrome, including flat nasal bridge, epicanthal folds, and upslanting palpebral fissures. (From Zitelli BJ, Davis HW. *Atlas of Pediatric Physical Diagnosis.* 5th ed. Philadelphia: Mosby; 2007.)

Ectodermal Dysplasia

Inheritance pattern: X-linked recessive, autosomal dominant, autosomal recessive

Gene(s): Ectodermal dysplasia 1 *(EDA1)*[24]; ectodysplasin 1 (ectodysplasin A receptor; *EDAR)*[25]; muscle segment homeobox homolog 1 *(MSX1)*[26]; paired box gene 9 *(PAX9)*[27]; *WNT10A*[28]; tumor protein p63 (TP63)[29]

General manifestations: Sparse hair; dry skin; absence of sweat glands; normal mental status; eyes sensitive to light; may overheat easily;[21] dysplastic and slow-growing nails[21]

Craniofacial/dental manifestations: Full lips; small nose; hypodontia; conical or malformed teeth; deficient alveolar ridge; relatively flat palate

Dental treatment considerations: There are more than 150 forms of the ectodermal dysplasia syndrome that affect one or more of the tissues derived from the ectoderm (Figs. 17.19 and 17.20). Although the best-known condition is the X-linked hypohidrotic form, there are also autosomal dominant and autosomal recessive forms with symptoms that range from mild with hypodontia only to a more severe form with many structures affected, in addition to a cleft lip and palate and anomalies of the fingers (ectrodactyly–ectodermal dysplasia–clefting syndrome caused by mutations in *TP63*). Children with hypohidrotic ectodermal dysplasia frequently lack most primary and permanent teeth. This leads to underdevelopment of the alveolar ridges and makes the fabrication of dentures more challenging.

When ectodermal dysplasia is inherited as an X-linked or autosomal dominant disorder, parents are usually familiar with the disorder because other family members may have been affected. However, the disorder may also be caused by a new mutation or inherited as an autosomal recessive trait. When this happens, the family may be completely unaware of the manifestations of this disorder. It is not uncommon for the dentist to be the first person to recognize ectodermal dysplasia in a child. Parents become concerned when their child has few if any erupted teeth by 2 to 3 years of age and often seek a dentist's advice. At this age, it is usually possible to assess the developing teeth using maxillary and mandibular occlusal radiographs. These will establish whether the dental development is delayed, if the primary teeth are missing, or if there is some other process that is interfering with tooth eruption. If primary teeth are not present, the child should be referred to a medical geneticist and/or genetic counselor for a thorough evaluation.

Dentists can provide a great service to children with ectodermal dysplasia by fabricating dentures at a young age and by educating the family about future treatment options. Dentures can be fabricated for young children as soon as they are cooperative enough to tolerate impressions. Because of their tendency to overheat, the use of protective stabilization for extended lengths of time in a very young child is contraindicated. As these children grow and mature, other options become available to them including implants and implant-retained dentures. Frequently bone grafts must be done before placing implants because of the reduced thickness and height of the alveolar ridge. Guidelines for the treatment of these patients at various ages are available from the National Foundation for the Ectodermal Dysplasias (NFED). The publication *Dental Guide to the Ectodermal Dysplasias* is available from NFED (https://view.flipdocs.com/?ID=10011422_390125). This organization provides information and support to families who have children with ectodermal dysplasia. Grants are available from

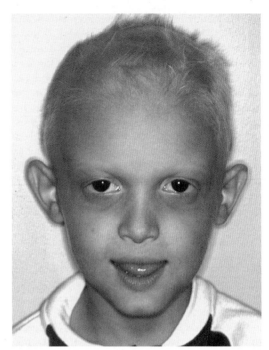

• **Figure 17.19** A child with ectodermal dysplasia showing sparse hair. (From Proffit WR, Fields HW, Sarver DM. *Contemporary Orthodontics*. 5th ed. St Louis: Mosby; 2013.)

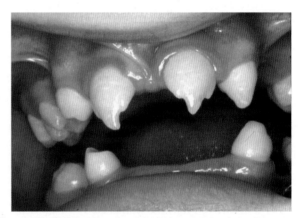

• **Figure 17.20** Dentition of a child with ectodermal dysplasia demonstrating missing lower incisors and malformed central incisors.

NFED for families to help defray the cost of dental treatment and for researchers to better understand the many forms of ectodermal dysplasia.

Isolated Hypodontia

Inheritance pattern: Autosomal dominant

Gene(s): MSX1, PAX9, EDA, AXIN2, EDAR, EDARADD, WNT10A, GREM2, and *TFAP2B*

General manifestations: One or more developmentally missing teeth. Not associated with other systemic manifestations.

Craniofacial/dental manifestations: Agenesis of one or more primary or permanent teeth

Dental treatment considerations: Isolated or nonsyndromic hypodontia or tooth agenesis is one of the most common developmental disorders in humans. It has been reported to be associated with genetic and environmental factors. The prevalence of hypodontia ranges from 1.6% to 9.6% depending on studied populations. It is more common in the permanent dentition than in the primary dentition. Excluding the third permanent molars, the most common missing teeth are the mandibular second premolars, maxillary lateral incisors, and maxillary second premolars. Isolated hypodontia has been reported to be caused by mutations in *MSX1, PAX9, EDA, AXIN2, EDAR, EDARADD, WNT10A, GREM2,* and *TFAP2B*.[30] Variable expression can be found in families with hypodontia. It is important to note that microdontia can be a form of hypodontia, which would explain why a parent with microdontia may have children with hypodontia. A panoramic radiograph is an important diagnostic tool for patients with dental anomalies including hypodontia.

Dental treatment considerations are governed by the age of the patient, the ability to tolerate the steps involved in appliance fabrication, and the long-term plans for tooth replacement including fixed or removable prostheses and/or implants.

Cleidocranial Dysplasia

Inheritance pattern: Autosomal dominant or new mutation
Gene(s): Runt-related transcription factor 2 (*RUNX2*)[31]
General manifestations: Moderate short stature; normal intelligence; partial to complete absence of clavicles
Craniofacial/dental manifestations: Frontal bossing; brachycephaly; late closure of fontanels; hypertelorism; delayed eruption of permanent teeth; supernumerary teeth; impacted teeth
Dental treatment considerations: The dental manifestations of this disorder can be extremely challenging and should be approached by a multidisciplinary team including a pediatric dentist, oral surgeon, orthodontist, and prosthodontist (Fig. 17.21). The pediatric dentist often serves as the case manager who brings the team together and facilitates communication among the other specialists and the patient's family. Children with cleidocranial dysplasia may have as many as 60 supernumerary teeth or as few as 1. Surgical removal of these extra teeth must be done with the appropriate timing and frequently involves multiple surgeries during childhood and adolescence. Once the supernumerary teeth have been removed, orthodontic forces are usually required to bring the permanent teeth into position. The timing of orthodontic treatment is crucial because appropriate anchorage must be established in advance, and often the first permanent molars are impacted.

It is possible that the delayed eruption of permanent teeth (and delayed exfoliation of primary teeth) will be the initial sign that something is abnormal in the child's development. Because this is a relatively rare disorder and its general characteristics are not life threatening, it may go undetected by the child's physician. Again, this is an opportunity for dentists to provide a service to their patients by recognizing the potential for a genetic condition and referring the child to a medical geneticist for a definitive diagnosis. Evaluation of a child with retained primary teeth should include a panoramic radiograph and possibly a cone beam computed tomography scan for enhanced localization and position of teeth.[32]

Williams-Beuren Syndrome

Inheritance pattern: Autosomal dominant or new mutation; can be chromosome 7q11.23 deletion syndrome[33]
Gene(s): 7q11.23 region, elastin *(ELN)*, LIM domain kinase 1 *(LIMK1)*, replication factor C *(RFC2)*[34]
General manifestations: Cardiovascular anomalies (supravalvular aortic stenosis); infantile hypercalcemia; outgoing personality; intellectual disability; hoarse voice
Craniofacial/dental manifestations: Stellate pattern in the iris[35]; hypodontia; enamel hypoplasia; prominent lips; wide mouth
Dental treatment considerations: Children and adults with Williams-Beuren syndrome can provide both fun and a challenge to your practice (Fig. 17.22). Their charming, friendly personality endears them to everyone. However, their hypersensitivity to sound and easy distractibility can make it necessary to spend extra time and patience during dental treatment. Because of the frequent cardiovascular anomalies associated with this disorder, it is essential to determine if there is a need for subacute bacterial endocarditis prophylaxis before dental treatment. If the parent is unsure about this, the dentist should contact the child's cardiologist and document the physician's advice in the patient's record.

Fragile X Syndrome

Inheritance pattern: X-linked
Gene(s): Fragile X mental retardation-1 *(FMR1)*[36,37]
General manifestations: Intellectual disability; autism in 60%; macroorchidism[21]
Craniofacial/dental manifestations: Macrocephaly; prognathism; large ears
Dental treatment considerations: Fragile X syndrome is documented as the cause of intellectual disability in almost 6% of males with intellectual disability (Fig. 17.23). In the dental clinic, treatment issues primarily center around the child's behavior and ability to tolerate dental procedures. This is further

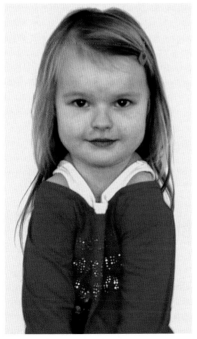

• **Figure 17.21** A child with cleidocranial dysplasia. (From Cobourne MT, DiBiase AT. *Handbook of Orthodontics*. Edinburgh: Mosby; 2010.)

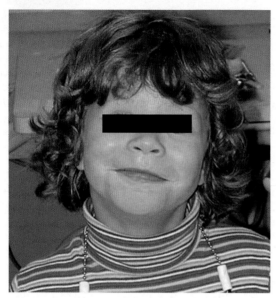

• **Figure 17.22** Facies of a child with Williams-Beuren syndrome.

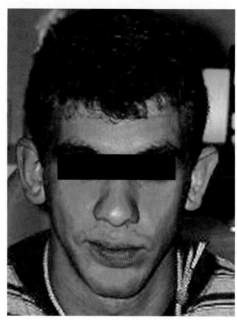

• **Figure 17.23** A young man with fragile X syndrome.

complicated in children who also have autism. As is true for many persons with special needs, their oral health is the responsibility of a parent or other care provider. For this reason, it is important for the dentist to provide the caregiver with the information and tools required to assess and maintain good oral hygiene and healthy dietary practices for these children.

Osteogenesis Imperfecta

Inheritance pattern: Autosomal dominant, autosomal recessive or sporadic
Gene(s): Type I collagen *(COL1A1, COL1A2)*[38]; cartilage-associated protein *(CRTAP)*[39]; prolyl 3-hydroxylase 1 *(LEPRE1)*[39]; peptidyl-prolyl isomerase B *(PPIB)*[40]
General manifestations: Moderate to severe bone fragility; short stature; normal intelligence; hearing impairment in adulthood; hyperextensible joints; deformity of limbs
Craniofacial/dental manifestations: Triangular facies; blue sclera; occasional dentinogenesis imperfecta; delayed eruption of teeth
Dental treatment considerations: Osteogenesis imperfecta is a heterogeneous disorder resulting from both quantitative and qualitative defects in type I collagen and from mutations in at least 10 other genes. Many of the newly identified genes are noncollagenous in nature, thus contributing to a greater understanding of bone biology. There are more than 12 subtypes of osteogenesis imperfecta, with symptoms that range from mild to severely deforming to lethal.[41] Osteogenesis imperfecta type I is the mildest form and may go undiagnosed until the child's first bone fracture. In some cases, parents of children with an undiagnosed mild form of osteogenesis imperfecta have been accused of child abuse when an unreported previous fracture is detected radiographically. It is important for a physician to rule out osteogenesis imperfecta when questions of previous fractures are being evaluated. Osteogenesis imperfecta type II is lethal at birth or shortly thereafter, and dental professionals are not likely to have exposure to children with this form of the disease. The most severe, deforming variety of osteogenesis imperfecta is type III. These children have extreme bone fragility and by childhood may have had as many as 30 fractures. They

are frequently not ambulatory and have a history of surgeries that includes placement of rods in their legs and spine. Osteogenesis imperfecta type IV is intermediate in severity between type III and type I. These children have moderate short stature, bone fragility, and significant bone deformity. Sclera is normal, and often dentinogenesis imperfecta is present in children with osteogenesis imperfecta type IV. Type V is mild to moderate in severity, type VI is moderate, and types VII and VIII are moderate to severe or lethal.[39] Dental treatment for patients with osteogenesis imperfecta should be approached with great care and with guidance from the parent to determine what the child can tolerate. Active or passive immobilization of patients with osteogenesis imperfecta is not recommended for obvious reasons. If behavior at a young age makes treatment in the traditional dental setting infeasible, other options such as general anesthesia should be considered. When a child with dentinogenesis imperfecta presents in a dental office, especially when there is no history of this disorder in the family, the dentist should consider the possibility that the child also has osteogenesis imperfecta. A referral to a medical geneticist for evaluation is appropriate if there is any doubt about the diagnosis.

Dentinogenesis Imperfecta

Inheritance pattern: Autosomal dominant or sporadic
Gene(s): Dentin sialophosphoprotein *(DSPP)*[42]
General manifestations: Normal intelligence; good general health unless in combination with osteogenesis imperfecta
Craniofacial/dental manifestations: Both primary and permanent teeth are affected; teeth are blue-gray or brown; susceptible to extreme wear; and pulpal obliteration and dental abscesses
Dental treatment considerations: The severity of this disorder varies considerably from one child to another both within and between families (see Fig. 17.15). In addition, the appearance of the primary dentition does not reliably predict the appearance of the permanent dentition. Primary teeth generally are more severely affected than the permanent ones. In the primary dentition, stainless steel crowns are frequently used to prevent

excessive wear of the molars. This should be initiated once wear is apparent on the molars. For some children this may occur as early as 2 years of age, whereas for others it may occur later. Abscessed primary teeth require pulp therapy but may need to be extracted if significant pulpal obliteration has occurred. Esthetic concerns on the part of the child or parent can be addressed in the primary dentition using esthetic anterior crowns or partial overdentures. In the permanent dentition, bleaching procedures have been used to lighten the color of the teeth, followed by anterior composite or porcelain veneers. As adults, most individuals require full-coverage crowns and frequently root canal therapy. Every effort should be made to maintain the teeth as long as possible to maximize the treatment options for the individual as an adult. Consultation with other dental specialists to assist in planning for future treatment is recommended. If parents report a history of bone fractures, the child should be referred for a medical evaluation to rule out osteogenesis imperfecta.

Amelogenesis Imperfecta

Inheritance pattern: Autosomal dominant, autosomal recessive, X-linked, sporadic

Gene(s): Amelogenin *(AMG)*[43]; enamelin *(ENAM)*[44]; family with sequence similarity, member H *(FAM83H)*[45]; matrix metalloproteinase 20 *(MMP-20)*[46]; kallikrein 4 *(KLK-4)*[47]

General manifestations: Normal intelligence; good general health

Craniofacial/dental manifestations: Enamel defects that affect both dentitions; appearance is variable depending on subtype; teeth may be sensitive, susceptible to wear; there may also be taurodontism in molars or an anterior open bite.

Dental treatment considerations: There are three major categories of amelogenesis imperfecta and 14 subtypes. More in-depth discussion of the subtypes can be found in Chapter 3. Dental treatment considerations require that the clinician understand the characteristics of the different subtypes before developing a treatment plan. In general, treatment concerns fit into a few general categories. With most subtypes, the teeth are susceptible to attrition and require full crown coverage to minimize wear. In the primary dentition, this is usually accomplished by placing stainless steel crowns on all the primary molars. A combination of veneers and full-coverage cast crowns may be used in the permanent dentition. Frequently transitional restorations must be made during the adolescent years until the permanent teeth are fully erupted. Other concerns with this group of disorders include tooth sensitivity, esthetics, susceptibility to dental caries, and malocclusion. It is not unusual for there to be delayed or partial eruption of permanent premolars and molars requiring gingival surgery to expose the crowns and orthodontic forces to move them into place before restoration. Because of the many complicated issues involved in treating patients with amelogenesis imperfecta, it is recommended that such patients be treated by a team of dental specialists who have had experience with this disorder. When that is not an option because of geographic or other constraints, every effort should be made to consult colleagues who have had experience with this disorder before treatment (see Fig. 17.16).

Treacher Collins Syndrome

Inheritance pattern: Autosomal dominant or sporadic

Gene(s): Treacher Collins–Franceschetti syndrome 1 *(TCOF1)*[48]

General manifestations: Normal intelligence; conductive deafness; pharyngeal hypoplasia; occasional congenital heart defect

Craniofacial/dental manifestations: Downslanting palpebral fissures; malar hypoplasia; lower eyelid coloboma; mandibular hypoplasia; malformation of external ear; cleft palate or submucous cleft

Dental treatment considerations: The severe micrognathia in some patients with Treacher Collins syndrome contributes to dental crowding and may make intubation difficult if treatment under general anesthesia is required (Fig. 17.24). Frequently orthognathic surgery is required during childhood or adolescence. Dental practitioners should consult with the child's physician to confirm the absence of other medical conditions such as congenital heart defects that might dictate modifications in how dental treatment is delivered.

Van der Woude Syndrome

Inheritance pattern: Autosomal dominant or sporadic

Gene(s): Interferon regulatory factor 6 *(IRF6)*[49]; Grainyhead-like 3 *(GRHL3)*[50]

General manifestations: Normal intelligence; good general health

Craniofacial/dental manifestations: Lower lip pits; cleft lip/palate; cleft uvula; hypodontia; occasional ankyloglossia

Dental treatment considerations: Cleft lip and/or palate may occur as a solitary finding or as part of a syndrome (Fig. 17.25). It is estimated that approximately 70% of children with Van der Woude syndrome have mutations in the gene *IRF6*.[50] Recently mutations in the gene *GRHL3* were found to lead to almost identical orofacial clefting phenotypes as seen in *VWS1* and has since been designated as *VWS2.* Children with Van der Woude syndrome may have lower lip pits alone or in combination with cleft lip and/or cleft palate. Because the symptoms are limited and affected individuals have normal intelligence, this disorder could be confused with nonsyndromic cleft lip/palate. It is important that children with cleft lip/palate or with

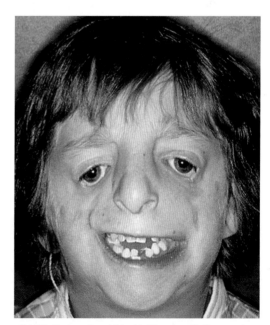

• **Figure 17.24** Facies of a child with Treacher Collins syndrome. (From Nanci A. Ten Cate's Oral Histology: Development, Structure, and Function. 8th ed. St Louis: Mosby; 2013.)

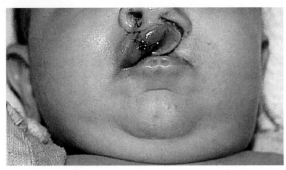

• **Figure 17.25** Cleft lip/palate in a child with Van der Woude syndrome.

lip pits only be seen and evaluated by a craniofacial anomalies team to determine the cause and heritability of their disorder. In addition, this type of team approach is important for providing coordinated, timely treatment of children with cleft lip/palate. Many hospitals have cleft lip/palate or craniofacial teams that include specialists from the following disciplines: plastic surgery, craniofacial and/or oral surgery, pediatric medicine, pediatric dentistry, orthodontics, speech pathology, audiology, prosthodontics, social work, and medical genetics.

Isolated (Nonsyndromic) Orofacial Clefts

Inheritance pattern: Autosomal dominant or nonmendelian inheritance pattern with gene–environment interactions
Gene(s): MSX1, TBX22, TP63, and *IRF6*
Craniofacial/dental manifestations: Cleft lip with or without cleft palate
Dental treatment considerations: Orofacial clefting—a group of anatomic birth defects where there is a gap or break in normal structures of the mouth—is one of the most common human developmental disorders, affecting 1 in every 600 newborns worldwide. The prevalence is high in East Asian and Native American (3.6 per 1000 births) populations and low in African-ancestry populations (0.3 per 1000 births). Orofacial clefts can be isolated or syndromic. There are more than 300 syndromes with orofacial clefting as part of the phenotype. The etiology of orofacial clefting is complex and heterogeneous, with both genetic and environmental influences. Isolated cleft lip/palate has been reported to be associated with mutations in a number of genes, including *MSX1, TBX22, TP63,* and *IRF6.* Environmental factors include maternal smoking and consumption of phenytoin, retinoic acid derivatives, alcohol, and folate antagonist drugs during pregnancy. Isolated cleft lip with or without cleft palate and cleft palate only are two different entities. Cleft lip with or without cleft palate may be present in the same families but not with cleft palate alone. Isolated mixed types of clefts in the same families can be seen in families with *IRF6* and *TP63* mutations. Orofacial clefting exhibits phenotypic variability in terms of severity and the orofacial structures that are affected. The microforms of cleft lip with or without cleft palate include small defects of lip and/or alveolar arch, scar-like ridges above the lip, and defects of the superior orbicularis oris muscle, which can be visualized only by ultrasonography.[51] The microforms of cleft palate consist of bifid uvula and submucous palatal clefts. The ability to detect the microforms is crucial in identifying the carriers of the mutations.

Hypophosphatasia

Inheritance pattern: Autosomal dominant, autosomal recessive, or sporadic
Gene(s): "Tissue nonspecific" isoenzyme of alkaline phosphatase *(TNSALP)*[52]
General manifestations: Normal or short stature; bone fragility; bowed lower extremities
Craniofacial/dental manifestations: Premature loss of teeth (most commonly primary incisors) due to lack of cementum; craniosynostosis
Dental treatment considerations: There are four forms of hypophosphatasia ranging from mild to lethal. The milder form that presents in childhood after 6 months of age results in premature loss of primary teeth and craniosynostosis. All types demonstrate decreased levels of serum alkaline phosphatase. Although this is a relatively rare disorder, dentists should be aware of its existence so that an appropriate referral can be made. Frequently the first sign of this disorder is the premature loss of a mandibular primary incisor without a history of trauma. The exfoliated tooth typically has no root resorption, and histologic analysis will show a lack of cementum. In the mild form of this disorder, the dental manifestations may be the only symptoms.

Apert Syndrome

Inheritance pattern: Autosomal dominant with complete penetrance. Most cases are sporadic. The majority of sporadic cases are associated with older paternal age
Gene(s): Fibroblast growth factor receptor 2 *(FGFR2)*[53]
General manifestations: Intellectual disability, ocular proptosis, hypertelorism, strabismus, symmetric syndactyly of hands and feet, and moderate to severe acne during adolescence
Craniofacial/dental manifestations: Acrobrachycephaly as a result of craniosynostosis, especially of coronal sutures; flat occiput; wide midline calvarial defect extending from glabella to posterior fontanel; midface underdevelopment leading to relative mandibular prognathism and severely crowded teeth; highly arched palate with lateral palatal swellings; depressed nasal bridge; and cleft soft palate or bifid uvula
Dental treatment considerations: Most of these patients require orthodontic treatment with orthognathic surgery to move the maxilla forward; even with intellectual disability, most patients cooperate well enough in the dental office to tolerate orthodontic treatment.

Crouzon Syndrome

Inheritance pattern: Autosomal dominant with variable expression. The majority of sporadic cases are associated with older paternal age.
Gene(s): Fibroblast growth factor receptor 2 *(FGFR2)*[54]
General manifestations: Most of these patients are intellectually normal; conductive hearing loss; cervical spine anomalies; calcification of stylohyoid ligaments.
Craniofacial/dental manifestations: Craniosynostosis; increased digital markings on skull radiographs; hypertelorism; exotropia; ocular proptosis secondary to shallow orbits is a consistent feature resulting in exposure conjunctivitis and keratitis; underdeveloped maxilla leading to crowding of maxillary teeth, ectopic eruption of the maxillary first permanent molars, and posterior crossbite; lateral palatal swellings.

Dental treatment considerations: Most of these patients require orthodontic treatment with orthognathic surgery to move the maxilla forward; patients with Crouzon syndrome usually cooperate well in the dental office.

Genetic Testing

The majority of genetic tests available today are used to diagnose specific inherited disorders such as cystic fibrosis, Huntington disease, or fragile X syndrome. These tests are typically ordered and interpreted by medical geneticists or genetic counselors. Genetic tests for inherited disorders involve screening for specific mutations or chromosomal disruptions. A second category of genetic tests screen for genetic risk factors for various disorders that have a genetic component. This includes disorders such as familial breast cancer and Alzheimer disease. Testing positive for one of these risk factors does not guarantee that one will get the disease, but it does indicate that an individual is at increased risk of developing the disease. This information allows one to make changes in his or her life to decrease additional risk factors for that disease.

In recent years DNA sequencing technologies have advanced significantly, allowing whole-genome sequencing for an individual using a saliva sample at the cost of less than $1000 (https://www.genome.gov/sequencingcosts/). Other technologies that have improved the ability to detect disease-causing mutations include whole-exome sequencing and microarray-based comparative genomic hybridization (CGH).[55]

Identification of genetic risk factors for dental caries and for periodontal disease is the goal of a number of dental researchers. It is conceivable that in the near future in-office genetic tests will be available to predict the caries risk or periodontal disease risk of an individual patient. Using the results of these tests, the dentist will be able to develop a targeted prevention plan to minimize the severity of disease for that individual.

Ethical, Legal, and Social Implications of the Human Genome Project

In the past, patients have not been denied dental insurance because of preexisting dental disease, and a thorough dental examination is not usually required for a patient to qualify for dental benefits. The result is that dentists may not be aware of the potential for discrimination to which some patients are susceptible because of their health history. Genetic testing that identifies a person's risk for disease before he or she has any manifestations of the disease introduces a new level of information about an individual's health and insurability that has not been available in the past. In many cases, the ethical, legal, and social implications of the information learned from the Human Genome Project are still being evaluated.

References

1. Slavkin HC. From phenotype to genotype: enter genomics and transformation of primary health care around the world. *J Dent Res.* 2014;93(7 suppl):3S–6S.
2. Nybo Andersen A-M, Urhoj SK. Is advanced paternal age a health risk for the offspring? *Fertil Steril.* 2017;107(2):312–318.
3. Gelehrter T, Collins FS. *Principles of Medical Genetics.* Baltimore: Williams & Wilkins; 1990.
4. Muncie HL, Campbell JS. Alpha and beta thalassemia. *Am Fam Physician.* 2009;80(4):339–344.
5. Mandal A, Leger R, Graham L, et al. An overview of human genetic disorders with special reference to African Americans. *J Bioprocess Biotech.* 2015;5:10.
6. Boraas JC, Messer LB, Till MJ. A genetic contribution to dental caries, occlusion and morphology as demonstrated by twins reared apart. *J Dent Res.* 1988;67:1150–1155.
7. Conry JP, Messer LB, Boraas JC, et al. Dental caries and treatment characteristics in human twins reared apart. *Arch Oral Biol.* 1993;38:937–943.
8. Vieira AR, Marazita ML, Goldstein-McHenry T. Genome-wide scan finds suggestive caries loci. *J Dent Res.* 2008;87:435–439.
9. Lewis DDSJ, Shaffer JR, Feingold E, et al. Genetic association of *MMP10, MMP14* and *MMP16* with dental caries. *Int J Dent.* 2017;2017:8465125.
10. Shaffer JR, Carlson JC, Stanley BO, et al. Effects of enamel matric genes on dental caries are moderated by fluoride exposure. *Hum Genet.* 2015;134(2):159–167.
11. Stanley BO, Feingold E, Cooper M, et al. Genetic association of MPPED2 and ACTN2 with dental caries. *J Dent Res.* 2014;93(7):626–632.
12. Eckert S, Feingold E, Cooper M, et al. Variants on chromosome 4q21 near PKD2 and SIBLINGs are associated with dental caries. *J Hum Genet.* 2017;62(4):491–496.
13. Lim DH, Maher ER. Human imprinting syndromes. *Epigenomics.* 2009;1(2):347–369.
14. Loke YJ, Hannan AJ, Craig JM. The role of epigenetic change in autism spectrum disorders. *Front Neurol.* 2015;6:107.
15. Sidhu H, Capalash N. UHRF1: the key regulator of epigenetics and molecular target for cancer therapeutics. *Tumour Biol.* 2017;39(2):1010428317692205.
16. Kaminsky Z, Wilcox HC, Eaton WW, et al. Epigenetic and genetic variation at SKA2 predict suicidal behavior and post-traumatic stress disorder. *Transl Psychiatry.* 2015;5:e627.
17. Schulz S, Immel UD, Just L, et al. Epigenetic characteristics in inflammatory candidate genes in aggressive periodontitis. *Hum Immunol.* 2016;77(1):71–75.
18. Leppig KA, Werler MM, Cann CI, et al. Predictive value of minor anomalies. Association with major malformations. *J Pediatr.* 1987;110:531–537.
19. Marden P, Smith D, McDonald MJ. Congenital anomalies in the newborn infant, including minor variations. *J Pediatr.* 1964;64:357–371.
20. Méhes K, Mestyan J, Knoch V, et al. Minor malformations in the neonate. *Helv Paediatr Acta.* 1973;28:477–483.
21. Jones K, Jones MC, Del Campo M. *Smith's Recognizable Patterns of Human Malformation.* Philadelphia: Saunders; 2013.
22. Rakhshan V. Congenitally missing teeth (hypodontia): a review of the literature concerning the etiology, prevalence, risk factors, patterns and treatment. *Dent Res J (Isfahan).* 2015;12(1):1–13.
23. Gorlin RJ, Cohen MM, Hennekam RCM. *Syndromes of the Head and Neck.* New York: Oxford University Press; 2001.
24. Kere J, Srivastava AK, Montonen O, et al. X-linked anhidrotic (hypohidrotic) ectodermal dysplasia is caused by mutation in a novel transmembrane protein. *Nat Genet.* 1996;13:409–416.
25. Monreal AW, Ferguson BM, Headon DJ, et al. Mutations in the human homologue of mouse dl cause autosomal recessive and dominant hypo-hidrotic ectodermal dysplasia. *Nat Genet.* 1999;22:366–369.
26. Vastardis H, Karimbux N, Guthua SW, et al. A human MSX1 homeodomain missense mutation causes selective tooth agenesis. *Nat Genet.* 1996;13:417–421.
27. Stockton DW, Das P, Goldenberg M, et al. Mutation of PAX9 is associated with oligodontia. *Nat Genet.* 2000;24:18–19.
28. Kantaputra P, Sripathomsawat W. WNT10A and isolated hypodontia. *Am J Med Genet.* 2011;155A:1119–1122.
29. Celli J, Duijf P, Hamel BCJ, et al. Heterozygous germline mutations in the p53 homolog p63 are the cause of EEC syndrome. *Cell.* 1999;99:143–153.
30. Yin W, Bian Z. The gene network underlying hypodontia. *J Dent Res.* 2015;94(7):878–885.

31. Mundlos S, Otto F, Mundlos C, et al. Mutations involving the transcription factor CBFA1 cause cleidocranial dysplasia. *Cell*. 1997;89:773–779.

32. Kim K, Ruprecht A, Jeon K, et al. Personal computer-based three-dimensional computed tomographic images of the teeth for evaluating supernumerary or ectopically impacted teeth. *Angle Orthod*. 2003;73:614–621.

33. Pober BR. Williams-Beuren syndrome. *N Engl J Med*. 2010;362:239–252.

34. Osborne LR, Martindale D, Scherer SW, et al. Identification of genes from a 500-kb region at 7q11.23 that is commonly deleted in Williams syndrome patients. *Genomics*. 1996;36:328–336.

35. Holmstrom G, Almond G, Temple K, et al. The iris in Williams syndrome. *Arch Dis Child*. 1990;65:987–989.

36. Crawford DC, Acuna JM, Sherman SL. FMR1 and the fragile X syndrome: human genome epidemiology review. *Genet Med*. 2001;3:359–371.

37. Kremer EJ, Pritchard M, Lynch M, et al. Mapping of DNA instability at the fragile X to a trinucleotide repeat sequence p(CCG)n. *Science*. 1991;252:1711–1714.

38. Byers PH, Wallis GA, Willing MC. Osteogenesis imperfecta: translation of mutation to phenotype. *J Med Genet*. 1991;28:433–442.

39. Shapiro JR, Sponsellor PD. Osteogenesis imperfecta: questions and answers. *Curr Opin Pediatr*. 2009;21(6):709–716.

40. van Dijk FS, Nesbitt IM, Zwikstra EH, et al. PPIB mutations cause severe osteogenesis imperfecta. *Am J Hum Genet*. 2009;85:521–527.

41. Marini JC, Reich A, Smith SM. Osteogenesis imperfecta due to mutations in non-collagenous genes: lessons in the biology of bone formation. *Curr Opin Pediatr*. 2014;26(4):500–507.

42. Zhang X, Zhao J, Li C, et al. DSPP mutation in dentinogenesis imperfecta Shields type II. *Nat Genet*. 2001;27:151–152.

43. Lagerstrom M, Dahl N, Nakahori Y, et al. A deletion in the amelogenin gene (AMG) causes X-linked amelogenesis imperfecta (AIH1). *Genomics*. 1991;10:971–975.

44. Rajpar MH, Harley K, Laing C, et al. Mutation of the gene encoding the enamel-specific protein, enamelin, causes autosomal-dominant amelogenesis imperfecta. *Hum Mol Genet*. 2001;10:1673–1677.

45. Kim JW, Lee SK, Lee ZH, et al. FAM83H mutations in families with autosomal-dominant hypocalcified amelogenesis imperfecta. *Am J Hum Genet*. 2008;82:489–494.

46. Kim JW, Simmer JP, Hart TC, et al. MMP-20 mutation in autosomal recessive pigmented hypomaturation amelogenesis imperfecta. *J Med Genet*. 2005;42:271–275.

47. Hart PS, Hart TC, Michalec MD, et al. Mutation in kallikrein 4 causes autosomal recessive hypomaturation amelogenesis imperfecta. *J Med Genet*. 2004;41:545–549.

48. The Treacher Collins Syndrome Collaborative Group. Positional cloning of a gene involved in the pathogenesis of Treacher Collins syndrome. *Nat Genet*. 1996;12:130–136.

49. Kondo S, Schutte BC, Richardson RJ, et al. Mutations in IRF6 cause Van der Woude and popliteal pterygium syndromes. *Nat Genet*. 2002;32:285–289.

50. Peyrard-Janvid M, Leslie EJ, Kousa YA, et al. Dominant mutations in GRHL3 cause Van der Woude syndrome and disrupt oral periderm development. *Am J Hum Genet*. 2014;94:23–32.

51. Marazita ML. Subclinical features in non-syndromic cleft lip with or without cleft palate (CL/P): review of the evidence that subepithelial orbicularis oris muscle defects are part of an expanded phenotype for CL/P. *Orthod Craniofac Res*. 2007;10(2):82–87.

52. Henthorn PS, Raducha M, Fedde KN, et al. Different missense mutations at the tissue-nonspecific alkaline phosphatase gene locus in autosomal recessively inherited forms of mild and severe hypophosphatasia. *Proc Natl Acad Sci USA*. 1992;89:9924–9928.

53. Wilkie AOM, Slaney SF, Oldridge M, et al. Apert syndrome results from localized mutations of FGFR2 and is allelic with Crouzon syndrome. *Nature Genet*. 1995;9:165–172.

54. Reardon W, Winter RM, Rutland P, et al. Mutations in the fibroblast growth factor receptor 2 gene cause Crouzon syndrome. *Nature Genet*. 1994;8:98–103.

55. Zhang C, Cerveira E, Romanovitch M, et al. Array-based comparative genomic hybridization (aCGH). *Methods Mol Biol*. 2017;1541:167–179.

The Primary Dentition Years:
Three to Six Years

The dental needs of those in the 3- to 6-year-old age group can be dramatically different from one child to the next. Most children are caries-free because of fluoride, home care, the establishment of a dental home, and preventive treatments like sealants. Some children have at most only very modest decay. The problem for dentistry is that there are still children who, for a variety of reasons, need restorative care for multiple teeth. These needs are often extensive and include full-coverage crowns and pulp therapy. The majority are from low-income and minority families. Access to care is difficult. These children may have lost teeth and arch length from extractions and damaging interproximal decay. They now need space maintenance and, in some instances, the regaining of space.

The oral habits acquired by children in the first 3 years, which may have been of no concern to the parent or clinician, become of concern now. Although the clear majority of children have outgrown these habits, some have difficulty in stopping them. Often the detrimental effects of these habits are discernable even by the untrained eye. Behavior guidance and hospital dentistry are included in this section because most patient management problems that a dentist will encounter will probably occur in this age group. Fortunately most children in this age group, with their growing communication skills, are a delight to work with.

18

The Dynamics of Change

ERIN L. GROSS AND ARTHUR J. NOWAK

In our society the years between the ages of 3 and 6 are often referred to as the preschool years, and children at these ages are called preschoolers. Preschoolers undergo enormous change physically, cognitively, emotionally, and socially.

Physical Changes

Body

By the third birthday the average boy is 39 inches tall and weighs about 35 pounds, while the average girl is 38.6 inches tall and weighs nearly a pound less. Growth slows during the preschool years, and children gain approximately 5 pounds and 3 inches in height each year. More important than a child's weight or height during this time is the maintenance of their rate of growth. Children who are tall or heavy at age 2 years are very likely to remain tall or heavy at age 5 years, and children who are short or light at age 2 years are very likely to be short or light at age 5 years.[1] Similar to the growth of younger children (described in Chapter 13), body elongation continues to be apparent during the preschool years. Head growth seems slow, whereas limb growth seems extremely rapid. Trunk growth can be regarded as intermediate, and the protuberant, pudgy abdomen of the toddling 2-year-old gradually disappears between the ages of 3 and 4 years.

A variety of other body changes take place during these years. Both the heart rate and the respiration rate slow down and blood pressure rises. Because of a change in the rate of the growth of the muscular system around age 4, approximately 75% of a child's acquired weight during the fifth year of development is the result of muscle acquisition.[2] The cartilage in the skeletal system is being increasingly replaced by bone, and all the bones of the body become more calcified and harder.

Craniofacial Changes

The head and face continue to grow during the period from ages 3 to 6. However, Fig. 18.1 shows that the percentage of increase in facial growth becomes greater than cranial growth around age 3.[3] This change has important effects on a child's craniofacial structures and appearance. Preschoolers' faces become larger, wider, longer, and more detailed as compared with the faces of newborns. During this stage of life, one begins to see the effects of the impending eruption of permanent teeth.[4]

Vann and colleagues[5] reported the results of a study reviewing cephalometric analysis of the primary dentition in 4-year-old children. They compared 17 cephalometric norms from a sample of 32 white children of North American ancestry with those of adults. There were no statistical differences between males and females. The investigators drew the following conclusions based on information given in Table 18.1:

1. The primary incisors are more upright than the permanent incisors (compare UI-SN and UI-F in Table 18.1).
2. The similarity of angle SNA in children (82.9 degrees) and adults (82.0 degrees) supports the concept that the nasion and point A move forward in relation to the sella, so that angle SNA is no different in preschool children and adults.
3. Angles SNB and SNPg in children measure 78.1 and 77.4 degrees, respectively, whereas in adults they measure 80.0 and 83.0 degrees. The ANB angle is greater in children (4.9 degrees) than in adults (2.0 degrees).

The soft tissue prominence of the nose and, to some extent, the mandible continues to increase consistently with some reduction in overall facial convexity (Fig. 18.2).[5] It is hard to judge the underlying skeletal configuration based on the soft tissue in this age group. Vertically, there is a lowering of the palatal vault with sutural growth and apposition on the oral side of the palate and resorption on the nasal side. There is an even greater lowering of the lowest point of the chin, but the mandibular plane (lower border of the mandible) stays parallel to its original orientation. This occurs because condylar growth exceeds the vertical maxillary growth, which prevents opening of the mandibular plane angle.

There is considerable growth in the transverse direction during this time as well (Fig. 18.3).[5] Remember that transverse growth comes to an end earlier than growth in other dimensions, so attention to problems in this dimension is important. Transverse maxillary growth during this period is largely the result of midpalatal sutural changes, whereas the growth of the body and angles of the mandible are the result of apposition and resorption.

Posterior maxillary and mandibular growth (sutural growth in the maxilla and endochondral growth in the mandible) help to

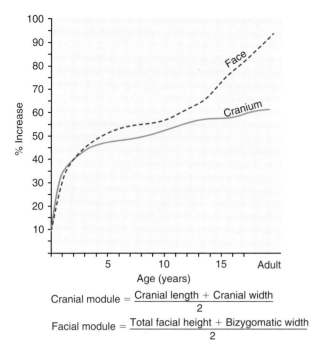

$$\text{Cranial module} = \frac{\text{Cranial length} + \text{Cranial width}}{2}$$

$$\text{Facial module} = \frac{\text{Total facial height} + \text{Bizygomatic width}}{2}$$

• **Figure 18.1** Comparison of cranial and facial modules (males). Increase in cranial and facial modules during growth. (Redrawn from Ranly DM. *A Synopsis of Craniofacial Growth*. Norwalk, CT: Appleton & Lange; 1988. Data from Scott JH. The growth of the human face. *Proc R Soc Med.* 1954;47:5.)

TABLE 18.1	Cephalometric Angles: A Comparison Between Preschoolers (4 to 5 Years) and Adults	
	Vann (N = 32)[a]	Adult[b]
SNA	82.9	82.0
SNB	78.1	80.0
SNPg	77.4	83.0
ANB	4.9	2.0
FNA	89.1	88.0
FNB	84.4	87.0
FNPg	85.5	88.0
IMPA	85.2	92.0
FMIA	65.9	65.0
UI-SN	92.4	104.0
UI-F	97.6	110.0
1-1	148.4	130.0
M	67.5	69.0
Y axis	58.5	59.0
OCC-SN	18.8	14.5
SN-MP	35.3	32.0
FMA	29.2	25.0

[a]All children in this study were between their fourth and fifth birthdays.
[b]Generally accepted adult norms borrowed from Downs, Steiner, and Tweed.
From Vann WF, Dilley GJ, Nelson RM. A cephalometric analysis for the child in the primary dentition. *ASDC J Dent Child.* 1978;45:45–52.

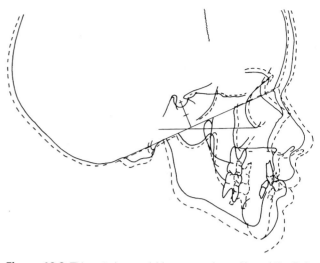

• **Figure 18.2** This anterior cranial base superimposition of the Bolton standard for 3- and 6-year-olds demonstrates the magnitude of antero-posterior and vertical skeletal growth during this period as well as the change in soft tissue. (Redrawn from Broadbent BH Sr, Broadbent BH Jr, Golden WH. *Bolton Standards of Dentofacial Developmental Growth*. St Louis: Mosby; 1975.)

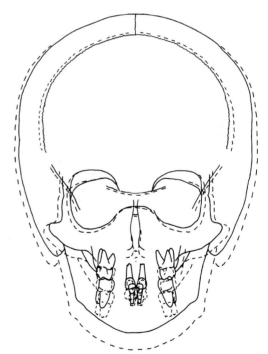

• **Figure 18.3** This anterior cranial base superimposition of the Bolton standard for 3- and 6-year-olds demonstrates the magnitude of transverse and vertical skeletal growth during this period. (Redrawn from Broadbent BH Sr, Broadbent BH Jr, Golden WH. *Bolton Standards of Dentofacial Developmental Growth*. St Louis: Mosby; 1975.)

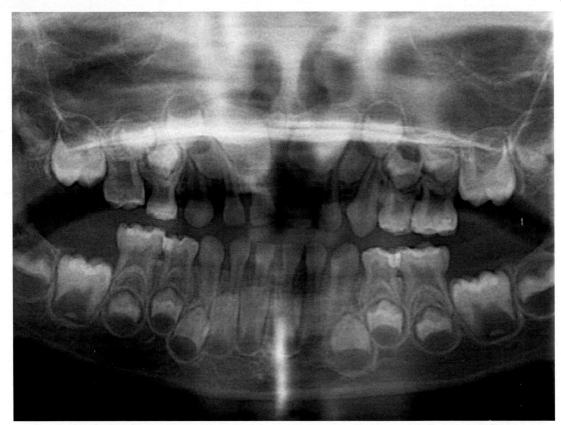

• **Figure 18.4** This panoramic radiograph shows the alteration in arch length required to accommodate the permanent teeth.

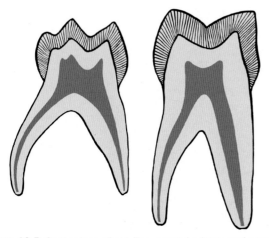

• **Figure 18.5** Comparison of maxillary second primary and permanent molars, linguobuccal cross-section. (Modified from Finn SB. *Clinical Pedodontics*. 4th ed. Philadelphia: Saunders; 1973.)

accommodate the emerging permanent first molars. There is some appositional growth at the dentoalveolar ridges as the permanent anterior teeth erupt.

Consistent with eruption of the new permanent teeth is the continued eruption of the primary teeth. Often the magnitude of this vertical change is unappreciated. It is also obvious that the permanent anterior teeth will occupy a more anterior and protrusive position in the face.

Dental Changes

Table 13.5 presents a chronology of the human dentition. This table demonstrates that the entire primary dentition has erupted and completed root development by 3 years of age. This is a relatively stable period for the primary dentition. Changes in the dental arches will occur with the eruption of the permanent teeth, but during this period, there is little change in primary incisor spacing, intercanine distance, or arch width. Arch length decreases slightly when posterior spaces close before eruption of the permanent molars.[6] Although the primary dentition is stable, this is a significant period of time for the development of the crowns of the permanent dentition (Fig. 18.4), which will erupt soon. Resorption of the roots of the primary incisors will begin for most children during the end of this period.

When the permanent dentition erupts, some obvious differences in morphology between it and the primary dentition will become apparent (Fig. 18.5). *Wheeler's Dental Anatomy and Physiology*[7] described the following essential differences:

1. The crowns of primary anterior teeth are wider mesiodistally in comparison with their cervicoincisal length than are the crowns of the permanent teeth.
2. The roots of the primary anterior teeth are narrower mesiodistally. Narrow roots with wide crowns present a morphologic appearance at the cervical third of the crown and root that differs markedly from that of the permanent anterior teeth. When the teeth are examined from the mesial or distal aspects, a similar situation in the root and crown measurement at the cervix is observed. The cervical ridge of enamel at the cervical third of

the crown, labially and lingually, is much more prominent in the primary teeth than in the permanent teeth.

3. The crowns and roots of the primary molars are more slender mesiodistally at the cervical third than those of the permanent molars.

4. The cervical ridge buccally on the primary molars is much more pronounced, especially on both the maxillary and mandibular first molars.

5. The roots of the primary molars are relatively more slender and longer than the roots of the permanent molars. They also flare more apically, extending beyond the projected outlines of the crowns. This flaring allows room between the roots for the development of permanent tooth crowns before it is time for the primary molars to lose their anchorage.

6. The buccal and lingual surfaces of the primary molars are flatter above the cervical curvatures than those of the permanent molars.

7. The primary teeth are usually lighter in color than the permanent teeth.

Cognitive Changes

Language is developing rapidly during this time, and children in this age group can speak in sentences of at least five words, follow basic grammar rules, tell stories, and be understood by strangers.[8] The preschooler's power of reasoning is also growing substantially. The simplistic "Why?" questions of the 2-year-old are replaced by more sophisticated and specific inquiries, such as, "How did it get so big?" and "Where did it come from?"

In Piaget's categorization of cognitive intelligence, the years between the ages of 3 and 6 are called preoperational.[9] The preoperational phase of cognitive development begins at the end of the sensorimotor period, around 18 to 24 months of age, and lasts until age 6 or 7 years. Piaget called the first part of this phase preconceptual and concluded that it lasted until about the age of 4.[10] During the preconceptual phase, the child's mind and mental prowess develop at a rapid rate. The child's mind acquires the ability to play and fantasize using mental imagery, which is much different from the earlier sensorimotor period, when the child was restricted to actions with real objects. However, the child in the preconceptual stage still generalizes all entities. For example, any bird is a bird. Use of more specific nouns like "robin," "quail," or "heron" must await a later level of development. If the child masters both the words "chicken" and "bird," he or she will not understand that a chicken is also a bird.

The preconceptual mind is also *centered*. Centration was defined by Piaget as the process of focusing all thought and reasoning of any mental problem on only one aspect of the whole of the structure and disregarding all other features.[9] Piaget used a dramatic experiment to prove this assumption. He found that children who watched him pour water from one of two identically filled tall, thin vases into a short, wide vase often asserted that the tall vase had more water in it than the short one. Children who made that assertion centered on the height of the water. Furthermore, the child's thought during these years is irreversible.[9] The child cannot mentally pour the water back from the short vase to the tall one to see that it would be at the same level as the water in the other tall vase.

After the preconceptual stage, the child enters a stage called the period of intuitive thought, which lasts until age 7. This is a period of growing sophistication in the child's abilities to group objects according to class, using more complex thoughts and images, and outgrowing the tendency toward centration. Late in this period the child can begin to acquire reading and writing skills. All of

this—combined with an increased vocabulary, longer attention span, control over impulses, and tolerance of separation from parents—demonstrates that the child is ready for school.

Emotional Changes

As discussed in Chapter 13, very young children fear strangers, separation from their parents, and new experiences. However, these fears have diminished by the third birthday to the point where these youngsters can take on new social situations without emotional consequences. The control of emotions, such as fear and frustration, develops dramatically between the ages of 3 and 6 and is paralleled by an equally dramatic socialization process. During these years, a child's concept of self-esteem and sense of gender identity emerge.[11]

One dramatic difference between the child from birth to age 3 and the child from ages 3 to 6 is the development of self-control.[11] Preschool children can be taught methods of self-control, such as distracting themselves when they become impatient or when they are receiving treatment from a dentist. They can be taught to monitor their own behavior. The conscience develops, and the child becomes capable of feeling guilty or anxious if and when he or she violates a moral norm.

An understanding of aggression is important for those who work with preschool children. Aggression is often caused by a child's inability to exert self-control, and there are two types. The first is called instrumental aggression; it is designed for achieving a goal, such as taking a toy from a sibling. The other is called hostile aggression; it is intended to cause hurt or pain to another person.[12] During the preschool years, the frequency of instrumental aggression should decline. Children who remain hostilely aggressive come from families in which parents and other children are also overtly aggressive. A parenting philosophy that is inconsistent and unclear in the enforcement of rules has also been linked with aggressive behavior in children.[13]

By the sixth birthday a child is not emotionally mature but is certainly emotionally complex. He or she is capable of feeling friendship and hostility, acting out aggression, and experiencing guilt and anxiety. This is a child who is susceptible to praise and can suffer hurt feelings. These children are also learning to relate to the emotions of other people.

Social Changes

Before the preschool years, children do not play together. They may play in parallel, but they are playing separately. However, the social transformations of preschoolers ensure that their lives will never be the same. They learn to take turns and play cooperatively, and they develop friendships.[8] They gain an understanding of how they relate to other people, including parents, siblings, peers, and authority figures.

There are many theories that attempt to explain the dramatic psychosocial transitions that take place in this age group. Psychoanalytic theory asserts that sexual fantasies and the guilt associated with them, which at first take the form of an unusual feeling for the parent of the opposite sex (Oedipus or Electra complex), force the child into identification with the parent of the same sex and into the adoption of a system of morality, complete with its code of values.[14] It is normal during this time for the child to favor the parent of the opposite sex. Behaviorists ascribe the assumption of typical gender roles and social values to the effects of reinforcement, both positive and negative, during this period. Social learning theories explain the changes during this period as the product of the influences of parenting and parental behavior. Some theorists believe that as the child becomes conscious of the reasons behind things, she or he is better able to recognize and be allegiant to the reasoning that underlies social order and values.

Regardless of the theoretical position one may subscribe to, it cannot be denied that the role of parents and the social environment is extremely powerful in the preschooler's life. We now know that toxic stress in early childhood can have lasting effects on health and behavior. Low socioeconomic status of a child's family is a well-recognized predictor of morbidities, yet there is significant individual variation. Boyce[15] described the "dandelion child," who will remain healthy no matter the environment, and the "orchid child," who is highly susceptible to suffering negative health outcomes when he or she had faced adversity. To give a child the best shot, parents must create a sense of safety and stability. Gopnik[16] compares being a parent to being a gardener. As gardeners, parents commit to caring for and loving their children, creating a space in which they can thrive.

References

1. Meredith HV. Selected anatomic variables analyzed for interage relationships of the size-size, size-gain, and gain-gain varieties. In: Lipsitt LP, Spiker CC, eds. *Advances in Child Development and Behavior*. Vol. 2. New York: Academic Press; 1965:221–256.
2. Thompson H. Physical growth. In: Carmichael L, ed. *Manual of Child Psychology*. 2nd ed. New York: John Wiley; 1954:292–334.
3. Broadbent BH Sr, Broadbent BH Jr, Golden WH. *Bolton Standards of Developmental Growth*. St Louis: Mosby; 1975.
4. Ranly DM. *A Synopsis of Craniofacial Growth*. New York: Appleton-Century-Crofts; 1980.
5. Vann WF, Gilley GJ, Nelson RM. A cephalometric analysis for the child in the primary dentition. *ASDC J Dent Child*. 1978;45(1):45–52.
6. Moorrees CF, Gron AM, Lebret LM, et al. Growth studies of the dentition: a review. *Am J Orthod*. 1969;55(6):600–616.
7. Ash MM Jr, Nelson SJ. *Wheeler's Dental Anatomy and Physiology*. 8th ed. St Louis: Saunders; 2003.
8. Shelov SP, Remer Altmann T, Hannemann RE. *Caring for Your Baby and Young Child: Birth to Age 5*. 6th ed. New York: Bantam Books; 2014.
9. Ginsburg H, Opper S. *Piaget's Theory of Intellectual Development*. 3rd ed. Englewood Cliffs, NJ: Prentice-Hall; 1988.
10. Watts J, Cockcroft K, Duncan N. *Developmental Psychology*. 2nd ed. Cape Town, South Africa: UCT Press; 2009.
11. Carey WB, Crocker AC, Coleman WL, et al. *Developmental-Behavioral Pediatrics*. 4th ed. Philadelphia: Saunders; 2009.
12. Anderson CA, Bushman BJ. Human aggression. *Annu Rev Psychol*. 2002;53:27–51.
13. Mussen PH, Conger JJ, Kagan J, et al. *Child Development and Personality*. 6th ed. New York: Harper and Row; 1984.
14. Elliot A. *Psychoanalytic Theory: An Introduction*. 3rd ed. London: Palgrave; 2015.
15. Boyce WT. The lifelong effects of early childhood adversity and toxic stress. *Pediatr Dent*. 2014;36(2):102–108.
16. Gopnik A. *The Gardener and the Carpenter: What the New Science of Child Development Tells Us About the Relationship Between Parents and Children*. New York: Farrar, Straus and Giroux; 2016.

19
Examination, Diagnosis, and Treatment Planning

ROCIO B. QUINONEZ, JOHN R. CHRISTENSEN, AND HENRY FIELDS

Diagnosis of Nonorthodontic Problems

For some dentists, the examination of the 3-year-old child represents a first dental experience, although the American Academy of Pediatric Dentistry recommends earlier examinations for diagnostic, preventive, and treatment purposes.[1] For a child who has not had an earlier dental examination, the new environment, new people, and manipulation of tissues can be a difficult or overwhelming experience.

An initial examination of a child this age can also be demanding for the dentist, who is faced with potential behavioral challenges, minimal to no clinical baseline, and the need to provide both immediate and long-term planning and treatment.

An early examination provides an opportunity to establish a course of dental health for years to come. Of particular interest in the examination of the 3- to 6-year-old are the following factors:

1. Limited existing health history
2. Minimal to no clinical baseline data
3. Behavioral unknowns
4. Primary dentition occlusion with limited predictive value
5. Preventive needs that must be assessed

All of the above must be addressed during evaluation of a child this age, especially if this is the child's initial dental visit.

Patient Records

The nature of health care record keeping in dentistry has evolved from a historical or financial repository to a vital working document. The bare essentials for a pediatric dental record are a health history, examination record, treatment plan, and series of visit notes. Health histories should allow for periodic updating and summary statement.[2] Parental or guardian consent should be obtained and recorded at the initial visit. Adjunctive records—such as study casts, preventive and dietary forms, or other analyses—also should be kept with the health care record. Similarly, in an era of electronic communication, emails, text messaging, and photos should be kept as part of the patient's record.

There are many possibilities for the dental examination record. Often practitioners opt for the standard form or template included in the electronic patient record employed in dental school. No clear-cut guidelines exist for choice of a pediatric dental tooth chart, but there are some basic requirements to satisfy medicolegal needs and to provide a complete developmental history. The examination record should do the following:

1. Adequately record developmental status and existing extra and intraoral conditions, including supporting structures, head, neck, and teeth
2. Record facial and occlusal status
4. Record oral hygiene, periodontal, and intraoral soft tissue status
5. Indicate findings from radiographic and other diagnostic tests
6. Establish a caries risk for the child that substantiates preventive and treatment recommendations

The tooth chart need not be anatomically correct; in many cases a diagram of teeth is of more value. Third-party reimbursement currently focuses on surfaces and tooth number, and the concept of diagramming caries extent on individual teeth is of little value, largely because at this time dentistry does not use a meaningful disease-based coding system.[3] It is critical that the charting system address both primary and permanent teeth so that each record entry provides an up-to-date developmental profile. In addition to a notation of the presence or absence of a tooth, the mobility of primary teeth and clinically evident tooth emergence should be noted in the pediatric dental chart. This helps to depict the child's developmental trajectory. Current child safety and forensic concerns strongly suggest making an initial chart of the dentition, including restorations and abnormalities.[4]

An assessment of soft and bony tissue should be noted. Periodontal probing of all teeth is not routine, but the dental chart should provide an area for noting deep pocketing or loss of attachment in some manner if present. The nature of this notation requires simply adequate baseline data to accomplish treatment and follow-up. Periodontal probing depths at six points per tooth is conventionally used during periodontal examination and may be considered in selective primary teeth.[5]

Many practitioners develop individual approaches to prevention that can be efficiently addressed on the examination record. A serial chart of oral hygiene performance or gingival scores can be helpful. Other helpful items on the examination record are vital signs, medical alerts and important allergies, behavior notes, and unusual findings. Reasons for deferring radiographic examination should be noted in the record. These data provide quick reference for the dentist at chairside.

Recent changes in patient privacy procedures, procedure coding, expected assessments, and dental disease risk assessment suggest the dental examination record (history and physical) should incorporate other measurement scales. These might include any or all of the following:

1. A caries risk assessment based on the Caries Assessment Tool of the American Academy of Pediatric Dentistry (see Chapter 14), or some other instrument that accounts for clinical and historical risk factors. This can be a list of factors or simply a choice of high, medium, or low risk.
2. An initial pain or behavioral assessment that provides the dentist with a sense of the child's cooperation or state of oral health upon initial examination. Some clinicians use a set of diagrammatic "faces" ranging from happy to sad (see Fig. 7.3). Others use a version of the Frankl behavior scale, which is a four-point selection ranging from definitely positive (score = 4) to definitely negative (score = 1). The Frankl scale offers the benefits of simplicity and behavior categories that are relevant to chairside dentistry.

The treatment plan should indicate the sequence of care and note the date on which each individual procedure was completed. Each visit note should indicate what was done and any notable occurrences. An up-to-date Current Dental Terminology (CDT) code should be attached to each procedure.

The History

The parent or guardian is the child's historian. The dentist must address both real and perceived problems. Parents may provide erroneous and unverified information simply because the information has not been tested by the health system. Two such examples are reported heart murmurs and allergies. Parents may have been informed of a murmur but are unaware of its seriousness. Parents also may confuse nausea with a true allergic reaction. The dentist may be required to address these concerns directly with a physician to obtain accurate information. In other situations, a long-established or past problem may have been forgotten or dismissed as unimportant. Such examples include inquiring about common chronic conditions that pose increased caries risk, including a history of (1) reflux (increased acid exposure), (2) ear infections requiring multiple courses of antibiotics (high in sucrose levels), (3) constipation resulting in frequent exposure to sweetened beverages (e.g., prune juice), and (4) reactive airway disease requiring steroid medication for control (increased xerostomia).

A general health history form can be used to determine a child's health background if attention is given to specific elements that relate to children. The dentist should be well versed in conditions that relate specifically to children. Table 19.1 provides a list of health items that are particularly common in the 3- to 6-year-old

group. The American Academy of Pediatric Dentistry offers a contemporary history form specifically designed for children that covers most childhood health issues.[6]

A short and noncontributory history was unusual in this age group in the past, but with the improvement in infant health practices and home care, immunization, and early medical intervention, many routine problems and illnesses have been prevented or resolved. On the other hand, a growing number of infants born prematurely survive who would have perished previously. Although some develop normally, a substantial number are physically or mentally compromised and require alternative and more complex health care approaches. Data suggest a "dose response," with decreased gestational age creating more adverse health outcomes at 3 to 5 years of age.[7] It is not uncommon in this age group to have parents note normal development or simply indicate a vague delay in speech or motor skills. This may occur because a disability has not been clearly diagnosed or the parent is reluctant to accept the fact that the child may have a problem.

The dentist's review of a checklist with annotations can be used to complete an accurate medical history. Medical histories should be updated every 6 months or prior to this time frame if changes arise. Medical histories completed electronically prior to the visit can facilitate its review and decrease the time spent in the office. Significant findings should be explained in the record. Any health history should be finalized by a summary of the status of the child, especially in the areas of drug allergies, surgical procedures, cardiac abnormalities, and developmental status. Many pediatric dental records are designed so that this summary appears on the examination form to preclude the need to go through the record for important information. This summary of positive responses is also a function of some electronic dental records. A dated notation also serves to confirm that the dentist has reviewed the history and made a decision about its impact on treatment at that point in time.

The dental history should be comprehensive. Many parents do not think about recording their child's dental history other than the eruption of the first tooth. The dental history should cover, at a minimum, past problems and care, fluoride experience, current hygiene habits, and an eruption-developmental profile. Table 19.1 addresses the essential elements of the dental history. The most contemporary approach to the dental history uses a developmental model that permits the parent to address age-specific issues. For example, the health history may ask about bottle use, weaning, access to sugar, and other dietary issues to cover a range of ages on one form. The checklist approach to the health history permits a "not applicable" choice when a child has outgrown a set of questions. This developmental approach provides an age-specific set of findings that can be converted to preventive instruction in the anticipatory guidance counseling by dental staff. Some pediatric dentists tailor the dental history to serve as a screen for caries and orthodontic, gingival, and injury risk factors, asking questions whose answers can later be addressed with take-home preventive messaging.

The Examination

The examination encompasses six major sections: behavioral assessment; general appraisal; and head and neck, facial, intraoral, and radiographic examinations.

Behavioral Assessment

The general appraisal and chairside examination provide an opportunity to observe behavior and assess potential cooperation of the

TABLE 19.1	Selected Health History Considerations With Common Findings in the 3- to 6-Year-Old Group	

Area of Concern	Common Findings
General Health	
Allergies	Probably related to food and other environmental allergens; may have allergy to medications such as antibiotics; rash is common manifestation; false allergies often reported
Asthma	May be reported; triggering factors usually known; medications also well known; impact of dental intervention usually not known
Bleeding	Parent may suggest excessive bruising without real problem
Blood transfusion	May have been performed at birth
Childhood infections	Immunizations will have occurred, or there is a clear history of having had a specific illness such as measles or chickenpox
Development	Poor parental knowledge for normal children; for those with developmental delays, a good history of diagnostic procedures and status
Heart	Functional murmur may exist, or parent may have been told of a murmur
Hypertension	Usually unknown unless child has chronic problem
Illnesses	Probable history of upper respiratory infections
Jaundice	Possible at birth
Medications	Probably has taken acetaminophen (Tylenol) as necessary; may have received amoxicillin or other antibiotic
Seizures	Possibly febrile; may be on seizure medication for only one seizure
Surgical procedures	Possible tonsillectomy or adenoidectomy; possible ear tubes; circumcision seldom noted as procedure
Dental Health	
Bottle use	Probably considered not to contribute to decay
Developmental/eruption	Knowledge may be limited to eruption dates of first teeth unless consistently very early or late
Fluoride	May know water status; possible vitamin with fluoride supplementation
Habits (thumbsucking)	Will be well known to parent if present
Home care	Usually confined to toothbrushing; may be largely left to child
Previous care	Possibly none; no dentist or care rendered
Reaction to care (behavior)	Possibly none; likely poor or tentative
Trauma to teeth and chin	Possible, but usually left untreated unless serious; commonly upper teeth and chin

This table suggests usual or common responses to questions asked of parents about the average child in this age group, but it does not suggest a norm or most frequent response for all children.

patient. A complete behavioral assessment is discussed in Chapter 24. It is noteworthy that preschool-age children with disruptive behavior are four times more likely to be at risk for developmental delays. When this is identified, the dental team should consider referral to the child's physician for further assessment.[8]

General Appraisal

The general appraisal addresses the child's physical and behavioral status. The classic areas of appraisal include gait, stature, and presence of gross signs and symptoms of disease. The normal 3- to 6-year-old is ambulatory, well coordinated in basic tasks, engaging, and physically healthy in appearance. Table 19.2 lists physical and behavioral milestones for the 3- to 6-year-old child. The dentist should incorporate these markers mentally into a profile for evaluation of the child's status. The general appraisal of the child is best

accomplished in the reception room or a similar nonthreatening environment. This appraisal should be followed by clarification of any abnormal findings and a discussion of potential behavioral problems with the parent.

The role of vital signs in the general appraisal is twofold. The first purpose is to identify abnormalities and the second is to satisfy the medicolegal role of providing baseline health data for emergency situations. Vital signs may be distorted if the child is upset or anxious. Taking vital signs of blood pressure, pulse, and respiration may be delayed until the child has become accustomed to the environment, but these data must be obtained before any drugs are administered. The child's weight should be recorded in a conspicuous location on the chart so the information is available in an emergency. Height should also be recorded and, together with weight, serve as an index of physical development. Because of concerns about childhood overweight (body mass index [BMI]

TABLE 19.2   Selected Developmental Characteristics of the 3- to 6-Year-Old Child

3-Year-Old	4-Year-Old	6-Year-Old
Intellectual Development		
Gives first and last name	Recognizes colors	Names 4 colors
Counts 3 objects	Counts 4 objects	Counts 10 objects
States own age and sex	Tells a story	Asks about the meaning of words
Gross/Fine Motor Skills		
Puts on shoes	Dresses without supervision	Dresses and undresses
Pedals tricycle	Balances on one foot	Hops on one foot
Copies a circle	Copies cross and square	Draws a triangle
Psychological		
The 3- to 6-year-old is in the *phallic* stage of development. During this period, the child undergoes *oedipal* conflicts, which may lead to opposite-sex parental preference. The child may exhibit some aggression with siblings. By age 6 years, the child may be ready to surrender some dependency on parents		
Dental Implications		
Needs maternal presence, especially during stress	May be difficult and aggressive	Should leave parent for treatment
Fear of separation	Responds to verbal direction	Proud of possessions
Visual fear	Auditory fear	Bodily harm fear
Physiologic Height (75th Percentile)		
Boys = 97.5 cm	Boys = 106 cm	Boys = 113 cm
Girls = 97 cm	Girls = 104.5 cm	Girls = 111.5 cm
(Growth rate for this period is approximately 6–8 cm per year)		
Weight (75th Percentile)		
Boys = 15.5 kg	Boys = 18 kg	Boys = 20 kg
Girls = 15.5 kg	Girls = 17.5 kg	Girls = 19.5 kg
(Growth rate for this period is approximately 2 kg per year)		
Pulse (90th Percentile)		
105 beats/min	100 beats/min	100 beats/min
Respiration (90th Percentile)		
30 breaths/min	28 breaths/min	26 breaths/min
Blood Pressure		
100/60 mm Hg	100/60 mm Hg	100/60 mm Hg

>85th percentile) and obesity (BMI >95th percentile),[9] the dentist should calculate a BMI for the child or enter height and weight on standardized growth curves and include these if referring the family to a physician for weight concerns. BMI is a valid measure beginning at age 2 years and can be determined by using an electronic BMI calculator.[10]

Examination of the Head and Neck

Examining a 3-year-old requires attention to both clinical findings and the patient's behavior in the dental setting. The 3-year-old has experienced previous medical examinations, but this may be the first dental examination. The provider has an excellent opportunity to complete a thorough dental examination while observing the child's behavior in a nonthreatening environment.

Table 19.3 outlines the elements and expectations for a thorough head and neck examination. The process begins with an orientation about what is to occur. The dentist should describe what will take place at each step in the examination. This tell-show-do technique, which involves explanation, demonstration, and finally completion of a step, is usually the way the diagnostic process is handled. Positive or negative responses from the child should be encouraged. Children should also be warned and supported before the dentist makes positional changes or begins intraoral manipulation. The knee-to-knee position, entailing the caregiver and dentist facing each other with the child's head on the dentist's lap, may be required in the case of an anxious child experiencing difficulty separating from his or her caregiver or for children with special health care needs.

Parental presence is always a matter of controversy. Initial parental involvement may be encouraged to allow a transition from a

TABLE 19.3	Elements of Head and Neck Examination		
Structure	Diagnostic Technique	Normal Characteristics	Selected Abnormal Findings/Possible Causes
Head			
Hair	Visualization	Quality Thickness Color	Dryness/malnutrition, ectodermal dysplasia Baldness/child abuse, self-abuse, chemotherapy Infestation/neglect
Scalp	Visualization	Skin color Dryness Ulceration	Scaling/dermatitis Sores/abuse, infection, neglect
Ears	Visualization Palpation Assessment of hearing	Intact and normally formed external ear and auditory canal Gross normal hearing	Malformed ears and canals/genetic malformation syndrome (e.g., Treacher Collins) Conductive and neurologic hearing loss/trauma, developmental disability
Eyes	Visualization Assessment of vision	Position and orientation in fact Movement of eyes Vision Reaction to light	Variation in separation and orientation/genetic malformation syndromes Cranial nerve damage/trauma, developmental disability
Nose	Visualization	Normal size, shape, function, and location	Malposition/genetic malformation syndrome (e.g., median facial cleft) Misshapen/ectodermal dysplasia, congenital syphilis, achondroplasia Discharge/URI, asthma, allergy Poor smell, cranial nerve damage
Lip	Visualization Assessment of function	Speech, closure Integrity Absence of lesions	Poor closure/lip incompetence Clefting/genetic clefting syndrome Asymmetry/Bell palsy or cranial nerve damage Ulceration/herpes infection
Temporomandibular joint	Visualization Palpation Auscultation	Symmetry in function Smooth movement Absence of pain Range of motion (maximum)	Deviation/trauma Crepitus, pain/temporomandibular joint disorder Limitation/arthritis, trauma
Skin	Visualization	Color Tone Moisture Absence of lesions	Edema/cellulitis, renal disorder Redness/allergic response Dryness/dehydration, ectodermal dysplasia Ulceration/infectious disease, abuse
Chin	Visualization	Absence of scar	Scar indicates previous mandibular trauma
Neck			
Lymph nodes	Palpation	Normal size, mobility	Increased size/infection, neoplasia Fixation/neoplasia
Thyroid	Palpation	Normal size	Increased size/goiter, tumor
Oral Cavity			
Palates	Visualization Palpation Assessment of function	Integrity Absence of lesion Normal function	Cleft/genetic syndrome Ulceration/herpes, mononucleosis, or other infection, abuse Petechiae/sexual abuse Deviation/cranial nerve damage
Pharynx	Visualization	Normal color	Normal size of tonsils Redness/URI, tonsillitis
Tongue	Visualization Palpation Assessment of function	Normal color Range of motion Absence of lesions	Redness/glossitis Ulceration/herpes, aphthous, or other infection, trauma Deviation/cranial nerve damage Limited movement/cerebral palsy

Continued

Structure	Diagnostic Technique	Normal Characteristics	Selected Abnormal Findings/Possible Causes
Floor of mouth	Visualization Palpation	Salivary function Absence of swelling Absence of lesions	Swelling/mucocele, sialolith Ulceration/aphthous ulceration or other infection, abuse
Buccal mucosa	Visualization Palpation	Absence of lesions Absence of swelling Salivary function	Ulceration/cheek bite, abuse Swelling/salivary gland Infection, mumps
Teeth	Visualization Palpation Percussion	Normal development Morphologic appearance Occlusion Color Integrity Mobility Hygiene	Absence/delayed eruption/congenital absence, genetic syndromes Extra teeth/supernumerary, cleidocranial dysplasia Abnormal morphologic appearance/microdontia, macrodontia, fusion Abnormal color/amelogenesis or dentinogenesis imperfecta, staining, pulpal necrosis, caries Fracture/trauma, abuse, caries Mobility/periapical infection, trauma, bone loss conditions, exfoliation Malposition/malocclusion, trauma Pain/periapical involvement

TABLE 19.3 Elements of Head and Neck Examination—cont'd

URI, Upper respiratory tract infection.

dentist-parent relationship to a more direct dentist-child relationship. This supported transition is important for children younger than 3 years of age but is less threatening for children near school age. Consideration of the patient's developmental stage rather than his or her chronologic age is indicated. Each child reacts differently to having a parent in the operatory, and the dentist must assess the benefit of that presence on the developing relationship he or she has with the child. It is within the parent's purview to request to be present during the examination and treatment, but it is within the practitioner's purview to choose not to treat the child under those circumstances. A growing number of practitioners allow parents in the treatment setting, and most data indicate that parents are a neutral factor for the child and may be perceived as a greater disadvantage for the dentist.[11,12] Advantages to parental presence, however, include the opportunity to teach positive oral health behaviors such as oral hygiene techniques or demonstrate the presence of disease progression.

The examination must evaluate the head and neck regions. It is critical to palpate and identify enlarged and fixed lymph nodes or other swellings. Many children of this age have swollen nodes, but the nodes are usually movable and confined to the lower face and jaws and only indicate minor infection. Swollen nodes in the neck and clavicular region are rarer and may suggest that the child has a more serious ailment.

Critical to a thorough examination of the head and neck is evaluation of form and function. The cranial nerves, speech, and mandibular function should be evaluated. However, a complete cranial nerve examination need not be performed because careful observation of sensory and motor function and the child's responses can indicate nerve status to a significant degree. Normal conversation can be used to identify gross speech disorders. While palpating the craniofacial structures, the dentist should talk with the child and observe his or her responses. Asking the child to open and demonstrate maximal opening and maximal intercuspation allows the child to perform simple tasks. Mandibular movements should

be observed for deviation and restriction of range of movement. The child should also be asked to move the mandible from side to side and to protrude it. Restriction of these movements may identify functional and morphologic problems that result from developmental anomalies or trauma.

Verbal responses also serve as behavioral signals of the child's adaptation. A child's cooperation, nonverbal communication, and physiologic responses often suggest stable, improving, or deteriorating behavior. Because the examination setting is nonthreatening, it provides a good opportunity to develop cooperation.

The manual examination should address any physical variations as well as the strength and mobility of structures. The visual aspect of the process should address color changes, asymmetry, and marked physiologic responses such as sweating or trembling.

Examination of the Face

A systematic facial examination is one portion of a complete orthodontic evaluation that describes skeletal and dental relationships in three spatial planes: anteroposterior, vertical, and transverse. The steps include a description of the overall facial pattern, the positions of the maxilla and mandible, and the vertical facial relationships. Next, the position of the lips is determined. Finally, facial symmetry is assessed, and the maxillary dental midline is located relative to the facial midline.

Overall Facial Pattern

First, the facial profile is evaluated in the anteroposterior plane. An assumption is made that the soft tissue profile reflects the underlying skeletal relationship. To begin the examination, the child should be seated upright, looking at a distant point. Three points on the face are identified: the bridge of the nose, the base of the upper lip, and the chin.

Line segments connecting these points form an angle that describes the profile as convex, straight, or concave (Fig. 19.1). A

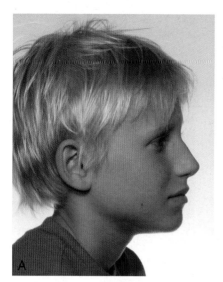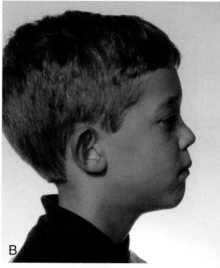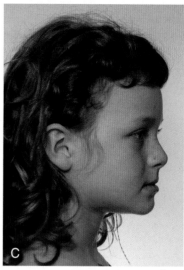

• **Figure 19.1** (A) A class I skeletal relationship is characterized by a well-balanced profile in the antero-posterior dimension. These relationships can be judged by mentally connecting the points of the bridge of the nose, the base of the upper lip (maxilla), and the soft tissue chin (mandible). This line should be slightly convex. (B) A class II skeletal relationship is characterized by a truly convex profile. (C) A class III skeletal relationship is characterized by a straight or concave profile.

well-balanced profile in this age group is slightly convex. A well-balanced profile in the anteroposterior dimension has an underlying skeletal relationship that is labeled class I (see Fig. 19.1A). This terminology is used because most class I skeletal relationships also have flush terminal plane or mesial step second primary molar relationships and Angle class I or end-to-end permanent first molar dental relationships if those teeth are erupted. Furthermore, the canine relationships usually will be class I, and there will be overjet of 2 to 5 mm. The Angle dental classification is described in a later section.

An assessment of the overall profile gives a general feeling for the skeletal relationships, but this evaluation does not diagnose the reason for the relationships. Some children in this age group have extremely convex profiles (see Fig. 19.1B). This is consistent with a class II skeletal relationship, and these patients usually have distal step second primary molar relationships and class II permanent first molar relationships if those teeth are erupted, class II canine relationships, and increased overjet. Other children have straight or concave profiles (see Fig. 19.1C). These are usually found with mesial step second primary molar relationships and class III permanent first molar relationships, class III canine relationships, and negative overjet.

Positions of the Maxilla and Mandible

If the profile is excessively convex or concave, the clinician can try to determine which skeletal component is contributing to the problem. This is a necessary step if orthodontic treatment is being considered. When the problem is known, the appropriate treatment can be tailored to the specific problem. It is extremely rare, however, to treat an anteroposterior problem in the primary dentition.

Specifically, in this diagnostic step, the anteroposterior positions of the maxilla and mandible are determined. A vertical reference line is extended from the bridge of the nose (the anterior aspect of the cranial base), and the position of other soft tissue points is noted relative to the reference line (Fig. 19.2). If the maxilla is properly oriented relative to other skeletal structures, the base of the upper lip will be on or near the vertical line. The soft tissue

chin will be slightly behind the reference line if the mandible is of proper size and in the correct position. If the maxilla is positioned significantly in front of the vertical reference line, the patient is said to exhibit maxillary protrusion. If the maxilla is substantially behind the line, the patient exhibits maxillary retrusion. The position of the mandible is described in the same way.

Thus, if the overall skeletal pattern is significantly convex (class II), the maxilla is positioned in front of the line (maxillary protrusion), the mandible is positioned behind the line (mandibular retrusion), or both. Class II skeletal relationships are sometimes caused by one jaw alone but are often the result of some combination of maxillary protrusion and mandibular retrusion.

Conversely, a facial pattern that is straight or extremely concave (class III) results when the maxilla is positioned behind the line (maxillary retrusion), the mandible is positioned in front of the line (mandibular protrusion), or both. Again, both jaws usually contribute to the skeletal dysplasia.

Some caution must be exercised because soft tissue profile relationships do not always accurately reflect the underlying skeletal relationships. Research has shown that the 3- to 6-year-old age group is especially difficult to classify accurately from a profile analysis.[13] In addition, vertical facial relationships influence the anteroposterior relationships. This interaction between the horizontal and vertical planes of space and its effect on the profile is discussed later.

Vertical Facial Relationships

The third portion of the facial examination is an evaluation of the vertical relationships. Proportionality is judged by dividing the face into thirds. The upper third extends from approximately the hairline to the bridge of the nose, the middle third from the bridge of the nose to the base of the upper lip, and the lower third from the base of the upper lip to the bottom of the chin (Fig. 19.3). These thirds are approximately equal, although the lower third will be slightly larger in well-proportioned faces.

Vertical problems tend to be manifest below the palate in the lower third of the face.[14] The short-faced person tends to have a lower facial third that is smaller than the other thirds (see

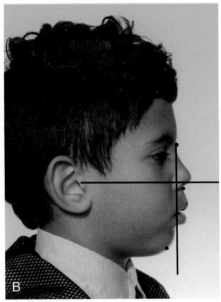
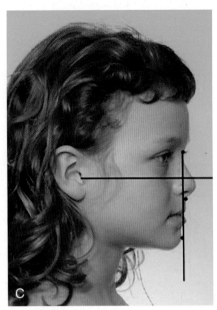

• **Figure 19.2** The contributions to the skeletal malocclusion can be estimated extraorally by determining the positions of the maxilla and mandible. A perpendicular reference line is established beginning at the soft tissue bridge of the nose. The positions of the maxilla and mandible are related to this line. If the base of the upper lip and nose are anterior to this line, the maxilla is protrusive. If these points are posterior to this line, the maxilla is retrusive. Similarly, the soft tissue chin is determined to be anterior (protrusive) or posterior (retrusive) to this line. (A) This patient has normal relationships for one younger than 6 years. (B) This patient has a significantly convex facial profile (class II), which results from a protrusive maxilla that is ahead of the line and a retrusive mandible that is posterior to the line. (C) This patient has a normal maxilla and a protrusive mandible.

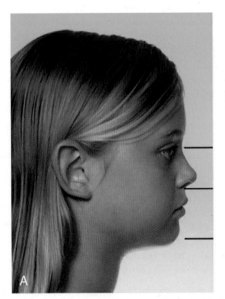
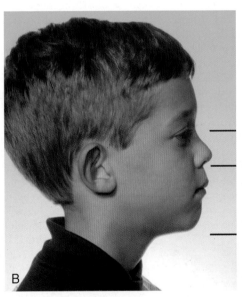
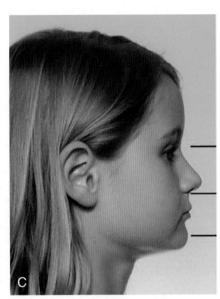

• **Figure 19.3** Vertical facial proportions can be evaluated by dividing the face into thirds and then comparing the middle third to the lower third. (A) In a well-proportioned face, the facial thirds are equal or the lower third is slightly larger. (B) A child with long lower facial third. (C) A child with short vertical facial dimensions has a proportionately smaller lower facial third.

Fig. 19.3C). The long-faced patient has a lower facial third that is larger than the other thirds (see Fig. 19.3B).

Lip Position

Next we advocate an evaluation of the anteroposterior lip position to give an estimation of the anteroposterior incisor position. Incisor position is grossly reflected in lip contour and posture. Lip posture is assessed by drawing an imaginary line from the tip of the nose to the most anterior point on the soft tissue chin. The lips normally lie slightly behind this line; however, in the 3- to 6-year-old child, the lower lip is generally 1 mm anterior to the line (Fig. 19.4). Two facts must be kept in mind. First, lip protrusion is characteristic

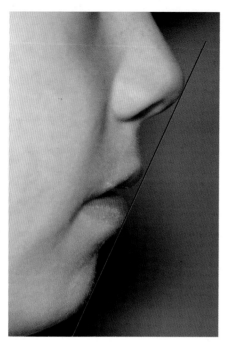

• **Figure 19.4** The anteroposterior position of the lips is determined by drawing a line from the tip of the nose to the most anterior point on the soft tissue chin. The upper lip normally should lie slightly behind the line, whereas the lower lip should lie slightly in front of this line in the 3- to 6-year-old child.

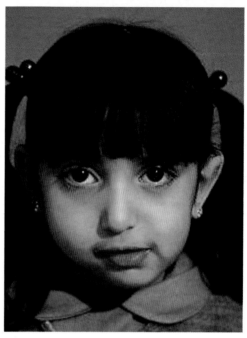

• **Figure 19.5** This patient exhibits marked asymmetry that is the result of a congenital fusion of the left condyle and coronoid process to the temporal bone.

of different ethnic groups, and lips that are considered protrusive in one group may not be considered protrusive in another. For example, African Americans and Asians tend to have more lip protrusion than do people of northern European descent. Second, the lips are evaluated in the context of the nose and chin. A large nose and chin can accommodate more protrusive lips, whereas a small nose and chin require less protrusive lips to be proportional.

Facial Symmetry

Transverse facial dimensions are examined to rule out true facial asymmetry. This is best evaluated with the patient reclining in the dental chair and the dentist seated in the 12 o'clock position. Hair is pulled away from the face; then a piece of dental floss can be stretched down the middle of the upper face to aid in judging the symmetry of the lower face. The mandible should be either at rest or in centric relation position. Maximal intercuspation or centric occlusion positions can be affected by dental interferences during closing.

All faces show a minor degree of asymmetry, but marked asymmetry is not normal (Fig. 19.5). Deviations or asymmetric positioning of the eyes, ears, or nose may be symptoms of cranial synostosis, an undiagnosed syndrome, or severe trauma. A child with these findings should be referred to appropriate professionals for a complete evaluation.

Asymmetry usually manifests in the lower facial third, whereas upper facial asymmetry is extremely rare. In this age group, a deviation of the midpoint of the mandible to one side or another may be due to true asymmetry, but it is most often indicative of a posterior crossbite and mandibular shift due to a dental interference. Posterior crossbites and mandibular shifts are two findings that are discussed later in the chapter.

The maxillary dental midline should be compared with the upper facial midline. This helps determine where the midline of the mandibular teeth is relative to the face when it is compared with the upper dental midline.

Intraoral Examination

The armamentarium for the intraoral examination includes a mirror, explorer, gauze, and periodontal probe. Additional materials are disclosing solution, dental floss, toothbrush, and scaler.

The intraoral examination begins with an excursion around the oral cavity, noting its general architecture and function. The fingers should be used to identify soft tissue abnormalities of the cheeks, lips, tongue, palate, and floor of the mouth before instruments are placed in the mouth. Children in this age group often permit oral inspection with "just fingers," and the dentist can use this technique as a springboard to obtain cooperation for the use of mirror and explorer. The mirror should be the first instrument introduced. This is usually readily accepted by the child owing to its familiarity and nonthreatening shape.

Young children are sometimes uncooperative. If they are, a decision must be made early about how to manage the behavior. Parental assistance can be used to obtain an examination of the oral cavity. Use of physical restraint by the dentist without parental consent is risky and should not be attempted.

An important portion of the intraoral examination is directed to the teeth. Each of the 20 primary teeth should be explored and scrutinized visually. Selective periodontal probing may be performed, but the yield is likely to be minimal because of the infrequency of irreversible attachment loss in the primary dentition.

Occlusal Evaluation

Another portion of the intraoral examination is the systematic analysis of the occlusion in three spatial planes. In addition, each dental arch is analyzed individually to describe arch form and symmetry, spacing and crowding, and the presence or absence of teeth. Arch analysis is best performed on diagnostic study models; however, diagnostic casts are usually not indicated in this age group unless there is some need to further study the intraoral findings or if tooth movement is contemplated.

Alignment

Dental arches can be categorized as either U-shaped or V-shaped. The mandibular arch is normally U-shaped, whereas the maxillary arch can be either shape. The dental arch should be symmetrical in the anteroposterior and transverse dimensions. Individual teeth are compared with their antimeres to determine if there is anteroposterior or transverse symmetry.

The ideal arch in the primary dentition has spacing between the teeth. Two types of spaces are identified. The first type, primate space, is located mesial to the maxillary canine and distal to the mandibular canine. Developmental space is the space between the remaining teeth (Fig. 19.6). Anterior spacing is desirable in the primary dentition because the permanent incisors are larger than their primary precursors. Although the presence of primate and developmental spacing does not ensure that the permanent dentition will erupt without crowding, these spaces usually alleviate some crowding during the transition from the primary to the mixed dentition. Crowding or overlapped teeth in the primary dentition may occur, although it is rare. True crowding in the primary dentition is usually not regarded as encouraging (Fig. 19.7). Crowding of isolated teeth, however, is sometimes due to space loss or indicative of a sucking habit. Lower anterior teeth can be tipped lingually into a crowded position as a result of constant pressure from a sucking habit.

Although it seems elementary, the clinician should carefully count the number of teeth in the mouth. Children in this age group should have all their primary teeth present. Those with delayed dental eruption may have either a very slow but normal sequence of eruption or some isolated eruption problem. To distinguish the two, the eruption sequence of the child is compared with the normal sequence of eruption, and the eruption pattern on the right side is compared with that on the left. If the sequence seems to be appropriate, dental development is probably slow. If, however, the patient's eruption pattern deviates from the normal sequence and there are differences between the contralateral sides of the mouth, further investigation is warranted to determine whether teeth are missing or are impeded from erupting. The maxillary lateral incisor is the most common missing tooth in the primary dentition.[15]

Counting the teeth also reveals the presence of supernumerary or extra teeth. Approximately 0.3% of children have supernumerary teeth in the primary dentition. The prevalence of fused and geminated teeth is approximately 0.1% to 0.5%.[15] One can usually distinguish fusion of two primary teeth from gemination without the aid of radiographs by counting the number of teeth. If two teeth are fused, there should be 9 teeth in the arch, one of which is very large, rather than 10 teeth. If gemination has occurred, there should be 10 teeth in the arch and one will be very large. A radiograph may be necessary to confirm the preliminary diagnosis of fusion or gemination. Fused primary teeth show two

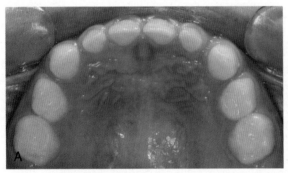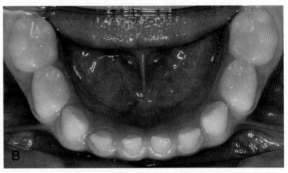

• **Figure 19.6** These maxillary (A) and mandibular (B) arches show primate spaces (mesial to the maxillary canines and distal to the mandibular canines) and developmental spacing (space between the remaining teeth).

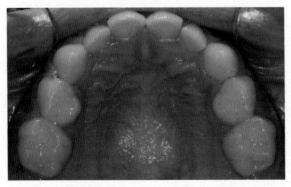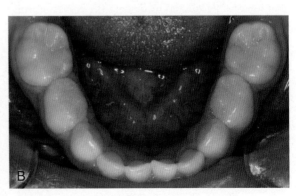

• **Figure 19.7** These maxillary (A) and mandibular (B) arches show a lack of primate and developmental spaces.

distinct and independent pulp chambers and canals with union of the dentin. Geminated primary teeth show two crowns and two pulp chambers connected to a single root and pulp canal (Fig. 19.8).

Anteroposterior Dimension

After the maxillary and mandibular arches have been examined for symmetry, spacing, and number of teeth, the relationship of the two arches to each other is examined. In the anteroposterior dimension, primary molar and canine relationships are determined and compared with the skeletal classification. In the primary dentition, molars are called flush terminal plane, mesial step, or distal step (Fig. 19.9). Primary canines are classified as class I, class II, class III, or end-to-end. These dental classifications generally reflect the skeletal classification.

Primary molar relationships, as described by the distal surfaces of the primary second molar, are worthy of attention not only because they describe the relationship of the primary mandibular teeth to the primary maxillary teeth but also because these surfaces guide the permanent molars into occlusion and determine the permanent molar relationships. Documenting primary molar relationships also allows one to follow the effects of growth or treatment.

Overjet, the horizontal overlap of the maxillary and mandibular incisors, is measured in millimeters (Fig. 19.10). It may be more helpful to describe overjet as ideal, excessive, or deficient rather than provide its measurement in millimeters.

Transverse Relationship

The transverse relationship of the arches is examined for midline discrepancies and posterior crossbites. The midline of each arch is compared with the other and with the midsagittal plane. Remember that the upper midline was evaluated to the facial midline during the facial evaluation.

A large midline discrepancy is unusual in the early primary dentition, and clinicians should be suspicious of a mandibular shift. The presence of a mandibular shift is often indicative of a posterior crossbite with a centric relation to centric occlusion shift.

If a posterior crossbite is encountered, the clinician should try to determine the cause. The majority of posterior crossbites are due to constriction of the maxillary arch. This is one situation in which diagnostic casts are helpful to aid in or confirm the diagnosis. After the arch at fault is identified, an attempt is made to determine whether the crossbite is bilateral or unilateral. If models are available, they can be measured to determine whether teeth are equidistant from the midpalatal raphe. If models are not available, the determination must be made clinically. The first step is to guide the mandible into centric relation. If teeth are in crossbite on both sides of the arch when the mandible is in centric relation, the child has a bilateral crossbite. If the teeth are in crossbite on only one side of the arch when the mandible is in centric relation, the crossbite is unilateral (Fig. 19.11). It is important to check that the mandible is in centric relation because a bilateral crossbite appears to be unilateral if the mandible shifts laterally

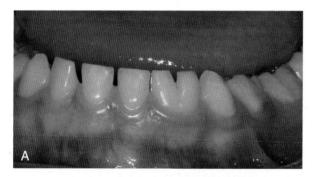
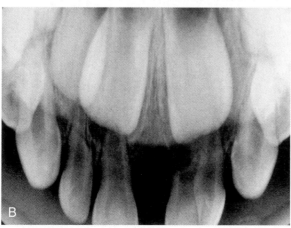
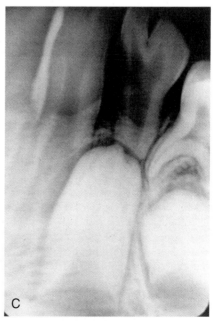

• **Figure 19.8** (A) This patient shows what appears to be a geminated lower left lateral incisor. Supporting radiographs are often necessary to distinguish fusion from gemination. (B) These fused primary teeth are joined only at the dentin and have independent pulp chambers and canals. (C) This geminated primary tooth has a large crown and a common pulp canal. ([B and C] Courtesy Dr. W.F. Vann.)

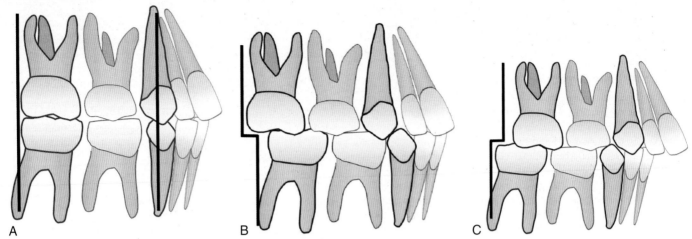

• **Figure 19.9** (A) In the primary dentition, an occlusion is classified per the relationship of the mandibular second molars and canines to the maxillary second molars and canines. In this example, the distal surface of the mandibular second molar is flush with the distal surface of the maxillary second molar. This primary molar relationship is called flush terminal plane. The long axis of the mandibular canine is coincident with the long axis of the maxillary canine. This is described as an end-to-end canine relationship. (B) In this example, the distal surface of the mandibular molar is mesial to the distal surface of the maxillary molar. This primary molar relationship is termed mesial step. The maxillary canine is positioned in the embrasure between the mandibular canine and the first molar. This is described as a class I canine relationship. (C) In this example, the distal surface of the mandibular molar is distal to the distal surface of the maxillary molar. This primary molar relationship is called distal step. The maxillary canine is positioned in the embrasure between the mandibular canine and the lateral incisor. This is described as a class II canine relationship.

into maximal intercuspation. The child shifts the jaw because the teeth do not fit well together, and the bite is uncomfortable because of dental interferences. A true unilateral crossbite that is due to a unilateral maxillary constriction in the primary dentition is rare but can occur.

Vertical Dimension

Overbite, the vertical overlap of the primary incisors, is measured and recorded in millimeters or as a percentage of the total height of the mandibular incisor crown (see Fig. 19.10) and is approximately 2 mm in the primary dentition. Deep bite is the complete or nearly complete overlap of the primary incisors. Anterior open bite, the absence of vertical overlap, is usually indicative of a sucking habit in this age group (Fig. 19.12). If the patient and parent deny the existence of a sucking habit, further investigation into the cause of open bite is needed. Skeletal malocclusion, ankylosed anterior teeth, condylar fracture or the sequelae of trauma, and degenerative diseases such as juvenile rheumatoid arthritis may account for the open bite and should be investigated.

Ankylosis, the fusion of tooth to bone, is common in the primary dentition (Fig. 19.13). Although an ankylosed tooth cannot erupt further, the unaffected adjacent teeth will continue to erupt. This creates the illusion that the ankylosed tooth is submerged in the bone. The prevalence of ankylosed teeth is between 7% and 14% in the primary dentition.[16,17] In addition, 50% of patients with an ankylosed tooth have more than one ankylosis. The following is a list of the most commonly ankylosed teeth in the primary dentition[16]:

1. Mandibular primary first molar
2. Mandibular primary second molar
3. Maxillary primary first molar
4. Maxillary primary second molar

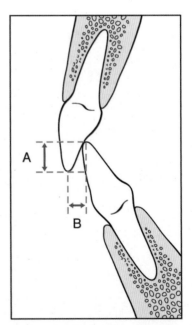

• **Figure 19.10** *A,* Overbite is the vertical overlap of the incisors and is measured from the incisal edge of one incisor to the other. Overbite can be recorded in millimeters or as a percentage of overlap of the total length of the mandibular incisor. *B,* Overjet is the horizontal overlap of the maxillary and mandibular central incisors and is measured from the most anterior point on the facial surfaces of these teeth. (Redrawn from Friedman MH, Weisberg J. The temporomandibular joint. In Gould JA ed. *Orthopedics and Sports Physical Therapy.* St Louis: Mosby; 1990.)

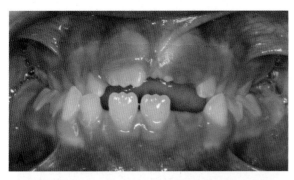

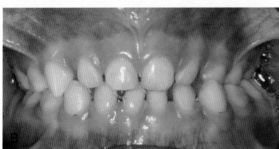

• **Figure 19.11** It is important to determine the patient's centric relation to identify the etiology of the problem and the treatment needs. (A) This patient has a bilateral posterior crossbite when the teeth are positioned in centric relation. (B) This patient has a unilateral posterior crossbite when the teeth are positioned in centric relation. Treatment approaches will be different for these two patients.

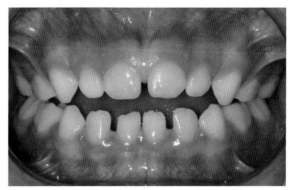

• **Figure 19.12** This patient exhibits an anterior open bite (the absence of vertical overlap). Anterior open bite, especially an asymmetric anterior open bite, is most commonly caused by a sucking habit in this age group.

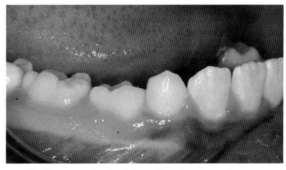

• **Figure 19.13** Ankylosis, the fusion of tooth to bone, is common in the primary dentition. This patient has an ankylosed primary mandibular first molar that is below the plane of occlusion.

A number of eruption and exfoliation problems have been blamed on ankylosed teeth. However, longitudinal studies indicate that ankylosed primary teeth exfoliate normally and allow normal eruption of succedaneous teeth.[17–19] An ankylosed tooth discovered during this developmental stage should not be removed routinely unless a large marginal ridge discrepancy develops between it and the unaffected adjacent teeth. If a marginal ridge discrepancy develops, the adjacent teeth may tip into the space occupied by the ankylosed tooth and cause space loss. A systematic review of ankylosed primary molars with permanent successors suggested removal of the ankylosed tooth in three situations. The first is if there is an altered eruption path of the permanent successor. The second situation is when the ankylosis is so severe that adjacent teeth begin to tip and create space loss. The last is when the exfoliation of the ankylosed tooth is significantly delayed.[19]

Supplemental Orthodontic Diagnostic Techniques

Diagnostic Casts

If diagnostic casts are necessary, the procedures outlined in Chapter 31 should be followed with children in the primary or mixed dentitions. Chapter 31 also includes a discussion of digital casts.

Radiographic Evaluation

Rarely would a cephalometric radiograph be needed in this age group, but those methods of analysis also are covered in Chapter 31. The dentist does require other radiographs to make a thorough diagnosis or problem list in the 3- to 6-year-old child. Children in this age range may find it difficult to cooperate with the radiographic procedures, in which case the radiographic examination should be deferred until behavior improves or can be managed. Introduction of the child to intraoral radiography can be managed as discussed in Box 19.1.

The general principle for any human radiation exposure is the ALARA principle, or "as low as reasonably achievable."[20] For the primary dentition, no radiographs are typically indicated when all proximal surfaces can be visualized and examined clinically. This includes both anterior and posterior teeth. When the proximal surfaces cannot be visualized and clinically examined, bitewing radiographs are indicated to determine the presence of interproximal caries (Fig. 19.14). Other projections are indicated in the following circumstances: history of pain, swelling, trauma, mobility of teeth, unexplained bleeding, disrupted eruption pattern, or deep carious lesions. These views include the maxillary (Fig. 19.15A) and mandibular (see Fig. 19.15B) periapical views and the maxillary (see Fig. 19.15C) and mandibular (see Fig. 19.15D) occlusal views. A complete full mouth survey (see Fig. 19.15E) is rarely obtained but may sometimes be necessary.

Pediatric (no. 0) films should be used most often in this age group with the exception of the pediatric occlusal films, which are no. 2 size, turned 90 degrees. The Snap-a-Ray (Rinn Corporation,

Elgin, IL) (Fig. 19.16) device has been used for film positioning in this age group with great success because of its small size and light weight. Other positioning instruments can be used, but some thought should be given to the size and weight of the instrument that must be placed intraorally. The patient should be adequately protected from unnecessary radiation. A lead apron and collar are necessary as it attenuates scattered radiation and provides protection for the thyroid and gonads. A 16-inch or longer cone further reduces skin exposure. Ideally, rectangular collimation should be used, but movement by children of this age may result in less than ideal radiographs with an extremely truncated beam. Before exposure of the radiographs, the ability of the child to cooperate must be assessed in order to prevent unnecessary radiation exposure. When parents assist, they must be adequately shielded and the parent must demonstrate the ability to stabilize the film and patient before exposure. Pregnancy (in the parent) is not a contraindication to obtaining radiographs when proper protection is used.[21] Dental personnel should refrain from holding films because of the risks of repeated exposure.

A concerned parent may ask about the frequency of taking films. The American Academy of Pediatric Dentistry[22] advises the use of radiographic exposure at a rate necessary to maximize detection of abnormalities while also minimizing exposure to ionizing radiation. Table 19.4 lists selection criteria for pediatric radiographs in the 3- to 6-year-old child. All radiographs should be obtained only after a clinical examination and history have been completed.

The advent of digital intraoral radiography has been both a benefit and a challenge for pediatric dental care, particularly for those in the 3- to 6-year-old age range. Two different systems predominate. The wired sensor is a solid-state x-ray detector that

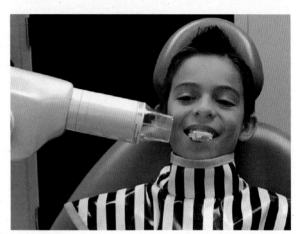

• **Figure 19.14** The proper technique for obtaining a posterior bitewing radiograph (no. 0 film) is critical because it is used frequently. The tube head should have a vertical angulation of +10 degrees and a horizontal angulation such that the face of the cone is parallel to the film packet; the beam is directed to the open embrasures. The film packet should be placed lingual to the teeth with the child biting on the tab. The film should be placed anteriorly to obtain a view of the distal surfaces of the canines. Asking the child to smile to show the teeth often helps to orient the beam and prevents overlap.

• BOX 19.1 Introducing a Child to Intraoral Radiography

1. Use tell-show-do introduction with a camera analogy. It helps to do a dry run, showing an unexposed packet of film and an exposed radiograph to explain the process using analogies including an overcoat or putting on a heavy blanket. By positioning the film and the x-ray machine, the dentist can also determine whether a child will cooperate for an exposure, preventing unproductive irradiation. Similarly, having the child bite on the Snap-a-Ray (Rinn Corporation, Elgin, IL) without a film provides a good precursor to obtaining the necessary images.
2. Consider the "preoperational" developmental stage of children at this age, or their ability to have one object represent another.[a] For example, have the x-ray head represent their favorite character that lives inside the x-ray head. You can say: "Say hello to Elmo who will come close and touch your cheek."
3. Match film size to comfort. Many children have difficulty with the film impinging on the lingual soft tissue of the mandible. In some cases, bending the anterior corners helps, but this may lower the diagnostic quality of the radiograph. Another technique is to place the film vertically to minimize anteroposterior size.
4. Obtain the least difficult radiograph first to acquaint the child with the procedures. Anterior occlusal films are usually easiest for very young children if indicated (e.g., tight contact or history of dental trauma).
5. Prepare all machine settings and ensure that the apparatus is positioned before positioning the film. Some children can hold a film for only a short period because of the gag reflex, discomfort, or a short attention span.
6. The lead apron and collar are often uncomfortable for a child, adding to the newness of the setting. Using analogies can help dispel some anxiety, such as describing the apron as an overcoat or putting on a heavy blanket since the air conditioning will come on.

[a]From Asokan S, Surendran S, Asokan S, et al. Relevance of Piaget's cognitive principles among 4-7 years old children: a descriptive cross-sectional study. J Indian Soc Pedod Prev Dent. 2014;32(4):292–296.

• **Figure 19.15** The following techniques are commonly used to obtain supplementary views. (A) Maxillary periapical view (no. 0 film). Vertical angulation: beam is at right angle to film; starting angle of +30 degrees. Horizontal angulation: face of cone is parallel to facial surface of teeth. Film placement: with film in jaw of holder, holder is placed between the maxillary and mandibular teeth with dimpled surface of film against the lingual surfaces of teeth. Child bites on larger sides of jaws. (B) Mandibular periapical view (no. 0 film). Vertical angulation: beam is at right angle to film; starting angle of ~5 degrees. Horizontal angulation: face of cone is parallel to facial surface of teeth. Film placement: with film in jaws of holder, holder is placed between the maxillary and mandibular teeth with dimpled surface of film against the lingual surfaces of teeth. Child bites on larger sides of jaws. (C) Maxillary occlusal view (no. 2 film). Vertical angulation: +60 degrees, with beam directed downward. Horizontal angulation: beam directed along midsagittal plane. Film placement: film packet is placed between maxillary and mandibular teeth so that it is parallel to floor. Film is oriented so that the long dimension extends to the right and left. The child bites gently on the film while seated upright. (D) Mandibular occlusal view (no. 2 film). Vertical angulation: ~15 degrees, with beam directed upward. Horizontal angulation: beam directed along midsagittal plane. Film placement: film packet is placed between the maxillary and mandibular teeth, and child is instructed to bite gently on the film. Patient is reclining so that the chin is extended. Bisecting angle technique is used. (E) A full mouth series comprising all of the above films. To minimize a child's exposure to radiation, dentists often reduce the number of films in a survey if tooth and supporting tissues can be viewed adequately on fewer films. (Courtesy Dr. Stephanie Furlong.)

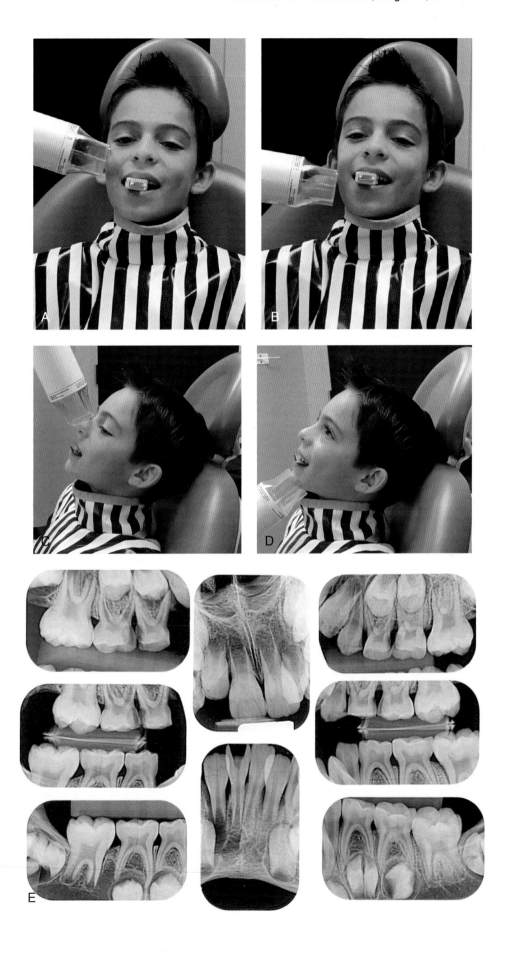

TABLE 19.4	Selection Criteria and Guidelines for Pediatric Radiographs in the 3- to 6-Year-Old Child	
Projection	**Criteria**	**Frequency**
Posterior bitewing	Proximal surfaces of posterior teeth cannot be examined clinically Child is cooperative	At initial examination if contacts closed Semiannually if interproximal surfaces have been restored, until child achieves low-risk status[a] or is caries-free; also 6–12-month intervals if child is at increased risk[b] Annually to 24-month interval if child is caries-free at initial bitewing examination
Posterior periapical	Suspected pathosis Confirmed pathosis Child is cooperative	As needed to diagnose and monitor treatment or patient condition
Anterior occlusal	Suspected pathosis Confirmed pathosis Child is cooperative	Same as above or as a caries-detecting radiograph if closed contacts preclude thorough examination

[a]Consider child cooperation in decision making.

[b]Increased risk for dental caries may be associated with (1) poor oral hygiene, (2) fluoride deficiency, (3) prolonged or inappropriate nursing, (4) high-carbohydrate diet, (5) poor family dental health, (6) developmental enamel defects, (7) developmental disability or acute medical problem, or (8) genetic abnormality.

Modified from American Dental Association, U.S. Department of Health and Human Services. *The Selection of Patients for Dental Radiographic Examination*; 2012.

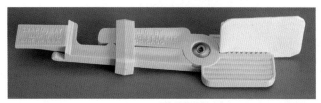

• **Figure 19.16** A Snap-a-Ray film holder. (From Boyd LRB. *Dental Instruments: A Pocket Guide.* 4th ed. St Louis: Saunders; 2012.)

requires a bulky nonflexible intraoral receptor because of the electronics. Sensors are available in typical dental film size and are wired to the computer using software to capture and display images. The phosphor plate system uses a flexible receptor much like a traditional dental film and is not attached to any device. The phosphor plates must be processed through a scanning or reading device to convert the image to digital format. Both systems have advantages and disadvantages.

1. The phosphor plates have some flexibility and are thinner, which is helpful in children and some adults for proper placement and patient comfort compared to the wired sensors.
2. Both systems require attention to infection control procedures because the receptors are intended to be reusable. Commercially available transparent plastic sleeves that are both inexpensive and disposable can be used to protect the patient.
3. Phosphor plates eventually succumb to the wear and tear of use in children, and image deterioration is common. Biting of films, common in young children and those unfamiliar with intraoral radiographic techniques, can quickly reduce the quality of images from phosphor plates. Bending and light exposure can also affect image quality.
4. Wired sensors are very expensive and require diligence in handling. Proprietary systems offer replacement warranties at far less than the cost of a new sensor.
5. Both systems rely on software, so computer malfunction can render a dental office unable to obtain radiographs.
6. Because of their bulk, wired sensors require the operator to develop new placement techniques, and they often require

purchase of product-specific alternative stabilizing devices that are different from those used with film.

7. The phosphor system requires a "development" step, like wet film technology, so it does not offer much in the way of time savings. Some processing systems for phosphor plates are cumbersome to use and require space. Wired sensors require storage that places minimal stress on sensor, wire, and attachments.

Treatment Planning for Nonorthodontic Problems

The process of diagnosing disease is based on clinical, historical, and supportive data. A problem list may be preferable to a series of diagnoses because the list represents a presumption that treatment will be provided. A synthesis of all data is required. The practical portions of the diagnostic process consider the following:

1. Existence of an abnormal state
2. Determination of cause
3. Alternatives or options to correct the problem
4. Anticipated benefits, immediate and long term
5. Problems or requirements for accomplishing treatment

A primary consideration is denoting an abnormal state, such as caries or a nonvital pulp. A problem list helps to separate abnormalities that need management from those that are simply identified. For example, a carious primary molar in a 6-year-old is a problem; a carious mandibular incisor is not if it is about to exfoliate. Identification of the cause of the abnormality is critical to determine short- and long-term treatment. A manageable cause most often results in both short- and long-term success. Caries is a largely environmental condition that can be managed with great likelihood of success in both the short and long term. On the other hand, dentinogenesis imperfecta is a genetic problem and has a guarded and limited prognosis.

For most patients, no single treatment plan is ideal. A variety of alternatives must be considered based on the child's health, cooperation, parental finances, and the anticipated benefits to be derived from the treatment. These issues are shared by dentist and parent. For example, extraction of carious primary teeth may be preferred to restoration if pulpal therapy is likely to be unsuccessful. Another example is the choice of a stainless steel crown rather than a three-surface amalgam restoration in a caries prone child because fewer surfaces will be left exposed to recurrent caries, and evidence supports recurrence of caries.[23,24]

A frank assessment of the cooperation and involvement in the child's treatment by the family must be considered. Dental treatment is necessarily a cooperative effort, with success resting on both personal and professional maintenance. The behavioral plan is critical to the success of the treatment plan in general. For the 3- to 6-year-old child, the methods of behavior guidance to be used must be included in the treatment plan for purposes of consent and often third-party payment.[25] The sequence of managing behavior, obtaining consent for medications, and providing reasonable alternatives to recommended procedures should be covered in discussion of the behavioral plan with the parents. Some dentists prefer to explain and obtain consent for all behavior procedures they might use at the initial case presentation to permit transition from one to the next during a treatment encounter.

Generally, acute infection and pain are managed first. Hopelessly involved teeth should be extracted, although this can be a challenging introduction to dental care for the young child. If numerous large lesions are present, they may be excavated and interim restorations placed. Use of glass ionomer cement, with its fluoride release, offers some additional preventive benefit. This "first aid" approach reduces the chance of caries progression, with its resultant pain; reduces difficulty in cleaning; and reduces deleterious oral flora. The introduction of silver diamine fluoride can also be considered part of the dental armamentarium when addressing dentinal caries (see Chapter 12).[26] For more definitive care, if teeth with deep lesions and chronic pulpal involvement are not painful, they can be incorporated in a treatment plan that proceeds by quadrant or sextant rather than being managed immediately.

All factors being equal, restorative care often is easiest in the maxillary posterior areas. The infiltration injections are easiest for patients to tolerate. The dentist can then move to the mandibular posterior sextants. Seldom are the mandibular anterior teeth involved unless rampant caries are present.

Finally, the maxillary anterior teeth can be approached. This is a good final selection because the injections are uncomfortable, and some families will not pursue all necessary care if the maxillary anterior teeth are restored first with a good esthetic result.

When restorative care is complete and the patient and parent demonstrate that they can maintain good oral health, orthodontic care, whether active or for space maintenance, can be considered. It is best if space maintenance can be implemented in the first 6 months after necessary extractions because space loss is most common during this period (see Chapter 26).

References

1. American Academy of Pediatric Dentistry. Guideline on perinatal and infant oral health care. Academy of Pediatric Dentistry Council on Clinical Affairs. *Pediatr Dent*. 2016;38(6):150–154.
2. American Academy of Pediatric Dentistry. Guidelines for record-keeping. Academy of Pediatric Dentistry Council on Clinical Affairs. *Pediatr Dent*. 2016;38(6):343–350.
3. World Health Organization. *International Statistical Classification of Diseases and Related Health Problems*. ICD-10: 10th Revision, 2016.
4. American Academy of Pediatric Dentistry. Policy on child identification programs. Academy of Pediatric Dentistry Council on Clinical Affairs, *Pediatr Dent*. 2016;38(6):32–33.
5. Armitage GC. Periodontal diagnoses and classification of periodontal diseases. *Periodontol 2000*. 2004;34(1):9–21.
6. American Academy of Pediatric Dentistry. Pediatric medical history. *Pediatr Dent*. 2016;38(6):428–430.
7. Boyle EM, Poulsen G, Field DJ, et al. Effects of gestational age at birth on health outcomes at 3 and 5 years of age: population based cohort study. *BMJ*. 2012;344:e896.
8. Szczepaniak D, McHenry MS, Nutakki K, et al. The prevalence of at-risk development in children 30 to 60 months old presenting with disruptive behaviors. *Clin Pediatr (Phila)*. 2013;52(10):942–949.
9. Barton M. Screening for obesity in children and adolescents: US Preventive Services Task Force recommendation statement. *Pediatrics*. 2010;125:361–367.
10. Centers for Disease Control and Prevention. About child and teen BMI. http://www.cdc.gov/healthyweight/assessing/bmi/childrens_bmi/about_childrens_bmi.html. Accessed August 31, 2017.
11. Marcum B, Turner C, Courts F. Pediatric dentists' attitudes regarding parental presence during dental procedures. *Pediatr Dent*. 1995;17(7):432–436.
12. Cox CJ, Krikken JB, Veerkamp JS. Influence of parental presence on the child's perception of, and behaviour, during dental treatment. *Eur Arch Paediatr Dent*. 2011;12(4):200–204.
13. Fields HW, Vann WF. Prediction of dental and skeletal relationships from facial profiles in preschool children. *Pediatr Dent*. 1979;1:7–15.
14. Fields HW, Vann WF. Prediction of dental and skeletal relationships from facial profiles in preschool children. *Pediatr Dent*. 1979;1:7–15.
15. Valachovic RW, Lurie AG. Risk-benefit considerations in pedodontic radiology. *Pediatr Dent*. 1980;2:128–146.
16. Brearly IL, McKibben DH. Ankylosis of primary molar teeth: parts I and II. *J Dent Child*. 1973;40:54–63.
17. Kurol J, Koch G. The effect of extraction on infraoccluded deciduous molars: a longitudinal study. *Am J Orthod*. 1985;87:46–55.
18. Messer LB, Cline JT. Ankylosed primary molars: results and treatment recommendations from an eight-year longitudinal study. *Pediatr Dent*. 1980;2:37–47.
19. Tieu LD, Walker SL, Major MP, et al. Management of ankylosed primary molars with premolar successors: a systematic review. *J Am Dent Assoc*. 2013;144:602–611.
20. White SC, Pharoah MJ. *Oral Radiology: Principles and Interpretation*. 7th ed. St Louis: Mosby; 2014.
21. Oral Health During Pregnancy Expert Workgroup. *Oral Health Care During Pregnancy. A National Consensus Statement*. Washington, DC: National Maternal and Child Oral Health Resource Center; 2012.
22. American Academy of Pediatric Dentistry. Guideline on prescribing dental radiographs for infants, children, adolescents, and persons with special health care needs. *Pediatr Dent*. 2016;38(6):355–357.
23. Innes NPT, Ricketts D, Chong LY, et al. Preformed crowns for decayed primary molar teeth. *Cochrane Database Syst Rev*. 2015;(12):CD005512.
24. Mata AF, Bebermeyer RD. Stainless steel crowns versus amalgams in the primary dentition and decision-making in clinical practice. *Gen Dent*. 2006;54(5):347–350.
25. American Academy of Pediatric Dentistry. Behavior guidance for the pediatric dental patient. *Pediatr Dent*. 2017;39(6):246–259.
26. Gao SS, Zhang S, Mei ML, et al. Caries remineralisation and arresting effect in children by professionally applied fluoride treatment—a systematic review. *BMC Oral Health*. 2016;16:12.

20

Prevention of Dental Disease

ARWA I. OWAIS AND ARTHUR J. NOWAK

With the eruption of all primary teeth, the preschool child enters a relatively short period of dental stability in preparation for the loss of the first primary tooth and the lengthy process of eruption of the permanent teeth. Historically, many preschoolers' first dental examination occurred during this period; however, with the increased awareness that home care should be established much earlier for all children, a child might have already established a dental home by this age. During this stage, instructions are reinforced for appropriate oral hygiene techniques and topical fluoride use. After taking into consideration the child's caries risk, adjustments in optimal systemic fluoride supplementation should be considered if the child is living in a nonfluoridated community.

Dietary management may now become a problem. This is the period of development of strong preferences for and aversions to specific foods. The effect of commercials from television, the Internet, and the press begins to take its toll. Children are frequently sent to a child care facility for a quasieducational experience, a babysitting service, or a true preschool developmental experience. Parental control of the quality and quantity of the diet is sometimes greatly sacrificed due to the fact that other care providers are often involved in preparing meals and snacks for the children.

When the end of the day is in sight and the children want to watch "just one more TV program," or play "just one more game," the daily supervised oral hygiene routine may be sacrificed for the quick 30-second unsupervised brushing. It is amazing how quickly parents assume that 4-year-old children can be responsible for their own oral hygiene when they cannot even comb their hair or print their name clearly.

Fluoride Administration

Dietary Fluoride Supplementation

Recommendations on the prescription of dietary fluoride supplementation for caries prevention were revised in 2013.[1,2] Dietary fluoride supplementation should be prescribed only for children who are at high risk of developing caries and whose primary source of drinking water is deficient in fluoride. Therefore the first step for the clinician is to determine if the child is at high caries risk as described in Chapters 14 and 15. If the child is at high risk for caries and drinks water that is deficient in fluoride, then fluoride supplementation should be considered (Table 20.1).[1,2]

The US Public Health Service (USPHS) currently recommends an optimal fluoride concentration of 0.7 mg/L. This replaces the earlier USPHS recommendation for fluoride concentrations of 0.7 to 1.2 mg which was based on outdoor air temperature of geographic areas.[3] The new recommendation, which was supported by the American Dental Association (ADA), does not change the ADA Council on Scientific Affairs' systematic review and clinical recommendation for the use of dietary fluoride supplements that was released in 2010 (see Table 20.1).

By 3 years of age, most children are able to chew and swallow tablets; therefore prescriptions for supplemental fluoride should be changed from liquid drops to chewable tablets to reflect this change in developmental status. The recommended supplemental fluoride dosage schedule also requires an increase in the amount of fluoride prescribed after a child reaches 3 years of age. The recommended daily dosage of supplemental fluoride is 0.5 mg for children aged 3 to 6 years who drink water containing less than 0.3 ppm of fluoride. The dosage is 0.25 mg for those whose water contains between 0.3 and 0.6 ppm fluoride. Children whose drinking water contains more than 0.6 ppm of fluoride do not require any supplementation. However, the potential for producing dental fluorosis on permanent anterior teeth will have diminished in this age group owing to substantial crown formation (see Chapter 15 for details on fluorosis). The practice of determining the fluoride levels of each child's drinking water before prescribing supplemental fluoride should continue. In the United States, information on the fluoride status of community water supplies, listed by state, county, and city, can be accessed on the Centers for Disease Control and Prevention (CDC) My Water Fluoride website (www.cdc.gov/oralhealth/).[4] If the fluoride level is unknown, then an analysis

TABLE 20.1   Clinical Recommendations for the Use of Dietary Fluoride Supplements

The expert panel convened by the American Dental Association Council on Scientific Affairs developed the following recommendations. They are intended as a resource for dentists and other health care providers. The recommendations must be balanced with the practitioner's professional judgment and the individual patient's needs and preferences.

Children are exposed to multiple sources of fluoride. The expert panel encourages health care providers to evaluate all potential fluoride sources and to conduct a caries risk assessment before prescribing fluoride supplements.

Recommendation	Strength of Recommendations
For children at low risk of developing caries, dietary fluoride supplements are not recommended, and other sources of fluoride should be considered as a caries-preventive intervention	D
For children at high risk of developing caries, dietary fluoride supplements are recommended according to the schedule presented in the next section of the table	D
When fluoride supplements are prescribed, they should be taken daily to maximize the caries-preventive benefit	D

Recommended American Dental Association Dietary Fluoride Supplement Dosing Schedule for Children at High Risk of Developing Caries

	AMOUNT OF FLUORIDE SUPPLEMENTATION AND STRENGTH OF RECOMMENDATIONS, ACCORDING TO FLUORIDE CONCENTRATION IN DRINKING WATER (PARTS PER MILLION[a])					
	<0.3		0.3 TO 0.6		>0.6	
Age	Fluoride Supplementation	Strength of Recommendations	Fluoride Supplementation	Strength of Recommendations	Fluoride Supplementation	Strength of Recommendations
Birth to 6 months	None	D	None	D	None	D
6 months to 3 years	0.25 mg/d	B	None	D	None	D
3–6 years	0.50 mg/d	B	0.25 mg/d	B	None	D
6–16 years	1.00 mg/d	B	0.50 mg/d	B	None	D

[a]1.0 part per million = 1 milligram per liter.
Strength of Recommendations: A, Directly based on category I evidence; B, directly based on category II evidence or extrapolated recommendation from category I evidence; C, directly based on category III evidence or extrapolated recommendation from category I or II evidence; D, directly based on category IV evidence or extrapolated recommendation from category I, II, or III evidence.
From Rozier RG, Adair S, Graham F, et al. Evidence-based clinical recommendations on the prescription of dietary fluoride supplements for caries prevention. A report of the American Dental Association Council on Scientific Affairs. *J Am Dent Assoc.* 2010;141(12):1480–1489.

can be requested from the local public health department, family dentist, or commercial laboratories.

Because parental compliance continues to play a key role in determining the effectiveness of these supplements, efforts to reinforce parental motivation should be made. One method of assessing parental compliance is to monitor the need to rewrite supplemental fluoride prescriptions at recall visits. The dosage of fluoride prescribed should be noted in each patient's record whenever a prescription is written. Parents who indicate no need for an additional prescription when the patient's record suggests that the previously prescribed supplement should have been consumed should be questioned about the number of tablets remaining. A large remaining supply suggests poor compliance.

Topical Fluoride Therapy

Topical fluorides have an increasingly important role in the 3- to 6-year-old group. The child's ability to appropriately use fluoride dentifrices increases throughout this period, although parental involvement at each brushing should continue. Professional topical applications are often applied during this interval, and their use should be based on caries risk assessment. One mode of topical application that is generally not recommended for the younger members of this age group is the use of fluoride mouth rinses, because most preschoolers are unable to avoid swallowing some of these solutions.[5]

Professional Applications of Fluoride

Topical application of highly concentrated forms of fluoride has been provided in clinical settings for many years. There is evidence that the use of 1.23% acidulated phosphate fluoride (APF) and 5% sodium fluoride varnish is effective in preventing dental caries in children 6 years and older. However, a recent report of the ADA Council of Scientific Affairs recommends only 2.26% fluoride varnish (5% sodium fluoride varnish) for children younger than 6 years because it does not have the risk of experiencing adverse events (particularly nausea and vomiting) associated with swallowing other forms of fluoride.[5] Fluoride varnish (Fig. 20.1) has become a popular topical agent for preschool children and individuals with special health care needs. It has been recommended for conditions

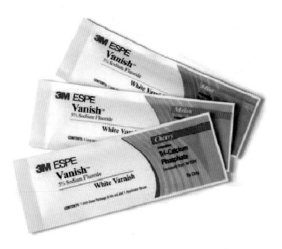

• **Figure 20.1** Example of a fluoride varnish. (Pictured: Vanish 5% sodium fluoride varnish. Courtesy 3M Science Applied to Life Inc., USA.)

in which decalcified enamel secondary to poor plaque removal or poor feeding practices is present.[6-8] A recent Cochrane review found that the application of fluoride varnish two to four times a year is associated with a substantial reduction in caries increment.[9] The American Academy of Pediatrics (AAP) has also endorsed the application of fluoride varnish in children up to 5 years of age.

In summary, the evidence-based approach to clinical recommendations should be integrated with the practitioner's professional judgment and the patient's needs and preferences.

Indications for Professional Topical Fluoride Applications

When and for whom topical application of fluoride should be provided in the dental office has been a source of some controversy. One school of thought invokes the argument that professional fluoride application is a primary preventive measure and should be provided to all children to minimize the potential for development of new carious lesions. Part of the historical basis for this approach relates to the lack of validated methods to predict whether an individual patient is likely to develop caries. Advocates of this philosophy tend to focus only on the potential benefits that might be achieved from topical fluoride application while ignoring the costs associated with providing the service.

Others feel that the decision to provide topical fluoride therapy should be based on the factors that have been shown to be associated with the risk of developing caries in groups or in individuals (e.g., access to fluoridated drinking water, use of other forms of topical fluoride, degree of spacing between teeth). Their approach is to consider the likelihood that each patient develops disease according to these caries risk factors and then to recommend professional topical fluoride therapy for those considered to be at significant risk for developing caries. Proponents of this philosophy tend to consider the costs associated with providing the service as well as the potential benefits. Caries risk assessment methods are available to help clinicians predict with accuracy which individuals are more likely to develop caries and therefore would benefit more from topical fluoride therapy.[10]

Cost-Benefit Considerations

In a private practice setting, the patient's willingness or ability to pay for different forms of treatment usually is an important factor in determining what types of services are provided. In the case of public programs or private third-party payers, the decision to provide reimbursement for various services may be based on a more formal analysis of the relationship between the costs and benefits associated with those services. The ratio of costs to benefits has historically been higher for topical fluoride applications provided in dental offices than for other types of preventive services or for the same services provided in other settings. Consequently, professional topical fluoride treatments have not been recommended as a public health measure because of their unfavorable cost-benefit ratio.

Documented changes in caries levels and patterns of decay in children in the United States have pushed these ratios even higher. Studies have reported that a substantial proportion of school-aged children in the United States are caries free and that a relatively small percentage of children account for a large percentage of all tooth decay.[11] In addition to the overall decline in the level of caries, there has been a decrease in the proportion of smooth-surface caries and a corresponding increase in the proportion of pit and fissure caries. The combination of these factors seems to be associated with a reduction in the effectiveness of concentrated topical fluoride therapy in terms of the actual number of surfaces saved from becoming carious during a given period.[12]

Changes of this nature have led some interested parties to call for a reexamination of the manner in which various preventive measures are provided. In an era when increased attention is being focused on measures for controlling all types of health care costs, some have proposed that consideration be given to making preventive dental services more cost-effective. One means of improving the cost-benefit ratio of topical fluoride therapy would be to provide this therapy in settings other than dental offices, such as school-based programs and home use. In addition, cost-effectiveness may be enhanced by targeting those children at high risk for developing caries.

A factor that has been repeatedly demonstrated to be associated with a reduction in both the risk of developing caries and the relative effectiveness of topical fluoride therapy is the availability of drinking water containing fluoride. Studies have shown that topical fluorides are considerably more effective in reducing the incidence of decay in nonfluoridated areas compared with fluoridated areas.[13] Therefore the cost of preventing a carious lesion in a fluoridated area by means of professional topical fluoride therapy is significantly greater than the cost of preventing a lesion in a nonfluoridated area. This suggests that, in fluoridated areas, topical fluoride treatments should be reserved for patients who have a history of moderate to high caries development or who are in proven high-risk categories. Those who do not seem to be particularly prone to developing caries, especially smooth-surface decay, would probably benefit more from other forms of prevention such as pit and fissure sealants. (See Chapter 33 for more details on pit and fissure sealants.)

The question of which preventive services should be provided for a particular child in the dental office remains an individual issue for dentists and their patients (or parents in the case of children). Accordingly, the final decision about professional preventive services must be based on the child's risk assessment and made by the child's parents once informed on the costs and expected benefits. However, the influence of third-party coverage for different

TABLE 20.2 Evidenced-Based Clinical Recommendations for Professionally Applied Topical Fluoride

Topical Fluoride Agent	AGE GROUP OR DENTITION AFFECTED			
	<6 Years (Primary Teeth)	6–18 Years (Mixed Dentition)	>18 Years (Permanent Teeth)	Adult Root Caries
Vanish, 2.26% fluoride	Every 3–6 months	Every 3–6 months	Every 3–6 months	Every 3–6 months
Varnish, 0.1% fluoride	Not recommended	Not recommended	Not recommended	Panel unable to make recommendation
Professionally applied 1.23% fluoride (APF) gel application	Not recommended	4 min every 3–6 months	4 min every 3–6 months	4 min every 3–6 months
Prophylaxis prior to 1.23% fluoride (APF) gel application	Not recommended	Not recommended	Not recommended	Panel unable to make recommendation
Fluoride foam (1.23% fluoride as APF)	Not recommended	Not recommended	Not recommended	Panel unable to make recommendation
Prophylaxis paste containing fluoride	Not recommended	Not recommended	Not recommended	Panel unable to make recommendation
Prescription-strength (0.5%) fluoride), home-use fluoride products (gel, paste)	Not recommended	Twice daily	Twice daily	Twice daily
Mouthrinse, 0.09% fluoride	Not recommended	At least weekly	Twice daily	Twice daily

Definitions for the Strength of Clinical Recommendations[a] Color Legend:

Strong	Evidence strongly supports providing this intervention
In Favor	Evidence favors providing this intervention
Weak	Evidence suggests implementing this intervention only after alternatives have been considered
Expert Opinion For[b]	Evidence is lacking; the level of certainty is low. Expert opinion guides this recommendation
Expert Opinion Against[b]	Evidence is lacking; the level of certainty is low. Expert opinion suggests not implementing this intervention
Against	Evidence suggests not implementing this intervention discontinuing ineffective procedures

[a]Definitions for the strength of clinical recommendations adapted from the US Preventive Services Task Force (USPSTF) system.
[b]The USPSTF system defines this category of evidence as "insufficient"; "grade I indicated that the evidence is insufficient to determine the relationship between benefits and harms (i.e., net benefit)." The corresponding recommendation grade "I" is defined as follows: "The USPSTF concludes that the current evidence is insufficient to assess the balance of benefits and harms of the service. Evidence is lacking, of poor quality, or conflicting, and the balance of benefits and harms cannot be determined."
APF, Acidulated phosphate fluoride.
Data from Weyant RJ, Tracy SL, Anselmo TT, et al. Topical fluoride for caries prevention: executive summary of the updated clinical recommendations and supporting systematic review. J Am Dent Assoc. 2013;144(11):1279–1291.

types of services can significantly affect this decision and ultimately the care received by the child.

The recommendations for professionally applied topical fluoride are that children 3 to 6 years of age should receive fluoride varnish applications every 3 to 6 months. Those children with high caries risk should receive the treatments more frequently (i.e., every 3 months) (Table 20.2).[5]

Prophylaxis Before Topical Fluoride Treatment

Another issue related to the effectiveness of professional topical fluoride therapy, which also has implications for lowering the cost-benefit ratio, concerns the need for the prophylaxis that has traditionally been provided before fluoride application. Research

in both laboratory and clinical trials has shown that the ability of a variety of topical fluoride agents to penetrate dental plaque and deposit fluoride in the enamel is not significantly reduced by the presence of an organic layer on the tooth surface. Therefore there is no added benefit from conducting prophylaxis prior to topical fluoride application.[14–17] On the other hand, prophylaxis is an excellent way to introduce children to the sensations associated with the use of a handpiece in the mouth. In addition, cleaning the teeth before an examination makes for a more thorough assessment.

Method of Application

The most popular professional topical fluoride agent currently in use for children up to age 6 years is 5% sodium fluoride varnish applied by primary health care providers. The ADA Council on Scientific Affairs recommends fluoride varnish in young children due to the fact that it poses fewer side effects than other topical fluoride products, because these children typically cannot expectorate properly.[5] Less time is required to place the varnish, and therefore the treatment may be more cost-effective than the use of a fluoride gel with trays.

Advantages of sodium fluoride varnish (see Fig. 20.1) include that it is easy to apply, in addition to being safe and effective. It can be applied by the primary care team and is covered by most insurance. A variety of 5% sodium fluoride varnish preparations are commercially available. The unit dose of 0.25 mL 5% NaF is recommended for use in preschool children. The application technique is covered in Chapter 15.

Considerations for Special Patients

As in any age group, some children require special consideration with respect to their need for fluoride therapy or the manner in which this therapy must be provided. Specifically, alternative approaches should be available for children with developmental disabilities or medical conditions that either place them at higher risk for caries or limit their ability to obtain fluoride in the usual manner. For example, fluoride varnish can be applied quickly, requires minimal cooperation, and is more convenient to those who may find it difficult to tolerate the trays used for other topical fluoride applications.

Another population of patients who require special consideration are those children being treated with irradiation or chemotherapy. These patients often experience ulcerative degeneration of the soft tissues, causing them to be extremely sensitive to preparations having a low pH (i.e., APF) or to certain flavoring agents. A diluted, neutral, nonirritating fluoride formulation should be provided for these patients. In addition, children with chronic renal failure may experience elevated serum fluoride levels for prolonged periods following ingestion of concentrated fluoride preparations owing to their kidney impairment. Because they also have been noted to have a lower incidence of caries than matched controls, systemic or professional topical fluorides are not recommended for these patients.[18] It is up to the clinician to use the best method of topical fluoride application that would be best for the individual patient.

ADAPTIVE DAILY ORAL HYGIENE FOR THE CHILD WITH SPECIAL HEALTH CARE NEEDS

Gayle J. Gilbaugh

Good oral health is an important aspect of every child's well-being and general health. For the child with special needs, it is both a health and a social issue. Lack of regular home care can lead to dental disease causing a painful and unsightly mouth. This can interfere with daily functions such as eating, sleeping, and making friends. A child with special health care needs does not need this additional burden. A healthy smile boosts the child's morale, enhances self-esteem, and is a part of total well-being.

Unfortunately, daily oral hygiene can be a challenge for children with special health care needs and their caregivers. Some children with disabilities may be capable of cleaning their own teeth, whereas others may find it physically and mentally difficult or impossible. In these cases a caregiver needs to provide some assistance.

Daily oral hygiene should be built into the schedule and require a minimum of frustration for the child and caregiver. The basic tooth cleaning concepts are the same as for any child and should be accomplished daily. For the child with special health care needs, achieving the goals may require some adaptations and a little ingenuity.

Historically there have not been many commercial oral care products that were tailored for people with special health care needs. However, nowadays a wide variety of cleaning devices, products, and adaptations are available for parents and caregivers, as shown in the second figure below. The following chart lists potential oral hygiene challenges and techniques or devices that may be of assistance while delivering care for individuals with special health care needs. All adaptations should be individualized according to the age and needs of a particular individual.

Potential Obstacle
Access to the child

Difficulty expectorating

Technique/Device
- Avoid small confined bathrooms
- Use a room with plenty of space for maneuvering
- Good light source
- Use pea-sized amount of toothpaste

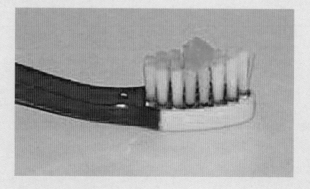

ADAPTIVE DAILY ORAL HYGIENE FOR THE CHILD WITH SPECIAL HEALTH CARE NEEDS—cont'd

Potential Obstacle	Technique/Device
	• A bulb syringe or portable power suction can be used for expectoration
	• Antimicrobial agents and fluoride can be applied with a toothbrush, cotton swab, or Toothette if indicated

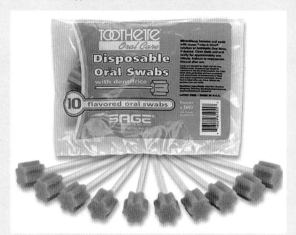

(Courtesy Sage Products, Cary, IL.)

Excessive gagging (high gag reflex)	• Use a toothbrush with a small compact head • Use a minimal amount of toothpaste • Avoid a supine position, keep the head elevated
Dry or chapped lips	• Apply petroleum jelly before brushing or flossing • Be gentle when stretching the lips
Unable to keep mouth open (hypertonic bite)	• Use a mouth prop • Commercial products are available or can be fabricated with several tongue depressors and adhesive tape • Position the mouth prop with care so that the lips are not caught underneath
Perioral sensitivity	• Desensitizing activities conducted several times a day can help the child to tolerate the daily oral hygiene regime • Consult with a speech-language pathologist or occupational therapist • Movements should be slow and gentle
Wheelchair bound	• Stand behind the wheelchair for the best view into the mouth • Carefully use your arm to support the patient's head against your body

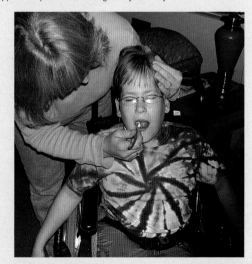

	• Sit behind the wheelchair and lock the wheels • Tilt the chair into your lap and use your arm to support the patient's head against your body
Difficulty sitting up	• Use a foam or beanbag chair to stabilize the child • Approach from behind and support the child's head with your arm • Lay the child on the bed or sofa with his or her head in your lap • Support the child's head and shoulders with your arm

Continued

ADAPTIVE DAILY ORAL HYGIENE FOR THE CHILD WITH SPECIAL HEALTH CARE NEEDS—cont'd

Potential Obstacle	Technique/Device
Uncontrollable movements	• One caregiver: have the child sit on the floor between the legs of the caregiver sitting on the sofa. The adult gently places his or her legs over the child's arms. Or, have the child lay on the floor with arms extended. The adult sits behind the child's head and gently places his or her legs over the child's arms.

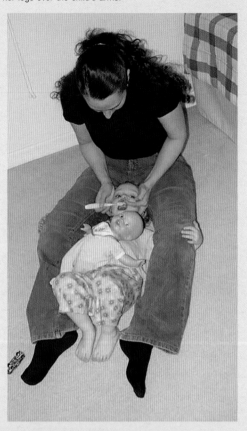

• Two caregivers: have the child lay on the bed or sofa with his or her head on your lap. The second caregiver can hold the child's hands or legs if needed.

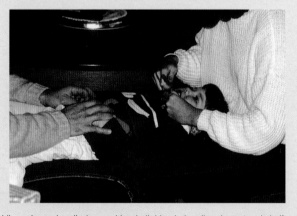

Difficulty grasping toothbrush	• Modify toothbrush by adding a larger handle (e.g., rubber ball, bicycle handle grip, or tennis ball)
	• Commercial toothbrushes with a large handle are available
	• Bend the toothbrush handle after holding under hot water
	• Attach a Velcro strap to the toothbrush handle to secure the toothbrush in the hand
Limited manual dexterity	• Power toothbrush

For additional information:
- *National Institute of Dental and Craniofacial Research: www.nidcr.nih.gov/OralHealth/Topics/DevelopmentalDisabilities*
- *National Maternal & Child Oral Health Resource Center: www.mchoralhealth.org/*
- *www.mchoralhealth.org/PDFs/SHCNfactsheet.pdf*
- *Autism Speaks: www.autismspeaks.org*
- *Dental Professionals' Tool Kit: www.autismspeaks.org/science/resources-programs/autism-treatment-network/tools-you-can-use/dental*

Dietary Management

A number of factors begin to emerge during the preschool period that can have a profound effect on the growth and development of children, as well as on their dental health. Following the large gains in growth during the first 3 years of life, the preschool child's rate of growth slows markedly. Therefore caloric requirements should be reduced accordingly, but a balanced diet need not be sacrificed. Because it is becoming common for both parents to be employed when a child reaches the age of 3 years, the management and control of the child's diet that had been maintained during the first 3 years of life may become threatened. When preschoolers are sent off to a babysitter, grandparents, or day care center, children are introduced to new environments, food selections, and management styles. It is no wonder that they become confused, begin to question routine dietary practices, and even stop eating foods that were once favorites.

By this time, they begin to be affected by what they see on television. The preschooler may be exposed to 2 to 8 (or more) hours of television on any day. Advertisements during this period are numerous, and unfortunately most are for food items, all of which the preschooler seems to want when he or she accompanies the parents to the market for the shopping.

Fortunately, children at this stage are still willing to try new foods. Parents need to experiment not only with new foods but also with the preparation of these foods. In addition, the presentation of foods is important. Appropriate amounts of a variety of colorful foods go a long way to increasing children's consumption at mealtime.

Although preschoolers seem to always be busy, they have an increasing amount of "idle" time because of their decreasing willingness to take a morning or afternoon nap. With more awake time available, snacking often increases as a reflection of comments heard on television, and the encouragement of peers. Appropriate snacking should be encouraged. Snacks heavy with salt, fats, or refined carbohydrates of a consistency that adheres to the teeth and oral tissues or dissolves slowly are more likely to lead to dental problems. Teachers and caretakers must be educated or told by parents or guardians about the kinds of snacks that are best for their children. On special occasions, such as birthday parties, Halloween, or Valentine's Day, a special treat of sweets can be allowed. At all other times, snacks should be selected from a list of foods that have been shown to be "friendly to teeth."

Fortunately, preschoolers are highly impressionable and can be greatly influenced by experiences within the family. Therefore mealtimes are important "classrooms" in which they learn and observe the feeding practices of older siblings and their parents. A friendly, congenial atmosphere at mealtime without threats ("You'd better eat all your food or you'll get no dessert") or badgering from siblings goes a long way toward establishing positive dietary practices.

It is because of these factors that the dentist may find it difficult to encourage parents to modify dietary practices when they are implicated in dental disease. Although many approaches are available to the dental team, no one approach is successful all the time. The approach used must be individualized to the personality of the practice, the willingness of the family to learn, and the specific dental problems encountered. Although caries is a multifactorial disease, it is essential to acknowledge that dietary sugars are the most important factor in causing this disease. Sugars provide a substrate for cariogenic oral bacterial to flourish and to generate enamel-demineralizing acids, consequently causing caries.

Quantitative analyses showed a strong relationship between sugar intake and the progressive lifelong development of caries.[19]

Although historically sucrose has been implicated as the major carbohydrate necessary for acid production, we now know that other simple carbohydrates can produce acid. This includes corn sweeteners which are commonly used in processed and convenience foods, as well as fructose and glucose which occur naturally in honey, fruits, and vegetables. Therefore it is no longer simply a matter of recommending that the patient reduce his or her sucrose intake. Over the years, sucrose has been appreciably replaced in the food industry with fructose and other sweeteners. The critical factor that remains is the potential for these foods to produce acid that lowers the pH in and around the tooth in the presence of plaque. Many foods have been tested and found to lower the pH of the interproximal plaque to 5.5 or lower (Box 20.1).[20]

Other critical cariogenic factors are the tendency of a food to adhere to the teeth, the rate at which a food dissolves, the potential for a food to stimulate saliva production, and the potential for a food to buffer the production of acid. It has been suggested that a food with a low cariogenic potential would have the following attributes[20]:
1. A relatively high protein content
2. A moderate fat content to facilitate oral clearance
3. A minimal concentration of fermentable carbohydrates
4. A strong buffering capacity
5. A high mineral content, especially of calcium and phosphorus
6. A pH greater than 6.0
7. The ability to stimulate saliva flow

Foods with "lower cariogenic potential" should be suggested to parents. At the same time, it is important to educate them to adhere to the required calorie intake of the young child.

Dietary Counseling

Although the dental profession recognizes the role of good nutrition and appropriate dietary practices in achieving and maintaining good oral health, promoting behavioral changes has been challenging. Fortunately, parents are now more aware of these issues and willing to listen, and many are even ready to make changes.

• BOX 20.1 Foods That Cause the pH of Interproximal Plaque to Fall Below 5.5

Apples, dried	Gelatin-flavored dessert
Apples, fresh	Grapes
Apple drink	Milk, whole
Apricots, dried	Milk, 2%
Bananas	Oatmeal
Beans, baked	Oranges
Beans, green canned	Orange juice
White bread	Pasta
Whole wheat bread	Peanut butter
Caramels	Potato, boiled
Cooked carrots	Potato chips
Cereals, presweetened and regular	Raisins
Chocolate milk	Rice
Cola	Sponge cake, cream-filled
Crackers, soda	Tomato, fresh
Cream cheese	Wheat flakes
Doughnuts	

Some excellent resources that provide information for families' nutritional requirements include the World Health Organization's *The WHO Guideline: Sugars Intake for Adults and Children*[21] presented in six languages, the 2015 to 2020[22] *Dietary Guidelines for Americans, 2015 to 2020,* and the preschoolers section in the MyPlate (Fig. 20.2).[23] These resources provide parents with practical information on eating and physical activity patterns that are focused on consuming fewer calories, making informed food choices, and being physically active to attain and maintain healthy weight, reduce risk of chronic disease, and promote overall health.

In families with a preschool child and no dental disease, the approach would be quite different from that recommended for families with a preschool child with dental disease. For all children the dentist should ask the parents the following questions during the initial interview to develop a baseline for further dietary assessment:

1. At what age was the child weaned from the breast or bottle?
2. If the child was still on the breast or bottle after 1 year of age, what was the frequency and duration of use?
3. When were solids introduced?
4. Were baby foods commercially prepared or homemade?
5. How many meals are served presently? Does the family eat together?
6. Who selects the menu and prepares the food?
7. Are snacks provided? Are they given at home, in nursery school, or by a babysitter? As a parent, do you choose the snacks? If not, do you know what they are?
8. Is the child a good eater? Does he or she eat a balanced diet? If not, what are the problem areas?
9. Does the child have any grandparents living at home? Or does the child spend appreciable time at the grandparents' home?
10. Are there any religious or ethnic preferences that would limit dietary choices?
11. What is the source of the water used for drinking and preparation of foods?
12. What is the child's daily liquid intake? How much of that liquid is derived from drinking water in your community?
13. How much time does the child spend daily watching television or in front of the computer/electronic devices?
14. How much play/physical activity does the child have daily?

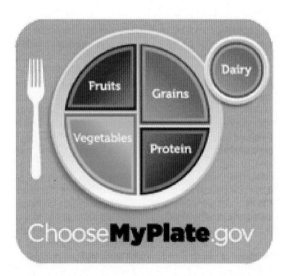

• **Figure 20.2** The US Department of Agriculture's newly released food guide, MyPlate. (Courtesy US Department of Agriculture.)

If the child has a disability, additional questions are indicated:

1. What dietary practices are modified because of the child's disability?
2. Are there additional nutritional requirements because of the disability?
3. Does the child feed herself or himself, or does she or he require assistance?
4. What medications are taken by mouth, and how often are they taken?
5. Does the child have difficulty with chewing and swallowing?
6. Does the child hold (ruminate) food in his or her mouth for long periods? Does he or she regurgitate food?

By being familiar with the *2015 to 2020 Dietary Guidelines* and the answers to these questions, the dentist and staff should have the basic background information on the nutritional requirements and dietary practices of the patient and his or her family. *The 2015 to 2020 Dietary Guidelines* provides five overarching guidelines including:

1. Follow a healthy eating pattern across the lifespan.
2. Focus on variety, nutrient density, and amount.
3. Limit calories from added sugars and saturated fats and reduce sodium intake.
4. Shift to healthier food and beverage choices.
5. Support healthy eating patterns for all.

In families with a preschool child who has no dental disease and evidence of sound dietary management, a word of positive reinforcement from the dentist is indicated. Dietary histories and counseling would seem to be counterproductive in this situation.

In families with preschool children who have caries or appear to be at high risk for caries, further assessment by the dentist is indicated. A dietary history should be obtained, from either the parent's recollection of the previous 24 hours or a written record of the next 3 to 7 days. Although the reliability of dietary histories is often questioned, in a spirit of trust and respect much can be learned.

Many dietary history forms are available commercially, or they can be easily made. Parents should be instructed on how to complete the history, making sure to list all foods eaten by the child at each meal, the amounts eaten, the types and quantities of food consumed between meals, and the liquid intake. Dietary or vitamin supplements and oral medications should also be listed.

Although the primary purpose of the dietary assessment in the dental office is to identify dietary patterns that are or may be potentially deleterious to oral health, the dentist should be aware of dietary intake and patterns that may greatly influence overall growth and development. In cases where diet-related problems are noted, the children should be referred for further assessment and counseling by a primary health care provider, dietician, or nutritionist.

With the dietary history available, the dentist can review the findings alone or with the parent:

1. How many times a day does the child eat?
2. Is there a diversified selection of foods? Are the meals well balanced?
3. Are recommendations regarding the four basic food groups being satisfied daily?
4. What is the frequency of snacking?
5. Are foods high in (refined) carbohydrates consumed frequently? Are they consumed during, after, or between meals?
6. Are snack foods of the kind that dissolve slowly or that adhere to the teeth?

After the problem areas have been identified, recommendations can be offered. Sweeping modifications of the family diet and dietary practices will be met with resentment, poor compliance, and negative results. A better approach would be to select one problem area, make a recommendation for change, wait a few weeks, and then evaluate the results. If results are positive, another area can be modified, and the family can then build on its successes.

Follow-up histories are indicated depending on the oral health status. Dietary counseling is only part of a comprehensive preventive program, although at times it is the most obvious area in need of adjustment. It can also be the most difficult area in which to obtain success.

A number of electronic nutrition analysis programs are available through the Internet. After a dietary history is entered, a number of analyses become available, including meal planning and recommendations for physical activity. To date, none is specific for evaluating diets that may contribute to oral disease in children.

Home Care

With the changes in the child's knowledge base, socialization, and maturation in growth and development taking place during this period, daily home care should be less difficult. Unfortunately, that usually is not the case. Parents tend to assume that their child can be more independent than he or she actually is. They also assume that the child's motor coordination has progressed to a point where adequate manipulation of a toothbrush and floss is within reach. Meanwhile, children at this age want to be independent; they like to brush their teeth themselves and do not want help from Mom and Dad.

A negotiated settlement has to be reached. For example, after meals the child can *brush* the teeth with minimal or no supervision, but at bedtime the parents will *clean* the teeth and massage the gums. Working together as a team, the parent and child can each carry out their identified responsibilities, developing a successful program that can be further monitored and modified by the dentist.

During this period, all the primary teeth are present. Spaces that were visible earlier may begin to close. Cleaning the mouth includes brushing the teeth, cleaning the tongue, and massaging the gingiva. This is a fine motor activity that most 3 to 6 year olds cannot perform completely without assistance. In addition, the lingual surfaces of the mandibular posterior teeth and the buccal surfaces of the maxillary posterior teeth are the most difficult to reach and to see if all the plaque has been removed.

As spaces are closing, the use of dental floss is indicated. Children from 3 to 6 years of age are unable to floss. Parents should be responsible for this activity. Care should be taken not to snap the floss into the interproximal gingiva, causing injury. Results of this injury may make the child less receptive to any oral hygiene procedures, including toothbrushing.

Visibility and accessibility can be greatly enhanced by correct positioning. Although most preschoolers want to stand at the sink, this is a difficult position from which parents can assist comfortably. Placing the child in a supine position periodically to improve visibility is recommended.

There are many improved designs in both manual and power toothbrushes. Parents have a large number of products from which to select. Sizes, shapes, colors, timers, and motivational characters are widely available from all manufacturers. Nevertheless,

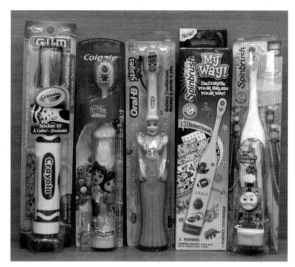

• **Figure 20.3** Examples of battery-powered toothbrushes designed for children ages 2 to 5 years. The brush features a popular character, which encourages brushing.

in this age group, parents must remain involved. The attention span of a typical 3- to 6-year-old is short, and with at least 100 surfaces on primary teeth to clean, they require parental assistance and supervision. Power toothbrushes have been shown to be as effective as manual toothbrushes and have the additional feature of being fun to use (Fig. 20.3). Therefore compliance is greatly increased.[24]

Application of a fluoride-containing dentifrice is recommended, although with parental supervision. A pea-sized amount of dentifrice should be placed on the brush and the child should be instructed to expectorate once brushing is completed. Larger amounts of dentifrice are not indicated. Studies have shown that preschoolers often swallow large amounts of dentifrice, which may contribute to development of fluorosis.[25] It is recommended that oral hygiene care should be performed regularly after meals. When circumstances prevent this, a thorough swishing of the mouth with water is recommended. At bedtime, oral hygiene is especially important because of the reduction in saliva production at night with an increase in acid production.

Toward the end of this period the preschool child begins to lose the primary teeth. The areas of exfoliation may be painful and the gingiva may be swollen, leading to discomfort. During these times the parent must maintain the oral hygiene habits to eliminate additional inflammation around exfoliating teeth.

Children with disabilities may require additional assistance because daily home care can be more challenging. Parents or caregivers should establish a daily routine because many individuals with special health care needs do best with routines. Allowing the child to hold a favorite item may have a calming effect. Encourage the parents to give verbal reassurance and brush in a slow, calm manner.

Depending on the disability and its severity, various positioning methods may be helpful for increasing visibility into the mouth and reducing excessive movement. For individuals with special health care needs incapable of independent brushing, the caregiver should take on that responsibility. See the "Adaptive Daily Oral Hygiene for the Child with Special Health Care Needs" box for additional adaptive strategies and techniques.

References

1. American Academy of Pediatric Dentistry. Guideline on fluoride therapy. *Pediatr Dent*. 2016;38(special issue):181–184.
2. Rozier RG, Adair S, Graham F, et al. Evidence-based clinical recommendations on the prescription of dietary fluoride supplements for caries prevention. A report of the American Dental Association Council on Scientific Affairs. *J Am Dent Assoc*. 2010;141(12):1480–1489.
3. Briss P, Bailey W, Barker LK, et al. U.S. Public Health Service recommendation for fluoride concentration in drinking water for the prevention of dental caries. *Public Health Rep*. 2015;130(4):318–331.
4. Division of Oral Health. My Water's Fluoride Web Application. U.S. Department of Health and Human Services, Centers for Disease Control and Prevention; 2016. http://www.cdc.gov/oralhealth/. Accessed August 7, 2017.
5. Weyant RJ, Tracy SL, Anselmo TT, et al. Topical fluoride for caries prevention: executive summary of the updated clinical recommendations and supporting systematic review. *J Am Dent Assoc*. 2013;144(11):1279–1291.
6. Seppa L, Leppönen T, Hausen H. Fluoride varnish versus acidulated phosphate fluoride gel: a 3-year clinical trial. *Caries Res*. 1995;28:327–330.
7. Weinstein P, Domoto P, Koday M, et al. Results of a promising open trial to prevent baby bottle tooth decay: a fluoride varnish study. *ASDC J Dent Child*. 1994;61:338–341.
8. Weintraub JA, Ramos-Gomez F, Jue B, et al. Fluoride varnish efficacy in preventing early childhood caries. *J Dent Res*. 2006;85:172–176.
9. Marinho VCC, Worthington HV, Walsh T, et al. Fluoride varnishes for preventing dental caries in children and adolescents. *Cochrane Database Syst Rev*. 2013;(7):CD002279.
10. American Academy of Pediatric Dentistry. Guideline on caries-risk assessment and management for infants, children, and adolescents. *Pediatr Dent*. 2016;38(special issue):142–149.
11. Dye A, Tan S, Smith V, et al. Trends in oral health status: United States, 1988-1994 and 1999-2004. *Vital Health Stat*. 2007;11(248):1–92.
12. Ripa LW. Professionally (operator) applied topical fluoride therapy: a critique. *Int Dent J*. 1981;31(2):105–120.
13. Centers for Disease Control and Prevention. Recommendations for using fluoride to prevent and control dental caries in the United States. *MMWR Recomm Rep*. 2001;50(RR–14):1–42.
14. Ripa LW, Leske GS, Sposato A, et al. Effect of prior tooth cleaning on bi-annual professional acidulated phosphate fluoride topical fluoride gel-tray treatments. Results after three years. *Caries Res*. 1984;18:457–464.
15. Johnston DW, Lewis DW. Three-year randomized trial of professionally applied topical fluoride gel comparing annual and biannual applications with/without prior prophylaxis. *Caries Res*. 1995;29(5):331–336.
16. Houpt M, Koenigsberg S, Shey Z. The effect of prior toothcleaning on the efficacy of topical fluoride treatment. Two-year results. *Clin Prev Dent*. 1983;5(4):8–10.
17. American Academy of Pediatric Dentistry. Guideline on the role of dental prophylaxis in pediatric dentistry. *Pediatr Dent*. 2011;33(special issue):151–152.
18. Crall JJ, Nowak AJ. Clinical uses of fluoride for the special patient. In: Wei SHY, ed. *Clinical Uses of Fluorides*. Philadelphia: Lea & Febiger; 1985:193–201.
19. Sheiham A, James WP. Diet and dental caries: the pivotal role of free sugars reemphasized. *J Dent Res*. 2015;94(10):1341–1347.
20. Schachtele CF, Jensen ME. Can foods be ranked according to their cariogenic potential? In: Guggenheim B, ed. *Cariology Today*. Basel: Karger; 1984:136–146.
21. World Health Organization (WHO). *Guideline: Sugars Intake for Adults and Children*. Geneva: WHO; 2015.
22. U.S. Department of Health and Human Services. Office of Disease Prevention and Health Promotion. Dietary guidelines; 2017. www.dietaryguidelines.gov. Accessed August 7, 2017.
23. U.S. Department of Agriculture. MyPlate, 2017. www.choosemyplate.gov. Accessed August 7, 2017.
24. Nowak AJ, Skotowski MC, Cugini M, et al. A practice based study of a children's power toothbrush: efficacy and acceptance. *Compend Contin Educ Dent*. 2002;23:25–32.
25. Levy SL, McGrady JA, Bhuridej P, et al. Factors affecting dentifrice use and ingestion among a sample of U.S. preschoolers. *Pediatr Dent*. 2000;22:389–394.

21
Dental Materials

KEVIN J. DONLY AND ISSA S. SASA

CHAPTER OUTLINE

Restorative materials used in pediatric restorative dentistry are commonly the same as those used in restorative dentistry in general. This chapter identifies commonly used materials in pediatric dentistry and provides information that applies specifically to their use. Many materials are available, and in many cases clinical considerations will dictate the choice of the appropriate material. Table 21.1 identifies the most commonly used materials in pediatric restorative dentistry and the relevant clinical considerations. Chapters 22, 33, and 40 discuss the specific clinical restorative techniques associated with these restorative materials.

Bases and Liners

The use of bases and liners is important in pediatric dentistry. Bases and liners are available to reduce marginal microleakage from the restoration and prevent sensitivity to the underlying tooth structure. Traditionally, preparations of calcium hydroxide, zinc oxide–eugenol, and zinc phosphate were the materials of choice. Currently, glass ionomer cement is also a common base.

Calcium Hydroxide

Calcium hydroxide cements are supplied in a visible light–cured system (Fig. 21.1A) and a two-paste system (Fig. 21.1B). A catalyst paste containing calcium hydroxide, zinc oxide, and zinc stearate in ethylene toluene sulfonamide reacts with a base paste containing calcium tungstate, calcium phosphate, and zinc oxide in glycol

salicylate to form an amorphous calcium disalicylate. The alkaline pH aids in preventing bacterial invasion. Studies have shown that calcium hydroxide "softens" under amalgam and resin-based composite restorations.[1,2] The results are attributed to hydrolysis of the calcium hydroxide by fluid contamination from dentinal tubules and microleakage. As hydrolysis occurs, occlusal forces cause apical displacement of the restoration, leading to discrepancies and breakdown at the restoration margin. Visible light–cured calcium hydroxide preparations have demonstrated clinical success[3] and may be less susceptible to hydrolysis. When calcium hydroxide is used, a less soluble high-strength base material such as glass ionomer may be placed to overlie the calcium hydroxide.

Zinc Oxide–Eugenol

Zinc oxide–eugenol cement (Fig. 21.2) contains zinc oxide, rosin, and zinc acetate in the powder. The rosin increases fracture resistance and the zinc acetate is effective in accelerating the reaction rate. The liquid is a preparation of eugenol, which reacts with the powder to form an amorphous chelate of zinc eugenolate. The zinc oxide–eugenol cements are used to provide a sedative effect in deep preparations, but their low compressive strength presents clinical limitations.

To strengthen zinc oxide–eugenol cements, acrylic resin and alumina reinforcers have been added. Although these cements are stronger, they remain weaker than the zinc phosphate and glass ionomer cements. When it was evaluated as a base, zinc oxide–eugenol demonstrated significant microleakage in comparison with glass ionomer cement.[4] Because of its sedative effects and years of clinical success, zinc oxide–eugenol remains the material of choice for the pulp chamber filling material following pulpotomies or pulpectomies in the primary dentition. Zinc oxide–eugenol cements should be used with caution under resin-based composite restorations because the eugenol can inhibit the polymerization of the resin. A glass ionomer cement base may be placed over zinc oxide–eugenol before the placement of resin-based composite in order to avoid polymerization.

Glass Ionomer Cement

Glass ionomer cement (Fig. 21.3) has become a commonly used basing agent. It has the ability to create a physicochemical bond to tooth structure and to release fluoride. Glass ionomer cement consists of calcium aluminosilicate glass particles mixed with polyacrylic acid. The initial reaction stage involves the ionization of polyacrylic acid, which leads to a change in the polymer chains from a coiled to a linear form. The hydrogen ions produced by

TABLE 21.1	Commonly Used Biomaterials in Pediatric Dentistry		
Materials	**Types Available**	**Composition**	**Clinical Considerations**
Intermediary bases	Calcium hydroxide Zinc oxide–eugenol[a]	Thin pastes of calcium hydroxide or zinc oxide and eugenol suspended in resins	Placed on small areas of cavity preparation deeper than ideal depth Placed on exposed dentin of preparations undergoing acid etching Used for direct pulp capping of permanent teeth Must not be left on enamel of preparations
Amalgam	Lathe-cut Spherical Admixed Unicompositional[a]	Silver (40%–74%) Tin (25%–30%) Copper (2%–30%) Zinc (0%–2%) Mercury (0%–3%)	A high copper (>6%) admixed or unicompositional, precapsulated alloy is recommended for restoration of pit and fissure and interproximal caries in posterior teeth
Stainless steel crowns	Straight sides Precontoured[a] Pretrimmed[a]	Iron (65%–73%) Chromium (17%–20%) Nickel (8%–13%) Manganese, silicon, and carbon (<2%)	Restoration of badly broken down teeth, usually posterior, must be well trimmed, contoured, polished, and cemented to ensure optimum gingival health
Filled resin-based composite	(Based on filler size) Traditional, 5–30 μm Microfill, 0.04–1 μm[a] Hybrids, 0.04–100 μm[a] (available as auto-cure or visible light–activated)[a]	Dimethacrylate (Bis-GMA) resin or urethane matrix with filler particles of quartz, silicates, or glass	Esthetic restoration of anterior teeth Available for use in class I and II restorations in posterior teeth Microfills provide most polishable surfaces and have excellent esthetics Hybrids demonstrate least shrinkage and wear and have good polishability and esthetics Visible light activation provides better polymerization control, better color stability, and less porosity than auto-polymerized resins
Cements	Glass ionomer[a] Reinforced zinc oxide and eugenol[a] Zinc oxide–eugenol	Silicate glass containing Ca, Al, F, polycarboxylic acid Zinc oxide reinforced with alumina, polymer, or eugenol Zinc oxide, eugenol	Primary use is cementation of stainless steel crowns May be used as a base Glass ionomer may be used as a liner for resins and conservative restorations in primary teeth Reinforced zinc oxide and eugenol most frequently used for obliterating primary pulp chambers following pulpotomy

[a]Types most frequently used.

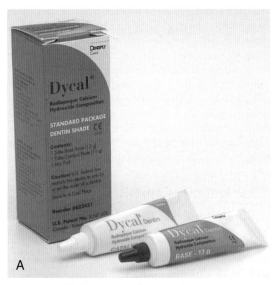
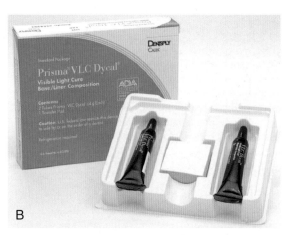

• **Figure 21.1** Calcium hydroxide cements. (A) Visible light–cured system (Dycal). (B) Two-paste system (Prisma VLC Dycal). (Courtesy DENTSPLY Caulk, Milford, DE.)

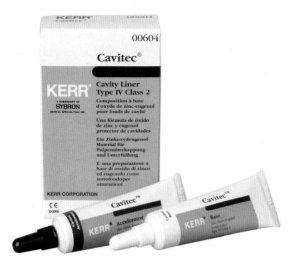

• **Figure 21.2** Zinc oxide–eugenol cement (Cavitec). (Courtesy Kerr Corporation, Orange, CA.)

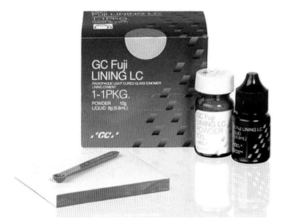

• **Figure 21.3** Glass ionomer cement (GC Fuji Lining LC). (Courtesy GC America, Alsip, IL.)

ionization attack the calcium aluminosilicate glass, which also contains fluoride, and causes the release of metal and fluoride ions. The majority of the metal cations (Ca^{2+}, Al^{3+}), divalent or trivalent, respectively, are bound by the ionized polymer to form cross-linked salt bridges. Calcium and aluminum ions bind to polyacrylic acid at the carboxyl groups, and a gel phase is precipitated to form a matrix of the hardening cement. Calcium carboxylates are formed first as a firm gel because of the rapid binding of calcium to the polyacrylic acid chains. This initial set has the property of being carvable, but at this stage the ionomer is very susceptible to water absorption. Likewise, the free aluminum ions are susceptible to diffusion from moisture contamination and thus are lost from the cement because they are unable to cross-link with the polyacrylic acid chains. Isolation of prepared teeth is recommended. Aluminum salt bridges are then formed with the polyacrylic acid matrix, and the cement hardens. The trivalent aluminum ions ensure a much stronger cross-linking than is possible with the calcium divalent bonds alone. The slower reaction of aluminum ions is attributed to the more stringent steric requirements imposed by a trivalent ion on a polyanion chain configuration.

Glass ionomer can bond to dentin by free hydrophilic carboxyl groups in the cement, promoting surface wetting to form hydrogen bonds at the tooth interface. At the same time, an ionic exchange occurs at the interface, with calcium ions being displaced by

phosphate ions. Some manufacturers recommend removing the smear layer, created during cavity preparation, with polyacrylic acid. This tooth "conditioning" provides an uncontaminated tooth surface for bonding. Because the setting reaction requires some moisture, it is critical not to desiccate the tooth after rinsing conditioning from the preparation.

Tartaric acid is added to the glass ionomer cement to accelerate the rate of hardening without decreasing the working time. Itaconic acid may be placed in glass ionomer mixtures to increase the reactivity of the polyacrylic acid to the glass, and polymaleic acid may be added to modify the reaction.

Studies have shown that glass ionomer bases and liners exhibit less marginal microleakage than zinc oxide–eugenol, zinc phosphate, and calcium hydroxide,[4,5] thereby preventing bacterial penetration. Fluoride is released from glass ionomer cement by dissolution and diffusion. Glass ionomer bases and liners have demonstrated the inhibition of secondary caries formation.[6–9] The fluoride released is taken up by both the enamel and dentin adjacent to the material.[10–13] This fluoride aids in creating an inhibition zone that is not susceptible to demineralization, when compared with areas adjacent to non–fluoride-releasing materials.[14,15]

Glass ionomer cements are supplied in anhydrous and hydrous forms. Due to the viscosity of the hydrous form, mixing the cement may be difficult. The anhydrous form has a longer shelf life because the polyacrylic acid is dehydrated and placed in the powder. It is critical that glass ionomer be mixed according to the manufacturer's instructions. If the cement is too thick it will not provide sufficient water to complete the reaction, and dentin sensitivity may be encountered; the necessary water will be obtained from the dentin, causing sensitivity due to hydraulic pressures created within the dentin.

Resin-modified glass ionomer cement preparations are available and can be light-cured.[16] Photoinitiated polymers have been placed in the glass ionomer cement formulation to provide light polymerization. Although these resin-modified glass ionomer cements can be light-cured, the material sets as a true cement, with an acid-base reaction taking place; therefore, given enough time, the material will chemically set without light curing.

Glass ionomer cement has a coefficient of thermal expansion similar to that of tooth structure; it can protect an underlying base and dentin, bonds to resin-based composite, and releases fluoride, which can inhibit secondary decay.

Dentin-Bonding Agents

Dentin-bonding agents have been incorporated into the restorative dentistry armamentarium. Previously, dentin- or enamel-bonding agents fell into two groups. The first was halophosphorus esters of 2,2-bis[4-(2-hydroxy-3-methacryloyloxypropyloxy)phenyl] propane (Bis-GMA). The second group was categorized as polyurethanes. The polyurethanes are halophosphorus esters of hydroxyethyl methacrylate (HEMA). Both of these dentin-bonding agents relied on a phosphate-calcium bond for retention.

Removal of the smear layer was found to increase the effectiveness of the dentin-bonding agents. The newer bonding agents include conditioning or primer components that remove or alter the smear layer over the dentin. This results in the creation of a mechanical bond by the infiltration of monomers into a zone of demineralized dentin, where the monomers polymerize and interlock with the dentin matrix.[17] A majority of the contemporary dentin-bonding agents are similar to those previously discussed or are composed of 4-methacryloxyethyl trimellitic anhydride.

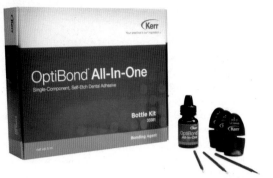

• **Figure 21.4** Self-etching bonding system (OptiBond All-In-One). (Courtesy Kerr Corporation, Orange, CA.)

Self-etching bonding systems (Fig. 21.4) have been developed to offer the convenience of etching and bonding simultaneously. Although research demonstrates adequate bonds to dentin and enamel, caution is advised. The products must be used as instructed by the manufacturer, particularly focusing on agitation of the product during placement and the recommended length of application time.[18,19]

Restorative Materials

Amalgam

Traditionally, amalgam was the material of choice for class I and class II restorations. Today amalgam continues to be an effective restorative material.[20,21] A 3-year study of the clinical performance of 260 amalgam restorations (86.4% class II) demonstrated 254 to be successful.[22] It is important to understand the clinical makeup and setting reaction of amalgam to correlate restoration successes and failures with the fundamental properties of the material.

Amalgamation

Dental amalgam consists of an alloy mix of silver, copper, tin, and, in some cases, zinc particles combined with mercury. The alloy particles have either a spherical or comminuted (lathe-cut) configuration. The unreacted alloy particles are termed the *silver-tin (gamma) phase*. These particles are combined with mercury, the mercury actually acting as a wetting agent of the alloy particles to initiate the setting reaction termed *amalgamation*. The particle surfaces react with mercury to form a cementing matrix, consisting of the gamma 1 and gamma 2 phases. The gamma 1 phase employs the binding of silver and mercury (Ag_2-Hg_3). The gamma 2 phase involves the binding of tin and mercury (Sn_7-Hg). The gamma 2 phase is responsible for early fracture and failure of the comminuted particle amalgam restorations. Tin cannot be eliminated from the alloy because of its importance in the setting reaction and control of dimensional change of amalgam. To avoid the detrimental gamma 2 phase, copper was introduced into the amalgamation reaction. The copper replaced the tin-mercury phase with a copper-tin phase (Cu_5-Sn_5). The copper-tin matrix decreases the corrosion of tin, preventing secondary weakening with subsequent fracture of the restoration.

The amount of mercury needed to complete the amalgamation reaction is contingent on the alloy composition and particle configuration but usually falls between 42% and 54% of the amalgam mix. When mercury exceeds 55%, there is a detrimental reduction in amalgam strength. Spherical alloy particles with the

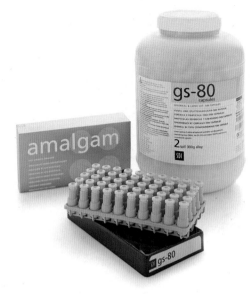

• **Figure 21.5** Preencapsulated amalgam (GS-80). (Courtesy SDI [North America], Bensenville, IL.)

addition of copper require less mercury than comminuted particles to complete the amalgamation process. It is important to point out that once amalgamation occurs, unreacted mercury is not available; the mercury is alloyed with silver, tin, or copper. Zinc is present in some alloy mixes to act as a scavenger for oxygen, which inhibits the formation of copper, silver, or tin oxides, thus weakening the amalgam restoration. Using preencapsulated amalgam (Fig. 21.5) and strictly following the manufacturer's recommendations for trituration and manipulation are critical in achieving restoration success.

Properties

Hardening amalgam may expand or contract depending on the type and manipulation of the material. The American Dental Association[23] requires that there be no more than 20 μm/cm of expansion or contraction after 24 hours.

The compressive strength required by the Council on Dental Materials and Devices[23] for amalgam is 11,600 psi (88 MN/m²) after 1 hour. Tensile strength is substantially lower; therefore cavity preparation design becomes critical. The preparation should have a design that allows the amalgam to be condensed as a "bulk" of material, avoiding shallow depths and a thin isthmus where fracture may occur. Comminuted and spherical low-copper amalgam demonstrates decreased marginal fracture resistance. This is partially due to the increased creep of these amalgams. Creep is the dimensional change that occurs when amalgam sustains a load during mastication, a result of the viscoelastic property of amalgam. The American Dental Association requires that an amalgam have a maximum of 5% creep to be certified.

Corrosion, a chemical or electrochemical deterioration of amalgam, occurs at the surface or subsurface. Deterioration may be due to pitting or scratching secondary to poor condensation, carving, or finishing of amalgam, which allows food or saliva components to attack the chemical matrix. Dissimilar metals in contact with each other can also cause corrosion as a result of a galvanic action that encourages the materials to go into solution. This leads to pitting and food entrapment within the pits, which subsequently causes further corrosion. The gamma 2 phase (tin-mercury) is most susceptible to corrosion; therefore the spherical high-copper amalgams are the least susceptible. Although extensive corrosion can lead to restoration failure, minimal corrosion in conjunction with creep allows open restoration margins to be packed full enough with corrosion by-products to significantly close these margins.

Condensation

Amalgam should be placed and condensed immediately after trituration, according to the manufacturer's recommendations. Placement of amalgam in small increments is appropriate. Condensation allows force to be applied for material adaptation with a minimum of excess mercury. Use of small condensers with firm pressure on small increments of amalgam minimizes voids within the final restoration. A delay in condensation should be avoided because the initial hardening that occurs after trituration but before condensation may make the effective removal of excessive mercury more difficult. This, in turn, decreases restoration's strength and increases the creep in the material. Moisture contamination should also be controlled because excess moisture causes delayed expansion, particularly in zinc-containing alloys. The use of isolation devices can prevent moisture contamination and isolate the working field effectively.

Finishing and Polishing

Finishing and polishing of the amalgam surface are highly recommended. Small scratches and pits can be removed with finishing burs, and abrasive stones and rubber points can be impregnated with abrasives. The final polish can be accomplished with a tin oxide compound. Care should be taken to use water when polishing to prevent the vaporization of mercury from the amalgam. Most amalgam restorations should not be polished for 24 hours, although the spherical high-copper amalgam can be polished almost immediately because its strength is obtained rapidly.

Resin-Based Composite

Resin-based composite (Fig. 21.6) has become one of the most widely used contemporary restorative materials over the past 30 years. Currently resin composite is used for sealants and for class I through V restorations in primary and permanent teeth.[24,25] Resin-based composite restorations have been accepted primarily because of their excellent esthetic qualities. Other advantages include relatively low thermal conductivity, preservation of tooth structure

in cavity preparation, and advances in the stability of compositional properties of the material.

Conventional resin based composites were viscous fluid nonvolatile monomers (Bis-GMA) that have filler particles incorporated into the resin. Bowen[26] formulated the Bis-GMA resin by synthesizing a dimethacrylate monomer, the product of the reaction between bisphenol A and glycidyl methacrylate. Many contemporary composite restorative materials contain dimethacrylate monomers (Bis-GMA) as the major component of the matrix phase. A relatively low-viscosity monomer (triethylene glycol dimethacrylate [TEGDMA]), which helps produce the desired handling qualities of the material, is an important component of the matrix phase. Fig. 21.7 schematically illustrates the chemical structure of Bis-GMA, and Fig. 21.8 illustrates the chemical structure of TEGDMA.

Incorporated into the monomer matrix are filler particles. A small number of available products contain urethane dimethacrylates rather than the Bis-GMA matrix. Initially, fused quartz and various glasses were incorporated into the Bis-GMA monomer as filler particles, providing a reinforced resin composite. The fillers were coated with a vinyl silane coupling agent, with the silane chemically bonding with the polymer matrix.[27] These particles were usually irregularly shaped to provide mechanical retention in the resin.

Composites available today contain quartz, colloidal silica, borosilicate glasses, and glasses containing barium, strontium, and zinc. Excluding quartz and colloidal silica, these filler particles give the material radiopacity, which is clinically advantageous during radiographic examination. Contemporary posterior resin-based composites contain a high percentage by volume of filler particles. This composition provides wear resistance and more stability.[28]

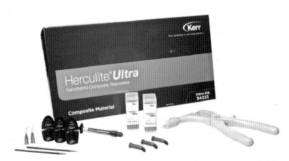

• **Figure 21.6** Resin-based composite system (Herculite Ultra). (Courtesy Kerr Corporation, Orange, CA.)

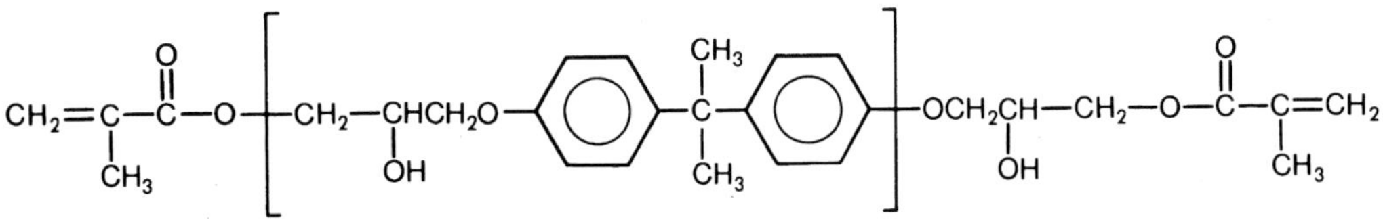

• **Figure 21.7** Chemical composition of 2,2-bis[4-(2-hydroxy-3-methacryloyloxypropyloxy)phenyl] propane (Bis-GMA).

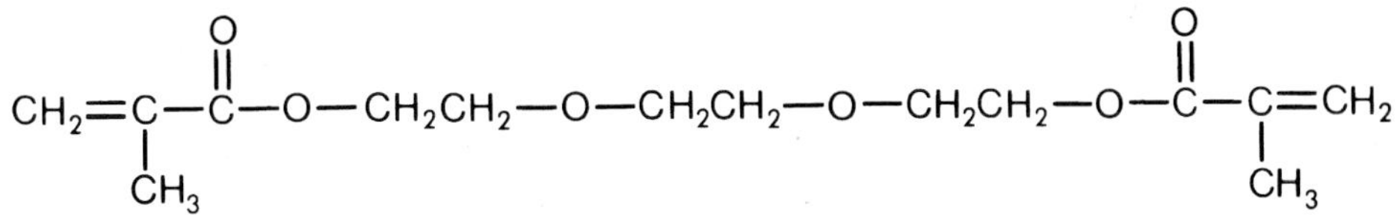

• **Figure 21.8** Chemical composition of triethylene glycol dimethacrylate (TEGDMA).

Thermal expansion and polymerization contraction are both reduced by increasing the volume percentage of filler particles. The increased filler content, needed for wear resistance, requires a decrease in matrix resin polymer, therefore allowing for a reduction in the amount of shrinkage that occurs upon polymerization. As the concentration of filler particles increases, the modulus of elasticity increases and tends to minimize shrinkage.[29]

Resin-based composites absorb water, yet hygroscopic expansion is very infrequently sufficient to compensate for polymerization shrinkage.[30,31] Therefore the incremental placement and polymerization of resin-based composite are critical during restorative care.[32-35]

Chemically Polymerized Resin-Based Composite

The traditional chemically activated resin-based composites form cross-links during copolymerization of methyl methacrylate and ethylene glycol dimethacrylate. The dimethacrylate monomers polymerize by means of free radical–initiated polymerization to form the organic matrix of a three-dimensional network. This highly viscous monomer can undergo free radical addition polymerization to provide a rigid cross-linked polymer. Usually the benzoyl peroxide present in one paste acts as the initiator, whereas a tertiary amine (dihydroxyethyl-*p*-toluidine) acts as the catalyst in the other paste.[36]

Visible Light–Polymerized Resin-Based Composite

Today most resin-based composites are visible light–activated materials (see Fig. 21.6). This allows for more controlled, incremental placement of material into a cavity preparation. The visible light–activated composites usually contain a diketone initiator (camphorquinone) and an amine catalyst (dimethylaminoethyl methacrylate). The diketone absorbs light at approximately 470 nm to form an excited state, which, together with the amine, results in ion radicals to initiate free radical polymerization.[37,38]

In attempts to reduce polymerization shrinkage, resin molecules longer than Bis-GMA have been placed in resin-based composites. An example would be EMA-6, which can be found in Filtek Z250 (Fig. 21.9; 3M ESPE Dental Products, St. Paul, MN).[39]

Problems that may be associated with light-activated resin-based composites include polymerization toward the light source, sensitivity of composite to ambient light, and variability in the

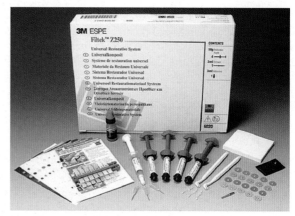

• **Figure 21.9** Resin-based composite with EMA-6 (Filtek Z250). (Courtesy 3M ESPE Dental Products, St Paul, MN.)

DENTAL LIGHT-CURING UNITS

Sharukh S. Khajotia and Fernando L. Esteban Florez

Dental light-curing units are handheld devices that are used for the polymerization of visible light–activated dental materials. The four types of light-curing units that are currently available include quartz-tungsten-halogen (QTH), light-emitting diode (LED), plasma arc curing (PAC), and Argon laser units.

QTH light-curing units are the most widely used and are made of a quartz bulb containing a tungsten filament in a halogen environment. QTH units emit ultraviolet irradiation and visible light (broad-spectrum), which is filtered to limit the wavelength output to between 400 and 500 nm while also minimizing heat. The intensity of light emitted by a QTH bulb ranges from 400 to 1200 mW/cm^2 and can decrease with use. The use of a radiometer is recommended for the routine monitoring of the light intensity, and permitting the built-in fan to cool the QTH bulb is recommended to facilitate optimal function of the unit.

LED light-curing units emit light in the blue part of the visible spectrum, typically between 440 and 490 nm, and do not emit heat. Therefore LED units do not require filters. They can be powered by rechargeable batteries because they require low wattage, and they are quieter than QTH units because they do not need a cooling fan. Initial versions of LED units emitted a lower intensity of light, whereas newer versions incorporate multiple LEDs with a variety of ranges of wavelengths to broaden the spectrum of the emitted light and increase the overall intensity in order to adequately polymerize all visible-light activated dental materials.

PAC light-curing units contain a xenon gas that is ionized to produce plasma. The high-intensity white light emitted is filtered to minimize heat and to limit the output to the violet-blue part of the visible spectrum (400–500 nm). Argon laser units emit the highest intensity and emit light at a single wavelength (approximately 490 nm). The higher costs associated with the use and maintenance of the PAC and Argon laser units has limited their widespread use in dentistry.

Visible light-activated dental materials contain an initiator such as camphorquinone (CQ) that absorbs light at the appropriate wavelength (approximately 470 nm for CQ). The free radicals necessary for the initiation of polymerization are generated when the initiator combines with an organic amine such as dimethylaminoethyl methacrylate (DMAEMA). The wavelength, intensity, and duration of exposure to light determine the number of photons absorbed by the initiator and therefore impact optimal polymerization. Factors such as light-curing unit intensity, angle of illumination, diameter of the tip of the light source, distance from the light source, and duration of exposure can significantly affect the number of free radicals formed, thereby making this system highly technique sensitive. Initiators other than CQ are also used in visible light-activated materials. Because they absorb light at different wavelengths than CQ, it is critical that the light-curing unit used emits light at the requisite wavelength for that particular initiator.

Newer light-curing units have higher intensities, typically greater than 1000 mW/cm^2, which permit either shorter durations of cure for a given depth of cure or increased depth of cure for a given duration of cure. The use of these higher intensity lights can, however, produce higher shrinkage stresses within the restoration. It is important to remember that the type of light-curing unit and curing mode used impact the polymerization kinetics, polymerization shrinkage, and associated stresses, microhardness, depth of cure, degree of conversion, color change, and microleakage in visible-light activated restorations. Lastly, precautions such as protective eyewear and light shields are critical for the safety of the patient and clinic personnel when using dental light-curing units.

depth of polymerization due to the intensity of light penetration. Polymerization toward the light source may cause the resin-based composite to pull away from the walls of the preparation. Sensitivity of resin-based composite to ambient light may cause initial polymerization before placement of the material into the preparation. Variability in the depth of light penetration, differences in curing light intensity, diameter of the tip of the light source, and time of light exposure can result in variations of polymerization. The benefits of light-activated resin composites include ease of manipulation, control of polymerization, and lack of need for mixing. Since mixing is not required with light-activated composites, it is less likely that air will be incorporated and form voids in the mixture.

Bulk-Fill Resins

Extensive efforts have been made over the last decade to develop low shrinkage resin-based composites through advances in filler technology and monomer chemistry.[40,41]

Conventionally the maximum incremental thickness of resin-based composite that provided adequate light penetration and polymerization was defined as 2 mm.[42,43] Use of these conventional materials requires a layering technique that is time consuming and has the potential to introduce voids, thus increasing the risk of failure.[44] The risk of failure presents itself clinically by allowing the ingress of bacteria, ultimately leading to secondary caries, pulpal inflammation, necrosis, or postoperative sensitivity.

Recently a new class of resin composite materials, the bulk-fill resin composites, has been introduced. Clinical recommendations suggest that these materials have a greater depth of cure, which allows them to be placed in 4-mm bulk increments and still have adequate polymerization.

This innovative technology is based on changes in monomer chemistry by modifying the Bowen monomer (Bis-GMA: 2,2 bis [4-(2-hydroxy-3-methacryloxypropoxy) phenyl] propane) to create monomers with lower viscosity.[45–48] This new modification is achieved by incorporating hydroxyl-free Bis-GMA aliphatic urethane dimethacrylate or highly branched methacrylates.[49] The outcomes of these changes in monomer and composite organic matrix have been shown to reduce polymerization shrinkage stresses over 70%.[45,46,50]

Resin-Based Composite Wear

Early resin-based composites, used for posterior restorations, exhibited excessive occlusal wear. Studies have shown that when conventional composites are placed in high stress concentration areas, excessive wear occurs.[51–54] Further investigations pursued factors that might influence the rate of wear, such as the size and hardness of the filler particles, the amount of porosity within the material, and the method of polymerization.[55] It was found that the ceramic filler particles nearly always remained intact. There was no evidence of wear on the particles themselves; they were found to be hard enough to cause wear of the surrounding unfilled resin during mastication until the resin matrix gradually wore away from the particles. Once a critical portion of the filler particle was exposed, it was easily dislodged. Although there seemed to be a correlation between the size of the filler particle and its hardness (larger particles possessing a more critical hardness), substantially larger particles were found to accelerate the wear. Therefore the hardness of particles is not necessarily the most significant factor affecting wear. The ideal material would have particles that have adequate hardness, are distributed within minimal unfilled resin, and have the least abrasion potential during mastication.[28,56] Thus, more recently, nanoparticles have been introduced as filler particles.

Porosity has been shown to be a major factor in the wear rate of posterior resin-based composites.[55,57] All resin restorations contain a certain degree of porosity and voids. These defects can be minimized by careful placement technique and polishing of the material. Because light-cured composites do not require mixing, they contain fewer voids. Problems of wear appear to be improved with newer composites. Composite resins are vacuum-packed to decrease porosity. It is important to note that mixing shades for esthetics may increase the porosity. This problem is created from the incorporation of air during the mixing process. Current posterior resin-based composites show minimal wear. This has been achieved by incorporating a variety of particle sizes into the polymer matrix. The increased filler content decreases the amount of matrix resin polymer. The mechanism of wear is hypothesized to be due to the loss of the resin matrix. Increasing wear resistance is believed to be possible because the filler particles are closely packed, thereby leaving little unfilled resin exposed.

Marginal Adaptation

The use of resin-based composites for restoring posterior teeth has historically presented the problem of marginal leakage at the resin-tooth interface.[54,58] This marginal leakage caused teeth with posterior resin-based composite restorations to be more prone to secondary caries than teeth with amalgam restorations. Failure of the composite to bond to the cavity preparation walls and voids in the restorative material have been identified as the causes of inadequate marginal adaptation. This problem has been reduced by (1) using contemporary posterior resin-based composites, which contain a high volume of filler that decreases polymerization shrinkage; (2) using an enamel bevel; (3) using newer dentin-bonding agents and glass ionomer cements; and (4) acid etching the enamel.

Formulations

Enamel-Bonding Agents

The use of phosphoric acid (35% to 50%) results in an acid-etched surface on enamel that creates an effective mechanical bond with the Bis-GMA enamel-bonding agent. Enamel-bonding agents (Fig. 21.10) are placed over the acid-etched enamel before composite placement. The bonding agents are merely unfilled dimethacrylates and are used because their low viscosity allows easy penetration of the etched enamel surface. The resin matrix of the resin-based composite will then chemically bond to the bonding agent.

Sealants

The use of pit and fissure sealants has been effective in preventing occlusal caries for almost five decades.[59–61] Traditional sealants are hydrophobic and are composed of a Bis-GMA resin structure used in resin-based composites. The Bis-GMA monomer is diluted with low-weight dimethacrylate monomer to make the sealant material a fluid that can easily penetrate the pits and fissures of occlusal surfaces. A new generation of resin-based sealants is formulated with hydrophilic resins that behave favorably in the moist environment (Fig. 21.11). These materials contain no Bis-GMA or bisphenol A derivatives, have better adaptation to tooth structure, and provide a better seal.

Although the use of sealants is an excellent preventive technique, initially there were concerns that caries could occur at sealant margins or where the sealant had partially broken away. The concept of adding fluoride-releasing resins was examined for caries inhibition and found to be effective in vitro.[62,63] Most sealants currently in use contain fluoride and are light-cured. Two component systems that self-polymerize are also available.

Microfilled Resin–Based Composite

Microfilled resin–based composite (Fig. 21.12A) has silane-treated colloidal silica filler particles in a Bis-GMA resin. Traditional microfilled composites contained approximately 50% (by volume) filler particles. Because of the high percentage of resin matrix, the particle configuration, and the small particle size (<1 μm in diameter), this resin composite is easily polished and reaches a high luster. Microfilled composites are recommended for restorations that are highly visible yet encounter minimal stress during mastication. The low percentage of filler results in a decrease in strength

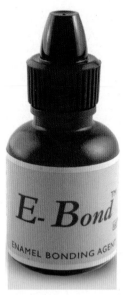

• **Figure 21.10** Enamel bonding agent (E-Bond). (Courtesy Danville Materials, San Ramon, CA.)

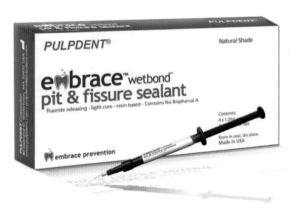

• **Figure 21.11** Pit and fissure sealant (EMRACE WetBond). (Courtesy Pulpdent Corporation, Watertown, MA.)

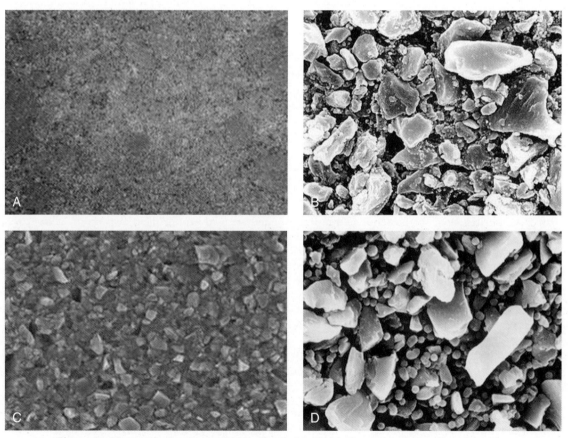

• **Figure 21.12** (A) Microfill material. (B) Macrofill material. (C) Hybrid material. (D) Nanofill material. (From Freedman G. *Contemporary Esthetic Dentistry.* St Louis: Mosby; 2012.)

and an increase in wear. To compensate for polymerization shrinkage, some of the Bis-GMA resin in the composite is prepolymerized by the manufacturer.

More highly filled (>70% by volume) microfilled resin–based composites are available and can be effectively used in areas where greater wear and stress is anticipated.

Macrofilled Resin–Based Composite

Macrofilled resin–based composite (Fig. 2.12B) has silane-treated filler particles (approximately 80% by volume) in a Bis-GMA resin. The particle sizes are much larger than those found in microfilled systems. Although these particles are larger than those found in the microfilled composites, they are smaller than the conventional resin-based composite particles. The high filler-particle percentage increases wear resistance. Because most of these resin composites are used for posterior restorations, the material is usually radiopaque from the filler type.

Hybrid Resin–Based Composite

Hybrid resin–based composites (Fig. 21.12C) have a combination of small and large particles, representing the size of the particles found in microfilled and macrofilled resin–based composites, respectively. The high percentage of filler particles provides strength and wear resistance, yet the smaller filler particles allow for particles to arrange in close proximity to each other, which can provide minimal polymerization shrinkage and improved polishability compared with macrofilled composite. These resin-based composites are considered for restorations that may have stress-bearing areas during mastication but must have a well-polished surface.

Nanofilled Resin–Based Composite

Since the introduction of resin-based composites, the size of filler particles has become smaller. More recently, nanofilled composites (Fig. 21.12D) that contain very small filler particles have been introduced. These resin composites offer the strength of a highly filled resin as well as polishability due to the small particles.

Glass Ionomer

Anterior Restorations

Preparations of glass ionomer cements are available in various shades that can be used for anterior restorations.[64,65] The use of glass ionomer for anterior restorations is limited to class III and class V preparations. The low fracture resistance and strength of mechanical bonding to enamel make its use impractical for class IV restorations. Retention of glass ionomer restorations in the restoration of class V preparations, where the gingival margin is not in enamel, may demonstrate favorable retention when restored with a glass ionomer rather than a resin-based composite. The fluoride release from glass ionomer restorations has been shown to inhibit the development of secondary caries.[66–69]

Posterior Restorations

The major disadvantage of glass ionomer cement as a posterior restorative material is its susceptibility to fracture and wear. Metal particles have been added to glass ionomer cement to increase their strength and wear resistance for posterior restorations. Fracture resistance remains a concern, and critical decisions should be made when using the material for posterior restorations. Investigations have demonstrated the clinical success of resin-modified glass ionomer cement as a posterior restorative material in the primary dentition.[66,70,71] Again, fluoride release and bonding capabilities are advantages of the glass ionomer cements.

Compomers

Compomers are recommended for use as a pediatric dental restorative material.[72–75] Compomers are actually a cross between resin-based composite and glass ionomer cement.

The compomers were developed in the hope of bringing the favorable properties of resin-based composite—such as wear resistance, color stability, and polishability—to the glass ionomers. An acid-base reaction takes place within the compomer material but is not the primary setting reaction; therefore visible light–polymerization is necessary to complete the setting reaction. Compomers are used with methacrylate primers that bond to enamel, dentin, and the compomer restorative material; therefore manufacturers consider the etching of tooth structure before restoration placement optional.

Cements

Cements are frequently used in pediatric dentistry. Their primary use is for the cementation of stainless steel crowns and orthodontic bands. Zinc oxide–eugenol and glass ionomer are the cements most commonly used. These cements were previously discussed in the section "Bases and Liners." The particles in glass ionomer cement are usually larger than those found in glass ionomer bases. There is less particle surface area available for reaction in the cement; therefore the cement sets more slowly than the base, allowing more working time. The importance of accuracy in the liquid/powder ratio of glass ionomer cement has been discussed. Encapsulated, premeasured cement is available and may be considered for clinical use. Automix syringe tips are available for the resin-modified glass ionomer materials as well.

Bioactive cements have more recently become available in the marketplace. These cements have glass particles incorporated into a resin matrix and have the advantage of bonding to tooth structure. The cements release calcium and fluoride. Manufacturers recommend these cements for cementing stainless steel, porcelain, and zirconia crowns.

The various cements most commonly used in pediatric dentistry and their clinical considerations are noted in Tables 21.1 and 21.2.

Monolithic Zirconia

Monolithic zirconia was introduced to dentistry almost two decades ago; more recently, it has been used for complete coverage crowns. The zirconia ceramic crown is very strong in flexural and compressive strength.[76] A highly polished, glossy surface is very favorable to gingival tissue.[76] Monolithic zirconia crowns are now available for the esthetic restoration of primary anterior and posterior teeth. An in vitro study has demonstrated that natural teeth opposing zirconia crowns have a more favorable wear than natural teeth opposing porcelain crowns.[77] Currently, manufacturers recommend the use of resin-modified glass ionomer cement for zirconia, including bioactive cements (Bio Cem, NuSmile, Houston, TX; Ceramir, Doxa Dental Inc., Chicago, IL; Activa Bio Active Cement, Pulpdent Corporation, Watertown, MA).

| TABLE 21.2 | Comparison of Dental Cements |

Cement	Composition	Working Time	Setting Time	Compressive Strength	Bond Strength to Dentin	Release of Fluoride	Pulpal Response	Removal of Excess
Ideal	—	Medium	Short-medium	Very high	High	Yes	None	Easy
Glass ionomer	Silicate glass containing Ca, Al, F Polycarboxylic acid	Short-medium	Short	High	Medium	Yes	Low	Moderate
Bioactive	—	High	Medium	High	High	Yes	None	Moderate
Zinc oxide and eugenol	Zinc oxide Eugenol	Long	Medium	Low-medium	None	No	None	Easy
Reinforced zinc oxide and eugenol	Zinc oxide reinforced with alumina or polymer eugenol	Long	Medium-long	Low-medium	None	No	None	Easy

Modified from Farah JW, Powers JM. Cements. *Dent Advisor*. 1985;2(1):3.

References

1. Donly KJ, Wild TW, Jensen ME. Posterior composite class II restorations: in vitro comparison of preparation designs and restoration techniques. *Dent Mater*. 1990;6:88–93.
2. Pereira JC, Manfio AP, Franco EB, et al. Clinical evaluation of Dycal under amalgam restorations. *Am J Dent*. 1990;3:67–70.
3. Straffon LH, Corpron RL, Bruner FW, et al. Twenty-four-month clinical trial of visible-light activated cavity liner in young permanent teeth. *J Dent Child*. 1991;58:124–128.
4. Manders CA, Garcia-Godoy F, Barnwell GM. Effect of a copal varnish, ZOE or glass ionomer cement bases on microleakage of amalgam restorations. *Am J Dent*. 1990;3:63–66.
5. Heys RJ, Fitzgerald M. Microleakage of three cement bases. *J Dent Res*. 1991;70:55–58.
6. Donly KJ, Ingram C. An in vitro caries inhibition of photopolymerized glass ionomer liners. *ASDC J Dent Child*. 1997;64:128–130.
7. Garcia-Godoy F, Jensen ME. Artificial recurrent caries in glass ionomer–lined amalgam restorations. *Am J Dent*. 1990;3:89–93.
8. Hicks MJ, Flaitz CM, Silverstone LM. Secondary caries formation in vitro around glass ionomer restoration. *Quintessence Int*. 1986;17:527–532.
9. Jensen ME, Wefel JS, Hammesfahr PD. Fluoride-releasing liners: in vitro recurrent caries. *Gen Dent*. 1991;39:12–17.
10. Diaz-Arnold AM, Holmes DC, Wistrom DW, et al. Short-term fluoride release/uptake of glass ionomer restoratives. *Dent Mater*. 1995;11:96–101.
11. Forsten L. Fluoride release and uptake by glass ionomers and related materials and its clinical effect. *Biomaterials*. 1998;19:503–508.
12. Forsten L. Resin-modified glass ionomer cements: fluoride release and uptake. *Acta Odontol Scand*. 1995;53:222–225.
13. Skartveit L, Tveit AB, Tøtdal B, et al. In vivo fluoride uptake in enamel and dentin from fluoride-containing materials. *ASDC J Dent Child*. 1990;58:97–100.
14. Donly KJ. Enamel and dentin demineralization inhibition of fluoride-releasing materials. *Am J Dent*. 1994;7:275–278.
15. Griffin F, Donly KJ, Erickson RC. Caries inhibition of three fluoride-releasing liners. *Am J Dent*. 1992;5:293–295.
16. Mitra SB. Property comparisons of a light-cure and a self-cure glass ionomer liner. *J Dent Res*. 1989;68A(Abstract 740):274.
17. Erickson RL. Mechanism and clinical implications of bond formation for two dentin bonding agents. *Am J Dent*. 1989;2:117–123.
18. Garcia-Godoy F, Donly KJ. Dentin/enamel adhesives in pediatric dentistry. *Pediatr Dent*. 2002;24:462–464.
19. Swift EJ. Dentin/enamel adhesives: review of the literature. *Pediatr Dent*. 2002;24:456–461.
20. Fuks A. The use of amalgam in pediatric dentistry. *Pediatr Dent*. 2002;24:448–455.
21. Osborne JW, Summitt JB, Roberts HW. The use of dental amalgam in pediatric dentistry: review of the literature. *Pediatr Dent*. 2002;24:439–447.
22. Osborne JW. Three-year clinical performance of eight amalgam alloys. *Am J Dent*. 1990;3:157–159.
23. Council on Dental Materials and Devices. Revised American Dental Association Specification No. 1 for Alloy for Dental Amalgam. *J Am Dent Assoc*. 1977;95:614–617.
24. Burgess JO, Walker R, Davidson BS. Posterior resin-based composite: review of the literature. *Pediatr Dent*. 2002;24:465–479.
25. Donly KJ, Garcia-Godoy F. The use of resin-based composite in children. *Pediatr Dent*. 2002;24:480–488.
26. Bowen RL. Dental filling material comprising vinyl-silane treated fused silica and a binder consisting of the reaction product of bisphenol and glycidyl methacrylate; 1962. U.S. Patent #3066112A.
27. Phillips RW, Swartz ML, Norman RD. *Materials for the Practicing Dentist*. St Louis: Mosby; 1969:182–191.
28. Bayne SC, Taylor DF, Sturdevant JR, et al. Protection theory for composite wear based on 5-year clinical results. *J Dent Res*. 1988;67 (Abstract 60):120.
29. Ruyter IE. Polymerization and conversion in composite resins. In: Taylor DF, ed. *Proceedings of the International Symposium on Posterior Composite Resins* (Chapel Hill, NC, October 1982). Chapel Hill, NC: University of North Carolina; 1984:255–286.
30. Asmussen E. Composite restorative resins. Composition versus wall to wall polymerization contraction. *Acta Odontol Scand*. 1975;33:337–344.
31. Bowen RL, Rapson JE, Dickson G. Hardening shrinkage and hygroscopic expansion of composite resins. *J Dent Res*. 1982;61:654–658.
32. Donly KJ, Jensen ME. Posterior composite polymerization shrinkage in primary teeth: an in vitro comparison of three techniques. *Pediatr Dent*. 1986;8:209–212.
33. Eick DJ, Welch FH. Polymerization shrinkage of composite resins and its possible influence on postoperative sensitivity. *Quintessence Int*. 1986;77:103–111.
34. Jorgensen KD, Asmussen E, Shimokobe H. Enamel damage caused by contracting restorative resins. *Scand J Dent Res*. 1975;83:120–122.
35. Segura A, Donly KJ. Posterior composite polymerization shrinkage recovery following hygroscopic expansion. *J Oral Rehabil*. 1993;20:495–499.

36. Craig RG. Chemistry, composition and properties of composite resins. *Dent Clin North Am.* 1981;25:219–239.

37. Ruyter IE. Monomer systems and polymerization. In: Vanherle G, Smith DC, eds. *Posterior Composite Resin Dental Restorative Materials.* Utrecht, Netherlands: Peter Szulc; 1985:109–135.

38. Smith DC. Posterior composite dental restorative material: materials development. In: Vanherle G, Smith DC, eds. *Posterior Composite Resin Dental Restorative Materials.* Utrecht, Netherlands: Peter Szulc; 1985:47–60.

39. Z250. *Material Safety Data Sheet.* St Paul, MN: 3M ESPE.

40. Weinmann W, Thalacker C, Guggenberger R. Siloranes in dental composites. *Dent Mater.* 2005;21:68–74.

41. Van Dijken JWV, Lindberg A. Clinical effectiveness of a low shrinkage composite. A five-year study. *J Adhes Dent.* 2009;11:143–148.

42. Pilo R, Oelgiesser D, Cardash HS. A survey of output intensity and potential for depth of cure among light-curing units in clinical use. *J Dent.* 1999;27:235–241.

43. Flury S, Hayoz S, Peutzfeldt A, et al. Depth of cure of resin composites. Is the ISO 4049 method suitable for bulk-fill materials? *Dent Mater.* 2012;28:521–528.

44. El-Safty S, Silikas N, Watts DC. Creep deformation of restorative resin-composites intended for bulk-fill placement. *Dent Mater.* 2012;28:928–935.

45. Burgess J, Cakir D. Comparative properties of low-shrinkage composite resins. *Compend Contin Educ Dent.* 2010;31:10–15.

46. Ilie N, Hickel R. Investigations on a methacrylate-based flowable composite based on the SDR technology. *Dent Mater.* 2011;27:348–355.

47. Czasch P, Ilie N. In vitro comparison of mechanical properties and degree of cure of bulk-fill composites. *Clin Oral Investig.* 2013;17:227–235.

48. Peutzfeldt A. Resin composites in dentistry: the monomer systems. *Eur J Oral Sci.* 1997;105:97–116.

49. Moszner N, Fischer UK, Angermann J, et al. A partially aromatic urethane as a new substitute for Bis-GMA in restorative composites. *Dent Mater.* 2008;24:694–699.

50. Giachetti L, Bertini F, Bambi C, et al. A rational use of dental materials in posterior direct resin restorations in order to control polymerization shrinkage stress. *Minerva Stomatol.* 2007;56:129–138.

51. Eames WB, Strain JD, Weitman RT, et al. Clinical comparison of composite, amalgam, and silicate restorative materials. *J Am Dent Assoc.* 1974;89:1111–1117.

52. Leinfelder KF, Sluder TB, Santos JF, et al. Five-year clinical evaluation of anterior and posterior restorations of composite resin. *Oper Dent.* 1980;5(2):57–65.

53. Osborne JW, Gale EN, Ferguson GW. One-year and two-year clinical evaluation of composite resin vs. amalgam. *J Prosthet Dent.* 1973;30:795–800.

54. Phillips RW. Observations on a composite resin for class II restorations: two-year report. *J Prosthet Dent.* 1972;28:164–169.

55. Leinfelder KF, Roberson TM. Clinical evaluation of posterior composite resins. *Gen Dent.* 1983;31:276–280.

56. Jaarda MJ, Wang RF, Lang BR. A regression analysis of filler particle content to predict composite wear. *J Prosthet Dent.* 1997;77:57–67.

57. Phillips RW, Lutz F. Status reports on posterior composites. Council on Dental Materials, Instruments, and Equipment. *J Am Dent Assoc.* 1983;107:74–76.

58. Derkson GD, Richardson AS, Waldman RJ. Clinical evaluation of composite resin and amalgam posterior restorations: two year results. *J Can Dent Assoc.* 1983;4:277–279.

59. Ripa LW. Sealants revisited: an update of the effectiveness of pit-and-fissure sealants. *Caries Res.* 1993;27(suppl 1):77–82.

60. Simonsen RJ. Retention and effectiveness of dental sealants after fifteen years. *J Am Dent Assoc.* 1991;122:34–42.

61. Wright JT, Crall JJ, Fontana M, et al. Evidence based clinical practice guideline for the use of pit and fissure sealants: a report of the American Dental Association and the American Academy of Pediatric Dentistry. *J Am Dent Assoc.* 2016;147(8):672–682.

62. Hicks MJ, Flaitz CM. Caries-like lesion formation around fluoride-releasing sealant and glass ionomer. *Am J Dent.* 1992;5:329–334.

63. Jensen ME, Wefel JS, Triolo PT, et al. Effect of a fluoride-releasing fissure sealant on artificial enamel caries. *Am J Dent.* 1990;3:75–78.

64. Berg JH. Glass ionomer cements. *Pediatr Dent.* 2002;24:430–438.

65. Croll TP, Nicholson JW. Glass ionomer cements in pediatric dentistry: review of the literature. *Pediatr Dent.* 2002;24:423–429.

66. Donly KJ, Segura A, Kanellis M, et al. Clinical performance and caries inhibition of resin-modified glass ionomer cement and amalgam restorations. *J Am Dent Assoc.* 1999;130:1459–1466.

67. Ewoldsen H, Herwig L. Decay-inhibiting restorative materials: past and present. *Compend Contin Educ Dent.* 1998;19:981–992.

68. Souto M, Donly KJ. Caries inhibition of glass ionomers. *Am J Dent.* 1994;7:122–124.

69. ten Cate JM, van Duinen RN. Hypermineralization of dentinal lesions adjacent to glass-ionomer cement restorations. *J Dent Res.* 1995;74:1266–1271.

70. Croll TP, Bar Zion Y, Segura A, et al. Clinical performance of resin-modified glass ionomer cement restorations in primary teeth: a retrospective evaluation. *J Am Dent Assoc.* 2001;132:1110–1116.

71. Mjör IA, Dahl JE, Moorhead JE. Placement and replacement of restorations in primary teeth. *Acta Odontol Scand.* 2002;60:25–28.

72. Hickel R. Glass ionomer, cements, hybrid-ionomers and compomers. Long term clinical evaluation. *Trans Acad Dent Mater.* 1996;9:105–112.

73. Marks LA, Weerheijm KL, van Amerongen WE, et al. Dyract versus Tytin class II restorations in primary molars: 36 months evaluation. *Caries Res.* 1999;33:387–392.

74. Peters MCRB, Roeters FJM. Clinical performance of a new compomer restorative in pediatric dentistry. *J Dent Res.* 1994;73A(Abstract 34):106.

75. Roeters JJ, Frankenmolen F, Burgersdijk RC, et al. Clinical evaluation of Dyract in primary molars: 3-year results. *Am J Dent.* 1998;11:143–148.

76. Malkondu Ö, Tinastepe N, Akan E, et al. An overview of monolithic zirconia in dentistry. *Biotechnol Biotechnol Equip.* 2016;30:644–652.

77. Jung YS, Lee JW, Choi YJ, et al. A study on the in-vitro wear of the natural tooth structure by opposing zirconia on dental porcelain. *J Adv Prosthodont.* 2010;2:111–115.

22
Restorative Dentistry for the Primary Dentition

WILLIAM F. WAGGONER AND TRAVIS NELSON

CHAPTER OUTLINE

Pediatric restorative dentistry is a dynamic combination of ever-improving materials and tried-and-true techniques. Many aspects of primary teeth restoration have not changed for decades. In 1924 G.V. Black outlined several steps for the preparation of carious permanent teeth to receive an amalgam restoration.[1] These steps have been adopted, with slight modification, for the restoration of primary teeth. Restorative techniques for the primary dentition using amalgam and stainless steel crowns (SSCs) have remained relatively consistent for decades (Fig. 22.1). However, with an increased use of adhesive restorative materials and bonding systems, there has been a shift to more conservative preparations and restorations. Materials such as glass ionomers, resin ionomer products, and improved resin-based composite systems have been developed that are having a profound impact on the restoration of primary teeth. In addition, premilled zirconia crowns (ZCs) now offer an esthetic alternative to SSCs. Unfortunately, long-term clinical data (i.e., longer than 3 years) regarding many of these newer materials are limited; but even so, many clinicians are successfully using these materials with increasing frequency.

The clinician can stay with the proven, successful materials of the past, such as amalgam and stainless steel, or move to newer, more esthetic materials that offer advantages such as bonding to tooth structure, fluoride release, improved esthetics, reduction of mercury exposure, and conservation of tooth structure. None of the esthetic materials have the track record and proven durability of amalgam or stainless steel, but when they are placed appropriately, they can provide useful restorations for the lifespan of the primary tooth. This chapter will provide information on both the new and the traditional restorative techniques. For the interested reader, in 2014 the American Academy of Pediatric Dentistry sponsored a Pediatric Dentistry Restorative Symposium Conference. The published proceedings[2] include extensive and up-to-date literature reviews and discussion of pediatric restorative techniques at a greater depth than can be included in this chapter. In addition, a more detailed discussion of dental materials used in pediatric restorative dentistry can be found in Chapter 21.

Instrumentation and Caries Removal

Nearly all instrumentation for restorative procedures is carried out with the high-speed handpiece (100,000 to 300,000 rpm, either electric or air turbine) combined with coolant. The coolant may be water spray or air alone. A water spray coolant is often recommended for high-speed instrumentation; however, there is some evidence that air coolant alone may be used without creating irreversible pulpal damage,[3,4] and use of both coolant techniques is taught in many pediatric dental residency programs.[5] There are some instances when a water spray coolant is absolutely necessary. This is especially true when removing old amalgam restorations or using diamond burs. Regardless of the coolant used, intermittent cutting at intervals of a few seconds with light, brushing strokes should be done to prevent excessive heat generation. Protective masks and eyewear should always be worn when using the high-speed air turbine handpiece.

The low-speed handpiece (500 to 15,000 rpm) is most frequently used primarily for caries removal and occasionally for polishing and finishing procedures. As with high-speed instrumentation, light pressure and brushing strokes should be used when using the low-speed handpiece. Use of hand instrumentation is minimal in most operative preparations in the primary dentition and is usually limited to final caries removal.

Although use of a handpiece for caries removal and cavity preparation is by far the most popular and frequently used method, there are at least three other methods of treating carious teeth. These are air abrasion, laser treatment, and chemomechanical methods. With these methods, tooth preparations move from the

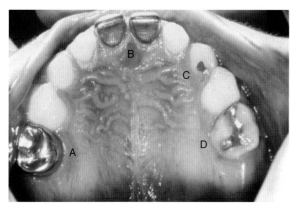

• **Figure 22.1** Traditionally restored primary dentition demonstrating stainless steel crown *(A)*, preveneered steel crowns *(B)*, class III amalgam *(C)*, and class II amalgam *(D)*. *Note:* All white, esthetic alternatives now exist for each of these restorations.

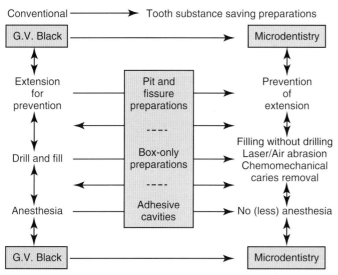

• **Figure 22.2** Cavity preparation continuum. (Courtesy Dr. Luc Martens, Ghent, Belgium.)

generated during the procedure, and the fact that it does not completely eliminate the need for conventional handpieces are three disadvantages of the system that seem to keep it from gaining widespread use. Laser techniques have also become popular with some dental operators. Lasers can be used in children for soft tissue surgery, caries prevention, caries diagnosis, biostimulation and pain control, hemostasis during pulpotomy procedures, and cavity preparation.[8] An erbium:YAG laser can be used in restorative dentistry for minimally invasive preparation of pits and fissures and hypoplastic teeth, cavity preparation of all classes (I thorough V), treatment of deep dentinal caries, and laser-assisted pulp capping. Some of the advantages of using lasers for cavity preparation include (1) better patient acceptance because they are quiet, (2) no vibration and minimal need for use of anesthetic, (3) minimally invasive cavity preparation because of the selective absorption of laser light by carious tissue, (4) production of very clean cavity preparations free of a smear layer, (5) minimal thermal increase in the pulp chamber, and (6) the production of cavity preparations with a macroroughened surface that increases surface bonding area for better adhesion of resin-based materials. Some disadvantages include (1) a longer learning curve; (2) higher equipment costs ($30,000 to $60,000 for an erbium:YAG laser); (3) need for specialized training; and (4) possible need for a traditional handpiece to complete the process, depending on the cavity size and preparation needed.[9] Chemomechanical caries removal is a noninvasive technique that eliminates infected dentin via a chemical agent by means of dissolution. Instead of drilling, a chemical agent such as Carisolv (MediTeam AB, Göteberg, Sweden) or Papacarie (F&A Laboratorio Farmaceutico Ltd., São Paulo, Brazil) is applied to the carious dentin and assisted by hand instruments to remove soft carious material. This method usually does not require anesthesia, it preserves sound tooth structure, and it relies on bonded restorative materials for final restoration. Drawbacks to this method include an increase in operator time to remove caries, only certain carious lesions are suitable for its use, a handpiece may still be necessary to gain access to the dentinal or interproximal areas, and few long-term data are available to confirm long-term success of the method.[10]

One final aspect to be considered when discussing tooth preparation is the use of magnification during operative procedures. Up until the 1990s the use of magnification for dental procedures by most practitioners came only with increasing age and failing eyesight, but now the use of magnifying loupes or microscopes for most dental procedures is taught from the beginning of most dental school training. Loupes are available in a wide range of magnification, but generally a set of loupes with a 2.5× to 3.5× magnification is recommended for restorative dentistry. The use of magnification for completing restorative procedures has several advantages, such as an increase in productivity, an increase in the level of excellence and confidence in dental treatment, an increase in visual diagnostic abilities, and perhaps most importantly, improvement in operator posture and comfort to help prevent musculoskeletal disorders brought about by poor operator positioning.[11] Use of magnification during cavity preparation has not yet become the standard of care, but it is highly recommended and will likely become the standard of care in the next few years.

Anatomic Considerations of Primary Teeth

Although some primary teeth resemble their permanent successors, they are not miniature permanent teeth. Several anatomic differences must be distinguished before restorative procedures are begun (Box 22.1; Fig. 22.3).

traditional, conventional preparations used by G.V. Black to much more conservative, "tooth-saving" preparations, known as microdentistry or minimally invasive dentistry. Depending on the type of carious lesions, method of instrumentation, and restorative material to be used, the clinician can opt for a conventional G.V. Black type of cavity preparation or for a much more conservative micropreparation. Fig. 22.2 illustrates a continuum of cavity preparation based on size and instrumentation.

Air abrasion uses a stream of purified aluminum oxide particles (27 to 50 µm) that are forced under pressure (40 to 120 psi) through a fine-focused nozzle onto the tooth surface. This cuts through enamel and dentin quickly, and it can also abrade or roughen a tooth surface.[6] Originally introduced into dentistry by R. Black in 1945,[7] air abrasion virtually disappeared from the dental environment by the early 1960s and was reintroduced in the early 1990s. Air abrasion offers some advantages over conventional handpieces. There is an absence of vibration and noise, caries excavation can often be done without the need for local anesthesia, and tooth preparation can be very fast. It is best suited for use with adhesive restorations that require minimal tooth preparation and less rigid classic cavity design than does amalgam. The cost of the air abrasion unit ($2000 to $5000), the dust that can be

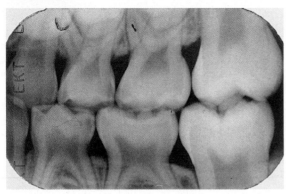

• **Figure 22.3** Note the difference in enamel thickness. The enamel of the primary molars is approximately half the thickness of the enamel of the first permanent molars. Also note the interproximal caries requiring restoration on the distal surface of the mandibular first primary molar and between the maxillary first and second primary molars.

• BOX 22.1 Anatomic Differences Between Primary and Permanent Teeth

1. Primary teeth have thinner enamel and dentin thickness than permanent teeth (see Fig. 22.3).
2. The pulps of primary teeth are larger in relation to crown size than permanent pulps.
3. The pulp horns of primary teeth are closer to the outer surface of the tooth than permanent pulps. The mesiobuccal pulp horn is the most prominent.
4. Primary teeth demonstrate greater constriction of the crown and have a more prominent cervical contour than permanent teeth.
5. Primary teeth have broad, flat proximal contact areas.
6. Primary teeth are whiter than their permanent successors.
7. Primary teeth have relatively narrow occlusal surfaces in comparison with their permanent successors.

• BOX 22.2 Advantages of Rubber Dam Use

1. Better access and visualization are gained by retracting soft tissues and providing a dark contrasting background to the teeth.
2. Moisture control is superior to other forms of isolation.
3. The safety of the child is improved by preventing aspiration or swallowing of foreign bodies and by protecting the soft tissues.
4. Placement generally results in decreased operating time.
5. Many children tend to become quieter and relaxed with a rubber dam in place. The dam seems to act as a separating barrier, so that movements in and out of the oral cavity are perceived by the child as being less invasive than without the dam in place.
6. With a rubber dam in place, a child becomes primarily a nasal breather. This enhances nitrous oxide administration when it has been deemed necessary from a behavioral standpoint.

Isolation in Pediatric Restorative Dentistry

Rubber Dam

The use of the rubber dam is indispensable in pediatric restorative dentistry. Numerous advantages have been listed for its use, all allowing for provision of the highest quality of care (Box 22.2). Most pediatric restorative procedures can be completed with the rubber dam in place. The few situations in which it may not be used include the following: (1) in the presence of some fixed orthodontic appliances; (2) when a very recently erupted tooth will not retain a clamp; and (3) in a child with an upper respiratory infection, congested nasal passage, or other nasal obstruction. However, even poor nasal breathers may tolerate the rubber dam if a small (2- to 3-cm) hole is cut in the dam in an area away from the operative quadrant. This allows for some mouth breathing.

Preparing for Placement of the Rubber Dam

The rubber dam is available in an assortment of colors and may even be scented or flavored. Virtually all rubber dams are made of latex, although a latex-free rubber dam material is available (Hygienic Corporation, Akron, OH) for use in latex-sensitive patients. A 5 × 5-inch medium-gauge rubber dam is best suited for use in children. Rubber dams are available in which a disposable rubber dam frame is manufactured already attached to the dam (Handidam, Aseptico, Woodinville, WA), eliminating the need for a separate dam frame. The darker the dam, the better the contrast between the teeth and dam. The holes should be punched so that the rubber dam is centered horizontally on the face and the upper lip is covered by the upper border of the dam, but the dam does not cover the nostrils. One method of proper hole placement is seen in Fig. 22.4A and B.

Punch the minimal number of holes necessary for good isolation of all teeth to be restored. For single class I or V restorations, only the tooth being restored may be isolated. If interproximal lesions are being restored, at least one tooth anterior and one tooth posterior to the tooth being restored should be isolated. This allows better access, more ease in placing a matrix, and visualization of adjacent marginal ridges for appropriate carving of the restoration.

When isolating several teeth, instead of punching numerous holes in the dam, some clinicians will simply punch two holes approximately one-half inch apart and cut the rubber dam with scissors connecting the two holes. This is called the "slit technique" and allows for very quick placement of the rubber dam. Because there is no rubber dam material interproximally, moisture control is not as dependable with this placement technique, but it is often still adequate, especially for isolation of maxillary quadrants.

Proper clamp selection is one of the most critical aspects of good rubber dam application. Box 22.3 lists the most frequently used clamps and their areas of utilization. Incisors usually require ligation with dental floss for stabilization instead of a clamp.

After selecting an appropriate clamp, place a 12- to 18-inch piece of dental floss on the bow of the clamp as a safety measure (Fig. 22.5). This is necessary for easy retrieval of the clamp if it is dislodged from the tooth and falls into the posterior pharyngeal area.

Before trying the clamp on the tooth, floss the contacts through which the rubber dam will be taken. If floss cannot be passed through the contact because of defective restorations or other factors, modification of the contacts or rubber dam will be necessary before placement. Next, using the rubber dam forceps, place the clamp on the tooth, seating it from a lingual to buccal direction. Be certain that the jaws of the clamp are placed below the height of contour and are not impinging on the gingival tissues. After seating the clamp, remove the forceps and place a finger on the buccal and lingual jaws of the clamp and apply gingival pressure to ensure that the clamp is stable and has been seated as far gingivally as possible.

Placement of the Rubber Dam

The punched rubber dam should be lightly stretched onto the rubber dam frame prior to placement of the clamp. This holds

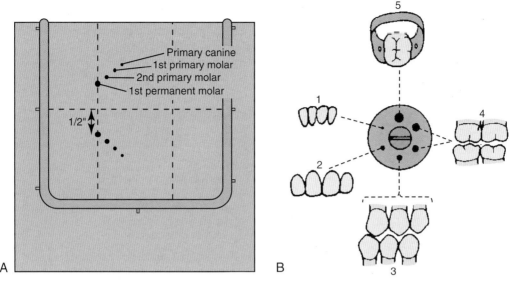

• **Figure 22.4** Preparation of the rubber dam. (A) The Young frame is applied to the rubber dam. The upper limit of the frame coincides with the upper edge of the rubber dam material. The dam is divided vertically into thirds, and the area inside the frame is divided in half horizontally. The holes for each tooth are placed as indicated, at a 45-degree angle 3 to 4 mm apart. (B) The rubber dam punch table with corresponding teeth and hole sizes. ([B] Modified from The DAE Project. *Instructional Materials for the Dental Health Professions: Rubber Dam.* New York: Teachers College Press, Teachers College, Columbia University; 1982:42.)

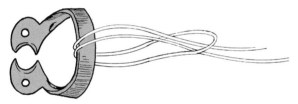

• **Figure 22.5** A floss safety through the bow of the rubber dam clamp allows for easy retrieval of the clamp, should it become dislodged from the tooth. (Modified from The DAE Project. *Instructional Materials for the Dental Health Professions: Rubber Dam.* New York: Teachers College Press, Teachers College, Columbia University; 1982:66.)

• BOX 22.3 Common Rubber Dam Clamps for Pediatric Restorative Dentistry

Partially erupted permanent molars: 14A, 8A[a,b,c]
Fully erupted permanent molars: 14, 8[b,c]
Second primary molars: 26, 27,[c] 3[a,b]
First primary molars/bicuspids/permanent canines: 2, 2A,[a,b] 207, 208[c]
Primary incisors and canines: 0,[a] 00,[b] 209[c]

[a]*Ivory, Heraeus-Kulzer, South Bend, IN.*
[b]*Hygienic Corp., Akron, OH.*
[c]*Hu-Friedy Mfg. Co., Chicago, IL.*
"A" clamps have jaws angled gingivally to seat below subgingival heights of contour.

---

the corners of the dam out of the line of the operator's vision during placement. If the material is stretched too tightly, tension is too great and the clamp may be dislodged when the material is stretched over the bow of the clamp. Next, pull the floss attached to the clamp through the most posterior hole in the dam that has been punched for the clamped tooth. Instruct the child to open

the mouth widely and consider placement of a mouth prop. With the index fingers, stretch the most posterior hole of the rubber dam over the bow and wings of the clamp. Sometimes when isolating the most posterior maxillary molars, the bow of the clamp rests very close to the anterior border of the ramus when the mouth is opened wide. This makes slipping the dam material over the bow difficult, but when one simply asks the child to close the mouth slightly, the ramus will move posteriorly and allow the material to slide between the bow and the ramus.

If necessary, adjust the tension of the rubber dam on the frame. Next, stabilize the rubber dam around the most anterior tooth. This may be done by placing a wooden wedge interproximally, by stretching a small piece of rubber dam through the contact, or by ligating with dental floss. To ligate, place floss (12 to 18 inches) around the cervix of the tooth and have the dental assistant hold the floss gingivally on the lingual with a blunt instrument. Draw the floss tightly around the tooth from the buccal and tie a surgical knot below the cervical bulge. Do not cut the ends of the ligature tie, because the long ends remind the operator that the ligature is present. After anterior stabilization, all other teeth can be isolated for which holes have been punched. A blunt hand instrument can be used to invert the rubber dam into the gingival sulcus around each isolated tooth.

Removing the Rubber Dam

To remove the rubber dam when restorative procedures are complete, first rinse away all debris and cut and remove any ligatures used for stabilization. Next, stretch the rubber dam so that the dam's interproximal septa may be cut with a pair of scissors. The clamp, frame, and dam are then removed as a unit with the rubber dam forceps. Inspect the dam and the mouth to see that no small pieces of dam material have been left interproximally. Gently massage the tissue around the previously clamped tooth, and rinse and evacuate the oral cavity.

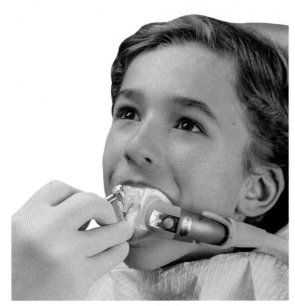

• **Figure 22.6** Isolite-alternate isolation system. (Courtesy Isolite Systems, Santa Barbara, CA. Used with permission.)

Alternative Isolation Systems

In recent years, novel isolation systems have been introduced to dentistry. These systems incorporate high-volume evacuation, a bite block, and protective barriers for the tongue and cheek. Some systems are made of transparent materials. This increases visibility and allows incorporation of illumination into the mouthpiece (Isolite, Isolite Systems, Santa Barbara, CA; Fig. 22.6). The mouthpieces are constructed of flexible polymer materials that are several millimeters thick but easily adapt to the mouth's contours and provide protection of the soft tissues. These systems reduce moisture and average oral humidity to levels that are similar to a rubber dam. As an added benefit, the design allows the operator to simultaneously work on opposing maxillary and mandibular quadrants. These systems also exhibit continuous evacuation, which may reduce the start/stop time required with the use of high-volume evacuators (HVEs) in four-handed dentistry. A comparison of alternative isolation systems with the rubber dam is found in Table 22.1.

Manufacturers produce mouthpieces in a variety of sizes to accommodate most patients. Two popular systems, Isolite and DryShield (DryShield, Fountain Valley, CA), require purchase of specific armamentarium for each dental unit that is equipped. Other systems such as Mr. Thirsty (Zirc, Buffalo, MN) connect directly to existing HVEs. Mouthpieces may be disposable (Isolite, Mr. Thirsty) or autoclavable and reusable (DryShield).

Placement of Alternative Isolation Systems

Step 1: Hold the control head with index finger and thumb. With your other hand, fold the cheek shield onto the tongue retractor. Gently slide the folded mouthpiece into the buccal vestibule on the side to receive treatment. Angle the mouthpiece to allow the lower edge of the tongue retractor to move along the buccal edge of the teeth.

Step 2: Move the bite block onto the occlusal surface of the teeth, just distal to the mandibular cuspid. Instruct the patient to "rest gently" on the bite block to secure.

TABLE 22.1	Contrasting the Rubber Dam With Alternative Isolation Systems	
	Rubber Dam	Alternative Isolation Systems (Isolite, DryShield, Mr. Thirsty)
Isolation		
Moisture control	+	+
Reduction of aerosol	+	+
Improves visibility of field	+	+
Continuous evacuation		+
Protection from debris and dropped instruments	++	+
Retracts gingival tissues	+	
Ability to isolate partially erupted teeth	+	++
Saves time	+	++
Illumination		+ (Isolite only)
Behavioral		
Reduces mouth breathing, may increase N₂O inhalation	+	
Reduces talking	++	+
Added noise		−
Challenge in sizing for some children/gagging		−
Local anesthesia required	−	
Implementation		
Cost for disposable supplies	Very low	Moderate
Cost for armamentarium	Low	High

Step 3: Place the cheek shield into the buccal vestibule. Move the isthmus onto the retromolar pad behind the maxillary tuberosity. Adjust the tongue retractor in the lingual vestibule as needed. Move the bite block distally to provide more vertical working room.

Behavioral Considerations When Using Alternative Isolation Systems

When used properly, both rubber dam and alternative isolation systems can provide good moisture control and protection of oral soft tissues. Although placement of rubber dams typically requires administration of local anesthetic, alternative isolation systems do not. This may lead users to believe that the alternative system is better tolerated by patients than are rubber dams. This observation may be especially true for sealants and other situations in which local anesthetic would not otherwise be used. However, for operative dentistry, local anesthetic is generally used. Therefore, when local anesthetic is applied, a rubber dam is perceived to be relatively comfortable and often presents as a less bulky isolation technique. In addition, compared with cotton roll isolation, research indicates that rubber dams may decrease stress when used with children. In contrast, a significant percentage of children expressed that they felt that the alternative isolation system mouthpiece stretched their mouth and made them feel as if they were going to gag. The effects on patient behavior of alternative isolation systems have not been well studied. Other factors to consider include greater noise when using alternative systems and the fact that rubber dams facilitate nose breathing, which can enhance the effect of nitrous oxide inhalation sedation.

Restoration of Primary Molars

The anatomy of the primary molars, with their fissured occlusal surfaces and broad, flat interproximal contact areas, makes them the most caries-susceptible primary teeth. The importance of primary molars in mastication and as maintainers of space for the succedaneous teeth, coupled with the development of suitable economic restorative materials, has shaped a philosophy of restoring and conserving primary molars, versus extraction or supervision of caries.

SSCs, ZCs, amalgam, and adhesive materials such as resin-based composites, resin-modified glass ionomers (RMGIs), polyacid-modified resin-based composites (compomers), and glass ionomers are the materials used in the restoration of primary molars. Although amalgam was historically the material of choice for intracoronal restorations, the use of adhesive materials for restoring posterior teeth continues to increase annually. It is estimated that more than 50% of intracoronal restorations placed are resin-based composites. Following is a discussion of primary molar restoration which has been divided topically based upon the number of tooth surfaces treated, with specific focus on differences encountered with different restorative materials.

Adhesive Materials in Primary Molars

As early as the mid-1960s, composite resins (now referred to as resin-based composites) were suggested as esthetic replacements for class I and class II amalgam restorations in molars. Initial results were promising, but clinical failures of the resin restorations began to occur after approximately 2 years, with the greatest problem being occlusal wear.[12] However, further improvements in resin-based composite materials, such as smaller filler particles, increases in material strength, and improvement of dentin-bonding agents, have led to improved clinical results. Currently there are still minimal long-term clinical data available on longevity of resin-based composite materials in primary teeth. However, there are several studies in teeth that demonstrate good performance over time.[13–17] For example, in a 5-year study comparing posterior composites and amalgams, Norman and colleagues[18] reported satisfactory results for both amalgam and composite. The only significant statistical differences were a poorer marginal integrity for the amalgam and a greater wear rate for the resin. However, the wear rate for the composite was well within the acceptable limits established by the American Dental Association (ADA) Council on Dental Materials. Roberts and associates also found no significant difference in clinical performance or wear of class II amalgam and resin-based composites restorations evaluated for 3 years.[19] Bernardo and colleagues, in a 7-year clinical study comparing amalgam and resin-based composite, found composite to be an acceptable restorative material.[20] However, amalgam demonstrated fewer failures than resin-based composites, particularly in restorations with three or more surfaces. In the Bernardo et al. study, recurrent decay was the main cause of failure of the posterior composite restorations. Evidence suggests that the risk of secondary caries in composite restorations is significantly greater than for amalgam, but amalgam is more prone to fracture than composites.[20,21] Another 5-year longitudinal study showed similar results, with no statistically significant difference in overall failure rate between composite and amalgam; however, composite restorations required seven times more repairs than amalgam.[17] The ADA's Council on Scientific Affairs has concluded that when used correctly in the primary and permanent dentition, the expected lifetimes of resin-based composites can be comparable to that of amalgam in class I, II, and V restorations.[22] It should be noted that these conclusions were based upon using the three-step etch, prime, and bond systems, and self-etching bond systems may not offer the same results.

The use of resin-based composite materials in primary molars offers the advantages of improved esthetics, elimination of mercury, low thermal conductivity, more conservation of tooth structure, easier reparability, and bonding of the restorative material to the tooth. Disadvantages include an exacting technique, incompatibility with moisture contamination during placement, increased operator time, potential marginal leakage, possible postoperative sensitivity, and a tendency for loose or open contacts.[23–25] The ADA has approved several resin-based composites for use in posterior teeth.

In addition to resin-based composites, polyacid-modified resin-based composites, also known as compomers (Dyract eXtra [Dentsply Sirona, York, PA]), RMGIs (Vitremer and Ketac Nano [3M ESPE, St. Paul, MN]), and glass ionomers (Ketac Fil Plus [3M ESPE]), have all been suggested and studied for use in primary molar restorations. Several clinical studies have evaluated compomer use in primary molars[26–31] and likewise found them to provide useful, predictable restorations. RMGI cement has also been evaluated in several clinical studies.[32–34] It seems that these restorations demonstrate more color change and occlusal wear than resin-based composites or compomers but still function well in class I, II, III, and V restorations. Glass ionomer cements have also been used in restoring primary molars but with less satisfactory results than the other adhesive materials.[34,35] Use of glass ionomers for multisurface or large restorations in primary molars, except for teeth with a very limited lifespan, is generally not recommended or indicated.

Amalgam Use in Primary Molars

Although use of adhesive restorative materials continues to rise, amalgam remains the restorative material of choice for many clinicians. Favorable handling properties, good longevity, and less technique sensitivity make this material a good option for restoration of primary posterior teeth. However, it should be noted that concerns have been raised about exposure of dentists, patients, and the environment to mercury in amalgam. This has led to the use of amalgam for cavity restoration to be banned in several European countries. Current scientific information continues to support the use of amalgam as a restorative material,[36] but for a more detailed discussion of the controversy the reader is referred to Chapter 21.

General Principles for Intracoronal Restoration of Primary Posterior Teeth

Class I Restorations

Amalgam Preparation Design

The classic G.V. Black outline form is the basis for both adhesive and amalgam class I preparations. For amalgam, it includes all retentive fissures and carious areas but is as conservative as possible (Fig. 22.7).

Ideal pulpal floor depth is 0.5 mm into dentin (approximately 1.5 mm from the enamel surface). The length of the cutting end of the no. 330 bur is 1.5 mm, so this becomes a good tool for gauging cavity depth. The cavosurface margin should be placed out of stress-bearing areas and should have no bevel. To help prevent stress concentration, the outline form should be composed

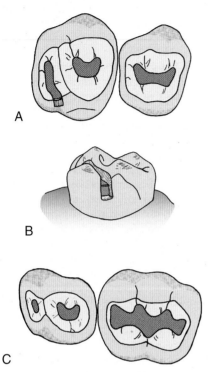

A

B

C

• **Figure 22.7** G.V. Black class I amalgam cavity preparations. (A) Maxillary right second and first primary molars (occlusal view). (B) Maxillary second primary molar, lingual view of distolingual groove preparation. (C) Mandibular right first and second primary molars (occlusal view).

of smoothly flowing arcs and curves, and all internal angles should be rounded slightly. When a dovetail is placed in the second primary molars, its buccolingual width should be greater than the width of the isthmus to produce a locking form to provide resistance against occlusal torque, which may displace the restoration mesially or distally. The isthmus should be one-third of the intercuspal width, and the buccolingual walls should converge slightly in an occlusal direction. The mesial and distal walls should flare at the marginal ridge so as not to undercut ridges. Oblique ridges should not be crossed unless they are undermined with caries or are deeply fissured. Primary mandibular second molars often exhibit buccal developmental pits. When carious, these should be restored with a small teardrop- or ovoid-shaped restoration, including all the adjacent susceptible pits and fissures. The steps of preparation and restoration of class I amalgam restorations are listed in Box 22.4.

Adhesive Restoration Preparation Design

In large part, class I adhesive restorations follow the same preparation principles as amalgam restorations. However, adhesive materials adhere to noncarious pits and fissures and can be placed successfully in shallower preparations. Therefore the preparation design for adhesive materials is typically more conservative and may incorporate elements of restorative and sealant techniques. This is referred to as a conservative adhesive restoration (CAR).

Conservative Adhesive Restorations for Primary Teeth. CAR is an updated term given to a restoration technique first described by Simonsen and Stallard in 1977[37] and refined in 1985[38] as preventive resin restoration (PRR). This restoration combines the preventive approach of sealing susceptible pits and fissures with conservative class I cavity preparation of caries occurring on the same occlusal surface. Instead of the traditional amalgam cavity preparation's "extension for prevention" beyond the area of decay into the adjacent pits and fissures, the CAR or PRR limits cavity preparation to the discrete areas of decay. These preparations are filled with an adhesive material, usually resin-based composite or compomer, and then the entire occlusal surface is sealed. This results in a restoration that conserves tooth structure and is both therapeutic and preventive. Note that "preventive resin restoration" is the nomenclature that

---

• **BOX 22.4** **Steps of Preparation and Restoration of Class I Amalgam Restorations**

1. Administer appropriate anesthesia and place the rubber dam.
2. Using a no. 330 bur in the high-speed turbine handpiece, penetrate the tooth parallel to its long axis in the central pit region and extend into all susceptible fissures and pits to a depth 0.5 mm in dentin.
3. Remove all carious dentin. Use a large, round bur in the slow-speed handpiece or a sharp spoon excavator.
4. Smooth the enamel walls and refine the final outline form with the no. 330 bur.
5. Rinse and dry the preparation, and inspect for (1) caries removal, (2) sharp cavosurface margins, and (3) removal of all unsupported enamel.
6. Triturate the amalgam, and place one carrier load of amalgam into the preparation.
7. Using a small condenser, immediately begin condensation of the amalgam into the preparation, condensing small overlapping increments with a firm pressure until the cavity is slightly overfilled.
8. Following condensation, use a ball burnisher to begin the initial contouring of the amalgam by pushing the excess amalgam up and away from the margins. Then carving of most alloys can begin almost immediately. A small cleoid-discoid carver works very well for carving primary restorations. Always keep part of the carving edge of the instrument on the tooth structure so that overcarving of the cavosurface

margin does not occur. Remove all amalgam flash from cavosurface margins. Keep the carved anatomy shallow. Placing deep anatomy in primary teeth (i.e., grooves) can weaken the restoration by creating a thin shelf of amalgam at the cavosurface margin and also by reducing the bulk of amalgam in the central stress-bearing areas, both leading to fracture.
9. When the amalgam has begun its initial set and resists deformation, begin to burnish the amalgam. Burnishing is done with a small, round burnisher, which is lightly rubbed across the carved amalgam surface to produce a satin-like appearance. Besides smoothing, burnishing creates a substructure with fewer voids and reduces finishing time.
10. A wet cotton pellet can be wiped across the burnished amalgam for a final smoothing (optional).
11. Remove the rubber dam, and check the occlusion. Children must be cautioned before the rubber dam is completely removed that they must not close their teeth into occlusion until instructed to do so. With articulating paper, check the restoration for occlusal irregularities, instructing the child to close gently. Make necessary adjustments with the carver.
12. Rinse the oral cavity and massage the soft tissue around the previously clamped tooth.

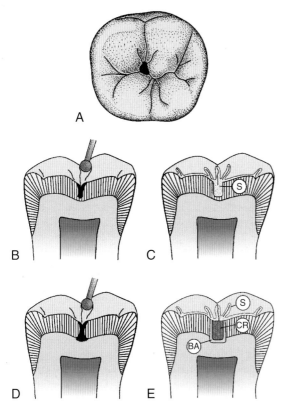

Table 22.2

Summary of Differences in Restorative Materials

	Adhesive Restorations	Amalgam
Technique	Highly technique sensitive	Less technique sensitive
Isolation	Critical	Important
Preparation design	Material properties allow for smaller, shallower preparations	Material properties require larger, more aggressive preparations
Noncarious pits and fissures	Noncarious pits and fissures can simply be sealed	Noncarious pits are included in preparation design for classic amalgams Contemporary techniques incorporate sealing over noncarious pits
Retention	Minor mechanical retention is prudent, as less enamel exists in primary teeth for bonding	Mechanical retention must be incorporated into preparation design

• **Figure 22.8** (A) The occlusal surface of a mandibular second primary molar with a small, discrete area of decay in the central pit. (B) A small bur (no. $\frac{1}{4}$ or $\frac{1}{2}$ round or Fissurotomy) is used to remove the decay, which is confined to the enamel. (C) A filled sealant *(S)* is applied into the preparation and over all susceptible pits and fissures. This is considered a sealant procedure. (D) In this diagram, the caries extends into the dentin. Again, a small round bur is used to conservatively remove the decay. (E) A bonding agent *(BA)* and resin-based composite *(CR)* material are placed in the preparation. Then a sealant *(S)* is applied over all the remaining susceptible pits and fissures.

has been historically used; however, this terminology has been replaced by "conservative adhesive restoration" to reflect the fact that other adhesive materials, besides resins, may be used in these restorations. CAR will be the term used to describe this technique in this chapter.

The CAR is ideally suited for minimal carious lesions in teeth that would otherwise lose a considerable amount of tooth structure if the extension for prevention treatment were followed.[39] Houpt and colleagues[40] reported 79% retention of CARs in permanent molars after 9 years and concluded that the CAR was a successful conservative alternative to treatment of minimal occlusal caries. Although long-term retention studies of CARs in primary teeth are lacking, with retention rates of CARs and sealants in permanent teeth being very similar, it is not unreasonable to believe that retention rates of CARs in primary teeth would also be similar to sealant rates.

Teeth that are suitable for CARs are those that demonstrate small, discrete regions of decay, often limited to a single pit (Fig. 22.8). As with sealants, the ability to isolate the tooth and keep it dry throughout the procedure is the single most important indication. Amalgam or RMGIs, being less sensitive to technique and moisture, would be the restorative materials of choice if the tooth cannot be kept dry. Many CARs do not require

anesthesia because of the minimal tooth preparation; however, soft tissue anesthesia may be necessary for comfort in placing the rubber dam.

Table 22.2 describes the differences between the two types of restorative materials.

Common Errors With Class I Restorations

Some frequent errors made in class I restorations are (1) preparing the cavity too deep; (2) undercutting the marginal ridges (particularly critical for amalgam); (3) carving the anatomy too deep; (4) not removing amalgam flash from cavosurface margins; (5) undercarving/undercontouring, which leads to subsequent fracture or tooth sensitivity from hyperocclusion; and (6) not including or sealing all susceptible fissures. Note that for amalgam an alternative to including all the susceptible fissures is to confine the amalgam preparation to the area of decay and seal the rest of the tooth with a pit and fissure sealant. Sealing over restorative materials significantly decreases microleakage[41] and increases the longevity of the restoration.[42,43]

Liners and Bases in Primary Teeth

Neither liners nor bases are very widely used in primary teeth, but various bases and liners are discussed in Chapter 21. Thin liners such as calcium hydroxide do not provide thermal insulation, and recent evidence suggests that calcium hydroxide may hydrolyze gradually,[44] leaving a small void underneath the restoration and ultimately weakening it.[45] Therefore use of calcium hydroxide is discouraged. Placement of bases in primary teeth is also uncommon, but when necessary, use of a glass ionomer or an RMGI material is recommended.

Class II Restorations

General Considerations

The outline form for several class II amalgam preparations is shown in Fig. 22.9. As with class I restorations, amalgam requires a larger and more specific form than adhesive materials. To prepare the

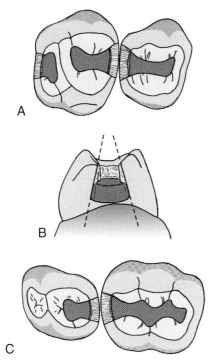

• **Figure 22.9** G.V. Black class II amalgam cavity preparations. (A) Maxillary right second and first primary molars (occlusal view). (B) Mandibular second primary molar (proximal view); note occlusal convergence of proximal walls. (C) Mandibular right first and second primary molars (occlusal view).

class II restoration, the guidelines given for the class I preparation should be followed during the preparation of the occlusal portion. Preparation of the proximal surface requires additional steps during both preparation and restoration. Placement of an interproximal wedge prior to and during preparation is highly desirable to achieve a slight separation of teeth and consequently a tighter interproximal contact of the final restoration. The wedge also protects the interproximal gingival tissue during instrumentation and thereby reduces the likelihood of hemorrhage into the proximal box during instrumentation.

Amalgam Restoration Preparation Design. For the class II amalgam, the proximal box should be broader at the cervical portion than at the occlusal portion. The buccal, lingual, and gingival walls should all break contact with the adjacent tooth, just enough to allow the tip of an explorer to pass. The buccal and lingual walls should create a 90-degree angle with the enamel. The gingival wall should be flat, not beveled, and all unsupported enamel should be removed. Ideally, the axial wall of the proximal box should be 0.5 mm into dentin and should follow the same contour as the outer proximal contour of the tooth. Because occlusal forces may permit a concentration of stress within the amalgam around sharp angles, the axiopulpal line angle is routinely beveled or rounded. No buccal or lingual retentive grooves should be placed in the proximal box. The mesiodistal width of the gingival seat should be 1 mm, which is approximately equal to the width of a no. 330 bur.

In primary teeth, many practitioners limit class II amalgam restorations to relatively small two-surface restorations. Three-surface (MOD) restorations may be done, but studies have shown that SSCs are a more durable and predictable restoration for large multiple surface restorations in primary teeth.[46,47] Messer and

Levering[48] reported that SSCs placed in 4-year-old and younger children showed a success rate approximately twice that of class II amalgams, for each year up to 10 years of service. Roberts and Sherriff[49] reported that after 5 years, one-third of class II amalgams placed in primary teeth had failed or required replacement, whereas only 8% of SSCs required retreatment. In the preschool child with large proximal carious lesions, SSCs are preferred to amalgams because of their durability. Similar-sized lesions in teeth that are within 2 or 3 years of exfoliation may be restored with amalgam because the anticipated lifespan is fairly short.

Adhesive Restoration Preparation Design. The steps in preparation and restoration of a primary or permanent molar with composite resin are very similar to those followed for restoration with amalgam but with a few alterations. For resin-based composites, absolute moisture control is a must, making a rubber dam almost mandatory. Tooth preparations for class II resin-based composites have undergone a tremendous evolution over the years, with many peculiar shapes and designs suggested. Unlike amalgam preparations, which have been well defined for years, there is no current consensus about the precise design of a class II preparation for a primary molar to receive an adhesive material. A 2001 survey of pediatric dentistry departments in North American dental schools found that 57% of the dental schools teach a conservative "box-only" preparation (with and without retention grooves), whereas 36% use and teach the traditional G.V. Black amalgam preparation.[50] Leinfelder[51] recommended that a class II preparation be primarily restricted to the region of the caries, with little to no occlusal extensions. He also states that extending the proximal box line angles in "self-cleansing" areas is not necessary and in fact creates a larger restoration that is more prone to occlusal wear. In recent years, dentin-bonding agents and adhesive restorative materials have improved dramatically, suggesting that under the right circumstances the slot preparation (Fig. 22.10) may be used effectively.[26,52–54] Although evidence indicates that the technique can be successful, experience suggests that a conservative preparation that incorporates mechanical retention such as a small dovetail or a cavosurface margin bevel[55] to increase surface area for bonding should improve retention and overall success of the restoration. Beveling not only increases the surface area to be etched but also removes the aprismatic layer of enamel which may not etch well and may leave islands of unetched enamel that can act as pathways for bacterial leakage and/or reduce resin bond strength to the enamel.[13]

Matrix Application

Matrices are placed for interproximal restorations to aid in restoring normal contour and contact areas and to prevent extrusion of restorative materials into gingival tissues. Many types of matrix bands are available for use in pediatric dentistry. Regardless of the type of matrix band used, after it is in place and a wedge firmly inserted, a small ball burnisher can be used to burnish the band in the area of the contact point against the adjacent tooth. This will help provide a tight proximal contact.

1. T band: allows for multiple matrices; no special equipment is needed.
2. Sectional matrices (e.g., Strip-T, Denovo Dental, Inc., Baldwin Park, CA; Palodent Plus Sectional Matrices, Dentsply Sirona): allow for multiple matrix placement, are very easy to use, are not circumferential, must be held in place by a wedge.
3. AutoMatrix (Dentsply Sirona): allows for multiple matrix placement, is very easy to use, requires special tightening and removal tools.

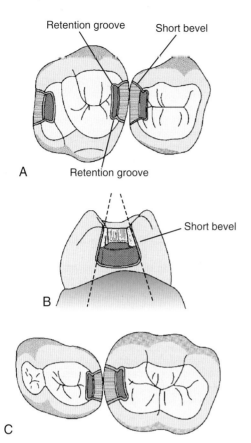

• **Figure 22.10** Modified class II cavity preparations for adhesive restorative materials. Note the short bevel around the preparations and small retention groves. (A) Maxillary right second and first primary molars (occlusal view). (B) Mandibular second primary molar (proximal view); note occlusal convergence of proximal walls. (C) Mandibular right first and second primary molars (occlusal view).

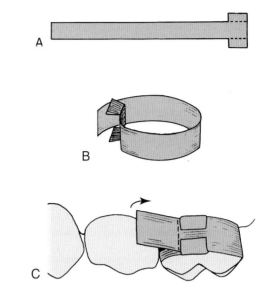

• **Figure 22.11** (A) The T-band matrix. (B) The T band is formed into a circle, and the extension wings are folded down to secure the band. (C) The T band is adapted to fit the tooth tightly and is trimmed with scissors, and the free end is bent back.

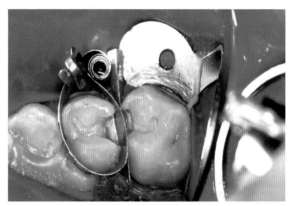

• **Figure 22.12** A sectional matrix (Strip-T, Denovo) is placed onto a mesioocclusal preparation of the second primary molar. An AutoMatrix (Dentsply Sirona) is seen placed on the distoocclusal preparation of the first primary molar. The matrix can be tightened to draw the band more closely to the tooth. A wedge secures both in place.

4. Tofflemire matrix: is used infrequently because it does not fit primary tooth contour well and is difficult to place as multiple matrices.

T bands are available in different sizes, contours, and materials. A straight, narrow, brass T band will work in almost all pediatric restorative procedures. The T-band matrix (Fig. 22.11) is formed by folding the band back on itself in the form of a circle and by folding over the extension wings of the "T" to make an adjustable loop. The band is contoured and positioned onto the tooth with the folded extension wings on the buccal surface. The free end of the band is drawn mesially to pull the band snugly against the tooth. The extension folds are then grasped firmly with a pair of Howe no. 110 pliers and removed from the tooth. The band should then be tightened an additional 0.5 to 1.0 mm, and the free end should be bent back over the vertical folds and cut with scissors to a length of 5 to 6 mm. The band is then reseated onto the tooth and wedged. It must fit below the gingival margin of the preparation and must also be at least 1 mm higher than the marginal ridge of the adjacent tooth. The T band is removed by opening the extension wings with an explorer or spoon excavator and allowing the band to open. Scissors are then used to cut one end of the band close to the restored proximal surface, the wedge is removed, and the band is then drawn buccally or lingually through the contact.

There are many commercially available sectional matrices or "matrix pieces." One commonly used in pediatrics is the Strip-T matrix. They are stainless steel matrix strips approximately one-half inch long that do not encircle the prepared tooth but rather fit only in the prepared proximal area. For small class II preparations, they are very simple to place and use. After placement, they must be firmly wedged to stay in place. They are not recommended for proximal preparations that extend beyond the line angles; a circumferential matrix (or SSC) is more appropriate in that instance.

AutoMatrix is a preformed loop of stainless steel matrix material that is placed on the tooth (Fig. 22.12) and tightened with a special tightening tool that comes with the kit. A small pin automatically keeps the tightened matrix tightly bound around the tooth. To remove the matrix, this small pin is clipped (another special tool) and the matrix is easily loosened and removed.

Placement of Restorative Materials in Class II Restorations

Amalgam. The steps of preparation and restoration of class II amalgam restorations are listed in Box 22.5.

• BOX 22.5 **Steps of Preparation and Restoration for Class II Amalgam Restorations**

1. Administer appropriate anesthesia, and place the rubber dam.
2. Place a wooden wedge in the interproximal area being restored (optional). This retracts the gingival papilla during instrumentation, keeps the operator from cutting the interseptal rubber dam material and underlying gingiva, and creates some prewedging, which helps to ensure a tight proximal contact of the final restoration.
3. Using a no. 330 bur in the high-speed turbine handpiece with a light, brushing motion, prepare the occlusal outline form at ideal depth.
4. To prepare the proximal box, begin at the marginal ridge by brushing the bur buccolingually in a pendulum motion and in a gingival direction at the dentin-enamel junction. Continue until contact is just broken between the adjacent tooth and the gingival wall and the wedge is seen. If the gingival wall is made too deep, the cervical constriction of the primary molar will create a very narrow gingival seat. The widest buccolingual width of the box will be at the gingival margin. Take care not to damage the adjacent proximal surface.
5. Remove any remaining caries with a sharp spoon excavator or with a round bur in the low-speed handpiece.
6. Round the axiopulpal line angle slightly. Because of the shape of the no. 330 bur, all other internal line angles will automatically be gently rounded.
7. Remove the wedge placed at the beginning of the treatment and place a matrix band.
8. While holding the matrix band in place, forcefully reinsert the wedge between the matrix band and the adjacent tooth, beneath the gingival seat of the preparation. The wedge is placed with a pair of Howe pliers or cotton forceps from the widest embrasure. The wedge should hold the band tightly against the tooth but should not push the band into the

proximal box. It may be necessary to trim the wedge slightly to achieve a proper fit.
9. Triturate the amalgam. With the amalgam carrier, add the amalgam to the preparation in single increments, beginning in the proximal box.
10. Using a small condenser, condense the amalgam into the corners of the proximal box and against the matrix band to ensure the reestablishment of a tight proximal contact. Continue filling and condensing until the entire cavity is overfilled.
11. Use a small round burnisher to begin the initial contouring of the amalgam. Carving of the occlusal portion is performed with a small cleoid-discoid carver, as in class I restorations. The marginal ridge can be carved with the tip of an explorer or with a Hollenback carver.
12. Carefully remove the wedge and the matrix band. Drawing the band in a buccal-lingual direction, as opposed to an occlusal direction, will be less likely to damage the marginal ridge of the newly placed restoration during withdrawal.
13. Remove excess amalgam at the buccal, lingual, and gingival margins with an explorer or Hollenback carver. Check to see that the height of the newly restored marginal ridge is approximately equal to the adjacent marginal ridge.
14. Gently floss the interproximal contact to check the tightness of the contact, to check for gingival overhang, and to remove any loose amalgam particles from the interproximal region.
15. Do a final burnish of the restoration, and use a wet cotton pellet held with the cotton pliers for final smoothing if necessary.
16. Remove the rubber dam carefully.
17. Check the occlusion for irregularities with articulating paper, and adjust as needed.

Adhesive Restorations. If an RMGI base or liner is to be used, it should be placed and cured before the etching or adhesive steps. For details regarding specifics of adhesive systems, refer to Chapter 40. The preparation should be etched for 15 to 20 seconds with an acid gel. The etchant should extend well beyond the cavosurface margin to cover any susceptible pits and fissures not included in the preparation. After thoroughly rinsing the etch from the tooth, a dentin-bonding agent is applied and cured. Several self-etching bonding systems are now available that eliminate the separate etching and rinsing steps. However, not all self-etching systems can be used successfully in primary teeth, and clinical studies are lacking as to their effectiveness.[13] Following application of the adhesive, many clinicians will place a flowable resin-based composite as a cavity liner. Although not mandatory, it appears that use of a thin (0.5 to 1 mm) flowable liner reduces the voids at the cervical cavosurface margin in class II restorations[56] and may consequently reduce microleakage. The flowable material may be cured before placement of the packable material, but best marginal sealing likely comes from placement of the packable composite over a thin, uncured flowable liner.

Many resin-based composites and compomers are prepackaged in small ampules that can be injected directly into the preparation. A plastic instrument or a condenser can be used to pack or condense the composite into the preparation. No more than a 2- to 4-mm depth of composite should be polymerized at one time. There is some debate about whether resin-based composites should be placed in bulk or incrementally. It appears that one of the primary concerns is that the curing light must penetrate to the full depth of the material. Limiting the depth of material placed to 2 to 4 mm per increment should ensure full polymerization. Incremental placement may also reduce polymerization shrinkage, a suspected cause of dentin-bonding agent failure and postoperative

sensitivity. Complete curing or polymerization of the material is very important to the success of the restoration. Undercuring may lead to a weakened restoration prone to failure under masticatory forces. When placing the final increment of packable resin, slightly overfill the preparation with material and use a ball burnisher to push the material toward and up over the enamel margins. This will remove excess material and effectively act as a carver. Do not use a cleoid-discoid carver on resin-based composite material. Use the tip of the explorer to carve the marginal ridge away from the matrix band. Remember to always move the instrument from material to tooth, pushing the material toward the margins. If you move instruments from tooth to restoration, you will likely pull material away from the margins, leaving a gap. After final cure of the restoration, remove the wedge and matrix band and cure the restoration one more time, directing the light toward the proximal from a buccal or lingual approach. Finishing can begin immediately following polymerization. The occlusal surface is grossly contoured with round, high-speed carbide finishing burs or fine-finishing diamond burs. Gross contouring of proximal surfaces is accomplished with flame-shaped, high-speed carbide finishing burs and with garnet disks, where accessible. Final finishing can be completed with a white stone or with rubber abrasive points to eliminate surface irregularities and final polishing with a composite polish or gloss. Fine abrasive disks or strips are used for final polishing of accessible proximal margins. The application of a surface sealant after polishing may serve to reduce occlusal wear and contraction gaps.[57]

Adjacent or Back-to-Back Class II Restorations

Amalgam. Adjacent interproximal lesions are not uncommon in the primary dentition. From the standpoint of time and patient management, it is desirable to restore these lesions simultaneously.

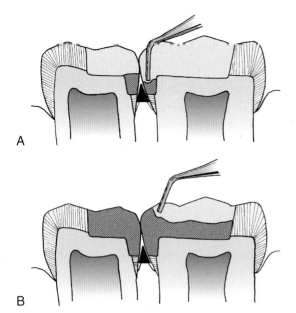

• **Figure 22.13** "Back-to-back" amalgam preparations. (A) After wedging, begin condensing the adjacent proximal boxes alternately. (B) Continue condensing the amalgams alternately until both preparations are slightly overfilled.

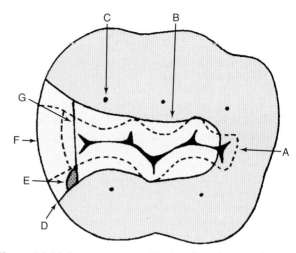

• **Figure 22.14** Common errors with class II amalgam cavity preparations. (A) Failure to extend occlusal outline into all susceptible pits and fissures. (B) Failure to follow the outline of the cusps. (C) Isthmus cut too wide. (D) Flare of proximal walls too great. (E) Angle formed by the axial, buccal, and lingual walls too great. (F) Gingival contact with adjacent tooth not broken. (G) Axial wall not conforming to the proximal contour of the tooth, and the mesiodistal width of the gingival floor is greater than 1 mm. (Modified from Forrester DJ, Wagner M, Fleming J. *Pediatric Dental Medicine*. Philadelphia: Lea & Febiger; 1981.)

Preparation for adjacent proximal restorations is identical to those previously described. A matrix is placed on each tooth and is properly wedged. T bands, sectional matrices, or automatrices are preferable because multiple matrix holders are difficult to place side by side. Condensation of the amalgam should be done in small increments, alternately in each preparation, so that the restorations are filled simultaneously (Fig. 22.13). Condensation pressure toward the matrix will help to ensure a tight interproximal contact. Carve the marginal ridges to an equal height, and carefully remove the wedge and matrix bands one at a time. Final carving is like that described for solitary class II restorations.

Adhesive Restorations. Placement of adjacent back-to-back class II resin-based composite restorations is acceptable and encouraged when there are two adjacent carious lesions to be restored, but the method is different from that of placing back-to-back amalgam restorations. After the preparations are completed, matrix bands or segmental matrices are placed on both preparations and a wedge is forcefully inserted between the two bands. Be certain that the placement of the matrices allows a convexity to the proximal surface of both teeth. Sometimes the matrices are placed such that if the resin material were placed into the preps, one proximal surface would be vastly overcontoured and the adjacent surface vastly undercontoured. This will result in two poorly contoured restorations. This can be prevented by carefully placing the matrices and observing their contour before resin placement; or by putting the matrix on one tooth, restoring it completely, and then placing the matrix band on the second tooth and restoring it. However, it is possible to place both matrices and restore simultaneously. With two matrix bands in place, etch and bond both preparations. To avoid voids in the proximal box, put the tip of the composite ampule in the bottom of the box against the gingival floor and slowly back fill the box. Next completely fill, contour, and polymerize one of the restorations. To ensure a tight contact between the two restorations, after the first restoration is polymerized, use a small ball burnisher and burnish the matrix band against the newly placed restoration

in the area where you want to create the contact point. Then add, contour, and polymerize the resin-based composite material in the second preparation. Remove the wedge and bands, and finishing and polishing procedures are identical to single restoration placement.

Common Problems With Class II Restorations

Class II restorations are prone to many of the errors discussed previously for class I restorations. In addition to these considerations, it is important to recognize that the proximal box of a class II preparation is a feature that can contribute to recurrent decay or restoration loss. Indeed, most restorative problems in pediatric dentistry result from a failure to prepare and restore the teeth in a way that considers their anatomic or morphologic structural characteristics (Fig. 22.14). Marginal failure in the proximal box, usually owing to an excessive flare of the cavosurface margin, is a common issue with class II restorations. Failure to remove all caries during preparation and leaving material voids due to inadequate condensation also contribute to restoration failure.[58,59] Failure of adhesive restorations may also result due to deviation from manufacturer recommendations for light cure time and maximum material depth.

Finishing of Adhesive and Amalgam Restorations

Finishing and polishing of adhesive restorations is standard practice and is described in detail previously. On the other hand, polishing of amalgams is no longer routinely recommended. Historically, polishing of amalgams was advocated to (1) eliminate surface scratches and blemishes, which act as centers of corrosion, (2) remove any remaining amalgam flash not carved away, and (3) refine the anatomy and occlusion. However, good burnishing and carving during placement eliminates most of the need for polishing. Although there are no contraindications to amalgam polishing, there is little evidence that polishing amalgam restorations contributes to their clinical success or longevity; thus this procedure has generally fallen out of favor.

Full Coronal Coverage of Primary Molars

Preformed metal crowns, also referred to as stainless steel crowns (SSCs), were introduced to pediatric dentistry by Humphrey in 1950.[60] Since then, they have become an invaluable restorative material and treatment of choice for badly broken down primary teeth. As mentioned previously, they are generally considered superior to large, multisurface amalgam or adhesive restorations and have a longer clinical lifespan than two- or three-surface restorations.[46–48,61,62] The crowns are manufactured in different sizes as a metal shell with some preformed anatomy and are trimmed and contoured as necessary to fit individual teeth.

There are two commonly used types of SSCs:

1. Precontoured crowns (e.g., 3M ESPE Stainless Steel Crowns, Minneapolis, MN; and Acero 3S crowns [Acero Crowns, Seattle, WA]): This type of crown is by far the most popular and their use is recommended. Their anatomy more closely resembles a natural tooth. These crowns are prefestooned and precontoured. Some trimming and contouring may be necessary but usually is minimal. If trimming of these crowns becomes necessary, the precontour will be lost and the crown will fit more loosely than before trimming.

2. Pretrimmed crowns (e.g., Unitek stainless steel crowns [3M ESPE] and Denovo Crowns): These crowns have straight, noncontoured sides but are festooned to follow a line parallel to the gingival crest. They still require contouring and some trimming. These are good crowns but require much more time and effort for placement and are not widely used.

The biggest parental complaint about SSCs is their esthetics. Unfortunately, there are no tooth-colored, durable SSCs available; however, there are other esthetic full coverage options which have been gaining in popularity since 2010. One such option is a premade ZC for primary teeth (Fig. 22.15). There is still not a lot of clinical information available about zirconia ceramic crowns for primary teeth; however, ZCs in adults have been shown to be very esthetic, durable, stain resistant, biocompatible, and retentive,[63] so it is anticipated that their performance in children will be similar. Although zirconia is a very hard material, it appears that ZCs do not cause excessive wear on the enamel of opposing teeth.[64] Like SSCs, these primary ZCs come in six premade sizes and can be prepared, fit, and cemented in a 20- to 30-minute visit. Their indications and placement will be discussed later. Two other esthetic full coverage alternatives which are not widely used are resin-bonded posterior strip crowns (Space Maintainers Laboratory, Chatsworth, CA) and a preveneered molar crown which is an SSC with a composite veneer overlay on the buccal and occlusal surfaces (e.g., NuSmile Primary Crowns, Houston, TX; and Cheng Crowns, Exton, PA). Because of their infrequent use, they will not be discussed in chapter.

SSCs are by far the most frequently used full coverage crown in the primary dentition, but the use of ZCs is increasing in popularity. The indications for use of both are listed in Box 22.6. The steps of preparation and placement of SSCs and ZCs are listed in Box 22.7 and are shown in Fig. 22.16.

Special Considerations for Primary Crown Placement[65]

Placement of Adjacent Crowns. When quadrant dentistry is practiced, it often is necessary to place SSCs or ZCs on adjacent teeth. The tooth preparation and crown selection for placing multiple crowns are similar to that previously described for single crowns. However, there are several areas of consideration as follows:

- Prepare occlusal reduction of one tooth completely before beginning occlusal reduction of the other tooth. When reduction of two teeth is performed simultaneously, the tendency is to underreduce both.

- Insufficient proximal reduction is a common problem when adjacent crowns are placed. Contact between adjacent proximal surfaces should be broken, producing approximately 1.5-mm separation at the gingival level.

- Both crowns should be trimmed, contoured, and prepared for cementation simultaneously. It is generally best to begin placement and cementation of the more distal tooth first. However, most importantly, the sequence of placement of crowns for cementation should follow the same sequence as when the crowns were placed for final fitting. Sometimes crowns will seat quite easily in one placement sequence and will seat with great difficulty if the sequence is altered.

Preparing Crowns in Areas of Space Loss. Frequently, when the tooth structure is lost because of caries, a loss of contact and drifting of adjacent teeth into space normally occupied by the tooth to be restored occurs. When this happens, the crown required to fit over the buccolingual dimension will be too wide mesiodistally to be placed and a crown selected to fit the mesiodistal space will be too small in circumference. Placing ZCs in areas of space loss can be extremely challenging and may be a contraindication to their placement. This is because the ZCs cannot be reshaped and the only way to get them to fit in areas of space loss is extensive

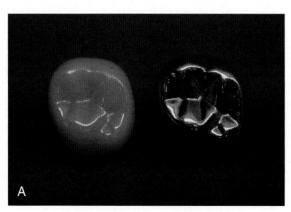
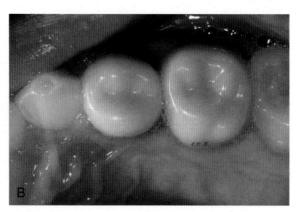

• **Figure 22.15** (A) A zirconia primary molar crown and a molar stainless steel crown. (B) Zirconia crowns on first and second primary molars.

HALL TECHNIQUE OF STAINLESS STEEL CROWN PLACEMENT

N. Sue Seale

The Hall technique (HT) of stainless steel crown (SSC) placement represents a remarkable change over the past 10 years in the use of SSCs. The technique, first practiced in 1988 by N. Hall, a general practitioner in Scotland, used a novel technique where a crown was fitted and cemented over a caries affected primary molar without local anesthetic (LA), caries removal, or tooth preparation.[1,2] There have been a number of investigations, both retrospective and prospective, published about SSCs placed with the HT,[2–5] and the authors all concluded that HT was a predictable restorative option with low retreatment rates.

The technique is simple. On the day of crown placement, the child should be seated in the dental chair and kept in an upright position because no rubber dam is used and the airway must be protected. No LA is administered. The dentist chooses the smallest SSC that will seat over the unprepared tooth. It should cover all cusps with a feeling of "spring back," and there should be no attempt to seat the crown during try-in. The chosen SSC is then filled with glass ionomer (GI) cement and seated over the caries affected primary molar, initially using finger pressure and then the child's own occlusal force if necessary. Excess cement is removed, and occlusal pressure maintained by having the child bite on a cotton roll until the cement sets. Occlusion is allowed to adjust to the increased occlusovertical dimension over time. Because the HT of SSC placement requires no tooth preparation, occasionally orthodontic spacers are needed in the interproximal areas of the tooth to be crowned to create the spacing necessary to allow easy placement of the crown. The spacers are left in place for several days prior to the crown appointment.[1,6]

The HT has been controversial since its introduction into the United States due to the initial open bite created by cementing the SSC over an unprepared tooth and because all caries-affected dentin is sealed in the tooth under the SSC. However, studies show the open bite resolved within the first month,[3,7] and sealing caries-affected dentin in teeth is much like an indirect pulp cap, which has abundant good evidence that it works so long as the seal is maintained and the pulpal status is properly diagnosed pretreatment.[8,9] To that end, high-quality radiographs showing the furcation and a thorough clinical history for symptoms are mandatory in selecting teeth to receive the HT of SSC placement.

Despite the controversy associated with the HT, there are definitely indications for its use in the United States. Young, uncooperative children who have open, active caries in their primary molars, but who have no funding for treatment in the operating room or who are placed on long wait lists to receive such treatment, can be treated on an interim basis with the HT. Newly erupting permanent molars with enamel hypoplasia and early destruction of the occlusal surfaces can be treated with the HT until the tooth erupts sufficiently to receive a more definitive restoration. The HT of SSC placement can be used much as interim therapeutic restoration (ITR) with GI has been used in the past. It provides an interim approach for large lesions where the tooth is badly broken down, and IRT with GI would not have the strength to protect the tooth.

As the HT receives increased use and more well-designed prospective studies evaluate its long-term effectiveness, there may be more acceptance of it, and more uses may become evident.

References

1. Innes N, Evans D, Hall N. The Hall technique for managing carious primary molars. *Dent Update*. 2009;36:472–478.
2. Innes NP, Stirrups DR, Evans DJ, et al. A novel technique using preformed metal crowns for managing carious primary molars in general practice—a retrospective analysis. *Brit Dent J*. 2006;200:451–454.
3. Innes NP, Evans DJ, Stirrups DR. The Hall technique: a randomized controlled clinical trial of a novel method of managing carious primary molars in general dental practice: acceptability of the technique and outcomes at 23 months. *BMC Oral Health*. 2007;7:18.
4. Innes NP, Evans DJ, Stirrups DR. Sealing caries in primary molars: randomized control trial, 5-year results. *J Dent Res*. 2011;90: 1405–1410.
5. Ludwig KH, Fontana M, Vinson LA, et al. The success of stainless steel crowns placed with the Hall technique: a retrospective study. *J Am Dent Assoc*. 2014;145:1248–1253.
6. *Hall Technique Guide, A Users Manual*. Version 3, University of Dundee, Scotland.
7. van der Zee V, van Amerongen WE. Influence of preformed metal crowns (Hall technique) on the occlusal vertical dimension in the primary dentition. *Eur Arch Paediatr Dent*. 2010;11:225–227.
8. Falster CA, Araujo FB, Straffon LH, et al. Indirect pulp treatment: in vivo outcomes of an adhesive resin system vs calcium hydroxide for protection of the dentin-pulp complex. *Pediatr Dent*. 2002;24:241–248.
9. Ricketts DN, Lamont T, Innes NP, et al. Operative caries management in adults and children. *Cochrane Database Syst Rev*. 2013;(3):CD003808.

• BOX 22.6   Indications for Use of Full Coverage Primary Crowns

1. Restoration of primary or young permanent teeth with extensive carious lesions. These include primary teeth with extensive decay, large lesions, or multiple surface lesions. First primary molars with mesial interproximal lesions are included in the category because the morphologic appearance that the tooth exhibits results in inadequate support for mesial interproximal restorations.
2. Restoration of hypoplastic primary or permanent teeth.
3. Restoration of primary teeth following pulpotomy or pulpectomy procedures.
4. Restoration of teeth with hereditary anomalies such as dentinogenesis imperfecta or amelogenesis imperfecta.
5. Restorations in disabled individuals or others in whom oral hygiene is extremely poor and failure of other materials is likely.
6. As an abutment for space maintainers or prosthetic appliances (stainless steel crowns only, not zirconia).
7. Strong consideration should be given to the use of full coverage restorations in children who require general anesthesia for dental treatment and demonstrate a high caries risk.

Data from Seale NS. The use of stainless steel crowns. Pediatr Dent. 2002;24(5):501–505.

circumferential tooth reduction. For SSCs a larger crown, which will fit over the tooth's greatest convexity, is selected and an adjustment is made to reduce mesiodistal width (Fig. 22.17). This adjustment is accomplished by grasping the marginal ridges of the crown with Howe utility pliers and squeezing it, thereby reducing the mesiodistal dimension. Considerable recontouring of proximal, buccal, and lingual walls of the crown with the no. 137 or no. 114 pliers will be necessary (Fig. 22.18). If difficulty in crown placement is still encountered, additional tooth reduction of the buccal and lingual surfaces and selection of another, smaller crown may be necessary. When the area of space loss is in the region of the distal surface of a mandibular first primary molar and difficulty

• BOX 22.7 Steps for Preparation and Placement of Stainless Steel Crowns and Zirconia Crowns on Primary Molars

Several different preparation designs have been advocated for stainless steel crowns (SSCs) over the years. Only one such preparation, requiring minimal tooth reduction for SSCs, is discussed here. Necessary adjustments for zirconia crown preparation, fitting, and cementation are noted for each step.

1. Evaluate the preoperative occlusion. Note the dental midline and the cusp-fossa relationship bilaterally.

2. Administer appropriate local anesthesia, ensuring that all soft tissues surrounding the tooth to be crowned are well anesthetized, and place a rubber dam. Because gingival tissues all around the tooth may be manipulated during crown placement, it is important to obtain lingual or palatal, as well as buccal or facial anesthesia.

3. Reduction of the occlusal surface is carried out with a no. 169L taper fissure bur or a football diamond in the high-speed handpiece. Make depth cuts by cutting the occlusal grooves to a depth of 1.0–1.5 mm, and extend through the buccal, lingual, and proximal surfaces. Next, place the bur on its side and uniformly reduce the remaining occlusal surface by 1.5 mm, maintaining the cuspal inclines of the crown (see Fig. 22.15). Establish access to decay with a no. 330 or 169L bur in the high-speed handpiece. Then remove decay with a large, round bur in the low-speed handpiece or with a spoon excavator. **Note:** *If a zirconia crown is going to be placed, slightly more occlusal reduction (1.5–2 mm) will be necessary.*

4. Proximal reduction is also accomplished with the taper fissure bur or thin, tapered diamond. Contact with the adjacent tooth must be broken gingivally and buccolingually, maintaining vertical walls with only a slight convergence in an occlusal direction. Proximal reduction should be approximately 1 mm. The gingival proximal margin should have a feather-edge finish line. Care must be taken not to damage adjacent tooth structure. **Note:** *For placement of a zirconia crown, proximal reduction should be at least 1.5 mm mesially and distally but also ending in a feather-edge.*

5. Round all line angles, using the side of the bur or diamond. The occlusobuccal and occlusolingual line angles are rounded by holding the bur at a 30- to 45-degree angle to the occlusal surface and sweeping it in a mesiodistal direction. For SSCs, buccolingual reduction is often limited to this beveling and is confined to the occlusal one-third of the crown. If problems are later encountered in selecting an appropriate crown size or in fitting a crown over a large mesiobuccal bulge, more reduction of the buccal and lingual tooth structure may become necessary. **Important Note:** *If a zirconia crown is being placed, circumferential reduction including the buccal and lingual surfaces is definitely necessary and all bulges and heights of convexity must be removed, especially on the mesiobuccal. The buccal and lingual proximal line angles are rounded by holding the bur parallel to the tooth's long axis and blending the surfaces together. All angles of the preparation should be rounded to remove corners. Avoid an overtapered preparation.*

6. Selection of an SSC crown begins as a trial-and-error procedure. The goal is to place the smallest crown that can be seated on the tooth and to establish preexisting proximal contacts. (*Helpful hint:* Size 4 is a frequently used crown size for molar SSCs.) The selected SSC is tried on the preparation by seating the lingual first and applying pressure in a buccal direction so that the crown slides over the buccal surface into the gingival sulcus. Friction should be felt as the crown slips over the buccal bulge. Some teeth are an "in-between" size, so that one crown size is too small to seat and the next larger size fits very loosely, even after contouring. Further tooth reduction, especially on the buccal and lingual surfaces, may be necessary in these cases to seat the smaller crown. After seating a crown, establish a preliminary occlusal relationship by comparing adjacent marginal ridge heights. If the crown does not seat to the same level as the adjacent teeth, the occlusal reduction may be inadequate; the crown may be too long; a gingival proximal ledge may exist; or contact may not have been broken with the adjacent tooth, preventing a complete seating of the crown. An extensive area of gingival blanching around the crown indicates that the crown is too long or is grossly overcontoured. Some crowns may need to be trimmed slightly for a better fit. Crown and bridge trimming scissors, a heatless stone

mounted on the low-speed straight handpiece, and a rubber wheel can be used to neatly trim and smooth an SSC. A properly trimmed crown should extend approximately 1 mm into the gingival sulcus. The margins of the finished, trimmed steel crown consist of a series of curves or arcs as determined by the marginal gingiva of the tooth being restored. There should be no corners, jagged angles, right angles, or straight lines found on these margins (see Fig. 22.16). **Note:** *Selection of zirconia crowns is also trial and error; however, when a zirconia crown does not seat completely onto a tooth, the crown cannot be adjusted and more tooth preparation is required until the crown slides over the preparation and is completely seated when compared with adjacent teeth. If the crown fits very loosely, a smaller crown should be selected. If it does not seat completely, further reduction of the tooth will be necessary. Often the zirconia crown does not seat well because of a gingival ledge on the preparation. Do not force a zirconia crown onto the preparation. The thin zirconia margins will not flex and may break if forced over a ledge or bulge.*

7. Contour and crimp the SSC to form a tightly fitting crown. Contouring involves bending the gingival one-third of the crown's margins inward to restore anatomic features of the natural crown and to reduce the marginal circumference of the crown, ensuring a good fit. Contouring is accomplished circumferentially with a no. 114 ball-and-socket pliers (see Fig. 22.17A) or with a no. 137 Gordon pliers. Final close adaptation of the crown is achieved by crimping the cervical margin 1 mm circumferentially. The no. 137 pliers may be used for this; special crimping pliers, such as no. 800-417 (3M ESPE; see Fig. 22.17B), are also available. A tight marginal fit aids in (1) mechanical retention of the crown, (2) protection of the cement from exposure to oral fluids, and (3) maintenance of gingival health. After contouring and crimping, firm resistance should be encountered when the crown is seated. After seating the crown, examine the gingival margins with an explorer for areas of poor fit. Observe the gingival tissue for blanching, and examine the proximal contacts. When removing the crown, a scaler or amalgam carver can be used to engage the gingival margin and dislodge the crown. A thumb or finger should be kept over the crown during removal so that movement of the crown is controlled. **Note:** *There is no contouring, crimping, or trimming a zirconia crown.*

8. The rubber dam is removed and the crown replaced so that the occlusion may be checked. Examine the occlusion bilaterally with the patient in centric occlusion. Look for movement of the crown occlusogingivally with biting pressure, and check for excessive gingival blanching. After the rubber dam is removed, special care must be taken when handling the crown in the mouth. A 2 × 2-inch gauze pad should be placed posterior to the tooth being crowned to prevent the crown from dropping into the oropharynx.

9. If the SSC was trimmed, final smoothing and polishing of the crown margin should be performed before cementation to ensure there are no jagged edges.

10. Rinse and dry the SSC inside and out, and prepare to cement it. Any number of cements, including glass ionomer, polycarboxylate, or self-curing resin ionomer cement, can be used. A glass ionomer cement is preferred for SSCs. The crown is filled approximately two-thirds with cement, with all inner surfaces covered. **Note:** *Before cementation, the inside of a zirconia crown should be free of contamination. Salivary and hemorrhagic by-products will adhere to the surface of zirconia and cannot be simply washed away. If the crown has been in contact with blood or saliva it is advisable to clean the interior by sandblasting, or use of a decontaminating agent such as Ivoclean (Ivoclar Vivadent, Amherst, NY). This will ensure maximum cement retention. A light activated resin-modified glass ionomer or bioactive cement is recommended for cementation of zirconia cement.*

11. Dry the tooth with compressed air and seat the SSC completely. Cement should be expressed from all margins. The handle of a mirror or the flat end of a band pusher may be used to ensure complete seating, or the patient may be instructed to bite on a tongue blade. Before the cement sets, have the patient close into centric occlusion and confirm that the

occlusion has not been altered. *Note: For zirconia crowns make sure the preparation is free of saliva and blood, and seat the crown gently, tack cure the cement (if light activated), and carefully removed excess cement while keeping the crown stabilized with finger pressure. After cement removal, finish curing the cement from buccal, lingual, and occlusal directions.*

12. Cement must be removed from the gingival sulcus. Excessive glass ionomer cement can be removed immediately with a wet gauze and/or

water spray. The interproximal areas can be cleaned by tying a knot in a piece of dental floss and drawing the floss through the interproximal region. A scaler may be needed to remove hardened cement.

13. Rinse the oral cavity well, and reexamine the occlusion and the soft tissues before dismissing the patient. *Note: You cannot adjust the occlusion of an SSC, and it is extremely difficult to adjust a zirconia crown. If the occlusion requires adjustment, consideration should be made to adjusting the tooth opposing the crown.*

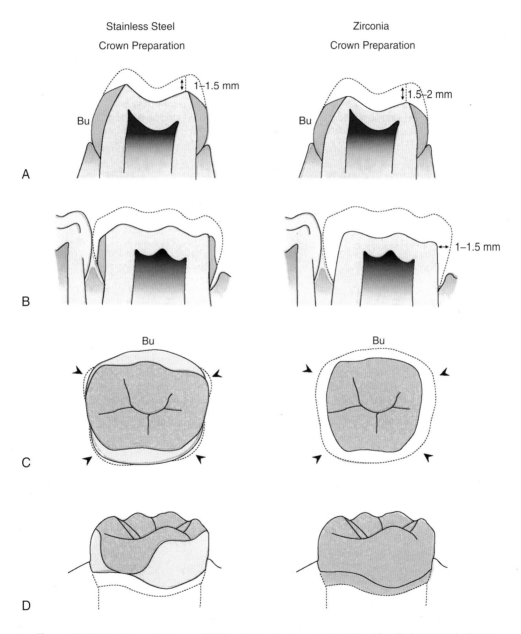

• **Figure 22.16** Stainless steel crown (SSC) and zirconia crown preparation. Mandibular second primary molar. (A) Proximal view. Note there is more occlusal reduction for zirconia crowns. *Bu,* Buccal. (B) Buccal view. Note feather-edge gingival margins on both crown preps but more proximal reduction for zirconia. (C) Occlusal view. Note for SSCs the line angles are just rounded, but circumferential reduction is necessary for the zirconia. (D) Mesiolingual view. For SSCs, lingual and buccal reduction is limited to beveling of the occlusal third, but for zirconia it extends subgingivally to a feather-edge.

is encountered finding the appropriate size crown because of the space loss, another alternative exists. Select a maxillary first primary molar crown for the opposite side of the mouth and try it on the mandibular tooth. Owing to the space loss, often the mandibular tooth preparation resembles a maxillary tooth and therefore is more suited for placement of the maxillary crown. By selecting the maxillary crown for the opposite side of the mouth, the crown's gingival margin contour in the area of the mesiobuccal cervical bulge fits the mandibular mesiobuccal cervical bulge. If several millimeters of space have been lost, it may be necessary to extract the tooth and place a space maintainer rather than struggle to place a crown on a compromised tooth preparation.

Restoration of Primary Incisors and Canines

Indications for restoration of primary incisors and canines are generally based on the presence of (1) caries, (2) trauma, or (3) developmental defects of the tooth's hard tissue. Adhesive materials,

usually resin-based composites or resin ionomer products, are placed into class III and class V restorations in primary anterior teeth. Class IV restorations may also be done; however, if a great deal of tooth structure has been lost, full coverage with a crown will provide a superior restoration.

Class III Adhesive Restorations

Class III adhesive restorations on primary incisors are very challenging to do well (Fig. 22.19). Caries often extend subgingivally, making good isolation and hemorrhage control difficult. Because of the large size of the pulps of these teeth, the preparations must be kept very small. A simple slot preparation may be used, which merely removes decay and has a short cavosurface bevel.[66] However, in children, especially those with bruxism, experience has revealed that retention of class III restorations solely with acid etching can be inadequate, and additional mechanical retention may be required. Retention can be gained with retentive locks on the facial or lingual

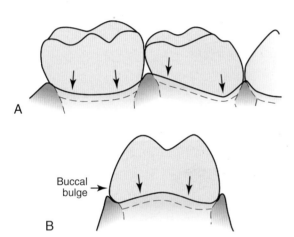

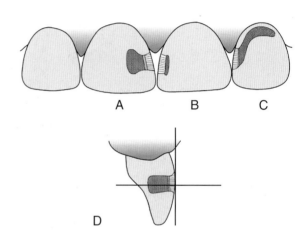

• **Figure 22.17** (A) The buccal gingival contour of the second primary molar *(left)* has been described as a smile, and the buccal gingival contour of the first primary molar has been described as a stretched-out S. Note the contour in the region of the mesiobuccal bulge of the first primary molar. The gingival contour of all the lingual surfaces (not pictured) is a smile. (B) The proximal gingival contour of primary molars has been described as a frown because the shortest occlusocervical heights are approximately midpoint buccolingually.

• **Figure 22.19** Class III cavity preparations (*A, B, C*: labial view). Note that a short bevel is placed on the cavosurface margin of all three preparations. (*A*) Slot preparation with a dovetail (a frequently used class III preparation). The dovetail provides additional retention. (*B*) Slot preparation, used for very small class III carious lesions. (*C*) Modified slot preparation, used when extensive gingival decalcification is evident adjacent to interproximal caries. (*D*) The interproximal box is placed perpendicular to a line tangent to the labial surface.

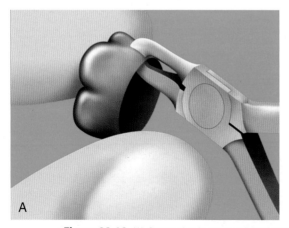

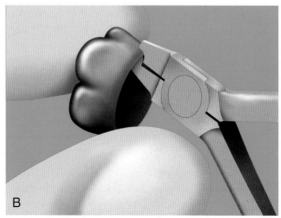

• **Figure 22.18** (A) Contouring is accomplished with a no. 114 pliers. (B) Final crimping is accomplished with a no. 800-417 pliers. (Courtesy 3M ESPE, St. Paul, MN.)

surface and by beveling the cavosurface margin to increase the surface area of the enamel etched.[67,68] It has been suggested that preparing the entire facial surface by 0.5 mm and veneering the surface for additional bonding can significantly improve retention of class III restorations.[69]

Restoring the distal surface of primary canines (Fig. 22.20) requires a preparation slightly different from that for incisors. The proximal box is directed at a different angle toward the gingiva.

Either amalgam or adhesive materials may be used as the restorative material in this location. The preparation, except for a short cavosurface bevel for resin materials, is identical regardless of the restorative material chosen. A dovetail may be placed on the facial surface, except when amalgam is chosen for a maxillary canine; in that situation, the dovetail is placed on the palatal surface. The steps in preparation and placement of a class III composite restoration are listed in Box 22.8.

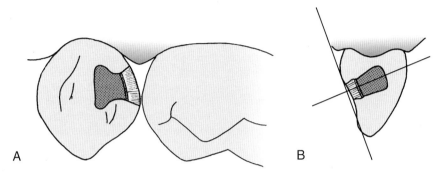

A   B

• **Figure 22.20** Class III preparation for primary canines. (A) The dovetail is usually placed on the lingual surface of maxillary canines and on the labial surface of mandibular canines. A short bevel (not shown) is placed on the cavosurface margin of preparations to be restored with resin-based composite. (B) The proximal box is placed perpendicular to a line tangent to the surface on which the dovetail is placed.

• BOX 22.8 **Steps in Preparation and Placement of a Class III Adhesive Restoration**

1. Administer appropriate anesthesia, and place the rubber dam. Ligation of individual teeth with dental floss provides the best stability.
2. Place a wooden wedge interproximally to minimize gingival hemorrhage by depressing the papilla and protecting it from the bur.
3. Create access, and remove caries with a no. 330 bur or no. 2 round bur in the high-speed handpiece, using a facial access. The axial wall is ideally placed 0.5 mm into dentin. A round bur in the low-speed handpiece can be used to remove deep decay. The gingival and lingual walls should just break contact with the adjacent tooth. It is not necessary to break contact with the incisal wall of the preparation to maintain adequate tooth structure.
4. To enhance retention, a dovetail or lock may be placed on the labial or lingual surface. The lock should not extend more than halfway across the labial surface and is kept in the middle horizontal third of the tooth; or may extend across the cervical, if there is presence of cervical decalcification.
5. Place a short bevel (0.5 mm) at the cavosurface margin. This may be accomplished with a fine, tapered diamond or with a flame-shaped composite finishing bur.
6. Clean and dry the preparation with water and compressed air.
7. Place a plastic or sectional metal matrix. Most plastic matrices will first have to be cut in half horizontally because they are manufactured for permanent teeth and are too wide for primary teeth. The matrix is placed interproximally, and a wedge is reinserted. **Note:** *A resin strip crown form can be trimmed to cover the preparation only (not the entire crown) to create a custom matrix, which often is easier to use than a matrix strip.*
8. If using a two-step bonding agent, etch the preparation for 15–20 seconds. An acid gel is preferable. Etching aids in retention and ensures improved marginal integrity and reduced marginal leakage. After etching, rinse and dry the preparation well. If a self-etching bonding agent is used, this step is eliminated.
9. Place a dentin-bonding agent in the preparation with a small brush. Gently blow compressed air into the preparation to disperse a thin layer

of bonding agent evenly over both dentin and enamel. Polymerize the bonding agent.

10. With a plastic instrument or a pressure syringe, place the composite in the preparation. Pull the matrix tightly around the cavity preparation with finger pressure and hold until cured. Hold the visible light as closely as possible to the composite and polymerize per the manufacturer's instructions. The light should be directed from both the facial and the lingual surfaces to ensure complete polymerization. Avoid looking directly at the polymerization light when it is turned on.
11. Finishing and polishing can be performed immediately following polymerization. The smoothest and most desirable surface of a composite is that which remains after a properly adapted matrix is removed; however, it is difficult to adapt a matrix so accurately that additional adjustment to the margins is unnecessary. Gross finishing or contouring can be performed with fine-grit diamonds or with carbide finishing burs. A flame carbide finishing bur (12–20 flutes) is excellent for finishing the facial and interproximal surfaces. The lingual surface is best finished with a round or pear-shaped carbide finishing bur. A lubricated, pointed white stone may also be used for smoothing. Composite polishing gloss may be used for final polishing to create a luster-like appearance. Final interproximal polishing of the restoration is completed with sandpaper strips. These strips will be best used if they are cut into thin strips 2–3 mm in width. Mounted abrasive disks can be used to finish the facial and lingual surfaces. As an optional step, after polishing is completed, an unfilled resin glaze may be added to the polished restoration. The glaze provides a better marginal seal and a smooth, finished surface. Before adding the glaze, the restoration and surrounding enamel should first be etched for 15–20 seconds to remove surface debris. After rinsing and drying, the resin is painted onto the restoration and is polymerized. Care should be taken not to bond adjacent teeth together with the resin glaze.
12. When finishing is completed, remove the rubber dam and floss the interproximal areas to check for overhangs and to remove excess glaze material.

Class V Restorations for Incisors and Canines

Class V restorations may be adhesive materials (most frequently) or amalgams. They are most often needed on the facial surface of canines. To prepare these restorations, penetrate the tooth in the area of caries with a no. 330 bur until dentin is reached (approximately 1 mm from the outer enamel surface). Move the bur laterally into sound dentin and enamel, thus establishing the walls of the cavity. The pulpal wall should be convex, parallel to the outer enamel surface. The lateral walls are slightly flared near the proximal surfaces to prevent undermining of the enamel. The final external outline is determined by the extent of caries. Mechanical retention in the preparation can be achieved with a no. 35 inverted cone bur or a no. ½ round bur, creating small undercuts in the gingivoaxial and incisoaxial line angles. For resin-based composites, a short bevel is placed around the entire cavosurface margin. Etching, bonding, material placement, and finishing are like that described for class III adhesive restorations, except that no matrix is used.

Full Coronal Coverage of Incisors

Indications[70]

The indications for full coverage of incisors are as follows:

- Incisors with large interproximal lesions, or large lesions covering a single surface (e.g., lingual surfaces in nursing caries)
- Incisors that have received pulp therapy
- Incisors that have been fractured and have lost an appreciable amount of tooth structure
- Incisors with multiple hypoplastic defects or developmental disturbances (e.g., ectodermal dysplasia)
- Discolored incisors that are esthetically unpleasing

- Incisors with small interproximal lesions that also demonstrate large areas of cervical decalcification (i.e., high caries risk)

It is a challenging task to repair extensively destroyed anterior teeth with restorations that are durable, retentive, and esthetic (see Fig. 22.19). There are several methods of providing full coronal coverage to primary incisors, but adhesive resin–based composite crowns (Strip Crowns [3M ESPE]) (see Fig. 22.19B), preveneered SSCs (e.g., Kinder Krowns [Kinder Krowns, St. Louis Park, MN], NuSmile Primary Crowns [NuSmile Crowns]), and preformed primary ZCs (e.g., EZ Pedo, Loomis, CA; NuSmile ZR Crowns) are the most popular methods. A survey published in 2010 of pediatric dentists reported that 46% of respondents preferred strip crowns for treatment of decayed primary incisors, and 41% preferred veneered crowns.[71] This survey was published prior to the widespread introduction of zirconia primary crowns, which have gained much popularity. Other considerably less popular options include plain SSCs and open face SSCs (see Fig. 22.19C). All have shortcomings (Table 22.3) but may still be used in certain situations. Plain SSCs provide a very durable restoration but are esthetically unpleasing to most parents. Open-face crowns[72] are used by some clinicians because their retention is superior to that of adhesive resin crowns; however, esthetic results are compromised. A very esthetic and frequently placed crown is the adhesive resin–based composite crown or "strip" crown. Studies have shown that these crowns demonstrate clinically satisfactory results with good durability and have high parental acceptance.[73,74] Preveneered crowns are both esthetic and durable but may show some metal and can demonstrate chipping of the veneer. As stated earlier in the chapter, there is still not a lot of clinical information available about zirconia ceramic crowns for primary teeth; however, ZCs in adults have been shown to be very esthetic, durable, stain resistant, biocompatible, and

ALTERNATIVE RESTORATIVE TREATMENT

Michael J. Kanellis

Atraumatic restorative treatment (ART) is a minimally invasive treatment technique for restoring teeth by means of hand instrumentation for decay removal and fluoride-releasing adhesive materials (glass ionomer) for filling.[1] ART has been promoted by the World Health Organization as a means of delivering care in underdeveloped countries that do not have electricity or access to sophisticated dental equipment.[2,3] In 2001 the American Academy of Pediatric Dentistry (AAPD) adopted a policy on ART, referring to it as "alternative restorative treatment." The AAPD policy acknowledged that "not all dental disease can be treated by 'traditional' restorative techniques" and recognized ART as "a useful and beneficial technique in the treatment and management of dental caries where traditional cavity preparation and placement of traditional dental restorations are not possible."[4] In 2008 the AAPD further refined their policy and included the technique in a broader discussion of "Interim Therapeutic Restorations" (ITR).[5] The use of ART in developed countries has led to modifications of the technique that allow for the occasional use of a slow speed handpiece and follow-up care that may include placement of a traditional restoration. Modifications of the technique have led to a call by Frencken (developer and early pioneer of the ART technique) for "adherence to its original description."[6]

There are several potential advantages to ART when used with young children. Because hand instrumentation is used, the noise and vibration of dental handpieces is eliminated.

Also eliminated is the need for acid etching, water coolant, and the accompanying high-velocity suction. Caries removal using hand instrumentation also often eliminates the need for local anesthesia. Because instrumentation is kept to a minimum, treatment can easily be carried out in

the knee-to-knee position. The use of a fluoride-releasing restorative material helps to prevent further decay.

The use of ART in combination with silver diamine fluoride, known as SMART (silver modified atraumatic restorative treatment) has been recommended because this combined approach kills bacteria prior to sealing a cavity with glass ionomer.[7]

References

1. Frencken JE, Pilot T, Songpaisan Y, et al. Atraumatic restorative treatment (ART): rationale, technique, and development. *J Public Health Dent.* 1996;56(3):135–140.
2. Phantumvanit P, Songpaisan Y, Pilot T, et al. Atraumatic restorative treatment (ART): a three-year community field trial in Thailand—survival of one-surface restorations in the permanent dentition. *J Public Health Dent.* 1996;56(3):141–145.
3. World Health Organization. Revolutionary new procedure for treating dental caries. Press Release WHO/28. April 7, 1994.
4. American Academy of Pediatric Dentistry Council on Clinical Affairs. Policy on alternative restorative treatment (ART). *Pediatr Dent.* 2005–2006;27(suppl 7):30.
5. American Academy of Pediatric Dentistry Council on Clinical Affairs. Policy on interim therapeutic restorations (ITR). *Pediatr Dent.* 2010–2011;32(6 Special Issue):39.
6. Frencken JE, Leal SC. The correct use of the ART approach. *J Appl Oral Sci.* 2010;18(1):1–4.
7. Fa BA, Jew JA, Wong A, et al. Silver modified atraumatic restorative technique (SMART): an alternative caries prevention tool. *Stoma EDU J.* 2016;3(2).

ALTERNATIVE RESTORATIVE TREATMENT—cont'd

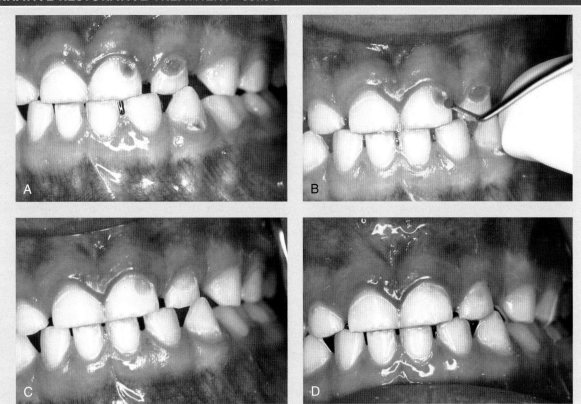

(A) Facial caries evident on incisors and cuspid. (B) Spoon excavator positioned for decay removal. (C) Following caries removal with spoon excavator. (D) Teeth restored with glass ionomer restorative material.

TABLE 22.3 Comparison of Full Coverage Techniques for Primary Incisors

Technique	Esthetics	Durability	Time for Placement	Selection Criteria
Resin (strip) crowns[a]	Very good initially; may discolor over time	Retention dependent on amount of tooth structure present and quality of acid etch. Can be dislodged fairly easily if traumatized	Time required for optimum isolation, etching, placement, finishing	When esthetics is a great concern. Adequate tooth structure remains for etching/bonding. Child is not highly prone to trauma. Gingival hemorrhage is controllable
Zirconia ceramic crowns[a]	Very good	Ceramic is very durable, rarely chips or breaks	Like a preveneered crown (prep must fit the crown form)	Adequate tooth structure remains, similar to a strip crown. Esthetics of great concern
Prefabricated veneered steel crowns	Very good	Good; however, facings may occasionally chip or fracture	Comparable to strip crowns; however, must make tooth fit the crown, which adds time	Esthetics is a concern. Hemorrhage difficult to control. Children with history of bruxism
Steel crowns[b]	Very poor	Very good; a well-crimped, cemented crown is very retentive and wears well	Fastest crown to place	Severely decayed teeth. Esthetics of no concern. Unable to control gingival hemorrhage. Need to place restoration quickly because of inadequate cooperation or time
Open-face steel crowns	Good; however, usually some metal shows	Good; like steel crowns, are very retentive; however, facings may be dislodged	May take the longest to place because of two-step procedure: 1. Crown placement 2. Composite placement	Severely decayed teeth. Durability needed: active, accident-prone child or severe bruxism evident

[a]Restoration of choice esthetically.
[b]Avoid using because of esthetics.

Preparation and Placement of Adhesive Resin–Based Composite Crowns (Pediatric Strip Crowns [3M ESPE]) With Considerations for Preveneered and Zirconia Crowns

1. Administer appropriate anesthesia.
2. Select the shade of resin-based composite to be used. Then place and ligate the rubber dam.
3. Select a primary incisor celluloid crown form with a mesiodistal width approximately equal to the tooth to be restored.
4. Remove decay with a large round bur in the low-speed handpiece. If pulp therapy is required, do it now.
5. Reduce the incisal edge by 1.5 mm using a tapered diamond or a no. 169L bur.
6. Reduce the interproximal surfaces by 0.5–1.0 mm (Fig. 22.21). This reduction should allow a crown form to slip over the tooth. The interproximal walls should be parallel, and the gingival margin should have a feather-edge.
7. Reduce the facial surface by at least 1.0 mm and the lingual surface by at least 0.5 mm. Create a feather-edge gingival margin. Round all line angles. *Note: For preveneered and zirconia crowns, interproximal reduction will be greater (approximately 1.5 mm), as will facial (1–1.5 mm) and lingual reduction (0.5–1 mm).*
8. Place a small undercut on the facial surface in the gingival one-third of the tooth with a no. 330 bur or no. 35 inverted cone. When the resin material polymerizes, engaging the undercut, this serves as a mechanical lock. *Note: This is not required for preveneered or zirconia crowns, but also not contraindicated.*
9. Trim the selected plastic crown form by cutting away excess material gingivally with crown-and-bridge scissors, and trial fit the crown form. A properly trimmed crown form should fit 1 mm below the gingival crest and should be of comparable height to adjacent teeth. Remember that maxillary lateral incisor crowns are usually 0.5–1.0 mm shorter than those of central incisors. *Note: Preveneered and zirconia crowns are tried on until a crown slides passively over the preparation. If either will not seat passively, more tooth reduction will be necessary until it does seat. Because neither of these crowns flex when being placed onto a preparation, they must not be forced to seat, which could lead to fracture.*
10. After the celluloid crown is adequately trimmed, punch a small hole in the lingual surface with an explorer to act as a vent for the escape of

trapped air as the crown is placed with resin onto the preparation. At this point hemorrhage must be well controlled so as not to interfere with bonding or esthetics. *Note: If the zirconia crown has been contaminated with blood or saliva during try-in, it should be either air abraded internally or cleaned with a zirconia decontaminant (IvoClean, Ivoclar Vivadent, Amherst, NY).*
11. If a self-etching bonding agent is not used, etch the tooth with acid gel for 15–20 seconds. Rinse and dry the tooth; then apply a dentin-bonding agent to the entire tooth and polymerize. *Note: This is not required for preveneered or zirconia crowns.*
12. Fill the crown form approximately two-thirds full with a resin-based composite material, and seat onto the tooth. Excess material should flow from the gingival margin and the vent hole. While holding the crown in place, remove the gingival excess with an explorer. *Note: Preveneered crowns are usually cemented with a glass ionomer cement, and zirconia crowns should be cemented with a resin-modified glass ionomer or bioactive cement. A light-activated cement may be used with zirconia crowns. The light will penetrate the zirconia.*
13. Polymerize the material. Be certain to direct the curing light from both the facial and lingual directions. *Note: For preveneered and zirconia, allow the cement to set and clean away all excess.*
14. Remove the celluloid form by using a composite finishing bur or a curved scalpel blade to cut the material on the lingual surface, and then peel the form from the tooth.
15. Remove the rubber dam and evaluate the occlusion.
16. Little finishing should be required on the facial surface. A flame carbide finishing bur can be used to finish the gingival margin should any irregularities be noted upon tactile examination with an explorer. A round or pear-shaped finishing bur may be used for final contouring of the lingual surface. Abrasive disks are used for final polishing of areas of the crown that require contouring. *Note: For preveneered crowns the proximal-incisal corners may be contoured slightly to give a slightly less "boxy" appearance. Adjustments to zirconia crowns' occlusion or contour are extremely difficult and usually are not attempted.*

retentive,[63] so it is anticipated that their performance in children will be similar. There is no question that they provide a very esthetic restoration.

The steps for preparation and placement of resin crowns are listed in Box 22.9 and shown in Fig. 22.22. Because all the anterior crown types have similarities in preparation and placement, noted differences for the veneered and ZCs are also listed in Box 22.9.

Preparation and Placement of Veneered Steel Crowns and Zirconia Primary Crowns

Veneered SSCs for primary incisors and canines (Fig. 22.23) provide a one-step esthetic restoration that, unlike resin-based composite crowns or open-face crowns, can be placed in the presence of hemorrhage without affecting the final esthetic result.[70] They can be placed on teeth with little remaining tooth structure. In addition, when moisture control is difficult and the resin crowns cannot be placed, these crowns may offer a good alternative because they are less sensitive to moisture.

Veneered SSCs have at least three limitations: (1) crimping is limited primarily to the lingual surfaces, which does not allow as close an adaptation; however, this does not appear to diminish retention because they can be retained as well as crimped anterior SSCs[77]; (2) each crown costs approximately $18 to $20, compared

with approximately $5 to $6 for strip crown forms, making an inventory much more costly; and (3) if the veneer fractures, usually replacing the crown, rather than repairing the fracture, will provide the fastest, most esthetically pleasing result.

One study found fractures or wear of the veneer in approximately 14% of crowns,[75] with canines most likely to be affected. This percentage is slightly less than the incidence of fractures reported with strip crowns.[74] Parental acceptance for these crowns has also been reported to be very high, with more than 90% of parents reporting they were satisfied or very satisfied with their child's veneered crowns.[76]

Zirconia primary crowns similarly cannot be crimped at all, have a comparably high inventory cost ($18 to $22/crown), and cannot be repaired in the mouth; however, these crowns are less likely to fracture or chip than preveneered crowns. The most obvious advantages of ZCs are their excellent esthetics, color stability, and durability.[77]

The preparation for both veneered steel crowns and ZCs is very similar to that of a resin crown (see Box 22.9), except that no facial undercut is required (although it can still be used); in addition, the amount of reduction of all tooth surfaces needed is considerably greater. A coarse tapered diamond bur is best for the incisal, proximal, and facial tooth reduction, with a football diamond

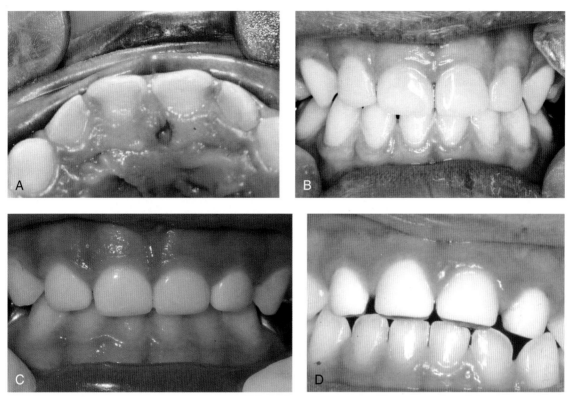

• **Figure 22.21** Full coronal coverage of primary incisors. (A) Multiple interproximal carious lesions in primary incisors. (B) The incisors restored with adhesive resin–based composite crowns (strip crowns). (C) Zirconia primary crowns (NuSmile ZR crowns, NuSmile, Houston, TX). (D) Preveenered crowns (NuSmile Signature crowns). ([A] and [B] Courtesy Dr. Ari Kupietzky, Jerusalem, Israel.)

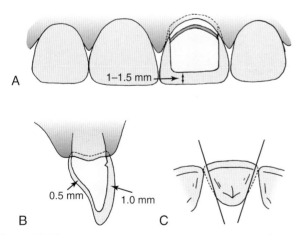

• **Figure 22.22** Adhesive resin–based composite crown (strip) preparation. (A) Labial view. (B) Proximal view. (C) Incisal view. The proximal slice should be parallel to the natural external contours of the tooth. *Note:* The crown preparation for the preveneered and zirconia crowns are very similar to this, except for slightly more overall tooth reduction.

bur used to reduce the lingual surface. When preparing a tooth for a veneered or ZC, the operator must keep in mind that the preparation must be made to fit the crown because the resin-based composite facing is too brittle to permit additional manipulation and the ZCs will not flex over convexities. Therefore preparation of an incisor for a veneered or ZC is an ongoing process. After the preparation is completed, select a crown and try it on the tooth.

If a crown is tried on the tooth and it does not quite fit, more tooth reduction will be necessary to allow the crown to slide onto the preparation so that the margins are subgingival. Neither type of crown should be forced onto the preparation but should be fit with only finger pressure. Too much force during seating can weaken or chip the resin veneer or break the gingival margin of the ZCs. A snug, but passive, sleeve-like fit of the crown over the tooth is recommended.[78] Veneered crowns do not generally require trimming, and ZCs cannot be trimmed. Crimping of veneered crowns is minimal and limited to the lingual surface only. Veneered crowns are best cemented with a glass ionomer cement and may need to be held in place as it sets. ZCs are best cemented with an RMGI or bioactive cement to maximize retention to the zirconia surface. An important note about ZCs: It is strongly recommended that hemorrhage and saliva be well controlled prior to cementing a ZC. Both may interfere with the bond of the RMGI cement to both the tooth and/or the zirconia. Although some of the zirconia manufacturers place internal retentive grooves inside the crown for added mechanical retention of the cement, not all do. Zirconia that has been contaminated with blood and/or saliva may lose much of its reactivity to bond well with cements.[79] For this reason, one ZC company (NuSmile ZR Crowns, NuSmile) provides a pink try-in crown that is used for fitting to the prep. After the appropriate fit is determined, the try-in crown is exchanged for a noncontaminated white crown which is filled with cement and placed on the tooth. The try-in crown may be autoclaved and used multiple times. If a ZC is contaminated by saliva or blood, it should be cleaned internally by either air abrasion (sandblasting) or the use of a cleansing agent specifically for zirconia (Ivoclean, Ivoclar Vivadent, Amherst, NY).

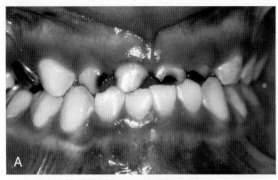
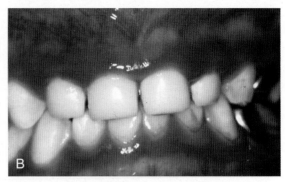

• **Figure 22.23** (A) Extensive caries in primary incisors. (B) Veneered crowns (NuSmile) restoring the four incisors.

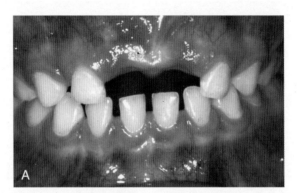

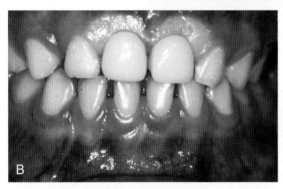
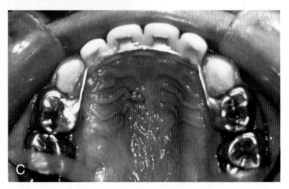

• **Figure 22.24** Prosthetic replacement of primary anterior teeth. (A) Edentulous space following extraction of two primary incisors. (B) Fixed prosthetic appliance replacing the two incisors in place. (C) Example of a fixed prosthetic appliance replacing four incisors. *Note:* Stainless steel crowns are used on the first primary molars as abutments. These provide better retention and durability than orthodontic bands.

Nonveneered SSCs are not frequently used to restore maxillary primary incisors because of the poor esthetics. However, they may be used on severely decayed canines and mandibular incisors, where esthetics is less noticeable.

Prosthetic Replacement of Primary Anterior Teeth

Premature loss of maxillary primary incisors because of extensive caries, trauma, or congenital absence requires consideration for providing a prosthetic tooth replacement for the child.[80] In most instances, prosthetic replacement of primary incisors is considered an elective procedure. Space maintenance in this region is not generally necessary. The most common reason for placement of a prosthetic appliance is parental concern about esthetics.

Lack of compliance in appliance wear and care by the young child is the greatest limitation of and contraindication for these appliances. If a young child decides that he or she does not like the appliance, he will find a way to remove it from his mouth and will usually discard it. Education of the parents regarding this fact is essential before the decision to construct an appliance is made. Another contraindication for prosthetic replacement is the presence of an anterior deep bite.

Prosthetic appliances may be either fixed or removable (Fig. 22.24), and many different designs are used for both. A fixed appliance will almost always be preferred to a removable appliance in preschool children because of compliance issues. When constructing either type, it is best to allow at least 6 to 8 weeks following the tooth loss before fabrication. This allows for good healing and gingival shrinkage. However, appliances can be placed the same day the extractions are done, and the gingival tissue seems to heal and adapt very well around the prosthetic appliance.

One fixed appliance design is a Nance-like device, constructed with two bands or, preferably, steel crowns on primary molars that are connected by a palatal wire to which the replacement teeth are attached. These prosthetic appliances can be fabricated by any laboratory but are commercially available through some commercial laboratories such as Space Maintainers Laboratory. This appliance is cemented onto the molars and is not easily removed by the child. It requires minimal adjustment.[81] The teeth can be made to sit directly on the ridge of the edentulous space (preferred), or acrylic gingiva can be added. Disadvantages of this appliance include (1) possible decalcification around the bands, (2) more difficulty in home cleaning, and (3) bending of the wires with fingers or sticky foods, which may create occlusal interferences and the need for adjustments. Potential loosening of the bands resulting from continual torquing of bands by the movement of the wire during normal chewing may necessitate frequent recementation.

The removable appliance is a Hawley-like device that replaces the teeth and uses circumferential and ball clasps on the molars. These appliances require the most compliance of any of the prosthetic replacements. They are not indicated in children younger than 3 years. Clasps will need adjustment, the frequency of which depends on the child's handling of the appliances. The greatest advantages of these appliances are that the appliance can be removed for daily cleaning and that adjustments are easily made by the dentist without having to remove and recement bands.

References

1. Black GV. *A Work on Operative Dentistry*. Vol. 11. ed 5. Chicago: Medico-Dental Publishing; 1924.
2. Donly KJ. Update in Pediatric Dentistry Restorative Symposium. *Pediatr Dent*. 2015;37(2):98.
3. Bhaskar SN, Lilly GE. Intrapulpal temperature during cavity preparation. *J Dent Res*. 1965;44(4):644–647.
4. Bouschor CF, Matthews JL. A four-year clinical study of teeth restored after preparation with an air turbine handpiece with air coolant. *J Prosthet Dent*. 1966;16(2):306–309.
5. Kupietzky A, Vargas G, Waggoner WF, et al. Use of coolant for high-speed tooth preparation: a survey of pediatric dentistry residency program directors in the United States. *Pediat Dent*. 2010;32(3):212–217.
6. Goldstein RE, Parkins FM. Air-abrasive technology: its new role in restorative dentistry. *J Am Dent Assoc*. 1994;125:551–557.
7. Black R. Technique for nonmechanical preparation of cavities and prophylaxis. *J Am Dent Assoc*. 1945;39:953–965.
8. Martens LC. Laser physics and a review of laser applications in dentistry for children. *Eur Arch Paediatr Dent*. 2011;12(2):61–67.
9. Olivi G, Genovese MD. Laser restorative dentistry in children and adolescents. *Eur Arch Paediatr Dent*. 2011;12(2):68–78.
10. Ganesh M, Parikh D. Chemomechanical caries removal (CMCR) agents: review and clinical application in primary teeth. *J Dent Oral Hyg*. 2011;3(3):34–45.
11. Valachi B. *Practice dentistry pain free: evidence-based strategies to prevent pain and extend your career*. Portland, OR: Posturedontics; 2008:102–110.
12. Leinfelder KF, Sluder TB, Santos JR, et al. Five-year clinical evaluation of anterior and posterior restorations of composite resin. *Oper Dent*. 1980;5:57–65.
13. Donly KJ, Garcia-Godoy F. The use of resin-based composite in children: an update. *Pediatr Dent*. 2015;37(2):136–143.
14. Cunha RF. A thirty-month clinical evaluation of a posterior composite resin in primary molars. *J Clin Pediatr Dent*. 2000;24(2):113–115.
15. Fuks AB, Araujo FB, Osorio LB, et al. Clinical and radiographic assessment of class II esthetic restorations in primary molars. *Pediatr Dent*. 2000;22(6):479–485.
16. Rastelli FP, Vieira RS, Rastelli MCS. Posterior composite restorations in primary molars: an in vivo comparison of three restorative techniques. *J Clin Pediatr Dent*. 2001;25(3):227–230.
17. Soncini JA, Maserejian NN, Trachtenberg F, et al. The longevity of amalgam versus compomer/composite restorations in posterior primary and permanent teeth. Findings from the New England Children's Amalgam Trial. *J Am Dent Assoc*. 2007;138(6):763–772.
18. Norman RD, Wright JS, Rydberg RJ, et al. A 5-year study comparing a posterior composite resin and an amalgam. *J Prosthet Dent*. 1990;64(5):523–529.
19. Roberts MW, Folio J, Moffa JP, et al. Clinical evaluation of a composite resin system with a dental bonding agent for restoration of permanent posterior teeth: a 3-year study. *J Prosthet Dent*. 1992;67:301–306.
20. Bernardo M, Luis H, Martin MD, et al. Survival and reasons for failure of amalgams versus composite posterior restorations placed in a randomized clinical trial. *J Am Dent Assoc*. 2007;138(6):775–783.
21. Hickel R, Kaaden C, Paschos E, et al. Longevity of occlusally-stressed restorations in posterior primary teeth. *Am J Dent*. 2005;18(3):198–211.
22. Statement on posterior resin-based composites. ADA Council on Scientific Affairs; ADA Council on Dental Benefit Programs. *J Am Dent Assoc*. 1998;129(11):1627–1628.
23. Posterior composite resins. Council on Dental Materials, Instruments, and Equipment. *J Am Dent Assoc*. 1986;112(5):707–709.
24. Posterior composite resins: an update. Council on Dental Materials, Instruments, and Equipment. *J Am Dent Assoc*. 1986;113(6):950–951.
25. Leinfelder KF, Vann WF. The use of composite resins on primary molars. *Pediatr Dent*. 1982;4(1):27–31.
26. Duggal MS, Toumba KJ, Sharma NK. Clinical performance of a compomer and amalgam for the interproximal restoration of primary molars: a 24-month evaluation. *Br Dent J*. 2002;193(6):339–342.
27. Gross LC, Griffen AL, Casamassimo PS. Compomers as class II restorations in primary molars. *Pediatr Dent*. 2001;23(1):24–27.
28. Kramer N, Frankenberger R. Compomers in restorative therapy of children: a literature review. *Int J Paed Dent*. 2007;17(1):2–9.
29. Marks LAM, Faict N, Welbury RR. Literature review: restorations of class II cavities in the primary dentition with compomers. *Eur Arch Paediatr Dent*. 2010;11(3):109–114.
30. Mass E, Gordon M, Fuks AB. Assessment of compomer proximal restorations in primary molars: a retrospective study in children. *ASDCJ Dent Child*. 1999;66(2):93–97.
31. Qvist V, Poulsen A, Teglers PT, et al. The longevity of different restorations in primary teeth. *Int J Paediatr Dent*. 2010;20(1):1–7.
32. Croll TP, Bar-Zion Y, Segura A, et al. Clinical performance of resin-modified glass ionomer cement restorations in primary teeth. *J Am Dent Assoc*. 2001;132(8):1110–1116.
33. Donly KJ, Segura A, Kanellis M, et al. Clinical performance and caries inhibition of resin-modified glass ionomer cement and amalgam restorations. *J Am Dent Assoc*. 1999;130(10):1459–1466.
34. Hübel S, Mejàre I. Conventional versus resin-modified glass ionomer cement for class II restorations in primary molars. A 3-year clinical study. *Int J Paediatr Dent*. 2003;13(1):2–8.
35. Qvist V, Laurberg L, Poulsen A, et al. Longevity and cariostatic effects of everyday conventional glass ionomer and amalgam restorations in primary teeth: three-year results. *J Dent Res*. 1997;76:387–1396.
36. Fuks AB. The use of amalgam in pediatric dentistry: new insights and reappraising the tradition. *Pediatr Dent*. 2015;37(2):125–132.
37. Simonsen RJ, Stallard RE. Sealant-restorations utilizing a dilute filled resin: one year results. *Quintessence Int*. 1977;8(6):77–84.
38. Simonsen RJ. Conservation of tooth structure in restorative dentistry. *Quintessence Int*. 1985;16(1):15–24.
39. Simonsen RJ. The preventive resin restoration: a minimally invasive, nonmetallic restoration. *Compend Contin Educ Dent*. 1987;8(6):428–435.
40. Houpt M, Fuks A, Eidelman E. The preventive resin (composite resin/sealant) restoration: nine-year results. *Quintessence Int*. 1994;25(3):155–159.

41. dos Santos PH, Pavan S, Assunção WG, et al. Influence of surface sealants on microleakage of composite resin restorations. *J Dent Child.* 2008;75(1):24–28.

42. Fernández E, Martín J, Vildósola P, et al. Can repair increase the longevity of composite resins? Results of a 10-year clinical trial. *J Dent.* 2015;43(2):279–286.

43. Moncada G, Fernández E, Martín J, et al. Increasing the longevity of restorations by minimal intervention: a two-year clinical trial. *Oper Dent.* 2008;33(3):258–264.

44. Pereira JC, Manfio AP, Franco EB, et al. Clinical evaluation of Dycal under amalgam restorations. *Am J Dent.* 1990;3:67–70.

45. Donly KJ, Wild TW, Jensen ME. Posterior composite class II restorations: in vitro comparison of preparation designs and restorative techniques. *Dent Mater.* 1990;6:88–93.

46. Dawson LR, Simon JF, Taylor PP. Use of amalgam and stainless steel restorations for primary molars. *ASDC J Dent Child.* 1981;48(6):420–422.

47. Randall RC. Preformed metal crowns for primary and permanent molar teeth: review of the literature. *Pediatr Dent.* 2002;24(5):489–500.

48. Messer LB, Levering NJ. The durability of primary molar restorations: II. Observations and predictions of success of stainless steel crowns. *Pediatr Dent.* 1988;10(2):81–85.

49. Roberts JF, Sherriff M. The fate and survival of amalgam and preformed crown molar restorations placed in a specialist pediatric dental practice. *Br Dent J.* 1990;169(10):237–239.

50. Guelmann M, Mjor IA, Jerrel GR. The teaching of class I and II restorations in primary molars: a survey of North American dental schools. *Pediatr Dent.* 2001;23(5):410–414.

51. Leinfelder KF. A conservative approach to placing posterior composite resin restorations. *J Am Dent Assoc.* 1996;127(6):743–748.

52. Marks LAM, Weerheijm LK, van Amerongen WE, et al. Dyract versus Tytin class II restorations in primary molars: 36 months evaluation. *Caries Res.* 1999;33(5):387–392.

53. Marks LAM, van Amerogen WE, Kreulen CM, et al. Conservative interproximal box-only polyacid modified composite restorations in primary molars, twelve-month clinical results. *ASDC J Dent Child.* 1999;66(1):23–29.

54. Welbury RR, Shaw AJ, Murray JJ, et al. Clinical evaluation of paired compomer and glass ionomer restorations in primary molars: final results after 42 months. *Br Dent J.* 2000;189(2):93–97.

55. Garcia-Godoy F. Resin-based composites and compomers in primary molars. *Dent Clin North Am.* 2000;44(3):541–570.

56. Chuang SF, Jin YT, Chang CH, et al. Influence of flowable composite lining thickness on class II composite resins. *Oper Dent.* 2004;29(3):301–308.

57. Lacy AM, Young DA. Modern concepts and materials for the pediatric dentist. *Pediatr Dent.* 1996;18(7):469–475.

58. Fuks AB. The use of amalgam in pediatric dentistry. *Pediatr Dent.* 2002;24(5):448–455.

59. Myers DR. Factors producing failure of class II silver amalgam restorations in primary molars. *ASDC J Dent Child.* 1977;44(3):226–229.

60. Humphrey WP. Use of chromic steel in children's dentistry. *Dent Surv.* 1950;26:945–947.

61. Einwag J, Dunninger P. Stainless steel crown versus multisurface amalgam restorations: an 8-year longitudinal study. *Quintessence Int.* 1996;22(5):321–323.

62. Seale NS, Randall R. The use of stainless steel crowns: a systematic literature review. *Pediatr Dent.* 2015;37(2):147–162.

63. Miyazaki T, Nakamura T, Matsumura H, et al. Current status of zirconia restoration. *Prosth Res.* 2013;57:236–261.

64. Johnson-Harris D, Chiquet B, Flaitz C, et al. Wear of primary tooth enamel by ceramic materials. *Pediatr Dent.* 2016;38(7):519–522.

65. Nash DA. The nickel-chromium crown for restoring posterior primary teeth. *J Am Dent Assoc.* 1981;102(1):444–449.

66. Trairatvorakul C, Piwat S. Comparative clinical evaluation of slot versus dovetail class III composite restorations in primary anterior teeth. *J Clin Ped Dent.* 2004;28(2):125–130.

67. Croll TP, Berg J. Simplified primary incisor proximal restorations. *Pediatr Dent.* 2003;25(1):67–70.

68. McEvoy SA. A modified class III cavity preparation and composite resin filling technique for primary incisors. *Dent Clin North Am.* 1984;28(1):145–155.

69. Piyapinyo S, White GE. Class III cavity preparation in primary anterior teeth: in vitro retention comparison of conventional and modified forms. *J Clin Pediatr Dent.* 1998;22(2):107–112.

70. Waggoner WF. Restoring primary anterior teeth. *Pediatr Dent.* 2002;24(5):511–516.

71. Queis H, Atwan S, Pajtas B, et al. Use of anterior veneered stainless steel crowns by pediatric dentists. *Pediatr Dent.* 2010;32(5):413–416.

72. Helpin ML. The open-face steel crown restoration in children. *ASDC J Dent Child.* 1983;50(1):34–38.

73. Kupietzky A, Waggoner WF. Parental satisfaction with bonded resin composite strip crowns for primary incisors. *Pediatr Dent.* 2004;26(4):337–340.

74. Kupietzky A, Waggoner WF, Galea J. Long term photographic and radiographic assessment of bonded resin composite strip crowns for primary incisors: results after 3 years. *Pediatr Dent.* 2005;27(3):221–225.

75. MacLean JK, Champagne CE, Waggoner WF, et al. Clinical outcomes for primary anterior teeth treated with preveneered stainless steel crowns. *Pediatr Dent.* 2007;29(5):377–381.

76. Champagne C, Waggoner W, Ditmyer M, et al. Parental satisfaction with preveneered stainless steel crowns for primary anterior teeth. *Pediatr Dent.* 2007;29(6):465–469.

77. Waggoner WF. Restoring primary anterior teeth: updated for 2014. *Pediatr Dent.* 2015;37(2):163–170.

78. Waggoner WF. Clinical tips for restoration of primary anterior teeth with preveneered anterior stainless steel crowns. *J Pediatr Dent Care.* 2003;9(3):25–29.

79. Yang B, Lange-Jansen HC, Schamberg M, et al. Influence of saliva contamination n zirconia bonding. *Dent Materials.* 2008;24(4):508–513.

80. Steffen JM, Miller JB, Johnson R. An esthetic method of anterior space maintenance. *J Dent Child.* 1971;38(3):154–157.

81. Waggoner WF, Kupietzky A. Anterior esthetic fixed appliances for the preschooler: considerations and a technique for placement. *Pediatr Dent.* 2001;23(2):147–150.

23

Pulp Therapy for the Primary Dentition

ANNA B. FUKS, ARI KUPIETZKY, AND MARCIO GUELMANN

CHAPTER OUTLINE

Maintaining the integrity and health of the oral tissues is the primary objective of pulp treatment. Premature loss of primary teeth can lead to malocclusion and esthetic, phonetic, and functional problems; these in turn may be transient or permanent. It is important to attempt to preserve pulp vitality whenever possible; however, when this is not feasible, the pulp can be entirely eliminated without significantly compromising the function of the tooth.[1,2]

This chapter provides a concise review of the normal histologic characteristics of the primary pulp, and describes briefly the dentinogenesis process and the factors affecting the dentin-pulp complex response to stimuli. Finally, it discusses the biological basis and rationale for the various modalities of pulpal treatment for the primary dentition.

Histology

The pulp of a primary tooth is histologically similar to that of a permanent tooth. The dental pulp is a specialized connective tissue of mesenchymal origin surrounded by tubular dentin walls occupying the pulp chamber and the root canal.

The odontoblasts are cells responsible for the synthesis and deposition of the collagen-rich dentin organic matrix, which is further mineralized around the pulp tissue. Therefore dentin and the pulp remain closely associated during tooth development throughout life and are commonly referred as the *dentin-pulp complex*. The odontoblasts line the periphery of the pulp space and extend their cytoplasmic processes into the dentinal tubules. These cells have several junctions, which allow intercellular communication and help maintain the relative position of one cell to another. Below the odontoblastic layer is the cell-free zone that contains an extensive plexus of unmyelinated nerves and blood capillaries. The large blood vessels and nerves are located in the core of the pulp and are surrounded by loose connective tissue.[2,3] Although this description is correct during active dentinogenesis, it is now accepted that the size of the odontoblasts and the content of their cytoplasmic organelles vary throughout their life cycle and are closely related to their functional activity. The relationship between the size of the odontoblasts and their secretory activity can be demonstrated by differences in their size in the crown and in the root and may express different dentinogenic rates in these two areas of the tooth.[4]

The odontoblasts are highly specialized cells that extend cytoplasmic processes into the dentinal tubules, where they contribute to the main part of the pulp-dentin complex. When this complex is damaged by injury (disease or operative procedures), it reacts in an attempt to defend the pulp.

The Pulp-Dentin Complex

Dentinogenesis in Healthy State

The inner enamel epithelium and its associated basement membrane have an important role in direct odontoblastic cytodifferentiation. They present bioactive molecules, including growth factors immobilized on the basement membrane that send signals to the cells of the dental papilla, inducing the differentiation of the ectomesenchymal cells into odontoblasts.[3] These cells express specific gene products that will form the highly mineralized extracellular matrix of dentin. Hydroxyapatite forms the main inorganic part of dentin, whereas the organic components consist mostly of type I collagen.[5] During the postmitotic state, the odontoblasts line the formative surface of the matrix and start secreting primary dentin. At the initiation of dentinogenesis, during mantle dentin formation, mineralization is achieved through the mediation of matrix vesicles. Mantle dentin is the first dentin to be formed, has an approximate thickness of 80 to 100 μm, and is almost free of developmental defects.[2]

When mantle dentin formation is completed and the odontoblasts form a tightly packed layer of cells, the matrix of dentin is produced exclusively by the odontoblasts. Although the other cells of the pulp (in the subodontoblastic layer and in the pulp core) support dentinogenesis, they do not have a direct role in primary dentin secretion.[6,7] As the matrix is secreted, the odontoblasts move pulpally, leaving a single cytoplasmic process embedded in a dentinal tubule in the matrix. These tubules, which increase in density near the pulp, confer the property of permeability on the dentin, a feature that has significant clinical importance.[4]

After secretion of the bulk of dentin during primary dentinogenesis, physiologic secondary dentin is secreted at a much slower rate throughout the life of the tooth, leading to a slow reduction in the size of the pulp chamber.[8] The original postmitotic odontoblasts, responsible for primary dentinogenesis, survive for the life of the tooth, unless subjected to injury. These cells remain in a resting stage after primary dentinogenesis, and the physiologic secondary dentin formation represents a basal level of cell activity in the resting tooth stage.[4]

Dentinogenic Response to Injury

In pathologic conditions, such as in mild carious lesions or traumatic injuries, the secretory activity of the odontoblasts is stimulated to elaborate tertiary dentin. This will lead to focal secretion of new matrix at the pulp-dentin interface and possibly within the tubules, contributing to the histologic appearance of dentinal sclerosis at the injury site and to a decrease in dentin permeability.[3,9] Thus the formation of tertiary dentin is much faster than the physiologic secondary dentin formation, so this tertiary deposition is regarded as an important defense mechanism of the pulp-dentin complex in response to either pathologic or physiologic insults (attrition).

The nature and quality of the tertiary dentin depend on its tubular structure and influence the dentin permeability of the area. Thus, in case of a mild injury, the odontoblasts responsible for the primary odontogenesis can frequently survive the challenge and are stimulated to secrete reactionary dentin beneath the injury site.[10] Because the original odontoblasts are responsible for this matrix secretion, there will be tubular continuity and communication with the primary dentin matrix (Fig. 23.1A).[9] Reactionary dentin might be considered an extension of physiologic dentinogenesis. However, since it is a pathologic response to injury, it should be regarded as distinct from the primary and secondary dentinogenesis. When the injury is severe, the odontoblasts beneath the injury may die; however, if suitable conditions exist in the pulp, a new generation of odontoblast-like cells may differentiate from underlying pulp cells, secreting a reparative dentin matrix. Since this dentin is formed by a new generation of cells, there will be discontinuity in the tubular structure, with a subsequent reduction in permeability (see Fig. 23.1B).[11]

A critical question concerns the factors responsible for triggering the stimulation of odontoblastic activity. Although there is still much to learn regarding the molecular control of cell activity in general, and of odontoblastic activity in particular, one family of growth factors, the transforming growth factors (e.g., TGF-β) superfamily, has been reported to have extensive effects on the mesenchymal cells of many connective tissues.[12]

During tooth development, the odontoblasts secrete TGF-β, and some remain sequestered in the dentin matrix. The sequestered TGF-β may be released during any process leading to tissue dissolution, like dental caries formation or the use of acid etching, for example. Thus dentin matrix should be considered not as an inert dental hard tissue but rather as a potential tissue store of a cocktail of bioactive molecules (particularly growth factors) waiting to be released, if appropriate tissue conditions prevail.[2,3]

In contrast to reactionary responses, reparative dentinogenesis represents a more complex sequence of biological processes. The migration and differentiation of pulpal progenitor cells must take place, creating a new generation of odontoblast-like cells, before matrix secretion. A series of stereotypic wound-healing reactions occurs in the pulpal connective tissue, including vascular and cellular inflammatory reactions. In vitro and in vivo experiments on reparative odontogenesis demonstrate that the noninflamed pulp constitutes an appropriate environment where competent pulp cells (potential preodontoblasts) can differentiate into new odontoblast-like cells, forming reparative dentin.[13,14]

Factors Affecting Dentin-Pulp Complex Response to Stimuli in Primary Teeth

Although the life span of the primary teeth is shorter and the dentin is thinner when compared with permanent teeth, the dentin-pulp complex response to dental caries in human primary teeth is similar to that of permanent teeth, including a reduction in the number of the odontoblasts and an increase in the number of inflammatory cells. These are found under the very deep lesions and are less numerous at more distant regions, being almost absent in the radicular apical pulp.[15]

The primary dentition is frequently subjected to stimuli such as trauma or caries with associated pulp inflammation.[16] The same

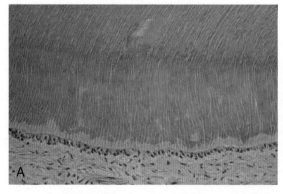
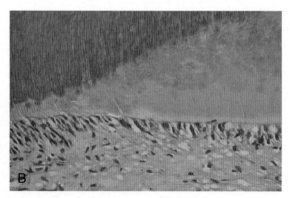

• **Figure 23.1** (A) Histologic section showing tubular continuity in reactionary dentin. (B) Histologic section showing lack of continuity in the reparative dentin. (Courtesy Carlos Alberto S. Costa, DMD, PhD.)

factors affect the dentin pulp responses in both primary and permanent teeth to external stimuli.

The Deleterious Effects of Bacterial Infiltration at the Restorative Materials Margins

A significant number of studies have implicated the presence of bacteria and their products as responsible for the induction of the most severe forms of pulpal inflammation.

The involvement of bacteria in the inflammatory reaction was demonstrated by the spontaneous healing of pulp exposures in germ-free animals[17] and cavity surfaces that were sealed with zinc oxide–eugenol (ZOE) cement to prevent any bacterial contamination.[18] The presence of bacteria in cavities with a remaining dentin thickness (RDT) less than 0.25 mm stimulates more severe pulp inflammatory reaction than in similar cavity preparations in the absence of bacteria.[19] Thus the presence of bacteria always increases the mean grade of pulpal inflammation, regardless of the RDT.[20] These authors also observed that the presence of bacteria in class V cavities resulted in a significant decrease in the number of odontoblasts per unit area; this effect was more pronounced in deep cavities with RDT less than 0.5 mm than cavities with RDT greater than 0.5 mm. One can conclude that the ability to maintain an effective seal to protect the pulp from recurrent injury resulting from bacterial microleakage is a decisive factor in the clinical success of restorative products.[21]

However, some studies have shown pulpal inflammation in the absence of bacteria,[22] clearly indicating that other factors are also responsible, even to a lesser extent, for pulp injury after restorative treatment.

The Protective Role of the Remaining Dentin Thickness

In vivo, the cavity RDT was found to be an important factor mediating pulpal inflammatory activity, particularly when the RDT was reduced below 0.25 mm.[19] In class V cavities prepared in human teeth, the protective tertiary dentin area increased with decreasing RDT until 0.25 mm.[19] With an RDT below 0.25 mm, a significant decrease in the number of odontoblasts was observed together with minimal reactionary dentin repair.[23] The RDT significantly modifies the pulpal response: the thicker the RDT, the lower the pulpal reaction.[17] The presence of an RDT over 500 μm (0.5 mm) delays the diffusion of noxious materials to the dental pulp and allows the odontoblasts to secrete a reactionary dentin, increasing the total distance between the restorative material and the pulp. Any additional decrease in the dentin thickness below 500 μm results in a significant reduction in the number of odontoblasts. The differentiation of odontoblast-like cells from progenitor pulp cells, which migrate to the injury site and secrete reparative dentin, may compensate for this reduction. This reparative dentin decreases the dentin permeability and increases the distance between the restorative material and the pulp, protecting it from noxious products. Thus the RDT appears to provide an important protective barrier against bacterial infiltration, toxins, or any noxious material applied onto the dentin.

Based on the RDT, three situations can be considered:

1. Initial carious lesions are present or cavity preparation is shallow (RDT greater than 500 μm): A localized reactionary dentin is secreted facing the restoration site and intratubular mineralization occurs, resulting in pulp protection by significantly decreasing dentin permeability. It has been suggested that this stimulation may be due to signaling molecules (e.g., transforming growth factors of the β family [TGF-β1], bone morphogenetic protein-2 [BMP-2]) liberated from the dentin during demineralization (see Fig. 23.1A).[24,25]

2. Carious lesion progression implies a deep cavity preparation (RDT less than 500 μm): These lesions may lead to partial odontoblast disintegration. Depending on the pulpal inflammatory state, progenitor/stem cells can migrate to the injury site and differentiate to yield a new generation of odontoblast-like cells. These cells are responsible for the deposition of a specific type of tertiary dentin termed *reparative dentin* (see Fig. 23.1B).[26,27]

3. During a subsequent restorative process, deep cavity preparations with RDTs between 250 and 40 μm lead to poor tertiary dentin repair activity.[19] This results from impaired odontoblast dentin secretory activity due to cellular injury.[28] Murray et al. demonstrated that the mean number of intact odontoblasts found beneath this kind of cavity preparation was 36% lower than the number found beneath similar preparations with an RDT between 500 and 250 μm. This inability of odontoblasts to provide adequate pulpal repair and pulpal protection after deep cavity cutting has been supported by observations of a persistent inflammatory pulpal response and odontoblast displacement following cavity cutting.[28]

Clinical Pulpal Diagnosis

Currently, very little or no correlation exists between clinical diagnostic findings and the histopathologic status of the pulp.[29] Technologically advanced tests and tools to indicate the vitality condition of the pulp, such as laser Doppler flowmetry and pulse oximetry, are available. However, when providing dental care for very young children and/or patients with special health care needs, these technologies may lead to unreliable responses, due to potential lack of cooperation.

Comprehensive medical history, thorough extra- and intraoral examinations, pain characteristics, and sensibility tests complemented by selected radiographs will provide the clinician with essential information regarding the pulp status of a particular tooth or teeth in question. In addition, the source of the discomfort (e.g., trauma or caries, the presence of large, deep, or failed restorations) also plays a critical role in pulpal diagnosis and, subsequently, on the prognosis of the treatment to be provided.

Medical History

When treating a medically compromised child, a more careful approach should be taken.[30] Despite the lack of evidence, for severely immunocompromised patients, the American Academy of Pediatric Dentistry (AAPD) recommends cautious considerations when treating deep carious lesions with close proximity to the pulp. The risk of potential infections, which might be life threatening, drives most clinicians to consider a more radical approach, such as extraction, rather than a more conservative treatment option to preserve the tooth in the arch. In these cases, when pulpally treated teeth are present, close monitoring for signs of pulp degeneration is recommended.[31]

Extra- and Intraoral Examination

The presence of extraoral facial swelling, redness, and/or submandibular lymphadenopathy may indicate the presence of an acute dentoalveolar abscess. In severe situations, facial cellulitis may involve the infraorbital space, resulting in partial/total closure of

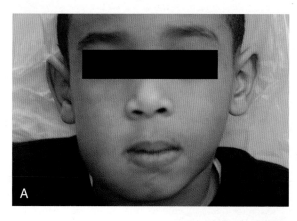
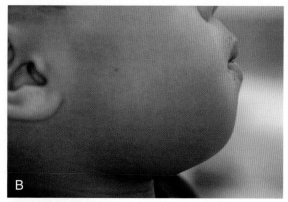
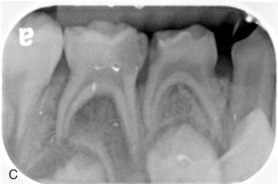

• **Figure 23.2** (A) Six-year-old male with facial swelling caused by deep carious lesion and infection involving tooth #K. (B) Lateral view of same patient, showing redness and extent of cellulitis. (C) Periapical radiograph taken prior to extraction of the affecting tooth.

the eye, limited mouth opening, fever, and malaise. Hospital admission for intravenous antibiotics may be necessary (Figs. 23.2A–C and 23.3A–C). Careful intraoral and radiographic examination seeking teeth with deep carious lesions or deep restorations must be performed. Diagnosis of pulp necrosis is then reached, and the treatment decision of extraction or root canal therapy is based on the restorability of the tooth, the severity of the infection, assessment of bone loss, lesion proximity to the succedaneous tooth follicle, and patient cooperation.[32]

When examining hard tissues, teeth with questionable diagnoses should be evaluated for abnormal mobility and sensitivity to percussion. The presence of open proximal carious lesions between adjacent teeth creates a space that can serve as a reservoir causing food impaction, providing false-positive response to percussion test (inflammation of interdental papilla rather than acute pulpal inflammation) (Fig. 23.4A and B).

Pain Characteristics

Young children are not good historians. For this group, parents are better prepared to report existing symptoms. Stimuli-related responses that cease when the insult is removed (provoked or elicited pain) generally indicate a favorable, reversible status of the pulp that could lead to a more conservative treatment approach such as indirect pulp therapy (IPT) or pulpotomy. Complaints of persistent, lingering, or throbbing pain, disturbing sleep and preventing regular activity, are generally referred to as "spontaneous pain." This most probably indicates an irreversible status of the pulp. The information in combination with clinical examination and

radiographic image(s) will lead the clinician to treatment options such as pulpectomy or extraction (Fig. 23.5A and B).

Sensibility Tests

Sensibility tests, sometimes called vitality or pulp tests, such as thermal and electric pulp test (EPT), are valuable diagnostic aids in endodontics. However, sensibility and percussion tests are not indicated in primary teeth, due to inconsistent results.[33] Younger patients may also be more anxious and less reliable because of the subjective nature of the test.[34] To avoid disruptive behavior, when performing percussion and palpation tests in young children, the tip of the finger should be gently used in combination with the tell-show-do (TSD) technique.[1] The clinician should start the test with a contralateral nonaffected tooth to familiarize the patient with a normal response to the stimuli.

Preoperative Diagnosis of Deep Caries Lesions

When facing deep carious lesions (Fig. 23.10) affecting the primary dentition, limitations exist regarding the determination of the vitality status of the pulp. Percussion and palpations tests, combined with bitewing and selected periapical radiographs, are complementary information that must be obtained. Good quality bitewing radiographs showing the furcation area clearly are essential for an accurate diagnosis. However, in young children in primary and early mixed dentition, especially when using size #0 or #1 films, visibility of the apical third of the primary molar roots and the apical formation of first permanent molars is not always possible. In

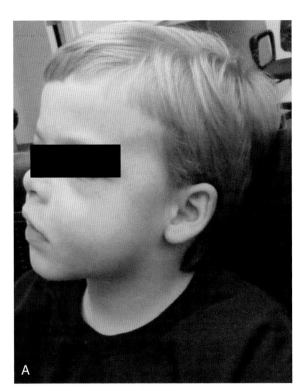
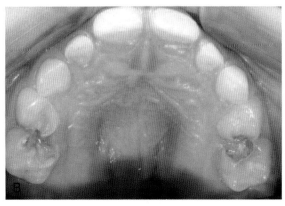
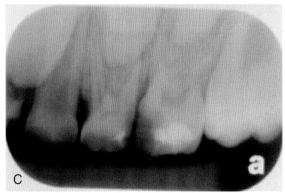

• **Figure 23.3** (A) Five-year-old male with facial swelling caused by a primary maxillary tooth. Note swelling involving the left eye. (B) Clinical view of grossly decayed teeth #I and #J. (C) Periapical radiograph of affected teeth. Extraction of #I and #J was the treatment of choice to resolve the infection. (Courtesy Abi Adewumi, BDS, FDSRCS [Eng].)

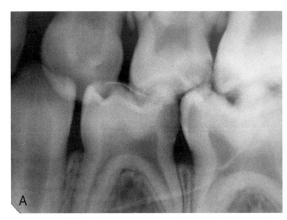
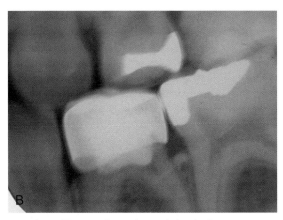

• **Figure 23.4** (A) Mandibular first and second primary molars with extensive caries and alveolar bone resorption due to food impaction. The history of spontaneous pain associated with tenderness to percussion may suggest pulp involvement. (B) The same teeth after restoration of the contact point with a stainless steel crown and an amalgam filling. The symptoms disappeared and bone regeneration is evident. (Courtesy Diana Ram, DDS.)

these situations, a periapical radiograph should be obtained to rule out the presence of internal resorption or periapical involvement.

Integrity and continuity of the lamina dura, together with the presence of trabecular bone in the bifurcation area of primary molars, are indicative signs of a vital pulp. Due to anatomical differences and the superposition of images, clear visualizations of these structures may be difficult to obtain in the maxillary arch.[30] In asymptomatic primary teeth, the amount of sound dentin (at least 1.0 mm) separating the deepest layer of the caries lesion and

the pulp horn can also play an important role when determining if a conservative approach such as IPT is recommended.[35] A clinical attempt to possibly assess the pulpal diagnosis status of deep caries lesions affecting primary molars using interim therapeutic restorations has been advocated.[36] For asymptomatic teeth or teeth with reversible pulpal inflammation, to preserve dental structures and avoid further damage to the pulp, conservative approaches such as stepwise excavation and incomplete caries removal should be considered.[37] Stepwise excavation is a two-step, complete caries

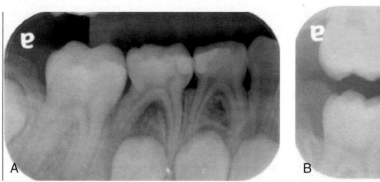
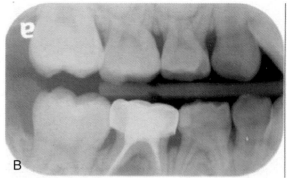

• **Figure 23.5** (A) Healthy 6-year-old patient with history of spontaneous pain for 2 days pointing to tooth #T. (B) Upon opening, tooth found to be necrotic. Root canal treatment with Vitapex paste performed, followed by a final restoration. (Courtesy Rosa Barnes, DDS.)

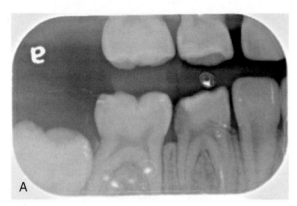
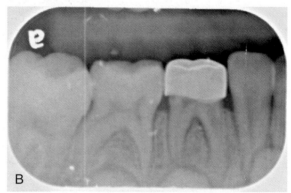

• **Figure 23.6** (A) Asymptomatic tooth #L selected for indirect pulp treatment. (B) Inadequate stainless steel crown coverage resulted in treatment failure after 1-year. (Courtesy Shawn Hanway, DMD.)

removal technique, with the goal of preventing pulp exposure.[38] Incomplete caries removal or selective removal of soft dentin follows the same conservative concept; however, the main difference implies leaving a layer of soft dentin at the pulpal/axial wall followed by a definitive, leakage-free restoration placed at the same appointment.[39] The goal is to prevent bacteria penetration and caries progression from occurring, which could lead to treatment failure (Fig. 23.6A and B). A more detailed explanation is discussed later in the "Vital Pulp Therapy for Normal Pulp/Reversible Pulpitis" section.

Operative Diagnosis

There are instances when a final diagnosis can only be achieved by direct evaluation of the pulp tissue, and a decision about treatment is made accordingly. The quality (color) and the amount of bleeding from a direct exposure of the pulp tissue must be assessed; profuse bleeding or purulent exudate indicates irreversible pulpitis or pulpal necrosis. Based on these observations, the treatment plan may be confirmed or changed. For example, if a formocresol pulpotomy is planned, the nature of the bleeding from the amputation site should be normal (red color and hemostasis evident in less than 5 minutes with mild cotton pellet pressure). If bleeding persists, a more radical treatment should be undertaken (pulpectomy or extraction). Excessive bleeding is an indication that the inflammation has reached the radicular pulp. Conversely, if a pulp polyp is present and bleeding stops normally after coronal pulp amputation, a pulpotomy may be performed instead of a more radical procedure (Fig. 23.7A–E).[40] Direct pulp capping (DPC) of carious

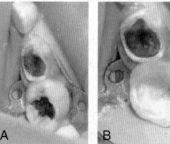
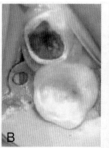
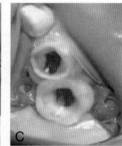
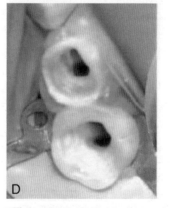
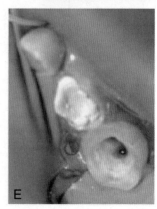

• **Figure 23.7** (A) First and second primary molars with extensive caries. (B) Pulp exposure after complete caries removal. (C) Extensive bleeding after pulp amputation; the color of the blood is bright red. (D) Bleeding stopped, indicating the tooth is appropriate for a pulpotomy. (E) The pulp stumps are covered with a zinc oxide–eugenol paste. (Courtesy Nathan Rozenfarb, DMD.)

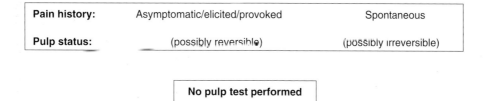

Pain history:	Asymptomatic/elicited/provoked	Spontaneous
Pulp status:	(possibly reversible)	(possibly irreversible)

No pulp test performed

(nonreliable)

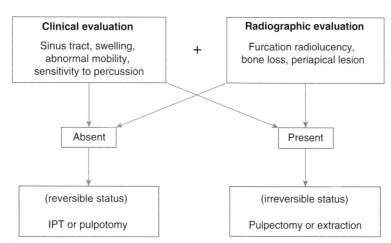

Clinical evaluation
Sinus tract, swelling, abnormal mobility, sensitivity to percussion

\+

Radiographic evaluation
Furcation radiolucency, bone loss, periapical lesion

Absent → (reversible status) IPT or pulpotomy

Present → (irreversible status) Pulpectomy or extraction

• **Figure 23.8** Pulpal diagnosis tree for deep carious lesions in primary teeth. *IPT*, Indirect pulp therapy.

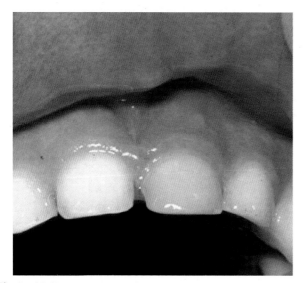

• **Figure 23.9** Luxation injury affecting tooth #F resulted in grayish discoloration and pulp necrosis with sinus tract.

exposed primary teeth is not recommended, due to questionable prognosis.[31]

A schematic diagram for pulpal diagnosis in primary teeth affected by deep carious lesions is presented in Fig. 23.8.

Trauma

Traumatic injuries to the primary dentition can have an impact on the vitality status of the pulp. Discoloration of the crown may indicate internal changes in the pulp canal. Yellow and grayish colors are the most commonly found sequelae of traumatic injuries. Periapical radiographs will aid in the diagnosis and determination of treatment if needed. Teeth diagnosed with pulp canal obliteration (yellowish) are vital and should be periodically monitored.

Teeth with light/dark gray discoloration may or may not be necrotic. If asymptomatic with no signs of soft tissue and/or periapical pathology, teeth should be only monitored.[41] The presence of a sinus tract in combination with grayish discoloration of the tooth is a pathognomonic of pulp necrosis (Fig. 23.9).

Correlation Between Histopathologic Status of the Pulp and Deep Caries

In primary teeth, very few studies investigated the correlation between caries depth and the degree of pulpal inflammation. Eidelman and Ulmansky[42] assessed the histologic appearance of the pulp of decayed, extracted, nonrestorable primary incisors affected by early childhood caries. Caries removal was performed, which may or may not have resulted in pulp exposures. When pulp exposure did not occur, pulps were more likely to be normal. It was concluded that the absence of pulp exposure could be a good indicator of a normal histologic status of the pulp. In cases when the pulp was exposed, most teeth had inflammation confined to the coronal pulp and were considered good candidates for pulpotomy. Kassa et al.[43] investigated the pulp inflammation status of extracted primary molars with occlusal and proximal caries. They found that when decay extended to more than 50% of dentin thickness, more extensive pulpal inflammation was noted for proximal caries lesions than for occlusal ones with similar depth.

Integration of the gathered clinical and radiographic information will give the clinician a direction to achieve the most accurate diagnosis possible. Clinical pulpal diagnosis continues to be a field

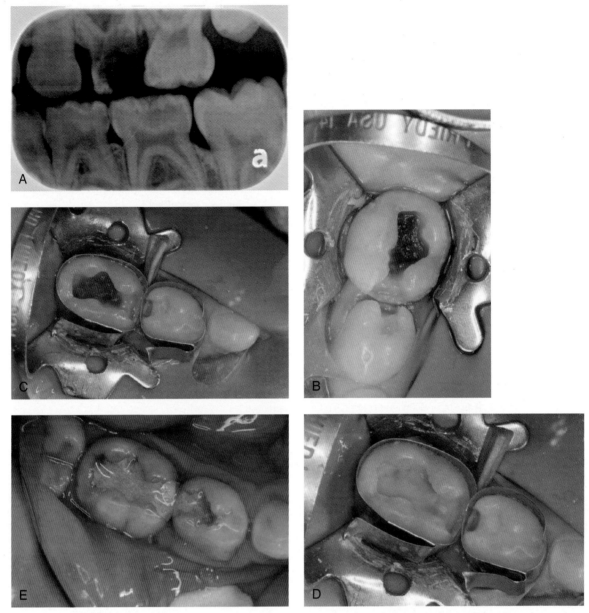

• **Figure 23.10** (A) Bitewing radiograph showing deep carious lesion affecting asymptomatic tooth #K. (B) Incomplete caries removal on the pulpal floor (tooth #K) leaving peripheral cavity walls caries-free. (C) Cavity preparations ready to be restored. (D) Resin-modified glass ionomer placed on pulpal floor as protective base. (E) Final restorations. (Courtesy Ary Kupietzky, DMD, MS.)

where more investigation is needed to develop conclusive tests to help the clinician with accurate decision-making.

Pulp Treatment Procedures

The most important and also the most difficult aspect of pulp therapy is determining the health of the pulp or its stage of inflammation so that an appropriate decision can be made regarding the best form of treatment. Different pulp treatment modalities have been recommended for primary teeth. They can be classified into two categories: vital pulp therapy for primary teeth diagnosed with a normal pulp or reversible pulpitis (pulp protection, IPT, DPC and pulpotomy) and nonvital pulp therapy for primary teeth diagnosed with irreversible pulpitis or necrotic pulp (pulpectomy and root filling). When the infection cannot be arrested by any of the methods listed, bony support cannot be regained, and the tooth is not restorable, extraction is the treatment of choice (see Fig. 23.8).

Vital Pulp Therapy for Normal Pulp/Reversible Pulpitis

Complete removal of all carious tissue followed by "extension for prevention" to place the margins of the restoration in areas less vulnerable to caries was considered the gold standard 150 years ago.[39] A paradigm shift in carious lesions treatment has occurred, and in 1997 Fusyama[44] suggested that in the superficial layer, grossly denatured *infected* dentin should be removed, while in the underlying layer, partially demineralized caries-*affected* dentin (containing intact, undenatured collagen fibrils amenable to remineralize) should be preserved during caries excavation.[45,46] These terms are now considered outdated, particularly the term *infected*, which conveys the idea that dental caries is an infectious or communicable disease that needs to be cured by removing bacteria.[47] Presently, managing a carious lesion includes several options, from the complete surgical excision, where no visible carious tissue is left prior to placement of the restoration, to the opposite extreme, where no caries is removed and noninvasive methods are used to prevent progression of the lesion.[48,49]

A group of cariology experts from 12 countries met in 2015 (the International Caries Consensus Collaboration—ICCC) to discuss issues of relevance to cariology researchers, dental educators, and the clinical dentistry community.[39]

In describing the clinical manifestation of caries, these experts agreed that it would be ideal to relate the visual, clinical appearance of the lesion directly to what is taking place histopathologically.[50,51] Although this is not so straightforward, histopathologic investigations of the relationship between the visual appearance of the carious tissue and several parameters such as bacterial invasion, degree of demineralization, and softness of dentin helped develop an understanding of the carious process. As histologic terms are less helpful when communicating with dentists in the clinical setting, and for practical purposes when trying to describe which carious tissue should be removed, the ICCC[39] described the different physical properties associated with the different status of dentin as follows:

Soft dentin will deform when a hard instrument is pressed onto it and can be easily scooped up (e.g., with a sharp excavator), with little force being required.

Leathery dentin does not deform when an instrument is pressed onto it, but it can still be lifted without much force. There might be little difference between *leathery* and *firm* dentin, while leathery is a transition in the spectrum between soft and firm dentin.

Firm dentin is physically resistant to hand excavation, and some pressure needs to be exerted through an instrument to lift it.

Hard dentin: A pushing force needs to be used with a hard instrument to engage the dentin. Only a sharp cutting-edge instrument or a bur will lift it. A scratchy sound or "cri dentinaire" can be heard when a straight probe is taken across the dentin.

As dental caries is a biofilm disease, the ICCC suggests both prevention of new lesions and management of existing lesions should focus primarily on control or management rather than tissue removal. Noncavitated (cleansable) lesions can be managed with biofilm removal (toothbrushing) and/or remineralization. Cavitated (noncleansable) dentin carious lesions cannot be managed by biofilm removal, and remineralization and restorative interventions are indicated.[47]

To remove carious tissue in teeth with vital pulps and without signs of irreversible pulp inflammation, several strategies are available, based on the previously mentioned level of hardness of the remaining dentin.[48] The decision among these strategies will be guided by the depth of the lesion and by the dentition (primary or permanent).

Nonselective removal to hard dentin (complete excavation or complete caries removal) uses the same criteria for carious tissue removal both peripherally and pulpally, and only hard dentin is left. This is considered overtreatment and is no longer advocated (ICCC).

Selective removal to firm dentin leaves leathery dentin pulpally, while the cavity margins are left hard after removal. This is the treatment of choice for both dentitions in shallow or moderately cavitated dentinal lesions (radiographically extending less than the pulpal third or quarter of dentin).

Selective removal to soft dentin is recommended in deep cavitated lesions (radiographically extending into the pulpal third or quarter of dentin). Soft carious tissue is left over the pulp to avoid exposure and further injury to the pulp, while peripheral enamel and dentin are prepared to hard dentin to allow a tight seal and a durable restoration. Selective removal to soft dentin reduces the risk of pulp exposure significantly when compared with nonselective removal to hard or selective removal to firm dentin.

Stepwise removal is carious tissue removal in two stages. Soft carious tissue is left over the pulp on the first step, and the tooth is sealed with a provisional restoration that should be durable to last up to 12 months to allow changes in the dentin and pulp to take place. In reentering, after removing the restoration, as the dentin is drier and harder, caries removal is continued. There is some evidence that in such deep lesions the second step might be omitted, as it increases the risk of pulp exposure.[52,53]

The second step also adds additional cost, time, and discomfort for the patient; there is also enough evidence that it is not considered necessary for primary teeth, and selective removal to soft dentin should be carried out.[53]

Protective Base

Guidelines published by the AAPD recommend placement of a protective base or liner on the pulpal and axial walls of a cavity preparation to act as a protective barrier between the restorative material and the tooth.[31] Dentin is permeable and allows the movement of materials from the oral cavity to the pulp and vice versa. It was believed for several years that pulp inflammation was caused by the toxic effects from dental materials.[54] However, there is sufficient evidence to show that pulpal inflammation resulting from dental materials is mild and transitory, with adverse reactions occurring as the result of pulpal invasion by bacteria or their toxins.[18,19,55] Continued marginal leakage with secondary recurrent caries is probably the most common cause of pulp degeneration under restorations. In deep cavities, the dentin covering the pulp is thin, and the tubules are large in diameter and packed closely together. This dentin is extremely permeable and should be covered with a material that seals dentin well, usually glass ionomer cement.[56]

The materials most recently used as cavity sealers are those that have demonstrated multisubstrate bonding ability to bond the restorative material to the tooth. These include resin cements, glass ionomers, and dentin-bonding agents. The benefits of using these materials to bond composite to tooth structure is a well-documented and accepted procedure.[56] However, employing them with amalgam is more controversial. Mahler and colleagues[57] observed no difference between amalgam restorations placed with and without bonding after 2 years, and concluded that the use of bonding agents under traditional amalgam fillings should not be recommended. *Thus protective liners or bases should only be placed in deep cavities approaching the pulp.*

Indirect Pulp Treatment (Selective Removal to Soft Dentin)

IPT is recommended for teeth that have deep carious lesions approximating the pulp but have no signs or symptoms of pulp degeneration. In this procedure, the deepest layer of the remaining carious dentin is covered with a biocompatible material. This results in the deposition of tertiary dentin, increasing the distance between the remaining soft dentin and the pulp, and in the deposition of peritubular (sclerotic) dentin, which decreases dentin permeability. It is important to remove the carious tissue completely from the dentinoenamel junction and from the lateral walls of the cavity to achieve optimal interfacial seal between the tooth and the restorative material, thus preventing microleakage.

As previously described, IPT *(selective removal to soft dentin)* is recommended in deep cavitated lesions (radiographically extending into the pulpal third or quarter of the dentin). Soft carious tissue is left over the pulp to avoid exposure and further injury, while peripheral enamel and dentin are prepared to hard dentin, to allow a tight seal and a durable restoration. Selective removal to soft dentin reduces the risk of pulp exposure significantly when compared with nonselective removal to hard dentin or selective removal to firm dentin (see Fig. 23.9A–E). Clinical experience and a good understanding of the process of caries progression can allow for better control of the "partial removal caries (selective removal to soft dentin)" step. A large round bur (no. 6 or 8) can provide better results than spoon excavators.[58] The ultimate objective of this treatment is to maintain pulp vitality[59] by (1) arresting the carious process, (2) promoting dentin sclerosis (reducing permeability), (3) stimulating the formation of tertiary dentin, and (4) remineralizing the carious dentin.

A chemomechanical approach to caries excavation known as Carisolv (Medi Team Dental, Savedalen, Sweden) has been developed. A gel made of three amino acids and a low concentration of sodium hypochlorite is rubbed into the carious dentin with specially designed hand instruments. With Carisolv, sound and carious dentin are clinically separated, and only carious dentin is removed, resulting in a more conservative preparation. When a bur is used, healthy tissue is frequently removed. The main drawback to this technique is the time needed to complete the procedure, because it is a much slower process than removing caries with a bur.[60]

Another chemomechanical product has been developed in Brazil under the commercial name of Papacarie (Fórmula & Ação, São Paulo, SP, Brazil). This product is a gel containing papain, an enzyme similar to human pepsin, that acts as a debriding agent with no harm to healthy tissue. No statistical difference was observed in a clinical study after 6 to 18 months when papain was compared with conventional caries removal in primary teeth.[61]

It is current knowledge that, in the appropriate metabolic state of the dentin-pulp complex, a new generation of odontoblast-like cells might differentiate and form tubular tertiary dentin (reparative dentinogenesis).[8,62] It must be emphasized that under clinical conditions, the matrix formed at the pulp-dentin interface often comprises reactionary dentin, reparative dentin, or fibrodentin formation. It is impossible to distinguish these processes in vivo, and the process might also be indistinguishable at both biochemical and molecular levels.

Presently, the materials most commonly used in IPT (selective removal to soft dentin) are calcium hydroxide, glass ionomer, and mineral trioxide aggregate (MTA). Many historical studies have examined the interaction between tooth tissues and calcium hydroxide, and more recently with MTA. The main soluble component from MTA has been shown to be calcium hydroxide. The clinical response of the tooth to both materials is based on comparable mechanisms involving the dissolution of calcium hydroxide and release of calcium and hydroxyl ions, raising the pH of the environment well above 7.0. Because dentin contains a large store of potentially bioactive molecules, it has been considered that the interaction of a high pH material, such as calcium hydroxide or MTA, may cause the release of some of these molecules. This action is similar to that occurring during the demineralization of dentin during a caries attack, where the pH of the local environment is low.[63]

When resin-modified glass ionomers are placed into a cavity preparation or on an exposed pulp, their initial pH within the first 24 hours is approximately 4.0 to 5.5. Therefore the glass ionomer demineralizes the adjacent dentin, releasing ions and potentially the sequestered bioactive materials as well. The pulpal response to glass ionomer is favorable when a layer of dentin remains between the material and the pulp.

Studies of DPC with glass ionomer show that both patient tolerance and clinical success rates are lower with ionomer than calcium hydroxide. This finding suggests that the acidic environment created by the glass ionomer is more damaging to the pulp than the basic environment of calcium hydroxide or MTA.[19,56]

Dentin-bonding agents have been recommended for use in DPC[64] and IPT.[65] However, there are some concerns regarding IPT (selective removal to soft dentin) with these materials.[63] Nakajima and coworkers[66] found a significant loss of bond strength to human carious dentin when compared with sound dentin. This finding leads one to further question the integrity of the bond and subsequent ability to prevent bacterial invasion of a carious substrate.

Contrary to previous beliefs, IPT can also be an acceptable procedure for primary teeth with reversible pulp inflammation, provided that the diagnosis is based on a good history and proper clinical and radiographic examination and the tooth has been sealed with a leakage-free restoration.[67]

The value of taking a good history complemented by a careful clinical and radiographic examination cannot be overstated when trying to reach an accurate diagnosis. However, sometimes this cannot be achieved, and the prognosis of the tooth will be affected. Fig. 23.11A and B show the treatment outcome of two mandibular first primary molars in the same patient. The tooth treated with an MTA pulpotomy presents internal root resorption, whereas its antimere, restored conservatively with a composite over an IPT, looks normal. These findings were probably attributable to the preoperative status of the pulp. The radicular pulp of the pulpotomized tooth was probably chronically inflamed at the time of treatment but could not be disclosed even by operative diagnosis.

Success rates of IPT have been reported to be higher than 90% in primary teeth, and thus its use is recommended in patients whose preoperative diagnosis suggests no signs of pulp degeneration. Ricketts and colleagues[68] concluded that "in deep lesions, partial caries removal is preferable to complete caries removal to reduce the risk of carious exposure." Several articles reported the success of this technique in primary teeth.[58,69–72] The overall success of IPT (selective removal to soft dentin) has been reported to be higher than the success rates of DPC or pulpotomy, the alternative pulp treatments for primary molars with deep dentinal caries.[58,69–73] One can conclude that, on the basis of these biological changes and the growing evidence of the success of IPT in primary teeth, *we can recommend IPT* (selective removal to soft dentin) *as the most appropriate treatment for symptom-free primary teeth with deep caries, provided that a proper, leakage-free restoration can be placed.*

A recent systematic review and meta-analysis on primary tooth vital pulp therapy[74] demonstrated that the "highest level of success and quality of evidence supported IPT and the pulpotomy

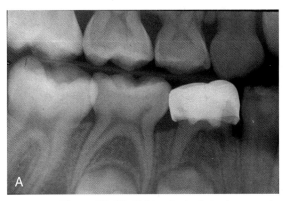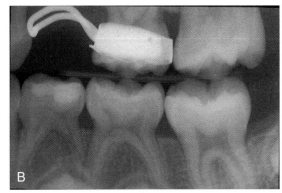

• **Figure 23.11** (A) Mandibular first primary molars of the same patient 3 years after treatment of deep caries. Tooth treated with mineral trioxide aggregate pulpotomy. Internal resorption is evident. (B) Contralateral tooth treated conservatively with indirect pulp treatment and a composite restoration. The pulp looks normal.

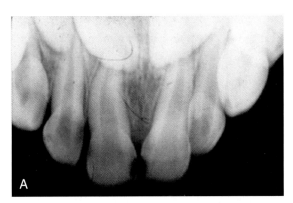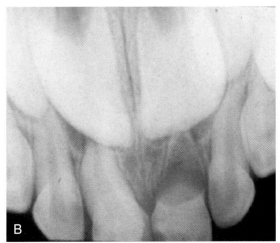

• **Figure 23.12** (A) Maxillary primary central incisor treated by direct pulp capping with CaOH₂ following pinpoint iatrogenic pulp exposure. (B) Extensive internal resorption was evident 6 months later.

techniques of MTA and FC for the treatment of deep caries in primary teeth after 24 months. DPC showed similar success rates to IPT and MTA or FC pulpotomies, but the quality of evidence was lower."

New experimental strategies use bioactive molecules such as enamel matrix protein (Emdogain [Straumann Canada Limited, Burlington, Ontario]) or TGF-β to stimulate tertiary dentin formation and decrease dentin permeability. However, these are not yet in clinical use.[3]

Direct Pulp Capping

DPC is carried out when a healthy pulp has been inadvertently exposed during an operative procedure. The tooth must be asymptomatic, and the exposure site must be pinpoint in diameter and free of oral contaminants. A calcium hydroxide medicament is placed over the exposure site to stimulate dentin formation and thus "heal" the wound and maintain the vitality of the pulp.[2] The effectiveness of TGF-β and BMPs in inducing reparative dentinogenesis in pulp capping situations in vivo[75–77] provides the basis for development of a possible new generation of biomaterials. Because the specificity of these growth factors to induce reparative processes is not clear, more studies are required to fully explain the kinetics of growth factor release and the sequence of growth factor–induced reparative dentinogenesis.

DPC of a carious pulp exposure in a primary tooth is not recommended but can be used with success on immature permanent teeth. The direct pulp cap is indicated for small mechanical or traumatic exposures when conditions for a favorable response are optimal. Even in these cases, the success rate is not particularly high in primary teeth. Failure of treatment may result in internal resorption (Fig. 23.12A and B) or acute dentoalveolar abscess. Kennedy and Kapala[78] claim that the high cellular content of the primary pulp tissue may be responsible for the increased failure rate of DPC in primary teeth. These authors believe that undifferentiated mesenchymal cells may differentiate into odontoclasts, leading to internal resorption, a principal sign of failure of DPC in primary teeth.

Some investigators advocate the use of dentin-bonding agents for DPC.[64,79] The rationale for this is based on the belief that if an effective, permanent seal against bacterial invasion is provided, pulp healing will occur. Animal research has shown the good compatibility of mechanically exposed pulps to visible light–activated composite when bacteria are excluded.[18] Araujo and associates[80] reported good clinical and radiographic results in cariously exposed primary teeth 1 year after acid etching and capping with a bonding agent and restoration with a resin-based composite. Based on these reports, Kopel[81] proposed a "revisitation" of the DPC technique in primary teeth. He suggested "gently wiping the dentin floor and the exposed pulp with an antibacterial solution such as chlorhexidine or a fixative such as formocresol or a weak glutaraldehyde solution," replacing calcium hydroxide with dentin-bonding agents. In another publication a year later, Araujo and colleagues[82] examined histologically primary molars with microexposures that were successfully treated with a composite acid etch technique and then extracted or exfoliated. These authors observed microabscesses adjacent to the exposure site, and no dentin bridge was formed in any specimen. These results were confirmed by Pameijer and Stanley,[83,84] who concluded that "the belief that any material placed on an exposed pulp will allow bridge formation as long as the cavity is disinfected is a fallacy." In a review on pulp capping with dentin-adhesive systems, Costa and coworkers[85] reported that self-etching adhesive systems led to inflammatory reactions, delay in pulpal healing, and failure of dentin bridging in human pulps capped with bonding agents. They state that vital pulp therapy using acidic agents and adhesive resins seems to be contraindicated.

Although guidelines published by the AAPD do not recommend DPC for caries exposed primary teeth,[31] promising results (over 90% success) of recent clinical trials may challenge that policy in the near future.[86–88] MTA, bonding agents, and enamel derivate protein (Emdogain), with or without prior rinsing of the exposed pulp with saline or an antibacterial solution such as sodium hypochlorite or chlorhexidine, were compared with calcium hydroxide as capping agents. Regardless of the methodology used, very strict inclusion criteria were common to all tested teeth: absence of clinical and radiographic signs and symptoms such as swelling, abnormal mobility, presence of fistula, spontaneous pain, sensitivity to percussion, and furcation involvement. In addition, all exposed pulps had to be limited to 1.0 mm or less. In only one study, rubber dam isolation was not used,[88] and bonding agents' techniques were compared with calcium hydroxide as pulp protection. Relative isolation did not interfere with the outcome. A high success rate was only obtained when phosphoric acid and non-rinse conditioners did not directly contact the pulp. Restorations of the treated teeth were performed with amalgam only,[88] amalgam and resin-based materials followed by a sealant coverage,[86] and stainless steel crowns.[87] Coll et al.[74] reported that up to 24 months, "DPC showed similar success rates to IPT and MTA or FC pulpotomies, but the quality of evidence was lower." When long-term results (beyond 24 months) of these procedures are available, more definitive conclusions can be drawn regarding this technique for primary teeth.

Presently, DPC in primary teeth should still be viewed with some reservations. However, this treatment could be recommended for exposed pulps in older children, 1 or 2 years before normal exfoliation. In these children, a failure of treatment would not require the use of a space maintainer following extraction, as it would in younger children.

Pulpotomy

As stated previously, recent evidence suggests that IPT (selective removal to soft dentin) is preferred over the traditional pulpotomy. All efforts should be made to avoid pulpal exposure when treating deep carious lesions. However, when the carious process has reached the pulp or in incidences of direct pulpal exposure during excavation of a carious lesion, the pulpotomy procedure is indicated and is the treatment of choice.

The pulpotomy procedure is based on the rationale that the radicular pulp tissue is healthy or is capable of healing after surgical amputation of the affected or infected coronal pulp.[1,2] The presence

of any signs and/or symptoms of inflammation extending beyond the coronal pulp is a contraindication for a pulpotomy. Thus, a pulpotomy is contraindicated when any of the following are present: swelling (of pulpal origin), fistula, pathologic mobility, pathologic external root resorption, internal root resorption, periapical or interradicular radiolucency, pulp calcifications, or excessive bleeding from the amputated radicular stumps. Other signs, such as a history of spontaneous or nocturnal pain or tenderness to percussion or palpation, should be interpreted carefully (see Fig. 23.4A and B).

The ideal dressing material for the radicular pulp should (1) be bactericidal, (2) be harmless to the pulp and surrounding structures, (3) promote healing of the radicular pulp, and (4) not interfere with the physiologic process of root resorption. A good deal of controversy surrounds the issue of pulpotomy agents, and unfortunately the "ideal" pulp dressing material has not yet been identified. A decade ago, the most commonly used pulp dressing material was formocresol (Buckley solution: formaldehyde, cresol, glycerol, and water). Primosch and associates[89] reported in 1997 that the majority of the predoctoral pediatric dental programs in the United States advocated the use of either full-strength formocresol (22.6% of programs) or a one-fifth dilution of formocresol (71.7% of programs) as the preferred pulpotomy medicament for vital primary teeth. However, more recent surveys have shown that formocresol is no longer the most commonly taught medicament for pulpotomy. In the United States, a 2008 survey detected a trend away from the teaching of 1:5 diluted formocresol, with more using ferric sulfate (FS) for pulpotomy; still, 22% of programs recommended full-strength formocresol.[90]

Conversely, in Brazilian dental schools, the pulpotomy agent that students are most frequently taught to use is diluted formocresol.[91] A study surveying the teaching practices in the United Kingdom and Ireland showed a preference for FS, with 93% of respondents advocating its use for pulpotomy.[92] Evidently, philosophies and approaches to pulpotomy agents vary among countries and regions, and even among dental schools. Issues regarding the selection of pulpotomy medicaments will be discussed later in this chapter.

Pulpotomy Technique

Before local anesthesia administration, a thorough clinical examination should be repeated, including visual examination of the vestibulum, palpation, and percussion of the involved and neighboring teeth. After local anesthesia has been given and the rubber dam placed, all superficial caries should be removed before pulpal exposure to minimize bacterial contamination following exposure. The roof of the pulp chamber should be removed by joining the pulp horns with bur cuts. This procedure is usually accomplished using a no. 330 bur mounted in a water-cooled high-speed turbine. The coronal pulp is then amputated using either a sharp excavator or a slowly revolving large round bur. This procedure should be done carefully to prevent further damage to the pulp and perforation of the pulpal floor. Care must be taken to ensure that all the coronal pulp tissue has been removed. Tags of tissue remaining under ledges of dentin may continue to bleed, masking the actual status of the radicular pulp stumps and thus obscuring a correct diagnosis (Fig. 23.13A).

Following coronal pulp amputation, one or more cotton pellets should be placed over each amputation site, and pressure should be applied for a few minutes. When the cotton pellets are removed, hemostasis should be apparent, although a minor amount of wound bleeding may be evident (see Fig. 23.13B). Excessive bleeding that persists in spite of cotton pellet pressure and a deep purple color

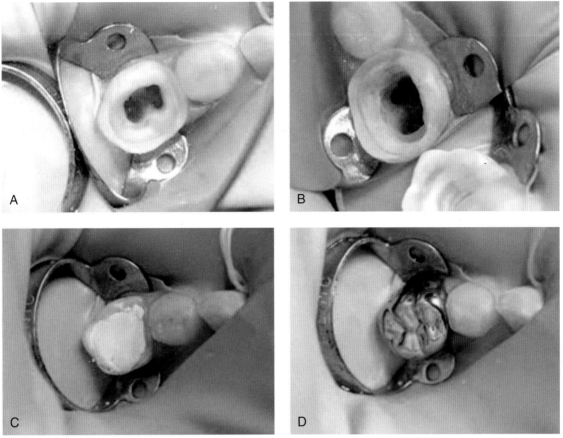

• **Figure 23.13** Pulpotomy technique steps. (A) Pulp chamber after coronal pulp amputation; wide access opening prevents leaving tissue tags. (B) After hemostasis and formocresol application, the tissue at the entrance of the canals shows dark color, a sign of tissue fixation. (C) The pulps stumps are covered by a zinc oxide–eugenol base. (D) The tooth is restored with a stainless steel crown. (Courtesy Nathan Rosenfarb, DDS.)

of the tissue may indicate that the inflammation has extended to the radicular pulp. Such signs indicate that the tooth is not a good candidate for formocresol pulpotomy, and pulpectomy or extraction should be done. No intrapulpal local anesthesia or other hemostatic agent should be used to minimize hemorrhage, because bleeding is a clinical indicator of the radicular pulp status. Following hemostasis, a cotton pellet moistened with Buckley solution (full concentration or one-fifth solution) is placed over the pulp stumps for 5 minutes. However, a study has suggested that a 1-minute exposure to full-strength formocresol is sufficient and comparable in clinical success to the 5-minute technique.[93] When the pellet is removed, the amputation site should appear dark brown (when a full concentration of formocresol is used) or dark red (when the one-fifth dilution is employed). In both cases, very little or no hemorrhage is present. A base of ZOE (either plain or reinforced) is placed over the amputation site and lightly condensed to cover the pulpal floor. A second layer is then condensed to fill the access opening completely (see Fig. 23.13C). The final restoration is preferably a stainless steel crown, which should be placed at the same appointment (see Fig. 23.13D). Holan and coworkers[94] observed that pulpotomized primary molars could be successfully restored with one-surface amalgams if their natural exfoliation is expected within 2 years or less. However, if placing the final restoration is not possible, the ZOE base will serve as an acceptable interim restoration until the stainless steel crown can be placed.

The MTA and FS procedures are essentially the same with either of the medicaments used in place of formocresol. The MTA is prepared as per manufacturer's instructions. MTA paste is applied to cover the exposed radicular pulp surface with a margin of not less than 1 mm beyond the pulp dentin interface. When using FS, the amputated pulps at the canal orifices are wiped with 15.5% solution of FS (Astringedent) for 10 to 15 seconds. Next, Astringedent is flushed from the pulp chamber with water. In all cases, if bleeding does not stop, then one should proceed to primary molar root canal therapy or extraction.

Guelmann and colleagues[95] analyzed the success rates of emergency pulpotomies in primary molars. They concluded that the low success rate (53%) of the pulpotomies during the first 3 months could be attributed to undiagnosed subclinical inflammation of pulps, whereas long-term failures might be associated with microleakage of the temporary restorations.

Clinical and radiographic studies have demonstrated that formocresol pulpotomies have success rates ranging from 70% to 97%.[96–99] The use of a one-fifth dilution of formocresol has been advocated by several authors[96,97] because of its reportedly equal effectiveness and potential for less toxicity. This solution is prepared by making a diluent of three parts glycerin and one part water.

Four parts of this diluent are then mixed with one part Buckley solution to make the one-fifth dilution.

Although many studies have reported the clinical success of formocresol pulpotomies, an increasing body of literature has questioned the use of formocresol. Rolling and Thylstrup[99] demonstrated that its clinical success rate decreased as follow-up time increased. Furthermore, the histologic response of the primary radicular pulp to formocresol appears to be unfavorable. A classic study claims that, subsequent to formocresol application, fixation occurs in the coronal third of the radicular pulp, chronic inflammation in the middle third, and vital tissue in the apical third.[100] Others report that the remaining pulp tissue is partially or totally necrotic.[101] Several reports have questioned the safety of formocresol,[102,103] and most authorities now agree that formocresol is at least potentially mutagenic, carcinogenic, and toxic when used in high concentrations and under specific conditions in animal studies. However, there are no documented cases of systemic distribution or pathologic tissue changes associated with the use of formocresol in humans.[104] The doses used in animal models far exceed those used in clinical practice; normal clinical doses carry little risk for patients. Indeed, a study examined the presence of formocresol in the plasma of children undergoing oral rehabilitation involving pulp therapy under general anesthesia, and showed that formaldehyde and cresol were undetectable above baseline plasma concentration in subjects receiving pulpotomy treatment under general anesthesia.[105] The authors concluded that the levels present were far below those recommended by the US Food and Drug Administration (FDA). It is unlikely that formocresol, when used in the doses typically employed for a vital pulpotomy procedure, poses any risk to children. Nevertheless, amid the controversies and concerns, efforts have increased to find a substitute medicament.

Potential Substitutes for Formocresol

Glutaraldehyde (GA) has been proposed as an alternative to formocresol because it is a mild fixative and is potentially less toxic. Because of its cross-linking properties, penetration into the tissue is more limited, with less effect on periapical tissues. The short-term success of 2% GA as a pulpotomy agent has been demonstrated in several studies.[106–111] However, longer-term success rates matching those of formocresol have not been reported. Fuks and associates[107] reported a failure rate of 18% in human primary molars 25 months after pulpotomy, using a 2% concentration of GA. In the same study sample at 42 months follow-up, the authors noted that 45% of the teeth that underwent pulpotomy with GA resorbed faster than their controls.[109]

Some biological materials have been proposed as pulp dressings, on the theoretical basis that they would promote physiologic healing of the pulpotomy wound. Varying levels of success in early experimental studies have been reported with freeze-dried bone[112] autolyzed, antigen-extracted, allogeneic dentin matrix[113]; allogeneic BMP,[14] a fully synthetic nanocrystalline hydroxyapatite paste[114]; enriched collagen solutions[115]; and Biodentine, a calcium-silicate–based material.[116] Clinical studies have reported promising results using FS, a hemostatic agent, in pulpotomized human primary teeth.[117,118] Fuks and colleagues[119] reported a success rate of 93% in teeth treated with FS and 84% in those where diluted formocresol (DFC) was employed. These teeth were followed up from 6 to 35 months. In a preliminary report of the same study, a much lower success rate was described (77.5% for the FS group and 81% for the DFC teeth), with internal resorption evident in five teeth treated with FS and four teeth fixed with DFC.[118] This discrepancy can be explained by an excessively severe interpretation of the

initial findings. Areas listed initially as internal resorption on the preliminary report remained unchanged after 30 months, and thus were reassessed as normal in the last evaluation (Fig. 23.14).[118] Success rates comparable to those of formocresol were also reported by Smith and coworkers.[120] A higher percentage of internal resorption using FS and formocresol was reported by Papagiannoulis[121] after a longer follow-up time; comparable results were seen in shorter postoperative examinations. A recent systematic review and meta-analysis concluded that pulpotomies performed with either formocresol or FS in primary molars have similar clinical and radiographic success, and that FS may be recommended as a suitable replacement for formocresol.[122] Based in these studies, FS can still be an appropriate and inexpensive solution for pulpotomies in primary teeth.

Preliminary studies have investigated the use of 5% sodium hypochlorite (NaOCl) as a primary molar pulpotomy agent. A pilot study by Vargas and colleagues[123] showed promising results after a 12-month period, and a retrospective study[124] confirmed these findings. Both studies concluded that clinical and radiographic success rates for NaOCl pulpotomies are comparable to FS and formocresol pulpotomies. In a recent prospective study[125] comparing NaOCl with formocresol examined treatment outcomes after 1 year, NaOCl demonstrated clinical and radiographic success comparable to formocresol pulpotomies. However, further studies with longer observation periods are needed before NaOCl may be recommended for routine use when performing pulpotomies on primary teeth, as demonstrated in a study[126] evaluating outcomes after 18 months which found the success rate of NaOCl as being significantly less than formocresol.

An evidence-based proven alternative to formocresol with reported success rates equal and even surpassing those of formocresol and all other pulpotomy agents is MTA.[127] MTA was developed by Torabinejad at Loma Linda University in the 1990s, first described in the dental scientific literature by Lee and colleagues[128] in 1993, and approved by the FDA in 1998. It is a mixture of a refined Portland cement (PC), dicalcium silicate, tricalcium silicate, tricalcium aluminate, gypsum, and tetracalcium aluminoferrite; bismuth oxide is also added, making the material radiopaque. Both in vitro and in vivo investigations have shown that MTA has many positive properties such as excellent biocompatibility, an alkaline pH, radiopacity, a high sealing capacity, and the ability to induce the formation of dentin, cement, and bone.[129]

In a preliminary study comparing MTA with formocresol, with follow-ups ranging from 6 to 30 months, none of the MTA-treated teeth showed a clinical or radiographic pathologic process. Pulp

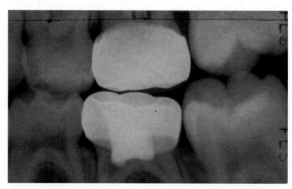

• **Figure 23.14** Mandibular second primary molar presenting internal root resorption following pulpotomy with ferric sulfate. The area remained unchanged for 30 months.

canal obliteration was detected in 13% of the teeth treated with formocresol and in 41% of those treated with MTA. A radiograph of two primary molars treated with MTA is presented in Fig. 23.15. Internal root resorption, a finding seen both in FS- and DFC-treated teeth in other studies,[119,121] was not observed in MTA-treated teeth in the preliminary report.[130] Longer clinical studies have since been published with high success rates.[131–137] Holan and associates[138] investigated MTA effects in 33 pulpotomized molars during a median follow-up evaluation period of 38.2 months, reporting a success rate of 97%. Farsi and coworkers[139] compared the effect of MTA in 60 pulpotomized molars with those of formocresol followed during 2 years and noted a success rate of 100%.

When MTA was first commercialized, it had a gray coloration; but in 2002 a new white formula was created to improve on the dark color properties exhibited by the gray preparation. White MTA has smaller particles and does not contain tetracalcium aluminoferrite or iron, both were found in gray MTA. Cardoso-Silva and colleagues[140] compared the results of gray and white MTA pulpotomies in a sample of 233 primary molars, with a maximum follow-up period of 84 months. The gray MTA had 100% radiographic success, and the white had a 93% success rate. Another interesting finding was that gray MTA showed a significantly higher number of dentine bridge formation than white MTA. MTA is commercially available as ProRoot MTA (DENTSPLY Tulsa Dental Products, Tulsa, OK), and more recently as MTA-Angelus (Angelus Soluções Odontológicas, Londrina, Brazil), but its price is very high. Since the material cannot be kept once the envelope is opened, its clinical use in pediatric dentistry practice becomes almost prohibitive. Indeed, a Cochrane review[141] concluded that among possible pulpotomy agents, two medicaments may be preferable: MTA or formocresol. However, the authors state that the cost of MTA may preclude its routine clinical use. Consequently, great interest has been focused on the evolution of PC as an alternative to MTA, and several experimental studies have compared both materials.

PC differs from MTA by the absence of bismuth ions and the presence of potassium ions. Both materials have comparable antibacterial activity and almost identical properties macroscopically, microscopically, and by x-ray diffraction analysis. A recent study[142] compared the success rates of PC, MTA, formocresol, and enamel matrix derivative in primary molar pulpotomies and found similar clinical and radiographic effectiveness after 24 months. However,

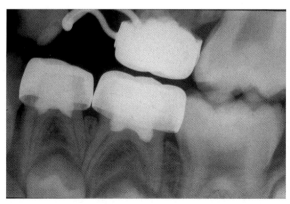

• **Figure 23.15** Mandibular first and second primary molars 36 months after pulpotomy with mineral trioxide aggregate. Pulp canal obliteration is evident in the distal root of the second molar; both procedures were rated as successful.

before routine clinical use of PC can be recommended, further studies with large samples and long follow-up assessments are needed.

Newer bioactive cements such as Biodentine have been used as pulpotomy agents with promising results. A recent 18-month follow-up randomized clinical study found similar results when Biodentine was compared with ProRoot MTA.[143]

Nonpharmacotherapeutic approaches to pulpotomy include the treatment of radicular pulp tissue by electrocautery or laser to eliminate residual infectious processes. Although these techniques are currently being used by a number of practitioners, no long-term controlled clinical studies are available to evaluate their success, and studies have shown conflicting results.[144–146]

In summary, the search for alternatives to formocresol as a pulp dressing in primary tooth pulpotomies has yet to reveal an ideal agent or technique. Until such an agent is found, formocresol (either in a one-fifth dilution or full strength), FS, or MTA can be used as capping agents in primary tooth pulpotomies.[147]

The systematic review and meta-analysis on primary tooth vital pulp therapy,[74] mentioned previously, will be the evidence-based material to be used in the new Guideline for Pulp Therapy for Primary Teeth for the AAPD. This review demonstrated that the "highest level of success and quality of evidence supported IPT and the pulpotomy techniques of MTA and FC for the treatment of deep caries in primary teeth after 24 months. Direct pulp capping showed similar success rates to IPT and MTA or FC pulpotomies, but the quality of evidence was lower." The comparable success rates for all three vital pulp therapy techniques (IPT, DPC, and pulpotomy) provide more latitude in treatment choices for the practitioner in managing a vital primary tooth with deep caries.

Nonvital Pulp Therapy for Irreversible Pulpitis or Necrotic Pulp: Pulpectomy and Root Filling

The pulpectomy procedure is indicated in teeth that show evidence of chronic inflammation or necrosis in the radicular pulp. Conversely, pulpectomy is contraindicated in teeth with gross loss of root structure, advanced internal or external resorption, or periapical infection involving the crypt of the succedaneous tooth. The goal of pulpectomy is to maintain primary teeth that would otherwise be lost. However, clinicians disagree about the utility of pulpectomy procedures in primary teeth. Difficulty in the preparation of primary root canals that have complex and variable morphologic features and uncertainty about the effects of instrumentation, medication, and filling materials on developing succedaneous teeth dissuade some clinicians from using the technique. The behavior management problems that sometimes occur in pediatric patients have surely added to the reluctance among some dentists to perform root canal treatments in primary teeth. These problems notwithstanding, the success of pulpectomies in primary teeth has led most pediatric dentists to prefer them to the alternative of extractions and space maintenance.

Certain clinical situations may justify pulpectomy, even with the knowledge that the prognosis may not be ideal. An example of such a case is pulp destruction of a primary second molar that occurs before the first permanent molar erupts. A premature extraction of the primary second molar without placement of a space maintainer usually results in mesial eruption of the first permanent molar with subsequent loss of space for the second premolar (Fig. 23.16A and B). Although a distal shoe space maintainer could be used, maintaining the natural tooth is definitely the treatment of choice. Therefore, a pulpectomy in a primary second molar is preferable, even if that tooth is maintained only

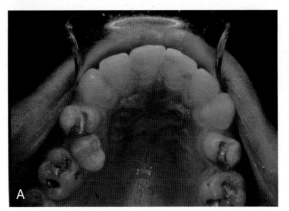
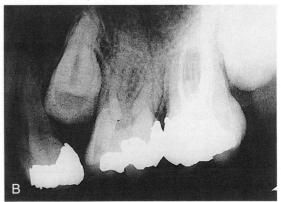

• **Figure 23.16** (A) Occlusal view of the permanent dentition following bilateral premature extractions of the maxillary primary second molars. The right second bicuspid erupted ectopically, and the left is impacted. (B) Radiograph of the area showing the impacted left premolar. (Courtesy Ilana Brin, DMD.)

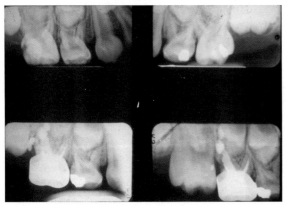

• **Figure 23.17** Nonvital maxillary second primary molar, treated by pulpectomy with zinc oxide–eugenol (ZOE). *Top left,* Before pulpectomy. *Top right,* Contralateral vital tooth. *Bottom left,* Excess of ZOE in palatal and distobuccal canals. *Bottom right,* Primary tooth successfully retained until eruption of first permanent molar.

until the first permanent molar has adequately erupted and is followed eventually by extraction of the primary second molar and placement of a space maintainer (Fig. 23.17A–D).

Root Canal Filling Materials

Developmental, anatomic, and physiologic differences between primary and permanent teeth call for differences in the criteria for root canal filling materials. The ideal root canal filling material for primary teeth should resorb at a rate similar to that of the primary root, be harmless to the periapical tissues and to the permanent tooth germ, resorb readily if pressed beyond the apex, be antiseptic, fill the root canals easily, adhere to their walls, not shrink, be easily removed if necessary, be radiopaque, and not discolor the tooth.[148] No material currently available meets all of these criteria. Several investigators assessed clinically and radiographically different root filling materials.[149–155] These studies had no controls, and their relevance is limited.

The filling materials most commonly used for primary pulp canals are ZOE paste, iodoform-based paste, calcium hydroxide, and calcium hydroxide and iodoform in combination.[2]

Zinc Oxide–Eugenol Paste. ZOE is a commonly used filling material for primary teeth in the United States. Camp[156] introduced

the endodontic pressure syringe to overcome the problem of underfilling, a relatively common finding when thick mixes of ZOE are employed. However, underfilling is frequently clinically acceptable. Primary teeth frequently present with interradicular radiolucent areas but without periapical lesions, and they sometimes even have some vital pulp at the apex (Fig. 23.18A and B). Conversely, overfilling may cause a mild foreign body reaction, and it has also been associated with increased failure rate when compared with underfilling or flush finishing.[157] Success rate with this material varied between 65% and 100%, with an average of 83%, and no significant difference could be observed when ZOE was compared with other calcium hydroxide and/or iodoform pastes.[157–161]

Another disadvantage of ZOE is that it may remain in the alveolar bone for a long time, although it is not certain that this has a clinically significant effect (Fig. 23.19A and B).

Iodoform-Based Pastes. Several authors have reported the use of Kri paste (Pharmachemie, Zurich, Switzerland), which is a mixture of iodoform, camphor, parachlorophenol, and menthol. It resorbs rapidly and has no undesirable effects on succedaneous teeth when used as a pulp canal medicament in abscessed primary teeth. Further, Kri paste extruded into periapical tissues is rapidly replaced with normal tissue.[157] Sometimes the material is also resorbed inside the root canal (Fig. 23.20A and B).

A paste developed by Maisto has been used clinically for many years, with good results reported.[162,163] This paste has the same components as the Kri paste, with the addition of zinc oxide, thymol, lanolin, and calcium hydroxide.

Although not very popular, calcium hydroxide, in a ready-mixed paste delivered via syringe or in a combination of two pastes (base and catalyst), has also been used as root canal filling in primary teeth. Clinical studies report an average success rate of 88%.[160,161] When iodoform and silicone oil were added to calcium hydroxide, a new paste, Vitapex (Neo Dental Chemical Products, Tokyo) or Diapex (DiaDent Group International, Burnaby, British Columbia, Canada), as commercialized in North America, has been clinically and histologically investigated.[164] These authors found that this material is easy to apply, resorbs at a slightly faster rate than that of the roots (complete resorption of the excess paste is expected within 2 to 8 weeks[164]), has no toxic effects on the permanent successor, and is radiopaque. For these reasons, Machida[148] considers the calcium hydroxide–iodoform mixture to be a nearly ideal primary tooth filling material.

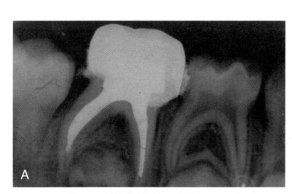
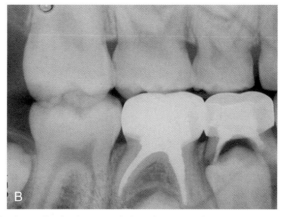

• **Figure 23.18** (A) Mandibular second primary molar immediately after completion of root canal treatment with Endoflas. Note the interradicular radiolucent area and filling slightly short of the apex on the distal canal. (B) The same tooth 3 years later showing healing of the lesion. (Courtesy Moti Moskovitz, DMD.)

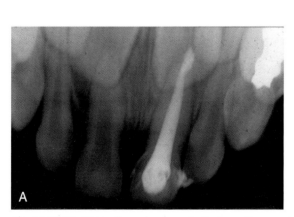
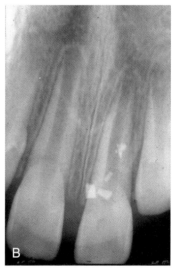

• **Figure 23.19** (A) Maxillary primary central incisor with excessive zinc oxide–eugenol (ZOE) immediately after pulpectomy. (B) Permanent successor of the root-treated primary tooth showing remnants of ZOE in the alveolar bone. (From Fuks AB, Eidelman E. Pulp therapy in the primary dentition. *Curr Opin Dent*. 1991;1:556–563.)

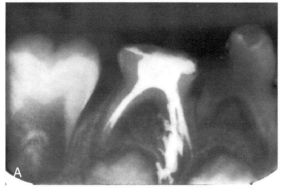
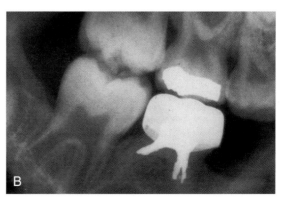

• **Figure 23.20** (A) Mandibular second primary molar pulpectomy with Kri paste. Note the excess of material immediately after treatment. (B) Nine months after treatment, the material has resorbed considerably and the lamina dura appears normal. (Courtesy Gideon Holan, DMD.)

Another preparation with similar composition is available in the United States under the trade name Endoflas (Sanlor Laboratories, Cali, Colombia). The results of root canal treatments using Endoflas in a student's clinic reported similar results to those observed with Kri paste.[153] A complete review of filling materials for primary root canals has been published by Kubota and associates.[165] A recent systematic review indicated that Vitapex has better results when compared with ZOE.[141]

The goals of the "lesion sterilization technique" are to sterilize the lesion and avoid use of mechanical instrumentation in the canal. In an effort to eliminate bacteria and promote disinfection of oral infections, a mixture of three antibacterial drugs (metronidazole, ciprofloxacin, and minocycline) in a ratio of 1:3:3 with propylene glycol has been suggested.[166] A high success rate has been reported treating carious lesions with or without pulpal and periapical involvement, but concerns about spreading resistant bacteria have been raised.[166,167] Thus this technique should be recommended for revascularization of immature, necrotic, permanent teeth, and its success has been widely documented in the endodontic literature.[168-170] See Chapter 34 for a comprehensive discussion of this technique.

Pulpectomy Technique

The pulpectomy procedure should be performed as follows: An access opening should be prepared similar to the methods used in a pulpotomy, but the walls may need flaring more to facilitate access of the canal openings for broaches and files.[156] Each canal orifice of the roots should be located and a properly sized barbed broach selected. Primary molar roots are usually curved to allow for the development of the succedaneous tooth. During instrumentation, these curves increase the chance of perforation of the apical portion of the root or the coronal one-third of the canal into the furcation.[171] The instruments should be slightly bent to adjust to the curvature of the canals, thus preventing perforations on the outer and inner portions of the root (Fig. 23.21).

The broach is used gently to remove as much organic material as possible from each canal. Endodontic files are selected and adjusted to stop 1 or 2 mm short of the radiographic apex of each canal, as determined by a radiograph (Fig. 23.22). This is an arbitrary length but is intended to minimize the chance of apical over-instrumentation that may cause periapical damage. The removal of organic debris is the main purpose for filing. The canal should be periodically irrigated to aid in removing debris. A sodium hypochlorite and/or a chlorhexidine solution should be used to ensure optimal decontamination of the canal(s).[154] However, because of the possibility that sodium hypochlorite solution could be forced into the periapical tissues, it should be used very carefully and with the minimum irrigation pressure.[172] Sterile saline rinses should follow each chemical irrigant. The canal is dried with appropriately sized paper points. Other methods of canal preparation use nickel-titanium (Ni-Ti) instrumentation,[151,173,174] laser therapy,[175] and ultrasonic instrumentation.[176,177] Advantages of these techniques may include better cleaning and shaping of the canal, promoting a more uniform paste fill. Disadvantages include equipment cost and the learning curve necessary to become proficient with the techniques.

When a ZOE mixture is used, several filling techniques may be employed. For large canals, as in primary anterior teeth, a thin mixture can be used to coat the walls of the canal, followed by a thick mixture that can be manually condensed into the remainder of the lumen. An endodontic plugger or a small amalgam condenser is useful for compacting the paste at the level of the canal orifice. Care should be taken not to overfill the canal. In primary molars, some of the canals may be quite small and difficult to fill. Commercial pressure syringes have been developed for this purpose. An alternative technique is to use a disposable tuberculin syringe or a local anesthetic syringe, in which the anesthetic capsule is emptied, after which the canal is dried and filled with ZOE paste.

When the root canal is filled with a resorbable paste such as Kri, Maisto, or Endoflas, a Lentulo spiral mounted on a low-speed turbine can be used, facilitating introduction of the material into the canal. When the canal is completely filled (observed by difficulty in introducing more paste), the material is compressed with a cotton pellet. Excessive extruded material is rapidly resorbed (see Fig. 23.19A and B).

Vitapex (Diapex) is packed in a very convenient and sterile syringe, and the paste is injected into the canal with disposable plastic needles. This technique is particularly easy to use for primary incisors but less practical for narrow canals of primary molars.[152]

Regardless of the root filling material used, an immediate postoperative periapical radiograph should be taken with two purposes:
1. Evaluate the quality of the fill and consider prescribing antibiotics in cases of excessive overfill.
2. Provide a baseline for assessing and comparing the success of the root canal treatment in follow-up visits.

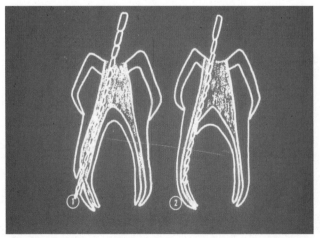

• **Figure 23.21** Perforations on the convex (1) and concave (2) aspects of a root of a primary molar caused by injudicious use of root canal instruments.

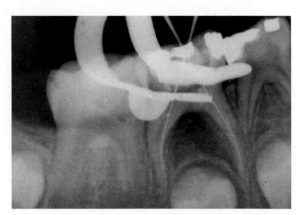

• **Figure 23.22** Radiographic determination of the length of the canals.

Criteria for Radiographic Success

Another point to consider is the criteria for radiographic assessment. Traditionally, root treatments were considered successful when no pathologic resorption associated with bone rarefaction was present.[149,158] Payne and associates[178] claim that most clinicians are prepared to accept pulp-treated primary teeth that have a limited degree of radiolucency or pathologic root resorption (Po), in the absence of clinical signs and symptoms. This is contingent on the assurance that the parent will contact the dentist if there is an acute problem and the patient will return for recall in 6 months. According to Payne and colleagues,[178] most of the pulp therapy studies in the existing literature have considered such teeth to be "successfully treated." These criteria seem to be more suitable for pediatric dentist practices and have been adopted clinically by Fuks and coworkers.[153] These authors, despite describing a low overall success rate (69%) because it did not include teeth in which the pathologic lesion was not completely healed (Po), extracted only one tooth (Px), whereas the remaining (Po) teeth were left for follow-up.

Adverse effects of root canal treatment of primary teeth may occur. Disturbances of the development of permanent tooth bud, radicular cysts, and deviation in the eruption of the permanent tooth have been documented.[179]

Regardless of the pulp treatment performed, treatment success relies on a leakage-free restoration.

Summary

Pulp therapy for the primary dentition includes a variety of treatment options, depending on the vitality of the pulp. Vital pulp therapy is performed when vital pulp remains, because the potential for recovery exists once the irritation has been removed. Pulpectomy is indicated in teeth showing evidence of chronic, irreversible inflammation or necrosis in the radicular pulp.

References

1. Fuks AB. Pulp therapy for the primary dentition. In: Pinkham JR, ed. *Pediatric Dentistry: Infancy Through Adolescence*. Philadelphia: Saunders; 2005.
2. Fuks A, Hebling J, Costa CAS. The primary pulp: developmental and biomedical background. In: Fuks AB, Peretz B, eds. *Pediatric Endodontics*. Switzerland: Springer International Publishing; 2016.
3. Tziafas D, Kodonas K. Differentiation potential of dental papilla, dental pulp, and apical papilla progenitor cells. *J Endod*. 2010;36:781–789.
4. Smith AJ. Dentin formation and repair. In: Hargreaves KM, Goodies HE, eds. *Seltzer and Bender's Dental Pulp*. Chicago: Quintessence; 2002.
5. Lesot H, Osman M, Ruch JV. Immunofluorescent localization of collagens, fibronectin, and laminin during terminal differentiation of odontoblasts. *Dev Biol*. 1981;82:371–381.
6. Linde A, Goldberg M. Dentinogenesis. *Crit Rev Oral Biol Med*. 1993;4:679–728.
7. Torneck CD. Dentin-pulp complex. In: Ten Cate AR, ed. *Oral Histology, Development, Structure and Function*. 2nd ed. St Louis: Mosby; 1985.
8. Baume LJ. The biology of pulp and dentine. In: Myers HM, ed. *Monographs in Oral Science*. Basel, Switzerland: Karger; 1980.
9. Mjor IA, Heyeraas KJ. Pulp–dentin and periodontal anatomy and physiology. In: Orstavik D, Pitt Ford TR, eds. *Essential Endodontology*. London: Blackwell; 1998.
10. Smith AJ, Cassidy N, Perry H, et al. Reactionary dentinogenesis. *Int J Dev Biol*. 1995;39:273–280.
11. Byers M, Narchi M. The dental injury model: experimental tools for understanding neuroinflammatory interactions and polymodal nociceptors functions. *Crit Rev Oral Biol Med*. 1999;10:4–39.
12. Messagne J. The transforming growth factor-beta family. *Annu Rev Cell Biol*. 1990;6:597–641.
13. O'Kane S, Ferguson MWJ. Transforming growth factor betas and wound healing. *Int J Biochem Cell Biol*. 1997;29:63–78.
14. Nakashima M. Induction of dentine in amputated pulp of dogs by recombinant human bone morphogenetic proteins-2 and -4 with collagen matrix. *Arch Oral Biol*. 1994;39:1085–1089.
15. Di Nicolo R, Guedes-Pinto AC, Carvalho YR. Histopathology of the pulp of primary molars with active and arrested dentinal caries. *J Clin Pediatr Dent*. 2000;25:47–49.
16. Furseth Klinge R. Further observations on tertiary dentin in human deciduous teeth. *Adv Dent Res*. 2001;15:76–79.
17. Kakehashi S, Stanley HR, Fitzgerald RJ. The effect of surgical exposures of dental pulp in germ free and conventional laboratory rats. *Oral Surg Oral Med Oral Pathol*. 1965;20:340–349.
18. Cox CF, Keall CL, Keall HJ, et al. Biocompatibility of surface-sealed dental materials against exposed pulps. *J Prosthet Dent*. 1987;57:1–8.
19. Murray PE, About I, Franquin JC, et al. Restorative pulpal and repair responses. *J Am Dent Assoc*. 2001;132:482–491.
20. About I, Murray PE, Franquin JC, et al. Pulpal inflammatory responses following non-carious class V restorations. *Oper Dent*. 2001;26:336–342.
21. Qvist V. Correlation between marginal adaption of composite resin restorations and bacterial growth in cavities. *Scand J Dent Res*. 1980;88:296–300.
22. Qvist V, Staltze K, Qvist J. Human pulp reactions to resin restorations performed with different acid-etch restorative procedures. *Acta Odontol Scand*. 1989;47:253–263.
23. About I, Murray PE, Franquin JC, et al. The effect of cavity restoration variables on odontoblast cell numbers and dental repair. *J Dent*. 2001;29:109–117.
24. Camps J, Dejou J, Remusat M, et al. Factors influencing pulpal response to cavity restorations. *Dent Mater*. 2000;16:432–440.
25. Sloan AJ, Smith AJ. Stimulation of the dentine-pulp complex of rat incisor teeth by transforming growth factor-beta isoforms 1-3 in vitro. *Arch Oral Biol*. 1999;44:149–156.
26. Tecles O, Laurent P, Zygouritsas S, et al. Activation of human dental pulp progenitor/stem cells in response to odontoblast injury. *Arch Oral Biol*. 2005;50:103–108.
27. Goldberg M, Smith AJ. Cells and extracellular matrices of dentin and pulp: a biological basis for repair and tissue engineering. *Crit Rev Oral Biol Med*. 2004;15:13–27.
28. Murray PE, About I, Lumley PJ, et al. Cavity remaining dentin thickness and pulpal activity. *Am J Dent*. 2002;15:41–48.
29. Levin LC, Law AS, Holland GR, et al. Identify and define all diagnostic terms for pulpal health and disease status. *J Endod*. 2009;35:1645–1657.
30. Camp JH. Diagnosis dilemmas in vital pulp therapy: treatment for the toothache is changing, especially in young, immature teeth. *Pediatr Dent*. 2008;30:197–205.
31. American Academy of Pediatric Dentistry Reference Manual. Guideline on pulp therapy for primary and immature permanent teeth. *Pediatr Dent*. 2016-17;38(Reference Manual):280–288.
32. Guelmann M. Clinical pulpal diagnosis. In: Fuks AB, Peretz B, eds. *Pediatric Endodontics*. Switzerland: Springer International Publishing; 2016.
33. Malmgren B, Andreasen JO, Flores MT, et al. Guidelines for the management traumatic dental injuries: 3. Injuries in the primary dentition. *Dent Traumatol*. 2012;28:174–182.
34. Jespersen JJ, Hellstein J, Williamson A, et al. Evaluation of dental pulp sensibility tests in a clinical setting. *J Endod*. 2014;40:351–354.

35. Reeves R, Stainley HR. The relationship of bacteria penetration and pulpal pathosis in carious teeth. *Oral Surg Oral Med Oral Pathol.* 1966;22:59–65.

36. Coll JA, Campbell A, Chalmers NI. Effects of glass ionomer temporary restorations on pulpal diagnosis and treatment outcomes in primary molars. *Pediatr Dent.* 2013;35:416–421.

37. Maltz M, Jardim JJ, Mestrinho HD, et al. Partial removal of carious dentine: a multicenter randomized controlled trial and 18-month follow-up results. *Caries Res.* 2013;47:103–109.

38. Bjørndal L. Indirect pulp therapy and stepwise excavation. *Pediatr Dent.* 2010;30:225–229.

39. Innes NP, Frencken JE, Bjørndal L, et al. Managing carious lesions: consensus recommendations on terminology. *Adv Dent Res.* 2016;28:49–57.

40. Fuks A, Guelmann M, Kupietzky A. Current developments in pulp therapy for primary teeth. *Endod Topics.* 2012;23:50–72.

41. Holan G. Long-term effect of different treatment modalities for traumatized primary incisors presenting dark coronal discoloration with no other signs of injury. *Dent Traumatol.* 2006;22:14–17.

42. Eidelman E, Ulmansky M. Histopathology of the pulp in primary incisors with deep dentinal caries. *Pediatr Dent.* 1992;14:372–375.

43. Kassa A, Day P, High A, et al. Histological comparison of pulpal inflammation in primary teeth with occlusal or proximal caries. *Int J Paediatr Dent.* 2009;19:26–33.

44. Fusyama T. The process and results of revolution in dental caries treatment. *Int Dent J.* 1997;47(3):157–166.

45. ten Cate JM. Remineralization of caries lesions extending into dentin. *J Dent Res.* 2001;80:1407–1411.

46. Yoshiyama M, Tay FR, Doi J, et al. Bonding of self-etch and total etch adhesives to carious dentin. *J Dent Res.* 2002;81:556–560.

47. Schwendicke F, Frencken JE, Bjorndal L, et al. Managing carious lesions: consensus recommendations on carious tissue removal. *Adv Dent Res.* 2016;28:58–67.

48. Ricketts D, Lamont T, Innes NPT, et al. Operative caries management in adults and children. *Cochrane Database Syst Rev.* 2013;(3):CD003808.

49. Green D, Mackenzie L, Banerjee A. Minimally invasive long-term management of direct restorations; the '5 Rs". *Dent Update.* 2015;42:413–426.

50. Ogawa K, Yamashita Y, Ichijo T, et al. The ultrastructure and hardness of the transparent human carious dentin. *J Dent Res.* 1983;62:7–10.

51. Corralo D, Maltz M. Clinical and ultrastructural effects of different liners/restorative materials on deep carious dentin: a randomized clinical trial. *Caries Res.* 2013;47:243–250.

52. Maltz M, Garcia R, Jardim JJ, et al. Randomized trial of partial vs. stepwise caries removal. *J Dent Res.* 2012;91:1026–1031.

53. Schwendicke F, Dörfer CE, Paris S. Incomplete caries removal: a systematic review and meta-analysis. *J Dent Res.* 2013;92:306–314.

54. Stanley HR. Pulpal responses to ionomer cements—biological characteristics. *J Am Dent Assoc.* 1990;120:25–29.

55. Brannstrom M. Communication between the oral cavity and the dental pulp associated with restorative treatment. *Oper Dent.* 1984;9:57–68.

56. Hilton TJ. Keys to clinical success with pulp capping: a review of the literature. *Oper Dent.* 2009;34:615–625.

57. Mahler DB, Engle JH, Simms LE, et al. One-year clinical evaluation of bonded amalgam restorations. *J Am Dent Assoc.* 1996;127:345–349.

58. Falster CA, Araujo FB, Straffon LH, et al. Indirect pulp treatment: in vivo outcomes of an adhesive resin system vs calcium hydroxide for protection of the dentin-pulp complex. *Pediatr Dent.* 2002;24:241–248.

59. Eidelman E, Finn SB, Koulourides T. Remineralization of carious dentin treated with calcium hydroxide. *J Dent Child.* 1965;32:218–225.

60. Ericson D, Zimmerman M, Raber H, et al. Clinical evaluation of efficacy and safety of a new method for chemo-mechanical removal of caries. A multi-centre study. *Caries Res.* 1999;33:171–177.

61. Motta LJ, Bussadori SK, Campanelli AP, et al. Randomized controlled clinical trial of long-term chemo-mechanical caries removal using Papacarie gel. *J Appl Oral Sci.* 2014;22:307–313.

62. Bjørndal L, Darnnavan T. A light microscopic study of odontoblastic and non-odontoblastic cells involved in tertiary dentinogenesis in well-defined cavitated carious lesions. *Caries Res.* 1999;33:50–60.

63. Ferracane JL, Cooper PR, Smith AJ. Can Interaction of materials with the dentin-pulp complex contribute to dentin regeneration? *Odontology.* 2010;98:2–14.

64. Kanca J III. Replacement of a fractured incisor fragment over pulpal exposure: a case-report. *Quintessence Int.* 1993;24:81–84.

65. Casagrande L, Falster CA, Di Hipolito V, et al. Effect of adhesive restorations over incomplete dentin caries removal: 5-year follow-up study in primary teeth. *J Dent Child (Chic).* 2009;76:117–122.

66. Nakajima M, Sano H, Burrow MF, et al. Bonding to caries affected dentin. *J Dent Res* (special issue). 1995;36(Abstract 74):194.

67. Fuks AB. Current concepts in vital primary pulp therapy. *Eur J Paediatr Dent.* 2002;3:115–120.

68. Ricketts DNJ, Kidd EAM, Innes N, et al. Complete or ultraconservative removal of decayed tissue in unfilled teeth. *Cochrane Database Syst Rev.* 2006;(3):CD003808.

69. Al-Zayer MA, Straffon LH, Feigal RJ, et al. Indirect pulp treatment of primary posterior teeth: a retrospective study. *Pediatr Dent.* 2003;25:29–36.

70. Farooq NS, Coll JA, Kuwabara A. Success rates of formocresol pulpotomy and indirect pulp therapy in the treatment of deep dentinal caries in primary teeth. *Pediatr Dent.* 2000;22:278–286.

71. Marchi JJ, de Araujo FB, Froner AM, et al. Indirect pulp capping in the primary dentition: a 4-year follow-up study. *J Clin Pediatr Dent.* 2006;31:68–71.

72. Straffon LH, Loos P. The indirect pulp cap: a review and commentary. *J Israel Dent Assoc.* 2000;17:7.

73. Straffon LH, Corpron RL, Bruner FW, et al. Twenty-four-month clinical trial of visible-light activated cavity liner in young permanent teeth. *ASDC J Dent Child.* 1991;58:124–128.

74. Coll JA, Seale NS, Vargas K, et al. Primary tooth vital pulp therapy: a systematic review and meta-analysis. *Pediatr Dent.* 2017;39:217–225.

75. Hu CC, Zhang C, Qian Q, et al. Reparative dentin formation in rat molars after direct pulp capping with growth factors. *J Endod.* 1998;24:744–751.

76. Rutheford RB, Wahle J, Tucker M, et al. Induction of reparative dentine formation in monkeys by recombinant human osteogenic protein-1. *Arch Oral Biol.* 1993;38:571–576.

77. Tziafas D, Alvanou A, Komnenou A, et al. Effects of recombinant basic fibroblast growth factor, insulin-like growth factor-II and transforming growth factor-beta 1 on dog dental pulp cells in vivo. *Arch Oral Biol.* 1998;43:431–444.

78. Kennedy DB, Kapala JT. The dental pulp: biological considerations of protection and treatment. In: Braham RL, Morris E, eds. *Textbook of Pediatric Dentistry.* Baltimore: Williams & Wilkins; 1985.

79. Kashiwada T, Takagi M. New restoration and direct pulp capping systems using adhesive composite resin. *Bull Tokyo Med Dent Univ.* 1991;38:45–52.

80. Araujo FB, Barata JS, Garcia-Godoy F. Clinical and radiographic evaluation of the use of an adhesive system over primary dental pulps. *J Dent Res* (special issue). 1996;75:280(Abstract 2101).

81. Kopel HM. The pulp capping procedure in primary teeth "revisited. *ASDC J Dent Child.* 1997;64:327–333.

82. Araujo FB, Barata JS, Costa CAS, et al. Clinical, radiographical and histological evaluation of direct pulp capping with a resin in primary teeth. *J Dent Res* (special issue). 1997;76:179(Abstract 1327).

83. Pameijer CH, Stanley HR. The disastrous effects of the "total etch" technique in vital pulp capping in primates. *Am J Dent.* 1998;Spec No:S45–S54.

84. Pameijer CH, Stanley HR. Pulp capping with "total etch" and other experimental methods. *J Dent Res.* 1999;78:219(Abstract 911).

85. Costa CA, Hebling J, Hanks CT. Current status of pulp capping with dentin adhesive systems: a review. *Dent Mater.* 2000;16:188–197.

86. Demir T, Cehreli ZC. Clinical and radiographic evaluation of adhesive pulp capping in primary molars following hemostasis with 1.25% sodium hypochlorite: 2-year results. *Am J Dent.* 2007;20: 182–188.

87. Garrocho-Rangel A, Flores H, Silva-Herzog D, et al. Efficacy of EMD versus calcium hydroxide in direct pulp capping of primary molars: a randomized controlled clinical trial. *Oral Surg Oral Med Oral Pathol Oral Radiol Endod.* 2009;107:733–738.

88. Tuna D, Olmez A. Clinical long-term evaluation of MTA as a direct pulp capping material in primary teeth. *Int Endod J.* 2008;41:273–278.

89. Primosch RE, Glomb TA, Jerrell RG. Primary tooth pulp therapy as taught in predoctoral pediatric dental programs in the United States. *Pediatr Dent.* 1997;19:118–122.

90. Dunston B, Coll JA. A survey of primary tooth pulp therapy as taught in US dental schools and practiced by diplomates of the American Board of Pediatric Dentistry. *Pediatr Dent.* 2008;30: 42–48.

91. Bergoli AD, Primosch RE, de Araujo FB, et al. Pulp therapy in primary teeth—profile of teaching in Brazilian dental schools. *J Clin Pediatr Dent.* 2010;35:191–195.

92. Chaollai A, Monteiro J, Duggal MS. The teaching of management of the pulp in primary molars in Europe: a preliminary investigation in Ireland and the UK. *Eur Arch Paediatr Dent.* 2009;10: 98–103.

93. Kurji ZA, Sigal MJ, Andrews P, et al. A retrospective study of a modified 1-minute formocresol pulpotomy technique part 2: effect on exfoliation times and successors. *Pediatr Dent.* 2011;33: 139–143.

94. Holan G, Fuks AB, Keltz N. Success of formocresol pulpotomy in primary molars restored with crown vs. amalgam. *Pediatr Dent.* 2002;24:212–216.

95. Guelmann M, Fair J, Turner C, et al. The success of emergency pulpotomies in primary molars. *Pediatr Dent.* 2002;24: 217–220.

96. Fuks AB, Bimstein E. Clinical evaluation of diluted formocresol pulpotomies in primary teeth of school children. *Pediatr Dent.* 1981;3:321–324.

97. Morawa A, Straffon LH, Han SS, et al. Clinical evaluation of pulpotomies using dilute formocresol. *ASDC J Dent Child.* 1975;42:360–363.

98. Ranly DM, Garcia-Godoy F. Current and potential pulp therapies for primary and young permanent teeth. *J Dent.* 2000;28: 153–161.

99. Rolling I, Thylstrup A. A 3-year clinical follow-up study of pulpotomized primary molars treated with the formocresol technique. *Scand J Dent Res.* 1975;83:47–53.

100. Berger JE. Pulp tissue reaction to formocresol and zinc oxide–eugenol. *ASDC J Dent Child.* 1965;32:13.

101. Langeland LK, Dowden W, Langeland K. Formocresol, "mummification," tissue disintegration, microbes, inflammation, resorption and apposition. *J Dent Res* (special issue). 1976;55(Abstract):268.

102. Fuks AB, Bimstein E, Bruchim A. Radiographic and histologic evaluation of the effect of two concentrations of formocresol on pulpotomized primary and young permanent teeth in monkeys. *Pediatr Dent.* 1983;5:9–13.

103. Myers DR, Pashley DH, Whitford GM, et al. Tissue changes induced by the absorption of formocresol from pulpotomy sites in dogs. *Pediatr Dent.* 1983;5:6–8.

104. Boj JR, Marco I, Cortes O, et al. The acute nephrotoxicity of systemically administered formaldehyde in rats. *Eur J Paediatr Dent.* 2003;4:16–20.

105. Kahl J, Easton J, Johnson G, et al. Formocresol blood levels in children receiving dental treatment under general anesthesia. *Pediatr Dent.* 2008;30:393–399.

106. Davis MJ, Myers R, Switkes MD. Glutaraldehyde: an alternative to formocresol for vital pulp therapy. *ASDC J Dent Child.* 1982;49:176–180.

107. Fuks AB, Bimstein E, Guelmann M, et al. Assessment of a 2% buffered glutaraldehyde solution in pulpotomized primary teeth of schoolchildren. *ASDC J Dent Child.* 1990;57:371–375.

108. Fuks AB, Cleaton-Jones P, Michaeli Y, et al. Pulp response to collagen and glutaraldehyde in pulpotomized primary teeth of baboons. *Pediatr Dent.* 1991;13:142–150.

109. Fuks AB, Bimstein E. Glutaraldehyde pulpotomies in primary teeth of school children: 42 month results. *J Dent Res* (special issue). 1991;70:473(Abstract 1654).

110. Garcia-Godoy F. A 42-month clinical evaluation of glutaraldehyde pulpotomies in primary teeth. *J Pedod.* 1986;10:148–155.

111. Goyal P, Pandit IK, Gugnani N, et al. Clinical and radiographic comparison of various medicaments used for pulpotomy in primary molars: a randomized clinical trial. *Eur J Dent.* 2016;10: 315–320.

112. Fadavi S, Anderson AW, Punwani IC. Freeze-dried bone in pulpotomy procedures in monkey. *J Pedod.* 1989;13:108–122.

113. Nakashima M. Dentin induction of implants of autolyzed antigen extracted allogeneic dentin in amputated pulp in dogs. *Endod Dent Traumatol.* 1989;5:279–286.

114. Shayegan A, Atash R, Petein M, et al. Nanohydroxyapatite used as a pulpotomy and direct pulp capping agent in primary pig teeth. *J Dent Child (Chic).* 2010;77:77–83.

115. Fuks AB, Michaeli Y, Sofer-Saks B, et al. Enriched collagen solution as a pulp dressing in pulpotomized teeth in monkeys. *Pediatr Dent.* 1984;6:243–247.

116. El Meligy OA, Allazzam S, Alamoudi NM. Comparison between biodentine and formocresol for pulpotomy of primary teeth: a randomized clinical trial. *Quintessence Int.* 2016;47:571–580.

117. Fei AL, Udin RD, Johnson R. A clinical study of ferric sulfate as a pulpotomy agent in primary teeth. *Pediatr Dent.* 1991;13: 327–332.

118. Fuks AB, Holan G, Davis J, et al. Ferric sulfate versus formocresol in pulpotomized primary molars: preliminary report. *J Dent Res* (special issue). 1994;73:885(Abstract 27).

119. Fuks AB, Holan G, Davis JM, et al. Ferric sulfate versus diluted formocresol in pulpotomized primary molars: long-term follow up. *Pediatr Dent.* 1997;19:327–330.

120. Smith NL, Seale NS, Nunn ME. Ferric sulfate pulpotomy in primary molars: a retrospective study. *Pediatr Dent.* 2000;22:192–199.

121. Papagiannoulis L. Clinical studies on ferric sulfate as a pulpotomy medicament in primary teeth. *Eur J Paediatr Dent.* 2002;3: 126–132.

122. Peng L, Ye L, Guo X, et al. Evaluation of formocresol versus ferric sulfate primary molar pulpotomy: a systematic review and meta-analysis. *Int Endod J.* 2007;40:751–757.

123. Vargas KG, Packham B, Lowman D. Preliminary evaluation of sodium hypochlorite for pulpotomies in primary molars. *Pediatr Dent.* 2006;28:511–517.

124. Vostatek SF, Kanellis MJ, Weber-Gasparoni K, et al. Sodium hypochlorite pulpotomies in primary teeth: a retrospective assessment. *Pediatr Dent.* 2011;33:327–332.

125. Ruby JD, Cox CF, Mitchell SC, et al. A randomized study of sodium hypochlorite versus formocresol pulpotomy in primary molar teeth. *Int J Paediatr Dent.* 2013;23:145–152.

126. Farsi DJ, El-Khodary HM, Farsi NM, et al. Sodium hypochlorite versus formocresol and ferric sulfate pulpotomies in primary molars: 18-month follow-up. *Pediatr Dent.* 2015;37:535–540.

127. Shirvani A, Asgary S. Mineral trioxide aggregate versus formocresol pulpotomy: a systematic review and meta-analysis of randomized clinical trials. *Clin Oral Investig.* 2014;18:1023–1030.

128. Lee S, Monsef M, Torabinejad M. Sealing ability of a mineral trioxide aggregate for repair of lateral root perforations. *J Endod.* 1993;19:541–544.

129. Mitchell P, Pitt Ford T, Torabinejad M, et al. Osteoblast biocompatibility of mineral trioxide aggregate. *Biomaterials.* 1999;20: 167–173.

130. Eidelman E, Holan G, Fuks AB. Mineral trioxide aggregate vs. formocresol in pulpotomized primary molars: a preliminary report. *Pediatr Dent.* 2001;23:15–18.

131. Sushynski JM, Zealand CM, Botero TM, et al. Comparison of gray mineral trioxide aggregate and diluted formocresol in pulpotomized primary molars: a 6- to 24-month observation. *Pediatr Dent.* 2012;34:120–128.

132. Noorollahian H. Comparison of mineral trioxide aggregate and formocresol as pulp medicaments for pulpotomies in primary molars. *Br Dent J.* 2008;204:E20.

133. Fernandez CC, Martinez SS, Jimeno FG, et al. Clinical and radiographic outcomes of the use of four dressing materials in pulpotomized primary molars: a randomized clinical trial with 2-year follow-up. *Int J Paediatr Dent.* 2013;23:400–407.

134. Erdem AP, Guven Y, Balli B, et al. Success rates of mineral trioxide aggregate, ferric sulfate, and formocresol pulpotomies: a 24-month study. *Pediatr Dent.* 2011;33:165–170.

135. Moretti AB, Sakai VT, Oliveira TM, et al. The effectiveness of mineral trioxide aggregate, calcium hydroxide and formocresol for pulpotomies in primary teeth. *Int Endod J.* 2008;41:547–555.

136. Sonmez D, Sari S, Cetinba T. A comparison of four pulpotomy techniques in primary molars: a long-term follow-up. *J Endod.* 2008;34:950–955.

137. Subramaniam P, Konde S, Mathew S, et al. Mineral trioxide aggregate as pulp capping agent for primary teeth pulpotomy: 2 year follow up study. *J Clin Pediatr Dent.* 2009;33:311–314.

138. Holan G, Eidelman E, Fuks A. Long-term evaluation of pulpotomy in primary molars using mineral trioxide aggregate or formocresol. *Pediatr Dent.* 2005;27:129–136.

139. Farsi N, Alamoudi N, Balto K, et al. Success of mineral trioxide aggregate in pulpotomized primary molars. *J Clin Pediatr Dent.* 2005;29:307–311.

140. Cardoso-Silva C, Barbería E, Maroto M, et al. Clinical study of mineral trioxide aggregate in primary molars. Comparison between grey and white MTA—a long term follow-up (84 months). *J Dent.* 2011;39:187–193.

141. Smaïl-Faugeron V, Courson F, Durieux P, et al. Pulp treatment for extensive decay in primary teeth. *Cochrane Database Syst Rev.* 2014;(8):CD003220.

142. Yildirim C, Basak F, Akgun OM, et al. Clinical and radiographic evaluation of the effectiveness of formocresol, mineral trioxide aggregate, portland cement, and enamel matrix derivative in primary teeth pulpotomies: a two year follow-up. *J Clin Pediatr Dent.* 2016;40:14–20.

143. Rajasekharan S, Martens LC, Vandenbulcke J, et al. Efficacy of three different pulpotomy agents in primary molars: a randomized control trial. *Int Endod J.* 2017;50:215–228.

144. Elliott RD, Roberts MW, Burkes J, et al. Evaluation of the carbon dioxide laser on vital human primary pulp tissue. *Pediatr Dent.* 1999;21:327–331.

145. Gupta G, Rana V, Srivastava N, et al. Laser pulpotomy-an effective alternative to conventional techniques: a 12 months clinicoradio-graphic study. *Int J Clin Pediatr Dent.* 2015;8:18–21.

146. Fernandes AP, Lourenço Neto N, Teixeira Marques NC, et al. Clinical and radiographic outcomes of the use of low-level laser therapy in vital pulp of primary teeth. *Int J Paediatr Dent.* 2015;25:144–150.

147. Marghalani AA, Omar S, Chen JW. Clinical and radiographic success of mineral trioxide aggregate compared with formocresol as a pulpotomy treatment in primary molars: a systematic review and meta-analysis. *J Am Dent Assoc.* 2014;145:714–721.

148. Machida Y. Root canal therapy in deciduous teeth. *Nihon Shika Ishikai Zasshi.* 1983;36:796–802.

149. Garcia-Godoy F. Evaluation of an iodoform paste in root canal therapy for infected primary teeth. *ASDC J Dent Child.* 1987;54:30–34.

150. Flaitz CM, Barr ES, Hicks MJ. Radiographic evaluation of pulpal therapy for primary anterior teeth. *ASDC J Dent Child.* 1989;56:182–185.

151. Barr ES, Flatiz CM, Hicks MJ. A retrospective radiographic evaluation of primary molar pulpectomies. *Pediatr Dent.* 1991;13:4–9.

152. Nurko C, Ranly DM, Garcia-Godoy F, et al. Resorption of a calcium hydroxide/iodoform paste (Vitapex) in root canal therapy for primary teeth: a case report. *Pediatr Dent.* 2000;22:517–520.

153. Fuks AB, Eidelman E, Pauker N. Root fillings with Endoflas in primary teeth: a retrospective study. *J Clin Pediatr Dent.* 2002;27:41–45.

154. Moskovitz M, Sammara E, Holan G. Success rate of root canal treatment in primary molars. *J Dent.* 2005;33:41–47.

155. Primosch RE, Ahmadi A, Setzer B, et al. A retrospective assessment of zinc oxide-eugenol pulpectomies in vital maxillary primary incisors successfully restored with composite resin crowns. *Pediatr Dent.* 2005;27:470–477.

156. Camp JH. Pulp therapy for primary and young permanent teeth. *Dent Clin North Am.* 1984;28:651–668.

157. Holan G, Fuks AB. Root canal treatment with ZOE and KRI paste in primary molars: a retrospective study. *Pediatr Dent.* 1993;15:403–407.

158. Mani SA, Chawla HS, Tewari A, et al. Evaluation of calcium hydroxide and zinc oxide eugenol as root canal filling materials in primary teeth. *ASDC J Dent Child.* 2000;67:142–147.

159. Mortazavi M, Mesbahi M. Comparison of zinc oxide and eugenol, and Vitapex for root canal treatment of necrotic primary teeth. *Int J Paediatr Dent.* 2004;14:417–424.

160. Ozalp N, Saroğlu I, Sönmez H. Evaluation of various root canal filling materials in primary molar pulpectomies: an in vivo study. *Am J Dent.* 2005;18:347–350.

161. Trairatvorakul C, Chunlasikaiwan S. Success of pulpectomy with zinc oxide-eugenol vs calcium hydroxide/iodoform paste in primary molars: a clinical study. *Pediatr Dent.* 2008;30:303–308.

162. Mass E, Zilberman U. Endodontic treatment of infected primary teeth, using Maisto's paste. *ASDC J Dent Child.* 1989;56:117–120.

163. Tagger E, Sarnat H. Root canal therapy of infected primary teeth. *Acta Odontol Pediatr.* 1984;5:63–66.

164. Nurko C, Garcia-Godoy F. Evaluation of a calcium hydroxide/iodoform paste (Vitapex) in root canal therapy for primary teeth. *J Clin Pediatr Dent.* 1999;23:289–294.

165. Kubota K, Golden BE, Penugonda B. Root canal filling materials for primary teeth: a review of the literature. *ASDC J Dent Child.* 1992;59:225–227.

166. Takushige T, Cruz EV, Asgor Moral A, et al. Endodontic treatment of primary teeth using a combination of antibacterial drugs. *Int Endod J.* 2004;37:132–138.

167. Prabhakar AR, Sridevi E, Raju OS, et al. Endodontic treatment of primary teeth using a combination of antibacterial drugs: an in vivo study. *J Indian Soc Pedod Prev Dent.* 2008;26(suppl 1):S5–S10.

168. Iwaya S, Ikawa M, Kubota M. Revascularization of immature permanent tooth with apical periodontitis and sinus tract. *Dent Traumatol.* 2001;17:185–187.

169. Banchs F, Trope M. Revascularization of immature permanent teeth with apical periodontitis: new treatment protocol? *J Endod.* 2004;30:196–200.

170. Shah N, Logani A, Bhaskar U, et al. Efficacy of revascularization to induce apexification/apexogenesis in infected, nonvital, immature teeth: a pilot clinical study. *J Endod.* 2008;34:919–925.

171. Goering AC, Camp JH. Root canal treatment in primary teeth: a review. *Pediatr Dent.* 1983;5(1):33–37.

172. Klein U, Kleier DJ. Sodium hypochlorite accident in a pediatric patient. *Pediatr Dent.* 2013;35:534–538.

173. Silva LA, Leonardo MR, Nelson-Filho P, et al. Comparison of rotary and manual instrumentation techniques on cleaning capacity and instrumentation time in deciduous molars. *J Dent Child (Chic).* 2004;71:45–47.

174. Crespo S, Cortes O, Garcia C, et al. Comparison between rotary and manual instrumentation in primary teeth. *J Clin Pediatr Dent.* 2008;32:295–298.

175. Soares F, Varella CH, Pileggi R, et al. Impact of Er,Cr:YSGG laser therapy on the cleanliness of the root canal walls of primary teeth. *J Endod*. 2008;34:474–477.
176. Canoglu H, Tekcicek MU, Cehreli ZC. Comparison of conventional, rotary, and ultrasonic preparation, different final irrigation regimens, and 2 sealers in primary molar root canal therapy. *Pediatr Dent*. 2006;28:518–523.
177. da Costa CC, Kunert GG, da Costa Filho LC, et al. Endodontics in primary molars using ultrasonic instrumentation. *J Dent Child (Chic)*. 2008;75:20–23.
178. Payne RG, Kenny DJ, Johnston DH, et al. Two-year outcome study of zinc oxide-eugenol root canal treatment for vital primary teeth. *J Can Dent Assoc*. 1993;59:528–530.
179. Moskovitz M, Tickotsky N. Pulpectomy and root canal treatment (RCT) in primary teeth: techniques and materials. In: Fuks AB, Peretz B, eds. *Pediatric Endodontics*. Switzerland: Springer International Publishing; 2016.

24
Behavior Guidance of the Pediatric Dental Patient

JANICE A. TOWNSEND AND MARTHA H. WELLS

CHAPTER OUTLINE

Pediatric dentistry is an age-defined specialty and is distinguished by the art of behavior guidance. Whether introducing a toddler to dentistry or continuing to care for a middle-aged patient with intellectual disability, behavior guidance is essential to the delivery of quality dental care while building a trusting and positive relationship.

Treating children can be one of the most rewarding experiences a dentist will encounter. With the proper mind-set, training, and environment, dentistry for children should be enjoyable for both the child and practitioner. The concept of behavior management has evolved over the years from the notion of "dealing with" the child to building a relationship with the child, parent, and dentist that is focused on meeting the child's oral health care needs. Hence the terminology has also evolved from behavior management to behavior guidance. While *behavior guidance* is the preferred term, *behavior management* will also be used in this chapter when referring to previously published works on the subject. The American Academy of Pediatric Dentistry (AAPD) defines behavior guidance as "the process by which practitioners help patients identify appropriate and inappropriate behavior, learn problem solving strategies, and develop impulse control and self-esteem."[1] The overall goal is the delivery of quality, safe dental care in an environment that is as pleasant as possible for children and which promotes a positive attitude toward oral health and future dental care. Dental treatment makes great demands on children, and they need the help of a caring practitioner to be able to cope with these demands. Dentists of every personality type can successfully treat children, and like all other aspects of dentistry, behavior guidance is a skill that requires practice, self-reflection, and effort to improve.

Understanding the Child Patient: Review of Child Development

To understand behavior guidance is to understand the child and potential sources of poor cooperation and fear. Children are not little adults, and children of different ages have a unique understanding of the world around them. Communication must be adapted to meet their developmental needs. It is beyond the scope of this chapter to fully review all theories of child and personality development; however, a few concepts are necessary for a full discussion of behavior guidance.

Cognitive Development

The term *cognitive development* describes the evolving ability of children to think, understand, and assign meaning to their experiences.[2] Developmental theory is often presented in stages, which are periods of relatively stable behavior. The age that children reach a stage is variable, but the sequence is typically constant among healthy children. Jean Piaget's stages of child development can help the clinician gain the perspective of the child patient, as summarized in Box 24.1, and are discussed further in the "Dynamics of Change" chapters (Chapters 13, 18, 30, and 37).

Learning Theory

Early learning theory asserts behavior is learned and the response to past behaviors influences future behaviors.[3] Fig. 24.1 illustrates how operant conditioning and reinforcement are relevant in pediatric dentistry. While this theory helps explain how some undesirable behavior can be extinguished, human behavior is more complex than the model of operant conditioning. Some children will not perform the desired behavior, even when both positive and negative stimuli are introduced. Moreover, this theory can also help explain how undesirable behavior can be inadvertently reinforced. For example, young children may perceive any adult attention as a type of positive reinforcement, and the parent and/or dentist may inadvertently reinforce inappropriate behaviors by verbally correcting the child.[3,4] The American Academy of Pediatrics recommends active ignoring of minor infractions, and the dentist may consider ignoring minor movements or intentional misbehavior.[5]

Temperament

It is common to see widely varying behavior in families with shared environment and genetics, and this additional influence is thought to be temperament. Temperament is used to describe traits that manifest early in life and are stable and consistent across different settings.[6] Chess and Thomas classified children according to nine temperament categories and formulated three constellations of temperament made up of various combinations of the individual categories that had significance: easy temperament, difficult temperament, and slow-to-warm-up temperament, as described in Box 24.2.[7]

Studies have shown that temperament, as measured by established psychological tools, can be significantly associated with behavior at a dental visit. Aminabadi et al. found a correlation between

---

• BOX 24.1 Stages of Cognitive Development

Sensorimotor Stage (birth to 24 months)
Infants use senses and motor abilities to understand the world and have little to no meaningful verbal communication other than single word commands. This is not to say that children are not aware of their surroundings; they are hyperaware of people around them as they reach this age and are perceptive to nonverbal communication.

Preoperational Stage (2–5 years)
Children begin to use language in similar ways to adults and can form mental symbols and words to represent objects. Language is concrete and literal and has limited logical reasoning skills. Children tend to perceive the world from their own perspective or be "egocentric."

Concrete Operational Stage (6–11 years)
Children demonstrate increased logical reasoning skills and can see the world from different points of view. They still have a difficult time with abstract ideas and benefit from concrete instructions.

Formal Operations (11+ years)
Children can think about abstractions and hypothetical concepts and reason analytically.

Data from Yates T. Theories of cognitive development. In: Lewis M, ed. Child and Adolescent Psychiatry: A Comprehensive Textbook. 2nd ed. Philadelphia: Lippincott Williams and Wilkins; 1996:134–155.

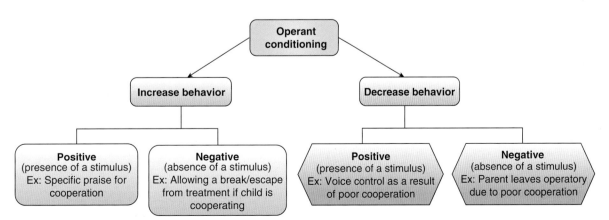

• **Figure 24.1** Operant conditioning and pediatric dentistry. Positive and negative reinforcement can be used to improve cooperation.

Temperament Categories

1. Activity level
2. Rhythmicity
3. Approach or withdrawal
4. Adaptability
5. Threshold of responsiveness
6. Intensity of reaction
7. Quality of mood
8. Distractability
9. Attention span and persistence

Temperament Classification

1. Easy temperament: biological regularity, quick adaptability to change, tendency to approach new situations versus withdraw, predominantly positive mood of mild or moderate intensity.
2. Difficult temperament: biological irregularity, withdrawal tendencies to the new, slow adaptability to change, frequent negative emotional expressions of high intensity.
3. Slow-to-warm-up temperament: this category comprises withdrawal tendencies to the new, slow adaptability to change, and frequent negative emotional reactions of low intensity. Such individuals are often labeled "shy."

Data from Chess S, Thomas A. Temperament. In: Lewis M, ed. Child and Adolescent Psychiatry: A Comprehensive Textbook. 2nd ed. Philadelphia: Lippincott Williams and Wilkins; 1996:170–181.

uncooperative dental behavior and high scores on temperament subscales of anger, irritability, fear, reaction, reactivity, and shyness.[8] Impulsivity and negative emotionality have also been more commonly found in children with behavior management problems.[9] These temperament profiles (impulsivity and negative emotionality) are a poor fit with the demands and formal structure of a dental visit. Patients with dental behavior management problems are less likely to have a balanced temperament profile than control groups.[10]

Coping

Coping is the ability to manage threatening, challenging, or potentially harmful situations and is crucial for well-being. Coping strategies may be behavioral or cognitive. Behavioral coping efforts are overt physical or verbal activities, whereas cognitive efforts involve the conscious manipulation of one's thoughts or emotions.[11] An example of behavioral coping is the use of self-statements focusing on competence, such as "I am a brave boy," which can help children tolerate uncomfortable situations for a longer period of time.[12] Effective coping strategies enable the individual to perceive some sense of control over the stressful event. Typically, older children have a more extensive coping repertoire than younger children. Girls have also been reported to use more emotional and comfort-seeking strategies when faced with a stressful event, but boys use more physical aggression and stalling techniques. However, coping skills vary greatly among individuals. Studies involving venipuncture show that lower pain scores were associated with children who reported using behavioral coping strategies.[11] Coping skills in patients with dental anxiety can be improved through cognitive behavioral therapy.[13]

Factors Influencing Child Behavior

Child behavior in pediatric dentistry is typically studied in terms of dental fear and/or anxiety and dental behavior management

problems. Dental fear and/or anxiety is the feeling the patient has regarding dentistry, whereas behavior management problems are the experiences the dentist has treating the patient.[14] Pediatric dental behavior management problems and fear are different entities, but because of their significant association, they will be discussed together as we explore variables related to uncooperative behavior.

Demographics

Most studies find that negative behavior in the dental office is most intense in younger children and decreases as children grow older.[15–17] Dental anxiety also decreases as the child grows older, as does needle phobia,[14,18–21] most likely due to maturing communication and coping skills. However, it is important to assess the patient's degree of psychological development because that may be more important than chronologic age when predicting disruptive behavior.[22]

The role of gender in dental anxiety and misbehavior is not as clear. The majority of studies found increased anxiety in females, particularly after children pass early school age,[15,21,23–25] while others found no difference.[16,18,19,22,26] Klingberg and Broberg[14] concluded in a 2007 review of the literature that a clear trend exists, with girls being both more dentally anxious and exhibiting more behavior management problems, which was in contrast with an early 1982 review where no clear difference in gender was found.[27] This may be in part due to increased willingness for females to verbalize fears because of cultural norms for gender.

Environment

The influence of environment on health or social determinants of health has been an area of recent interest. Toxic stress is the "result of strong, frequent, or prolonged activation of the body's stress response systems in the absence of the buffering protection of a supportive adult relationship."[28] This type of stress may be a result of child abuse and neglect, exposure to violence, poverty, or maternal depression.[28] Exposure can begin prenatally and can result in lasting changes to the neural architecture, resulting in persistent developmental and physiologic harm and increasing risks for lifelong chronic diseases.[28,29] Evidence suggests individual differences are present in physiologic reactivity to stress, as measured by the amount of corticotropin hormone released in stressful situations.[29] Some children, dubbed *dandelion children*, are low reactors and exhibit little physiologic change when presented with toxic stress, but other children, dubbed *orchid children*, exhibit extreme physiologic changes (i.e., high reactors).[29]

Studies have linked dental anxiety and resultant behavior management problems to socioeconomic status and household characteristics.[9,19,23] Explanations for this behavior may include increased caries history and resultant invasive treatment and/or lack of access to dentists with experience treating children.[30] Behavior management problems have also been linked to single parent homes,[9] possibly due to increased economic and social pressures in these environments. Emerging areas of study are the correlation between dental behavior and residence in an area at high risk for toxic stressors such as violence and low socioeconomic status.

Culture may be defined as a system of shared beliefs, values, customs, and behaviors that members of society use to cope with their world; it is a shared system of attitudes and feelings.[31] Children are increasingly influenced by culture once they reach the formal operations stage of cognitive development. Although

TABLE 24.1	Parenting Styles
Parenting Style	**Description**
Authoritative	High parental responsiveness/affection and high parental demand for obedience; warmth and involvement, reasoning/induction, democratic participation
Authoritarian	Low parental responsiveness/affection but high parental demand for obedience; clear parental authority, unquestioning obedience and punitive strategies
Permissive	High parental responsiveness/affection but low parental demand for obedience; tolerance, tendencies to ignore child's misbehavior; child shares in the decision-making process with parent generally accepting child's decisions
Neglecting	Low parental responsiveness and low parental demand

cooperation may be greater in cultures that place great stress on obedience, dental anxiety (typically based on behavior) may be overlooked.[31]

Parenting styles may also affect child behavior. Baumrind defined three specific parenting styles—(1) authoritative, (2) authoritarian, and (3) permissive—and a fourth, neglecting, has since been added (Table 24.1).[32,33] Positive behavior has been associated with children of authoritative parents compared with children of authoritarian and permissive parents.[34] Aminabadi et al. found a positive correlation between authoritative parenting style and positive child behavior and a correlation between permissive parenting and negative behaviors.[35] Most likely, this parenting style is associated with improved behavior because it reinforces adult authority so that a child will follow commands of the dentist, but the style also offers parental nurturing and support for any anxiety the child may have about the dental visit. Krikken et al. did not find an impact on child behavior and anxiety associated with parenting style, although for one group of children, they did find increased anxiety with authoritarian parenting style.[36]

Dental Fear

The relationship between dental fear and negative behavior is not straightforward, and it would be an oversimplification to attribute all misbehavior to dental fear. The etiology of dental fear in children is multifactorial and a product of previous experience, generalized fear, and familial anxiety.[17]

Between 9% and 20% of children and adolescents exhibit dental fear and anxiety,[14] although Baier et al. found a 20% prevalence.[17] Dental fear has been found in most but not all children with behavior management problems.[9] While the odds are increased that children who exhibit negative behavior have dental fear, and children who have dental fear may exhibit negative behavior, not all uncooperative children report dental fear.[17] Children who report being fearful by various measurement tools are twice as likely to behave negatively than children who are not fearful.[17]

Pinkham classifies fears of dentistry as realistic and theorized fears.[37] Realistic fears are previous bad experiences, fears acquired

from siblings and peers, and the fear of the needle, while an example of a theorized fear is the fear of being electrocuted by the x-ray tube.[17] Dental fear is a worldwide problem and a universal barrier to oral health services; fears acquired in childhood through direct experience with painful treatment or vicariously through parents, friends, and siblings may persist into adulthood.[38]

Dental fear has been attributed to lack of trust in the dentist and lack of control over a traumatic event.[38] Dental techniques that help the patient regain trust and control, such as use of signaling, may prevent or alleviate these fears. Regarding specific procedures, the dental injection is the most feared procedure, followed by "drilling" and "tooth scaling."[23] Other common fears are "feeling the needle" and "seeing the needle."[24] Needle phobia, however, does not imply a high level of children's dental anxiety and diminishes with increasing age.[20]

Dental fear and anxiety have also been linked to increased general fears.[23] Dental fear itself may be a manifestation of another disorder, such as fear of heights and flying, claustrophobia, and other fears.[38] Dental fear and anxiety may also be linked to general behavioral problems, and children at risk of developing internalizing disorders (i.e., separation anxiety disorder, generalized anxiety disorder, obsessive-compulsive disorder) are more likely to exhibit dental fear.[14]

Irregular dental visits and increased length of time since the last dental visit are significantly associated with increased dental anxiety.[21,23] Unfortunately, the cycle of avoiding dental care, having increased need for invasive and emergent dental needs, and having a painful experience that reinforces avoidance can be observed in childhood and adolescence.

Pain

The child in pain will almost always exhibit behavior guidance challenges. Pain is an inherently subjective experience and should be assessed and treated as such. Pain has sensory, emotional, cognitive, and behavioral components that are interrelated with environmental, developmental, sociocultural, and contextual factors.[39] Tissue damage is not required to provoke pain, and reports of pain should not be casually dismissed. It is counterproductive to argue with the child that a sensation is "uncomfortable but does not hurt," especially in young children who are unable to describe levels of pain and experience noxious stimuli dichotomously (i.e., either "yes, it hurts" or "no, it does not hurt"). Introduction to new experiences through the tell-show-do (TSD) technique can prevent patients from interpreting new sensations as painful.

Although adequate management of pain is considered fundamental in providing dentistry for children, this has not always been the case. Historically, childhood pain has routinely been denied and undertreated.[39] Milgrom and coworkers[40] found in a 1994 survey that "many dentists believe dental care for children is not particularly painful but only unpleasant, and a substantial proportion denies the reality of child dental pain. Some dentists tend to believe children confuse pressure with pain or knowingly present false or exaggerated responses, possibly in an attempt to escape the dental environment."

One advantage to the highly fluid nature of pain is that, just as anxiety can upregulate pain perception, many of our behavior management strategies such as relaxation and distraction can downregulate pain. Hypnosis and mental imagery strategies can help patients modulate their own pain.[41] This topic is discussed in more detail in Chapter 7.

Parental Anxiety

The dental anxiety of children is influenced by their family and peers.[23] Parental anxiety, especially maternal anxiety, is influential on the child's development of anxiety.[20,21] Corkey and Freeman[22] found the mother's dental anxiety status, the length of time since the mother's last dental visit, her regularity of dental attendance, and her dislike of restorations were all significantly related to child dental anxiety status. The study concluded that maternal dental anxiety status and maternal psychiatric morbidity were both closely related to child dental anxiety status.[22] Although the mother is the primary source of fear, recent studies have suggested fathers can also affect their children.[42]

Setting the Stage for Successful Behavior Guidance

The Dental Office

Offices that exclusively treat children have a wide array of décor, from a child-friendly theme to office artwork or the presence of video games. Creating the child-friendly environment in an office that treats both children and adults can be more challenging, but a poster on the ceiling of the operatory or a few stuffed animals can make the child patient more at ease. It is important to send the message that this is a place that children have come before and are welcome.

Many offices have new patient packets or websites that familiarize parents with office policies and set expectations that may include letters directly to the children or activities for the children to prepare them for the visit. Parents should be encouraged not to put too much emphasis on the visit, because this may lead to negative stress. A preexposure visit to the office for healthy children may provide little benefit[43] but should be considered for patients with special health care needs such as autism spectrum who benefit from familiarity and routine.

Scheduling

Conventional wisdom states that very young children are usually at their best early in the day. They may be able to tolerate a prophylaxis visit that is minimally demanding in the afternoon, but may be too tired later in the day for an operative appointment with higher levels of stress. Studies have not verified this and have actually found decreased negative behavior for restorative treatment in afternoon visits versus morning.[15] However, the dentist may want to schedule these patients when staff have the most energy, and if a patient does have a difficult operative visit, reappointing for a morning visit might be beneficial before resorting to advanced behavior guidance techniques.

Typically dentists believe that a child needs an introductory visit to the office before performing an invasive procedure. Feigal refers to this examination or examination and prophylaxis only appointment as a "preconditioning appointment" and claims it helps ease children into the dental experience with as little stress as possible.[44] However, Brill[45] showed no difference in behavior between children who had an initial nonthreatening dental visit and those who had a first restorative treatment visit. Thus emergent or urgent treatment should not be delayed on these grounds alone.

The Dentist and the Dental Team

The successful behavior guidance of a child is dependent on the dentist's ability to communicate with the parent, child, and staff.[26] Dentists who treat children can have a variety of personalities and still be effective. Some are very extroverted and emotive, providing an energetic atmosphere that makes children feel included and special. Other dentists tend to be quiet and gentle to put patients at ease. This flexibility is beneficial because some children need upbeat encounters, and others need quiet ones.[41] As long as the underlying message is kindness and regard for the child's well-being, dentists with almost any personality type can be successful at treating children.

The dentist's appearance should be neat and professional. Traditional attire such as a white coat need not be avoided, because a few studies have shown parents and children to prefer it.[46,47] In addition, protective gear required for universal precautions has not been shown to increase fear in children.[48]

The dental team should be a reflection of the office philosophy. The entire team should display a positive, friendly attitude toward the patient. Training in communication, multicultural awareness, child development, behavior guidance, and informed consent for auxiliaries can help them become an integral part of successful behavior guidance.[49] Using the same euphemisms and terms by staff can help provide stability for the child.

Patient Assessment

To improve the child's experience, it is important that the dentist gain familiarity with the child before treatment. At a minimum, the dentist should inquire about previous dental visits and the patient's behavior at these visits. Previous disruptive behavior in the dental situation and previous extraction is significantly associated with dental anxiety status.[21,22] Generally, it is helpful to ask parents how they feel the child will cooperate today, and it may also be helpful to ask how the patient copes with medical visits. Although this assessment is not always correct, it can help the dentist get a better sense of the child and parental expectations.

A number of questionnaires and surveys that can help the dentist gather more information about the fear, anxiety, and temperament of the child patient are available, although their clinical efficacy is unknown. A simple facial images scale with smiling, neutral, and frowning faces has been validated in children as young as 3 years to assess dental anxiety.[50] The dental subset of the Children's Fear Survey Schedule has been used to determine fear in younger children,[18] and the Emotionality, Activity, and Sociability (EAS) Temperament Survey can gauge for temperament types more prone to distress, particularly shyness.[51]

Often much can be learned from observing patients as they play in the waiting room, interact with parents, and respond to the initial approach of dental personnel.[52,53]

Parents in the Operatory

Contemporary parents overwhelmingly would like to accompany their children in the operatory.[54,55] The most recent survey of AAPD members found that the majority of respondents had parents back for all procedures except for sedations.[56]

Having parents in the operatory provides an opportunity for immediate communication on changes in treatment plan, oral hygiene instructions, and postoperative instructions from the dentist rather than an intermediary. Also, it reduces the possibility of a parental misunderstanding or disagreement regarding how the child was treated. Finally, some dentists feel that the relationship with the parents is as important as the relationship with the children to establish trust. In historic studies, no increase in negative behavior was noted when parents were present as passive observers.[57,58] Recent studies suggest either no difference in behavior[59] or improved behavior and reduced anxiety when parents are present.[60,61]

If parents are to remain in the operatory, then the dentist should prepare them to best assist with treatment. A dentist may ask a parent to be a "silent observer" so that the child can focus on the dentist's voice and requests. Moreover, parents should be informed that natural parent behaviors such as reassurance can contribute to child distress behavior and should be avoided.[62] Jain et al.[63] found the majority of parents were compliant with written and verbal instructions to remain a silent observer during dental procedures. However, most dentists report that they do use parental help with basic communication, reinforcement, and occasional stabilization.[56] Dentists must have clear policies that are communicated to parents before treatment about their presence in the operatory and their role. Parents can use this information to decide if the practice is best for their needs.

The dentist should use caution in determining if siblings should observe an operative visit, especially one with local anesthesia. Also, it is best to have only one parent in the operatory to reduce distraction and the occasional disagreement between parents.

Setting Parent Expectations

Before any procedure, the dentist should inform the parent of reasonable expectations of the child's behavior based on their assessment and discuss how this behavior will be managed. Gaining a valid informed consent from the parents before treatment is critical. Parents should also be warned that behavior at the examination visit may deteriorate with the added demands of restorative procedures. Positive acceptance of operative treatment by preschool children tends to decrease over the appointments, indicating a negative "appointment effect" in younger children.[18] This means that sometimes more urgent needs should be treated first instead of starting with simple procedures and completing complex procedures at subsequent visits. In addition, children who have invasive procedures may exhibit more negative behavior at recall visits than those who do not receive restorative treatment in between recall visits.[64]

Review of Behavior Guidance Techniques

Discrete behavior guidance techniques have been described in the literature and are listed in the AAPD guidelines[1] but are rarely used in isolation. The experienced practitioner weaves almost all of them into a visit to help guide the patient through challenges and to reward cooperative behavior. Although these techniques seem intuitive and may be used by the dentist not instructed in behavior guidance, consciously practicing them can help improve skills and success with children. The dentist should formulate a behavior guidance treatment plan for the total patient's well-being, including short-term and long-term goals of this treatment.[65]

Basic Behavior Guidance

Communication and Communicative Guidance

The foundation for all basic behavior guidance is communication. The dental appointment involves a series of requests from the

dentist and responses from the child. Requests and commands for the child patient are best when they are direct, brief, literal, and appropriate for the child's level of understanding. Avoid "don't" commands in toddlers and preschoolers as they have less developed language processing skills and are more likely to make impulse errors in communication.[4,66] These commands may prompt the unwanted behavior they are intended to avoid.[4,66] Extensive explanations are ineffective and can erode the authority of the dentist. Sarcasm and belittling of the patient have no place in dentistry for children.

In order to achieve cooperation and success, the dentist should establish open lines of communication with the child and preserve them throughout the appointment. When communicating with children it is important to use a relaxed tone of voice, acknowledge their interests, and talk to them at an appropriate developmental level.[67]

Communication should come primarily from the dentist who must establish a relationship of trust through verbal and nonverbal techniques. The dentist must be aware of any off-putting nonverbal habits they have, such as sighing or avoiding eye contact, because patients and parents quickly perceive and interpret them negatively.[49] The exercise of video recording oneself during patient interactions can alert the practitioner to undesired habits that may interfere with the message.

To achieve success, it is important that the dentist phrase requests in a manner that encourages compliance and gives the child choices when possible. For example, the dentist may not give the child the choice of whether they want topical anesthetic but can ask if the patient wants strawberry or bubble gum flavor to preserve a sense of control.[23] If a patient does not comply with a request, then it is often necessary to rephrase the request in a manner that encourages compliance. The behavior guidance technique of voice control and nonverbal communication is effective in rephrasing requests.

In providing dentistry for the child patient, the focus of all conversation should be the child. A discussion with the dental assistant or parent does nothing to encourage cooperation from the child and may provoke undesired behavior for attention. A child-focused conversation provides distraction for the child.

One question often asked is how truthful to be with the child patient when the dentist is fearful that the truth may cause the child to object to a procedure that is otherwise tolerated. The obvious example of this is when the child patient asks, "Am I getting a shot?" One way to cope with a difficult question like this may be to use a euphemism, such as "We don't have shots here, but I am going to use some sleepy juice so your tooth doesn't hurt." Other dentists are more direct in explaining the need for the local anesthetic, and in one study, showing the syringe was associated with similar behavior outcomes as concealing it.[68] Clinicians must use their best judgment to honor the trust of the child while helping the child cope with the procedure as much as possible.

Tell-Show-Do

The technique known as tell-show-do (TSD) is one of the most intuitive yet essential behavior management techniques. In TSD, the patient is introduced to the dental environment in a nonthreatening way that can be comprehended. First the child is told about the procedure or instrument in a child-friendly manner. For example, the rubber dam may be called a "trampoline." Next the child is shown what will happen or what will be used, and allowed to see, touch, or smell the material or instrument, or watch a demonstration of the procedure. For example, once the child is told about the explorer, the dentist may use it to feel the child's fingernail (Fig.

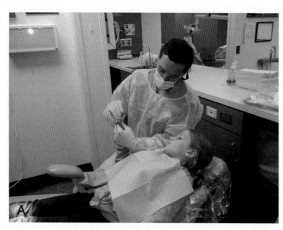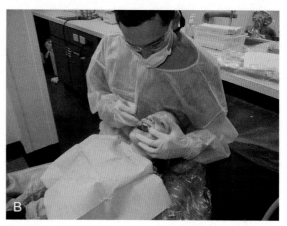

• **Figure 24.2** Tell-show-do. (A) The patient is told about the explorer and shown how it will be used on the teeth in a nonthreatening manner. (B) The explorer is immediately introduced into the mouth and the teeth are examined.

TABLE 24.2	Common Euphemisms for Tell-Show-Do
Device	Euphemism
Rubber dam	Trampoline, raincoat
High-speed handpiece	Mr. Whistle
Slow-speed handpiece	Mr. Bumpy
Rubber dam clamp	Tooth ring, tooth hugger
High volume suction	Mr. Thirsty
Saliva ejector	Straw
Amalgam restoration	Silver star
Stainless steel crown	Princess hat
Curing light	Flashlight
Etch	Blue shampoo
Sealant or composite	Tooth paint
Cement	Tooth glue
Nitrous hood	Astronaut mask

24.2). Finally, the child experiences the procedure, instrument, or material. This technique works best with children capable of communication and is very successful in all but very young toddlers. The dentist would be advised to not overlook this useful technique in older children and adolescents to help allay fear. This technique is almost universally acceptable to children, parents, and dentists.[69–73] However, some children have expressed concern it could increase anxiety, and they were concerned about seeing the tools.[74] One way to avoid anxiety over seeing the instruments is to cover all of the tools with the patient napkin, except nonthreatening items like the mirror and a toothbrush.

Many of a dentist's actions are psychologically neutral. The sensation is present but their pain- or fear-inducing qualities are interpretations added onto the sensation, usually through previous experience or by influencing figures such as parents and siblings. TSD and euphemisms, such as those shown in Table 24.2, allow the dentist to define new sensations.

A common mistake that novice clinicians make is showing the child a number of different instruments and materials before starting any procedure. This can overwhelm the patient, increase anxiety, and delay treatment. It is best for the practitioner to apply TSD to one procedure at a time and work through the various steps of the procedure.

TSD is the foundation for a new technique in the AAPD guidelines, ask-tell-ask.[1] In this technique, the patient is asked about feelings toward planned procedures and informed about the procedure using appropriate language. After this TSD component is completed, the patient is once again asked how he or she feels about the procedure. If the patient continues to have concerns, the dentist should attempt to address them or reconsider his or her behavior guidance plan.

Nonverbal Behavior Guidance

Nonverbal communication is the reinforcement and guidance of behavior through appropriate contact, posture, facial expressions, and body language.[1] Children constantly receive nonverbal cues to interpret the world around them, and these cues work synergistically with words and style to communicate with children.

The conscientious practitioner can use this form of communication to help shape ideal behavior in the child patient.[75] Smiling, making eye contact, and an upbeat tone of voice convey to the child that the practitioner is confident that the child will enjoy the visit. A practitioner must remember that personal protective equipment (PPE) such as a mask and eye protection may hide the practitioner's facial expressions and should not walk into the operatory to greet a patient in PPE. Nonverbal cues are important for the young child, and smiles and a friendly pat on the arm may help the toddler with limited verbal skills feel more comfortable. Children between the ages of 7 and 10 years who were patted on the upper arm or shoulder displayed less fidgeting behavior than their counterparts who did not receive this touch; they also reported greater enjoyment of the visit.[76]

The dentist may choose to sit down and have the preschool patient approach him or her, versus running the risk of being intimidating through height. This technique is called "leveling." If a child is misbehaving, a stern facial expression and more upright posture can convey authority and regain the child's attention and compliance.

One must recognize that very young patients may misinterpret nonverbal cues. Wilson and associates[77] found that 3-year-old patients were significantly less accurate than 6- and 9-year-olds at correctly identifying emotions associated with facial expressions depicted in photographs. Three-year-old patients were significantly more likely to confuse happy and angry for sad.[77] The dentist should be especially careful with patients of this age to make verbal and nonverbal communication as clear as possible.

Positive Reinforcement

Positive reinforcement is a way to recognize the cooperation of the child patient and promote future positive behavior through rewards. Positive reinforcement is universally accepted[69,74,75,78] and contributes to the child's overall sense of accomplishment with successfully completing a dental procedure. Social positive reinforcement is most effective and best when it is specific to the behavior that is cooperative. The patient will be pleased by a comment such as "You are being such a great patient today." However, children are more likely to continue the desired behavior if the praise is more specific, such as "Thank you for sitting so still and opening your mouth so wide." Such a focused comment often motivates a child to continue to sit still and open a bit wider. Complimenting the child in front of parents and dental assistants, again being specific to the positive behaviors the child exhibits, is a great way to boost the child's self-esteem and memories of the visit.

Rewards such as a small toy or sticker also provide positive reinforcement, as shown in Fig. 24.3. These items are concrete, and the child can take them home and show them off as a source of pride and accomplishment. It should be noted that these prizes will not have the same meaning or reinforcement of positive dental behavior without accompanying social reinforcement.

Some question whether positive reinforcement is appropriate in all circumstances. For example, should children receive a reward if they do not exhibit cooperative behavior, or will this reinforce bad behavior? This is determined by the individual philosophy of the practitioner and should be consistently enforced. A practitioner may find one positive aspect of the child's behavior during the appointment and give a sticker for that aspect. For example, "Thank you for coming to see me today. I appreciate you sitting in the chair and opening your mouth wide for me, and this sticker is for being so good at that. I think next time if you can sit still the entire time, you'll get two stickers."

Sometimes what parents intend to be positive reinforcement becomes negative. They may preemptively offer children multiple, large rewards, such as going to a fast food restaurant and getting a prize at a toy store. The notion that the ordeal they are going to experience merits these rewards can increase the anxiety of the children and cause them to view the upcoming treatment as threatening. Preparing the parent prior to the operative appointment and asking him or her not to make large promises to the child before the visit can avoid this situation. If the child indeed displays adequate cooperation, the parent can surprise the child with such a treat, providing irregular reinforcement.

Distraction

Of all the pediatric behavior guidance techniques, distraction has the most research to support its efficacy. A Cochrane review of psychological interventions for needle-related procedural pain in children found strong evidence supporting distraction.[79] Dental visits are challenging, and distraction is an effective technique to promote coping. The nursing literature has shown that parental reassurance during immunizations was related to increased need for restraint, increased verbal pain, and increased information-seeking, whereas children with parental-assisted distraction exhibited better behavior and less fear.[80]

The most basic form of distraction is conversation with the dentist. Storytelling can be related to the procedure, such as telling a child you are chasing "sugar bugs" while using the high-speed handpiece. One former student would chase away all the different colors of sugar bugs and then knock down their house. Other stories may be totally unrelated to dentistry to take them away from the experience, such a shopping trip with a cartoon character or a story about pets. Counting is also a very popular form of distraction for some children.[75] Physical distraction such as asking a child to rotate different feet during the injection can be helpful, and games such as guessing favorite colors or teachers' names are a fun way to take a child's mind off of the procedure. The dentist may enlist the help of an auxiliary in distracting the patient, either by telling a story or playing a game. One study that used a poster and a story by the auxiliary during dental treatment found decreased anxious or disruptive behavior.[81] Parents may also be utilized during distraction, and when trained properly to avoid distress-promoting behavior, they can make a strong contribution to coping strategies, as shown in Table 24.3.[41,62,80,82]

Early studies using television program or music distraction did not show a significant impact on behavior.[83,84] In recent years a number of quality studies have shown that wraparound eyewear is effective in reducing uncooperative behavior.[85–87] This increase in success may be due to the ability of this type of eyewear to block out upsetting stimuli and to use popular and engaging programs.

Voice Control

Voice control is a means of obtaining compliance from a child patient, with the dentist modulating tone and/or volume to gain the patient's attention and cooperation.[88] The term *voice control* is unique to pediatric dentistry. In voice control, instructions should be firm, definite, and convincing; to be most successful, the facial expression must mirror the message.[88]

Typically the practitioner of voice control will make a request in a normal tone. If this request is not honored, the dentist can rephrase it in a firmer tone. The volume may become louder, or sometimes reduced to a whisper to get the patient's attention. More importantly, the command should be repeated slowly and clearly. This technique is most acceptable to the child, dentist, and parent when it is followed by positive reinforcement for improved

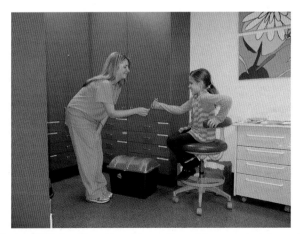

• **Figure 24.3** Social and tangible positive reinforcement at the end of the appointment.

TABLE 24.3	Distress-Promoting Behaviors Often Employed by Parents	
Distress-Promoting Behavior	**Example**	**Alternative**
Uninformative reassuring	"Don't worry, Billy. Everything will be okay."	"You are a brave boy! Going to the dentist will be easy for such a brave boy."
Giving control to the child when there really is not a choice	"Are you ready to start now?"	"It is time to get your teeth counted!"
Apologizing	"I'm sorry this is taking so long, honey."	Use distraction: "What do you want to do when we leave? Would you like to go to the park? I know the slide is your favorite!"
Displaying empathy	"I know it hurts."	Reframe it: "Let's play a game! It's called the tooth dance. Your tooth is going to wiggle, wiggle, wiggle—look, its dancing!"
Making confusing statements	"Bonnie, you can do anything but move."	Use clear directions: "Bonnie, keep your hands in your lap."
Making demands to the provider	"Johnny does better if you give him choices. Don't just tell him what to do." "Don't lie to my child; he knows he's going to get a shot."	The parent may need to be a silent observer.

behavior and the previously positive tenor of the appointment is reestablished. This reinforces the dentist as the coach who helps guide the patient to proper behavior.

Voice control can be considered an aversive technique because parents may interpret this as punishing the child by "yelling at him or her." This is not an accurate reflection of the true intent of voice control. Human nature values the approval of others, and a change to a negative tone signals disapproval. Therefore the benefit of voice control may be the withdrawal of positive reinforcement as much as the introduction of an aversive technique. Others argue that voice control is still in the linguistic domain of behavior guidance and simply a way of rephrasing the previous request in a way that gets the patient's attention.[53] Although voice control can be effective at normal and reduced volume, Greenbaum and colleagues[89] found that the loud voice was most effective at minimizing disruptiveness. Furthermore, the children reported a more positive experience when loud voice control was used.[89] Voice control may not be effective for a child who is constantly verbally chastised.

Parents [69,78,90] and children [74,91] may find voice control objectionable, and parents should be informed of the possibility of its use before the appointment. One explanation might be "I would like to keep your child as safe as possible and provide the best quality dentistry. If your child begins behavior that will interfere with this and does not comply with requests, I will change my tone to sound more firm to get his attention, just like you would if he were about to do something that would hurt him." Most parents will consent with proper explanation.[71]

Positive Previsit Imagery

Positive previsit imagery is a new technique added to the AAPD guidelines.[1] This technique has its foundation in social learning theory and involves showing children positive images of dentistry prior to the visit.[92] Two studies have shown that exposing children to positive images of dentistry significantly reduced anxiety compared to neutral pictures,[92,93] while one other study failed to find a significant difference.[94]

Direct Observation

Direct observation uses social learning theory and the concept of modeling to improve behavior by allowing a child to observe a cooperative patient undergoing dental treatment.[1] *Modeling* refers to learning by observation. In addition to helping children acquire new behaviors, it can help extinguish fear behavior through the process of "vicarious extinction," where children observe other children undergoing experiences that they fear and become less afraid. For example, a younger or fearful patient typically watches a cooperative sibling undergo a procedure to extinguish fears. Greenbaum and Melamed note that it is particularly efficacious as a preventive measure to use with children who have had no prior exposure to dental treatment.[95] This observation can be live or in video form, and Melamed et al. found significantly less disruptive behavior when children watched a video of a child who displays coping and cooperative behavior during a dental appointment and is rewarded,[96,97] but Paryab and Arab found no difference.[98] In addition, a parent can be the model, as Farhat-McHayleh et al. found lower heart rates in children if they observed their mother as the live model.[99]

Memory Restructuring

A child's memory of an event is influenced by the information he or she receives after the event.[100] If a parent reminds the child of an unpleasant dental experience, memories of the visit can become more negative. Memory restructuring has been suggested as a tool to prevent dental fear after an aversive experience.[101] This technique has four specific elements. First, a *visual reminder* such as a happy picture of the child at a dental appointment is shown to the child, and second, the child is asked if the parent was told how brave the child was during the dental visit. The child is enlisted in role-play to tell the dentist what the parent was told. This is the *verbalization* component where the child reports behaving well. Then the dentist praises the child with specific, *concrete examples* of the cooperative behavior, such as sitting very still. Finally, the child is asked to demonstrate the behaviors again to satisfy the *sense of accomplishment*. Pickrell et al., in a study of 6- to 9-year-old patients, found this technique improved child behavior and changed memories of fear.[101]

Parental Presence/Absence

The child's desire for parental presence can become an important adjunct to behavior management. If a child is behaving poorly, then the dentist can request that the parent leave until the child becomes cooperative. This is an effective way to encourage communication for the child unwilling to interact with the dentist. For this technique to work properly, parents must be willing to comply when they are asked to leave, and parents should consent in advance to leave the operatory if asked. Parents may feel more comfortable with this is if they are told that they do not have to leave the room; moving just out of the line of vision of the child is sufficient. When the child cooperates, the dentist should offer praise, and the parent should return promptly.

Nitrous Oxide

The use of nitrous oxide/oxygen (N_2O/O_2) is a form of pharmacologic behavior management that is discussed in detail in Chapter 8. It has been found to have a significant effect on reducing mild to moderately anxious and uncooperative child behavior, and does facilitate coping at subsequent visits, even if it is not used at those visits.[102,103] It is important to understand that the use of N_2O/O_2 is only effective if accompanied by communicative behavior management techniques. N_2O/O_2 is used to improve the child's ability to cope so that he or she is more receptive to techniques such as TSD, positive reinforcement, and distraction. The child must have some coping skills and an appropriate temperament to be receptive to nitrous oxide sedation. Nelson et al. found that children with high effortful control (the ability to inhibit negative reactions and focus on a task and persist even if it is difficult) were more successfully sedated with nitrous oxide.[104] Generally N_2O/O_2 is readily accepted by parents.[69,71]

Alternative Communicative Techniques

Escape

Escape gives children the ability to take a break from the demands of the dental visit. Typically escape is the cessation of activity in the mouth, not getting up from the chair. Two different types of escape have been discussed: contingent and noncontingent. Escape from unpleasant or undesirable events is one of the most common and powerful sources of motivation, and plays a major role in behavior management problems such as temper tantrums.[105] Contingent escape is given when a patient complies with a request or exhibits cooperative behavior. One often used form of this is "If you can hold still until I count to 10, we can take a break." Allen and associates[106,107] have demonstrated success with this procedure in preschool-aged disruptive children. Advantages of this technique are its nonaversive nature, and it generally takes no more time than other behavior guidance techniques.[106,107]

Noncontingent escape is given regardless of behavior; it is granted at a predetermined interval. Studies have shown similar improvements in behavior with contingent and noncontingent escape.[108] Practically, noncontingent escape is difficult to carry out consistently, but the concept of breaks is very effective with children. If the handpiece is stopped for any reason, it can be rephrased as a break.

Desensitization

Desensitization is exposure to fear-invoking stimuli in a progressive manner, beginning with the least disturbing.[109] Patients self-identify their fears, are taught relaxation techniques, and are gradually exposed to the situations that they identify. Studies in adult patients with small sample sizes show that this technique is effective long term in reducing dental fear.[110,111] Case reports have described successful desensitization of adolescents with dental fear and patients with special health care needs.[112,113]

Deferred Treatment

An often overlooked alternative is to simply defer treatment. When behavior is an obstacle to safe, high-quality care, and treatment needs are not urgent, deferring treatment is an alternative to advanced behavior guidance.[1] Treatment of patients with pain, infection, or advanced carious lesions should not be deferred, but care of small carious lesions, application of sealants, and space maintenance can often wait until patient cooperation improves. Parents must be aware that ideal treatment is being deferred because of patient behavior, and they must understand the potential consequences. There must also be a designated plan of observation so that treatment can be implemented if the condition worsens. This is often termed "active surveillance."

Advanced Behavior Guidance Techniques

For some children, basic behavior guidance is inadequate to permit safe, high-quality dental care. This may be due to the young age of the child, special health care needs, extreme defiance, or fearfulness. In these cases it is important to engage the parents to discuss risks, benefits, and alternatives of advanced behavior guidance so that they can make an informed decision for their child.

Protective Stabilization

Protective stabilization is defined as "any manual method, physical or mechanical device, material, or equipment that immobilizes or reduces the ability of a patient to move his or her arms, legs, body, or head freely."[114] It is used to decrease risk of injury during treatment and may be classified as either active or passive.[115] In active stabilization, the parent, dentist, or assistant helps stabilize the patient; typically this is carried out only for a very short period of time or in times of unexpected, physically uncooperative behavior. This type of stabilization is less effective in preventing untoward movement and has been associated with more injuries compared with passive immobilization in adult patients with intellectual disability.[116]

Passive protective stabilization is the use of a device to restrict patient movement for patient safety. Devices used commonly are Papoose Boards (Olympic Medical Corporation, Seattle, WA) or Rainbow Wraps (Specialized Care Co Inc., Hampton, NH), as shown in Fig. 24.4. These devices have fabric wraps to help reduce the movement of arms and legs. Often this technique is employed when patient behavior unexpectedly deteriorates during an appointment, and the appointment must be brought to a safe conclusion or in emergency settings.[115] Protective stabilization may also be used during a sedation appointment to prevent untoward movements by the sedated child. The risks of protective stabilization are physical or psychological harm, loss of dignity, and violation of patient's rights.[117]

Protective stabilization is among the most controversial of behavior guidance techniques. Parents tend to rate both active and passive immobilization as unacceptable,[69,70,73,118] and many pediatric dentists find its use rarely acceptable for routine dental treatment.[56] Parents did rank active immobilization more favorable if the dental assistant performed it or if it was performed by the dentist for the

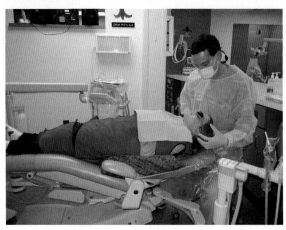

• **Figure 24.4** Medical stabilization with a papoose board.

injection only.[70] It is important to note that in these studies, parents were shown videos of various procedures with little or no explanation. Frankel[119] found that after the use of a papoose board immobilization device for the treatment of uncooperative children, 90% of mothers approved of its use, 96% thought it was necessary to perform the dentistry, 78% did not think it had a later negative effect on the child, and 86% were willing to use it with their next child. The author pointed out that the technique was positively presented in a warm and caring office environment, whereas other studies have only shown videos with no personal experience and no explanation.[119]

Separate AAPD guidelines exist for the use of protective stabilization, and any dentist using this technique should thoroughly review them.[115] As with all advanced techniques, the clinician must be trained in its use (beyond the predoctoral dental school curriculum) and specific informed consent should be obtained, documented, and reviewed at each appointment. Use of protective stabilization should be documented including type of device, duration, indication, presence of parent or reason for his or her absence, and untoward outcomes. Contraindications include patients who cannot be immobilized safely due to medical, psychological, or physical conditions.[115]

Sedation and General Anesthesia

Sedation is a pharmacologic behavior management technique described in more depth in Chapter 8. As with nitrous oxide, sedation is an adjunct to the child's innate coping. Children under sedation should be arousable, interactive, and benefit from communicative behavior guidance techniques. Children with no coping skills, such as those who are very young or who have medical or developmental disabilities, may benefit from general anesthesia. Studies that look at behavior following these modalities support them as effective ways of protecting the developing psyche of patients. McComb and associates[120] concluded that treatment with oral sedation had no significant effect on future dental behavior at a recall exam performed 2 to 34 months later. Other studies have found more positive behavior in children after treatment under general anesthesia versus conscious sedation.[121,122]

Parents have previously expressed poor acceptance of sedation and general anesthesia for their children's dental care, but this view has changed dramatically in the last decade.[41,72] Lawrence and coworkers found it to be the least acceptable behavior management technique, even with explanation of the need for the procedure.[72] More recently, however, Eaton and associates[69] found sedation or

general anesthesia to be the third most acceptable technique after TSD and nitrous oxide. In addition, most parents view sedation as safe and may request sedation for their cooperative child before the dentist has the opportunity to attempt basic behavior guidance techniques.[123] However, the dentist must take into account the risks of sedation, the extent of treatment needs, and the cooperation of the patient before deciding to use an advanced behavior guidance technique.

Mouth Props in Dentistry for Children

Mouth props are routinely used in dentistry to improve the quality of dental care and the comfort and safety of the patient. They can help prevent fatigue from the mouth staying open during long visits, as well as accidental patient closing that may cause trauma or moisture contamination of the area being treated. The AAPD Guidelines on Behavior Guidance[1] state that the use of a mouth prop on a compliant child is not considered stabilization. However, the use of a mouth prop on an uncooperative child has been interpreted as protective stabilization that requires informed consent.

Multiple types of mouth props are used in pediatric dentistry, as shown in Fig. 24.5, and they all have specific indications, advantages, and disadvantages. The McKesson style of mouth props (Hu-Friedy, Chicago, IL) is a rubber, wedge-shaped device and generally well accepted by patients. Uncooperative patients may easily dislodge this device, and it is not adjustable. Also, these devices typically occlude half of the mouth and can make the approach for an inferior alveolar block difficult. Although unlikely, aspiration of these mouth props is a possibility, and they should be tied with 18 inches of floss and secured extraorally.

Molt adjustable mouth props (Hu-Friedy) can also be used. Their appearance may intimidate children, but with TSD they are well accepted. The child can be told that they have a "popcorn popper" in their mouth to explain the clicking noise of opening the mouth prop. The practitioner must use caution because rapid opening of the mouth prop on anterior teeth can luxate or avulse them. Anterior teeth can also be avulsed if the patient reaches up and pulls the appliance out of the mouth before it is released.

Soft foam mouth props (Specialized Care Co., Hampton, NH) may be used on children with special needs; they are less rigid and easier to place in a patient who refuses to open, and they are also less likely to damage anterior teeth than rigid mouth props. Caution should be used with these because they are easily deformed. It is advisable to replace these mouth props with McKesson rubber props once adequate opening is obtained, to avoid breaking a mirror or injuring a patient with an instrument.

Loose primary teeth can be dislodged and possibly swallowed or aspirated with any type of mouth prop. It is advisable to check the dentition as a precaution before using any mouth prop.

Documenting Behavior and Use of Behavior Management Techniques

The behavior of the child patient is an important component of the visit that must be documented. A variety of scales for behavior exist, and a commonly used one is the Frankl score, as shown in Table 24.4.[124]

Qualitative comments, in addition to a quantitative score to record behaviors, can help in planning future management strategies for a child. The comments should be objective and nonjudgmental about the child and parents. Words like "overindulged" or "spoiled"

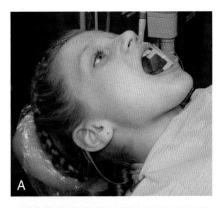
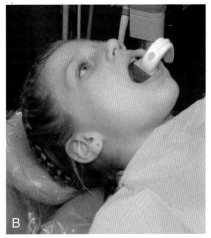
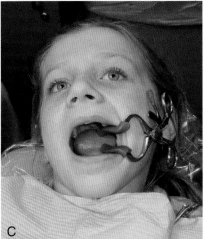
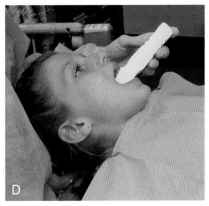

• **Figure 24.5** Mouth props. (A) McKesson style mouth prop. (B) Mouth prop with extra oral handle. (C) Molt mouth prop. (D) Disposable foam mouth prop.

TABLE 24.4	**Frankl Behavior Rating Scale**[a]	
Behavior Score	**Classification**	**Description**
Frankl 4	Definitely positive	Good rapport with the dentist Interested in the dental procedures Laughing and enjoying the situation
Frankl 3	Positive	Accepting of treatment but at times cautious Willing to comply with the dentist, at times with reservation, but patient follows the dentist's directions Cooperative
Frankl 2	Negative	Reluctant to accept treatment Uncooperative Sullen, withdrawn
Frankl 1	Definitely negative	Refusal of treatment Crying forcefully Fearful

[a]For children who are too young to cooperate, the term *precooperative* is preferred.

are subjective, should be avoided, and may offend parents on review of the record.

Behavior guidance techniques should be documented. Typically communicative techniques do not need to be recorded, but it is helpful to include particularly effective techniques as a reminder for future visits. Pharmacologic and advanced techniques must be recorded specifically. The monitoring and recording requirements for nitrous oxide, sedation, and general anesthesia should comply with state regulations. If active immobilization is used, it is important to record who immobilized the patient, what body part was immobilized, for what part of the procedure, and for how long. If passive immobilization is used, the type of device and the approximate time it is used should be recorded.[115] It is also prudent to document that an updated verbal consent was obtained in addition to the written consent obtained before use.

Role of Behavior Management in Society

Dentists do not care for children in a vacuum. Sheller[49] notes that society, parents and their children, the insurance industry, regulatory bodies, legal system, dental staff, and the education, expectations, and choices of dentists all influence the options available for child patient management.

Changes in Society and Parenting

Many societal changes in the last two decades have impacted the nature of parenting in America. The changing economic and social climate has produced different types of families. A trend is for families to live increasingly isolated and disconnected lives. This is due to young families moving away from extended family members, an increased incidence of single parents, and free-time limitations caused by the work schedules of dual-income or single parent families.[125] Economic stress has added to the loss of emotional and practical support. Stressed parents have been reported to implement:

1. Inconsistent (sometimes lax or overreactive) parenting
2. More negative communications
3. Decreased monitoring/supervision of children
4. Unclear rules and limits on children's behavior
5. More reactive and less proactive behavior
6. Increasingly harsh discipline

All of these factors can contribute to a decline in the quality of the parent-child relationship.[125] The rise of violence in the media, both in entertainment and journalism, contributes to a culture that seems to endorse or at least "model" poor behavior control and glamorizes aggression, which may result in more defiant behavior in children.[67]

In a survey of the American Academy of Pediatric Dentistry on behavior management techniques, 85% of practitioners indicated that they believed that parenting styles have changed during their years in practice. They most frequently indicated parents are "less willing to set limits for their children" and are "less willing to use physical discipline."[126] A large majority (88%) of diplomates of the American Board of Pediatric Dentistry reported that parenting styles had "absolutely or probably changed" during their practice time. Ninety-two percent reported that changes were "probably or definitely bad," and 85% felt that these changes had resulted in "somewhat or much worse" patient behavior.[127]

Changing Parental Perspectives of Behavior Management

Parents have been routinely queried as to their opinions on acceptability of behavior guidance techniques. Table 24.5 shows the results of past studies in America on parental preference of behavior guidance techniques.

Over the last two decades, aggressive physical management techniques, specifically hand-over-mouth and passive restraint, have decreased in acceptability, and pharmacologic techniques have increased in acceptability.[69] Positive reinforcement and TSD are acceptable for nearly all dental procedures. More aversive techniques such as physical restraint during the injection or the use of the papoose board may only be acceptable to parents for certain procedures like the injection or an extraction.[70]

Two areas for further research are the influences of social class and ethnicity on the acceptability of management techniques. Havelka and coworkers[71] found that high social status groups were more accepting than low social status groups of active restraint and TSD but less accepting of using a papoose board and general anesthesia. Scott and Garcia-Godoy[73] found that Hispanic parents had favorable attitudes toward verbal techniques, such as TSD and voice control, and unfavorable attitudes toward physical management techniques, such as papoose board, hand-over-mouth, and active restraint.

Third-Party Reimbursement

A concern for dentists is lack of reimbursement for the time and skill needed to manage the behavior of a child patient effectively. Third-party insurers play an increasingly influential role on practice decisions and are skeptical about paying for services that cannot be measured.[49] How this dynamic will affect dentists' choices of behavior guidance techniques is unknown. Third-party reimbursement for general anesthesia for dental procedures for young children is largely dependent on state regulations. Currently 37 states require medical insurance to cover general anesthesia for dental procedures when deemed medically necessary.[128]

Informed Consent

Informed consent is vital to ensure that the parent is adequately informed about proposed treatment; alerted to risks, benefits, and alternatives; and most importantly becomes an active part of the oral care plan. Medical sociologists have noted a shift toward a

TABLE 24.5 Techniques Ranked by Parental Acceptance in Four Similar Studies

Ranking	Murphy et al.[148] (1984)	Lawrence et al.[72] (1991)	Eaton et al.[69] (2005)	Patel et al.[118] (2016)
1	Tell-show-do	Tell-show-do	Tell-show-do	No basic behavior guidance techniques were surveyed
2	Positive reinforcement	Nitrous oxide	Nitrous oxide	Sedation
3	Mouth prop	Voice control	GA	GA
4	Voice control	Active restraint	Active restraint	Active restraint
5	Physical restraint, dentist	Hand-over-mouth	Oral premedication	Passive restraint
6	Physical restraint, assistant	Papoose board	Voice control	
7	Hand-over-mouth	Oral premedication	Passive restraint	
8	Sedation	GA		
9	General anesthesia (GA)			
10	Papoose board			

Modified from Patel M, McTigue DJ, Thikkurissy S, Fields HW. Parental attitudes toward advanced behavior guidance techniques used in pediatric dentistry. *Pediatr Dent.* 2016;38(1):30–36.

consumerist position on health care, and parents are overwhelmed with information, sometimes false, on dentistry.[49] It is important that parents fully understand and trust the treatment plan for their child. Allen and coworkers[129] found that, compared with video or written presentation, the oral method of delivering information to parents about child behavior guidance techniques was the best method to ensure that the average parent felt informed and was likely to consent.

Informed consent should be obtained by the practitioner, and written documentation of informed consent is superior to oral consent only.[130] However, one must not mistake the signing of forms for true informed consent. Informed consent is a process of understanding that relies on honest communication from the practitioner and willingness to understand by the parent. Misrepresentations for behavior guidance techniques can cause conflict in the parent-dentist relationship and have legal consequences.[130]

It is important that dentists make it clear to parents what level of cooperation is required of their child to be treated and that parents make clear which guidance techniques are acceptable. Clinicians should work to understand the parents' reasoning behind their decisions to individualize the plan for the patient and family.[67] This is an area where the investment of time and patience can prevent future problems, because malpractice complaints have been reported to occur more frequently when a good relationship between the provider and patient is lacking.[131]

Typically only a parent or legal guardian can provide informed consent for a minor patient. Some states, however, provide an exception for emancipated minors, so clinicians must be aware of the laws where they practice. It is also important to note that informed consent can be withdrawn at any time, and a practitioner must comply as soon as possible to safely end the procedure.[130]

Adair and colleagues[126] reported that 42% of pediatric dentists give parents a single printed form that describes at least some of the behavior guidance techniques they use. In this study, the majority of practitioners did not obtain consent for the use of most communicative techniques and obtained only oral consent for passive and active immobilization for unsedated children.[126] However, current AAPD guidelines recommend written consent if protective stabilization is used, and this is best obtained on a separate day.[115] If unanticipated behavior necessitates use of immobilization, immediate intervention is indicated to ensure safety, and then written informed consent should be obtained, as well as consent for alternative methods such as sedation if further treatment is necessary.[1] Box 24.3 shows the method used at the Louisiana State University Department of Pediatric Dentistry to inform parents about various behavior guidance techniques. This form is accompanied by a separate treatment plan that lists the specific techniques that will be employed. Additional consents are obtained for medical immobilization, sedation, and general anesthesia.

Putting It All Together

Behavior Guidance for the Infant/Toddler

Children less than 30 months of age can usually only respond to simple commands such as "sit in the chair" or "open your mouth."[37] At this age they are entirely dependent on parents and have little verbal language. Typical fears of the 2-year-old child are strangers, loud sounds, sudden movement, and falling. Having the parents involved is critical because children in this group are typically very

---

• BOX 24.3 Description of Patient Management Techniques for Informed Consent at Louisiana State University

LSU School of Dentistry Pediatric Dental Consent Information
In order to provide the best dental care of your child, we would like to inform you more about the practice of dentistry for children and risks associated with this practice.

Patient Management
It is our intent that all professional care provided in our dental clinic shall be of the best possible quality we can provide for each child. Providing high-quality care in a safe manner can be difficult if the child lacks the ability to cooperate. All efforts will be made to obtain the cooperation of the children by the use of warmth, friendliness, kindness, and understanding. There are several behavior management techniques that are used by pediatric dentists to gain the cooperation of children to eliminate disruptive behavior or prevent patients from causing injury to themselves due to uncontrollable movements. This includes:
1. **Tell-Show-Do:** The dentist or assistant explains to the child what is to be done, shows an example on a tooth model or the child's finger, and then the procedure is done to the child's tooth.
2. **Positive Reinforcement:** The dentist rewards the child who displays cooperative behavior with compliments, praise, a pat on the shoulder, or a small prize.
3. **Voice Control:** The attention of the disruptive child is redirected by a change in the tone and volume of the dentist's voice.
4. **Mouth Props:** A device is placed in the child's mouth to prevent closure of the child's teeth on dental equipment.

5. **Hand and/or Head Holding by Dentist, Dental Assistant, or Parent:** An adult keeps a child's body still so the child cannot grab the dentist's hand or sharp dental tools. This is to ensure patient safety.
6. **Medical Immobilization:** The child is placed in a restraining device made of cloth and Velcro. This is to ensure that the child is not hurt by his or her own movements. *Your child's doctor will discuss the specific consents should medical immobilization be required for dental treatment.*
7. **Nitrous Oxide Sedation:** Nitrous oxide ("laughing gas") is a medication breathed through a nose mask to relax a nervous child and enable him/her to better tolerate dental treatment. The child will remain awake but is expected to be relaxed and calm. The nitrous oxide is breathed out of the child's body within a few minutes of being turned off. We recommend an adult hold the child's hand as they leave the clinic.
8. **Oral Sedation:** Sedative drugs may be recommended to help your child receive quality dentistry in a safe manner if other behavior management techniques do not work. *Your child will not be orally sedated without you being further informed and obtaining your specific consent for this procedure. Your child's doctor will discuss the specific instructions and consents should your child need to be sedated for dental treatment.*
9. **General Anesthesia:** The dentist performs the dental treatment with the child anesthetized in the hospital operating room. *Your child will not be given general anesthesia without you being further informed and obtaining your specific consent for this procedure. Your child's doctor will discuss the specific instructions and consents should your child need to be sedated for dental treatment.*

LSU, Louisiana State University.
Modified from The LSU Health Sciences Center, School of Dentistry, New Orleans, LA.

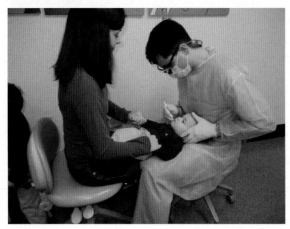

• **Figure 24.6** Knee-to-knee examination technique with parent controlling the child's arms.

attached to parents. Older toddlers can be introduced to the office by letting them see and touch things.[105] Examination of children this age typically takes place on the parent's lap in the "knee-to-knee" position, using gentle active restraint from the dentist and parent (Fig. 24.6). Parents should be informed that patients may not cooperate for treatment, even for a simple examination, at this age. It is important to set appropriate expectations for behavior before any intervention. Patients with dental caries requiring treatment are a challenge at this age because of their poor coping skills, and advanced management techniques are usually indicated. Caries should be stabilized with interim restorative techniques or silver diamine fluoride treatment if possible until behavior improves. If severe caries are present, then advanced behavior guidance techniques are indicated.

Behavior Guidance for the Preschooler

Language improves dramatically during these years (ages 3 to 5), improving the success of basic behavior guidance.[37] By age 4 years, all children should be competent in the domain of language, unless an abnormality is present in their psychological development. Musselman[132] describes these children as "great talkers," and they take pride in their clothes and activities.

At this age, clear communication by the dentist is critical. These children may need more time and patience than others, but the outcomes can be the most rewarding. An undemanding, introductory appointment with emphasis on TSD is especially beneficial. Younger children in this age group may be startled by the chair moving back, so it is advisable to have the chair in a supine position at the beginning of the appointment or to have the dentist present the experience of the chair going back as a "spaceship ride." These patients will respond best to clear, single-step instructions, followed by positive reinforcement. Even though a toothbrush may adequately remove deposit at this age, use of the rotary prophy cup with child's toothpaste may desensitize the child to the handpiece and give insight into compliance for planned operative treatments. Appointments should be short and efficient so as to not overwhelm the child's coping abilities.

Children in this age group are increasingly seeking to establish independence, and they take pride in their accomplishments. Four-year-olds have been called "bossy" and may try to impose their will on the experience.[132] Enlisting the child to assist you

with specific tasks such as holding the mirror or cotton rolls can help bring about cooperative behavior through distraction.

Behavior Guidance for the School-Aged Child

School provides children with the experience of separating from parents, responding to instructions from strangers, and cooperating in a structured environment. However, these new experiences may be a source of stress for the child, which can manifest in the dental environment.[132] Nash[133] suggests three skills that can be used for effective communication with children: (1) reflective listening, (2) self-disclosing assertiveness (i.e., "I cannot see the teeth when the mouth is closed"), and (3) descriptive praise. In addition, this age group is especially receptive to play and humor. Playing games and telling jokes can be useful to build rapport and make the visit more enjoyable.[134] These techniques are appropriate in all age groups but are especially helpful in this age group of patients as they become more sophisticated in their relationships with adults outside the home.

Behavior Guidance for the Adolescent

Adolescents can be a very enjoyable group to treat. They are approaching adulthood with unique personalities and are on their way to establishing and achieving goals. However, it is a mistake to view this group as adults. Adolescents have complex pressures regarding peers, personal appearance, and struggles for independence, and the behavior they exhibit in the dental chair is typically influenced by events outside the office. Adolescents still have fears of dental procedures and should be managed in a compassionate manner. Listening with empathy is the most effective behavior guidance technique with adolescent patients. Physical techniques such as muscle relaxation, deep breathing, and progressive exposure have been shown to be successful in the treatment of phobic adolescents.[112]

Behavior Guidance for the Child With Previous Negative Dental Experiences

Children with previous negative dental experiences present one of the greatest challenges to the practitioner. It is important to gather as much information about the previous experience from the parent as possible. This interview is best conducted out of the child's hearing to prevent reviving past memories, but this can be difficult, as these children typically need parental support. Parents should be discouraged from reminding the child of previous difficult dental experiences, because Barton and colleagues[135] argue that the memories are not always easily recalled by the child. The purpose of this interview is to try to get a sense of the child's coping skills and temperament and to avoid past triggers.

In communicating with the child, it helps to emphasize the office as a pleasant area for children and that you are interested and confident in treating the child patient. Even if the child has no dental needs, an introductory appointment such as an exam and prophylaxis can help extinguish fears and promote positive memories with this environment. It can help to emphasize that you are doing something new and different so the child's previous experience is distinguished from this one. Again, the previous experience should not be brought up again. The practitioner should not jump to advanced behavior techniques based solely on a previous bad experience at another office. Sometimes the child can be treated successfully by a compassionate dentist using communicative techniques in a new environment, and nitrous oxide can be a helpful adjunct in retraining fearful patients.

Behavior Guidance for the Child With Special Health Care Needs

Children with special health care needs require additional consideration with behavior guidance. Children with special health care needs have been excluded from a number of studies evaluating nonpharmacologic behavior guidance, so evidence in this area is lacking. Various sources report that predoctoral dental education is inadequate to prepare dentists to treat patients with special health care needs.[136,137]

Dental fear assessment is challenging in this population, but one study of adults with a range of cognitive, motor, psychological, and medical conditions found that 42% had some level of dental fear and also found caregivers accurately estimated fear.[138] A question should be included on the medical history to gauge the child's development or education level to let the provider know if intellectual disability is present. An interview with the primary caregiver is the best way to predict cooperation, and questions should include level of cognitive ability (i.e., milestones, grade level), cooperation in medical settings, triggers for uncooperative behavior, soothing strategies, adherence to schedule, current therapies, and other beneficial accommodations. When possible, the child should also be asked about any concerns in the dental setting. Marshall et al. found that in children with autism spectrum disorders (ASD), cooperation for dental appointments was predicted by parental report of toilet training, toothbrushing, haircuts, academic achievement, and language.[139]

Dentists should communicate with children who have special health care needs at a level appropriate for their cognitive development. The dentist should not assume patients with conditions that impair communication, such as cerebral palsy, are intellectually disabled. Patients with ASD may be using applied behavior therapy and may benefit from a dental visit "social story" or picture book that allows them to rehearse procedures in a developmentally appropriate manner.[140] A sensory-adapted dental environment that uses relaxing lights and music has been recommended for children with developmental disabilities.[141] Children with balance disorders such as Down syndrome may accept the chair more easily if it is already reclined.

Communicative behavior guidance techniques should be used with short, one-step instructions for patients with intellectual disabilities (Box 24.4). Applied behavioral therapy using familiarization and repetitive tasking has been successful in patients with autism.[142] Any physical disabilities should be considered in positioning and

• **BOX 24.4 Communication With Patients Who Have Intellectual Disabilities**

When an intellectually impaired patient wants to communicate with you:
- Use leveling.
- Remove distractions.
- Use declarative sentences.
- Use open-ended questions.
- Provide corrective feedback.
- Rephrase questions if needed.

Data from Harper DC, Wadsworth JS. A strategy to train health care professionals to communicate with persons with mental retardation. Acad Med. 1991;66:495–496.

communication. For example, distraction techniques that limit full visibility of surroundings, such as wraparound eyewear, may be disconcerting for children with hearing impairment.[143]

Protective stabilization is often used in the treatment of children with special needs to prevent untoward movements. Some children with cerebral palsy find this comforting because it helps them control their movements, but caution must be used to not forcefully extend contracted limbs. Children with ASD have been reported to find more comfort and cooperation in the security and weight of an immobilization device.[144] Parents of children with special health care needs may be more accepting of medical immobilization than parents of children without disabilities,[145] although one study found few differences between parents of disabled and fully abled children in their acceptance of management techniques.[146] Parents are more likely to be accepting of them if they have been used in the past.[147]

As with all children, the decision to use protective stabilization must be carefully considered, and parents must have all the necessary information to give informed consent. Pharmacologic management should be used for uncooperative patients with extensive treatment needs.

Conclusion

Sheller nicely summarizes the demands of dentistry for children by stating that "the task of pediatric dentists is the same as it was a generation ago: to perform precise surgical procedures on children whose behavior may range from cooperative to hostile to defiant."[49] Behavior guidance will remain the art of recognizing the complexities of children's and dentists' temperaments, parental attitudes, and varying treatment needs and creating an optimal treatment plan to best address the child's needs.

References

1. American Academy of Pediatric Dentistry. Guideline on behavior guidance for the pediatric dental patient. *Pediatr Dent.* 2016;38(special issue):185–198.
2. Piaget J. The stages of the intellectual development of the child. *Bull Menninger Clin.* 1962;26:120–128.
3. Baghdadi ZD. Principles and application of learning theory in child patient management. *Quintessence Int.* 2001;32(2):135–141.
4. Blum MJ, Williams GE, Friman PC, et al. Disciplining young children: the role of verbal instructions and reasoning. *Pediatrics.* 1995;96(2):336–341.
5. American Academy of Pediatrics. Committee on Psychosocial Aspects of child and family health: guidance for effective discipline. *Pediatrics.* 1998;101(4):723–728. Reaffirmed July 2014.
6. Thomas A, Chess S, Birch H, et al. A longitudinal study of primary reaction patterns in children. *Compr Psychiatry.* 1960;1:103–112.
7. Chess S, Thomas A. Temperament. In: Lewis M, ed. *Child and Adolescent Psychiatry: A Comprehensive Textbook.* 2nd ed. Philadelphia: Lippincott Williams & Wilkins; 1996:170–181.
8. Aminabadi NP, Puralibaba F, Erfanparast L, et al. Impact of temperament on child behavior in the dental setting. *J Dent Res Dent Clin Dent Prospects.* 2011;5(4):119–122.
9. Arnrup K, Broberg AG, Berggren U, et al. Lack of cooperation in pediatric dentistry—the role of child personality characteristics. *Pediatr Dent.* 2002;24(2):119–129.
10. Arnrup K, Broberg AG, Berggren U, et al. Temperamental reactivity and negative emotionality in uncooperative children referred to specialized paediatric dentistry compared to children in ordinary dental care. *Int J Paediatr Dent.* 2007;17(6):419–429.

11. Hodgins MJ, Lander J. Children's coping with venipuncture. *J Pain Symptom Manage.* 1997;13(5):274–285.
12. Curry SL, Russ SW, Johnsen DC, et al. The role of coping in children's adjustment to the dental visit. *J Dent Child.* 1988;55(3):231–236.
13. Shahnavaz S, Rutley S, Larsson K, et al. Children and parents' experiences of cognitive behavioral therapy for dental anxiety—a qualitative study. *Int J Paediatr Dent.* 2015;25(5):317–326.
14. Klingberg G, Broberg AG. Dental fear/anxiety and dental behaviour management problems in children and adolescents: a review of prevalence and concomitant psychological factors. *Int J Paediatr Dent.* 2007;17(6):391–406.
15. Taylor MH, Moyer IN, Peterson DS. Effect of appointment time, age, and gender on children's behavior in a dental setting. *ASDC J Dent Child.* 1983;50(2):106–110.
16. Holst A, Crossner C. Direct ratings of acceptance of dental treatment in Swedish children. *Community Dent Oral Epidemiol.* 1987;15(5):258–263.
17. Baier K, Milgrom P, Russell S, et al. Children's fear and behavior in private pediatric dentistry practices. *Pediatr Dent.* 2004;26(4):316–321.
18. Cuthbert MI, Melamed BG. A screening device: children at risk for dental fears and management problems. *ASDC J Dent Child.* 1982;49(6):432–436.
19. Dogan MC, Seydaoglu G, Uguz S, et al. The effect of age, gender, and socio-economic factors on perceived dental anxiety determined by a modified scale in children. *Oral Health Prev Dent.* 2006;4(4):235–241.
20. Majstorovic M, Veerkamp JS. Relationship between needle phobia and dental anxiety. *J Dent Child (Chic).* 2004;71(3):201–205.
21. Tickle M, Jones C, Buchannan K, et al. A prospective study of dental anxiety in a cohort of children followed from 5 to 9 years of age. *Int J Paediatr Dent.* 2009;19(4):225–232.
22. Corkey B, Freeman R. Predictors of dental anxiety in six-year-old children: findings from a pilot study. *ASDC J Dent Child.* 1994;61(4):267–271.
23. Bedi R, Sutcliffe P, Donnan PT, et al. The prevalence of dental anxiety in a group of 13- and- 14-year old Scottish children. *Int J Paediatr Dent.* 1992;2(1):17–24.
24. Peretz B, Efrat J. Dental anxiety among young adolescent patients in Israel. *Int J Paediatr Dent.* 2000;10(2):126–132.
25. Majstorovic M, Morse DE, Do D, et al. Indicators of dental anxiety in children just prior to treatment. *J Clin Pediatr Dent.* 2014;39(1):12–17.
26. Torriani DD, Ferro RL, Bonow MLM, et al. Dental caries is associated with dental fear in childhood: findings from a birth cohort study. *Caries Res.* 2014;48:263–270.
27. Winer GA. A review and analysis of children's fearful behavior in dental settings. *Child Dev.* 1982;43:1111–1133.
28. Shonkof JP, Garner AS, Committee on Psychosocial Aspects of Child and Family Health; Committee on early Childhood Adoption and Dependent Care; Section on Developmental and Behavioral Pediatrics. The lifelong effects of early childhood adversity and toxic stress. *Pediatrics.* 2012;129(1):e.232–e.246.
29. Boyce WT. The lifelong effects of early childhood adversity and toxic stress. *Pediatr Dent.* 2014;36(2):102–108.
30. Vignehsa H, Chellappah NK, Milgrom P, et al. A clinical evaluation of high- and low-fear children in Singapore. *ASDC J Dent Child.* 1990;57(3):224–228.
31. Folayan MO, Idehen EE, Ojo OO. The modulating effect of culture on the expression of dental anxiety in children: a literature review. *Int J Paediatr Dent.* 2004;14(4):241–245.
32. Baumrind D. Current patterns of parental authority. *Dev Psychol Monogr.* 1971;4:1–103.
33. Robinson C, Mandleco B, Olsen SF, et al. The parenting styles and dimensions questionnaire (PSDQ). *Handb Fam Meas Tech.* 2001;3:319–321.
34. Howenstein J, Kumar A, Casamassimo PS, et al. Correlating parenting styles with child behavior and careis. *Pediatr Dent.* 2015;37(1):59–64.
35. Aminibadi NA, Deljavan AS, Jamali Z, et al. The influence of parenting style and child temperament on child parent dentist interactions. *Pediatr Dent.* 2015;37(4):342–347.
36. Krikken JV, van Wijk AJ, ten Cate JM, et al. Child dental anxiety, parental rearing style and referral status of children. *Community Dent Health.* 2012;29(4):289–292.
37. Pinkham JR. Personality development: managing behavior of the cooperative preschool child. *Dent Clin North Am.* 1995;39(4):771–787.
38. Milgrom P, Weinstein P. Dental fears in general practice: new guidelines for assessment and treatment. *Int Dent J.* 1993;43(3 suppl 1):288–293.
39. American Academy of Pediatrics, American Pain Society. The assessment and management of acute pain in infants, children, and adolescents. *Pediatrics.* 2001;108(3):793–797.
40. Milgrom P, Weinstein P, Golletz D, et al. Pain management in school-aged children by private and public clinic practice dentists. *Pediatr Dent.* 1994;16(4):294–300.
41. Feigal RJ. Guiding and managing the child dental patient: a fresh look at old pedagogy. *J Dent Educ.* 2001;65(12):1369–1377.
42. Lara A, Crgo A, Romero-Maroto M. Emotional contagion of dental fear to children: the fathers' mediating role in parental transfer of fear. *Int J Paediatr Dent.* 2012;22(5):324–330.
43. Rouleau J, Ladouceur R, Dufour L. Pre-exposure to the first dental treatment. *J Dent Res.* 1981;60(1):30–34.
44. Feigal R. Pediatric behavior management through nonpharmacologic methods. *Gen Dent.* 1995;43(4):327–332.
45. Brill WA. Comparison of the behavior of children undergoing restorative dental treatment at the first visit versus the second visit in a private pediatric dental practice. *J Clin Pediatr Dent.* 2001;25(4):287–291.
46. Mistry D, Tahmassebi JF. Children's and parents' attitudes toward dentists' attire. *Eur Arch Paediatr Dent.* 2009;10(4):237–240.
47. Panda A, Garg I, Bhobe AP. Children's perspective on the dentist's attire. *Int J Paediatr Dent.* 2014;24(2):98–103.
48. Davis R, McKibben DH, Nazif MM, et al. Child reaction to protective garb at the first dental visit. *Pediatr Dent.* 1993;15(2):86–87.
49. Sheller B. Challenges of managing child behavior in the 21st century dental setting. *Pediatr Dent.* 2004;26(2):111–113.
50. Buchanan H, Niven N. Validation of a Facial Image Scale to assess child dental anxiety. *Int J Paediatr Dent.* 2002;12(1):47–52.
51. Quinonez R, Santos RG, Boyar R, et al. Temperament and trait anxiety as predictors of child behavior prior to general anesthesia for dental surgery. *Pediatr Dent.* 1997;19(6):427–431.
52. McTigue DJ, Pinkham J. Association between children's dental behavior and play behavior. *ASDC J Dent Child.* 1978;45(3):218–222.
53. Pinkham JR. Observation and interpretation of the child dental patients' behavior. *Pediatr Dent.* 1979;1(1):21–26.
54. Shroff S, Hughes C, Mobley C. Attitudes and preferences of parents about being present in the dental operatory. *Pediatr Dent.* 2015;37(1):51–55.
55. Peretz B, Zadik D. Attitudes of parents toward their presence in the operatory during dental treatments to their children. *J Clin Pediatr Dent.* 1998;23(1):27–30.
56. Wells M, McTigue D, Casamassimo P, et al. Gender shifts and effects on behavior guidance. *Pediatr Dent.* 2014;36(2):102–108.
57. Venham LL, Bengston D, Cipes M. Parent's presence and the child's response to dental stress. *ASDC J Dent Child.* 1978;45(3):213–217.
58. Pfefferle JC, Machen JB, Fields HW, et al. Child behavior in the dental setting relative to parental presence. *Pediatr Dent.* 1982;4:311–316.
59. Cox IC, Krikken JB, Veerkamp JS. Influence of parental presence on the child's perception of, and behavior during dental treatment. *Eur Arch Paediatr Dent.* 2011;12(4):200–204.
60. Vasiliki B, Konstantinos A, Vassilis K, et al. The effect of parental presence on the child's perception and co-operation during dental treatment. *Eur Arch Paediatr Dent.* 2016;17(5):381–386.
61. Pani SC, AlAnazi GS, AlBaragash A, et al. Objective assessment of the influence of the parental presence on the fear and behavior of

anxious children during their first restorative dental visit. *J Int Soc Prev Community Dent.* 2016;6(suppl 2):S148–S152.

62. Salmon K, Pereira JK. Predicting children's response to an invasive medical investigation: the influence of effortful control and parent behavior. *J Pediatr Psychol.* 2002;27(3):227–233.

63. Jain C, Mathu-Muju KR, Nash DA, et al. Randomized controlled trial: parental compliance with instructions to remain silent in the dental operatory. *Pediatr Dent.* 2013;35(1):47–51.

64. Brill WA. The effect of restorative treatment on children's behavior at the first recall visit in a private pediatric dental practice. *J Clin Pediatr Dent.* 2002;26(4):389–393.

65. Chambers DW. Behavior management techniques for pediatric dentists: an embarrassment of riches. *ASDC J Dent Child.* 1977;44(1):30–34.

66. Jones RN, Sloane HN, Roberts MW. Limitations of "don't" instructional control. *Behav Ther.* 1992;23:131–140.

67. Harper DC, D'Alessandro DM. The child's voice: understanding the contexts of children and families today. *Pediatr Dent.* 2004;26(2):114–120.

68. Brosnan MG, Curzon ME, Fayle S. The use of the local analgesia syringe in children. Should it be kept out of sight? A clinical trial of two methods of presentation. *Eur J Paediatr Dent.* 2002;3(2):68–72.

69. Eaton JJ, McTigue DJ, Fields HW, et al. Attitudes of contemporary parents toward behavior management techniques used in pediatric dentistry. *Pediatr Dent.* 2005;27(2):107–113.

70. Fields HW, Machen JB, Murphy MG. Acceptability of various behavior management techniques relative to types of dental treatment. *Pediatr Dent.* 1984;6(4):199–203.

71. Havelka C, McTigue D, Wilson S, et al. The influence of social status and prior explanation on parental attitudes toward behavior management techniques. *Pediatr Dent.* 1992;14(6):376–381.

72. Lawrence SM, McTigue DJ, Wilson S, et al. Parental attitudes toward behavior management techniques used in pediatric dentistry. *Pediatr Dent.* 1991;13(3):151–155.

73. Scott S, Garcia-Godoy F. Attitudes of Hispanic parents toward behavior management techniques. *ASDC J Dent Child.* 1995;65(2):128–131.

74. Davies EB, Buchanan H. An exploratory study investigating children's perceptions of dental behavioural management techniques. *Int J Paediatr Dent.* 2013;23:297–309.

75. Hamzah HS, Gao X, Yiu CKY, et al. Managing dental fear and anxiety in pediatric patients: a qualitative study from the public's perspective. *Pediatr Dent.* 2014;36(1):29–33.

76. Greenbaum PE, Lumley MA, Turner C, et al. Dentist's reassuring touch: effects on children's behavior. *Pediatr Dent.* 1993;15(1):20–24.

77. Wilson S, Flood T, Kramer N, et al. A study of facially expressed emotions as a function of age, exposure time, and sex in children. *Pediatr Dent.* 1990;12(1):28–32.

78. Peretz B, Karouba J, Blumer S. Pattern of parental acceptance of management techniques used in pediatric dentistry. *J Clin Pediatr Dent.* 2013;38(1):27–30.

79. Uman LS, Birnie KA, Noel M, et al. Psychological interventions for needle-related procedural pain and distress in children and adolescents. *Cochrane Database Syst Rev.* 2013;(10):CD005179.

80. Manimala MR, Blount RL. The effects of parental reassurance versus distraction on child distress and coping during immunizations. *Child Health Care.* 2000;29(3):161–177.

81. Stark LJ, Allen KD, Hurst M, et al. Distraction: its utilization and efficacy with children undergoing dental treatment. *J Appl Behav Anal.* 1989;22(3):297–307.

82. Dahlquist LM, Busby SM, Slifer KJ, et al. Distraction for children of different ages who undergo repeated needle sticks. *J Pediatr Oncol Nurs.* 2002;19(1):22–34.

83. Aitken JC, Wilson S, Coury D, et al. The effect of music distraction on pain, anxiety, and behavior in pediatric dental patients. *Pediatr Dent.* 2002;24(2):114–118.

84. Venham LL, Goldstein M, Goulin-Kremer E, et al. Effectiveness of a distraction technique in managing young dental patients. *Pediatr Dent.* 1981;3(1):7–11.

85. Hoge MA, Howard MR, Wallace DP, et al. Use of video eyewear to manage distress in children during restorative dental treatment. *Pediatr Dent.* 2012;34(5):378–382.

86. Ram D, Shapira J, Holan G, et al. Audiovisual video eyeglass distraction during dental treatment in children. *Quintessence Int.* 2010;41(8):673–679.

87. El-Sharkawi HF, El-Housseiny AA, Aly AM. Effectiveness of new distraction technique on pain associated with injection of local anesthesia for children. *Pediatr Dent.* 2012;34(2):e35–e38.

88. Pinkham JR, Paterson JR. Voice control: an old technique re-examined. *J Dent Child.* 1985;52:199–202.

89. Greenbaum PE, Turner C, Cook EW 3rd, et al. Dentist's voice control: effects on children's disruptive and affective behavior. *Health Psychol.* 1990;9(5):546–558.

90. Boka V, Arapostathis K, Vretos N, et al. Parental acceptance of behaviour-management techniques used in paediatric dentistry and its relation to parental dental anxiety and experience. *Eur Arch Paediatr Dent.* 2014;15(5):333–339.

91. Kantaputra PN, Chiewcharnvalijkit K, Wairatpanich K, et al. Children's attitudes toward behavior management techniques used by dentists. *J Dent Child (Chic).* 2007;74(1):4–9.

92. Fox C, Newton JT. A controlled trial of the impact of exposure to positive images of dentistry on anticipatory dental fear in children. *Community Dent Oral Epidemiol.* 2006;34(6):455–459.

93. Gangwal RR, Rameshchandra Badjatia S, Harish Dave B. Effect of exposure to positive images of dentistry on dental anxiety among 7 to 12 years old children. *Int J Clin Pediatr Dent.* 2014;7(3):176–179.

94. Ramos-Jorge ML, Ramos-Jorge J, Vieira de Andrade RG, et al. Impact of exposure to positive images on dental anxiety among children: a controlled trial. *Eur Arch Paediatr Dent.* 2011;12(4):195–199.

95. Greenbaum PE, Melamed BG. Pretreatment modeling. A technique for reducing children's fear in the dental operatory. *Dent Clin North Am.* 1988;32(4):693–704.

96. Melamed BG, Weinstein D, Katin-Borland M, et al. Reduction of fear-related dental management problems with use of filmed modeling. *J Am Dent Assoc.* 1975;90(4):822–826.

97. Melamed BG, Hawes RR, Heiby E, et al. Use of filmed modeling to reduce uncooperative behavior of children during dental treatment. *J Dent Res.* 1975;54(4):797–801.

98. Paryab M, Arab Z. The effect of Filmed modeling on the anxious and cooperative behavior of 4-6 years old children during dental treatment: a randomized clinical trial study. *Dent Res J (Isfahan).* 2014;11(4):502–507.

99. Farhat-McHayleh N, Harfouche A, Souaid P. Techniques for managing behaviour in pediatric dentistry: comparative study of live modelling and tell-show-do based on children's heart rates during treatment. *J Can Dent Assoc.* 2009;75(4):283.

100. von Baeyer CL, Marche TA, Rocha EM, et al. Children's memory for pain: overview and implications for practice. *J Pain.* 2004;5(5):241–249.

101. Pickrell JE, Heima M, Weinstein P, et al. Using memory restructuring strategy to enhance dental behaviour. *Int J Paediatr Dent.* 2007;17(6):439–448.

102. Nathan JE, Venham LL, Stewart M, et al. The effects of nitrous oxide on anxious young pediatric patients across sequential visits: a double-blind study. *ASDC J Dent.* 1988;55(3):220–230.

103. Veerkamp JS, Gruythusen RJ, Hoogstraten J, et al. Anxiety reduction with nitrous oxide: a permanent solution? *ASDC J Dent Child.* 1995;62(1):44–48.

104. Nelson TM, Griffith TM, Lane KJ, et al. Temperament as a predictor of nitrous oxide inhalation sedation success. *Anesth Prog.* 2017;64(1):17–21.

105. Kuhn BR, Allen KD. Expanding child behavior management technology in pediatric dentistry: a behavioral science perspective. *Pediatr Dent.* 1994;16(1):13–17.

106. Allen KD, Loiben T, Allen SJ, et al. Dentist-implemented contingent escape for management of disruptive child behavior. *J Appl Behav Anal.* 1992;25(3):629–636.

107. Allen KD, Stokes TF. Use of escape and reward in the management of young children during dental treatment. *J Appl Behav Anal.* 1987;20(4):381–390.

108. O'Callaghan PM, Allen KD, Powell S, et al. The efficacy of noncontingent escape for decreasing children's disruptive behavior during restorative dental treatment. *J Appl Behav Anal.* 2006;39(2):161–171.

109. Wolpe J. Reciprocal inhibition as the main basis of psychotherapeutic effects. *AMA Arch Neurol Psychiatry.* 1954;72(2):205–226.

110. Hakeberg M, Berggren U, Carlsson SG. A 10-year follow-up of patients treated for dental fear. *Scand J Dent Res.* 1990;98(1):53–59.

111. Coldwell SE, Getz T, Milgrom P, et al. CARL: a LabVIEW 3 computer program for conducting exposure therapy for the treatment of dental injection fear. *Behav Res Ther.* 1998;36(4):429–441.

112. Levitt J, Mcgoldrick P, Evans D. The management of severe dental phobia in an adolescent boy: a case report. *Int J Paediatr Dent.* 2000;10(4):348–353.

113. Fetner M, Cascio CJ, Essick G. Nonverbal patient with autism spectrum disorder and obstructive sleep apnea: use of desensitization to acclimatize to a dental appliance. *Pediatr Dent.* 2014;36(7):499–501.

114. Office of the Federal Register. Code of Federal Regulations. 42 Public Health, 482.13. 2010.

115. American Academy of Pediatric Dentistry. Guideline on protective stabilization for pediatric dental patients. *Pediatr Dent.* 2016;38(special issue):199–203.

116. Spreat S, Lipinski D, Hill J, et al. Safety indices associated with the use of contingent restraint procedures. *Appl Res Ment Retard.* 1986;7(4):475–481.

117. Nunn J, Foster M, Master S, et al. British Society of Paediatric Dentistry: a policy document on consent and the use of physical intervention in the dental care of children. *Int J Paediatr Dent.* 2008;18(suppl 1):39–46.

118. Patel M, McTigue DJ, Thikkurissy S, et al. Parental attitudes toward advanced behavior guidance techniques used in pediatric dentistry. *Pediatr Dent.* 2016;38(1):30–36.

119. Frankel RI. The Papoose Board and mothers' attitudes following its use. *Pediatr Dent.* 1991;13(5):284–288.

120. McComb M, Koenigsberg SR, Broder HL, et al. The effects of oral conscious sedation on future behavior and anxiety in pediatric dental patients. *Pediatr Dent.* 2002;24(3):207–211.

121. Fuhrer CT 3rd, Weddell JA, Sanders BJ, et al. Effect of behavior of dental treatment rendered under conscious sedation and general anesthesia in pediatric patients. *Pediatr Dent.* 2009;31(7):492–497.

122. Klaassen MA, Veerkamp JS, Hoogstraten J. Changes in children's dental fear: a longitudinal study. *Eur Arch Paediatr Dent.* 2008;9(suppl 1):29–35.

123. White J, Wells M, Arheart KL, et al. A questionnaire of parental perceptions of conscious sedation in pediatric dentistry. *Pediatr Dent.* 2016;38(2):116–121.

124. Frankl SN, Shiere FR, Fogels HR. Should the parent remain with the child in the dental operatory? *ASDC J Dent Child.* 1962;29(2):150–163.

125. Long N. The changing nature of parenting in America. *Pediatr Dent.* 2004;26(2):121–124.

126. Adair SM, Waller JL, Schafer TE, et al. A survey of members of the American Academy of Pediatric Dentistry on their use of behavior management techniques. *Pediatr Dent.* 2004;26(2):150–166.

127. Casamassimo PS, Wilson S, Gross L. Effects of changing U.S. parenting styles on dental practice: perceptions of diplomats of the American Board of Pediatric Dentistry. *Pediatr Dent.* 2002;24(1):18–22.

128. Pediatric Oral Health Research and Policy Center. An essential health benefit: general anesthesia for treatment of early childhood caries. http://www.aapd.org/assets/1/7/POHRPCTechBrief2.pdf. Accessed April 21, 2016.

129. Allen KD, Hodges ED, Knudsen SK. Comparing four methods to inform parents about child behavior management: how to inform for consent. *Pediatr Dent.* 1995;17(3):180–186.

130. Seale NS. Behavior Management Conference Panel III Report—legal issues associated with managing children's behavior in the dental office. *Pediatr Dent.* 2004;26(2):175–179.

131. Bross DC. Managing pediatric dental patients: issues raised by the law and changing views of proper child care. *Pediatr Dent.* 2004;26(2):125–130.

132. Musselman RJ. Considerations in behavior management of the pediatric dental patient. Helping children cope with dental treatment. *Pediatr Clin North Am.* 1991;38(5):1309–1324.

133. Nash DA. Engaging children's cooperation in the dental environment through effective communication. *Pediatr Dent.* 2006;28(5):455–459.

134. Wright GZ, Kupietzky A. Non-pharmacologic approaches in behavior management. In: Wright GZ, Kupietzky A, eds. *Behavior Management in Dentistry for Children.* 2nd ed. Ames, IA: John Wiley & Sons; 2014:81.

135. Barton DH, Hatcher E, Potter R, et al. Dental attitudes and memories: a study of the effects of hand over mouth/restraint. *Pediatr Dent.* 1993;15(1):13–19.

136. Weil TN, Inglehart MR. Dental education and dentists' attitudes and behavior concerning patients with autism. *J Dent Educ.* 2010;74(12):1294–1307.

137. Rutkauskas J, Seale NS, Casamassimo P, et al. Preparedness of entering pediatric dentistry residents: advanced pediatric program directors' and first-year residents' perspectives. *J Dent Educ.* 2015;79(11):1265–1271.

138. Martin MD, Kinoshita-Byrne J, Getz T. Dental fear in a special needs clinic population of persons with disabilities. *Spec Care Dentist.* 2002;22(3):99–102.

139. Marshall J, Sheller B, Williams BJ, et al. Cooperation predictors for dental patients with autism. *Pediatr Dent.* 2007;29(5):369–376.

140. Charles JM. Dental care in children with developmental disabilities: attention deficit disorder, intellectual disabilities, and autism. *J Dent Child.* 2010;77:84–91.

141. Shapiro M, Melmed RN, Sgan-Cohen HD, et al. Effect of sensory adaptation on anxiety of children with developmental disabilities: a new approach. *Pediatr Dent.* 2009;31(3):222–228.

142. Al Humaid J, Tesini D, Finkelman M, et al. Effectiveness of the D-TERMINED program of repetitive tasking for children with autism spectrum disorder. *J Dent Child.* 2016;83(1):16–21.

143. Fakruddin KS, Gorduysus MO, El Batawi H. Effectiveness of behavioral modification techniques with visual distraction using intrasulcular local anesthesia in hearing disabled children during pulp therapy. *Eur J Dent.* 2016;10(4):551–555.

144. Romer M. Consent, restraint, and people with special needs: a review. *Spec Care Dent.* 2009;29(1):58–66.

145. De Castro AM, de Oliveira FS, de Paiva Novaes MS, et al. Behavior guidance techniques in Pediatric Dentistry: attitudes of parents of children with disabilities and without disabilities. *Spec Care Dentist.* 2013;33(5):213–217.

146. Brandes DA, Wilson S, Preisch JW, et al. A Comparison of opinions from parents of disabled and non-disabled children on behavior management techniques used in dentistry. *Spec Care Dentist.* 1995;15(3):119–123.

147. Marshall J, Sheller B, Mancl L, et al. Parental attitudes regarding behavior guidance of dental patients with autism. *Pediatr Dent.* 2008;30(5):400–407.

148. Murphy MG, Fields HW, Machen JB. Parental acceptance of pediatric dentistry behavior management techniques. *Pediatr Dent.* 1984;6:193–198.

25

Periodontal Problems in Children and Adolescents

WILLIAM V. STENBERG, JR.

Children and adolescents are affected by a variety of periodontal diseases and conditions. Gingivitis is common, especially around puberty. Significant loss of periodontal attachment or alveolar bone is more unusual in young patients and can result from systemic disease or occur as isolated dental disease. In addition, gingival anatomic problems, such as lack of attached gingiva, can arise during development and may necessitate early management.

Gingivitis

Gingivitis is characterized by inflammation of the gingival tissues with no loss of attachment or bone. It occurs in response to the bacteria that live in biofilms at the gingival margin and in the sulcus.[1] The clinical signs of gingivitis include erythema, bleeding on probing, and edema. In the early primary dentition, gingivitis is uncommon. Younger children have less plaque than adults do and appear to be less reactive to the same amount of plaque. This can be explained both by differences in bacterial composition of plaque and by developmental changes in the inflammatory response. Gingivitis occurs in half the population by the age of 4 or 5 years, and the incidence continues to increase with age. The prevalence of gingivitis peaks at close to 100% at puberty, but after puberty it declines slightly and stays constant into adulthood.[2] Some children exhibit severe gingivitis at puberty, as shown in Fig. 25.1. Puberty-associated gingivitis is related to increases in steroid hormones.[3] The gingiva may be enlarged with granulomatous changes similar to those occurring in pregnancy. The peak prevalence of puberty-associated gingivitis is at age 10 years in girls and age 13 years in boys. Extensive gingivitis in 12-year-olds, as indicated by bleeding upon probing in more than 15% of sites, has been shown to negatively affect children in how they perceive their oral health as well as their daily lives.[4]

Certain local factors may be important contributors to gingivitis in children. Crowded teeth and orthodontic appliances may make oral hygiene more difficult and predispose to gingivitis. Mouth breathing may cause chronically dehydrated gingiva in the maxillary labial area and lead to a characteristic localized gingivitis as shown in Fig. 25.2. Inflammation, especially erythema, often occurs around erupting primary and permanent teeth.

Gingivitis is reversible and can be managed with improved oral hygiene. Appropriately sized toothbrushes, as well as toothpaste and floss flavored to appeal to children, may enhance compliance. Young children, especially those younger than 6 years of age, will require some parental assistance with their oral hygiene care. Older children and even some adolescents can benefit from some degree of parental supervision.

Gingival Enlargement

Chronic Inflammatory Gingival Enlargement

Longstanding gingivitis in young patients sometimes results in chronic inflammatory gingival enlargement, which may be localized or generalized. It commonly occurs when plaque is allowed to accumulate around orthodontic appliances, as shown in Fig. 25.3, or in areas chronically dried by mouth breathing. The interdental papillae and the marginal gingiva become enlarged, and the tissue is usually erythematous and bleeds easily. It may be soft and friable with a smooth, shiny surface (see Fig. 25.3A), or dense and fibrotic with a matted surface (see Fig. 25.3B). Inflammatory gingival enlargement often slowly resolves when adequate plaque control is instituted, unless the tissues are fibrotic; in such cases, gingivectomy is often required.

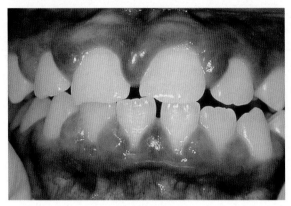

• **Figure 25.1** Puberty-associated gingivitis in a 13-year-old African-American boy. The dark pigmentation of the gingiva is a normal racial characteristic.

Drug-Induced Gingival Enlargement

Long-term therapy with certain systemic medications can produce an overgrowth of gingival tissue (Fig. 25.4).[5] It can occur after therapy with the anticonvulsant phenytoin (Dilantin), the immunosuppressant cyclosporine, or calcium channel blockers. The overgrowth is painless and differs from chronic inflammatory enlargement in that it is fibrous, firm, and pale pink, often with little tendency to bleed. The enlargement occurs first in the interdental region and may appear lobular. It gradually spreads to the gingival margin. The condition can become extreme, sometimes covering the crowns of the teeth and interfering with eruption or occlusion.

Drug-influenced gingival enlargement occurs slowly and may resolve to some degree when medication is discontinued. There appears to be a genetic component to susceptibility to gingival enlargement. The severity of the enlargement is also affected by both the adequacy of oral hygiene and the gingival concentration of the medication. If medication cannot be discontinued or changed, the enlargement can be surgically removed, but it will recur. Surgery is indicated when the appearance of the gingiva is unacceptable to the patient, when the enlargement interferes with comfortable functioning, or when enlargement produces periodontal pockets that cannot be maintained in a healthy state. Postoperative discomfort after gingivectomy can be considerable and should be

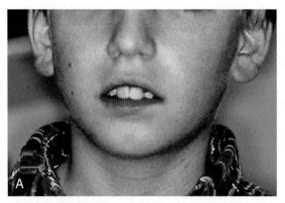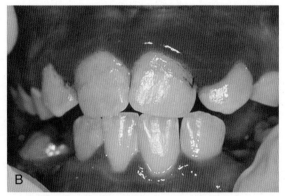

• **Figure 25.2** (A) The typical oral posture of mouth breathing. (B) The resultant gingivitis of the maxillary facial gingiva.

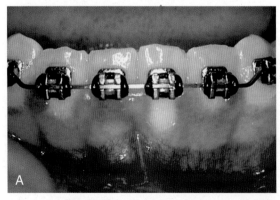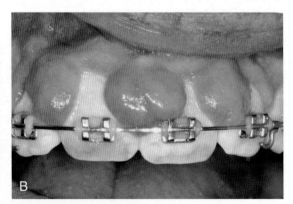

• **Figure 25.3** (A) Gingival enlargement (noted between lateral incisors and canines) in response to longstanding plaque accumulation on the mandibular incisors secondary to orthodontic appliances. Note uneven gingival margin and narrow gingiva on left mandibular central incisor, without root exposure ("pseudorecession"). (B) Gingival enlargement secondary to orthodontic appliances.

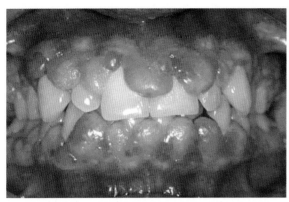

• **Figure 25.4** Severe gingival enlargement, secondary to cyclosporine and nifedipine therapy, in a teenaged kidney transplant patient.

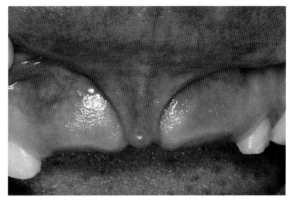

• **Figure 25.6** Prominent midline maxillary labial frenum in a child.

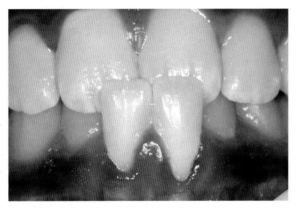

• **Figure 25.5** A reduction in the width of gingiva resulting from labial eruption of the mandibular central incisors. Localized recession has occurred on the left central incisor as the result of plaque accumulation in an area that was difficult to clean and had inadequate attached gingiva. The dark pigmentation of the gingiva is a normal racial characteristic.

carefully weighed against potential benefits for special needs patients who may not be able to give fully informed consent.

Anatomic Problems

Development and Defects of the Attached Gingiva

When teeth erupt, they pierce through an existing band of keratinized gingiva, and the width of this band and its relationship to the teeth change very little during subsequent growth and development. Deflections in the path of eruption, such as those due to crowding or overretention of primary teeth, may result in a narrowed band of attached gingiva.[6] This is particularly common when mandibular incisors erupt labial to the alveolar ridge, as shown in Fig. 25.5. If the band of attached gingiva is very narrow, even a small subsequent loss of attachment can result in a mucogingival defect (which occurs when the pocket depth exceeds the width of keratinized gingiva), and recession may occur, as shown in Fig. 25.5 (left central incisor). The loss of attachment and recession that occurs with a labially malpositioned tooth is often referred to as *stripping*. Other factors that may contribute to recession in children and adolescents are habit-related self-inflicted injury, oral piercings, and the use of smokeless tobacco.

A free gingival graft or connective tissue graft is indicated to stabilize and repair the gingiva of teeth with significant recession. Such grafts commonly use allogenic material or donor tissue from the patient's own palate. Surgical repair of lingual recession due to oral piercings can be performed but requires more complex treatment than typical labial gingival grafts.[7] Orthodontic movement of a labially malpositioned tooth in the direction of the alveolar ridge may produce a small increase in attached gingiva and place the tooth in a periodontally more stable position.

Frena

Periodontal examination of the pediatric patient should include evaluation of the frena. These are mucosal folds with enclosed muscle tissue that serve as attachments for the lips and tongue to the immobile tissue of the mandible and premaxilla. The three primary frena are the maxillary labial, mandibular labial, and lingual frena. Aberrant frena can be related to various problems at different stages of growth and development.

Abnormal frena can also be associated with various syndromic and nonsyndromic conditions. Therefore the clinician is advised to carefully evaluate the frena of pediatric patients. Hyperplastic frena have been associated with the Ellis-van Creveld syndrome, and multiple hyperplastic frena in females can be associated with the oral-facial-digital syndrome. The congenital absence of frena may indicate Ehlers-Danlos syndrome. It has also been associated with infantile hypertrophic pyloric stenosis. Even in otherwise healthy patients, the appearance of the frena can be variable. Therefore the clinician is advised not to use a frenum as the sole criteria in a diagnosis but correlate the presentation with other signs and symptoms.

Maxillary Midline Frenum

A prominent maxillary frenum, often accompanied by a large midline diastema, is a common finding in children (Fig. 25.6). It is often a cause for concern by parents and health care providers. In general, surgical treatment of this condition should be delayed until the maxillary canines have fully erupted, because they will often cause spontaneous closure of the diastema. If orthodontic therapy is necessary, consideration for surgery can usually be delayed until the completion of active treatment and is only necessary if the diastema presents an esthetic or functional problem at that time. Treatment has traditionally consisted of a Z-plasty procedure, but lasers are effective and are increasingly being used to provide this treatment.

The maxillary midline frenum can also present problems in nursing infants, a condition known as "lip tie." Studies have shown dramatic improvements in nursing ability in infants after surgical release of the maxillary midline frenum.[8]

Mandibular Labial Frenum

The mandibular labial frenum should normally attach between the mandibular central incisors at a level below the attached gingiva. A hypertrophic frenum, or one with an aberrant attachment near the free gingival margin, may be associated with gingival recession. In these cases, treatment is directed at the reconstruction of the attached gingiva and not at the frenum per se. Treatment options consist of periodontal plastic surgery, such as a free gingival graft with vestibular extension or a connective tissue graft. The frenum is relocated to a more apical position as a consequence of these procedures. This is very effective at providing root coverage and gingival stability, in addition to preventing reattachment of the frenum to the free gingival margin.

Lingual Frenum

A restrictive lingual frenum ("tongue tie") is often seen in children (Fig. 25.7). In approximately 3% of children, the attachment may limit normal tongue mobility (ankyloglossia), which can lead to discomfort or difficulties while nursing and can also impact the development of speech. Some studies have shown marked improvement in speech and language assessment in children who were treated for ankyloglossia and had preexisting speech difficulties.[9] Although lingual frenotomies may be indicated for infants with feeding issues, there are insufficient data to recommend prophylactic surgery in asymptomatic patients. Consultation with a speech pathologist is recommended if problems are suspected. Occasionally, the restrictive lingual frenum may impact the lingual gingiva (see Fig. 25.7). Treatment generally consists of a simple frenotomy, which can be performed with scissors or with lasers.

Periodontitis

Significant loss of periodontal attachment is common in adults, with chronic periodontitis (formerly called "adult-onset" periodontitis) affecting the majority of the population. When epidemiologic observations have been made, 20% of 14- to 17-year-olds in the United States are found to have attachment loss of at least 2 mm at one or more sites.[10,11] The number and severity of affected sites increase steadily with age, demonstrating that chronic periodontitis

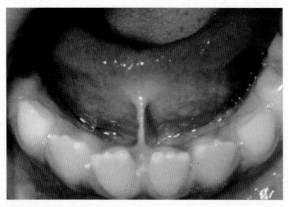

• **Figure 25.7** Restrictive lingual frenum in a child. Note the relationship of the frenum to the tip of the tongue and the lingual gingiva of the central incisors.

often begins in adolescence. Chronic periodontitis responds well to oral hygiene measures and can easily be arrested in its early stages when attachment loss is minimal and deep pockets have not developed.

Smoking is a major risk factor for periodontitis, and smoking among children and adolescents is no longer limited to traditional tobacco cigarettes. The use of e-cigarettes, which consists of inhaling noncombusted, electrically vaporized chemicals including nicotine, is known as "vaping." E-cigarette, hookah, and pipe tobacco use is increasing faster in younger age groups than use of traditional cigarettes. E-cigarettes are currently the most commonly used tobacco product among middle and high school students.[12] Candy-flavored electronic cigarettes have been shown to elicit a strong interest in smoking among children, and adolescents who begin with e-cigarettes are much more likely to start using traditional cigarettes and become heavy smokers. The misconception that e-cigarettes are a harmless alternative to smoking is common, but recent studies have demonstrated a causal link to periodontal destruction.[13] The effect of secondhand aerosol from e-cigarettes on infants and small children is unknown, but studies suggest that such exposure may also be harmful. The actual components of electronic cigarettes are toxic if ingested by small children, and calls to poison control centers have skyrocketed since their popularity has increased. More than 50% of such calls involved children aged 5 years and younger.[14]

Smoking is not limited to tobacco. With the recent legalization of medical marijuana in many states, the availability to children and adolescents has increased. The frequent use of cannabis (marijuana and hashish) is associated with deeper periodontal probing depths, more clinical attachment loss, and increased risk of developing severe periodontitis.[15] Smoking crack cocaine and other illicit drugs is also linked to periodontal destruction.[16] The potential for periodontal destruction, as well as the long-term effects of tobacco and other psychoactive compounds on the developing adolescent brain and body, are of great concern. Current and past smoking status should be determined as part of a periodontal assessment for young patients, including detailed questioning about nontraditional smoking and other tobacco use. Appropriate cessation counseling and/or referrals should be provided.

Aggressive Periodontitis

Rare, rapidly progressing forms of periodontitis also affect children and adolescents who are otherwise healthy. Aggressive periodontitis has localized and generalized forms and can occur in the permanent or the primary dentition.

Localized Aggressive Periodontitis in the Permanent Dentition

Localized aggressive periodontitis (LAP), formerly called *localized juvenile periodontitis,* is characterized by the loss of attachment and bone around the permanent incisors and first permanent molars. The radiographic appearance is distinctive (Fig. 25.8). The attachment loss is rapid, occurring at three times the rate of chronic disease. Inflammation in LAP is not as extreme as that occurring in periodontitis associated with systemic disease such as neutropenia, but both inflammation and plaque accumulation are often greater than those found in the typical teenager. The disease is usually detected in early adolescence but may begin as LAP of the primary dentition (discussed later). The prevalence of LAP is estimated to be approximately 1%, and in the United States it most commonly

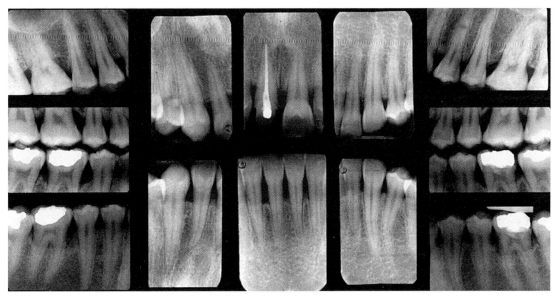

• **Figure 25.8** Radiographic appearance of localized aggressive periodontitis showing the typical bone loss pattern around first permanent molars and central incisors. Note the root canal treatment of the central incisor. Luxation injuries are common in these patients because of mobility of the incisors.

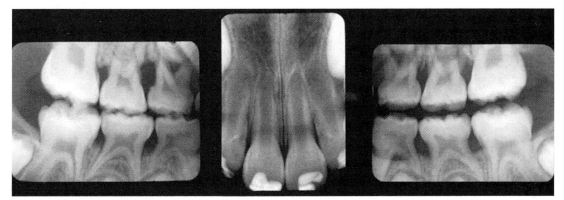

• **Figure 25.9** Radiographic appearance of localized aggressive periodontitis showing the characteristic loss of bone around the primary molars. In this patient the disease has not progressed to include the permanent teeth, as sometimes occurs.

occurs in the African-American population. Some cases appear to be inherited as an autosomal dominant trait, and LAP has been linked to a neutrophil chemotactic defect. LAP may progress to generalized aggressive periodontitis (GAP).

Despite the genetic component, LAP is clearly linked to the presence of high numbers of *Aggregatibacter actinomycetemcomitans,* and successful treatment outcomes correlate well with eradication of the bacteria. Treatment consists of local débridement in combination with systemic antibiotic therapy and microbiologic monitoring. Localized surgical intervention is often necessary to manage the residual defects. Systemic tetracyclines have been used with some success but should not be used in children under 9 years of age due to the potential for delayed bone growth and permanent tooth discoloration. Metronidazole alone or in combination with amoxicillin appears to be effective in arresting disease progression.[17]

Generalized Aggressive Periodontitis

GAP sometimes occurs in adolescents and teenagers. In young adults the same disease was formerly called *rapidly progressive periodontitis.*[18] GAP may affect the entire dentition and is not self-limiting. Heavy accumulations of plaque and calculus are found in GAP, and inflammation may be severe. GAP is not associated with high levels of *A. actinomycetemcomitans* but instead has a microbiologic profile closer to that of chronic disease. It should be managed aggressively with local therapy as well as systemic antibiotics.

Localized Aggressive Periodontitis in the Primary Dentition

LAP in the primary dentition (formerly called *localized prepubertal periodontitis* [LPP]) is characterized by localized loss of attachment in the primary dentition. It occurs in children without evidence of systemic disease. The disease is most commonly manifested in the molar area, where localized, usually bilaterally symmetric loss of attachment occurs (Fig. 25.9). In the United States LAP of the primary dentition occurs most commonly in the African-American population. It is usually accompanied by mild to moderate inflammation, and heavier than average plaque deposits may be visible.

It is commonly first diagnosed during the late primary dentition or early transitional dentition. LAP of the primary dentition may progress to LAP in the permanent dentition.

LAP in the primary dentition is associated with a bacterial infection and a specific, but minor, host immunologic deficit. Some cases are associated with systemic (genetic) diseases. Antibiotic therapy combined with local débridement appears to be an effective treatment regimen. Metronidazole is the antibiotic of choice for LAP of the primary dentition. Tetracyclines are contraindicated.

Necrotizing Ulcerative Gingivitis/Periodontitis

Necrotizing ulcerative gingivitis/periodontitis is characterized by the rapid onset of painful gingivitis with interproximal and marginal necrosis and ulceration. The incidence peaks in the late teens and early 20s in North America and Europe, but in less developed countries it is common in young children. Malnutrition, viral infections, stress, lack of sleep, and smoking have been reported as predisposing factors. Necrotizing ulcerative gingivitis/periodontitis is associated with high levels of spirochetes and *Prevotella intermedia*. Local débridement usually produces rapid resolution of the disease, but antibiotic therapy with penicillin or metronidazole may be indicated in patients with elevated body temperature.

Systemic Diseases and Conditions With Associated Periodontal Problems

Early loss of periodontal attachment in children is often a sign of systemic disease. Periodontitis may occur in the presence of defects in the immune system that result in susceptibility to infection such as leukocyte adhesion deficiency (LAD) or neutropenia,[1] developmental defects in the attachment apparatus as in hypophosphatasia, or from the invasion of neoplastic cells as in leukemia.

Diabetes

An increased risk and earlier onset of periodontitis occur in both insulin-dependent and non–insulin-dependent diabetes mellitus.[19] As many as 10% to 15% of teenagers with insulin-dependent diabetes mellitus have significant periodontal disease. Poor metabolic control increases the risk of periodontitis, and untreated periodontitis in turn worsens metabolic control of diabetes. Effective preventive regimens and early diagnosis and treatment of periodontitis are important for the overall health of patients with diabetes.

Down Syndrome

Down syndrome is accompanied by an increased susceptibility to periodontitis. Most Down syndrome patients develop periodontitis by 30 years of age, and it may first occur in the primary dentition.[20] Plaque levels are high in these patients, but the severity of periodontal destruction exceeds that attributable to local factors alone. Various minor immune deficits in patients with Down syndrome may be responsible for the increased susceptibility to periodontitis. Severe recession in the mandibular anterior region associated with a high frenum attachment is also common in Down syndrome.

Hypophosphatasia

Hypophosphatasia is a genetic disorder in which the enzyme bone alkaline phosphatase is deficient or defective. Phenotypes of hypophosphatasia can vary from premature loss of deciduous teeth to severe bone abnormalities leading to neonatal death.[21] In general, the earlier the presentation of symptoms, the more severe the disease. In mild forms the early loss of primary teeth may be the first and only clinical sign, as shown in Fig. 25.10. The early loss of teeth is the result of defective cementum formation, which affects attachment of tooth to bone. There currently is no treatment for the disease, but the dental prognosis for the permanent teeth is good. Typically, the primary incisors are exfoliated before the age of 4 years, the other primary teeth are affected to varying degrees, and the permanent dentition is normal. Hypophosphatasia can be diagnosed by a finding of low alkaline phosphatase levels in a serum sample.

Leukocyte Adhesion Deficiency

LAD, also called generalized prepubertal periodontitis,[22] is a rare, recessive genetic disease that leaves patients susceptible to bacterial infections, including periodontitis. Because of the high incidence of skin abscesses, recurrent otitis media, pneumonitis, and other bacterial infections of soft tissues, a diagnosis is usually made before dental symptoms appear. Dental symptoms are manifested early in the primary dentition. Bone loss is rapid around nearly all teeth, and inflammation is marked. Scrupulous oral hygiene measures are necessary to control the periodontitis associated with LAD.

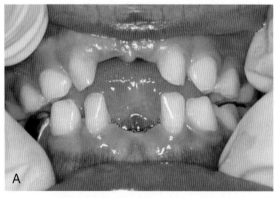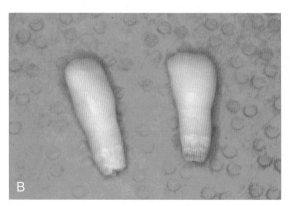

• **Figure 25.10** (A) The dentition of a 4-year-old child with early loss of upper and lower central incisors due to hypophosphatasia. (B) The lower incisors, exfoliated at 13 months of age. Note the incomplete root development at the time the teeth were exfoliated.

Neutropenia

Neutropenia is a hematologic disorder characterized by reduced numbers or complete disappearance of neutrophils from the blood and bone marrow. In addition to increased susceptibility to recurrent infections such as otitis media or respiratory and skin infections, patients with neutropenia generally suffer from severe gingivitis and pronounced alveolar bone loss. Periodontal therapy consists of rigorous local measures to control plaque, but patients are seldom able to maintain the level of oral hygiene necessary to prevent the development and progression of periodontal disease.

Papillon-Lefèvre Syndrome

Papillon-Lefèvre syndrome is a rare disease that has, as a symptom, the onset of severe periodontitis in the primary or transitional dentition. It is a genetic disorder that is easily identified on clinical examination by the finding of hyperkeratosis of the palms of the hands and soles of the feet. Severe inflammation and rapid bone loss are characteristic of the periodontitis. Therapy consists of aggressive local measures to control plaque formation. Successful treatment outcomes in children have been reported with antibiotic therapy.[23]

Histiocytosis

Langerhans cell histiocytosis (LCH), previously known as histiocytosis X, is a rare disorder of childhood that presents with histiocytic infiltration of bones, skin, liver, and other organs. In 10% to 20% of cases, the initial infiltrates occur in the oral cavity, usually in the mandible. Typical findings include gingival enlargement, ulcerations, mobility of teeth with alveolar expansion, and discrete, destructive lesions of bone that can be observed on radiographs. LCH may be diagnosed by biopsy. Therapy consists of local measures such as radiation and surgery to remove lesions and systemic chemotherapy for disseminated disease. The prognosis for disseminated early-onset disease is poor, with mortality rates exceeding 60%. On the other hand, mild localized LCH has an excellent prognosis. The lesions of LCH and the local therapy used to treat them may result in loss of teeth or arrested development of teeth.

Leukemia

Leukemias are the most common form of childhood cancer. Acute lymphoblastic leukemia (ALL) is the most common and has the best prognosis. Acute myeloid leukemia (AML) accounts for approximately 20% of childhood leukemias and has a poorer long-term survival rate. AML may present with gingival enlargement caused by infiltrates of leukemic cells. This presentation usually does not occur with ALL. The lesions associated with the gingival enlargement are bluish red and may sometimes invade bone. In addition to the gingival lesions, the patient may have fever, malaise, gingival or other bleeding, and bone or joint pain. AML may be diagnosed by a blood cell count. Anemia, abnormal leukocyte and differential counts, and thrombocytopenia are usually observed.

Periodontal Examination of Children

The periodontal health of children and adolescents should be assessed at each examination. The gingival tissues should be examined for redness, edema, bleeding, or enlargement. Oral hygiene may be assessed via a plaque index. Use of a disclosant provides an excellent oral hygiene instruction tool and a plaque index provides a method for monitoring and documenting oral hygiene practices. Calculus is not as common in young patients as it is in adults, but it is found in approximately 10% of children and approximately one-third of teenagers. Patients of all ages should always be checked for calculus during periodic examinations, and deposits, when noted, should be removed.

Particularly after the eruption of permanent teeth, attachment levels should be determined by periodontal probing. Probing of the permanent incisors and first permanent molars provides a diagnostic screening for LAP. Because erupting teeth can be probed all the way to the cementoenamel junction, transient deep pockets are a normal finding in the transitional dentition and must be distinguished from true attachment loss by locating the cementoenamel junction.

When radiographs are available, bone levels should be examined. Normal crestal height should be within 1 to 2 mm of the cementoenamel junction.[24] After permanent teeth have erupted, the patient should also be examined for deficiencies in the width of attached gingiva and areas of recession should be noted.

References

1. Tatakis DN, Kumar PS. Etiology and pathogenesis of periodontal diseases. *Dent Clin North Am*. 2005;49:491–516.
2. Matsson L. Factors influencing the susceptibility to gingivitis during childhood: a review. *Int J Paediatr Dent*. 1993;3:119–127.
3. Mombelli A, Gusberti FA, van Oosten MA, et al. Gingival health and gingivitis development during puberty. A 4-year longitudinal study. *J Clin Periodontol*. 1989;16:451–456.
4. Tomazoni F, Zanatta F, Tuchtenhagen S, et al. Association of gingivitis with child oral health-related quality of life. *J Periodontol*. 2014;85:1157–1565.
5. Dongari A, McDonnell HT, Langlais RP. Drug-induced gingival overgrowth. *Oral Surg Oral Med Oral Pathol*. 1993;76:543–548.
6. Andlin-Sobocki A, Bodin L. Dimensional alterations of the gingiva related to changes of facial/ lingual tooth position in permanent anterior teeth of children. A 2-year longitudinal study. *J Clin Periodontol*. 1993;20:219–224.
7. Parra C, Jeong Y, Hawley C. Guided tissue regeneration involving piercing-induced lingual recession: a case report. *Int J Periodontics Restorative Dent*. 2016;36:869–875.
8. Pransky SM, Lago D, Hong P. Breastfeeding difficulties and oral cavity abnormalities: the influence of posterior ankyloglossia and upper-lip ties. *Int J Pediatr Otorhinolaryngol*. 2015;79(10):1714–1717.
9. Messner A, Lalakea M. The effect of ankyloglossia on speech in children. *Otolaryngol Head Neck Surg*. 2002;127(6):539–545.
10. Armitage GC. Development of a classification system for periodontal diseases and conditions. *Ann Periodontol*. 1999;4:1–6.
11. Bhat M. Periodontal health of 14-17-year-old US schoolchildren. *J Public Health Dent*. 1991;51:5–11.
12. Singh T, Arrazola RA, Corey CG, et al. Tobacco use among middle and high school students—United States, 2011–2015. *MMWR Morb Mortal Wkly Rep*. 2016;65:361–367.
13. Sundar IK, Javed F, Romanos GE, et al. E-cigarettes and flavorings induce inflammatory and pro-senescence responses in oral epithelial cells and periodontal fibroblasts. *Oncotarget*. 2016;7:77196–77204.
14. Chatham-Stephens K, Law R, Taylor E, et al. Centers for Disease Control and Prevention (CDC). Notes from the field: calls to poison centers for exposures to electronic cigarettes—United States, September 2010-February 2014. *MMWR Morb Mortal Wkly Rep*. 2014;63(13):292–293.
15. Shariff J, Ahluwalia K, Papapanou P. Relationship between frequent recreational cannabis (marijuana and hashish) use and periodontitis in adults in the United States: National Health and Nutrition Examination Survey 2011 to 2012. *J Periodontol*. 2017;88(3):273–280.

16. Antoniazzi R, Zanatta F, Rösing C, et al. Association between periodontitis and the use of crack cocaine and other illicit drugs. *J Periodontol.* 2016;87(12):1396–1405.
17. Saxen L, Asikainen S. Metronidazole in the treatment of localized juvenile periodontitis. *J Clin Periodontol.* 1993;20:166–171.
18. Position paper: epidemiology of periodontal diseases. American Academy of Periodontology. *J Periodontol.* 1996;67:935–945.
19. de Pommereau V, Dargent-Pare C, Robert JJ, et al. Periodontal status in insulin-dependent diabetic adolescents. *J Clin Periodontol.* 1992;19:628–632.
20. Reuland-Bosma W, van Dijk J. Periodontal disease in Down's syndrome: a review. *J Clin Periodontol.* 1986;13:64–73.
21. Chapple IL. Hypophosphatasia: dental aspects and mode of inheritance. *J Clin Periodontol.* 1993;20:615–622.
22. Watanabe K. Prepubertal periodontitis: a review of diagnostic criteria, pathogenesis, and differential diagnosis. *J Periodontal Res.* 1990;25:31–48.
23. Ishikawa I, Umeda M, Laosrisin N. Clinical, bacteriological, and immunological examinations and the treatment process of two Papillon-Lefèvre syndrome patients. *J Periodontol.* 1994;65:364–371.
24. Sjodin B, Matsson L. Marginal bone level in the normal primary dentition. *J Clin Periodontol.* 1992;19:672–678.

26

Space Maintenance in the Primary Dentition

CLARICE S. LAW AND HENRY FIELDS

General Considerations

Management of premature tooth loss in the primary dentition requires careful thought by the clinician because the consequences of proper or improper space maintenance may influence dental development well into adolescence.[1] Early loss of primary teeth may compromise the eruption of succedaneous teeth if there is a reduction in the arch length. On the other hand, timely intervention may save space for the eruption of the permanent dentition. The key to space maintenance in the primary dentition is in knowing which problems to treat.[2]

Premature tooth loss in this age group is best thought of in terms of anterior (incisors and canines) and posterior (molars) teeth. The causes and treatment of missing teeth differ in these two regions. Anterior tooth loss is due primarily to trauma and tooth decay. Children in this age group are still developing gross motor skills, so injuries to the primary incisors are common. In addition, despite efforts at promoting preventive care, a number of children still suffer from early childhood caries.[3,4] These decay patterns result in both anterior and posterior tooth loss. The majority of posterior tooth loss is due to dental caries; rarely are primary molars lost to trauma. If no space loss has occurred immediately after tooth loss, space maintenance is appropriate because the permanent successor will not erupt for several years. If space loss has occurred, a comprehensive evaluation is required to determine whether space regaining or no treatment is indicated. This type of evaluation and decision-making is described in the discussions of the mixed dentition (see Chapter 31) because most attempts at regaining space are made at that time.

Missing primary incisors are usually replaced for four reasons: space maintenance, function, speech, and esthetics. These reasons merit consideration. There is little evidence to support the concept that early removal of a primary incisor will result in space loss in most situations.[5] There may be some redistribution of space between the remaining incisors, but there is no net loss of space. Intuitively, this makes sense because there is no apparent movement or drifting of teeth when developmental spacing is present in the primary dentition. The exceptions seem to be when incisors are lost prior to the eruption of the primary canines or if there is crowding in the anterior segment.

Poor masticatory function has also been proposed as a reason for replacing missing primary incisors. Concerns have been expressed about a child's ability to eat after all maxillary incisors have been removed due to early childhood caries. There is little evidence to support this concern. Anecdotally, feeding has not proven to be a problem for children with missing incisors, and when given a proper diet, a child can continue to grow normally.

Some investigators have cited slowed or altered speech development as a justification for replacing missing maxillary incisors. This may be valid if the child has lost several teeth very early and is just beginning to develop speech. Many sounds are made with the tongue touching the lingual surfaces of the maxillary incisors, and inappropriate speech compensations may develop if these teeth are missing. However, if the child has already acquired speech skills, the loss of an incisor is not particularly important because any speech problems that may develop tend to be transient and resolve when the permanent incisors erupt.[5]

Probably the most valid reason for replacing missing incisors is esthetics. The literature regarding the attitudes of young children toward dental esthetics is controversial.[5] However, parents are more likely to express esthetic concerns. The difficulty is when parents wish to replace the teeth but the child's behavior does not allow the clinician to construct and place the appliance. If parents do not indicate a desire to replace missing anterior teeth, no treatment is certainly appropriate.

Loss of a primary canine as a result of trauma or decay is rare. Because it is so rare, there is some debate about whether space loss will occur if there is no space maintenance. If the clinician is concerned about future space loss, either a band and loop space maintainer or a removable partial denture may be placed if the patient is cooperative. These appliances may need to be remade when the permanent lateral incisor erupts. It is speculated that the upper or lower midline may shift to the affected side if no space maintenance is used, although there are no data to support or refute this claim.

Because loss of primary incisors is not typically associated with space loss and isolated loss of canines is rare, space maintenance during the primary dentition years is aimed primarily at the replacement of primary molars. Extraction of a primary molar can result in space loss. The tooth distal to the newly created space drifts mesial; more with loss of the second molar than the first molar. In fact, there is some evidence that loss of a primary first molar may not result in any overall space loss as long as the permanent first molar is well interdigitated with the opposing molar.[6] It seems that the occlusion keeps the molars from tipping or moving mesial. On the other hand, loss of a primary second molar has a high probability of space loss due to unhindered mesial drift of the permanent first molar. There is also evidence that the tooth mesial to the affected molar can drift distal into the space; this is more common with the primary first molar than the second.[7] Thus loss of space or arch length can occur from both directions (Fig. 26.1). Space loss can even occur without losing a primary tooth if interproximal cavitations are not treated, resulting in loss of the interproximal contact. Similarly, space loss can also occur when teeth adjacent to an ankylosed tooth continue to erupt and tip over the ankylosed molar due to the loss of a contact point.

Space maintenance begins with good restorative dentistry. The dentist should strive for ideal restoration of all interproximal contours. Early restoration of interproximal caries ensures that no space loss occurs. However, in some instances, large carious lesions may make ideal restoration of the tooth impossible, and space loss is inevitable. Even if the pulpal tissues have been compromised, pulp therapy should be initiated and the tooth maintained, if at all possible, because the natural tooth is still superior to the best space maintainer available; it is functional, the correct size, and exfoliates appropriately. In cases of ankylosis the tooth should be maintained until space loss is imminent; it is then extracted and the space maintained. Ankylosed teeth show limited vertical change in the primary dentition years.

Teeth lost during the primary dentition years can cause later-than-normal eruption of the succedaneous teeth. This means that the appliances should be monitored, adjusted, and possibly replaced over a longer period of time. Abutment teeth for appliances may exfoliate or interfere with adjacent erupting teeth. Abutment teeth are also at greater risk of decay and decalcification due to the

appliance. These aspects of care should be considered during treatment planning.

Space Maintaining Appliances

The *Code on Dental Procedures and Nomenclature (Code) CDT 2017* lists four categories for space maintenance appliances[8]: fixed unilateral, fixed bilateral, removable unilateral, and removable bilateral. There is no specificity for the stage of dentition during which these are used. Unilateral appliances are used to maintain space for a single missing tooth. Fixed unilateral appliances include the band and loop, crown and loop, and the distal shoe. Interestingly, the distal shoe has a code in the CDT distinct from the fixed unilateral appliances. Removable unilateral appliances are rarely mentioned in the literature and, if so, mainly with cautions against use due to their small size. Bilateral appliances maintain space for two adjacent teeth or in cases where one or more teeth are missing in different quadrants within the same arch. The Nance appliance, transpalatal arch (TPA), and passive lingual arch or lower lingual holding arch are included as examples of fixed bilateral space maintainers. Removable bilateral appliances are more commonly used than unilateral designs particularly in cases where multiple teeth have been lost prematurely. These generally consist of variations on the Hawley type retainer.

Fixed Unilateral Appliances

One of the most common appliances used in the primary dentition is the band and loop. It is frequently used to maintain space for unilateral loss of the primary first molar before or after eruption of the permanent first molar (Fig. 26.2). It consists of a band that is cemented to the primary second molar with the loop contacting the distal surface of the primary canine. The appliance provides resistance to the pressure of the early mesial shift that occurs as the permanent first molar begins its eruption, as well as the distal drift of the adjacent canine. The band and loop can also be used to provide space maintenance for premature loss of a primary second molar but requires the permanent first molar be erupted sufficiently to fully seat a band. In some cases a variation called the reverse band and loop is used to hold the space of the missing primary second molar. The band is seated on an intact primary first molar with the loop extending distally to contact the mesial

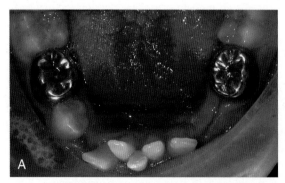
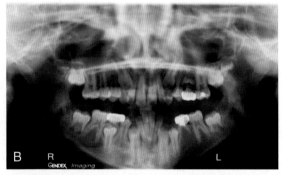

• **Figure 26.1** Premature loss of the primary first molar can result in loss of space from both directions. The primary mandibular second molar drifts mesially, and the primary canine drifts distally, but predominantly there is movement from the anterior in the posterior direction for the mandibular arch. (A) Arch perimeter has been lost on both sides. (B) Panoramic radiograph shows the canine and two premolars attempting to erupt into the limited space on the patient's right. The left mandibular second premolar is missing.

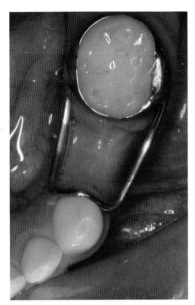

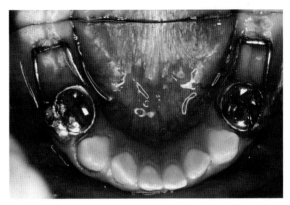

• **Figure 26.4** The distal shoe appliance is used to maintain the space of a primary second molar that has been lost prematurely before the eruption of the permanent first molar. A stainless steel extension is soldered to the distal end of the band and 36-mil loop; this extension is positioned 1 mm below the mesial marginal ridge of the unerupted permanent first molar. The extension serves to guide the eruption of the permanent first molar.

• **Figure 26.2** The band and loop appliance is used to maintain the space after the premature loss of a single tooth. The band and loop appliance is indicated when there is unilateral loss of a primary first molar before or after the eruption of the permanent first molar. The loop is constructed of 36-mil round wire and is soldered to the band.

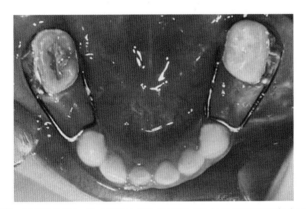

• **Figure 26.3** If both primary first molars are lost prematurely in the mandibular arch and the permanent incisors have not erupted, bilateral band and loop appliances are used to maintain space. A lingual arch is not indicated in this situation because it may interfere with the subsequent eruption of the permanent mandibular incisors.

surface of the permanent molar. Overall, the band and loop appliance is inexpensive and easy to fabricate. However, its use requires continuous supervision and care, and it does not restore the occlusal function of the missing tooth.

The band and loop appliance is also commonly used in the primary dentition for bilateral loss of primary molars before the eruption of the permanent incisors (Fig. 26.3). More discussion on this will take place in the subsequent section on fixed bilateral appliances. A variation of the band and loop appliance that is not highly recommended is the crown and loop appliance. The crown and loop technique requires preparation of the abutment tooth for a stainless steel crown followed by soldering of a space-maintaining wire directly to the crown. Care and maintenance of the crown and loop is more difficult than for the band and loop if there is damage or if modifications are required. If the solder joint fails and the wire breaks loose, there is no way to repair the

crown and loop appliance intraorally. The crown must be cut off, a new crown fitted, and the wire resoldered. It is much easier to restore the abutment tooth with a stainless steel crown and then make a band and loop that fits the crown.

The distal shoe appliance is used to maintain the space of a primary second molar that has been lost before the eruption of the permanent first molar (Fig. 26.4). An unerupted permanent first molar drifts mesial within the alveolar bone if the primary second molar is lost prematurely. The result of the mesial drift is loss of arch length and possible impaction of the second premolar.

There are many problems associated with the distal shoe appliance. Because of its cantilever design, the appliance can replace only a single tooth. In addition, the occlusal convergence of the crown of the primary first molar makes proper band fit difficult and increases band fragility. In some cases, cutting the top off a stainless crown and trimming the gingival margin to resemble a band will work best. Occlusal function should not be restored because of this lack of strength. Finally, histologic examination shows that complete epithelialization does not occur after placement of the appliance.[9] Because the epithelium is not intact, the distal shoe appliance is contraindicated in medically compromised patients and patients at risk for infective endocarditis.

The distal shoe can have modifications. It can also be fabricated with the crown and distal shoe modification in design. Although feasible, like the crown and loop, it is difficult to modify and repair. The reverse band and loop described previously can be used as a substitute for the distal shoe, with the appliance designed so that the wire of the loop rests on the soft tissue (sometimes with mild pressure) approximately where the distal surface of the lost primary second molar was located. The goal is to minimize mesial movement of the unerupted permanent first molar. To date, there are several case reports but no clinical trials to support this recommendation.

Fixed Bilateral Appliances

The second category of appliances used to maintain posterior space in the primary dentition consists of fixed bilateral appliances. These appliances are indicated when teeth are lost in both quadrants of the same arch or multiple teeth have been lost within a quadrant.

The lower lingual holding arch is commonly used in the mandibular arch during the mixed dentition period. However, because the permanent incisor tooth buds develop and erupt lingual to their primary precursors in the lower arch, a mandibular lingual arch is not recommended in the primary dentition; the wire resting adjacent to the primary incisors might interfere with the eruption of the permanent dentition (Fig. 26.5). Instead, two band and loop appliances are recommended when there is bilateral tooth loss in the mandibular arch. When the permanent molars and incisors erupt, a lower lingual holding arch can be considered as a replacement for the band and loop appliances.

A maxillary fixed bilateral appliance is feasible in the primary dentition because the appliance can be constructed to rest away from the incisors. Two types of lingual arch designs are used to maintain maxillary space—the Nance arch and TPA. These appliances use a large wire (0.036 inches) to connect the banded primary teeth on both sides of the arch distal to the extraction site. The difference between the two appliances is where the wire is placed in the palate. The Nance arch incorporates an acrylic button that rests directly on the palatal rugae. In some cases the acrylic button may irritate the palatal tissue. The TPA is made from a wire that traverses the palate directly without touching it (Fig. 26.6). Although the TPA is a cleaner appliance and is easier to construct, many clinicians think it allows the teeth to move and tip mesially, resulting in space loss.

Fixed bilateral appliances can also be options for children who have had incisors extracted (Fig. 26.7). Prosthetic primary teeth can be affixed to a lingual arch extending from banded molars to serve as replacements for the missing incisors. These appliances, often called Groper fixed anterior bridges or pediatric partials, generally address esthetics but can serve functional purposes if posterior teeth have been extracted. Because the permanent incisors erupt much sooner than canines and premolars, appliances serving dual functions as esthetic incisor replacements and posterior space maintainers will require alternate options in the mixed dentition.

Removable Appliances

Removable appliances make up the third category of appliances used to maintain space in the primary dentition (Fig. 26.8). Like

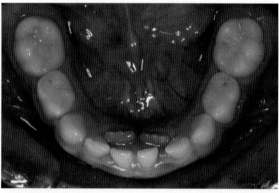

• **Figure 26.5** Lingual eruption of the permanent mandibular incisors is not uncommon. A mandibular lingual arch is not recommended as a space maintainer in the primary dentition because it may interfere with the eruption of these incisors. Bilateral band and loop appliances are recommended when both primary mandibular first molars are lost prematurely.

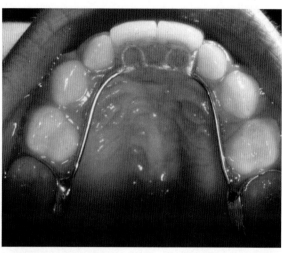

• **Figure 26.7** A fixed (as shown here) or removable partial denture can be used to replace missing anterior teeth in the primary dentition. In most cases the partial denture is placed for esthetic reasons rather than to prevent space loss in the anterior dental arch.

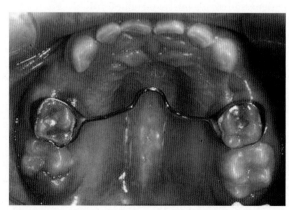

• **Figure 26.6** The transpalatal arch (TPA) is a fixed lingual arch appliance used to maintain space following bilateral loss of maxillary teeth. The TPA is more hygienic than the Nance appliance because it consists of only the 36-mil palatal wire, but it can allow the abutment teeth to tip mesially in some cases, resulting in space loss.

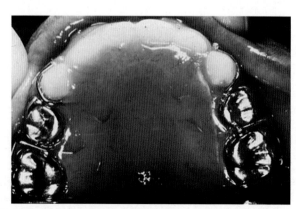

• **Figure 26.8** A removable partial denture is used to maintain space in the primary dentition when more than one tooth in a quadrant is lost. This appliance is an alternative to the lingual arch with teeth attached. In the patient portrayed here, only anterior teeth have been replaced.

fixed bilateral appliances, removable appliances are typically used when more than one tooth has been lost in a quadrant. The removable appliance is often the only alternative because there are no suitable abutment teeth and because the cantilever design of the distal shoe or the band and loop appliance is too weak to withstand occlusal forces over a two-tooth span. Removable appliances can also be an alternative to fixed bilateral appliances for the replacement of missing incisors. Not only can the partial denture replace more than one tooth, but it also replaces occlusal function.

Two drawbacks of the appliance are retention and compliance. Retention is a problem because primary canines do not have large undercuts for clasp engagement. If multiple tooth loss is unilateral, retention problems can be overcome by placing sturdy retention clasps on the opposite side of the arch. However, if multiple teeth are lost bilaterally, retention problems are almost inevitable.

The problem of compliance is closely related to that of retention. Children aged 3 to 6 years will not tolerate an ill-fitting appliance and may not use it. In fact, some children will not tolerate a retentive appliance. The dentist is then resigned to waiting until the permanent teeth (molars) erupt so that they can be used as abutments for a conventional lingual arch appliance. Partial dentures occasionally require clasp adjustment and acrylic modification to maintain good retention and allow eruption of the underlying or adjacent permanent teeth. Some children are compliant in wearing an appliance but not in cleaning the appliance and the underlying tissue. This can result in decay, tissue irritation, and hyperplasia.

Fabrication and Laboratory Considerations

The classic method of constructing a fixed appliance is a two- or three-visit process. If there is tight interproximal contact of the molars, the first visit is to place separators. If there is interdental spacing the first appointment involves fitting a band and obtaining an impression. The final appointment is to deliver the appliance.

The initial step in constructing a fixed appliance is to select and fit a band on the abutment tooth or teeth (Fig. 26.9). The next step is to obtain an impression of the banded tooth and edentulous area. Alginate impression material is most commonly used. A quarter-arch tray may be used for the unilateral appliances. The next step varies depending on the office or laboratory preference. The band(s) is removed from the tooth with a band remover and stabilized in the impression. The impression is poured in stone with the band(s) in place. An alternative approach is to pour the dental casts without the band(s) in place and send the appropriately sized band(s) to the laboratory to be seated by the technician during appliance fabrication. Other offices obtain only impressions and ask the laboratory to fit bands and fabricate the appliance on the dental cast. Intraoral scanning may also be used. A digital scan provides information to print a three-dimensional (3D) model on which the appliance is constructed. The dentist, an in-office technician, or a commercial dental laboratory will bend a 0.036-inch wire into the appropriate appliance.

The appliance is commonly delivered in a separate visit. First, it is tried in and adjusted to fit. The interior of the band is cleaned thoroughly, and the cement is loaded along the gingival margin. If the cement is loaded on the occlusal side, there is a risk there

WORKING WITH THE DENTAL LABORATORY

Steven H. Gross

Dental laboratory technology is a science and an art. Because each dental patient's needs are different, the duties of a dental laboratory technician are comprehensive, varied, and an important part of your dental team. There are steps a dental office can take to make sure their lab work is returned on time and the fit is ideal. The following are recommendations for the dental team.

Comprehensive Signed Prescription

Each prescription should include a due date and a patient appointment date. A detailed and unambiguous prescription will ensure that the laboratory provides the dentist and patient with a properly fabricated appliance. If there is a problem in meeting the due date, the lab can call and choose a delivery method to ensure on-time delivery.

Accurate Models

An accurate yellow stone cast that captures all the teeth and soft tissues of interest is the most importation step to ensure an excellent fitting appliance. It has been suggested that 30% of all models, impressions, and digital scans sent to laboratories are inadequate for appliance fabrication. Having each cast poured and inspected by the doctor for bubbles or distortion before the patient is released would be good practice to improve appliance quality. Air bubbles or holes on tooth surfaces are unacceptable. Good-quality impression materials such as alginate or polyvinyl siloxane (PVS) are best. Compound impressions are the number one cause of distorted models and

should be avoided. Simple precautions can save the office valuable chair time, expense, and the inconvenience of calling a patient back for new impressions.

Bands

Most labs prefer that preformed bands not be poured-up on the model. Simply tape bands to the prescription slip and label the bands—right or left and upper or lower. Then take impressions without the bands in place. Teeth to be banded should be fully exposed. If they are not, it is difficult for the lab to guarantee band and appliance fit.

Sending the Case

The office should provide the lab with an accurate wax construction bite. Each cast should be wrapped individually in foam. The casts should be carefully placed in a sturdy corrugated box—many labs will provide boxes with either a delivery company or a prepaid mailing label. It is best to pour models with as small a base as possible (or trim the casts) to save weight and extra cost.

Communication

Open communication with the laboratory is key to provide excellent care for the patient. The doctor and laboratory should be able to discuss cases openly and exchange ideas when there are questions on how to design an appliance. Open communication will lead to a long and mutually beneficial relationship.

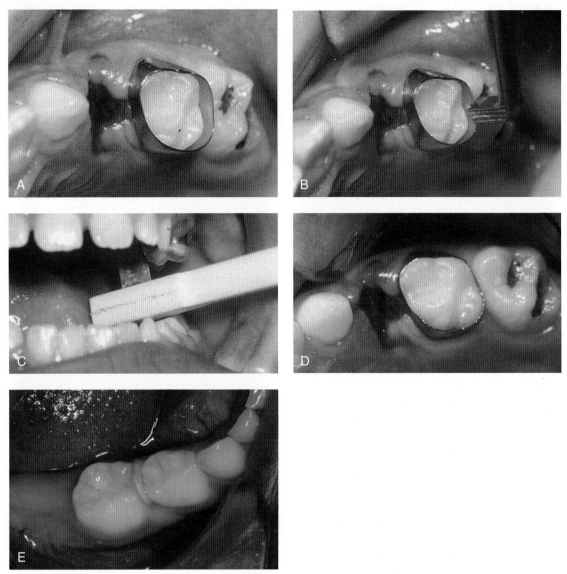

• **Figure 26.9** (A) The initial step in fabricating a band and loop device is to fit a band on the abutment tooth. Band selection is a trial-and-error procedure and continues until a band can be nearly seated on the tooth with finger pressure. (B) A band pusher is used to seat the band to a nearly ideal position. The dentist should maintain a good finger rest because soft and hard tissue injury can occur if the pusher slips without proper support. (C) Final occlusogingival position is achieved with a band biter. In the maxillary arch the band biter should be placed on the distolingual portion of the band for final positioning. In the mandibular arch the band biter should be placed on the distofacial portion of the band. (D) A properly fitted band is seated approximately 1 mm below the mesial and distal marginal ridges. (E) If a tight interproximal contact prevents the band from seating properly, orthodontic separators are placed to create space for the band material. The separators are removed within 7 to 10 days, and the band is fitted.

will be a void in the cement. Next, the band is placed on the clean, dry abutment tooth (teeth), and the excess cement is cleaned. There are several types of cement from which to choose, but glass ionomer cement is recommended. This type of cement releases fluoride over time to protect the tooth from demineralization. The appliance should be checked every 6 months to ensure it still fits properly, cement has not washed out, and the abutment teeth are nonmobile. Eruption of the permanent tooth is an easily recognized indication for removal.

The distal shoe has some variation in the process. The appliance can be constructed from an impression taken after removal of the primary second molar or from an impression taken before the

tooth is extracted. In the former situation the gingiva must be incised when the appliance is placed if the extraction site has healed. In the latter situation the construction cast must be modified to simulate loss of the primary second molar, but placement in the extraction site at the time of surgery is straightforward. The appliance is constructed very much like the band and loop. The primary first molar is banded and the loop extended to the former distal contact of the primary second molar. A piece of stainless steel is soldered to the distal end of the loop and placed in the extraction site. The stainless steel extension acts as a guide plane for the permanent first molar to erupt into proper position and should be positioned 1 mm below the mesial marginal ridge of

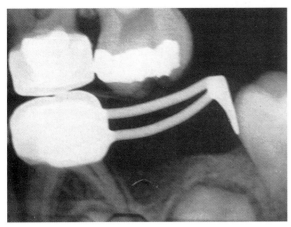

• **Figure 26.10** A periapical radiograph is recommended before cementing the distal shoe appliance to ensure that it is properly positioned in relation to the unerupted permanent first molar.

the unerupted first permanent molar in the alveolar bone. After the molar has erupted, the extension can be cut off or a new band and loop appliance can be constructed. To ensure that the stainless steel extension is in the proper position and in close proximity to the permanent first molar, a periapical radiograph is recommended before the appliance is cemented (Fig. 26.10).

An alternative to the two-step process is the prefabricated appliance, which comes in band and loop and distal shoe variations. These are fabricated intraorally and save chairside time and laboratory expense. There is extra chairside time and equipment needed to fit and place the appliances. These are a practical alternative to the traditional unilateral space maintainers but may lack durability.[10]

Summary

Space maintenance in the primary dentition should be considered in terms of anterior and posterior space loss. Space maintenance

is generally not required for missing primary incisors but can be placed if esthetic concerns are a factor. Posterior space maintenance is a necessity in this age group and should be undertaken when primary molars are lost prematurely and the space is adequate. The band and loop appliance is used most often; other appliances can be used as different situations dictate. Judicious space maintenance benefits the child patient and may prevent future alignment and crowding problems.

References

1. Proffit WR, Fields HW, Sarver DM. Treatment of nonskeletal problems in preadolescent children. In: *Contemporary Orthodontics*. 5th ed. St Louis: Elsevier; 2012.
2. Ngan PH, Fields HW. Orthodontic diagnosis and treatment planning in the primary dentition. *ASDC J Dent Child*. 1995;62(1):25–33.
3. National Institutes of Health, National Institute of Dental and Craniofacial Research. Dental caries (tooth decay) in children (age 2 to 11). https://www.nidcr.nih.gov/DataStatistics/FindDataByTopic/DentalCaries/DentalCariesChildren2to11.htm. Accessed August 16, 2017.
4. Centers for Disease Control and Prevention, National Center for Health Statistics. Oral and dental health. https://www.cdc.gov/nchs/fastats/dental.htm. Accessed August 16, 2017.
5. Holan G, Needleman HL. Premature loss of primary anterior teeth due to trauma—potential short- and long-term sequelae. *Dent Traumatol*. 2014;30(2):100–106.
6. Law CS. Management of premature primary tooth loss in the child patient. *J Calif Dent Assoc*. 2013;41(8):612–618.
7. Tunison W, Flores-Mir C, ElBadrawy H, et al. Dental arch space changes following premature loss of primary first molars: a systematic review. *Pediatr Dent*. 2008;30(4):297–302.
8. Reggiardo P. *Coding and Insurance Manual: A Comprehensive Resource for Reporting Pediatric Dental Services*. Chicago: American Academy of Pediatric Dentistry; 2016.
9. Mayhew MJ, Dilley GJ, Dilley DCH, et al. Tissue response to intragingival appliances in monkeys. *Pediatr Dent*. 1984;6(3):148–152.
10. Brill WA. The distal shoe space maintainer chairside fabrication and clinical performance. *Pediatr Dent*. 2002;24(6):561–565.

27

Oral Habits

CLARICE S. LAW, JOHN R. CHRISTENSEN, AND HENRY FIELDS

CHAPTER OUTLINE

The presence of an oral habit in a 3- to 6-year-old child is an important finding during the clinical examination. The most common oral habits—digit and pacifier sucking—generally cease spontaneously between 3 and 4 years of age at the beginning of the age range.[1] By 6 years of age, most children begin the transition into the permanent dentition, making habit cessation more important. Thus the 3- to 6-year age range is a very important period for facilitating the transition out of an oral habit. In this chapter, we will consider the various oral habits that may be associated with either malocclusion or oral health.

Thumb and Finger Habits

Thumb and finger habits make up the majority of oral habits. Approximately two-thirds of such habits end by 5 years of age, decreasing from a prevalence of approximately 30% at 12 months of age to approximately 10% at 5 years.[2] Dentists are often questioned about the kinds of problems these habits may cause if they are prolonged. The malocclusions caused by nonnutritive sucking may be more of an individual response than a highly specific cause-and-effect relationship. The types of dental changes that a digit habit may cause vary with the amount of force applied to the teeth (force magnitude), the manner in which the digit is positioned in the mouth (force direction), how much time the child engages in the habit (frequency in hours per day), and how long the habit persists (duration in months or years).

Research and clinical experience have shown that as little as 35 g of force can tip a tooth.[3] It is apparent that children vary in the amount of force applied during sucking. Some suck with a great deal of intensity, and others essentially rest the digit in their mouth. The frequency of digit sucking throughout a routine day will also have an impact on tooth movement. Clinical experience suggests that 4 to 6 hours of force per day is probably the minimum necessary to cause tooth movement.[3] Therefore a child who sucks intermittently with high force may not produce much tooth movement at all, whereas a child who sucks with less force but continuously (for more than 6 hours) can cause significant dental change, which is consistent with the equilibrium theory. However, it is the duration of time sucking (in months and years) that probably plays the most critical role in tooth movement caused by a digit habit.[1,2,4,5] The most frequently reported dental outcomes of an active digit habit are the following[3]:

1. Posterior crossbite
2. Anterior open bite
3. Increased overjet

Some studies have also reported differences in canine and molar relationship, but these are not present with the same frequency.

The maxillary arch constriction associated with a posterior crossbite is probably due to the change in equilibrium balance between the oral musculature and the tongue.[1,2,4,5] When the thumb is placed in the mouth, the tongue is forced down and away from the palate. The orbicularis oris and buccinator muscles continue to exert a force on the buccal surfaces of the maxillary dentition, especially when these muscles are contracted during sucking. Because the tongue no longer exerts a counterbalancing force from the lingual surface, the posterior maxillary arch collapses into crossbite (Fig. 27.1).

Anterior open bite, or the lack of vertical overlap of the upper and lower incisors when the posterior teeth are in occlusion, develops because the digit rests between the maxillary and mandibular incisors (Fig. 27.2). This prevents complete or continued eruption of the incisors, whereas the posterior teeth are free to erupt. Anterior open bite may also be caused by intrusion of the incisors. However, inhibition of eruption is easier to accomplish than true intrusion, which would be the result of a habit of greater duration.

Faciolingual movement of the incisors depends on how the thumb or finger is placed and how many fingers are placed in the mouth. Some consider this positional variable to be a confounding factor related to force and duration of the habit. Usually, the thumb is placed so that it exerts pressure on the lingual surfaces of the maxillary incisors and on the labial surfaces of the mandibular incisors (Fig. 27.3). A child who actively sucks can create enough force to tip the upper incisors facially and the lower incisors lingually. The result is an increased overjet and, by virtue of the tipping, decreased overbite.

Data on the amount of skeletal change are not clear. Some believe the maxilla and its alveolar process are moved anteriorly

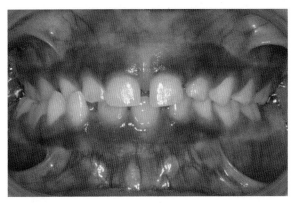

• **Figure 27.1** This patient exhibits a right maxillary posterior crossbite. A posterior crossbite is often the side effect of a thumb or pacifier habit because the tongue is displaced inferiorly and the orbicularis oris and buccinator muscles exert a force on the upper teeth. When there is no counterbalancing force from the tongue, the upper arch falls into crossbite.

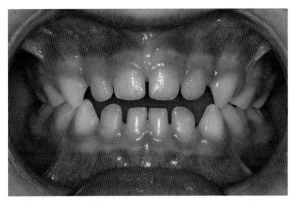

• **Figure 27.2** This patient's anterior open bite is a direct result of an active thumb sucking habit. An open bite results when the thumb impedes eruption of the anterior teeth, moves them facially, and allows the posterior teeth to erupt passively. Actual intrusion of the anterior teeth is possible but unlikely.

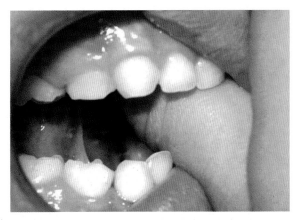

• **Figure 27.3** With most thumb-sucking habits, the thumb exerts pressure on the lingual surface of the maxillary incisors and on the facial surface of the mandibular incisors. This causes the maxillary incisors to tip facially and the mandibular incisors to tip lingually, resulting in increased overjet.

and superiorly.[6] Certainly, if the teeth are moved, some alveolar change occurs. Whether this is translated to the skeletal maxilla is not as well known. In one study a significantly higher percentage of distal step molar relationships in 5 year olds was noted among digit suckers compared with children with no sucking habit.[7]

Treatment

Timing of treatment must be gauged carefully. If parents or the child does not want to engage in treatment, it should not be attempted. The child should be given an opportunity to stop the habit spontaneously before the permanent teeth erupt. If treatment is selected as an alternative, it is generally undertaken between the ages of 4 and 6 years. Delay until the early school-age years allows for spontaneous discontinuation of the habit by many children, often through peer pressure at school. As long as the habit is eliminated before full eruption of the permanent incisors, the eruption process will spontaneously reduce the overjet and open bite as the permanent teeth occupy new positions. It is generally agreed that interception of a digit-sucking habit does no harm to the child's emotional development, nor does it result in habit substitution. However, the dentist should evaluate the child for psychological overtones before embarking on habit elimination. Such procedures might best be postponed for children who have recently undergone stressful changes in their lives, such as a new sibling, separation or divorce of parents, moving to a new community, or changing schools. Four different approaches to treatment have been advocated, depending on the willingness of the child to stop the habit. It is important to select the approach that is age appropriate and acceptable to parents to increase the odds of successful treatment.

Counseling

The simplest yet least widely applicable approach is counseling with the patient. This involves discussion between the dentist and the patient of the problems created by nonnutritive sucking. These adult-like discussions focus on the changes that have occurred because of the sucking and their impact on esthetics. Usually an appeal is made to the children on the basis of their maturity and responsibility. Clearly, this approach is best aimed at older children who can conceptually grasp the issue and who may be feeling social pressure to stop the habit. Some children are captured by this approach and successfully eliminate their habit.

Reminder Therapy

The second approach, reminder therapy, is appropriate for those who desire to stop the habit but need some help. The purpose of any treatment should be thoroughly explained to the child. An adhesive bandage secured with waterproof tape on the offending finger can serve as a constant reminder not to place the finger in the mouth (Fig. 27.4). The bandage remains in place until the habit is extinguished. There are some parents who are reluctant to use the bandage as a reminder. They are concerned that it may come off during sleep and the child may swallow or aspirate the bandage. Therefore some clinicians use a mitten or a tube sock to cover the fingers of the hand. This is especially useful during sleeping hours. Other commercial products such as shirts that cover the hand or plastic sleeves that cover the thumb are available. Another approach is to paint a commercially available bitter substance on the fingers that are sucked. However, sometimes this type of therapy is perceived as punishment and may not be as effective as a neutral

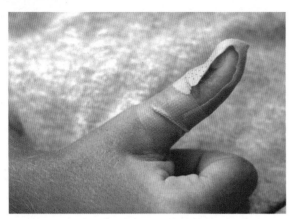

• **Figure 27.4** One or two adhesive bandages can be taped to a child's finger to serve as a reminder not to place the finger in the mouth. The bandage is worn until the child stops sucking the finger.

reminder. In conclusion, reminder therapy works by changing the sucking sensation enjoyed by the child.

Reward System

A third treatment for oral habits is a reward system. A contract is drawn up between the child and the parent or between the child and the dentist. The contract simply states that the child will discontinue the habit within a specified period of time and in return will receive a reward. The reward does not need to be extravagant but must be special enough to motivate the child. Praise from the parents and dentist has a large role. The more involvement the child takes in the project, the more likely it is that the project will succeed. Involvement may include placing stickers on a homemade calendar when the child has successfully avoided the habit for a specified period of time, for example, an afternoon or an entire day. At the end of the specified time period, the reward is presented with verbal praise for meeting the conditions of the contract (Fig. 27.5). The reward system is less successful if the child uses the habit to fall asleep. Reward systems and reminder therapy are often combined to improve the likelihood of success.

Adjunctive Therapy

If the habit persists after reminder and reward therapy and the child truly wants to eliminate the habit, adjunctive therapy that includes a method to physically interrupt the habit and remind the patient can be used. This type of treatment usually involves restraining the patient's arm in an elastic bandage or some equivalent so it cannot be flexed and the hand brought to the mouth.[8] Another treatment is to place an appliance in the mouth that physically discourages the habit by making it difficult to suck a thumb or finger. The dentist should explain to the patient and parent that the appliance is not a punishment but rather a permanent reminder not to place the finger in the mouth.

The elastic bandage method is usually applied only at night. The bandage is snugly, but not tightly, wrapped over the arm extending from below the elbow to above it. The elasticity of the material (not the tightness) straightens the child's arm as he falls asleep and removes the thumb from the mouth, preventing him from engaging in the habit while sleeping. Success over several weeks should be rewarded. The total program may take 6 to 8 weeks (anecdotally noted by success in children who have stopped habits while arms were casted for broken bones).

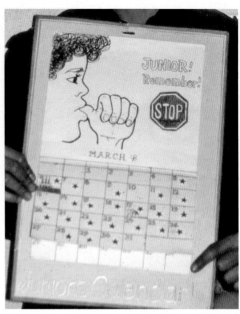

• **Figure 27.5** A personalized calendar can be used to motivate a child to stop a thumb sucking habit. Stick-on stars are applied to the calendar on days when the child has successfully avoided the habit. At the end of a month or a specified period of time, a reward and verbal praise can be provided for discontinuing the habit.

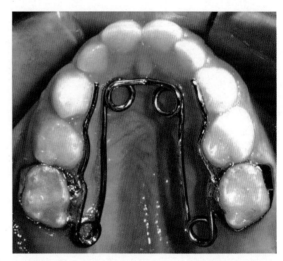

• **Figure 27.6** The quad helix is a fixed appliance used to expand a constricted maxillary arch. The anterior helices also discourage a sucking habit by reminding the child not to place a finger in the mouth. This appliance is often used in children in whom there is an active sucking habit and a posterior crossbite.

An intraoral appliance approach can also be used in the adjunct method. The two appliances used most often to discourage the sucking habit are the quad helix and the palatal crib. The quad helix is a fixed appliance commonly used to expand a constricted maxillary arch—a common finding accompanied by posterior crossbite in patients who practice nonnutritive sucking (Fig. 27.6). The helices of the appliance serve to remind the child not to place the finger in the mouth if they are placed in the area where the child places the thumb when sucking. The quad helix is a versatile appliance because it can correct a posterior crossbite and discourage a finger habit at the same time.

The palatal crib is designed to interrupt a digit habit by interfering with finger placement and sucking satisfaction. The palatal crib is generally used in children in whom no posterior crossbite exists. However, it may also be used as a retainer after maxillary expansion with a quad helix in a child who has not stopped sucking with the quad helix. For a palatal crib, bands are fitted on the permanent first molars or primary second molars. A heavy lingual arch wire (0.038 inches minimum) is bent to fit passively in the palate and is soldered to the molar bands. Additional wire is soldered onto this base wire to form a crib or mechanical obstruction for the digit. It is advisable to make a lower cast at the time the appliance is constructed so that the occlusion can be checked for interferences (Fig. 27.7). The parent and child should be informed that certain side effects appear temporarily after the palatal crib is cemented. Eating, speaking, and sleeping patterns may be altered during the first few days after appliance delivery. These difficulties usually subside within 3 days to 2 weeks. If the child is informed that the appliance is strictly a helpful reminder and not punishment, psychological implications of ending the habit are not an issue.[9] An imprint of the appliance usually appears on the tongue as an indentation. This imprint may persist for up to 1 year after the appliance is removed. The major problem with the palatal crib and, to a lesser degree, the quad helix is the difficulty of maintaining good oral hygiene. The appliance traps food and is difficult to clean thoroughly. Oral malodor and tissue inflammation can result.

Other appliances have been suggested to accomplish results similar to the quad helix and the palatal crib. The Bluegrass appliance places a Teflon roller in the most superior area of the palate and in the same general area as a Nance arch. The appliance is easier to clean, is less disruptive to eating and speech, and is reported to be as effective as a crib in discontinuing a habit.[10] The patient is encouraged to use the tongue to turn the roller, with the idea that the act of turning will act as a competing habit and decrease the need to suck a thumb or finger for oral gratification. The other advantage of the Bluegrass appliance is that it can be combined with a W arch to correct a transverse constriction if it is present (Fig. 27.8).

Adjunctive habit discouragement appliances should be left in the mouth for 6 to 12 months. The clinician should have the patient return at 1- or 2-month intervals to monitor how the child is doing with the habit and to encourage the patient if indicated. The palatal crib usually stops the child from sucking immediately but requires at least another 6 months of wear to extinguish the habit completely.[11] The quad helix also requires a minimum of 6 months of treatment. Three months is needed to correct the crossbite, and 3 months is required to stabilize the movement. A retrospective study of the Bluegrass appliance determined three of four patients stopped their habit at 36 weeks.[11]

Pacifier Habits

Dental changes created by pacifier habits are largely similar to changes created by thumb habits (Fig. 27.9). Anterior open bite and maxillary constriction (with posterior crossbite) occur consistently in children who suck pacifiers. Labial movement of the maxillary incisors may not be as pronounced as that accompanying a digit habit. Manufacturers have developed pacifiers that they claim are more like a mother's nipple and not as deleterious to the dentition as a thumb or conventional pacifier. Research results have not substantiated this statement.[8,12,13] Increased duration of pacifier habits is related to an increased prevalence of anterior open bite and reduced overbite and posterior crossbite.[6] It appears the

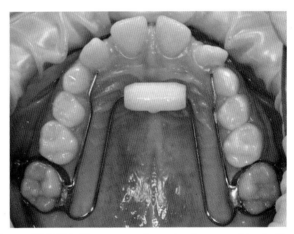

• **Figure 27.8** This Bluegrass appliance has been combined with a W arch to create an appliance that will help to stop a digit habit and at the same time correct the posterior constriction that has resulted from the habit. The Teflon roller is placed in the anterior portion of the palate to disrupt the habit and allow the tongue to turn the roller.

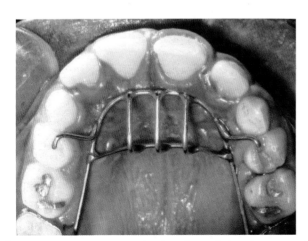

• **Figure 27.7** A palatal crib is a fixed appliance designed to stop a digit habit by mechanically interfering with digit placement and sucking satisfaction. The parent of the child should expect temporary disturbances in eating, speaking, and sleeping patterns during the first few days after use of the appliance.

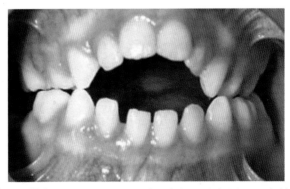

• **Figure 27.9** A pacifier can create dental changes that are nearly identical to those of a digit habit. The labiolingual movement of the incisors is usually not as pronounced as that associated with a digit habit.

longer the habit persists, the greater the odds for open bite and posterior crossbite become. There are minimal changes after 18 months of use, but changes become more pronounced after 36 months of use. Pediatricians and pediatric dentists should counsel parents about discontinuing the pacifier habit between 18 and 36 months.[14]

Pacifier habits appear to end earlier than digit habits. More than 90% were reported to end before 5 years of age and 100% by age 8.[9] Pacifier habits theoretically are easier to stop than digit habits because the pacifier can be discontinued gradually or completely withdrawn with discussion and explanation to the child. This type of control is obviously not possible with digit habits, which makes a notable difference in the degree of patient compliance required to eliminate the two types of habits. In a few cases the child may stop the pacifier habit and then start sucking a digit. Elimination of the subsequent finger habit may be necessary.

Several reports have demonstrated a relationship between early use of pacifiers and a reduced risk of sudden infant death syndrome (SIDS) in infants. A meta-analysis study supported the use of pacifiers during sleep.[15] The clinician should be prepared to discuss the role of the pacifier with parents in reducing SIDS. Early pacifier use may be beneficial, but the infant should be weaned from the pacifier around 18 to 36 months to prevent dental changes.

Lip Habits

Habits that involve manipulation of the lips and perioral structures are called lip habits. Those that might come to the attention of the dental professional are lip licking, lip biting, and lip sucking. The influence of each on the oral structures is varied, with effects on either soft tissues or malocclusion.

Lip licking is a relatively benign habit as far as dental effects are concerned. Red, inflamed, and chapped lips and perioral tissues are the most apparent signs associated with lip licking (Fig. 27.10). The condition increases in frequency during the dry winter season and is known as lip licking dermatitis. Little can be done to stop this habit effectively. Treatment is usually palliative and limited to moisturizing the lips, although some clinicians have used appliances to interrupt the habits.

Lip biting is included in the group of habits known as body-focused repetitive behaviors.[4] These habits have unknown causes, with possible genetic or neurobiologic origins, and are estimated to occur in 3% of adults in the United States. The most common outcome of lip biting, and the related behavior of cheek biting, is hyperkeratosis or ulcerations and sores, which can become infected. Treatment in the dental setting is palliative; with referral for cognitive behavioral therapy as an appropriate intervention for more severe cases.

Milder forms of lip biting and the related habit of lip sucking generally do not cause dental problems but certainly can maintain an existing malocclusion if the child engages in them with adequate intensity, frequency, and duration. Whether these habits can create a malocclusion is a question that is not easily answered. The most common presentation of lip sucking is the lower lip tucked behind the maxillary incisors (Fig. 27.11). This places a lingually directed force on the mandibular teeth and a facial force on the maxillary teeth. The result is a proclination of the maxillary incisors, a retroclination of the mandibular incisors, and increased overjet. This problem is most common in the mixed and permanent dentitions. Treatment depends on the skeletal relationship of the child and on the presence or absence of space in the arch. If the child has a class I skeletal relationship and an increased overjet that is solely the result of tipped teeth, the clinician can tip the teeth to their original or a more normal position with either a fixed or a removable appliance. If a class II skeletal relationship exists, a more involved growth modification procedure is needed to manage the malocclusion.

Tongue Thrust

Tongue thrust has been difficult to define as a habit. Review of the literature reveals different meanings, with some using the term "tongue thrust" to describe a passive anterior posture of the tongue and others describing an active thrust of the tongue forward on swallowing. The latter is often specifically described as an atypical swallow,[3] which can be further categorized as primary, with psychological origins for persistence, or secondary, with associated physical features.[16]

The atypical swallow pattern is considered to be normal during the early period of development. The tongue thrust characteristic of the infantile swallow decreases between 12 and 15 months as the primary molars erupt.[17] Between ages 3 and 5, prevalence can decrease from 55% to 35%, with prevalence between 5% and 15% reported for older children and adults.[18] When the atypical

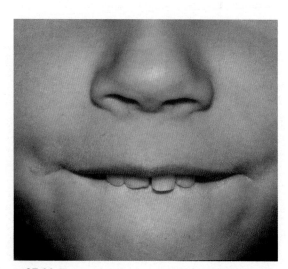

• **Figure 27.11** The most common habit involving the lips is tucking the lower lip behind the maxillary incisors. The lower lip forces the maxillary teeth facially and the mandibular teeth lingually, resulting in an increased overjet. In addition, the lower lip and other perioral tissues can become chapped and inflamed as a result of constant wetting.

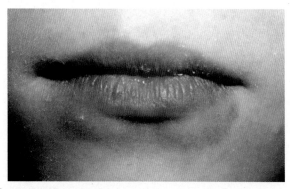

• **Figure 27.10** Red, inflamed, chapped lips and perioral tissues are often indicative of a lip sucking or licking habit. These problems are more common and severe during the winter months.

swallow is observed in older children and adults, it is often associated with prolonged breastfeeding, short frenulum, hypertrophic adenoids and tonsils, oral breathing, allergic rhinitis, and abnormal head lower jaw, and tongue posture.[18] Nonnutritive sucking habits beyond the age of 5 have also been associated with atypical swallowing patterns for 6- to 9-year-old children.[3,19]

In terms of malocclusion, tongue thrust has been correlated with posterior crossbite, open bite, and excess overjet.[18] There is no evidence suggesting that the atypical swallow causes malocclusion, with the frequency, duration, and force magnitude of the thrust insufficient to result in tooth movement.[20] Furthermore, epidemiologic data indicate that the percentage of persons with infantile and transitional swallowing patterns is greater than the percentage of persons with open bite,[18,19,21] indicating no simple cause-and-effect relationship between tongue thrusting and open bite. Thus atypical swallow is often thought of as an "opportunistic behavior" that adapts to the malocclusion rather than being the causative factor.[18,22] The passive anterior resting posture of the tongue is thought to have a greater influence on malocclusion than the atypical swallow, with the anterior open bite most commonly observed.[23]

Treatment of tongue thrust varies depending on the origin of the associated problems. If there is a concurrent nonnutritive sucking habit or history of mouth breathing, these issues should be managed first. Limited or interceptive orthodontics should be considered if the patient exhibits malocclusion. Myofunctional therapy is often suggested, but the body of evidence has not yet clearly demonstrated the effectiveness of the exercises.[22]

Mouth Breathing

Mouth breathing is difficult to label as a habit. Some persons may appear to be mouth breathers because of their mandibular posture or incompetent lips. It is normal for a 3- to 6-year-old to be slightly lip incompetent (Fig. 27.12). Mouth breathing may also be a transitional developmental finding. In children younger than age 8, the percentage of mouth breathers is approximately equivalent to the percentage of nasal breathers. After age 8, 35% of those without obvious allergic rhinitis or nasal congestion can continue to be mouth breathers.[24] Other studies suggest that the prevalence of habitual mouth breathing without clear signs of airway obstruction is between 9% and 10%.[24,25] However, many children are mouth breathers because of a suspected nasal airway obstruction, with one study indicating a 72% prevalence of mouth breathing due to tonsil or adenoid obstruction and 19% due to allergic rhinitis.[25]

In terms of the impact of mouth breathing on oral health, an association with gingival inflammation has been well established.[22] However, the association between mouth breathing and malocclusion is more complex. There is certainly a stereotype of "adenoid facies" associated with individuals with nasal obstruction, consisting of anterior open bite, constricted maxilla, and a class II malocclusion. And although there is a higher prevalence of these occlusal findings in children with nasal obstruction, the majority of children with airway issues do not fit the stereotype, suggesting that mouth breathing may have an environmental influence on those genetically susceptible to the hyperdivergent/dolichofacial, constricted, retrognathic growth pattern.[25]

For the dental professional, the most important thing to consider when encountering a child with a tendency toward mouth breathing is whether the child may be at risk for obstructive sleep apnea (OSA) or sleep disordered breathing. Upper airway obstruction that negatively impacts sleep can also affect growth, academic performance, and behavior.[26,27] There are also long-term health consequences to OSA, so appropriate referral and medical management are imperative.

Treatment is also complicated and not well reported in the literature. Some studies have shown that children treated with adenoidectomy for obstructed airway have shown improvements both in vertical patterns of growth[28] and in transverse dimensions.[29] However, this does not imply that turbinectomy or adenoidectomy is required to clear the nasal airway solely to change the facial growth pattern.[30,31] Recent advances in cone beam computed tomography (CBCT) may provide more answers to the relationship among craniofacial morphology, airway size, and function.[32]

Nail Biting

Nail biting (onychophagia), like lip biting, is often included among the body-focused repetitive behaviors, with a prevalence estimated between 20% and 30% of the general population.[19] It has been suggested that the habit is a manifestation of increased stress. Management may include habit counseling or even referral for behavior therapy. It is a rare habit in persons younger than 4 years. The incidence increases in the 4- to 6-year age group and continues to increase until adolescence.[33] The proportion of males to females is relatively equal up to age 10 years, but then male nail biters are predominant.[16,34,35] There have been suggestions that nail biting may be related to incisor malocclusion, but bacterial infections, gingivitis, and minor enamel fractures are more commonly associated.[34,35] There is no recommended protocol for the dental professional to address nail biting because dental complications are so mild.

Bruxism

Bruxism involves clenching or grinding of the teeth in repetitive jaw movements. Although it can occur throughout the day, it is usually

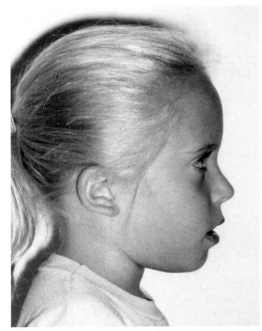

• **Figure 27.12** The normal relaxed lip posture in the 3- to 6-year-old child is for the lips to be slightly apart or incompetent. These children are often labeled mouth breathers because of this posture, but they may, in fact, be completely nasal breathers.

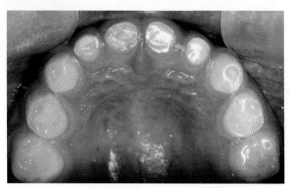

• **Figure 27.13** This patient's primary maxillary incisors and canines were worn more rapidly than normal owing to a habit of bruxism.

reported to occur during sleep in children. Most children engage in some bruxism that can result in moderate wear of the primary canines and molars. Rarely, with the exception of developmentally disabled persons, does the wear endanger the pulp by proceeding faster than secondary dentin is produced (Fig. 27.13). Masticatory muscle soreness and temporomandibular joint pain have also been attributed to bruxism. The exact cause of significant bruxism is unknown. Influences are multifactorial, with central nervous system activity, genetics, and psychosocial factors under investigation.[35] Traditional explanations center on local, systemic, and psychological factors.[34-36] The local theory suggests that bruxism is a reaction to an occlusal interference, high restoration, or some irritating dental condition. Systemic factors implicated in bruxism include intestinal parasites, subclinical nutritional deficiencies, allergies, and endocrine disorders. The psychological theory submits that bruxism is the manifestation of a personality disorder or increased stress. However, these attributions have been demonstrated only in children older than 6 years. There is no evidence that sleep bruxism and psychosocial factors are related in children younger than 5.[37] Children with musculoskeletal disorders (cerebral palsy) and severely developmentally disabled children commonly grind their teeth. These patients' bruxism is the result of their underlying physical and mental condition and is difficult to manage dentally.

Treatment for those with marked abrasion or persistent parents could be attempted with a "boil and bite" mouth guard that is inexpensive to purchase and remoldable as the dentition rapidly changes during the mixed dentition years. If this intervention is not successful, referral to appropriate medical personnel should be considered to rule out any systemic problems. If the habit is thought to be due to psychological factors, referral to a child development expert is warranted. Rarely, occlusal wear is so extensive that stainless steel crowns or other restorative options are needed to prevent pulpal exposure or eliminate tooth sensitivity.

Summary

The period of time between 3 and 6 years of age is an interesting transitional period for addressing potential oral habits. Digit and pacifier habits should be decreasing significantly by the end of this period. Preferably, a habit that has resulted in movement of the primary incisors or has inhibited their eruption or has resulted in posterior crossbite or maxillary constriction will have been eliminated before the permanent incisors erupt. If a habit that causes dental changes is not eliminated or spontaneously discontinued before the permanent incisors erupt, they too will be affected. On the other hand, these are not irreversible changes. If the habit is stopped

during the mixed-dentition years, the adverse dental changes will begin to reverse naturally. Appliance therapy may be required, but generally the teeth will move toward a more neutral position with the absence of the forces of the habit. If no dental changes have occurred, no treatment can be advocated on the grounds of dental health, but some patients and parents may want treatment because digit or pacifier habits become less socially acceptable as the child becomes older. The most important point to remember about any intervention is that the child must want to discontinue the habit for treatment to be successful.

Lip habits are not likely to be as prevalent during the primary dentition stage but may be observed as children transition into the mixed dentition stage. These habits generally do not have harmful oral effects nor influence malocclusion but in rare cases may be signs of psychological issues requiring interprofessional consultation.

Tongue thrust and mouth breathing may be commonly observed during the primary dentition period as normal developmental findings, but as children transition into the mixed dentition, these habits may be signs of other issues. Tongue thrust might indicate a myofunctional issue or malocclusion that should be addressed. Mouth breathing may be a sign of airway obstruction that could have negative health and growth effects and should also be addressed through interprofessional consultation.

Nail biting and bruxism have variable prevalence rates in the primary dentition. Neither habit is expected to have an impact on occlusion or tooth position, but both may affect the integrity of the teeth. Nail biting should be addressed with habit cessation counseling, and bruxism is generally expected to decrease in most cases.

References

1. Silva M, Manton D. Oral habits—part 1: the dental effects and management of nutritive and non-nutritive sucking. *J Dent Child*. 2014;81(3):133–139.
2. Bishara SE, Warren JJ, Broffitt B, et al. Changes in the prevalence of nonnutritive sucking patterns in the first 8 years of life. *Am J Orthod Dentofacial Orthop*. 2006;130(1):31–36.
3. Proffit WR, Fields HW, Sarver DM. *Contemporary Orthodontics*. 5th ed. St Louis: Elsevier; 2012.
4. Dogramaci EJ, Rossi-Fedele G. Establishing the association between nonnutritive sucking behavior and malocclusions: a systematic review and meta-analysis. *J Am Dent Assoc*. 2016;147(12):926–934.e6.
5. Duncan K, McNamara C, Ireland AJ, et al. Sucking habits in childhood and the effects on the primary dentition: findings of the Avon Longitudinal Study of Pregnancy and Childhood. *Int J Paediatr Dent*. 2008;18(3):178–188.
6. Larsson E. Dummy- and finger-sucking habits with special attention to their significance for facial growth and occlusion: 4. Effect on facial growth and occlusion. *Swed Dent J*. 1972;65:605–634.
7. Fukata O, Braham RL, Yokoi K, et al. Damage to the primary dentition resulting from thumb and finger (digit) sucking. *ASDC J Dent Child*. 1996;63:403–408.
8. Adair SM. The Ace Bandage approach to digit-sucking habits. *Pediatr Dent*. 1999;21:451–452.
9. Haryett RD, Hansen FC, Davidson PO. Chronic thumb-sucking: a second report on treatment and its psychological effects. *Am J Orthod Dentofacial Orthop*. 1970;57:164–178.
10. Haskell BS, Mink JR. An aid to stop thumb sucking: the "Bluegrass" appliance. *Pediatr Dent*. 1991;13(2):83–85.
11. Greenleaf S, Mink JR. A retrospective study of the use of the Bluegrass appliance in the cessation of thumb habits. *Pediatr Dent*. 2003;25(6):587–590.

12. Adair SM, Milano M, Dushku JC. Evaluation of the effects of orthodontic pacifiers on the primary dentitions of 24- to 59-month-old children: preliminary study. *Pediatr Dent*. 1992;14:13–18.

13. Bishara SE, Nowak AJ, Kohout FJ, et al. Influence of feeding and non-nutritive sucking methods on the development of the dental arches: longitudinal study of the first 18 months of life. *Pediatr Dent*. 1987;9:13–21.

14. Melink S, Vagner MV, Hocevar-Boltezar I, et al. Posterior crossbite in the deciduous dentition period, its relation with sucking habits, irregular orofacial functions, and otolaryngological findings. *Am J Orthod Dentofacial Orthop*. 2010;138(1):32–40.

15. Hauck FR, Omojokun OO, Siadaty MS. Do pacifiers reduce the risk of sudden infant death syndrome? A meta-analysis. *Pediatrics*. 2005;116(5):e716–e723.

16. The TLC Foundation for Body-Focused Repetitive Behaviors. Learn about BFRBs. http://www.bfrb.org/index.php. Accessed August 16, 2017.

17. Silva M, Manton D. Oral habits—part 2: beyond nutritive and non-nutritive sucking. *J Dent Child*. 2014;81(3):140–146.

18. Maspero C, Prevedello C, Giannini L, et al. Atypical swallowing: a review. *Minerva Stomatol*. 2014;63(6):217–227.

19. Stahl F, Grabowski R, Gaebel M, et al. Relationship between occlusal findings and orofacial myofunctional status in primary and mixed dentition. Part II: prevalence of orofacial dysfunctions. *J Orofac Orthop*. 2007;68(2):74–90.

20. Ovsenik M, Farčnik FM, Korpar M, et al. Follow-up study of functional and morphological malocclusion trait changes from 3 to 12 years of age. *Eur J Orthod*. 2007;29(5):523–529.

21. Ovsenik M. Incorrect orofacial functions until 5 years of age and their association with posterior crossbite. *Am J Orthod Dentofacial Orthop*. 2009;136(3):375–381.

22. Mason RM. Myths that persist about orofacial myology. *Int J Orofacial Myology*. 2011;37:26–38.

23. Kelly JE, Sanchez M, Van Kirk LE. An assessment of the occlusion of the teeth of children 6-11 years, United States. *Vital Health Stat 11*. 1973;130:1–60.

24. Warren DW, Hairfield WM, Dalston ET. Effect of age on nasal cross-sectional area and respiratory mode in children. *Laryngoscope*. 1990;100(1):89–93.

25. Souki BQ, Pimenta GB, Souki MQ, et al. Prevalence of malocclusion among mouth breathing children: do expectations meet reality? *Int J Pediatr Otorhinolaryngol*. 2009;73(5):767–773.

26. Ivanhoe JR, Lefebvre CA, Stockstill JW. Sleep disordered breathing in infants and children: a review of the literature. *Pediatr Dent*. 2007;29(3):193–200.

27. Owens JA. Neurocognitive and behavioral impact of sleep disordered breathing in children. *Pediatr Pulmonol*. 2009;44(5):417–422.

28. Peltomäki T. The effect of mode of breathing on craniofacial growth—revisited. *Eur J Orthod*. 2007;29(5):426–429.

29. Caixeta AC, Andrade I, Pereira TB, et al. Dental arch dimensional changes after adenotonsillectomy in prepubertal children. *Am J Orthod Dentofacial Orthop*. 2014;145(4):461–468.

30. Bresolin D, Shapiro CC, Shapiro PA, et al. Facial characteristics of children who breathe through the mouth. *Pediatrics*. 1984;73:622–625.

31. Wenzel A, Hojensgaard E, Henriksen JM. Craniofacial morphology and head posture in children with asthma and perennial rhinitis. *Eur J Orthod*. 1985;7:83–92.

32. Lenza MG, Lenza MM, Dalstra M, et al. An analysis of different approaches to the assessment of upper airway morphology: a CBCT study. *Orthod Craniofac Res*. 2010;13(2):96–105.

33. Wagaiyu EG, Ashley FP. Mouthbreathing, lip seal and upper lip coverage and their relationship with gingival inflammation in 11–14 year-old schoolchildren. *J Clin Periodontol*. 1991;18(9):698–702.

34. Halteh P, Scher RK, Lipner SR. Onychophagia: a nail-biting conundrum for physicians. *J Dermatolog Treat*. 2017;28:166–172.

35. Tanaka OM, Vitral RW, Tanaka GY, et al. Nailbiting, or onychophagia: a special habit. *Am J Orthod Dentofacial Orthop*. 2008;134(2):305–308.

36. Kuch EV, Till MJ, Messer LB. Bruxing and non-bruxing children: a comparison of their personality traits. *Pediatr Dent*. 1979;1:182–187.

37. Machado E, Dal-Fabbro C, Cunali PA. Prevalence of sleep bruxism in children: a systematic review. *Dental Press J Orthod*. 2014;19(6):54–61.

28

Orthodontic Treatment in the Primary Dentition

JOHN R. CHRISTENSEN AND HENRY FIELDS

The goals of orthodontic care in the primary dentition should be to treat conditions that predispose one to develop a malocclusion in the permanent dentition or to monitor conditions that are best treated later.[1] Some primary dentition problems can be effectively managed, and the result provides a long-term benefit. With other conditions, treatment should be deferred until intervention can provide a long-term benefit.

The clinician needs to differentiate skeletal problems from dental to fulfill these goals. Treatment of skeletal malocclusions in this age group is ordinarily deferred until a later age; the delay is generally for practical reasons rather than an inability to alter skeletal structure at this age. Three general reasons are offered for delaying treatment. First, the diagnosis of skeletal malocclusion is difficult in this age group. Subtle gradations of skeletal problems and immature soft tissue development make clinical diagnosis of all but the most obvious cases difficult. Second, although the child is growing at this stage, the amount of facial growth remaining when the child enters the mixed dentition years is sufficient to aid in the correction of most skeletal malocclusions. Third, any skeletal treatment at this age requires prolonged retention because the initial growth pattern tends to reestablish itself when treatment is discontinued. In essence, retention is active treatment over a sustained period of years to maintain the correction.

On the other hand, several dental problems merit attention during the primary dentition years. This chapter is devoted to these issues.

Skeletal Problems

Skeletal problems are addressed only if there is progressive asymmetry due to a functional disturbance.[2] The reason for treating these patients early is that treatment at a later time may be more difficult and complex if the child continues to grow asymmetrically and dental compensation increases. The goal of early treatment is to prevent the asymmetry from becoming worse or to alter growth so the asymmetry improves. Most progressive asymmetry patients are treated with removable functional appliances designed to alter growth by manipulating skeletal and soft tissue relationships and allowing differential eruption of teeth. Orthognathic surgery is a second treatment option for progressive asymmetry but is reserved for patients with severe asymmetry or those whose condition does not respond to functional appliance therapy. It may be necessary to operate a second time when the child is older because growth often tends to remain asymmetric even after surgical correction. Because diagnosis and treatment of progressive asymmetry are difficult, it is recommended to refer these cases to a specialist for evaluation and treatment.

Early evaluation of patients with dentofacial anomalies is also advocated. Dentofacial anomalies include several environmentally and genetically induced conditions that alter the relationship of the facial structures. Examples include cleft lip and palate, hemifacial microsomia, Crouzon and Apert syndromes, and mandibulofacial dysostosis (Treacher Collins syndrome). A specialist or specialty team works to minimize the facial disfigurement through early surgical and orthodontic intervention.

Dental Problems

Selected dental malocclusion in the primary dentition is readily managed by the practitioner who has knowledge of fixed and removable appliances. The key to successful orthodontic management is careful diagnosis and treatment planning. A comprehensive database should be obtained. In this age group, tooth movement usually is restricted to tipping teeth into proper position as in anterior crossbite correction. Rarely are orthodontic appliances indicated to move teeth bodily, but posterior crossbite correction is one of those.

Before specific treatment problems are discussed, the biology of tooth movement should be briefly reviewed. Two theories of tooth movement have been proposed to describe the mechanism of movement. The first is the "pressure-tension" theory. A force applied to a tooth causes alterations in the periodontal ligament and surrounding alveolar bone. This pressure creates reduced blood flow within the periodontal ligament, leading to limited cellular activity and disorganization of the ligament. On the tension side the stretching of fibers creates an increase in cellular activity resulting in elevated fiber production.[3] The pressure-tension theory is based on histologic studies of the periodontium. During the early stages of compression or pressure, cell-free zones are created (hyalinization). The body reacts to the hyalinization by recruiting macrophages, foreign body giant cells, and osteoclasts from nearby undamaged areas. These cells resorb the bone adjacent to the hyalinized periodontal ligament. The term used to describe this process is undermining resorption. The osteoblast also plays a significant role in tooth movement. In the area of periodontal ligament tension, osteoblasts begin to enlarge and produce new bone matrix. Other preosteoblasts are recruited to aid in bone deposition. Together, the cells work to break down the necrotic tissue and matrix on the pressure side of the tooth and build new bone and structure on the side of tension.

The second theory of tooth movement suggests that a force applied to a tooth is spread equally to all regions of the periodontal ligament. The alveolar bone is deflected, and this begins the changes seen in the periodontal ligament. This is called the bone-bending theory. Forces applied to teeth will bend bone, tooth, and solid structures of the periodontal ligament. Bone is far more elastic than the other tissues, so when bone is held in a deformed position bone turnover and production are initiated. The force applied to the tooth is dissipated within the bone by production of stress lines within the area of force application. Continuous force application like that delivered by an orthodontic appliance becomes a stimulus for cells to alter their normal activities. This altered activity modifies the shape and internal organization of the bone to accommodate these forces.

After force application, the tooth will move approximately the width of the periodontal ligament or until the hyalinization begins. After this small movement, the tooth will not move again for some 4 to 20 days. Movement will not occur until removal of the necrotic tissue is complete and bone resorption, both direct (from periodontal ligament) and indirect (adjacent marrow spaces), has occurred.

When the tooth has moved a certain distance, the force exerted by the orthodontic appliance diminishes to an amount below that necessary for tooth movement. During this time, remodeling is completed and the periodontal ligament and alveolar bone cells begin to return to their normal state. This reorganization period is necessary to prevent injury to the tooth and supporting structures. The clinical implication of cellular change, tooth movement, and cellular reorganization is that orthodontic appliances should be reactivated only at 4- to 6-week intervals with a light, continuous force to avoid injury to the periodontium. There is some biological basis for the recommendation of monthly visits during orthodontic treatment.

After tooth movement is complete, the patient enters the retention phase of treatment. Retention is the time period the teeth are held in their new position. Retention is necessary because teeth that have been moved orthodontically tend to move back or relapse into their original position after the appliance has been removed. Relapse may be due to many factors; however, gingival changes seem to be the primary factor. The gingival tissue does not regain its pretreatment shape like bone and periodontal ligament. The gingiva contains a network of gingival fibers that are compressed or stretched during tooth movement. The genes of both collagen and elastin are activated, and tissue collagenase is inhibited. This causes the extracellular matrix of the gingiva to become more elastic and at greater risk for relapse. Reorganization of the gingival tissues most likely requires a full year. Surgical treatment such as a gingival fibrotomy has been shown to increase stability, indicating

the role of gingival fibers in relapse.[4] This type of procedure is not performed in the primary dentition but may be required in the mixed or permanent dentitions. If surgical treatment is not performed, long-term retention is indicated to prevent relapse.[5] Other factors also influence postorthodontic tooth movement. Pressure from the orofacial musculature, postorthodontic facial growth, and the interdigitation of the teeth (or lack of) has been reported to contribute to orthodontic instability.[6]

Arch Length Problems

The most common arch length problem in the primary dentition is tooth loss. This is managed as outlined in Chapter 26 with space maintenance if the space is adequate. If space has been lost because of tooth loss, space regaining can be instituted. A notable situation in which to use space regaining is when the primary first molar is lost prematurely. The only realistic space regaining in the primary dentition is repositioning the primary second molar before the permanent first molar erupts. A removable appliance is best used for this purpose. A primary second molar can be repositioned approximately 1 mm per month using a removable appliance with multiple clasps and a finger spring (Fig. 28.1). Three millimeters of molar movement is a realistic extent of the treatment. The appliance is similar to the appliance used to reposition a permanent first molar. If a second primary molar is lost, timely placement of a distal shoe is required, to prevent space loss with the eruption of the permanent first molar.

Although inviting and seemingly intuitive, there is little relationship between the arch length (arch perimeter) in the primary and permanent dentitions.[7] This means that weak correlations do not support the early interventions advocated by some and described here. Early intervention is expanding the primary arches with either a fixed or a removable appliance. This treatment is provided to ensure space for the permanent teeth.[8] The expansion provides variable increases in arch width and arch perimeter and is associated with little long-term benefit.[9] This early approach to potential crowding remains controversial and unsubstantiated. It is also important to remember there is a potential to treat up to 4.5 mm of crowding in the late mixed dentition simply with the use of a passive lower lingual arch.[10]

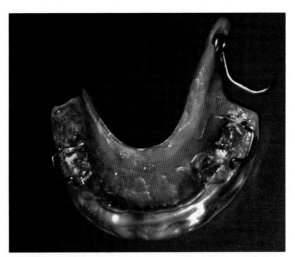

• **Figure 28.1** This appliance was designed to move the right molar distal. Note there are two retentive clasps to hold the appliance in place. The appliance would dislodge as the spring was activated without retention. This type of appliance can move a molar approximately 3 mm.

Incisor Protrusion and Retrusion

In addressing the anteroposterior plane of space, the clinician is mainly concerned with the position of the incisors, particularly the maxillary incisors. The majority of anteroposterior problems involve anterior crossbite, a condition in which the maxillary incisors occlude lingual to the mandibular incisors. A fixed lingual arch or a removable appliance can be used to correct the crossbite, but several things should be kept in mind when moving primary anterior teeth. First, the crowns are extremely short incisogingivally. This means overly aggressive activation of springs will cause them to slip down the lingual surface and not engage the crowns of the teeth. It is best to activate the springs in a facial and gingival direction with gentle activation. Second, the crowns of some primary first molars converge toward the occlusal surface. This makes banding or clasp retention challenging. Third, there are few or no undercuts on the anterior teeth that will engage a labial bow for retention. For this reason, if a labial bow in the primary dentition is not used for tooth movement, it probably should be discarded from the appliance prescription. Finally, because the primary teeth will be exfoliated near 6 to 7 years of age, it is not wise to consider moving a primary incisor much after 4 years of age. Because compliance can be a problem before age 4 years and because primary root resorption and tooth morphology are problems after age 4, few clinicians attempt treatment for anterior crossbites in the primary dentition.

If crossbite correction is indicated, a maxillary lingual arch can be designed to push directly on the incisors with reasonably heavy force (0.036-inch wire) or the lingual arch can have lighter forces delivered with attached finger springs (0.022-inch wire). Either way, the arch can be activated to tip maxillary teeth into proper position. The lingual arch is activated approximately 1 mm per visit because it is a heavy-gauge wire that exerts a heavy force. The auxiliary wires can be activated 2 mm (Fig. 28.2). In general, a tooth moves 1 mm per month during treatment. Therefore, if a tooth requires 3 mm of movement to be properly aligned, 3 months of treatment is necessary.

With a removable appliance, wire finger springs are incorporated into the palatal acrylic to move the teeth facially. Placing retentive clasps on the posterior teeth stabilizes the appliance. The finger springs are activated 1.5 to 2.0 mm per month. If the patient exhibits a positive overbite and overjet after treatment, retention is probably not necessary because the occlusion generally holds

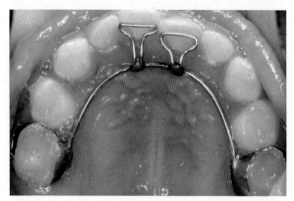

• **Figure 28.2** This patient's anterior crossbite involving the primary maxillary central incisors is being treated with a T spring soldered to a lingual arch. The spring is activated 1 to 2 mm per month until the incisors are tipped out of crossbite.

the tipped incisor in its new position. If there is no overbite, the appliance should be maintained until overbite is established to ensure that relapse does not occur.

The decision to correct an anterior crossbite in the primary dentition is a difficult one. The clinician should determine if the crossbite is skeletal or dental in nature. Other factors to consider are the number of teeth involved, the presence of a mandibular shift, and the age of the patient. There are few evidence-based studies to support or refute correction of a dental anterior crossbite in the primary dentition. In other words, would the crossbite self-correct with the exchange of the permanent incisors? Or, does the early correction maintain itself when the permanent incisors erupt? There are hints that self-correction is possible in dental causes of anterior crossbite.[11–13]

One further point should be made about anterior crossbite. In some cases of posterior crossbite or occlusal interference, a child positions the jaw forward (known as a mandibular shift) to achieve maximal intercuspation and an anterior crossbite results (usually called a pseudo class III malocclusion because the patient is often class I and shifts into a class III position). In this situation the patient positions the lower jaw forward only to obtain comfortable intercuspation as needed to function. This type of anterior crossbite is due to jaw posturing rather than tooth or jaw malposition. In these cases, treatment is directed to the posterior crossbite or the occlusal interference and not to the anterior crossbite. In some cases the interfering tooth is the one in crossbite.

Excessive overjet in the primary dentition is usually due to a nonnutritive sucking habit or to a skeletal mismatch between the upper and lower jaws. Most skeletal problems should not be treated at this time because of the tendency for abnormal growth patterns to recur. However, incisor protrusion as a result of a sucking habit can be addressed. Treatment is usually directed at eliminating the habit rather than correcting the incisor protrusion. Incisor protrusion usually corrects itself or is significantly reduced if the habit is discontinued and if the equilibrium between the tongue, lips, and perioral musculature is reestablished. The quad helix, palatal crib, and Bluegrass appliance are discussed in Chapter 27 and are the appliances of choice for habit therapy (see Figs. 27.6 to 27.8). Studies designed to determine how long the appliance must remain in place to terminate the habit effectively suggest a 6-month minimum.[14] The key to treatment is whether the patient and the parents both want to have the patient stop the habit. If one or neither is interested in discontinuing the habit, it is best to delay treatment until they are ready.

Posterior Crossbite

Posterior crossbite in the primary dentition is usually a result of constriction of the maxillary arch. Constriction often results from an active digit or pacifier habit, although there are many cases in which the origin of the crossbite is undetermined. The first step in managing a posterior crossbite is to establish whether there is an associated mandibular shift. If a mandibular shift is present, treatment generally should be implemented to correct the crossbite. Some authors have implicated a mandibular shift as the cause of asymmetric growth of the mandible.[15] The asymmetry is thought to occur because the condyles are positioned differently within each fossa. Muscle and soft tissue stretch exert forces on the underlying skeletal and dental structures that may alter normal growth and arch development. If no shift is detected, the mandible should grow symmetrically. It has been suggested to wait on treatment until the permanent molar erupts if there is no mandibular shift.[12] After the permanent molar erupts, the clinician can treat if it erupts in crossbite or continue to observe if there is no permanent molar crossbite or mandibular shift.

There are two basic approaches to the management of posterior crossbite in young children: (1) equilibration to eliminate mandibular shift and (2) expansion of the constricted maxillary arch. In a few cases the mandibular shift is due to interference caused by the primary canines. These cases can be diagnosed by repositioning the mandible and noting the interference. Selective removal of enamel with a diamond bur in both arches eliminates the interference and the lateral shift into crossbite. This type of treatment has evidenced-based support.[16]

In cases of bilateral maxillary constriction, expansion is recommended to correct the lateral shift. This situation should be managed as soon as it is diagnosed unless the permanent first molar is expected to erupt within 6 months. If permanent molar eruption is imminent, it is better to allow the permanent molars to erupt and incorporate these teeth into treatment if necessary. Both fixed and removable appliances can be designed to correct maxillary constriction, although fixed appliances are reliable and require little patient cooperation. A randomized prospective study of unilateral crossbite correction in the mixed dentition suggested the most successful intervention was with fixed appliances.[17]

Fixed appliances are variations of a lingual arch bent into the shape of a W. In fact, one of the most popular appliances used to treat crossbites is named the "W arch" (Fig. 28.3). Another popular appliance is the quad helix (see Fig. 27.6). The W arch is constructed of 0.036-inch wire that rests 1.0 to 1.5 mm off the palate to prevent soft tissue irritation. The W arch is expanded approximately 4 to 6 mm wider than its passive width, or so that one arm of the W is resting over the central grooves of the teeth when the other arm is seated. To move teeth preferentially in the anterior region of the mouth, the appliance is activated by bending the palatal portion of the arm near the solder joint, as demonstrated in Fig. 28.4. If more correction is needed in the molar region, the appliance is activated via bending of the anterior palatal portion. The appliance expands the arch approximately 1 mm per side per month.

The patient should return monthly to allow the dentist to check the progress of treatment and to reactivate the W arch if needed. The appliance can be activated intraorally by squeezing the wire with a three-pronged plier, although the force and direction of activation may be difficult to approximate, and unwanted tooth movement can result. Usually it is easier and more accurate to remove, activate, and recement the appliance. Expansion should continue until the crossbite is slightly overcorrected and the lingual cusps of the maxillary teeth occlude on the lingual inclines of the buccal cusps of the mandibular teeth. Most crossbites are corrected in 3 months, and the teeth are retained for an additional 3 months.

The quad helix is designed much like the W arch but incorporates more wire into the appliance, making it more flexible. It is constructed of 0.038-inch wire with two helices in the anterior palate and two helices near the solder joint in the posterior palate. The helices are wound away from the palate and can serve to remind the digit-sucking patient to refrain from the habit if they are positioned correctly where the patient places the finger or thumb. Therefore this is the preferred appliance for a patient with a finger habit and posterior crossbite. Because the quad helix has more wire than the W arch, it has a greater range of action and can be activated farther than the W arch while delivering an equivalent amount of force. Overcorrection and retention are also required for the quad helix.

Despite activation of the W arch or quad helix on one side only, teeth on both sides of the arch react to equivalent force. These types of fixed lingual arch type appliances have been shown to produce both skeletal and dental changes in the primary and mixed dentitions.[17]

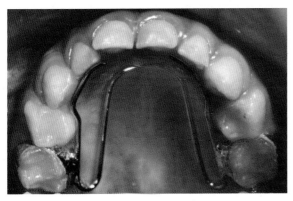

• **Figure 28.3** The W arch is a fixed appliance used to correct posterior crossbites in the primary dentition.

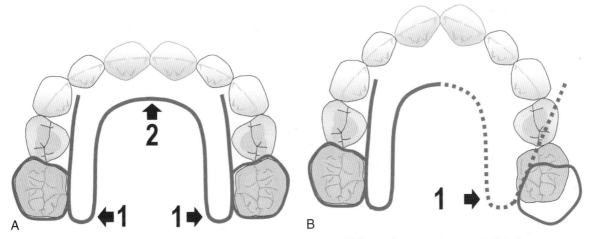

• **Figure 28.4** (A) The W arch can be activated in two spots. (B) The preferred way to move teeth in the anterior region of the mouth is to activate the W arch by bending the arm of the W in the area marked location *1.*

Continued

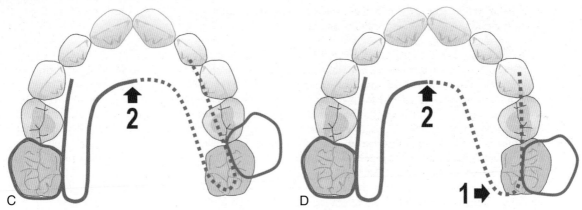

• **Figure 28.4, cont'd** (C) If the clinician wants to obtain more movement in the molar region, the appliance is activated by bending the anterior portion of the W in the area marked location *2*. (D) In general, the appliance is activated 3 to 4 mm beyond its passive width or to a position where one arm of the W extends over the central grooves of the teeth when the other arm is seated in place.

Open Bite

Vertical problems in the primary dentition usually are due to a finger or pacifier habit, and they result in an anterior open bite. Treatment for an anterior open bite that is due to a sucking habit is discussed in Chapter 27. Deep bite in the primary dentition is generally not corrected at this time. The depth of bite usually improves with the eruption of the permanent first molars if the problem is the result of dental malocclusion.

References

1. Ngan P, Fields HW. Orthodontic diagnosis and treatment planning in the primary dentition. *J Dent Child.* 1995;62:25–33.
2. Proffit WR, Fields HW, Sarver DM. Treatment of skeletal problems in children. In: *Contemporary Orthodontics.* 5th ed. St Louis: Mosby; 2012.
3. Kishnan V, Davidovitch Z. Cellular, molecular, and tissue-level reactions to orthodontic force. *Am J Orthod.* 2005;129:469.e1–469. e32.
4. Redlich M, Shoshan S, Palmon A. Gingival response to orthodontic force. *Am J Orthod Dentofacial Orthop.* 1999;116:152–157.
5. Lang G, Alfter G, Göz G, et al. Retention and stability—taking various treatment parameters into account. *J Orofacial Orthop.* 2002;63:26–41.
6. Melrose C, Millett DT. Toward a perspective on orthodontic retention? *Am J Orthod Dentofacial Orthop.* 1998;113(5):507–514.
7. Bishara SE, Khadivi P, Jakobsen JR. Changes in tooth size–arch length relationships from the deciduous to the permanent dentition: a longitudinal study. *Am J Orthod Dentofacial Orthop.* 1995;108: 607–613.
8. McInaney JB, Adams RM, Freeman M. A nonextraction approach to crowded dentitions in young children: early recognition and treatment. *J Am Dent Assoc.* 1980;101:251–257.
9. Lutz HD, Poulton D. Stability of dental arch expansion in the deciduous dentition. *Angle Orthod.* 1985;55:299–315.
10. Gianelly AA. Treatment of crowding in the mixed dentition. *Am J Orthod Dentofacial Orthop.* 2002;121:569–571.
11. Nagahara K, Murata S, Nakamura S, et al. Prediction of the permanent dentition in deciduous anterior crossbite. *Angle Orthod.* 2001;71(5): 390–395.
12. Dimberg L, Lennartsson B, Arnrup K, et al. Prevalence and change of malocclusions from primary to early permanent dentition: a longitudinal study. *Angle Orthod.* 2015;85:728–734.
13. Nagahara K, Suzuki T, Nakamura S. Longitudinal changes in the skeletal pattern of deciduous anterior crossbite. *Angle Orthod.* 1997;67(6):439–446.
14. Haryett RD, Hansen FC, Davidson PO. Chronic thumb-sucking. A second report on treatment and its psychological effects. *Am J Orthod.* 1970;57:164–178.
15. Primozic J, Richmond S, Kau CH, et al. Three-dimensional evaluation of early crossbite correction: a longitudinal study. *Eur J Orthod.* 2011;35(1):7–13.
16. Harrison JE, Ashby D. Orthodontic treatment for posterior crossbites. *Cochrane Database Syst Rev.* 2001;(1):CD000979.
17. Petrén S, Bondemark L. Correction of unilateral posterior crossbite in the mixed dentition: a randomized controlled trial. *Am J Orthod Dentofacial Orthop.* 2008;133(6):e790–e797.

29

Oral Surgery in Children

ABIMBOLA O. ADEWUMI

CHAPTER OUTLINE

In many ways, oral surgical procedures for children are similar to and possibly easier than those performed for adults. There are some important differences as well. The purpose of this chapter is to present basic techniques and surgical principles needed to perform oral surgical procedures safely and competently on children and adolescents. This chapter discusses the extraction of teeth, minor soft tissue procedures (e.g., biopsies and frenectomies), odontogenic infections, and the recognition and initial management of facial injuries and fractures. This chapter presents an overview of the principles of successful oral surgical procedures in children.

Preoperative Evaluation

The dentist treating the child patient must be careful to consider the entire patient and not focus only on the oral cavity. Important considerations in caring for the child patient include the following:
1. Obtaining a comprehensive medical history, with special emphasis on medical conditions that might complicate treatment, such as bleeding disorders
2. Obtaining appropriate medical and dental consultations
3. Anticipating and preventing emergency situations
4. Being fully capable of managing emergency situations when they occur (see Chapter 10)

In addition to the medical preoperative evaluation, it is important to perform a thorough dental preoperative evaluation, which includes taking appropriate preoperative radiographs. These often include two or more periapical radiographs of the same area to determine buccal, lingual, facial, or palatal relationships of impacted teeth. There are instances in which taking a three-dimensional radiograph is indicated (e.g., for locating supernumerary or impacted teeth, teeth adjacent to a cleft site, or in which conditions where ankyloses is suspected). Another preoperative consideration is the need for future space maintenance as a result of the premature loss of primary teeth (see Chapter 26). Failure to provide immediate space maintenance may allow for the mesial migration of permanent first molars after premature primary molar loss.

Tooth Extractions

Armamentarium

Many dentists choose to use the same surgical instruments for both child and adult patients. However, most pediatric dentists and oral and maxillofacial surgeons prefer the smaller pediatric extraction forceps, such as the no. 150S and 151S (Fig. 29.1), for the following reasons:
1. Their reduced size more easily allows placement in the smaller oral cavity of the child patient.
2. The smaller pediatric forceps are more easily concealed by the operator's hand.
3. The smaller working ends (beaks) more closely adapt to the anatomy of the primary teeth.

The choice of the proper instrumentation can also depend on special considerations unique to the child and the adolescent. The use of cow horn mandibular forceps is contraindicated for primary teeth, owing to the potential for injury to the developing premolars (Fig. 29.2). Great care must also be given to the routine use of elevators and forceps adjacent to large restorations such as chrome crowns and especially restorations adjacent to erupting single-rooted teeth that may easily become dislodged with the slightest force.

General Considerations

The manual technique used to perform extractions in the child patient is similar to the manual extraction technique used in the adult. The greatest difference is in patient management. It is essential that the dentist take the time to describe the ensuing procedure completely and accurately to the child. Many practitioners show the child a curette or other benign instrument and explain: "This spoon will walk around your sick tooth and wiggle and dance with it. If your tooth is really sick, then we will give it a big hug, and it will wiggle or dance right out!" The practitioner may give the child's shoulder or hand a squeeze to demonstrate that "big hug" so the child knows he or she may still feel some pressure. Alternatively, just before the actual extraction, the dentist can place the balls of the index finger and thumb in the area of the extraction and demonstrate to the child the types of pressures and movements that he or she will encounter during the extraction. This digital pressure should be firm enough to rock the child's head from side to side in the headrest. The dentist should be sure to obtain profound anesthesia because, once the patient has felt pain, it may be difficult to regain the child's confidence to a level in which he or she will behave in a manner that allows completion of the procedure. Advanced behavior guidance techniques and pharmacologic adjuncts such as nitrous oxide or sedation may be required in a more anxious child (see Chapter 8).

Several steps of the extraction procedure should be performed with every extraction. The dentist should consult with the parents

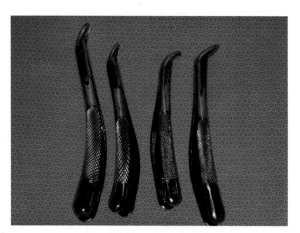

• **Figure 29.1** Extraction forceps: *left to right,* no. 150, no. 150S, no. 151S, no. 151.

before surgery in order to prepare them for the upcoming procedure. The entire surgical procedure and the expected postoperative recovery course should also be described. This allows the parents to make special postoperative arrangements, such as the need for a soft diet or child care support.

Several factors make it possible for the child patient to aspirate or swallow foreign objects during dental treatment. These factors include (1) the common practice of treating the child patient in a reclining position, (2) poor visibility as a result of the smaller opening into the oral cavity and the proportionately larger tongue of the child, and (3) the increased likelihood of unexpected movements by the child patient. To prevent this from happening, the patient should be positioned in the chair so that the upper jaw is at no more than a 45-degree angle with the floor (Fig. 29.3). If an angle greater than 45 degrees is preferred by the operator, the posterior oral airway should be protected by placing a gauze screen or performing the extraction with the use of a rubber dam.

The dentist should be placed in the position in which he or she can easily control the instrumentation, have good visual access to the surgical site, and control the child's head. Fingers of the nondominant hand of the dentist are then placed in the patient's mouth on either side of the tooth being extracted. The role of the nondominant hand is to help control the patient's head; to support the jaw being treated; to help retract the cheek, lips, and tongue from the surgical field; and to palpate the alveolar process and adjacent teeth during the extraction.

After the proper operator and nondominant hand positions are established, the actual extraction technique may begin. Variations in technique for individual teeth are discussed later in this chapter, but the following general principles apply to all extractions.[1,2] An instrument such as a dental curette or periosteal elevator is used to separate the epithelial attachment of the tooth to be extracted (Fig. 29.4). Then appropriate elevators may be used to luxate the tooth to be extracted, but great care must be used not to damage adjacent or underlying teeth. The appropriate forceps is then placed

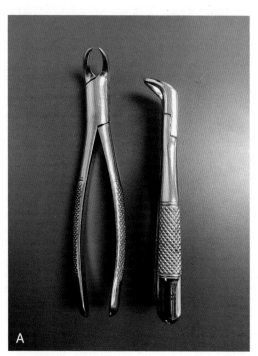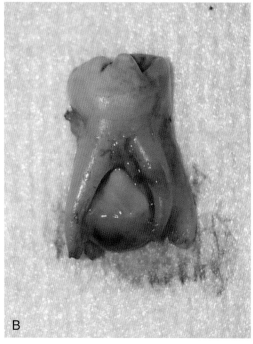

• **Figure 29.2** (A and B) The use of cow horn mandibular forceps is contraindicated for primary teeth, owing to the potential for injury to the developing premolars. ([B] Courtesy Gabriel Dominici.)

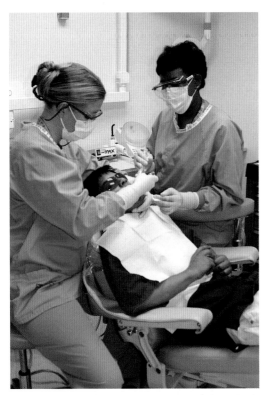

• **Figure 29.3** To help prevent aspiration of extracted teeth, the child is positioned so that the upper jaw is at a 45-degree angle to the floor.

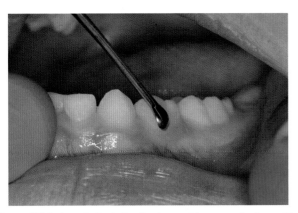

• **Figure 29.4** A periosteal elevator is used to separate the epithelial attachment of the tooth before extraction.

• BOX 29.1 Postoperative Instruction List for Patients

1. Bite on gauze for 30 minutes. Do not chew on the gauze.
2. Do not use a straw to drink for 24 hours.
3. Brush remaining teeth daily, but do not rinse or use a mouthwash on the day of the surgery.
4. Take pain medication as directed.
5. If pain increases after 48 hours or if abnormal bleeding continues, call our office.
6. To prevent bleeding and swelling, keep your head elevated on two or three pillows while you rest or sleep.
7. Do not spit. Spitting will cause bleeding. Excess saliva and a little bit of blood looks like a lot of bleeding.
8. If bleeding starts again, put a gauze pad, a clean wash cloth, or a damp tea bag over the bleeding area and bite on it with firm steady pressure for 1 hour. Do not chew on it.
9. Ice packs can be used immediately after surgery and for the next 24 hours to reduce swelling. Keep ice packs on for 10 minutes and off for 10 minutes.
10. Black and blue marks are bruises that often occur after surgery. Usually they are barely noticeable. Sometimes the skin is discolored. Do not worry about this.
11. Drink lots of liquid and eat anything you can swallow.
12. Call our office about any complications or if you need to change your appointment.

---

on the tooth to be extracted, usually seating the lingual or palatal beak first and then rotating the facial beak into proper position. The extraction is then performed via the proper forceps technique.

After the tooth is removed from its socket, the surgical site is evaluated visually and with the use of a curette. The curette should be used as an extension of the dentist's finger to palpate and evaluate the extraction site. No attempt should be made to scrape the extraction site. If a pathologic lesion such as a cyst or periapical granuloma is present at the apex of a permanent tooth socket, it should be gently enucleated. Aggressive manipulation of a curette in a primary tooth socket is contraindicated due to the potential for damage to the succeeding tooth bud. The operator should palpate both the facial and palatal or buccal and lingual aspects of the surgical site to feel for any bone irregularities or alveolar expansion. Any bone sharpness should be conservatively removed with either a rongeur or a bone file. Digital pressure should be sufficient to return the alveolus to its presurgical configuration if gross expansion has occurred.

Initial hemostasis must be obtained and is accomplished by having the child bite on an intraoral gauze pack. In the anesthetized, deeply sedated, or very young child, a pack that extends out of the oral cavity should be used to prevent swallowing of the gauze. The extraction site should also be evaluated for the need for sutures, although they are rarely indicated after extraction of primary teeth. An absorbable gelatin sponge (e.g., Gelfoam, Pfizer Inc., NY) is an alternative to sutures to aid hemostasis. Gelfoam is particularly useful when gingival and bony tissues immediately surrounding the extraction site are not grossly torn or damaged, but the sponge should not be inserted into the socket that has frank infection. The sponge is first folded or rolled between the operator's fingers and then inserted into the socket and held with mild pressure for a minute. The sponge is absorbed by the body over a 4- to 6-week period. Before the patient is dismissed, a written list of postoperative instructions should be given and explained to both the patient and the parents (Box 29.1). The postoperative instruction list should explain how to contact the dentist after hours in case of an emergency.

Maxillary Molar Extractions

Primary maxillary molars differ from their permanent counterparts in that the height of contour is closer to the cementoenamel junction and their roots tend to be more divergent and smaller in diameter. Because of the root structure and potential weakening of the roots during the eruption of the permanent tooth, root fracture in primary maxillary molars is not uncommon. Adequate local anesthesia must be obtained and can be accomplished through a maxillary infiltration and palatal injection or a greater palatine block (see Chapter 7). Another important consideration is the relationship of the primary molar roots to the succeeding premolar crown. If the roots encircle the crown, the premolar can be inadvertently extracted with the primary molar (Fig. 29.5). After the epithelial attachment is released, a no. 301 straight elevator is used to luxate the tooth (Fig. 29.6). The extraction is completed using a maxillary universal forceps (no. 150S). Palatal movement is initiated first, followed by alternating buccal and palatal motions with slow continuous force applied to the forceps. This allows expansion of the alveolar bone so that the primary molar with its divergent roots can be extracted without fracture. The tooth is delivered in the occlusobuccal direction.

Extraction of Maxillary Anterior Teeth

The maxillary primary and permanent central incisors, lateral incisors, and canines all have single roots that are usually conical. This makes them much less likely to fracture. Adequate local anesthesia must be obtained and can be accomplished through infiltration of the maxillary anterior vestibule as well as injecting into the incisive papilla (nasopalatine block) to anesthetize the lingual side of the teeth (see Chapter 7). Apply anterior forceps along the long axis of the tooth apical to the cementoenamel junction, followed by slight rotary and vertical movements. The motion simulates using a screwdriver to remove a nail (i.e., apical

thrust, twist, and pull). A no. 1 forceps is useful in the extraction of maxillary anterior teeth (Fig. 29.7).

Mandibular Molar Extractions

When extracting mandibular molars, the dentist must pay special attention to the support of the mandible with the nonextraction hand to prevent injury to the temporomandibular joints (Fig. 29.8). Adequate local anesthesia is obtained through an inferior alveolar block. Occasionally, supplemental injections like a long buccal block are necessary. Infiltration alone is not sufficient to obtain adequate anesthesia for extraction procedures (see Chapter 7). After luxation with a no. 301 straight elevator, a no. 151S forceps is used to extract the tooth with the same alternating buccal and palatal motions used to extract maxillary primary molars.

Extraction of Mandibular Anterior Teeth

The mandibular incisors, canines, and premolars are all single rooted. Therefore one must take great care that the forceps does not place any force on adjacent teeth because they can become easily luxated and dislodged. This also enables the dentist to use rotational movements in the extraction process, as described previously.

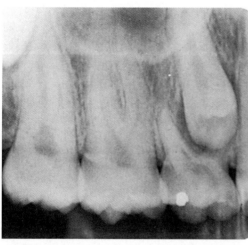

• **Figure 29.5** Primary molars with roots encircling the developing premolar may have to be sectioned to prevent accidental extraction of the premolar.

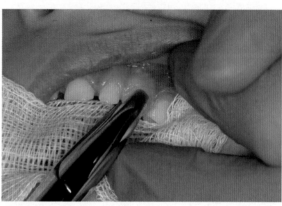

• **Figure 29.7** Rotational movements and buccolingual motions are used to extract primary incisors. The dentist's nondominant hand helps to control the child's head, supports the jaw being treated, retracts adjacent soft tissues, and palpates the alveolar process and adjacent teeth during extraction. Also note the gauze screen in the oral cavity to aid in preventing aspiration or swallowing of extracted teeth.

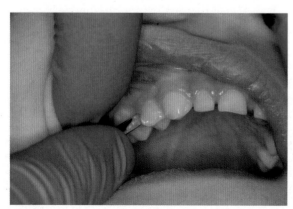

• **Figure 29.6** A no. 301 straight elevator is used to luxate the tooth. Extreme care is taken to prevent accidental luxation of adjacent teeth.

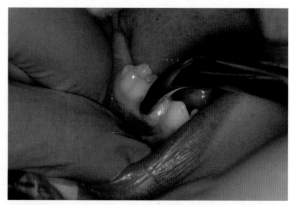

• **Figure 29.8** The nonextraction hand supports the mandible during extraction of mandibular molars.

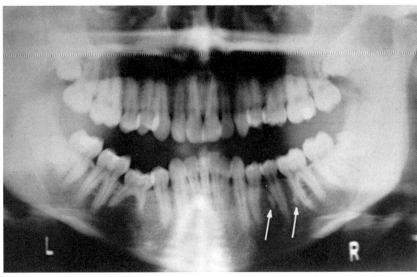

• **Figure 29.9** In this patient, unresorbed primary root tips *(arrows)* did not impede eruption of the succeeding premolar. Also note that the congenitally missing primary molar roots are not being resorbed and the occlusal surface of this tooth is well below the occlusal plane.

Management of Fractured Primary Tooth Roots

Any dentist who extracts deciduous molars occasionally has the opportunity to treat root fractures. After the root has fractured, the dentist must consider the following factors. Aggressive surgical removal of all root tips may damage the succedaneous tooth. On the other hand, leaving the root may increase the chance for postoperative infection and may increase the theoretical potential of delaying permanent tooth eruption, although most primary root tips will resorb. A commonsense approach is best. If the tooth root is clearly visible and can be removed easily with an elevator or root tip pick, the root should be removed. If several attempts fail or if the root tip is very small or is situated deep within the alveolus, the root is best left to be resorbed, most probably by the erupting permanent tooth. As a general rule, root tips greater than or equal to one-third of the root should be removed and tips less than a third may be left to prevent damage to the underlying successor. In some cases the root tips do not resorb but are situated mesially and distally to the succeeding premolar and do not impede its eruption (Fig. 29.9). A note of the root left in situ should be placed in the patient's records, the patient and parents should be notified that a root fragment has been retained, and they should be assured that the chance of unfavorable sequelae is remote.

If the preoperative evaluation indicates that a root fracture is likely or that the developing succedaneous tooth may be dislodged during the extraction, an alternative extraction technique should be used. In these cases the crown should be sectioned with a fissure bur in a buccolingual direction (Fig. 29.10) so that the detached portions of the crown and roots can be elevated separately.[1]

Soft Tissue Surgical Procedures

A number of soft tissue procedures occasionally must be performed for the child patient. Careful presurgical consideration should be given to the following:

1. Expected change in the condition with maturation
2. Optimal time (or patient age) for the procedure
3. Type of anesthetic or sedation required
4. Postoperative complications or sequelae
5. Expected results

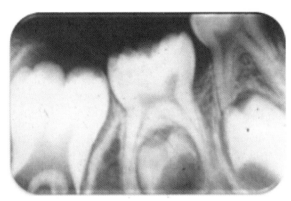

• **Figure 29.10** The crown should be sectioned with a fissure bur in a buccolingual direction down the midline of the tooth so that the detached portions of the crown and roots can be elevated separately.

Biopsies

Biopsy techniques in children are similar to those in adults. A very small lesion is probably best managed with an excisional biopsy, whereas lesions 0.5 cm or larger should probably have an incisional biopsy, especially if there is any doubt regarding the diagnosis of the lesion. Before performing a biopsy on a lesion, the dentist should consider the possibility that the lesion is vascular. Any such area should be palpated for intravascular turbulence (thrill), auscultated with a stethoscope for the presence of a bruit, and checked by needle aspiration for the presence of blood within the lesion. Biopsies should not be performed on vascular lesions until a thorough work-up has been completed.[3]

Some areas of the oral cavity, such as the mucosa and lips, are easily accessible, whereas other areas, such as the tongue, can be difficult and may require sedation or general anesthesia (GA) to accomplish the biopsy. The biopsy area should be carefully evaluated for proximity to important anatomic structures, such as the mental nerve or salivary ducts or their orifices. Resorbable sutures are preferred to prevent the necessity of removing sutures in the child patient. The disadvantage of some resorbable sutures is that the knot can be very hard to remove and irritating to the child. Soaking gut sutures in glycerin before their use softens them considerably.

Dentoalveolar Surgery for Impacted Canines

Procedures to uncover impacted canines have been associated with a high rate of success and may require referral to a specialist.[4] Preoperative radiographs are taken to accurately locate the canine in the alveolus. It is often necessary to take two or more periapical radiographs, using the buccal object rule to predict the labiopalatal position of an impacted tooth. More advanced diagnostic imaging such a cone beam computerized tomography (CBCT) is now recommended for accurate localization of the impacted canine prior to surgery. Great care must be taken not to disturb the root of the impacted canine because it is thought that the chance of ankylosis increases if the cementum is disturbed. If root development is not complete, the exposed canine may be allowed to erupt passively. If the impacted canine has complete root development or is poorly positioned, an orthodontic bracket or chain may be bonded to the exposed portion of the crown with resin to aid a more active eruption. The exposed canine can then be orthodontically positioned in the arch.

Facial Injuries

The dentist may be the first health care professional consulted for injuries to the teeth, lips, jaws, or soft tissues of the face. The dentist should be aware of potential problems with each type of injury and either treat the patient appropriately or make a referral to the appropriate specialist.

Initial care should be directed to pain control, hemorrhage control, patient reassurance, wound cleansing if possible, and tetanus prophylaxis when indicated. Care should be taken to account for all teeth. In cases of avulsion or crown fractures, in which teeth cannot be accounted for, chest or abdominal radiographs may be needed to locate swallowed or aspirated teeth, whereas soft tissue radiographs may be indicated to rule out crown fragments embedded through, for instance, a lip laceration (Fig. 29.11). See Chapter 16 for the radiographic technique. Traumatic injuries to the teeth are discussed in Chapters 16 and 35. A significant number of patients who present with facial trauma may also have acute life-threatening injuries such as chest or abdominal trauma or more significant head or neck injury. The dentist must ensure that there

is no loss of consciousness or no other serious injuries before addressing the facial injuries.

Soft tissue injuries of the face or oral cavity can usually be managed with primary closure. Great care must be taken to be certain that no foreign objects are left hidden within the wound. Gravel or dirt left embedded in the soft tissue may leave a permanent tattoo, especially in the facial region.

Puncture-type wounds often carry glass or debris deep within the wound. When there is doubt about the presence or absence of a foreign body in the soft tissue, a soft tissue radiograph may be helpful in identifying the presence of embedded material (see Fig. 29.11).

Small lacerations of the wet portion of the lips, gingivae, alveolar mucosa, or tongue usually heal very well even if left unsutured. A resorbable suture is most commonly used intraorally, especially in children because silk sutures have the disadvantage of the need for removal.

Large lacerations should be closed, regardless of their location, and multilayer wound closure may be indicated for very deep lacerations or for lacerations that extend from the face into the oral cavity (through-and-through lacerations). Principles of a layered closure include a watertight mucosal closure, followed by closure of the muscular, facial, subcutaneous, and skin layers as necessary. Facial lacerations are always reapproximated first at significant anatomic structures, such as the vermilion border, columella of the nose, or eyebrows. Malalignment of these structures produces a noticeable cosmetic defect. It is generally advisable to refer to an oral surgeon or a plastic surgeon if the laceration crosses the vermilion border of the lip.

Facial Fractures

The definitive treatment of facial fractures is best handled by an experienced dental practitioner, such as an oral maxillofacial surgeon. A thorough head and neck as well as facial exam is necessary to rule out an unsuspected fracture. Patients with maxillary or midface fractures may present with any or all of the signs and symptoms listed in Box 29.2. Patients with mandibular fractures may present with any or all of the signs or symptoms listed in Box 29.3.

Initial management of facial fractures should be directed toward the immobilization of fractured segments, early antibiotic therapy for open fractures, and pain control.[5] Definitive treatment should then be performed by a qualified specialist.

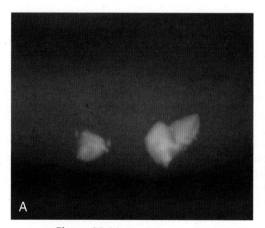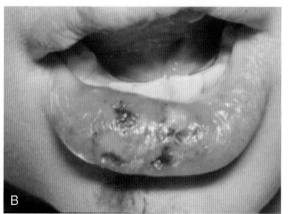

• **Figure 29.11** A soft tissue radiograph (A) may be indicated to rule out crown fragments embedded through a lip laceration (B).

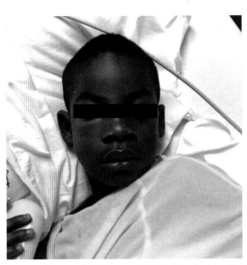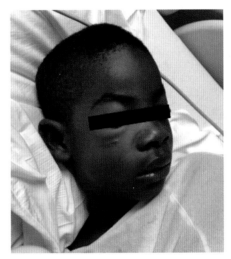

• **Figure 29.12** A child with right facial cellulitis and swelling due to an abscessed tooth.

Odontogenic Infections

Infections of odontogenic origin are common in child and adolescent patients. Classic signs and symptoms of infection include redness, pain, swelling, and local and systemic temperature increases (Fig. 29.12). Because of wider marrow spaces in the child, an odontogenic infection can rapidly spread through the bone, possibly resulting in damage to the erupting teeth. Most odontogenic infections in the child are not serious and can be easily managed by removing the source of infection with pulp therapy or removal of the involved tooth. Although uncommon, serious complications can occur when infection spreads beyond the dentition, including cellulitis, cavernous sinus thrombosis, brain abscess, temporary blindness, airway obstruction, and mediastinal spread of infection. Managing cellulitis can be challenging because it has a wide variability of clinical presentation due to the involvement of multiple anatomical structures, polymicrobial etiology, and differing disease progression.[6] Signs and symptoms of a more serious spread of infection include an elevated systemic temperature (102°F to 104°F), difficulty in swallowing, voice hoarseness, difficulty in breathing, nausea, fatigue, and sweating. The child with an odontogenic infection may become dehydrated as a result of his or her refusal to take fluids because of oral pain. Children who present with these symptoms often need management with hospitalization, intravenous (IV) fluids, and antibiotics.

Management of odontogenic infections is directed at providing prompt and adequate drainage of the infection. This can be accomplished in minor infections by way of a pulpectomy or extraction. Management of more serious odontogenic infections is best accomplished by surgical incision and drainage.[1] Research has shown that rapid treatment of the offending tooth along with IV antibiotics is significantly more cost effective and results in a shorter hospital admission than treating the infection with IV antibiotics alone.[6] It is often necessary to identify the causative organism or organisms to prescribe the most appropriate antibiotic (see Chapter 9). For outpatient therapy, oral penicillin remains the empirical choice for odontogenic infections[7]; however, amoxicillin may provide more rapid improvement in pain or swelling and better compliance because of the longer dosage interval.[8] For individuals with a penicillin allergy, clindamycin or azithromycin are recommended.[8] A 5- to 7-day course of treatment is generally recommended.[7] For inpatient therapy, common IV antibiotics used in the management of cellulitis are IV ampicillin/sulbactam, clindamycin, or penicillin with metronidazole.[8]

Ankyloglossia and Frenectomies

Ankyloglossia

Etymologically, "ankyloglossia" originates from the Greek words "agkilos" (curved) and "glossa" (tongue). The English synonym is "tongue-tie."[9] Ankyloglossia (AG) is a congenital anomaly characterized by an abnormally short lingual frenum, which may restrict tongue tip mobility.[10] AG can be either a classic anterior tongue-tie, a submucosal restriction, and/or a tethered superior labial frenum (upper lip-tie).[11]

Otolaryngologists (ear, nose, and throat specialists), oral surgeons, pediatricians, speech therapists, and lactation consultants may all voice different opinions regarding the various aspects of AG, and its definitions range from vague descriptions of a tongue that functions with a less-than-normal range of activity to a specific description of the frenum being short, thick, muscular, or fibrotic. The plethora and variety of AG definitions in the literature suggest the lingering controversy regarding this condition and its clinical significance. Associations between tongue-tie, lactation problems, speech disorders, and other oral motor disorders (e.g., problems with swallowing or licking) have also been inconsistent and are an ongoing source of controversy within the medical community.[12] One survey of otolaryngologists, pediatricians, speech pathologists, and lactation consultants reported significant disparities within and among these groups regarding their approaches to AG and their beliefs regarding its association with feeding, speech, and social problems. Unfortunately, dentists are similarly divided on the topic.[12] AG may reduce tongue mobility and has been associated with functional limitations in breastfeeding, swallowing, articulation, orthodontic problems including malocclusion, open bite, separation of upper/lower incisors, mechanical problems related to oral clearance, and psychological stress.[13]

Etiology of Ankyloglossia

The exact etiopathogenesis of tongue-tie is unknown[9]; however, one author has described the etiology of AG as follows: the tongue is fused to the floor of the mouth in early development. Cell death and resorption free the tongue, with the frenum left as the only remnant of initial attachment. The lingual frenulum typically becomes less prominent with the natural process of the child's growth: as the alveolar ridge grows in height and teeth begin to erupt. This process occurs during the first 6 months to 5 years of life.[12] There may be a genetic predisposition to AG, and an association between AG and some syndromes, such as X-linked cleft palate syndrome, have been observed.[12] AG has also been diagnosed in some rare syndromes such as van der Woude, orofaciodigital syndrome, and Beckwith-Wiedemann.[10,12] Nevertheless, most AGs are an isolated congenital anomaly that is observed in persons without any other congenital anomalies or diseases.[9,12] Prevalence ranges from 0.02% to 10.7%, depending on the definition of the authors, and is seen more often in males.

• BOX 29.4 Classifications of Ankyloglossia

Coryllos Classifications of Tongue-Tie

(Divided into four types, according to how close to the tip of the tongue the leading edge of the frenulum is attached)

Type 1: Attachment of the frenulum to tip of tongue
Type 2: Attachment is 2–4 mm behind tip of tongue/on or behind alveolar ridge
Type 3: Attachment to mid-tongue and the middle of the floor of the mouth, usually tighter and less elastic
Type 4: Attachment against base of tongue, thick shiny and inelastic

Kotlow Classifications of Upper Lip-Tie

Class I: No significant attachment
Class II: Attachment mostly into the gingival tissue
Class III: Attachment in front of the anterior papilla
Class IV: Attachment into the papilla or extending into hard palate

---

Classification of Ankyloglossia

AG can be observed at different ages with specific indications for treatment for each group.[10,14] The Hazelbaker assessment tool for lingual frenulum function (HATLFF) was developed to evaluate the severity of tongue-ties in newborns. It is based on the tongue's appearance and its functional aspects, and it uses a scoring system to classify babies' tongues into one of three categories: functionally impaired, acceptable, or perfect.[9] However, it is complex, lengthy, and has not been validated in a controlled manner.[12]

Ghaheri et al. described two simpler classifications of upper lip-tie and tongue-tie (Box 29.4).[11] Coryllos types 1 and 2, considered as "classical" tongue-tie, are the most common and obvious tongue-ties and probably account for 75%. Types 3 and 4 are less common and, because they are more difficult to visualize, are the most likely to go untreated. Type 4 is most likely to cause symptoms that are more significant for mother and infant.[15] Kotlow described upper lip-tie classification for infants.[16]

Ankyloglossia and Breastfeeding

Recognition of potential benefits of breastfeeding in recent years has resulted in renewed interest in functional AG sequelae. Of infants with AG, there is a reported 25% to 80% incidence of breastfeeding difficulties, including failure to thrive, maternal breast pain, poor milk supply, and refusing the breast. Infants with restrictive AG cannot extend their tongues over the lower gum line to form a proper seal and therefore use their jaws to keep the breast in the mouth. Depending on the audience, enthusiasm for surgical treatment varies.[13]

Typically reported problems related to poor latch include signs of frustration such as head-banging, maternal nipple pain, and signs of an unsatisfied baby (i.e., frequent or continuous feeds often with "fussing").[17] Francis et al. performed a systematic review of the surgical and nonsurgical treatments for infants with AG and breastfeeding outcomes, although the quality of the majority of the studies was very low. In the randomized controlled trials (RCTs) in which the mother self-reported improved breastfeeding, significant improvements for frenotomized infants versus nontreated infants were noted (96% vs. 3% and 78% vs. 47%, respectively).[13] Three RCTs used an observer to assess breastfeeding effectiveness, and in all of these studies the observer was blinded to the treatment. Among these, one study reported significant improvement in breastfeeding immediately after frenotomy compared with sham treatment. In contrast, of the remaining two RCTs, the independent blinded observers did not detect a difference in breastfeeding improvement immediately and 5 days following intervention. Regarding maternal nipple pain, similar results as those for breastfeeding have been found, with one RCT reporting significant improvement and others finding nonsignificant reductions in maternal discomfort between intervention and sham groups. Overall, a small body of evidence suggests that frenotomy may be associated with mother-reported improvements in breastfeeding and pain, but the strength of evidence on this topic is low. Future research could change our understanding of the effect of frenotomy on breastfeeding.[13]

Ankyloglossia and Nonbreastfeeding Issues

Nonbreastfeeding Outcomes

With only two comparative studies reviewed by Chinnadurai et al., both with significant methodologic limitations, evidence is insufficient to draw conclusions about the benefits of surgical interventions regarding nonbreastfeeding feeding (i.e., bottle) outcomes for infants and children with AG.[18]

Speech Outcomes

Speech concerns were the second most prevalent outcome described in the AG literature, specifically articulation and intelligibility. Poor-quality cohort studies have reported improved articulation and intelligibility with surgical AG treatment; however, other benefits to speech are unclear. Given the lack of good-quality studies, the strength of the evidence for the effect of surgical interventions to improve speech and articulation is insufficient. In a separate review, authors concluded that although there are some possible positive indications to treating tongue-ties, especially from the parents' perception, there is no substantial evidence to support prophylactic frenotomy on the basis of promoting subsequent speech development.[17]

Social Concerns

Possible social concerns related to reduced tongue mobility may include speech, oral hygiene, excessive salivation, kissing, spitting while talking, and self-esteem. With only one poor-quality comparative study, the evidence related to the ability of AG treatment to alleviate social concerns is currently insufficient.[18]

Surgical Treatment

Treatment options such as observation, speech therapy, frenotomy without anesthesia, and frenectomy under GA have all been suggested in the literature to correct an abnormal frenulum. The following techniques are of particular interest in pediatric dentistry: frenotomy and frenectomy.

Frenotomy Technique

The frenotomy procedure is defined as the cutting or division of the frenum. The discomfort associated with the release of thin and membranous frena appears to be brief and minor. Thus there is a paucity of literature regarding effective analgesia for frenotomy.[12] The procedure may be accomplished without local anesthesia; however, some practitioners highly recommend the use of topical lidocaine anesthetic gel and/or local anesthetic for pain control and to alleviate any parental concerns.[10] Benzocaine should be used with caution in infants, due to the concern for methemoglobinemia (see Chapter 7).[19] Release of the tongue-tie appears to be a minor procedure but may cause complications such as bleeding or infection or injury to Wharton duct. There is a risk that postoperative scarring may limit tongue movement even further, necessitating reoperation. From the limited literature, the incidence of complications appears to be rare.[12]

The infant is placed supine with the elbows held close to the body, and the parent or an assistant stabilizes the head. The tongue is lifted gently with sterile gauze and stabilized by the nondominant hand, exposing the frenum. The frenum is then divided with small sterile scissors at its thinnest portion. The incision begins at the frenum's free border and proceeds posteriorly, adjacent to the tongue (Fig. 29.13). This is necessary to avoid injury to the more inferiorly placed submandibular ducts in the floor of the mouth. There should be minimal blood loss (i.e., no more than a drop or two, collected on sterile gauze). If needed, bleeding can be controlled easily with a brief period of pressure applied with gauze. The incision is not sutured. Feeding may be resumed immediately. No specific follow-up care is required, except that breast milk is recommended for at least the next few feedings. Parents should be advised that a postoperative white fibrin clot might form at the incision site during the first few days. Follow-up in 1 to 2 weeks should show that the incision is completely healed.

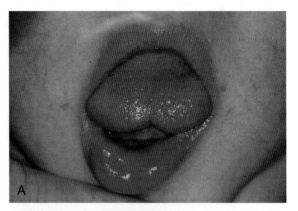
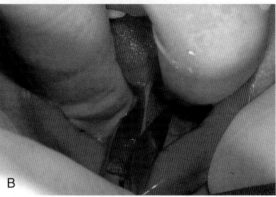
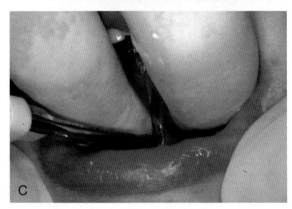

• **Figure 29.13** (A–C) Frenotomy procedure for an infant. (From Junqeira MA, Cunha NN, Costa e Silva LL, et al. Surgical techniques for the treatment of ankyloglossia in children: a case series. *J Appl Oral Sci.* 2014;22:241–248.)

When this technique's relative simplicity is weighted against the severity of the consequences of untreated cases or future treatment with the frenectomy procedure, pediatric dentists should consider the frenotomy technique.[10]

Frenectomy Technique

The frenectomy procedure[20] is defined as the excision or removal of the frenum, which can be accomplished by the conventional technique with a scalpel or by the use of a soft tissue laser. Frenectomy is the preferred procedure for patients with a thick and vascular frenum where severe bleeding may be expected, and in some cases, reattachment of the frenum by scar tissue may occur. The procedure in young children is often performed under GA. However, older children or adults may tolerate the procedure with the use of local anesthesia alone. The frenum is released in a similar

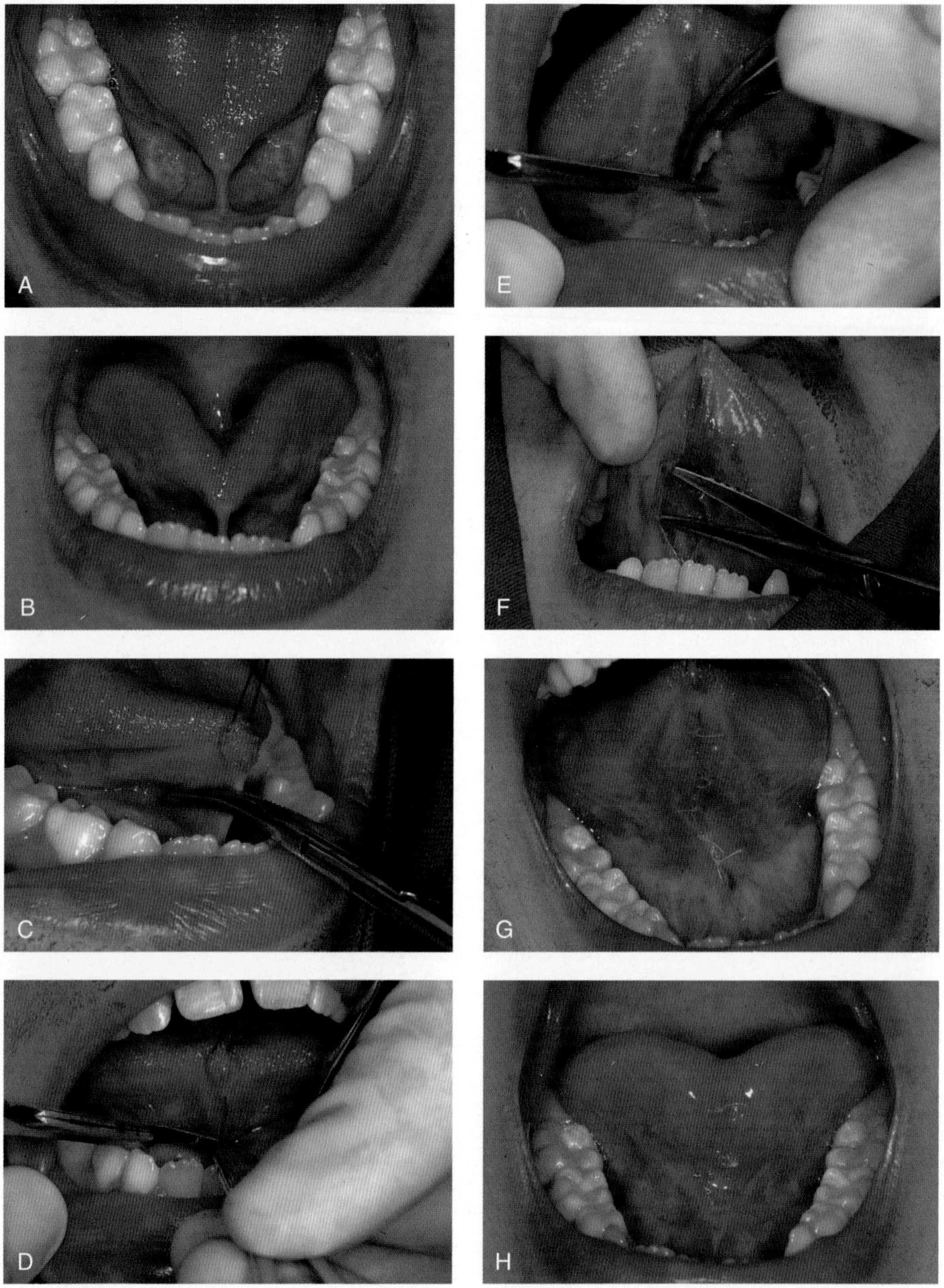

• **Figure 29.14** (A–H) Frenectomy procedure in an older child using a hemostat and a surgical blade. Wound closure is usually performed using a Z-plasty flap procedure. (From Junqeira MA, Cunha NN, Costa e Silva LL, et al. Surgical techniques for the treatment of ankyloglossia in children: a case series. *J Appl Oral Sci.* 2014; 22:241–248.)

manner as in the frenotomy technique, although occasionally limited division of the genioglossus may be required for adequate release (Fig. 29.14). The wound is sutured with a Z-plasty flap closure.[10] Studies that have compared the conventional technique with the use of various lasers have generally found that use of the laser energy negates the need for sutures, results in less bleeding during the procedure, and produces less postoperative discomfort and functional complications (eating and speech).[21–24] Although emerging research shows advantages to the use of laser energy, the laser technique requires some precautions. The practitioner must understand the type of laser being used and the appropriate settings and technique for that laser because multiple types of lasers are available (carbon dioxide, Nd:YAG, diode, etc.). In addition, the clinician and staff must be properly trained in laser safety for themselves and the patient.

Complications of Frenotomy/Frenectomy

Complications of the frenotomy/frenectomy procedure[20] include infection, excessive bleeding, recurrent AG due to excessive scarring, new speech disorders developing postoperatively, and glossoptosis (tongue "swallowing") due to excessive tongue mobility.

A clinician is encouraged to:

1. Examine the frenum attachment
2. Diagnose AG if it is present and evaluate its severity
3. Be aware of the benefits of intervention
4. Refer patients to a qualified surgeon if unable to perform a frenotomy or frenectomy

References

1. Sanders B. *Pediatric Oral and Maxillofacial Surgery*. St Louis: Mosby; 1979.
2. Kruger G. *Textbook of Oral and Maxillofacial Surgery*. 6th ed. St Louis: Mosby; 1984.
3. Gibilisco JA. *Oral Radiographic Diagnosis*. Philadelphia: Saunders; 1985.
4. Fifield CA. Surgery and orthodontic treatment for unerupted teeth. *J Am Dent Assoc*. 1986;113:590–591.
5. Rowe N, Williams J. *Maxillofacial Injuries*. Edinburgh: Churchill Livingstone; 1985.
6. Thikkurissy S, Rawlins JT, Kumar A, et al. Rapid treatment reduces hospitalization for pediatric patients with odontogenic-based cellulitis. *Am J Emerg Med*. 2010;28(6):668–672.
7. American Academy of Pediatric Dentistry. Guideline on use of antibiotic therapy for pediatric dental patients. *Pediatr Dent*. 2016;38(6):325–327.
8. Flynn T. What are the antibiotics of choice for odontogenic infections, and how long should the treatment course last? *Oral Maxillofac Surg Clin North Am*. 2011;23(4):519–536.
9. Suter VGA, Bornstein MM. Ankyloglossia: facts and myths in diagnosis and treatment. *J Periodontol*. 2009;80:1204–1219.
10. Kupietzky A, Botzer E. Ankyloglossia in the infant and young child: clinical suggestions for diagnosis and management. *Pediatr Dent*. 2005;27:40–46.
11. Ghaheri BA, Cole M, Fausel SC, et al. Breastfeeding improvement following tongue-tie and lip-tie release: a prospective cohort study. *Laryngoscope*. 2016;127(5):1217–1223.
12. Rowan-Legg A. Ankyloglossia and breastfeeding. Canadian Pediatric Society Position Statement. *Paediatr Child Health*. 2015;20(4):209–214.
13. Francis DO, Krishnaswami S, McPheeters M. Treatment of ankyloglossia and breastfeeding outcomes: a systematic review. *Pediatrics*. 2015;135(6):e1458–e1466.
14. Ferrés-Amat E, Pastor-Vera T, Ferrés-Amat E, et al. Multidisciplinary management of ankyloglossia in childhood. Treatment of 101 cases. A protocol. *Med Oral Patol Oral Cir Bucal*. 2016;21(1):e39–e47.
15. Coryllos E, Genna CA, Salloum AC. American Academy of Pediatrics section on breastfeeding. http://www2.aap.org/breastfeeding/files/pdf/BBM-8-27%20Newsletter.pdf. Accessed February 13, 2017.
16. Kotlow LA. Diagnosing and understanding the maxillary lip-tie (superior labial, the maxillary labial frenum) as it relates to breastfeeding. *J Hum Lact*. 2013;29(4):458–464.
17. Brookes A, Bowley DM. Tongue tie: the evidence for frenotomy. *Early Hum Dev*. 2014;90(11):765–768.
18. Chinnadurai S, Francis DO, Epstein RA, et al. Treatment of ankyloglossia for reasons other than breastfeeding: a systematic review. *Pediatrics*. 2015;135(6):e1467–e1474.
19. US Food and Drug Administration. Benzocaine and babies: not a good mix; 2015. https://www.fda.gov/ForConsumers/ConsumerUpdates/ucm306062.htm. Accessed September 21, 2017.
20. Junqeira MA, Cunha NNO, Costa e Silva LL, et al. Surgical techniques for the treatment of ankyloglossia in children: a case series. *J Appl Oral Sci*. 2014;22(3):241–248.
21. Medeiros Júnior R, Gueiros LA, Silva IH, et al. Labial frenectomy with Nd:YAG laser and conventional surgery: a comparative study. *Lasers Med Sci*. 2015;30:851–856.
22. Haytac MC, Ozcelik O. Evaluation of patient perceptions after frenectomy operations: a comparison of carbon dioxide laser and scalpel techniques. *J Periodontol*. 2006;77:1815–1819.
23. Akpinar A, Toker H, Lektemur Alpan A, et al. Postoperative discomfort after Nd:YAG laser and conventional frenectomy: comparison of both genders. *Aust Dent J*. 2016;61:71–75.
24. Gargari M, Autili N, Petrone A, et al. Using the diode laser in the lower labial frenum removal. *Oral Implantol*. 2012;5(2–3):54–57.

PART 4

The Transitional Years: Six to Twelve Years

Many changes will occur as a child ages from 6 to 12 years old. The physical changes will be dramatic, and the changes relating to facial form, occlusion, the advent of permanent teeth, and the esthetic appearance of these permanent teeth are the professional responsibility of the dentist. He or she must supervise the exfoliation of the 20 primary teeth present in the 6-year-old and eruption of the 28 permanent teeth that are found in most 12-year-olds. The dentist must establish a relationship with the patient and family to ensure that dental care is delivered within a trusting framework. The dentist must advocate preventive measures such as sealants, meticulous hygiene during orthodontics, additional fluoride products as needed, and nutrition counseling as these patients make their own food choices. The dentist must also provide answers to parents concerned about the appearance of their child, intercept those developing malocclusions, and when appropriate, refer those patients with malocclusions that need specialist care. The dentist who can deliver the child from age 6 years to adolescence with little to no amount of hard tissue disease, no remarkable soft tissue diseases, allegiance to prevention and developed home care habits, and harmonious dentofacial relationships has indeed mastered the ultimate obligations in treating this age group.

30

The Dynamics of Change

MAN WAI NG, ZAMEERA FIDA, AND HENRY FIELDS

Physical Changes

Body

The median (50th percentile) weight and height of 6-year-old boys in the United States are 47.5 pounds and 45.5 inches, respectively, whereas the same medians for girls are 46 pounds and 45 inches. By the time children reach age 12 years, boys will weigh 90 pounds and be 59 inches tall and girls will weigh 90.25 pounds and be 59.5 inches tall. This is a time of substantial continuous growth.[1]

During the period between the ages of 6 and 10 years, boys as a group are generally slightly taller than girls until around age 10 years. From age 10 years to around age 15 years, girls are slightly taller than boys. From a weight standpoint, boys are slightly heavier than girls until around age 11 years, when girls overtake boys in weight for a brief time. Although it is generally assumed that girls are a couple of years ahead of boys in their sexual and general maturation, this may be an overstatement due to the observability of the changes taking place. The real difference is actually about 1 year. This is because height and breast development are considered the main markers of female development compared with penis, scrotum, and height development in males. Nonetheless, the pregrowth spurt in males is steady and creates a larger platform upon which to launch the more robust, later spurt as compared with the pattern in females. This accounts for the larger terminal size of males, in general, to females.

Other growth and developmental changes that are noteworthy during these years are further increases in blood pressure, continuing decreases in the pulse rate, increased mineralization of the skeleton, and increases in muscular tissue. In addition, the lymphatic tissues reach a peak of development during these years, to the point where they exceed the amounts found in adults.

Craniofacial Changes

The period from ages 6 through 12 years represents a continuous progression of the growth in the head and neck. From age 5 to 10 years (approximately the age range of interest here), neural and cranial growth are found to be almost entirely complete (Fig. 30.1). During this same age span, the jaws (maxilla = A = 2 and mandible = B = 3 of Fig. 30.1) grow at a faster rate than the cranium.

Using the Bolton standards for illustrative purposes,[2] nasal projection and increased mandibular prominence are demonstrated (Fig. 30.2). The nasal cartilage and mandibular condyle continue to grow by endochondral bone formation for some time. The female mandibular growth spurt is most likely completed during this time period, whereas the mandibular growth spurt in males is yet to come. Growth modification can therefore be considered in this age group. Changes in cranial base length caused by endochondral bone formation at the sphenooccipital synchondrosis cease in early adolescence, but some appositional changes continue to occur at the basion and nasion. Vertically, there is a continued lowering of the palatal vault with sutural growth and apposition on the oral side of the palate and resorption on the nasal side as the intramembranous process of bone formation continues. Vertical facial growth is also complemented by dentoalveolar growth as the permanent teeth erupt and the alveolar ridges develop.

In the transverse plane, there is continued growth at the midpalatal suture. Most transverse palatal sutural growth is completed for females during this period when the first bridging of the suture occurs. Transverse appositional widening of the alveolar ridge occurs with eruption of the permanent teeth. Widening of the anterior arch accompanies lateral incisor eruption and is followed by width increases in the canines and premolars (Fig. 30.3).

The implications of these changes are that anteroposterior growth modification for class III problems should be attempted during this time. It seems there is more total facial change in this age group than in older patients.[3] For class II problems, growth modification can be attempted now or during early adolescence with equivalent results. Transverse changes should be completed using lingual arch–type appliances or rapid palatal expansion if greater forces are necessary to interrupt the stable midpalatal suture late in this age group. Vertical growth will continue in the face through late adolescence.

Growth Increments

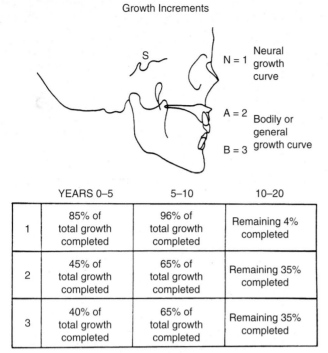

	YEARS 0–5	5–10	10–20
1	85% of total growth completed	96% of total growth completed	Remaining 4% completed
2	45% of total growth completed	65% of total growth completed	Remaining 35% completed
3	40% of total growth completed	65% of total growth completed	Remaining 35% completed

• **Figure 30.1** Differential growth center rates of craniofacial components. (From Behrents RG. *Growth in the Aging Craniofacial Skeleton*. Ann Arbor, MI: Center for Human Growth and Development, University of Michigan; 1985.)

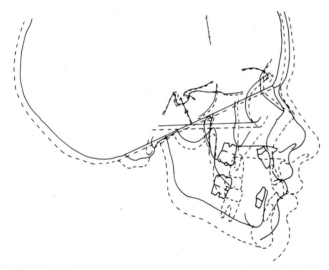

• **Figure 30.2** This anterior cranial base superimposition of the Bolton standard for 6- and 12-year-olds (*solid line* and *dashed line,* respectively) demonstrates the magnitude of anteroposterior and vertical skeletal growth during this period as well as the soft tissue change. (Redrawn from Broadbent BH Sr, Broadbent BH Jr, Golden WH. *Bolton Standards of Developmental Growth*. St Louis: Mosby; 1975.)

Dental Changes

Early during this period most children experience the eruption of all four first permanent molars and the exfoliation of the mandibular and maxillary primary central and lateral incisors. The permanent incisors erupt between the ages of 6 and 7 years (see Table 13.5). However, it is not unusual for the maxillary permanent lateral incisors to erupt later than age 7 years in some children. Eruption

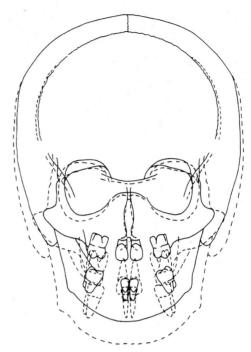

• **Figure 30.3** This anterior cranial base superimposition of the Bolton standard for 6- and 12-year-olds (*solid line* and *dashed line,* respectively) demonstrates the magnitude of transverse and vertical skeletal growth during this period. (Redrawn from Broadbent BH Sr, Broadbent BH Jr, Golden WH. *Bolton Standards of Developmental Growth*. St Louis: Mosby; 1975.)

of the anterior teeth should be carefully and easily observed by the practitioner for developmental and esthetic reasons.

Except for third molars, all of the permanent teeth usually have erupted by the end of the 12th year. Permanent tooth enamel formation is complete by age 8 years. In the mandibular arch (except for the first permanent molar), molars erupt in immediate succession, that is, centrals, laterals, canines, first and second premolars, and second permanent molars from 6 to 7 years through 11 to 13 years of age. The same sequence takes place in the maxillary arch except for the maxillary canine, which usually erupts after one or both premolars and at about the same time as or before the eruption of the second permanent molars (Fig. 30.4).

The mandibular central incisor roots are complete by age 9 or 10 years. The roots of the four first permanent molars, the maxillary central incisors, and the mandibular lateral incisors are usually complete by age 10 years. The roots of the maxillary lateral incisors are complete by age 11 years.[4]

Because the position of the dental lamina of the permanent teeth is located to the lingual side of all of the primary teeth (except for the dental lamina coming off the second primary molars for the three permanent molars), the anterior teeth develop in their vault or crypt lingual to and near the apex of the primary incisors. When the roots begin to form on the permanent teeth, the permanent teeth start to migrate to the oral cavity. Generally, they follow a pattern such that they come across the primary root, resorbing it and erupting slightly lingual to the location sustained by the primary tooth (Fig. 30.5). Ultimately the permanent teeth are usually angulated more buccally compared with their primary predecessors (Fig. 30.6). The developing premolars develop between the roots of the primary molars and continue to erupt in a slightly buccal position.

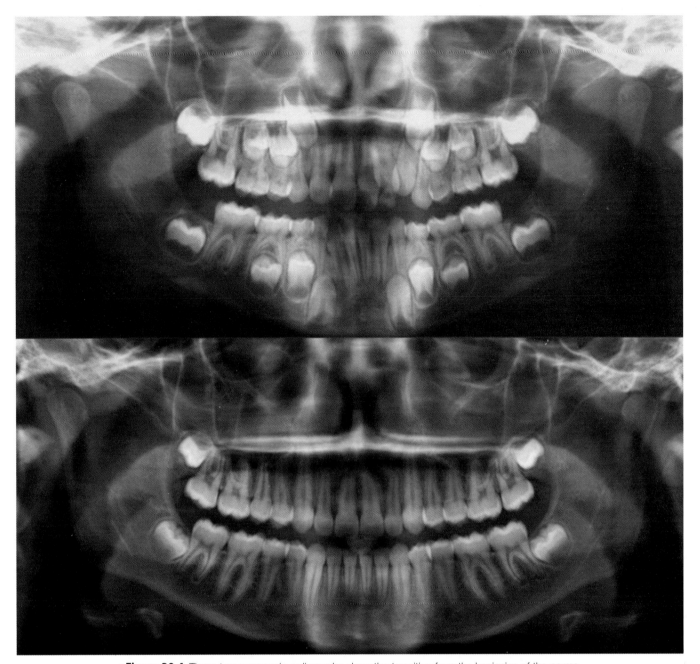

• **Figure 30.4** These two panoramic radiographs show the transition from the beginning of the permanent dentition to its completion with the exception of the third molars. Note that an upper left lateral supernumerary tooth was removed.

It is normal to find diastemas between the primary incisors. This helps provide space for the larger permanent incisors. The permanent canine in the maxillary arch is usually the last permanent tooth to erupt mesial to the first permanent molar. As the permanent canine begins to erupt, it migrates down the distal root surface of the maxillary lateral incisor and ultimately moves the crowns of the incisors mesially and will close moderate to small diastemas. This period of development has been called the "ugly duckling stage" (Fig. 30.7).[5]

Most of the eruption problems occur during this time period and the clinician should be checking for these at each exam. Ectopic eruption of permanent first molars, ectopic eruption of lateral incisors due to positioning or crowding, ectopic canine eruption, and transpositions all can be traced to this period of development. Obviously monitoring and intervention in these conditions are crucial to a normally developing dentition. The clinician should consider whether early and sustained crowding requires extraction of primary or permanent teeth or whether space maintenance should be considered to treat nonextraction. By the end of this period, most of the residual space resulting from either idiopathic spacing or leeway spacing has closed. Further eruption and drift occur in response to continued growth.

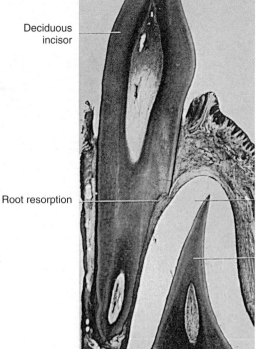

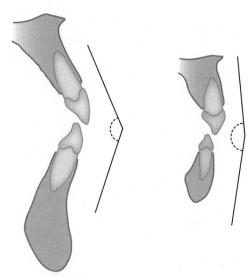

• **Figure 30.5** Resorption of the root of a primary incisor owing to pressure from the erupting successor. (From Bhaskar SN, ed. *Orban's Oral Histology and Embryology*. 11th ed. St Louis: Mosby; 1990.)

• **Figure 30.6** Angulation of permanent and primary incisors. (Redrawn from Moyers RE. *Handbook of Orthodontics*. 3rd ed. Chicago: Year Book; 1973.)

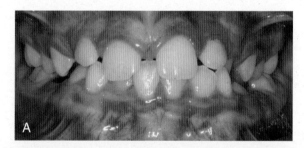

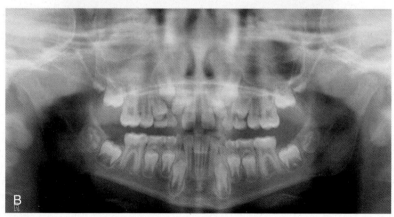

• **Figure 30.7** (A and B) The "ugly duckling" stage is typified by spacing between the permanent maxillary incisors. The roots of the incisors are tipped mesially by the erupting crowns of the permanent maxillary canines. As the canines erupt, they push the incisors together and close modest diastemas but not extensive ones.

Cognitive Changes

A book could easily be written describing the great cognitive acquisitions, adjustments, and sophisticated changes occurring in a child from age 6 to 12 years. Mental capacity alone grows extensively. Unquestionably the attention span of the child older than 7 years is substantially greater than that of the child younger than 5 years.

The school-age years of 6 to 12 are when a child becomes literate. Before age 6 years, few children can do much more than print their names. After age 12 years, most children have accomplished an appropriate approach to grammar and syntax and have the ability to produce increasingly sophisticated oral and written communications. In some parts of the world, it is not uncommon for a child to be fluent in a second language by age 12 years.

According to Piaget,[6] the ages between 6 and 12 years roughly approximate the third major developmental stage of cognition—that is, the phase of concrete operations. Piaget proposed the following four major periods of intellectual development:
1. *Sensorimotor:* birth to 18 months
2. *Preoperational:* 18 months to 7 years
3. *Concrete operations:* 7 to 12 years
4. *Formal operations:* 12 years and onward

So far we have presented a study of the child through the sensorimotor and preoperational stages. In the concrete operations stage, Piaget describes numerous sophisticated changes in the child's mental abilities. For instance, the 5-year-old may be able to walk "two blocks down, one block right to the second white house" to get to his or her aunt's residence, but the same 5-year-old could not draw this route on a piece of paper. However, by age 7 or 8 years, the child could portray the route on a self-drawn map. In other words, mental representations of actions become a part of the cognitive abilities of the child during these years. For the dentist who communicates with children, it will be helpful to design discussions based on the child's mental representation ability.

During the years from 6 to 12 (7 to 12 according to Piaget), children acquire the ability to understand the constancies between length, mass, number, and weight despite external differences. Relativity also emerges in the child's evaluation system. To the 4-year-old, the word *dark* means black. The 10-year-old can talk about a "dark" green car. In summary, the child between the ages of 6 to 12 years grows cognitively. By the age of 12 years, mind and mental prowess have matured, and real as well as theoretical or abstract information can be assimilated.

Emotional Changes

The period from 6 to 12 years is one of advancement toward the acceptance by the child of societal norms of behavior. Crying, tantrums, and other rages will, in normal children, be relinquished as possible modes to express frustration. Whereas the preschooler needs and perhaps demands immediate rewards and satisfaction, the child in the transitional years masters the emotional ability to delay gratification. This awareness of delay is reinforced by the child's schooling, and increasingly the child is guided toward the appropriate investment of his or her time in worthwhile activities. Homework, household chores, caring for pets, and extracurricular activities such as scouting, team sports, dance, and music lessons are some of the behaviors expected of this age group, which were almost impossible during the preschool years.

Another emotional refinement that is developed from age 6 to 12 years is the ability to use life's tasks to effectively stave off boredom. Previously, the preschooler immersed his mind in an activity until all his energy and attention were spent. Then, at the point of burnout, he looked to his parents or other attendants to find something else for him to do. Between ages 6 and 12 years, however, the need for adults to direct the child's attention rapidly recedes, and by age 12 years a child usually has a ledger of wants and desires, a sense of the time that should be spent in their pursuit, and an ability to set priorities for which wants and desires should come first or last.

In this age range, body image starts to become an emotional feature of the child's life. Unquestionably, for the majority of children, the importance of body image becomes most dramatic during adolescence, but its emergence certainly occurs during these years. Whereas the 6-year-old usually cares little about having ketchup on his face or mud on his pants, the 12-year-old may agonize over a blemish or wearing clothes that are not stylish. In summary, body appearance becomes a subject of emotional awareness and emphasis during these years. Unquestionably this has dental ramifications. A 6-year-old may be indifferent to the appearance of hypomineralized incisors or a malocclusion. By age 12 years, such conditions may account for a lack of smiling, social withdrawal, and a loss of self-esteem. Teasing and bullying may exacerbate the problem.

Although there certainly are exceptions, the majority of children from ages 6 to 12 years find overall emotional satisfaction only when they are accepted socially by their peers. Lack of acceptance, outright ostracism, teasing, and bullying can certainly be very damaging emotionally. During these years—with the help of parents, teachers, role models, and other significant individuals—it is important for the child to become emotionally resilient. The abilities to handle and recover from humiliation, frustration, loss, and disappointment should at least begin to emerge during these years. If they do not, then adolescence may become tumultuous years.

Social Changes

The period between ages 6 and 12 years is often called middle childhood. These years are clearly more complicated socially than the earlier years because of the demands of school, the increasing importance of peers, and the enormous expansion of the child's social environment. These years see the child intensifying his or her focus on and pursuance of existing interests and competencies while minimizing or eliminating others.

School is extremely important for this age group and represents an extrafamilial world that may reinforce social responses learned at home, provide new ones, and even discourage others. In school, children are expected to control themselves, cultivate good work habits, sit quietly for long periods of time, and comply with rules and expectations for personal conduct set by adults.[7]

Perhaps surprisingly, most children anticipate school positively and remain enthusiastic about their experiences there. It has also been noted that children's self-importance, self-control, and ability to be independent (e.g., getting their own breakfast) increase quickly during the first few months of school.[8] Unfortunately, self-confidence and motivation tend to decline later in the elementary school years, and this trend continues through adolescence. This may result in students avoiding certain courses or dropping out of school completely. Children may shy away from activities in which they are initially unlikely to succeed. However, if they are able to see that they can become competent with practice and development, supportive adults are able to help children manage their frustrations.[7]

The peer group that a child joins also can be a powerful socializing force. Sometimes the values of the peer group are antithetical to those of the teacher and parents. This presents a conflict for the child in that he or she may risk reprimand from authoritative adults or ridicule or rejection from his or her peers if he or she conforms to one or the other's expectations. It is important for parents to understand these conflicts and how socially influential peer pressure can be for children in this age group. It is also important to note that the child who eagerly accepts a peer value that disappoints her or his parents may in fact be doing so to gain the feelings of acceptance and nurturing that were not provided sufficiently at home.

One last factor marks the middle childhood years. This is the advent of increasingly stronger, more stable, and more meaningful friendships. Generally friendships are made with children of the same gender. Friends at this age level as a rule also share similar socioeconomic status, intelligence, maturity, and interests. At the same time, it is important to recognize that as closer bonds and friendships are defined, social cruelty and bullying also increase.

Dental Caries and Dietary Factors

Dental caries is the most common chronic disease of childhood. Even though caries prevalence in permanent teeth has remained relatively stable since the 1980s and some 60% of adolescents have dental caries, this disease still affects a majority of school-aged children in the United States.[9] See Chapter 12 for a discussion on the epidemiology of caries in the transitional dentition.

Why Dietary Factors Are Important to the Transitional Dentition

There is ample evidence linking dietary sugars to the etiology of dental caries.[10] As mentioned in Chapter 12, sugars (sucrose, fructose, glucose, and others) are among the major etiologic factors in dental caries. Sucrose has been labeled the "arch criminal of dental caries,"[11] but animal studies have shown that other sugars, notably glucose and fructose, are as cariogenic as sucrose.[12,13]

Sucrose

One of the first controlled studies to document sucrose as an etiologic factor was the Vipeholm study[14] near Lund, Sweden. A total of 436 inmates in a mental institution were given sugar in various forms to supplement the relatively sugar-free institutional diets. The sugar was offered as sucrose in solution or in retentive forms, such as sweetened bread and toffee. The sucrose in solution and the bread were introduced with meals, whereas the other forms were given between meals. The study showed that an increase in sucrose intake was associated with an increase in caries activity. Furthermore, this caries activity decreased when the sucrose-rich foods were discontinued. The cariogenic potential of the sucrose was enhanced when it was given between meals and in a more retentive form (caramels and toffees). The time required for the sugar to clear the oral cavity was closely related to the caries activity. The study also pointed out that caries formation varied among individuals and that caries formation continued in some individuals even after a return to low-sucrose diets. The subjects who received only 30 g of sucrose per day, all at mealtimes, developed an average of 0.27 new carious lesions per year. Those who ingested 330 g of sucrose per day (300 g in solution) developed 0.43 new carious surfaces per year. Lastly, subjects in the group who received 24 sticky toffees per day developed 4.02 new lesions per year. This group ingested 300 g of sucrose per day and 40% of it was consumed between meals. Although there were flaws in the design of this study, the magnitude of the differences in caries development are impressive. The questions regarding the ethics of this type of study ensure it will probably never be repeated.

Another study corroborating the role of sucrose was conducted with 3- to 14-year-olds who resided at Hopewood House in Bowral, New South Wales, Australia.[15,16] Almost all of these institutionalized children had lived there since infancy and were fed an almost pure vegetarian diet supplemented with milk and an occasional egg yolk. The vegetables were generally served raw, and refined carbohydrates were rigidly restricted. In spite of poor oral hygiene, the caries prevalence among the children was very low. Primary dentition involvement was almost nonexistent, whereas the caries prevalence of the permanent teeth was about one-tenth that of the mean score for other Australian children. Almost one-third of the children remained caries-free throughout the 5-year study. Children who left Hopewood House at an older age experienced a significant increase in dental caries.

Some still question the primary role of sucrose and other sugars in the etiologic development of caries.[17] Burt and Pai[18] concluded in their systematic review that the relationship between sugar consumption and caries is weaker but not eliminated in the modern era of fluoridation. Marshall and colleagues[19] conclude that the cariogenicity of a food is less dependent on the nature of the sugar than on the characteristics of the food and the nature of the exposure, primarily frequency. However, others remain convinced that free sugars (which include all mono- and disaccharides added to food and sugars naturally present in honey, syrup, fruit juices, and concentrates) are the primary factors facilitating the development of dental caries.[10,20]

Other Food Factors

There is evidence to show that both the frequency of intake of sugar-rich foods and drinks and the total amount consumed are related to dental caries. In addition, these two factors are closely related.[10] In a study of 5-year-old children in Iceland, Holbrook et al. found a threshold effect for the frequency of sugar consumption on caries development to be up to four times a day. Children reporting four or more episodes of sugar intake per day or three or more between-meal snacks per day had much higher caries rates. In 5-year-old children who developed three or more lesions, the sugar intake averaged 5.1 times per day compared with 2.1 times a day for children who developed less than three carious lesions.[21] The Vipeholm study also showed that caries development was low when sugars were consumed up to four times a day at mealtimes.[14] More frequent contact with sugars at mealtime and frequent between-meal snacks result in prolonged or multiple pH challenges to the teeth and possibly to longer oral clearance times. Yet several longitudinal studies have shown the amount of sugar intake to be more important than frequency.[10] Ismail et al. found a very high correlation between the frequency of consumption of sugary drinks between meals and the amount consumed. In addition, both the frequency and the amounts consumed were associated with higher caries risk.[22]

The multiplicity of food factors requires that estimations of the relative cariogenicity of foods be approached with caution. These factors include carbohydrate-sucrose concentration, retentiveness, oral clearance rate, detergent quality, texture, effect of mixing foods, sequence of ingestion, frequency of ingestion, and pH of the food itself. For example, most fruits will depress plaque pH by virtue of their own low pH. This occurs even though the low pH of the food inhibits natural fermentation of its sugar content. Low-pH fruits can also demineralize enamel by the direct action of their acids. At the same time, low-pH fruits stimulate a flow of saliva that buffers plaque pH drops; other foods, such as vegetables, stimulate salivary flow through the chewing reflex. On balance, however, there is not a strong case for a caries-protective effect from fruits and vegetables.[23] On the other hand, Moynihan and Petersen argued that dried fruits may potentially be more cariogenic, since the drying process breaks down the cellular structure of the fruit, thus releasing free sugars, and that dried fruits tend to have a longer oral clearance.[10]

In fact, stickiness or retentiveness is another food factor that has received much attention. Foods high in cooked processed starch content (e.g., breads, cereals, potato chips), judged by lay individuals to be relatively nonsticky, were much slower to clear the oral cavity, whereas those foods that were high in sucrose (e.g., caramels and jelly beans), judged as among the stickiest foods, exhibited a rapid clearance from the mouth.[24,25] However, epidemiologic studies have shown that in general starch is of low risk for dental caries. Consumers of high-starch/low sugar diets generally demonstrate low caries experience whereas consumers of low-starch/high sugar diets demonstrate high level of caries.[10] In the Hopewood House study, children consumed a high starch/low sugar diet and had low levels of caries.[15,16] Rugg-Gunn concluded that the cariogenicity of uncooked starch and cooked staple starchy foods such as rice, potatoes, and bread is low. On the other hand, finely ground and heat-treated starch can induce caries, but less so than sugars. Furthermore, the addition of sugar increases the cariogenicity of cooked starchy foods.[26]

Clearly no one cariogenicity test can account for all these factors except possibly trials in humans. Even in human trials, individual variations exist in plaque composition and amount, salivary buffering capacity, and enamel resistance to dissolution with or without the ability to remineralize.

Certain food components and factors may have cariostatic or caries-inhibiting effects. Phosphates, principally sodium metaphosphate, have been shown to reduce caries in animal studies.[27] The effect is probably local, related to buffering capacity, a reduction of enamel solubility, and other bacterial and biochemical properties. Unfortunately, clinical trials with phosphate supplements in human diets have not proved as effective.[28] Other animal studies[29] have shown that foods high in fat, protein, fluoride, or calcium may protect against caries. Such foods include cheese, yogurt, bologna, chocolate, and peanuts. Fats may protect by coating the teeth and reducing the retention of sugar and even plaque by changing the enamel's surface activity. Fats also may have toxic effects on oral bacteria and may decrease sugar solubility. Protein elevates the urea level in saliva and increases the buffering capacity of the saliva. Protein may also have an enamel-coating effect. Protein and fat in combination may raise plaque pH after exposure to carbohydrates. Tannins and other components of cocoa have been shown to suppress caries activity. The addition of fluoride to dietary sucrose in concentrations as low as 2 ppm has also been found to significantly reduce decay in rats.[30] Similar studies in humans have yet to be undertaken.

It has been proposed that the fibrous quality of some foods, such as celery or apples, may have a detergent effect on the teeth.[31] Such foods may remove gross debris during mastication, but they are ineffective at plaque removal. By requiring vigorous chewing, these foods may stimulate salivary flow, which in turn buffers plaque acid and promotes the remineralization of enamel.

Dietary Counseling

Stookey[32] has enumerated the attributes of the ideal snack as one that should (1) stimulate salivary flow by its physical form; (2) be minimally retentive; (3) be relatively high in protein and low in fat, have minimal fermentable carbohydrate, and have a moderate mineral content (especially calcium, phosphate, and fluoride); and (4) have a pH above 5.5 so as not to decrease oral pH, with a large acid-buffering capacity and a low sodium content. Certain foods, such as raw vegetables, meet most or all of these requirements. Present-day food technology should make it possible to create snacks that are nutritious and noncariogenic, but this will not happen until the food industry finds a reliable cariogenicity test and the incentives to invest in such production.

Based on evidence showing positive associations between sugars and caries, the World Health Organization (WHO) in 2015 issued guidelines calling for restricted sugar intake. The WHO guidelines include (1) a strong recommendation to reduce free sugar intake over the course of a lifetime, (2) a strong recommendation to limit free sugar intake to less than 10% of total energy (calories) consumed, and (3) a conditional recommendation to reduce the free sugar intake to less than 5% of total energy intake. The term *free sugar* refers to all mono- and disaccharides added to foods by the manufacturer, cook, or consumer plus sugars naturally present in honey, fruit juices, and syrups. The term "fermentable carbohydrates" refers to free sugars, glucose polymers, fermentable oligosaccharides, and highly refined starches. Less than 10% energy equates to less than 15 to 20 kg/person per year of sugar intake or less than 40 to 55 g/day.[33] Added sugar labeling and education are also included in the guidelines. What remains to be seen is how the findings will translate into public policies to induce positive behavior changes limiting the intake of sugars.[34]

In the meantime, we are left with the difficult but important task of working with families to improve the dietary habits of caries-susceptible children. The dental profession has an obligation to make dietary information available to them. Although it is neither feasible nor desirable to eliminate sugar completely from the diet, counseling and coaching should be provided to patients and families to lower the daily intake of free sugars, reduce the frequency of between-meal snacks, and limit sugars and processed cooked starches to mealtimes when salivary flow is higher. Lowering the frequency of fermentable carbohydrate ingestion is more important than reducing the total carbohydrate intake. Utilizing a risk-based chronic disease management approach[35,36] to addressing dental caries in clinical dental practice can be effective in assisting patients and their families to make sustainable changes in their dietary and oral hygiene practices and, in doing so, improving their caries risk (see the case study).

Summary

The period from ages 6 through 12 years is probably the most dynamic period for craniofacial, dental, emotional, and social changes in a child's growth. Growth modification and intervention related to dental eruption and space problems can be critical. All interventions are undertaken on a rapidly changing social and emotional substructure that can make success or failure precarious.

Effective counseling and coaching to establish and maintain healthy dietary habits as well as good oral hygiene are important to reduce the child's risk of developing dental caries.

References

1. Kuczmarski RJ, Ogden CL, Guo SS, et al. *CDC Growth Charts for the United States: Methods and Development*. Washington, DC: National Center for Health Statistics; 2000.
2. Broadbent BH Sr, Broadbent BH Jr, Golden WH. *Bolton Standards of Developmental Growth*. St Louis: Mosby; 1975.
3. Kapust AJ, Sinclair PM, Turley PK. Cephalometric effects of face mask/expansion therapy in Class III children: a comparison of three age groups. *Am J Orthod Dentofacial Orthop*. 1998;113(2):204–212.
4. Smith BH, Garn SM. Polymorphisms in eruption sequence of permanent teeth in American children. *Am J Phys Anthropol*. 1987;74:289–303.
5. Broadbent BH. The face of the normal child. *Angle Orthod*. 1937;7:183–208.
6. Piaget J. The stages of the intellectual development of the child. In: Marlowe BA, Canestrari AS, eds. *Educational Psychology in Context: Readings for Future Teachers*. Thousand Oaks, CA: Sage; 2006:98–106.
7. Eccles JS. The development of children ages 6 to 14. *Future Child*. 1999;9(2):30–44.
8. Stendler CB, Young N. Impact of first grade entrance upon the socialization of the child: changes after eight months of school. *Child Dev*. 1951;22:113–122.
9. Dye BA, Lopez G, Mitnik MS, et al. Trends in dental caries in children and adolescents according to poverty status in the United States from 1999 through 2004 and 2011 through 2014. *J Am Dent Assoc*. 2017;148:550–565.
10. Moynihan P, Petersen PE. Diet, nutrition and the prevention of dental caries. *Public Health Nutr*. 2004;7(1A):201–226.
11. Newbrun E. Sucrose, the arch criminal of dental caries. *J Dent Child*. 1969;36:239–248.
12. Koulourides T, Bodden S, Keller S, et al. Cariogenicity of nine sugars tested with and intraoral device in man. *Caries Res*. 1976;10:427–441.
13. Stephan RM. Effect of different types of human foods in dental health of experimental animals. *J Dent Res*. 1966;45:1551–1561.
14. Gustafsson B, Quensel CE, Lanke L, et al. The Vipeholm dental caries study: the effect of different carbohydrate intake on 436 individuals observed for five years. *Acta Odontol Scand*. 1954;11:232–264.
15. Sullivan HR, Goldsworthy NE. Review and correlation of the data presented in papers 1-6 (Hopewood House study). *Aust Dent J*. 1958;3:395–398.
16. Sullivan HR, Harris R. Hopewood House study 2. Observations on oral conditions. *Aust Dent J*. 1958;3:311–317.
17. Walker ARP, Cleaton-Jones PE. Sugar intake and dental caries: where do we stand? *ASDC J Dent Child*. 1989;56:30–35.
18. Burt BA, Pai S. Sugar consumption and caries risk: a systematic review. *J Dent Educ*. 2001;65:1017–1023.
19. Marshall TA, Eichenberger-Gilmore JM, Larson MA, et al. Comparison of the intakes of sugars by young children with and without caries experience. *J Am Dent Assoc*. 2007;138:39–46.
20. Sheiham A, James WPT. Diet and dental caries: the pivotal role of free sugars reemphasized. *J Dent Res*. 2015;94(10):1341–1347.
21. Holbrook WP, Arnadottir IB, Takazoe I, et al. Longitudinal study of caries, cariogenic bacteria and diet in children just before and after starting school. *Eur J Oral Sci*. 1995;103(1):42–45.
22. Ismail AI, Burt BA, Eklund SA. The cariogenicity of soft drinks in the United States. *J Am Dent Assoc*. 1984;109:241–245.
23. Bibby BG. Fruits and vegetables and dental caries. *Clin Prev Dent*. 1983;5:3–11.
24. Kashket S, van Houte J, Lopez LR, et al. Lack of correlation between food retention on the human dentition and consumer perception of food stickiness. *J Dent Res*. 1991;70:1314–1319.
25. Luke GA, Hough H, Beeley JA, et al. Human salivary sugar clearance after sugar rinses and intake of foodstuffs. *Caries Res*. 1999;33:123–129.
26. Rugg-Gunn AJ. *Nutrition and Dental Health*. Oxford: Oxford Medical Publications; 1993.
27. Nizel AE, Harris RS. The effects of phosphate on experimental dental caries: a literature review. *J Dent Res*. 1964;43:1123–1136.
28. Lilienthal B. Phosphates and dental caries. In: Myers H, ed. *Monographs in Oral Science*. Basel, Switzerland: Karger; 1976.
29. Featherstone JDB, Mundorff SA. *Identification of the Cariogenic Elements of Foods*. Final report for period September 1981–May 1984. Alexandria, VA: National Technical Information Service; 1984.
30. Mundorff SA, Glowinsky D, Griffin C. Fluoridated sucrose effect on rat caries. *J Dent Res*. 1986;65(special issue):282(abstract 1017).
31. Caldwell RC. Physical properties of foods and their caries-producing potential. *J Dent Res*. 1970;49:1293–1298.
32. Stookey GK. Developing the perfect snack food. In: Alfano MC, ed. *Changing Perspectives in Nutrition and Caries Research*. New York: Medcom; 1979.
33. Moynihan PJ, Kelley SAM. Effect on caries of restricting sugars intake: systematic review to inform WHO guidelines. *J Dent Res*. 2014;93(1):8–18.
34. Meyer BD, Lee JY. The confluence of sugar, dental caries, and health policy. *J Dent Res*. 2015;94(10):1338–1340.
35. Edelstein BL, Ng MW. Chronic disease management of strategies of early childhood caries: support from the medical and dental literature. *Pediatr Dent*. 2015;37(3):281–287.
36. Ng MW, Fida Z. Early childhood caries prevention and management. In: Berg JH, Slayton RL, eds. *Early Childhood Oral Health*. Hoboken, NJ: John Wiley & Sons; 2016.

31

Examination, Diagnosis, and Treatment Planning

SCOTT B. SCHWARTZ, JOHN R. CHRISTENSEN, AND HENRY FIELDS

3. *Development of skills in personal oral hygiene.* The child emerging from the middle school years should have acquired the skills and knowledge to conduct effective personal oral hygiene.
4. *Participation in health care decisions.* Historically, dentists are taught to see the school-aged child as a passive recipient of care; however, the current health care landscape has become a dynamic decision-making environment. The dentist should be prepared to manage issues and challenges related to parental consent versus patient assent as young children transition into their teenage years. Usually during this period, children begin to develop an image of themselves, aspects of which will relate to their facial and dental esthetics. Although this image may be influenced by their parents, it is often unique to the child's perspective. The development of this self-image may influence the compliance of the child and affect the desire to take responsibility for his or her own health.

The History

Elements of history taking and recording are discussed in Chapter 19. An important aspect of history taking in this group should be the involvement of the child. While the parent remains the historian of choice, the role of the child can evolve from being the listener into the active participant. By adolescence, the child can provide accurate, valuable information. Adolescents should be encouraged to become participants in relaying an accurate medical history, particularly through a well-developed physician-patient relationship. A health history form should address issues like those applicable to the younger child, but with different expectations. The differences in patient history for children in this age group in general include the following:

1. *Medical intervention has usually occurred.* Most children have a physician and may have experienced an emergency visit or some invasive procedure. School enrollment has required a physical examination and other treatment for most children.
2. *The health history is more involved.* By this time, most childhood-onset disorders have manifested themselves, but some may not have been noted. Therefore, it is important to continue to conduct a thorough systems review. Because more children are surviving early childhood cancer, additional attention should be given to determine the types of treatments encountered. Full body or smaller field radiation therapy, chemotherapy, and the use of bisphosphonates all carry risks related to tooth

Examination of the child in the transitional years presents a diagnostic dilemma of managing oral health at a dynamic stage of development. Although the preschooler's dentition is relatively stable, the child in the transitional years progresses from a full complement of primary teeth through a mixed dentition to a full permanent dentition excluding the third molars. Maintaining the ease and success of this transition constitutes the main challenge for the dentist treating this age group. A large part of this chapter is devoted to orthodontic considerations, but the other elements of significance in dental management of this age group should not be ignored. They are as follows:

1. *Preventive considerations related to dental sealants, nutrition, and fluoride intake.* The eruption of permanent teeth requires that a decision be made about sealant application. Entry into the more heterogeneous, less controlled environment of school places the child at risk for increased carbohydrate exposure. The child's access to fluoride in school, diet, and other sources makes regular reevaluation of fluoride exposure a necessity. Preventive strategies must be reviewed as caries risk factors change during this dynamic period.
2. *Prevention and management of trauma.* The school-aged child may be active in sports. For a period in the school years, the permanent maxillary incisors are at greater risk for traumatic injury, especially if they protrude.

development, eruption, and bone quality when considering surgical interventions and tooth movement.

3. *The dental history is evolving.* Children usually have undergone a dental visit as part of school enrollment. In the transitional years, the patient increases independence at school and in social venues. Diet history, caries risk, and the preventive regimen at home change significantly.

4. *The history should capture those children early on the curve of health experiences.* As children transition into this age group, sensitive topics may become relevant to the dentist. Some instances in which the involvement of an adolescent historian may have profound benefits for both health care provider and patient are (1) onset and frequency of sexual activity related to presence of various oral pathologies and pregnancy; (2) use of alcohol, tobacco, and other substances that can increase risk of disease; and (3) psychiatric issues such as anorexia nervosa and bulimia. Adolescents who are pregnant are more visible in the current social climate. Given the sensitive nature of the information that may be disclosed by the patient at this age, the dentist should try to provide appropriate space from parent or guardian to ensure the confidentiality of responses.

The Examination

As in younger children, the dental examination includes a behavioral assessment; general appraisal; and head and neck, facial, intraoral, and radiographic examinations.

Behavioral Assessment

Another advantage for the dentist is the child's emergence into a period when few children experience behavioral problems that cannot be resolved with simple, nonpharmacologic behavior guidance techniques. Even early in this period, many children can be reasoned with to accept dental treatment. The child who resists attempts at careful and compassionate explanations of care may require special attention and further evaluation from a medical provider. The rising awareness and prevalence of attention disorders and other conditions such as autism spectrum disorder pose new challenges for the dental provider. A thorough review of the patient's history should identify current pharmacologic and other therapeutic approaches to behavioral and psychological diagnoses. It is imperative that the dentist is familiar with the diagnostic criteria for such conditions and is prepared to implement a more nuanced approach to care. The next step is to "chair-test" the child, using the dentist's proven techniques of managing children. The technique used may be tell-show-do, positive reinforcement, voice control, or some other method that has worked consistently in the past. Remember that consent must be obtained from the parent if the behavior management technique used is not one that a reasonable parent would expect.[1] New environments, particularly the dental clinic, can exacerbate anxiety and behavior issues for any child, especially those with a previously identified behavioral diagnosis. If behavioral intervention fails, the dentist should consider further evaluation or referral. Some causes of extreme behavior problems in this age group include substance abuse, physical or sexual abuse, family problems, or a learning disability.

General Appraisal

The school-aged population provides a wide range of physical and emotional profiles, yet the general appraisal should be easier from

several standpoints. First, the school-aged child should have developed gross motor skills and any variations from normal should be obvious. For example, the toddler may be active but still clumsy. The school-aged child, even at the early end of this age group, can play with skill. Speech development should also well exceed that of the preschooler as should the child's emotional and intellectual status. This adaptation is really a manifestation of development of the brain and is one reason why schooling begins at this age.

One advantage available to the dentist who treats children in this age group is the host of health professionals with whom he or she can work if problems are noted. School placement often has identified problem areas and the appropriate therapy usually has been initiated. These professionals can assist in clarifying findings made during the dental visit. Table 31.1 lists some characteristics of the school-aged child that are important in the diagnostic process.

Determination of Developmental Status

Patients in early adolescence are clearly growing, but in the later stages growth slows dramatically and at some point, nearly ceases. The same is roughly true for facial growth. When patients are clearly growing, growth modification can be attempted. Many

TABLE 31.1	Selected Developmental Characteristics of the 6- to 12-Year-Old Child	
Intellectual Development		**Physical Development**
Demonstrates school readiness early in this period		Refinement of motor skills occurs as central nervous system develops
Should be able to read and write in this period		Spine straightens to improve posture
Becomes capable of logical thought		Sinuses enlarge
Psychological Development		Lymphoid system reaches high point of development
Acquires a sense of accomplishment for tasks		
Learns responsibility for actions		
Develops a sense of right and wrong		
Looks outside the home for standards or values		
Physiologic Development		
6-Year-Old	**9-Year-Old**	**12-Year-Old**
Height		
Boys = 121 cm	Boys = 140 cm	Boys = 154 cm
Girls = 119 cm	Girls = 137 cm	Girls = 157 cm
(Growth rate is approximately 6 cm/year in this period.)		
Weight (75th Percentile)		
Boys = 24 kg	Boys = 33 kg	Boys = 44 kg
Girls = 23 kg	Girls = 32 kg	Girls = 45 kg
(Growth rate is approximately 3–3.5 kg/year in this period.)		
Pulse (Average for Age)		
100 beats/min	90 beats/min	85–90 beats/min
Respiration (50th Percentile)		
23 breaths/min	20 breaths/min	18 breaths/min
Blood Pressure (Average for Age)		
105/60 mm Hg	110/65 mm Hg	115.65 mm Hg

clinicians believe that growth modification is easiest when the child is undergoing accelerated growth during the adolescent growth spurt.

This judgment on treatment timing would be much easier if a biological marker could be identified that provided definitive information about the developmental status of the patient. Growth modification could be started if the marker indicated that sufficient growth remained to alter skeletal relationships. To be clinically useful, this biological marker would have to be reliable, easily identified, recognized in both sexes, and closely correlated with the growth of the facial bones. Unfortunately, a single biological marker of this description is not available. Several clinical markers have been identified. However, studies have indicated that the relationship between the markers and facial growth, although statistically significant, is not so precise that growth can be predicted accurately. Because of the limited predictive value of the markers, one marker alone is seldom used; instead, several are combined with multiple evaluations.

Height and weight measurements are often used to determine the patient's growth status. Measurements are plotted on standardized growth charts to indicate the relative size of the patient. An average-sized child is located near the 50th percentile, and a large child is somewhere near the 90th percentile. A single measurement does not provide the clinician with all pertinent growth information, but it does give some idea about where the patient is developmentally compared with other children at this age.

A series of measurements, which may be available from the patient's physician or school nurse, provides much more information. The dentist should record height and weight measurements at each periodic visit. The measurements can be plotted in one of two ways. The first way is to plot the measurements on a cumulative growth chart (Fig. 31.1). This provides information about the patient's total amount of growth up to the last measurement. The normal growth curve is sigmoidal and the pubertal growth spurt corresponds to the steepest portion of the slope. Because growth charts are based on mean growth rates, the individual patient may show an accelerated or delayed growth spurt if his or her growth rate is not coincident with the mean growth rate. More importantly, some concern should be expressed if the patient is not following the percentiles (e.g., dropping from the 50th to the 40th to the 30th percentile over time). This suggests there may be a physical or psychological problem requiring medical attention.

Height and weight measurements can also be plotted as yearly growth increments rather than as total growth achieved up to that point (Fig. 31.2). By plotting measurements this way, changes in the growth rate can be easily identified. A sharp rise in height usually signals the start of the pubertal growth spurt and growth modification treatment should be initiated immediately if it is required.

Height and weight measurements also can be compared with the height and weight of the patient's natural parents and siblings. Although the interaction between environment and heredity is not clearly understood, there is some familial influence on ultimate size, and it may be possible to glean useful information from the comparison.

Hand-wrist radiographs have been used by some investigators to judge the skeletal age and development of the patient. The size and maturational stage of certain hand and wrist bones are compared with published standards of normal bone development and skeletal age.[2] Unfortunately, the correlation between the appearance of reliable bone markers (skeletal growth status) and mean maximal mandibular growth velocity is not perfect and should not serve as the only index of facial growth. There are several problems with this method of determining developmental status by the dentists. First, it requires an additional radiograph. Second, the ability to reliably read hand-wrist radiographs requires consistent practice that is rarely gained in routine patient care.

Another radiographic method that does not require additional radiation exposure is the use of cervical vertebral maturation from diagnostic cephalometric radiographs (Fig. 31.3). This method uses the maturation stages of the second through fourth cervical vertebrae (Fig. 31.4) to evaluate mandibular growth potential. It is claimed that the peak mandibular growth occurs between stages 2 and 3 in the five-stage method.[3] Timing treatment for growth modification during this period of growth, according to some, could enhance the treatment effects.[4] There is some disagreement regarding the reliability of this method but is has been shown to be highly reliable for making the determination whether a patient's mandibular growth rate is still increasing or has passed its peak (i.e., stage 1 or 2 vs. stage 3, 4, or 5). The stage of mandibular growth is the clinically relevant determination for the patient being considered for growth modification.[5]

Secondary sexual characteristics provide some information about the amount of growth the patient has yet to experience. In females, breast stage development and menarche are markers that can be used to assess developmental status. Breast development determination as an objective clinical evaluation is obviously not practical in the dental office and is of little clinical use. Menarche, however, can be determined from the health history questionnaire or from an interview at the initial patient examination. Unfortunately, the pubertal growth spurt precedes menarche by more than 1 year.[6] Therefore, menarche is basically used to decide whether growth modification is still feasible.

In males, there is no single indicator such as menarche by which to judge developmental status. The amount and texture of facial hair and the patient's general physical appearance are two highly variable indicators of male developmental status and maturity. Facial hair usually appears near or following peak statural growth.

For a person with an obvious skeletal problem, more than one cephalometric head film of the patient may be available. These head films can be superimposed to provide information about the amount and direction of growth that has occurred over time (see later discussion on cephalometric analyses and Fig. 31.53). Although past growth tendencies do not guarantee that the patient will continue to grow or will grow according to the same pattern, comparing head films provides a great deal of information about the patient's growth history. However, it is unlikely for the average patient to have a series of head films available for pretreatment review. It is sometimes beneficial to obtain a cephalometric head film on a parent if the patient closely resembles the parent. While not definitive, the film can provide a "blueprint" to predict the patient's growth.

The patient's developmental status can also be judged from the developmental stage of the dentition. Panoramic or periapical radiographs can be used to determine the stage of development of individual permanent teeth. The results can be compared with standards relating dental development to chronological age.[7] However, studies indicate that the relationship between dental age and skeletal maturation is weak and clinically useless.[8]

In summary, several biological markers are available by which the clinician can assess the developmental status of the patient. Unfortunately, no one marker by itself provides definitive information about the patient's growth potential. The most logical approach is to gather all available information and then make a judgment

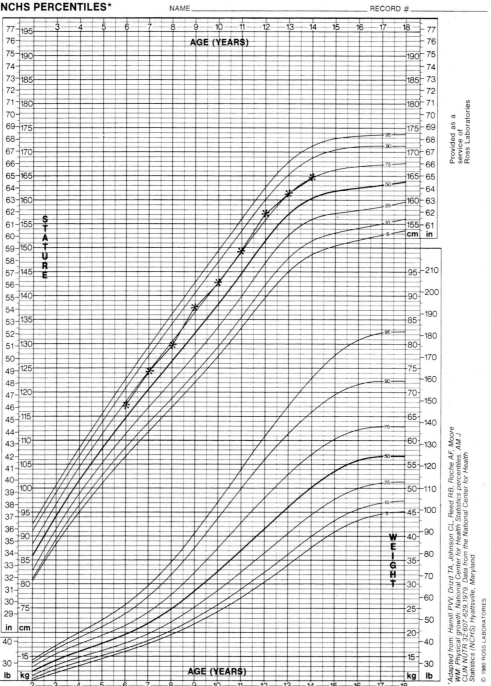

GIRLS: 2 TO 18 YEARS
PHYSICAL GROWTH
NCHS PERCENTILES*

NAME _____ RECORD # _____

• **Figure 31.1** A standardized growth chart is used to indicate the relative size of the patient. A single measurement does not provide the clinician with all pertinent growth information, but it does give some idea of the developmental level of the patient compared with other children at a particular time. A series of measurements plotted on a standardized growth chart provides much more information than a single measurement. The measurements may be plotted in two ways. In the cumulative growth chart method, illustrated here, asterisks plot the measurements. This chart shows the patient's total growth up to the last measurement. This female patient has been measured yearly, starting at age 6 years, and is roughly following the 75th percentile line. (Modified from Hamill PVV, Drizd TA, Johnson CL, et al. Physical growth: National Center for Health Statistics percentiles. *Am J Clin Nutr.* 1979;32:607–629. Data from the National Center for Health Statistics, Hyattsville, MD; Courtesy Ross Laboratories.)

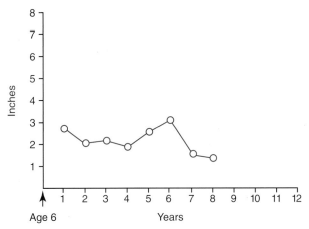

• **Figure 31.2** Growth information also can be plotted as yearly growth increments rather than as total growth achieved to a certain point. The growth data for the female patient described in Fig. 31.1 are plotted here incrementally, beginning at age 6 years. By plotting measurements this way, changes in the growth rate can be easily identified. A sharp rise usually signals the start of the pubertal growth spurt.

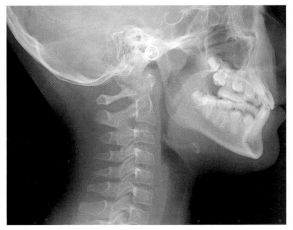

• **Figure 31.3** Another method used to gauge growth status is evaluation of the shape of cervical vertebrae 2, 3, and 4. These images are available on routine cephalometric radiographs and require no additional radiation. It appears they can be reliably read and are interpreted according to the stages described in Fig. 31.4.

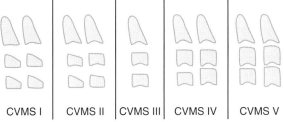

CVMS I   CVMS II   CVMS III   CVMS IV   CVMS V

• **Figure 31.4** The five stages of cervical vertebrae maturation are described in this diagram. These stages are equated with physical maturation, somatic growth, and mandibular growth. According to the reported data, peak mandibular growth is experienced before stage III. A concavity develops on the lower border of the third vertebra during stage II and a similar one develops on the lower border of the fourth vertebra during stage III. Vertebrae 3 and 4 undergo gradual transformation from horizontally rectangular shape to square to vertically rectangular shape during the maturation process. *CVMS,* Cervical vertebrae maturation stage. (Redrawn from Baccetti T, Franchi L, McNamara JA Jr. An improved version of the cervical vertebral maturation [CVM] method for the assessment of mandibular growth. *Angle Orthod.* 2002;72:316–323.)

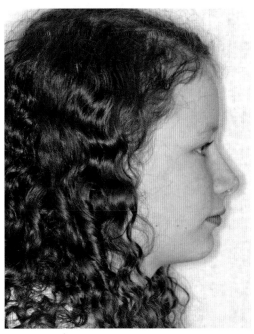

• **Figure 31.5** The ideal soft tissue profile for the bridge of the nose, the base of the upper lip, and the chin is slightly convex to straight in the anteroposterior dimension in the 6- to 12-year-old child. This child demonstrates that type profile and well-balanced vertical proportions with the lower face slightly larger than the middle facial third.

regarding the patient's growth potential and suitability for growth modification.

Head and Neck Examination

The head and neck examination should be completed in a manner similar to that outlined in Chapter 19.

Facial Examination

Facial examination of the 6- to 12-year-old child is a systematic examination of the face in three planes of space. It is essentially the same as the facial examination described in Chapter 19, and the reader should review that information if necessary. This section comments on findings that are particularly important for the 6- to 12-year-old.

In examination of the profile, one notes the anteroposterior and vertical dimensions of the face and the position of the lips and incisors relative to the face. The ideal soft tissue profile is slightly convex (Fig. 31.5), practically speaking a bit straighter with more mandibular contribution than that of the preschool-aged group. Most clinicians find that detection of anteroposterior skeletal problems is somewhat easier in this age group, possibly because of reduced soft tissue thickness. A mild mandibular deficiency in a 4-year-old child may have been difficult to diagnose initially, but it is more apparent at age 8 years and even more obvious at age 12 years. In most cases, skeletal relationships can be confirmed by the dental relationships (molar and overjet). That means that if the facial form (convex, straight, or concave) matches the dental relationships (respectively, class I molar and moderate overjet, class II molar and 5- to 6-mm overjet, or class III molar and zero or negative overjet), there is usually not much doubt about the skeletal relationships. If a skeletal problem exists, the source of the discrepancy is identified by comparing the position of the maxilla and mandible with a vertical reference line through soft tissue nasion (see Chapter 19, Figs. 19.1 and 19.2). This helps to direct treatment, if indicated, to the skeletal component at fault.

Again, in this age group, vertical profile assessment continues to concentrate on the proportionality of the middle and lower facial thirds. At this point, growth has increased the vertical linear facial dimensions, and the proportionality of the well-balanced face remains basically the same, but the lower facial third is slightly larger than the middle facial third. Research has indicated that vertical dysplasia usually is confined to the lower facial third in this age group.[9] Therefore the middle third can be compared with the lower facial third (see Fig. 31.5).

Incisor and lip position should be examined carefully in this age group. The child is entering the mixed dentition period, and the position of the erupted permanent incisors generally is reflected in the position of the lips. The upper lip gives a good indication of the underlying position of the maxillary incisor. The position of the lower lip also depends on the position of the maxillary incisor because the lower lip normally covers 1 to 2 mm of the maxillary incisal edge at rest. Therefore lip posture is a strong indicator of maxillary dental protrusion. Lip and incisor position should always be considered in the context of the nose and chin. A large nose and chin are more able to accommodate protrusive incisors and lips than are a small nose and chin. As a rule, for white children, the lips should be positioned on or slightly behind a line connecting the tip of the nose with the chin (Fig. 31.6). Most Asian and African American children have more incisor and lip protrusion than white children. When the incisors are fully erupted, it is possible to begin to consider their vertical position relative to the lips. This gives an indication of some critical esthetic relationships. Lips tend to grow vertically throughout the early adolescent years. It is not uncommon to see children early in this

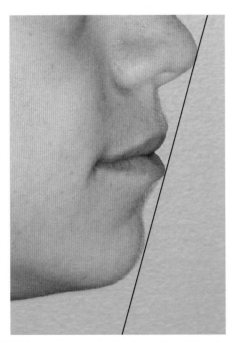

• **Figure 31.6** In this age group, the lips are positioned on or slightly behind a line connecting the tip of the nose with the soft tissue chin. Lip position must be considered in the context of the nose and chin. A large nose and chin are better able to accommodate protrusive lips than are a small nose and chin.

age group with incompetent lips (lips that do not approximate or have more than a couple of millimeters of separation at rest). The maximum display of incisors at rest and maximum lip incompetence occur around 11 years in females and 12 years in males.[10] Most children become more lip competent as they mature. Ideally a child shows about 2 mm of tooth below the relaxed lip line. At full smile, they show nearly the full tooth with the upper lip retracting to a couple of millimeters below the cervical area of the tooth. Gingival exposure of not more than 2 mm is considered esthetically acceptable for this age group. Of course, there can be much variation while still maintaining good esthetics, but these are generally accepted guidelines.

Intraoral Examination

The procedures used for oral examination are like those used in the preschool group and include charting of teeth and dental caries. Less emphasis on managing the child's behavior during the examination process is needed because these children are more cooperative. The areas of evaluation that require more emphasis are the periodontal, preventive, and orthodontic aspects.

Periodontal Evaluation

A thorough examination of this age group involves both periodontal probing and use of a gingival index (GI) if inflammation is a problem. If orthodontic treatment is a consideration, it may be delayed or the treatment plan altered if the periodontal tissues are not healthy. Orthodontic treatment initiated during periods of active gingival or periodontal disease may further compromise periodontal health because fixed appliances are difficult to keep clean, and existing inflammatory conditions are exacerbated, resulting in further loss of supporting structures. The periodontal examination should address the following aspects:

1. *Selective probing of anterior teeth and permanent first molars.* A periodontal probe is necessary to evaluate the health of the tissues properly (Fig. 31.7). The probe measures the depth of the sulcus and the amount of free marginal and attached gingiva. Bleeding upon probing is also an indication of active gingival disease. Sulcular depths of greater than 3 mm and attached gingiva of less than 1 mm indicate possible periodontal problems, and further evaluation is warranted. The likelihood of bone loss and apical migration of the attachment is low, but some children in this age group experience aggressive periodontitis. Erupting teeth usually have a deep sulcus until the crown is fully erupted. Gingival inflammation in early puberty may also confound pocket-depth measurements.

2. *Evaluation of tissue attachments, especially those of the lower anterior teeth.* Facial clefts and recession due to malpositioned teeth and inflammation, if identified early, can be successfully managed with tissue grafting, tooth movement, or a combination of both (Fig. 31.8). The amount of attached gingiva also should be considered in the context of the type of tooth movement being planned. Facial movement of a lower incisor with minimal attached gingiva may cause further loss of attachment, and an evaluation by a periodontist is indicated. Often simply proceeding cautiously will be acceptable, but in other instances a gingival grafting procedure may be considered. Lingual movement of the same incisor does not involve the risk of attachment loss and may even contribute to an increase in health or the amount of attached tissue. Last, the position of the frena and their height of attachment on the alveolar ridge should be determined via gentle manipulation of the lips and cheeks. Occasionally

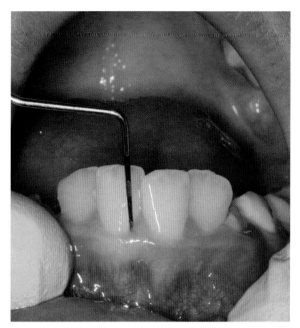

• **Figure 31.7** During examination of each arch, a periodontal probe is used to evaluate gingival health. Special attention should be paid to increased pocket depth, lack of attached gingiva, and bleeding upon probing. Orthodontic treatment that is initiated during periods of active gingival or periodontal disease may further compromise periodontal health.

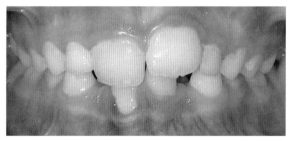

• **Figure 31.8** This labial gingival cleft is just beginning, probably caused by poor oral hygiene and the heavy occlusion on the prominent lower incisor. It should be evaluated before orthodontic treatment.

• **BOX 31.1** **Types of Frenal Attachments**

Mucosal—when the frenal fibers are attached up to the mucogingival junction.
Gingival—when the fibers are inserted within the attached gingiva.
Papillary—when the fibers are extending into the interdental papilla.
Papilla penetrating—when the frenal fibers cross the alveolar process and extend up to the palatine papilla.

---

frenal attachments near the crest of the ridge must be repositioned before or after orthodontic treatment because they pull on attached marginal tissue and compromise gingival health or prevent space closure. There are four types of frenal attachments (Box 31.1).[11] The first is mucosal. This is when the frenal fibers attach up to the mucogingival junction. When fibers insert within the attached gingival tissue, the frenal attachment is termed *gingival*. A papillary attachment is defined as fibers extending into the interdental papilla. Lastly, the papilla penetrating attachment occurs when the frenal fibers cross the alveolar

process and extend into the palatine papilla. Generally a frenum is indicated for removal when there is an aberrant attachment causing a midline diastema or when the frenum is attached so closely to the attached gingival tissue that there is inadequate gingival tissue covering the tooth or there is gingival recession.

3. *Identification of problem areas, such as mandibular and maxillary anterior teeth.* Calculus accumulation, inflammation secondary to anterior crowding, poor cleaning, and eruptive gingivitis are examples of localized problems that require specialized attention.

Numerous gingival indices exist to assess inflammation.[12] The GI[13] can be adapted for pediatric use. The GI uses the following scoring system: 0 = normal gingiva; 1 = mild inflammation: slight change in color, slight edema, no bleeding on probing; 2 = moderate inflammation: redness, edema, and glazing, or bleeding on probing; 3 = severe inflammation: marked redness and edema, tendency toward spontaneous bleeding, ulceration.

In the private practice setting, it may be easier to modify an existing index, using key teeth to provide baseline readings and progress. These readings can be recorded on the examination form adjacent to the data for the teeth being examined. Routine performance of full-mouth probing is not warranted.

Oral Hygiene Evaluation

The assessment of clinical needs and patient skills in oral hygiene is a part of the examination process. The history should reveal a pattern of personal care and the clinical examination should document the effectiveness of care and address problem areas in the oral cavity. A patient's brushing skills and dexterity in flossing can be judged at chairside and are generally directly correlated with classically difficult-to-clean areas such as plaque accumulation on teeth opposite to the side on which the brush is held, buccally placed canine teeth, and lingual surfaces. This information should be used to formulate an individual hygiene strategy. If orthodontic treatment is being considered, oral hygiene instructions should be given before orthodontic treatment is started and should be consistently reinforced during the treatment. In some cases it is prudent to delay orthodontic treatment until oral hygiene can be maintained at an acceptable level.

Occlusal Evaluation

The occlusal evaluation is organized around a systematic approach to alignment and the anteroposterior, transverse, and vertical planes of space.[14]

Alignment

The intraoral occlusal examination in the mixed dentition begins with an assessment of arch form and alignment characteristics. An ideal arch should be symmetric in the anteroposterior and transverse dimensions. Minor asymmetry may exist but is usually confined to the anterior region if there is inadequate space for eruption of the permanent incisors. Significant asymmetry is rare and is usually indicative of skeletal asymmetry or some type of oral habit or crossbite that has displaced the teeth and alveolus. The arch form is described as U or V shaped. Alignment problems are usually the result of a true arch length deficiency or a transitional arch length deficiency due to the size of the erupting permanent teeth. These are most common in the anterior portions of the arch but can occur anywhere. The type of alignment problem should be noted during the examination. The teeth can be tipped, bodily positioned, or rotated in their aberrant location. These types of positioning errors have definite implications for the type of treatment that can be recommended.

Tooth Number

After the form and symmetry of each arch have been characterized, it is imperative to count the number of permanent and primary teeth. A clinical examination and appropriate radiographs allow the practitioner to determine which teeth are present, developing, or missing. Disturbances in the initiation and proliferation stage of tooth development may lead to an abnormal number of teeth. Teeth that do not form are referred to as congenitally missing (Fig. 31.9). The most common missing teeth in the permanent dentition, apart from the maxillary and mandibular third molars, are the mandibular second premolar, maxillary lateral incisor, and maxillary second premolar in that order.[15] In general, the most distal tooth in a class of teeth is most liable to be congenitally missing. Some have looked at whether there is a genetic component to missing and impacted teeth. It is reported that patients with palatally impacted canines exhibit a higher incidence of missing permanent teeth than the general population and that several generations in the family will exhibit the same palatal impaction (Fig. 31.10).[16] Recent evidence suggests there are specific genes that cause specific

tooth loss when there is a mutation.[17] It is apparent that future genetic study may identify more genes that affect tooth development. The practical implication of a missing anterior tooth is to look elsewhere in the mouth for more eruption or tooth development issues (additional missing teeth, impaction, or transpositions).

Another cause of missing or malformed teeth is radiation therapy or chemotherapy. This can affect the formation and eruption of the teeth developing at the time or those in the field of the therapeutic beam. Generally patients treated with radiation before age 5 years will have more anomalies of dental development, but patients receiving chemotherapy and older patients who still have developing teeth are also likely affected (Fig. 31.11).[18]

Supernumerary teeth are teeth added to the normal complement of teeth. These teeth are found in about 2% of the population and are most often found in the maxillary midline region.[19] Midline supernumerary teeth are also called mesiodens (Fig. 31.12). Supernumerary teeth are also found distal to the maxillary molars and in the mandibular premolar regions.

Although not a tooth in the strictest sense, the odontoma is discussed in this section on tooth number. The odontoma is a benign mixed tumor of enamel and dentin that is diagnosed radiographically. Two types of odontomas are identified. Odontomas that resemble teeth are called compound odontomas; those that are irregularly shaped are labeled complex odontomas. Both types may interfere with normal tooth eruption and are usually treated by surgical removal before eruption problems arise but late enough to avoid surgical trauma to adjacent developing teeth (Fig. 31.13).

Tooth Structure

Disturbances in the morphodifferentiation and histodifferentiation stages of tooth development result in alterations of tooth size and shape. Each arch should be examined for generalized large (macrodontia) or small (microdontia) teeth and for localized tooth size discrepancies. Generalized large or small teeth usually can be aligned so that there is a compatible occlusal relationship if the teeth in both arches are equally affected. However, localized tooth size problems make it difficult to establish good dental relationships. Again, the most distal tooth in the dental class is the one most often affected. Undersized maxillary lateral incisors and mandibular second premolars are the most common isolated problems in tooth size (see Fig. 31.10A). These also appear to be genetically linked

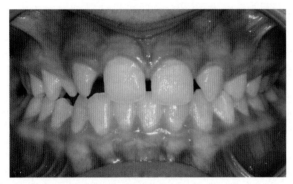

• **Figure 31.9** This patient is congenitally missing both permanent maxillary lateral incisors, and the permanent maxillary canines have spontaneously substituted in their places. The most common missing teeth in the permanent dentition, besides the third molars, are the maxillary lateral incisor and the mandibular second premolar.

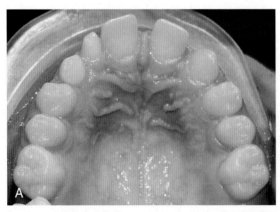
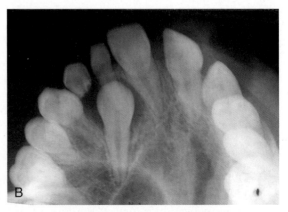

• **Figure 31.10** (A) The occurrence of multiple anomalies of tooth position, number, and shape linked by genetics is demonstrated in this patient who has an erupted peg-shaped permanent maxillary right lateral incisor and a retained primary maxillary right canine. (B) The occlusal radiograph shows the peg lateral, the missing permanent maxillary left lateral incisor, and the ectopically erupting permanent maxillary right canine.

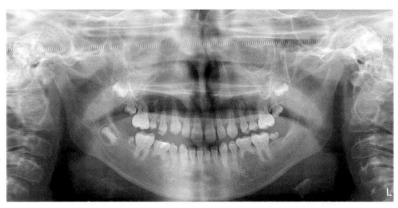

• **Figure 31.11** This patient was diagnosed with a primitive neuroectodermal tumor and was treated with radiation and chemotherapy from the ages of 2 to 4 years. The teeth developing during that time period are stunted, missing, or have arrested root development. Of interest, the third molars are developing normally because their development started after the end of the therapy.

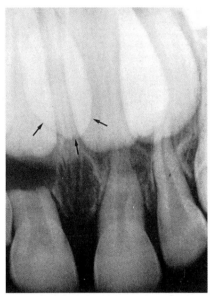

• **Figure 31.12** A midline supernumerary tooth, or mesiodens, is situated between the unerupted maxillary central incisors. Arrows indicate the position of the mesiodens, which can cause disturbances in eruption and adjacent tooth formation.

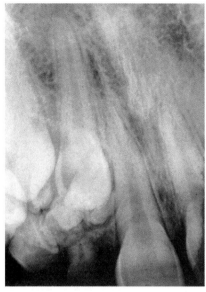

• **Figure 31.13** An odontoma is impeding the eruption of the maxillary right lateral incisor and canine. The odontoma should be surgically removed before eruption problems arise but late enough to avoid surgical trauma to the adjacent developing teeth. (Courtesy Dr. Phillip R. Parker.)

anomalies, so evaluating patients with peg laterals should include evaluation for palatally displaced canines, additional missing teeth, and transpositions. Sometimes complex orthodontic and restorative treatment is necessary to achieve a harmonious occlusal relationship and satisfy esthetic requirements when local tooth size problems exist. This type of treatment usually amounts to distributing space between the teeth so that when the teeth are restored to normal size and contour, they fit in a good occlusal relationship with good anterior esthetics (Fig. 31.14). Other times, treatment may mean reducing the mesiodistal dimension of oversized crowns through interproximal reduction (Fig. 31.15).

Teeth with abnormal crown and root morphologic characteristics may create occlusal problems. Careful clinical and radiographic examination is necessary to diagnose these problems. If the abnormality involves the crown (maxillary peg lateral or talon cusp), either the crown should be recontoured by addition of restorative material to increase its size or the talon cusp should be

reduced in size by selective equilibration to eliminate occlusal interference (Fig. 31.16). Both conditions usually require tooth movement before definitive restorative care to obtain an esthetically pleasing and functional result. Root structure abnormalities such as significant dilaceration may make orthodontic movement of teeth difficult (Fig. 31.17). Often the portion of the root apical to the irregularity is resorbed or remodeled during tooth movement. If a tooth with root abnormalities is scheduled for extraction, it may be prudent to refer the patient to a specialist because the abnormality will certainly complicate the extraction. Finally, fused or geminated teeth can pose difficulties due to their size. The clinician should consult with other dental specialists because the treatment will often involve a combination of endodontics, surgery, orthodontics, and restorative care.[20,21]

Clearly, in this age group four upper and lower incisors should be evident early on. When they are not, concern and follow-up are warranted. The clinician should recognize that it is highly

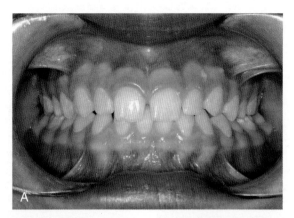

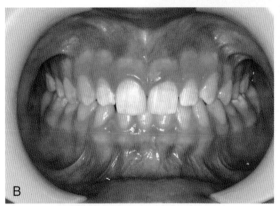

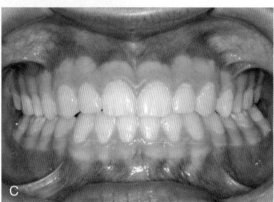

• **Figure 31.14** (A) In this case, a maxillary tooth size deficiency contributed to the diastema. If the space was closed with orthodontics, the resulting occlusion would not be correct. In addition, the tapered crown form of the central incisor would result in less than ideal esthetics. (B) Composite resin was added to the mesial surface of both central incisors before orthodontic treatment to correct the tooth size deficiency and give the teeth normal contour. (C) The orthodontic result shows excellent occlusion and esthetics.

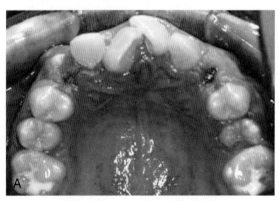

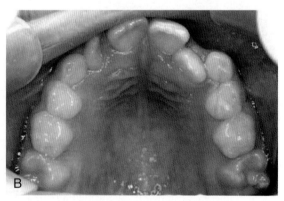

• **Figure 31.15** (A) The permanent maxillary right central incisor is substantially larger than the contra-lateral left central incisor. (B) The permanent maxillary left lateral incisor shown here in a lingual position is at least 2 mm larger than normal and the contralateral tooth. Isolated teeth such as these often require mesiodistal interproximal reduction to fit harmoniously in a final occlusion.

unusual for a child 9 years of age not to have all the upper and lower incisors (Fig. 31.18). If not present, the clinician should investigate why they are not and develop an appropriate treatment plan to address it. Likewise, maxillary permanent canines should be positively palpated or their existence confirmed radiographically by age 10 years. It appears that cone beam computed tomography (CBCT) images are superior to two-dimensional (2D) images for determining the status of canines and the adjacent teeth.[22] A sensible method, then, is to obtain a panoramic radiograph, which can reveal other related anomalies when missing anterior teeth (lateral incisors or canines) or peg-shaped lateral incisors are encountered. Then, depending on the findings, a small field of view CBCT may be indicated. These views can be supplemented with a traditional cephalometric digital image if required for limited or comprehensive orthodontic care. This exposes the patient to less radiation than would be delivered if a full field CBCT was initially obtained. The details of these examinations are noted later in the chapter.

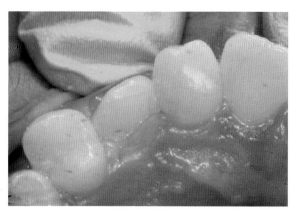

• **Figure 31.16** This patient has a talon cusp on the maxillary right lateral incisor. The enamel protuberance may have a pulp horn in it and cannot just simply be reduced by abrasion with a bur. These anomalies can cause interference in the occlusion and prohibit normal overbite and overjet. Usually, periodic gradual reduction with a bur will allow the pulp horn to recede, preserve tooth vitality, and improve the morphology toward a normal occlusion.

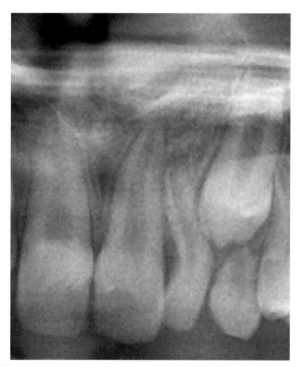

• **Figure 31.17** Root structure abnormalities, such as this dilacerated maxillary left lateral incisor, make orthodontic movement of teeth very difficult. A dilaceration of this magnitude makes the root more susceptible to apical resorption and complicates the final positioning of the crown and root.

Tooth Position

The position of erupted and unerupted permanent teeth in this age group should be noted and compared with the normal sequence and time of eruption. Minor asymmetry in dental eruption is normal, and there is little cause for concern if less than 6 months' difference in eruption exists between contralateral sides of the mouth. Five tooth positioning problems are associated with the mixed dentition: ectopic eruption, transposition, impaction, and primary failure of eruption, and the midline diastema. Interestingly, there appears to be a genetic component to some of these tooth

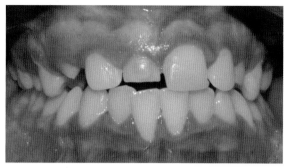

• **Figure 31.18** All permanent incisors should have erupted by 9 years of age. This patient has a retained primary maxillary central incisor and obvious eruption problems. This clinical sign should not be overlooked and has an impact on the developing dentition and the child's self-esteem.

position problems. Several studies have shown a genetic link between missing teeth, tooth anomalies, and altered eruption paths.[16,23–25] There seems to be clustering of these problems. If one of these conditions is identified, the clinician should examine the patient for these other related problems as mentioned earlier.

Ectopic eruption describes a path of eruption that causes root resorption of a portion or all of the adjacent primary tooth. Ectopic eruption is most often associated with the permanent maxillary first molar, mandibular lateral incisor, and maxillary canine.[26–28] In ectopic eruption of the permanent first molar, a portion of the erupting first molar resorbs the distal root of the primary second molar and is inhibited from erupting by the distal portion of the primary molar (Fig. 31.19). In many cases, the permanent molar spontaneously "jumps" or moves distally and erupts into the correct position. In other cases, the permanent molar lodges under the primary molar crown and no longer erupts. Usually, no pain or discomfort is associated with ectopic eruption unless communication develops between the oral cavity and the pulpal tissue of the primary molar, causing an abscess. Permanent molar ectopic eruption is often detected during clinical examination and confirmed with routine bitewing radiographs.

The prevalence of permanent first molar ectopic eruption is reported to be 3% to 4%.[29] Several possible causes of ectopic molar eruption have been proposed: (1) the maxillary teeth are larger than normal, (2) the maxilla is smaller than normal, (3) the maxilla is positioned further posteriorly than normal in relation to the cranial base, or (4) the angulation of the erupting maxillary permanent first molar is abnormal.[30,31] Although ectopic molar eruption may occur in the mandibular arch, it is more common in the maxilla.

Ectopic eruption of the permanent lateral incisor is most common in the mandibular arch. The erupting incisor resorbs all or a portion of the primary canine root because the path of eruption is abnormal, there is transitional crowding from the primary to the permanent dentition, or there is a true arch length deficiency. The diagnosis is generally signaled by premature primary canine exfoliation, often accompanied by a midline shift to the side of the ectopic eruption or impeded eruption of the lateral incisor, or it is discovered on an occlusal radiograph (Fig. 31.20).

The third common type of ectopic eruption occurs with maxillary permanent canine eruption and associated resorption of the permanent lateral incisor (Fig. 31.21). Studies have shown that if canines erupt from a more medial position in the dental arch and with a slightly more mesial horizontal path of eruption (an average of 10 degrees), there is a greater risk of lateral incisor resorption.

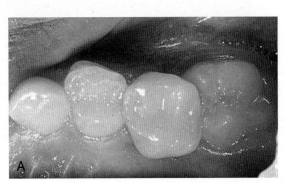
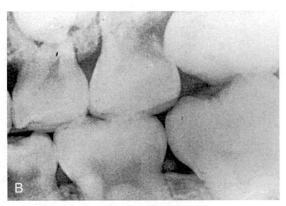

• **Figure 31.19** In ectopic eruption, the permanent first molar resorbs a portion of the distal root of the primary second molar. (A) In this case, the permanent first molar has lodged under the primary second molar crown. In other cases, the permanent molar spontaneously "jumps" or moves distally and erupts into the normal position. (B) The distal resorption of the primary molar root is evident on this radiograph.

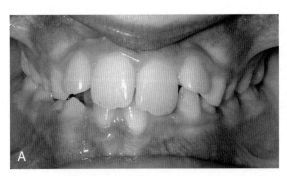
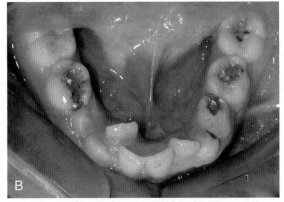

• **Figure 31.20** When a primary canine is lost because of ectopic eruption of a permanent lateral incisor, the midline often shifts to the side of the lost primary canine. (A) It is apparent from this view that the mandibular midline has shifted to the patient's right. (B) The permanent right lateral incisor is now blocked to the lingual as a consequence of the mandibular midline shift.

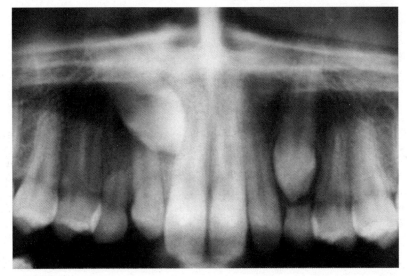

• **Figure 31.21** The maxillary right canine has erupted into the lateral incisor space and resorbed a portion of the root. This type of resorption is more common than believed, but often not to this extent.

It is recommended to remove the primary canine to promote more ideal canine eruption if the canine cusp on images is positioned medially to the midline of the lateral incisor.[26,32] Some investigations suggest additional treatment to improve canine position, such as primary canine removal in conjunction with maxillary expansion.[33]

A related phenomenon is lingual eruption of the permanent incisors, predominantly the mandibular incisors (Fig. 31.22). The prevalence of lingually erupting mandibular incisors is about 10%.[34] The cause of ectopic and lingually erupting incisors is not well established. One explanation suggests that ectopic and lingual eruption of the incisors results from an abnormal pattern of resorption. Alternatively, it has been suggested that lingual eruption is a variation of the normal eruption pattern because the lower incisor tooth buds form lingual to the primary incisors and may not migrate facially.

Transposition occurs when there is "a positional interchange of two adjacent teeth, especially their roots or the development or eruption of a tooth in a position occupied normally by a nonadjacent tooth."[25] Usually transpositions are observed later in the transitional dentition years. The early-stage transposition is uncommon but is the type of transposition observed in the early mixed-dentition years (Fig. 31.23). This usually is a transposition of the mandibular lateral incisor and canine.[24] The lateral incisor will show distal tipping, resorption of the primary canine (and sometimes the primary first molar), and rotation as it migrates. Other transpositions that are observed later in the transitional years are likely to be the mature mandibular lateral and canine, and the more prevalent transpositions of the maxillary canine and first premolar and maxillary canine and lateral incisor.[25]

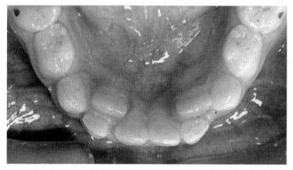

• **Figure 31.22** Ectopic eruption of the permanent lateral incisors is most common in the mandibular arch. In this example, the mandibular lateral incisors erupted lingual to their ideal position and the primary laterals are still present. In some cases, the lateral incisors erupt into a more normal position but cause premature exfoliation of the primary canine.

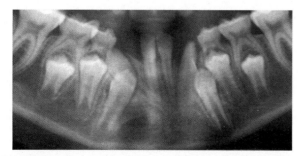

• **Figure 31.23** Early-stage transposition of the mandibular lateral incisors and the canines. Note that the permanent mandibular right lateral incisor has resorbed the primary canine and the primary first molar is about to be lost. If intercepted early, true transposition will not occur.

Tooth impaction, as noted earlier, is diagnosed during the clinical examination or from appropriate radiographs. Over-retained primary teeth, supernumerary teeth, severe crowding, or a failure in the eruption mechanism can cause impaction of the anterior teeth (Fig. 31.24A). Often the permanent tooth erupts if the over-retained primary tooth or supernumerary tooth is removed. If the tooth is impacted as a result of crowding, it is necessary to provide space either orthodontically or by extraction to allow eruption. Generally the last tooth to erupt in an arch or quadrant is impacted because the space is reduced or no longer available. This eruption mechanism or the aberrant eruption direction usually is the cause of impaction of the maxillary canine. The maxillary canine is most often the last tooth to erupt into the arch. It also erupts or travels the longest distance to take its place in the arch. These two factors combine to make the maxillary canine the most common impacted tooth in the maxillary arch and indeed the mouth (see Fig. 31.24B). Posterior tooth impaction is normally the result of inadequate arch length. Inadequate arch length is caused by a tooth–jaw size discrepancy or space loss as a result of premature primary tooth loss. If the arch length problem is generalized, either permanent teeth should be removed or the arch should be expanded to allow eruption of all the permanent teeth. Limited, localized crowding due to space loss can be treated by orthodontically regaining the lost space.

At times the permanent first molar fails to erupt or erupts partially. The dilemma for the clinician is to diagnose the problem. There seem to be three diagnoses for an unerupted permanent molar. The first is primary failure of eruption. Primary failure of eruption is an unusual eruption problem that affects the posterior teeth (Fig. 31.25). It is diagnosed when a tooth fails to erupt despite the presence of adequate space and the absence of overlying hard tissue that prevents eruption. Furthermore, all teeth distal to the affected tooth also fail to erupt. The cause of primary failure of eruption is unknown but appears to have a genetic component.[35–37] The second cause of an unerupted permanent molar is mechanical failure of eruption. Two characteristics distinguish mechanical failure of eruption from primary failure of eruption. The first is that some type of mechanical obstruction can explain the lack of eruption. The path of eruption is not clear like primary failure eruption. Obstruction can be from lack of space, a developmental problem with the tooth, or placement of the tongue. Removal of the obstruction will generally allow tooth movement. The other characteristic distinguishing primary from mechanical failure of eruption is that teeth distal to the affected tooth will erupt. This is difficult to determine early in treatment. Ankylosis of the tooth is the third diagnosis for an unerupted tooth. A tooth with ankylosis will not erupt even if there is space and the teeth distal are not affected.[38]

A small, maxillary midline diastema in the early mixed dentition is normal (Fig. 31.26). Typically it is caused by the position of the unerupted lateral incisors or canines (Fig. 31.27A). The unerupted teeth are positioned superior and distal to the roots of the central incisors, and they direct the central incisor roots toward the midline and the crowns toward the distal (see Fig. 31.27B). As the lateral incisors or canines erupt, the incisors upright themselves slowly and the midline space begins to close. Treatment to close a diastema is usually delayed until the permanent canines are fully erupted unless the space available for eruption of the lateral incisors or canines is severely limited or the esthetics are a compelling concern. If the diastema is larger than 2 mm, the cause may be a mesiodens (see Fig. 31.12), a localized tooth size problem, or abnormal incisor positioning. A mesiodens is usually discovered on radiographic examination, and its removal normally allows the diastema to close. A size mismatch between the upper and lower teeth may result

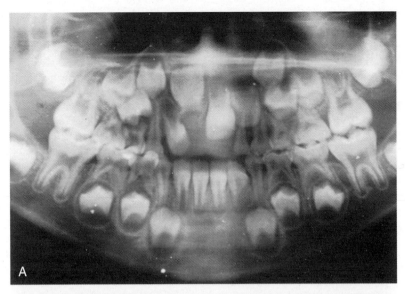

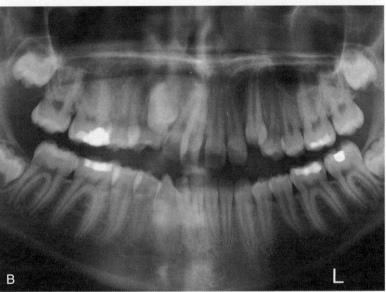

• **Figure 31.24** In the transitional years, tooth impaction in the anterior region is usually caused by over-retained primary teeth, supernumerary teeth, or severe crowding. In a few cases, a failure in the eruption mechanism is responsible for the delayed eruption. (A) In this case, the maxillary right central incisor is completely inverted and is directed toward the nasal cavity. (B) The ultimate sequela of a lack of space is illustrated by this impacted maxillary right canine even though the orientation of the tooth is correct. Note that the maxillary left canine will successfully erupt.

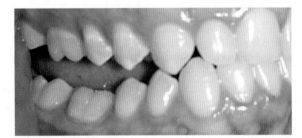

• **Figure 31.25** Primary failure of eruption usually presents as a posterior segment of open bite. It appears to cause eruption problems with all teeth posterior to the most anterior affected tooth in that quadrant. In this case, given the occlusal plane, it appears that the lower teeth are involved. Treatment can be challenging and the open bite must be closed surgically or prosthetically after growth has ceased.

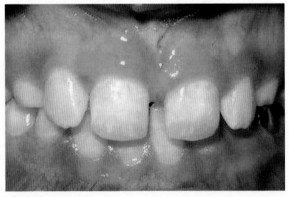

• **Figure 31.26** A small maxillary midline diastema is normal in the mixed dentition. The diastema tends to close with the eruption of the permanent maxillary lateral incisors and canines.

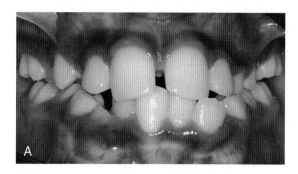

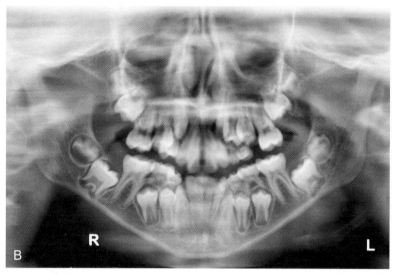

• **Figure 31.27** (A) The "ugly duckling" stage is evident when the crowns of the lateral incisors tip distally and open diastema between the anterior teeth. (B) The permanent canines are pushing against the roots of the permanent lateral incisors. Some of the anterior space will close with the eruption of the canines.

in a diastema. In this situation, the maxillary incisor crowns are small or excessively tapered, although the mandibular teeth may be too large in relation to the maxillary teeth. If large spaces are present, a combination of tooth movement and anterior restorations is required to correct the size discrepancy. Abnormal incisor positioning and protrusion also may result in a midline diastema. The abnormal positioning may be due to past or present finger habits or to abnormal eruption. The best treatment is to first eliminate the habit and then to retract the incisors orthodontically and consolidate space.

Anteroposterior Dimension

Permanent molar and canine relationships should be noted and compared with the anteroposterior skeletal relationships that were determined during the extraoral examination. Permanent molar and canine relationships are illustrated in Fig. 31.28. Dental relationships generally reflect the underlying skeletal relationships, including asymmetry, although it is feasible to have different dental and skeletal relationships if teeth are missing or have drifted. For example, a person with a class I skeletal relationship may have a class II molar relationship if there has been posterior space loss and the permanent maxillary first molar drifted forward into the space (Fig. 31.29).

If the permanent teeth are properly aligned in the alveolar bone at a normal angulation, overjet is a direct measurement of the relationship between the dental arches. Normal overjet is approximately 2 mm; therefore the discrepancy between the arches can be calculated by subtracting 2 mm from the measured overjet.

Incisor position is not always ideal, however, and estimates of dental arch discrepancies must be adjusted if both upper and lower anterior teeth are either protrusive or retrusive.

Transverse Relationship

Dental midline and posterior crossbite evaluation is conducted in the same manner described in Chapter 19. Usually dental midline deviations are either the result of simply moderate to severe crowding or ectopic eruption and tooth loss with a shift of the midline as teeth realign in the newly available space (see Fig. 31.20). Functional deviations of the mandible are identified by noting discrepancies between centric relation and centric occlusion. Posterior crossbites are determined to be either unilateral or bilateral. In the early mixed-dentition years, treatments for both skeletal and dental crossbites are essentially the same. As the child becomes older, it becomes more critical to identify whether a crossbite is due to skeletal or dental causes because the midpalatal suture becomes more interdigitated over time. The management of posterior crossbite in the complete permanent dentition varies according to whether the crossbite is skeletal or dental in origin and the estimate of whether the midpalatal suture is open, bridged, or closed.

Vertical Dimension

The vertical dental examination is concerned with overbite and open-bite measurements and ankylosis. Normal overbite in this age group is approximately 2 mm. If there is a deviation from normal, the clinician should try to determine if the deviation is due to a dental or a skeletal problem. If the facial examination

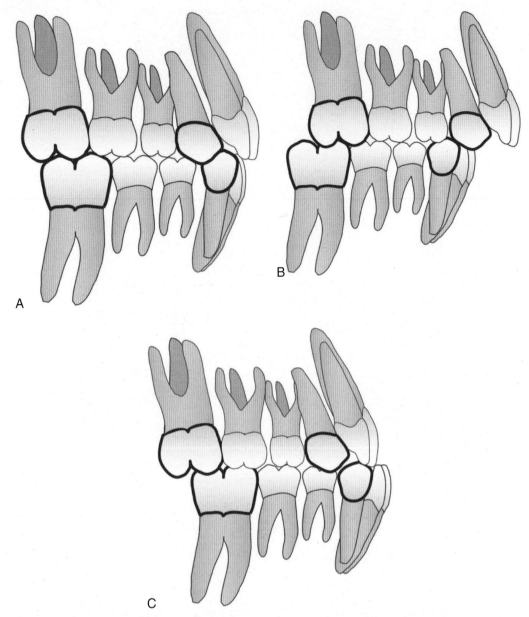

• **Figure 31.28** (A) In the permanent dentition, permanent molar and canine relationships are determined and compared with the anteroposterior skeletal relationships. To determine molar relationships, the position of the mesiobuccal cusp of the permanent maxillary first molar is related to the position of the facial groove of the permanent mandibular first molar. If the mesiobuccal cusp occludes in the facial groove, the molar relationship is called class I. The canine relationship is determined by the relationship of the maxillary canine to the embrasure between the mandibular canine and the first premolar (or primary first molar). If the maxillary canine occludes in the embrasure, the canine relationship is also called class I. (B) If the mesiobuccal cusp of the permanent maxillary first molar occludes mesial to the mandibular facial groove, the molar relationship is called class II. The canine relationship is called class II if the maxillary canine occludes mesial to the mandibular canine–first premolar embrasure. (C) If the mesiobuccal cusp of the permanent maxillary first molar occludes distal to the mandibular facial groove, the molar relationship is called class III. The canine relationship is class III if the maxillary canine occludes distal to the mandibular canine–first premolar embrasure.

revealed a vertical skeletal problem, it is sometimes reflected in the dental relationships. Treatment of the malocclusion varies with the source of the problem.

Ankylosis of the primary teeth can present several problems because of the magnitude of vertical dentoalveolar growth. Dental eruption and vertical growth of the alveolus may amount to as much as 10 mm from age 6 to 12 years. Thus ankylosis of a primary tooth at an early age may result in large marginal ridge discrepancies, tipping of adjacent teeth, and vertical bone loss. Most of these problems, with the exception of space loss, resolve when the permanent tooth erupts. Ankylosed teeth and associated problems are discussed in Chapter 19, and the reader is referred to that chapter for a more detailed discussion. One aspect of ankylosed primary teeth that must be addressed differently is when the primary tooth is ankylosed and the permanent tooth is missing. If the vertical occlusal step becomes exaggerated, and by definition the vertical bone level relative

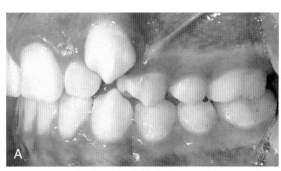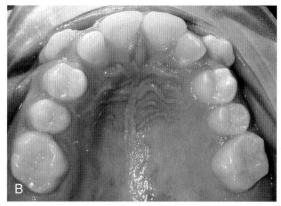

• **Figure 31.29** Space loss can cause dental relationships to not reflect skeletal relationships. (A) This patient had maxillary posterior space loss with mesial drift so that the molars are class II and not reflective of the skeletal class I relationships. (B) The space loss caused the permanent canines to erupt to the facial.

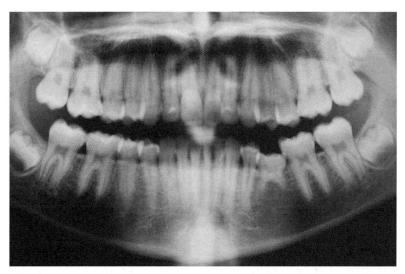

• **Figure 31.30** The ankylosed primary mandibular second molar demonstrates the alteration of bone level that can occur when ankylosed primary teeth without successors are maintained too long. Timely removal of the ankylosed tooth and treatment planning for orthodontic movement of the adjacent teeth or prosthetic replacement are critical.

to adjacent teeth is exaggerated, intervention is indicated. This is the case because there is no permanent tooth to erupt and bring alveolar bone with it. If the primary tooth is allowed to remain, its eventual extraction will leave a bony defect adjacent to the remaining permanent teeth (Fig. 31.30). Timely removal of the primary tooth and further treatment will have to be considered. A second option for treatment is to decoronate the primary molar rather than remove it in cases where there is no permanent successor. There still is loss of vertical height of the alveolus but decoronation seems to maintain the alveolar width. Loss of bone due to extraction of a primary tooth without a successor is more rapid and severe in the anterior than in the posterior areas of the mouth.

Supplemental Orthodontic Diagnostic Techniques

Photographs

Among the most basic diagnostic records routinely obtained are facial and intraoral photographs. There are several commercial

software programs available to the clinician to store and manipulate the images. A minimum of three extraoral images of the face are obtained: a frontal face with lips relaxed, a frontal face with posed smile, and a lateral face with lips relaxed. Five intraoral images consisting of a frontal, right and left lateral, and maxillary and mandibular occlusal views are obtained. These images are stored in a montage for study and to present during case reviews (Fig. 31.31). Some like to supplement these images with a three-quarter view with lip relaxed, a three-quarter view with posed smile, and a lateral view with a posed smile (Fig. 31.32).

Diagnostic Casts

Orthodontic treatment in the mixed dentition is more complex than treatment in the primary dentition. The clinician must consider the difference in size between the primary and permanent dentitions, the amount of space available for the permanent teeth, and the dental and skeletal status of the patient. This formidable job requires supplemental information to make accurate orthodontic diagnoses and to develop coherent treatment plans. Diagnostic study casts are an essential part of a thorough evaluation if

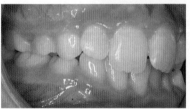
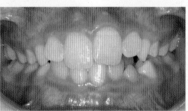
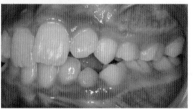

• **Figure 31.31** Digital images of pretreatment and posttreatment extraoral and intraoral views of orthodontic patients can be stored electronically in the patient record or printed as a hard copy. This method circumvents the problems of losing images to either poor photographic technique or filing methods.

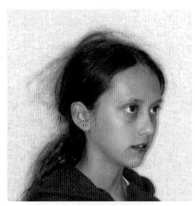
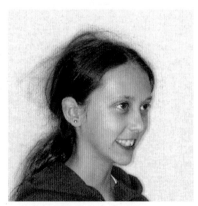
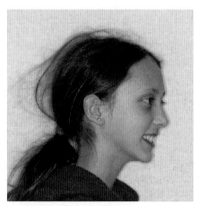

• **Figure 31.32** These three additional views are often obtained to evaluate facial esthetics and relationships. (A) The three-quarter view with lips relaxed. (B) The three-quarter view with a posed smile. (C) The lateral view with a posed smile.

problems are detected during the examination and definitive analysis or if treatment is required. These study casts can be conventional stone casts (Fig. 31.33) or digital representations of stone casts. In the former case, impressions are obtained using the following method.

An appropriate impression tray must be chosen. Properly fitted trays seat comfortably in the mouth and extend far enough posteriorly to cover the most distal tooth and either the maxillary tuberosity or the mandibular retromolar pad. The trays should be of a nonperforated variety that holds the impression material in

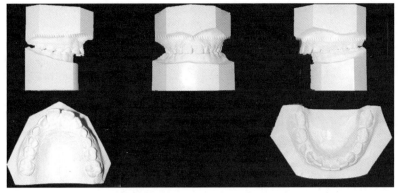

• **Figure 31.33** Views of plaster casts that have been trimmed so that the backs are flush in centric occlusion and the bases are trimmed symmetrically from the occlusal view so the intra-arch asymmetries are obvious.

the tray and expresses the excess material into the vestibule. Some semiperforated trays are now in use, but they must generate enough tissue pressure to reflect the tissue. When the soft tissue is displaced, it allows the dentoalveolar morphology to be clearly viewed on the cast. The trays also can be lined with wax that aids in tissue displacement and makes seating the tray into position more comfortable.

After the appropriate tray has been selected, the alginate is mixed and placed in one tray. For either arch, the tray should be rotated laterally into the mouth and firmly seated, first posteriorly against the palate or the retromolar pad. This technique limits the posterior flow of alginate and forces excess alginate anteriorly and laterally. The tray is then rotated and seated over the anterior teeth. Finally, the tray is held in place until the alginate has set. After the upper and lower impressions are obtained, a wax bite is made by placing a softened piece of base plate or other wax bite material between the teeth, having the patient close in centric occlusion. The wax is cooled with air and serves to orient the casts properly during trimming.

Impressions should be disinfected, wrapped in moist paper towels, and stored in sealed plastic bags or poured soon in white plaster because the alginate will dehydrate and distort if it is left exposed for more than a few minutes. The plaster is thoroughly mixed, usually using a vacuum spatulator to reduce bubbles, and then vibrated into the impression and flowed from one tooth to another to prevent air entrapment, which results in holes in the models. Separate plaster bases are poured, and the impressions are inverted on the bases when the plaster is partially set. After the plaster has set, the trays are separated carefully from the casts to prevent breaking the teeth.

The maxillary cast is trimmed so that the top of the base is parallel to the occlusal plane. The back of the upper cast is trimmed perpendicular to its top and the midpalatal raphe. The maxillary and mandibular casts are occluded, and the back of the mandibular base is trimmed parallel to the top of the maxillary cast. Finally, the sides of the casts are trimmed symmetrically, which allows the clinician to judge arch symmetry.

Alternatively for digital casts, impressions are obtained in a similar manner, but with a long-term stable alginate. The impressions are disinfected, wrapped in moist towels, bagged in plastic, and shipped to a commercial laboratory for pouring, and the resulting models are scanned. A digital representation of the casts is transmitted to the practitioner via the Internet. These digital images are less likely to be misplaced or broken and present no storage

problems. They can also be manipulated to view all relationships for analysis and imported to the patient's record as static images for electronic archiving or printing (Fig. 31.34). The digital casts also can be analyzed and measured like conventional casts (Fig. 31.35). Findings recorded during the clinical examination are reviewed and confirmed using the casts. Alignment and tooth position characteristics should receive special attention because appliance design must be appropriate for each rotation and displacement.

Advances in technology continue to change diagnostic records in dentistry. Intraoral scanners have been developed to construct a model of the teeth without making an impression. The scanner creates a three-dimensional (3D) reconstruction of the teeth and is as accurate as the traditional alginate impression. As this technology continues to improve, its use may surpass the traditional impression because patients do not like traditional impressions, mostly because of gagging issues. In addition to intraoral scanning of teeth, some are using the information gathered from a 3D cone beam scan to construct a model of the teeth. There is some question if the reconstructions from cone beam computerized tomography are as accurate as intraoral scanning and traditional impressions.[39] In general, they are probably accurate enough for diagnostic purposes but not appliance construction.

After the diagnostic casts are obtained, analyses should be performed to determine tooth size relationships and arch length adequacy. The tooth size analysis compares the size of the teeth in one arch with the size of the teeth in the other. Tooth size must be compatible to ensure that teeth fit together correctly after treatment. The arch length analysis is done to predict whether there is sufficient space available in the dental arch for the unerupted permanent teeth.

Tooth Size Analysis

The tooth size is calculated using Bolton's method.[40] Bolton selected 55 cases of excellent occlusion and measured the mesiodistal diameter of all teeth on the casts except for the permanent second and third molars. From the measurements obtained, Bolton determined that a certain ratio existed between the size of the upper and lower permanent teeth. A ratio could be determined for either the 6 anterior teeth or all 12 of the measured teeth in each arch by measuring the teeth manually (Fig. 31.36). Little constructed a table based on the Bolton ratios to simplify tooth size determinations (Fig. 31.37).[14] This analysis can be performed using the digital casts and the associated software (Fig. 31.38).

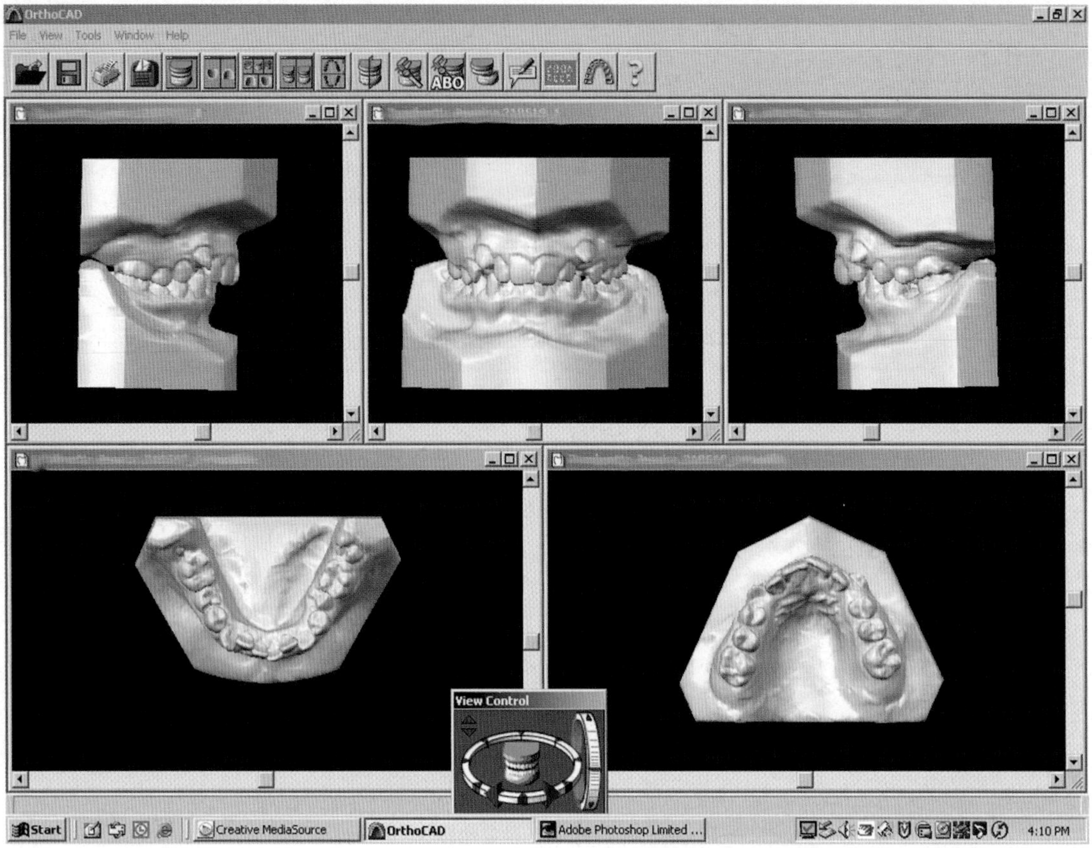

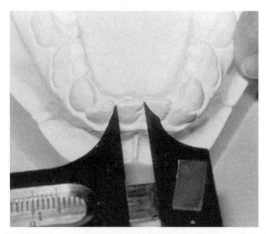

• **Figure 31.34** Digital casts can be displayed from the web or stored in image management software. The digital casts can be manipulated so that the casts can be separated or occluded and rotated or tipped to reveal all relationships. This prevents problems with loss and breakage of the casts and reduces the store space problems. (From Proffit WR, Fields HW, Sarver DM. *Contemporary Orthodontics.* 5th ed. St Louis: Elsevier; 2013.)

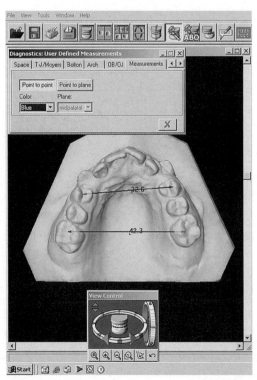

• **Figure 31.35** The digital casts can also be manipulated to examine relationships and measured electronically like conventional plaster casts so that arch dimensions can be evaluated. (Courtesy OrthoCAD by Cadent, Inc, San Yosa, CA.)

• **Figure 31.36** To complete the tooth size analysis developed by Bolton, the mesiodistal width of each permanent tooth (except for second and third molars) is measured with a Boley gauge or a needle-pointed divider. The measurements are added together to provide totals for the six anterior teeth and for the overall arch.

Ultimately, when tooth size problems are complex, diagnostic setups are required to determine which teeth should be positioned in specific orientations so that final diagnostic decisions can be made.

Several clinical situations contribute to tooth size discrepancy. Maxillary lateral incisors are commonly smaller than normal, resulting in a mandibular anterior tooth size excess (relatively speaking, the lower teeth are too large even though the problem is in the maxillary arch; see Fig. 31.14A). The size of the second premolar also varies highly. When significant tooth size discrepancies are discovered, the child is best referred to a specialist because simple tooth movement does not produce an esthetically satisfactory result or good occlusion. Management of tooth size discrepancies often requires a combination of tooth movement and restorative dentistry.

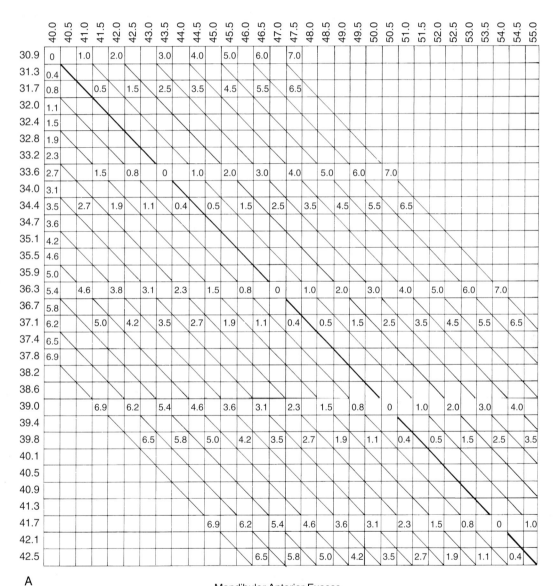

• **Figure 31.37** To use the table, the mesiodistal width of each permanent tooth (permanent first molar to permanent first molar) is measured with a needle-pointed divider or sharp Boley gauge. The widths of the teeth are summed. To determine whether there is an anterior (canine to canine) or overall (molar to molar) tooth size discrepancy, the intersection of the maxillary and mandibular totals is located on the appropriate table. (A) The width of the mandibular anterior teeth is indicated on the vertical axis, and the width of the maxillary anterior teeth is found on the horizontal axis. The intersection indicates whether a tooth size discrepancy exists and whether it is a maxillary or mandibular excess, and it indicates the size of the discrepancy in millimeters. Because there is some error in measuring the casts and some error in the analysis itself, tooth size discrepancies of 1.5 mm or less are not considered significant. *Continued*

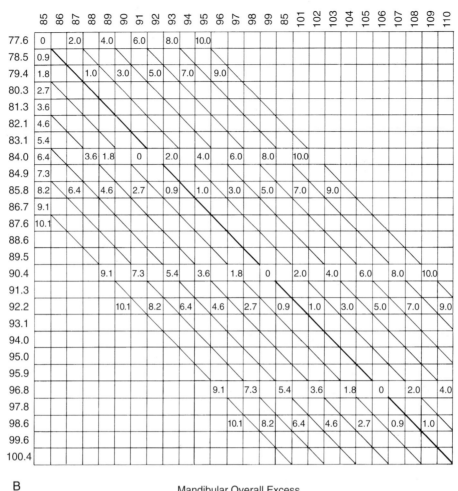

B   Mandibular Overall Excess

• **Figure 31.37, cont'd** (B) This table provides the same information for overall tooth size relationships. (Courtesy Dr. Robert Little. From Proffit WR, Fields HW Jr, eds. *Contemporary Orthodontics.* St Louis: Mosby; 1992.)

Space Analysis

The space analysis is normally completed in the mixed dentition and is used to predict the amount of space available for the unerupted permanent teeth. A number of different methods of space analysis exist; however, all space analyses have two features in common. First, the permanent first molars and the mandibular incisors must be erupted to allow one to perform the analysis. Second, the mandibular incisors (sometimes in addition to other measurements) are used to predict the size of the unerupted canines and premolars. The following four assumptions are made in calculating a space analysis:

1. *All permanent teeth are developing normally.* Although this seems obvious, the analysis is meaningless if teeth are congenitally missing.
2. *There is a correlation between the size of the erupted mandibular incisors and the remaining permanent teeth.* The prediction of unerupted tooth size is more accurate if the correlation is strong.
3. *The prediction tables are most valid for a specific population.* The ethnic background of the patients used in most space analysis studies is northwestern European. If the patient is not of northwestern European descent, the analysis should be interpreted with some caution.
4. *Arch dimensions remain stable throughout growth.* This assumption is made to simplify the procedure, although it is recognized that the intercanine width, intermolar width, and arch length dimensions do change with age and eruption of teeth. Skeletal growth patterns may also affect arch dimension stability. Patients with class II mandibular deficiency tend to have proclined mandibular incisors to compensate for the deficiency, whereas those with class III deficiency tend to have more upright or retroclined mandibular incisors.

Although several methods of space analysis exist, the Tanaka-Johnston analysis is most clinically useful because it requires no additional radiographs or tables to predict tooth size.[41] The first step in the Tanaka-Johnston analysis is to determine the available arch length. The distance from the mesial of the permanent first molar to the mesial of the contralateral permanent first molar is measured by dividing the arch into several segments (Fig. 31.39A). Each segment is measured over the contact points and incisal edges of

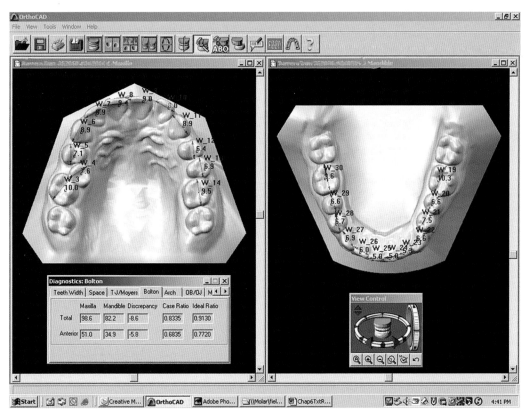

• **Figure 31.38** The tooth size analysis can be completed on conventional casts or electronically using digital casts. This screen capture shows that the teeth have been measured electronically using the cursor and mouse and then the analysis calculations performed by the software. (From Proffit WR, Fields HW, Sarver DM. *Contemporary Orthodontics.* 5th ed. St Louis: Elsevier; 2013.)

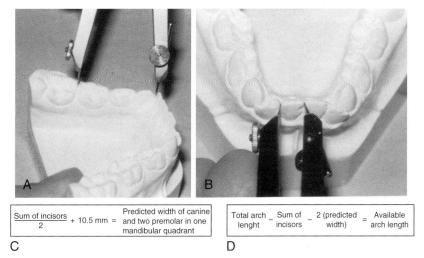

$$\frac{\text{Sum of incisors}}{2} + 10.5\ mm = \begin{array}{c}\text{Predicted width of canine}\\ \text{and two premolar in one}\\ \text{mandibular quadrant}\end{array}$$

C

$$\begin{array}{c}\text{Total arch}\\ \text{lenght}\end{array} - \begin{array}{c}\text{Sum of}\\ \text{incisors}\end{array} - \begin{array}{c}2\ (\text{predicted}\\ \text{width})\end{array} = \begin{array}{c}\text{Available}\\ \text{arch length}\end{array}$$

D

• **Figure 31.39** (A) The first step in the Tanaka-Johnston space analysis is to determine available arch length. This is accomplished by dividing the arch into several segments and measuring each segment over the contact points and incisal edges of the teeth. (B) The second step is to measure the width of the four mandibular incisors and add them together. (C) The mesiodistal width of the unerupted canine and premolars in one quadrant is calculated by using the previous formula. In the mandibular arch, 10.5 mm is used to determine the canine-premolar widths. In the maxillary arch, half the sum of the mandibular incisors is still used, but 11.0 mm is substituted for 10.5 mm because the unerupted permanent maxillary teeth are slightly larger. (D) The final step in the analysis is to subtract the width of the four incisors and the predicted canine-premolar width from the total arch length. The remainder is the available arch length. If the remainder is positive, there is adequate space in the arch. If the remainder is negative, the permanent teeth require more room to erupt than is available in the arch.

the teeth. The segments are added together to provide an approximation of total arch length. The second step in the analysis is measurement of the width of the four mandibular incisors (see Fig. 31.39B). The widths of the four incisors are added together to determine the amount of room necessary for ideal alignment. The mesiodistal width of the unerupted mandibular canine and premolars in one quadrant is predicted by adding 10.5 mm to half the width of the four lower incisors (see Fig. 31.39C). The final step in the space analysis is to subtract the width of the lower incisors and two times the calculated premolar and canine width (both sides) from the total arch length approximation (see Fig. 31.39D). If the result is positive, there is more space available in the arch than is needed for the unerupted teeth. If the result is negative, the unerupted teeth require more space than is available to erupt in ideal alignment.

The maxillary space analysis is conducted in the same way. Maxillary arch length is measured, the width of the maxillary incisors is determined, and 11.0 mm is added to half the width of the four lower incisors to predict the size of the unerupted maxillary canine and premolars in one quadrant. The incisor width and the predicted canine-premolar width are subtracted from the total arch length to determine the amount of space available in the maxillary arch. This analysis also can be performed using the digital casts and the associated software (Fig. 31.40).

After the arch length predictions are made, the clinician should return to the cast and decide whether the results make sense.

For example, if the arch appears to be crowded and the analysis predicts 5 mm of excess space, the analysis should be repeated or scrutinized for mistakes. Furthermore, the results should be considered in the context of the patient's soft tissue profile. The space analysis may indicate that the patient is moderately short of space, yet because he or she has very retrusive lips and incisors, the treatment of choice would be to expand the arch by moving the incisors facially to provide better lip support (Fig. 31.41). Conversely, an analysis may predict that there is no crowding, yet extractions are considered necessary because the patient has very protrusive teeth and lips (Fig. 31.42). Dental protrusion and dental crowding are actually manifestations of the same problem. Whether the arch is crowded or the incisors are protrusive depends on the interaction between the pressure of the resting tongue and the circumoral musculature.

Two factors must be considered when using the Tanaka-Johnston analysis. It tends to overpredict slightly the width of the unerupted teeth. This makes the extent of crowding appear more severe than it actually is. In addition, if the patient is not of northwestern European background, it is difficult to know whether the prediction is overstated or understated. An alternative method for determining available space is to measure arch length and incisor width as noted previously and then obtain periapical radiographs of the canines and premolars. The mesiodistal widths of the unerupted teeth are measured on the periapical films and then corrected for

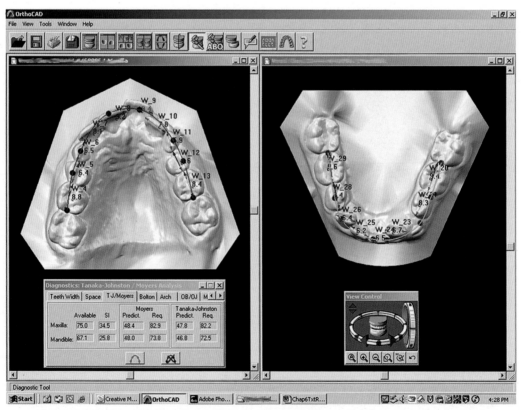

• **Figure 31.40** The software packages that support the digital casts provide for several methods of space analysis. Again, using the tooth dimensions measured from the casts, the analyses are calculated. The accuracy of the result is contingent on careful management of the cursor for tooth measurement and how the arch dimensions are defined by the arch form, which is shown here as the overlying arc on each arch. (From Proffit WR, Fields HW, Sarver DM. *Contemporary Orthodontics.* 5th ed. St Louis: Elsevier; 2013.)

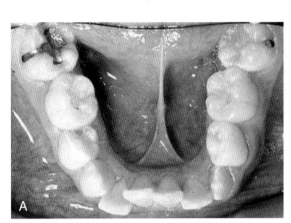
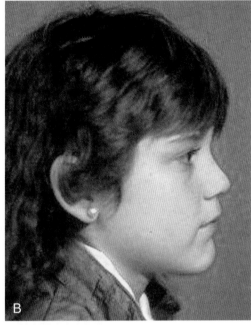

• **Figure 31.41** The results of the space analysis (A) are considered in the context of the patient's soft tissue profile. In this example, the space analysis indicates that the arch length is short. The profile analysis (B), however, indicates that the patient cannot tolerate further loss of lip support. It is more prudent in this case to expand the arch than to extract teeth to provide additional space.

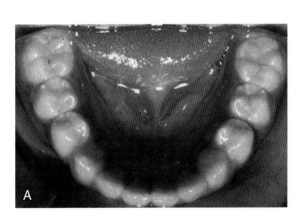
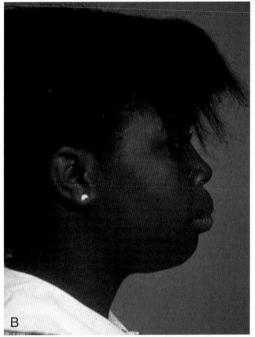

• **Figure 31.42** In this example, the space analysis (A) indicates that there is no shortage of arch length. The profile analysis (B), however, indicates that the patient has extremely protrusive lips and incisors. It is more prudent to extract teeth and retract the incisors and lips in this case. This figure illustrates the fact that dental crowding and dental protrusion are actually manifestations of the same problem.

magnification by comparing the width of erupted teeth on the films with the actual width of these teeth on the cast. With this technique, an individual space analysis can be performed for every patient. The disadvantages of this technique are that the patient is exposed to more radiation, and undistorted radiographs of the canines are difficult to obtain.

Analysis of Cephalometric Head Films

The facial profile analysis should be used by the clinician to gather basic information about the spatial relationships of the teeth and jaws. If the clinician identifies significant anteroposterior or vertical discrepancies, the patient should be evaluated by a specialist. At that time, a lateral cephalometric radiograph may be used to obtain a more precise assessment of the problem. Analysis of lateral cephalometric head films is an additional diagnostic aid used to determine the relationship between the skeletal and dental structures. The cephalometric head film is normally ordered when significant skeletal discrepancies exist and comprehensive orthodontic treatment is being considered. The cephalometric analysis is an adjunct to the facial profile analysis. It provides confirmation of the clinical examination and possibly more specific information about the contribution of each skeletal and dental component to the malocclusion. Therefore it must be viewed carefully.[42]

A large number of cephalometric analyses exist; however, the common goal of all analyses is to determine the size and position of the skeletal structures and the position of the teeth. The first step in the cephalometric analysis is to obtain a diagnostic head film. For the radiograph to be diagnostic, the head must be positioned in a cephalostat in a natural, relaxed posture. In other words, the patient's head should not be tipped up or down or to one side or the other. Incorrect positioning alters the perceived relationship of the skeletal structures and makes interpretation of the landmarks more difficult, even to the point of suspecting skeletal asymmetry. A mandibular deficiency may not be apparent if the patient's head is tipped upward. Natural head position is produced by having the patient look at the distant horizon and gradually assume a comfortable position by tipping the head up and down in smaller and smaller increments until he or she is comfortable. The teeth should be together in centric occlusion and the lips relaxed when the film is exposed.

After the head film is made, the radiograph should be screened for pathologic findings. Although cephalometric head films can have points identified and measurements made by hand, currently, landmarks are located on a computer screen using a mouse and dedicated cephalometric software that can construct the tracing (Fig. 31.43). The software generates linear and angular

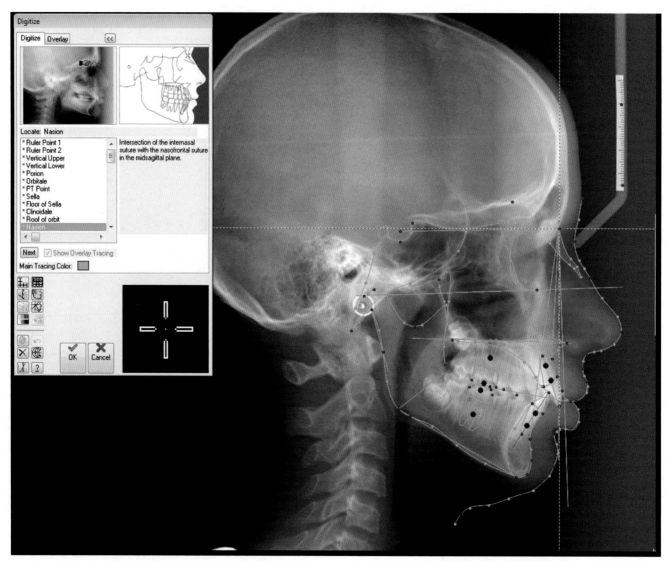

• **Figure 31.43** Current technology allows the clinician to digitize the critical points and have the measurements performed electronically by the software package (Dolphin Imaging and Management Solutions, Chatsworth, CA). This procedure can be performed with a personal computer and mouse using a digital radiographic image. The computer will provide various representations of traced landmarks and anatomy as well as lines and planes.

measurements, and a graphic image of the face constructed from the digitized landmarks provides the basis for the cephalometric analysis (Fig. 31.44). Depending on the sophistication of the program, the program can be used to simulate growth for the patient in yearly intervals or project treatment goals. In cases where there are multiple options for treatment, the software can demonstrate to patients how their face may change or look with each individual treatment.

The analysis should evaluate the position of the maxilla and mandible in relation to that of the cranial base and the relationship of the maxilla and mandible to each other. Analysis also should evaluate the position of the teeth in each jaw and the relationship of the upper teeth to the lower teeth. Vertical relationships between total, upper, and lower facial heights of the anterior face should be determined. Finally, the analysis should evaluate the soft tissue profile and the position of the lips in relation to the teeth, nose, and chin. A cephalometric analysis requires two reference lines to orient the position of the teeth and jaws. Historically, the Frankfort horizontal plane has been used as the horizontal reference line because it was thought to be parallel to the true horizontal plane when the patient was looking at a distant point. The Frankfort horizontal plane connects the upper rim of the external auditory meatus (porion) with the inferior border of the orbital rim (orbitale; Fig. 31.45). Although the Frankfort horizontal plane is not always parallel to the true horizontal plane, it is still the most widely used horizontal reference line. The vertical reference line can be either a true perpendicular (to the horizon) through the nasion (the bony bridge of the nose) or a line perpendicular to the Frankfort plane through the nasion. The position and size of the maxilla and mandible are evaluated by comparing A point (maxilla) and pogonion (mandible), anterior points on these structures, to the vertical reference line. Normal maxillary position and size should place A point near the vertical line (Fig. 31.46).

The pogonion is normally 5 mm behind the vertical plane with a well-positioned mandible in a preadolescent patient.[43]

Angular and linear measurements can be used to compare the position of the maxilla with that of the mandible. The angle formed by connecting A and B points with nasion has traditionally been used to describe the position of the two jaws (Fig. 31.47). In normally related jaws, the angle is between 2 and 5 degrees. Larger positive values suggest a class II relationship, whereas negative values indicate class III tendencies. The difference between the size of the lower and upper jaws, as determined from the Harvold measurements, can also be used to relate the jaws.[44]

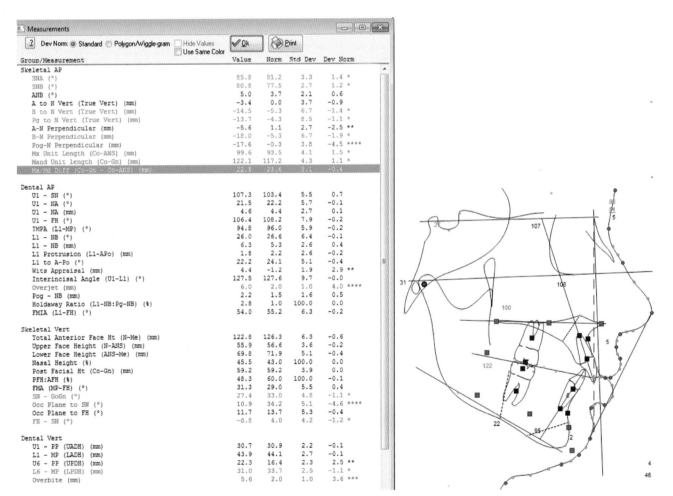

• **Figure 31.44** Printouts of computer-generated cephalometric analyses often take a form similar to the ones illustrated here (Dolphin Imaging and Management Solutions, Chatsworth, CA). The resulting measurements can even be combined with a graphic image of the face. The content can be customized by altering the anatomic landmarks and measurements to provide those most useful to the individual clinician.

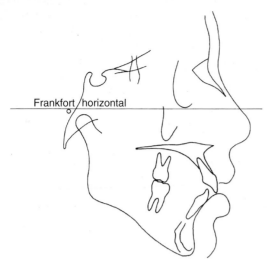

• **Figure 31.45** Cephalometric analysis requires two reference lines to orient the position of the head and teeth. Historically, the Frankfort horizontal plane has been used as the reference line because it is felt to be parallel to the true horizontal when the patient is looking at the horizon. The Frankfort horizontal plane is constructed by connecting the upper rim of the external auditory meatus (porion) with the inferior border of the orbital rim (orbitale). The vertical reference line is either a true perpendicular line to the nasion, the bony bridge of the nose, or a line perpendicular to the Frankfort plane through the nasion.

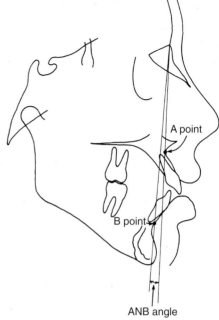

• **Figure 31.47** The relative positions of the maxilla and mandible are also compared by using an angular measurement. In normally related jaws, the angle formed by connecting A and B points with nasion (ANB) is between 2 and 5 degrees. Larger positive values suggest a class II relationship, whereas negative values indicate a class III tendency.

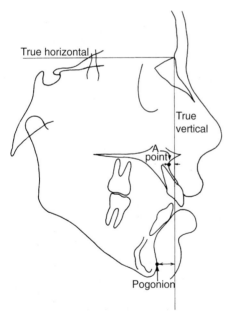

• **Figure 31.46** The position and size of the maxilla and mandible are evaluated by comparing the A point (maxilla) and pogonion (mandible) with a vertical reference line. In a well-positioned maxilla, the A point is located near the vertical reference line. The pogonion is normally 5 mm behind the vertical line in a properly positioned mandible.

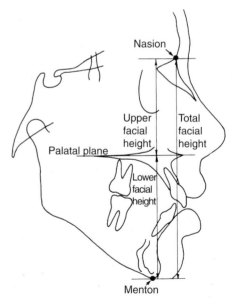

• **Figure 31.48** Vertical facial proportions are determined by measuring total, upper, and lower facial heights. Total facial height is normally measured from the nasion to the menton. The division between upper and lower facial height is made at the palatal plane (a line connecting the anterior and posterior nasal spines). The measurements are used to construct facial height relations or are compared with age-appropriate norms.

Vertical facial proportions can be measured in two ways. The most direct method of determining vertical proportions is to measure total, upper, and lower anterior facial heights and to construct facial height ratios or compare linear measurements with age-appropriate norms.[44,45] Total facial height is normally measured from nasion to menton. The division between the upper and lower facial heights is made at the anterior nasal spine (Fig. 31.48). The

upper facial height should compose approximately 45% of the total facial height in a well-proportioned face.[46] Vertical facial height can be indirectly determined from the mandibular plane angle (the angle between the mandibular plane and the Frankfort horizontal plane). A long-faced person tends to have a large mandibular plane angle, whereas a short-faced person has a smaller mandibular plane angle (Fig. 31.49).

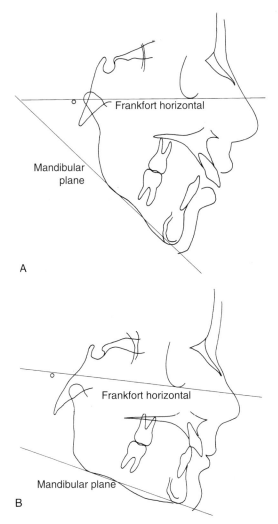

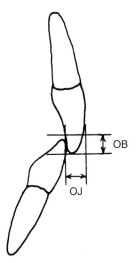

• **Figure 31.50** The position of the maxillary and mandibular incisors and indirectly the entire dentition is evaluated by measuring the overjet and overbite. Overjet *(OJ)* is a horizontal measure of the distance between the most anterior points on the facial surfaces of the maxillary and mandibular central incisors. Overbite *(OB)* is a vertical measure of the overlap between the incisal edges of the maxillary and mandibular incisors.

• **Figure 31.49** (A) Vertical facial height is determined indirectly from the mandibular plane angle (the angle between the mandibular plane and the Frankfort horizontal plane). This angle is usually approximately 24 degrees. A large mandibular plane angle is normally indicative of a long lower facial height. (B) Conversely, a small mandibular plane angle is indicative of a short lower facial height.

Maxillary and mandibular dental position is evaluated by measuring overjet, overbite, and the axial and bodily position of the incisors. Overjet and overbite are simple measurements taken from the facial surfaces and incisal edges of the incisors, respectively (Fig. 31.50). The axial and bodily position of the maxillary incisor is determined relative to the nasion–A point line; the mandibular incisor position is related to the nasion–B point line. Axial inclination is determined from the angle formed by the intersection of the long axis of the incisor with the appropriate nasion–A point or nasion–B point lines. Bodily position is a measure of linear distance from the facial surface of the incisor to the reference line (Fig. 31.51).[47]

A number of soft tissue analyses exist to describe the facial profile. The major problem with soft tissue analysis is that the head film is a static representation of a dynamic object. Lip position may be different on the head film depending on whether the patient was in a relaxed posture (as recommended) or was straining to put the lips together when the film was made. This makes clinical assessment of the profile all the more important.

Nevertheless, lip position is usually compared with the nose and chin. The Ricketts E line, which is convenient to use, is a line connecting the tip of the nose with the anterior contour of the chin (Fig. 31.52). In the permanent dentition, the upper lip is normally 1 mm behind the line and the lower lip is on the line or slightly behind it.[48]

It is important to realize that the numbers derived as norms serve as references and not as the diagnosis itself. Certain measurements may suggest a discrepancy, and this should be verified by the clinical examination. The clinician also should remember that hard and soft tissue analyses vary according to the ethnic background of the patient. Appropriate analyses and standards should be used. Serial cephalometric radiographs obtained before treatment, before and during treatment, or before and after treatment are often useful for evaluating growth, treatment progress, or treatment result, respectively.

Serial cephalometric head films can be superimposed to illustrate changes in jaw and tooth positions. The observed changes are a combination of tooth movement and growth, and it is difficult to differentiate one from the other. To superimpose head films, one must locate an area in the head that is relatively unchanged over the time period in question—that is, an area that is not affected by growth or treatment from which change can be determined. Traditionally, three superimpositions are made with each pair of serial cephalometric radiographs when growth and treatment changes are being evaluated.

The first superimposition illustrates overall changes in the face. The comparison is made by superimposing the structures of the anterior cranial base or along the sella-nasion line registering at the sella. The amount and direction of change in the soft tissue profile and position of the jaws are readily apparent (Fig. 31.53A). To demonstrate the amount and direction of dental change, structures of the maxilla and mandible are superimposed to eliminate all skeletal change from the evaluation (see Fig. 31.53B and C). In the maxilla, the zygomatic process and anterior palatal vault are superimposed to find the best fit. In the mandible, the inner surface of the mandibular symphysis, the outline of

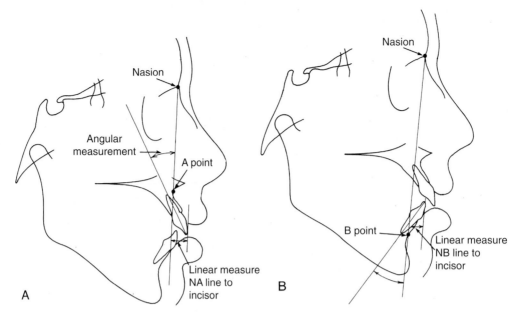

• **Figure 31.51** (A) The axial and bodily positions of the maxillary incisor are determined by making angular and linear measurements. Axial position is determined by drawing an angle formed by the intersection of the long axis of the incisor with the nasion–A *(NA)* point line. A large angle (more than approximately 22 degrees) suggests that the incisor is axially protrusive; a small angle suggests that the incisor is upright. The bodily position of the incisor is determined by measuring the linear distance between the facial surface of the incisor and the nasion–A point line. On the average, this distance is 4 mm. A large measurement suggests that the incisor is positioned too far anteriorly, whereas a small or negative measurement indicates that the incisor is positioned too far posteriorly in relation to the maxilla. (B) The position of the mandibular incisor is similarly evaluated, although the nasion–B *(NB)* point line is used as a reference line. For these measurements, the average inclination is 25 degrees and the average linear distance is 4 mm.

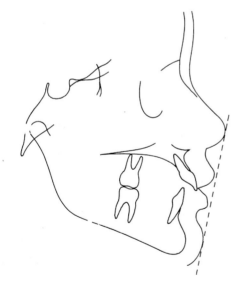

• **Figure 31.52** The Ricketts E line is a convenient reference line used to assess the position of the lips in relation to the nose and chin. In the permanent dentition, the upper lip is normally 1 mm behind a line connecting the tip of the nose to the anterior contour of the chin. The lower lip is usually on or slightly behind this line.

the mandibular canal, and the unerupted third molar crypts are superimposed.

CBCT is a relatively new technology that may replace the lateral cephalogram in the future or at least supplement the information gained from the cephalogram and the panoramic radiograph. The image produced from the radiographic scan allows the clinician to study the area of interest from multiple vantage points. Computer software can render the image in three dimensions so the patient and clinician can better understand the spatial relationships of the teeth and skeletal structures. There are several advantages of CBCT. For example, if a maxillary canine is impacted, traditional panoramic and cephalometric films yield information in two dimensions of a 3D situation. The clinician has historically gathered additional information from periapical radiographs, yet there is still some guesswork of where the canine is positioned. The cone beam scan can give the clinician precise information on the position of the impacted canine, its angulation, its proximity to other teeth, possible resorption of teeth, and the amount of bone surrounding the tooth. This allows the orthodontist and the surgeon to make a more detailed plan regarding the status of the impacted or ectopic tooth and the adjacent teeth. This can be translated into a surgical and orthodontic plan (Fig. 31.54). The main disadvantage of the cone beam scan is the amount of radiation the patient is exposed to compared with a traditional radiographic exam. However, this may change as the technology is improved and the scan time is reduced. A method to address this issue currently is to obtain truncated maxillary views (smaller fields of view) to reduce radiation, assuming this is the only area of interest (Fig. 31.55). Advocates of CBCT also point out that the traditional exam materials can be created out of the data set gathered from the scan. These exam materials include a cephalometric radiograph, a panoramic radiograph, and a virtual set of orthodontic models. Depending on the views and the specific machine and requested resolution, full scans may exceed truncated scans supplemented with traditional digital images, as mentioned earlier.

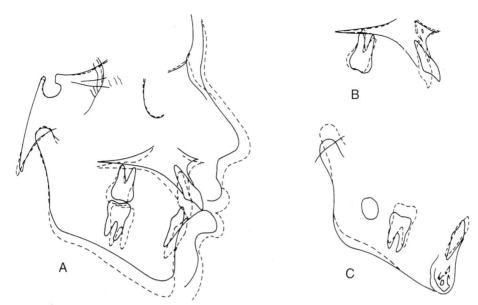

• **Figure 31.53** (A) Serial cephalometric head films are superimposed to illustrate changes in jaw and tooth positions during growth and orthodontic treatment. To assess overall change, a stable area within the head that is not influenced by growth or treatment is located. These overall changes in the face are illustrated by superimposing them on structures of the anterior cranial base. In this case, the solid line represents the patient before orthodontic treatment was initiated. The second or *dashed line* represents the patient after treatment was completed. During treatment, the maxilla moved slightly forward and downward. The horizontal position of the mandible remained virtually unchanged. However, the mandible did move vertically. The position of the lips improved during the treatment period as well. (B) To illustrate the amount and direction of dental change, structures in the maxilla and mandible are superimposed. In this case, the maxillary superimposition, based on a best fit of palatal morphologic appearance, shows that the incisor and molar were both tipped distally. In addition, there was a change in the vertical position of the incisor. The change in incisor and molar position contributed to an improvement in molar relationships and overjet reduction. (C) The mandibular superimposition, made by overlaying the inner aspect of the mandibular symphysis, the canal of the inferior alveolar nerve, and the unerupted third molar crypt, shows that both the incisor and molar erupted vertically.

Radiographic Evaluation

Transition into the mixed dentition requires modification of the basic pediatric survey. Some considerations for radiographs of children in this period are the following.

1. Identification of missing teeth, supernumerary teeth, and the developmental status of permanent anteriors and premolars require greater periapical coverage on films. The maxillary lateral incisors should be evident early in this period. The permanent second premolars are usually evident on radiographs at age 4 years, but they may not be apparent until age 8 years.
2. Absence of erupted maxillary lateral incisors that are of normal size and shape should be apparent early. If not, they should be confirmed with a panoramic radiograph. The reason for this approach is that the missing or peg-shaped lateral incisors are also associated with missing second premolars, distally erupting mandibular canines, palatally erupting maxillary canines, and transpositions of the canines and adjacent teeth.
3. Potential eruption problems may be diagnosed from the radiographs by study of the unerupted teeth. Ectopic eruption of permanent first molars has been discussed and is diagnosed from routine bitewing radiographs. Ectopic eruption of incisors and canine impaction, which are other maxillary eruption problems, are often diagnosed from panoramic radiographs but can be erroneously evaluated in this manner if only a panoramic radiograph is used (Fig. 31.56).[16,49]

If the canines cannot be palpated on the facial aspect of the alveolus at approximately 10 years of age, labial or palatal positioning of the canine is best determined using the panoramic radiograph to determine whether any of the other associated conditions are also present. The first step in determining the position of the canine is to closely examine the panoramic film and compare the size of the right and left canines. Similar to using a flashlight to create a shadow, the closer the object is to the light source (or radiation source), the larger the shadow cast. As the object moves away from the light source, the shadow is smaller. The panoramic beam comes from behind the head, so a palatal positioned canine is closer to the beam and will appear larger than the other canine on the panoramic film. Because of the rendering of a 3D object on a 2D film, this technique can still leave question as to the position of the canine.

To make detailed determinations regarding the position of the canines, other images may also be necessary. If orthodontic treatment is being considered and a cephalometric head film has been obtained, one may look at the cephalometric head film to determine the anteroposterior position of the canine. However, a truncated CBCT film may be the simplest and most decisive film used to supplement the panoramic radiograph (see Fig. 31.55).

CBCT has become an important imaging tool in dentistry. The use of CBCT imaging in the pediatric dental patient

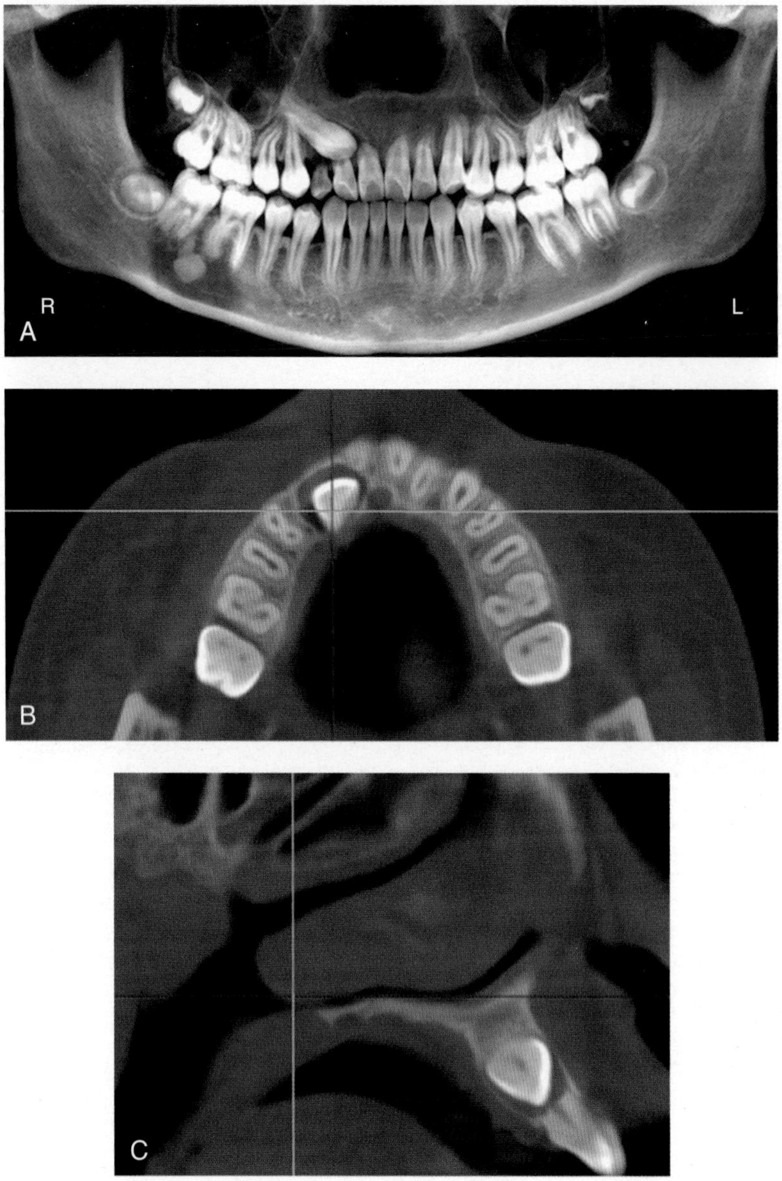

• **Figure 31.54** (A) A conventional panoramic reconstruction showing the ectopic eruption of the maxillary right canine. The root morphology of the maxillary right lateral and central incisors also looks suspicious. (B) Three-dimensional reconstruction of the patient from a small field of view cone beam computed tomography reveals that the canine is superior to the lateral and central incisors. (C) This view demonstrates the root resorption of the central incisor.

is very limited until patients begin to transition into permanent dentition. CBCT becomes more important in this age group. There has been debate on how much or how often this technique should be used. The debate has not been about the information gained but the amount of radiation needed to image the patient. Different machines expose the patient to varying amounts of radiation.[50] Newer machines have been introduced that not only reduce the amount of radiation needed to obtain an image but are also able to limit the size of the field to the area of interest so the radiation is diminished even further.

CBCT imaging is beginning to be used to assess the health of teeth, supporting structures, and temporomandibular joints (TMJs) after dental trauma. The image can establish not only if tooth and bone are intact or fractured but can

also determine the location and morphology of the fracture. Guidelines suggest that standard periapical and occlusal radiographs are sufficient for most cases, but as radiation exposure decreases, CBCT may become the standard technique. Images obtained shortly after trauma are used to assess the extent of the trauma and help determine the proper treatment. After the traumatic incident, CBCT imaging provides a tool to measure the effectiveness of the initial treatment and the current state of healing.

CBCT is also used to assess the volume of the airway in children with obstructive sleep apnea and other airway issues. Currently there is significant interest in this area to see if CBCT is a reliable screening, diagnostic, and treatment assessment tool. At this time, there is not sufficient evidence to provide a definitive answer.

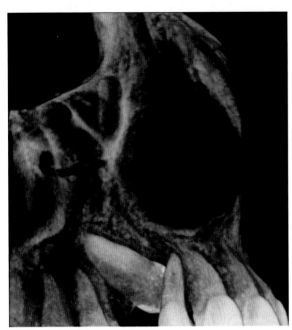

• **Figure 31.55** A truncated maxillary view (smaller fields of view) is a good way to visualize the position of impacted teeth and to reduce radiation to the patient. This type of information gives the clinician a very precise idea of the tooth position.

In orthodontics, CBCT is useful to locate impacted teeth with more precision than ever before. In the past, the surgeon would expose the impacted tooth and determine the orientation of the tooth and its position in relation to adjacent teeth. Now the dentist and surgeon can view the orientation of the tooth, its location, and its effect on other teeth prior to surgery. More importantly, the orthodontist can direct the surgeon to bond the tooth in a certain position to enhance the movement of the tooth and provide the most efficient force vector. CBCT images are also being used to plan orthognathic surgical procedures. The images provide a much clearer picture of the malocclusion and the type of skeletal movement necessary to correct the malocclusion. In addition, new software allows surgeons to complete virtual surgery prior to the actual surgery and have preformed bone plates and surgical splints that fit with increased accuracy. As cone beam technology becomes more sophisticated with smaller field size and decreased radiation exposure, the use of traditional 2D films will diminish.

4. Small palate size, especially early in the school-aged period, prevents or complicates maxillary periapical radiography via a long-cone film-stabilizing apparatus.
5. Greater anteroposterior length in the posterior occlusion requires more bitewing coverage.

In the early mixed-dentition period, all tooth-bearing areas should be surveyed. Supernumerary, missing, and impacted teeth are the most common issues revealed in the radiographic exam. The American Academy of Pediatric Dentistry recommends posterior bitewing films and a panoramic radiograph or posterior bitewing films and selected periapical radiographs. The panoramic radiograph offers the advantage of showing the TMJ. Definitive TMJ films are indicated when there are clinical signs of dysfunction or a history of TMJ abnormalities. If a more traditional intraoral film survey is considered, it should include appropriate anterior occlusal

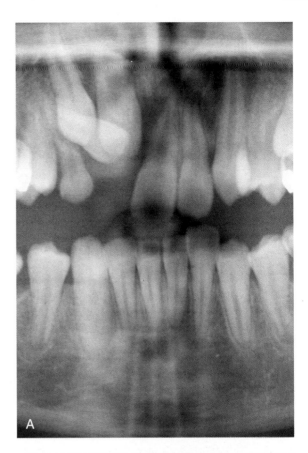

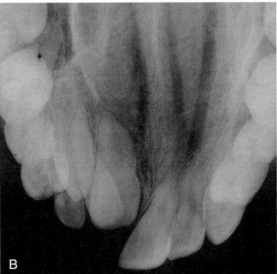

• **Figure 31.56** Often images of unerupted canines and lateral incisors are distorted on panoramic radiographs and can be better visualized on occlusal radiographs. (A) The panoramic radiograph shows little overlap of the maxillary left canine and lateral incisor. (B) The occlusal radiograph shows considerable overlap of the same canine and lateral incisor.

views, at least one periapical view in each posterior quadrant, and posterior bitewings (Fig. 31.57). The number of films should be dictated by the size of the tooth-bearing areas, the adequacy of tissue coverage by the size of films, and the needs of the child. A 12-film survey (four posterior periapical, two anterior occlusals, and two posterior bitewing films) should suffice for the older

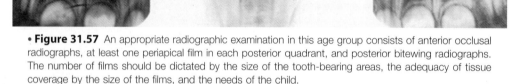

• **Figure 31.57** An appropriate radiographic examination in this age group consists of anterior occlusal radiographs, at least one periapical film in each posterior quadrant, and posterior bitewing radiographs. The number of films should be dictated by the size of the tooth-bearing areas, the adequacy of tissue coverage by the size of the films, and the needs of the child.

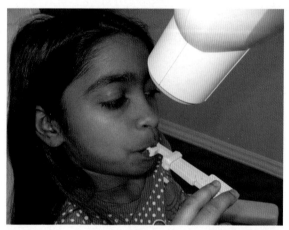

• **Figure 31.58** A film holding device similar to the device shown here can be used as an anterior film stabilizer. The prong end is used to hold a film in place by the child. A bisecting-angle technique is used.

school-aged child. It is difficult to determine whether a 12-film survey or a panoramic/bitewing combination yields a greater effective radiation dose. The variables of machine type, collimation, and film speed make determination difficult. There is discussion currently in the dental imaging literature on whether to switch from the concept of "as low as reasonably achievable" (ALARA) to "as low as diagnostically acceptable" (ALADA).[51]

Radiographic techniques used in the youngest in this age group may include modifications. The anterior area requires placement of the film positioner deeper in the palate to obtain proper orientation. A film holding device can be used with a bisecting-angle technique (Fig. 31.58). The bitewing technique used in this age group is essentially the same as that used in the preschooler. It may take more skill to open contacts by careful positioning of the

beam. Larger films may be preferable because they cover more area in each exposure.

Selection criteria also apply to this age group. Justification of a full-mouth survey of some type is based on the need to identify dental developmental problems and pathologic processes. The number of films made should reflect the adequacy of composite exposure provided by individual views, using the smallest number possible that still reveal all necessary areas. In the age range of 6 to 12 years, several film combinations are possible. No single set of projections is considered best.

Treatment Planning for Nonorthodontic Problems

The planning of care for this age group usually centers on orthodontic considerations, although many patients require additional treatment. Some elements of treatment planning that may have to be addressed but are only peripherally related to orthodontics include the following:

1. *Management of primary caries.* Within this age period, many primary teeth normally exfoliate. A decision to extract a tooth or restore it must be made with its remaining lifespan in mind as well as the length of time that the child will be without a replacement. Prosthetic replacement for a short time may not be indicated if adequate functional surfaces are available elsewhere and space maintenance is not indicated.
2. *Management of pathology.* Some forms of oral pathology, such as supernumerary teeth, odontomas, or missing teeth, are given definitive management in this period owing to the child's increased ability to cooperate and the impending effects of the problem.
3. *Prevention of dental disease.* The choice of sealants is made during this period to protect occlusal surfaces of the teeth. The clinician

must consider how to manage incipient smooth surface and interproximal lesions of permanent teeth. Topical fluoride regimens should be considered if the patient is determined to have a high caries risk. At the writing of this edition, new treatment modalities are being introduced to treat incipient and early caries. Silver diamine fluoride has been discussed earlier and may be used to treat sensitivity and decay in hypoplastic molars. A systematic review of the resin infiltration technique that uses acid pretreatment of interproximal surfaces followed by infiltration with resin into incipient or enamel-based lesions is effective in the short and medium term.[52,53]

4. *Health issues.* Children with disabilities or serious illnesses are in a transitional time. The child with cancer, orofacial clefting, cerebral palsy, or a host of other conditions may need special consideration in regard to such issues as lifespan, realistic functional requirements, retention of teeth for growth purposes, and the role of the appearance of teeth in social acceptance. Decisions regarding these issues are often complex, and input from parents, the child, and other professionals is helpful in decision-making. The dentist's role is to provide information about the need for care, the benefits anticipated, the alternatives to care (including no treatment), and the burden of maintenance of care. These special patients may challenge the dentist's skills in planning care, and they may require careful and frequent observation rather than treatment.

Regardless of the specific situation, dental and periodontal diseases are addressed first and stabilized. Restorative care is rendered next, and more definitive prosthodontic or orthodontic treatment is completed last.

References

1. Hagan PP, Hagan JP, Fields HW Jr, et al. The legal status of informed consent for behavior management technique in pediatric dentistry. *Pediatr Dent.* 1984;6:204–208.
2. Greulich WW, Pyle SI. *Radiographic Atlas of Skeletal Development of the Hand and Wrist.* Palo Alto, CA: Stanford University Press; 1959.
3. Baccetti T, Franchi L, McNamara JA Jr. An improved version of the cervical vertebral maturation (CVM) method for the assessment of mandibular growth. *Angle Orthod.* 2002;72:316–323.
4. Baccetti T, Franchi L, Toth LR, et al. Treatment timing for twin-block therapy. *Am J Orthod Dentofacial Orthop.* 2000;118:159–170.
5. Ballrick JW, Fields HW, Beck FM, et al. The cervical vertebrae staging method's reliability in detecting pre and post mandibular growth. *Orthod Waves.* 2013;72(3):105–111.
6. Marshall WA, Tanner JM. Puberty. In: Falkner F, Tanner JM, eds. *Human Growth: A Comprehensive Treatise.* Vol 2. New York: Plenum Press; 1986.
7. Moorrees CA, Fanning EA, Hunt EE Jr. Age variation of formation stages for ten permanent teeth. *J Dent Res.* 1963;42:1490–1502.
8. Chertkow S. Tooth mineralisation as an indicator of the pubertal growth spurt. *Am J Orthod Dentofacial Orthop.* 1980;77:79–91.
9. Fields HW, Proffit WR, Nixon WL, et al. Facial pattern differences in long-faced children and adults. *Am J Orthod Dentofacial Orthop.* 1984;85:217–223.
10. Dickens S, Sarver D, Proffit W. Changes in frontal soft tissue dimensions of the lower face by age and gender. *World J Orthod.* 2002;3:313–320.
11. Devishree S, Guijari SK, Shubhashini PV. Frenectomy: a review with the reports of surgical techniques. *J Clin Diagn Res.* 2012;6(9):1587–1592.
12. Ramfjord SP. The periodontal index. *J Periodontol.* 1967;38:602–610.
13. Loe N, Silness J. Periodontal disease in pregnancy. I. Prevalence and severity. *Acta Odontol Scand.* 1963;21:533–551.
14. Proffit WR, Fields HW, Sarver DM. *Contemporary Orthodontics.* 3rd ed. St Louis: Mosby–Year Book; 2000.
15. Polder BJ, Van't Hof MA, Van der Linden FP, et al. A meta-analysis of the prevalence of dental agenesis of permanent teeth. *Community Dent Oral Epidemiol.* 2004;32:217–226.
16. Pirinen S, Arte S, Apajalahti S. Palatal displacement of canine is genetic and related to congenital absence of teeth. *J Dent Res.* 1996;75(10):1742–1746.
17. Frazier-Bowers SA, Scott MR, Cavender A, et al. Mutational analysis of families affected with molar oligodontia. *Connect Tissue Res.* 2002;43(2–3):296–300.
18. Sonis AL, Tarbell N, Valachovic RW, et al. Dentofacial development in long-term survivors of acute lymphoblastic leukemia. A comparison of three treatment modalities. *Cancer.* 1990;66(12):2645–2652.
19. Küchler EC, Costa AG, Costa Mde C, et al. Supernumerary teeth vary depending on gender. *Braz Oral Res.* 2011;25(1):76–79.
20. Braun A, Appel T, Frentzen M. Endodontic and surgical treatment of a geminated maxillary incisor. *Int Endod J.* 2003;36:380–386.
21. Velasco LF, de Araujo FB, Ferreira ES, et al. Esthetic and functional treatment of a fused permanent tooth: a case report. *Quintessence Int.* 1997;28(10):677–680.
22. Botticelli S, Verna C, Cattaneo PM, et al. Two- versus three-dimensional imaging in subjects with unerupted maxillary canines. *Eur J Orthod.* 2011;33:344–349.
23. Baccetti T. Tooth anomalies associated with failure of eruption of first and second permanent molars. *Am J Orthod Dentofacial Orthop.* 2000;118:608–610.
24. Peck S, Peck L, Kataja M. Concomitant occurrence of canine malposition and tooth agenesis: evidence of orofacial genetic fields. *Am J Orthod Dentofacial Orthop.* 2002;122:657–660.
25. Garib DG, Alencar BM, Lauris JR, et al. Agenesis of maxillary lateral incisors and associated dental anomalies. *Am J Orthod Dentofacial Orthop.* 2010;137(6):732.e1.
26. Ericson S, Kurol J. Resorption of maxillary lateral incisors caused by ectopic eruption of the canines. A clinical and radiographic analysis of predisposing factors. *Am J Orthod Dentofacial Orthop.* 1988;94(6):503–513.
27. Kurol J, Bjerklin K. Ectopic eruption of maxillary first permanent molars: a review. *ASDC J Dent Child.* 1986;53(3):209–214.
28. Portela MB, Sanchez AL, Gleiser R. Bilateral distal ectopic eruption of the permanent mandibular central incisors: a case report. *Quintessence Int.* 2003;34(2):131–134.
29. Kimmel NA, Gellin ME, Bohannan HM, et al. Ectopic eruption of maxillary first permanent molars in different areas of the United States. *ASDC J Dent Child.* 1982;49:294–299.
30. Bjerklin K, Kurol J. Ectopic eruption of the maxillary first permanent molar: etiologic factors. *Am J Orthod.* 1983;84:147–155.
31. Pulver F. The etiology and prevalence of ectopic eruption of the maxillary first permanent molar. *J Dent Child.* 1968;35:138–146.
32. Ericson S, Kurol J. Early treatment of palatally erupting maxillary canines by extraction of the primary canines. *Eur J Orthod.* 1988;10:283–295.
33. Sigler LM, Baccetti T, McNamara JA Jr. Effect of rapid maxillary expansion and transpalatal arch treatment associated with deciduous canine extraction on the eruption of palatally displaced canines: a 2-center prospective study. *Am J Orthod Dentofacial Orthop.* 2011;139(3):e235–e244.
34. Gellin ME, Haley JV. Managing cases of overretention of mandibular primary incisors when their permanent successors erupt lingually. *ASDC J Dent Child.* 1982;49:118–122.
35. Frazier-Bowers SA, Puranik CP, Mahaney MC. The etiology of eruption disorders—further evidence of a 'genetic paradigm.' *Semin Orthod.* 2010;16(3):180–185.
36. Proffit WR, Vig KWL. Primary failure of eruption: a possible cause of posterior open-bite. *Am J Orthod Dentofacial Orthop.* 1981;80:173–190.

37. Rasmussen P, Kotsaki A. Inherited primary failure of eruption in the primary dentition: report of five cases. *ASDC J Dent Child.* 1997;64(1):43–47.

38. Frazier-Bowers SA, Koehler KE, Ackerman JL, et al. Primary failure of eruption: further characterization of a rare eruption disorder. *Am J Orthod Dentofacial Orthop.* 2007;131(5):578.e1.

39. Akyalcin S, Dyer DJ, English JD, et al. Comparison of 3-dimensional dental models from different sources: diagnostic accuracy and surface registration analysis. *Am J Orthod Dentofacial Orthop.* 2013;144(6):831–837.

40. Bolton WA. Disharmony in tooth size and its relation to the analysis and treatment of malocclusion. *Am J Orthod Dentofacial Orthop.* 1958;28:113–130.

41. Tanaka MM, Johnston LE. The prediction of the size of unerupted canines and premolars in a contemporary orthodontic population. *J Am Dent Assoc.* 1974;88:798–801.

42. Fields HW, Sinclair PM. Dentofacial growth and development. *ASDC J Dent Child.* 1990;57:46–55.

43. McNamara JA Jr. A method of cephalometric analysis. In: McNamara JA, Ribbens KA, Howe RP, eds. *Clinical Alteration of the Growing Face.* Monograph 12, Craniofacial Growth Series. Ann Arbor, MI: University of Michigan, Center for Human Growth and Development; 1983:81–105.

44. Harvold EP. *The Activator in Orthodontics.* St Louis: Mosby; 1974.

45. Isaacson JR, Isaacson RJ, Speidel TM, et al. Extreme variation in vertical facial growth and associated variation in skeletal and dental relations. *Am J Orthod Dentofacial Orthop.* 1971;41:219–229.

46. Wylie WL, Johnson EL. Rapid evaluation of facial dysplasia in the vertical plane. *Angle Orthod.* 1952;22:165–182.

47. Steiner CC. The use of cephalometrics as an aid to planning and assessing orthodontic treatment. *Am J Orthod Dentofacial Orthop.* 1960;46:721–735.

48. Ricketts RM. Perspectives in the clinical application of cephalometrics. *Angle Orthod.* 1981;51:115–150.

49. Jacobs SG. Localization of the unerupted maxillary canine: how to and when to. *Am J Orthod Dentofacial Orthop.* 1999;115(3):314–322.

50. Ludlow JB, Timothy R, Walker C, et al. Effective dose of dental CBCT—a meta analysis of published data and additional data for nine CBCT units. *Dentomaxillofac Radiol.* 2014;44(1):20140197.

51. Jaju PP, Jaju SP. Cone-beam computed tomography: time to move from ALARA to ALADA. *Imaging Sci in Dent.* 2015;45(4):263–265.

52. Tinanoff N, Coll JA, Dhar V, et al. Evidence-based update of pediatric dental restorative procedures: preventive strategies. *J Clin Pediatr Dent.* 2015;39(3):193–197.

53. Ammari MM, Soviero VM, da Silva Fidalgo TK, et al. Is non-cavitated proximal lesion sealing an effective method for caries control in primary and permanent teeth? A systematic review and meta-analysis. *J Dent.* 2014;42(10):1217–1227.

32

Prevention of Dental Disease

KECIA S. LEARY AND ARTHUR J. NOWAK

CHAPTER OUTLINE

The patient between 6 and 12 years of age presents an interesting professional challenge for the dentist. At the beginning of this period, the dentist is dealing with a patient who continues to depend on the parents but is now in a formalized school program for approximately 7 hours a day. By the end of this period, the dentist is dealing with a patient who has gained partial independence from his or her parents and is nearly ready for middle school or junior high school. These preteens are approaching puberty and its many physiologic, emotional, and social challenges.

In addition, a number of oral-facial changes are taking place throughout this period. Most of the primary teeth are replaced with permanent teeth. The alignment and occlusion of the teeth are developing, and the "adult face" is emerging. What "I" look like becomes important, as does the opinions of others, especially peers.

Diet and dietary practices are severely challenged by the educational environment and social pressures both during the day and after school hours. Requirements vary from year to year in this period. Prevalence of obesity increases greatly as opportunities to purchase high-calorie foods in schools, vending machines, and convenience stores may be combined with changes in physical activity. The growth pattern of the patient changes from slow progressive physical growth early in the period to substantial physical growth at the end of the period. The dietary requirements depend not only on growth and development but also on the level of physical and mental activity engaged in by the child. Snacking is a common practice during this period, and children are constantly prompted to think about food and eating.

Many changes in manual dexterity take place during this period. Although continuing gross motor development prevails, this is the period when fine motor skills begin to mature. During this period the child is challenging the parents for independence, especially in areas of personal hygiene, clothes selection, and dietary choices.

Conflicts emerge between the parents' desires and the child's wishes. It is a time when parents still have a strong daily influence on all types of activity, including oral care. With eruption of the permanent teeth, topical fluoride needs and occlusal sealants take on added importance. Orthodontic treatment is often initiated during this time frame. This can contribute to some specific challenges to oral hygiene. Periodic assessments and input by the dentist are important so that the child receives the optimal protection available.

Fluoride Administration

The period from 6 to 12 years is extremely important with regard to fluoride administration, for three major reasons: (1) the crowns of many permanent teeth continue to form during this period, (2) the posterior permanent teeth erupt and are at greater risk for developing caries until the process of "posteruptive maturation" has occurred, and (3) the child becomes increasingly responsible for the maintenance of their oral health. For the child at highest risk for caries, the optimal use of a selected fluoride therapy should be used to provide protection during this first phase of carious attack on those teeth that will constitute the permanent dentition.

Systemic Fluorides

Studies suggest that a substantial portion of the anticaries protection provided by water fluoridation in humans occurs during the preeruptive period.[1,2] Therefore pediatric dentists recommend drinking fluoridated water to help reduce dental caries activities.[3] Additional studies in laboratory animals have reported that daily doses of fluoride administered via gastric intubation during the period of tooth formation reduced the incidence of caries in these teeth after eruption.[4] Because systemically acquired fluoride may be deposited and redistributed in developing teeth during the mineralization phase, as well as during the subsequent period before eruption, current recommendations call for systemic fluoride supplements for children at high risk of developing caries and residing in areas where the water is fluoride deficient until they reach the age of 16 years.[5] This protocol should help to ensure maximum protection for the posterior teeth, which are more vulnerable to carious attack. Supplemental fluoride dosages remain constant for children between the ages of 6 and 16 years in areas where access to community water fluoridation is less than 0.6 ppm fluoride.[3] However, all sources of fluoride (systemic and topical) should be taken into consideration before prescribing systemic fluoride.[5]

Topical Fluorides

During the period from 6 to 12 years of age, the child should become increasingly responsible for the maintenance of his or her oral health. Many forms of topical fluoride are appropriate for children in this age group, including fluoride toothpastes, fluoride mouthrinses, and concentrated fluoride preparations for professional and home application.

Accumulating evidence continues to support the effectiveness and importance of frequent applications of agents that contain relatively low concentrations of fluoride. The two principal forms of these agents in the United States are fluoride toothpastes and fluoride mouthrinses. Daily prescription strength toothpaste and weekly prescription fluoride mouthrinses are recommended for those children who have been identified as high risk with moderate levels of evidence.[6]

Fluoride Toothpastes

The twice-daily use of a fluoride-containing dentifrice should form the foundation of the child's preventive dental activities. To maximize the effect of fluoridated toothpaste, rinsing after brushing should be kept to a minimum or eliminated altogether.[7] Although many toothpastes include fluoride in their formulations, products that have the Seal of Acceptance from the American Dental Association (ADA) should be recommended. The ADA Seal of Acceptance indicates that the product has been voluntarily submitted by the manufacturer and has met the ADA Council on Scientific Affairs' requirements for safety and efficacy. To qualify for the seal, toothpaste evaluation includes measurement of fluoride content, fluoride release, fluoride bioavailability in demineralized enamel, relative dentin abrasivity level, and other tests in accordance to dental standards. Currently, toothpastes with the ADA Seal include sodium fluoride (NaF), sodium monofluorophosphate (MFP), and stannous fluoride (SnF) as active ingredients. Parents should be advised that some over-the-counter toothpaste products may contain higher fluoride concentrations (e.g., 1500 ppm).[8] However, the majority of toothpastes sold in the United States are 1000 ppm.

Fluoride Mouthrinses

The use of fluoride mouthrinses increased considerably during the 1980s as a result of school-based mouth rinsing programs. The most popular preparations contain neutral NaF, although SnF and acidulated phosphate fluoride (APF) rinses also are available. Several fluoride mouthrinses, including many 0.05% NaF products, are available on an over-the-counter (nonprescription) basis.

Numerous clinical trials conducted in the 1960s and 1970s reported caries reductions in the 20%–40% range among children in nonfluoridated areas who rinsed either weekly with a 0.2% NaF rinse or daily with a 0.05% NaF product.[7] More recent studies, conducted since the overall decline in dental caries in children became evident, have reported that (1) the expected benefits from fluoride rinsing in terms of the actual number of tooth surfaces saved from becoming carious are generally less than previously reported, and (2) rinsing appears to have a greater effect in older children (10 years of age).[7] Nevertheless, the observation that fluoride rinsing provides greater protection to erupting teeth during the time when rinses are being applied provides a rationale for their use in some 6- to 12-year-old age groups. Rinses are particularly indicated for persons deemed to be at high risk for caries, such as those with fixed appliances, limited dexterity, or reduced salivary flow. They are not indicated for children who do not have the ability to expectorate without swallowing.[9]

Concentrated Agents for Professional Application or Home Use

Applications of more concentrated forms of fluoride should be considered for persons who are at elevated risk for dental caries, including those who cannot or do not make optimal use of the high-frequency, low-concentration forms of fluoride therapy. In general, this implies semiannual applications of concentrated fluoride gels or fluoride varnish applications (see Chapter 15).

Several fluoride gels and solutions, including combinations of APF and SnF, are available for home use. Practitioners should be aware that some of these products contain concentrations of fluoride that are similar to those found in fluoride toothpastes or over-the-counter rinses, and in most cases they have not undergone clinical testing. Some of these low-concentration products have also been advocated for professional application, but they are unlikely to be effective when used infrequently.[10] Therefore the advantage of these less concentrated products over commercially available fluoride toothpastes and mouthrinses is questionable. More concentrated fluoride gels (0.5% APF) have been shown to be effective in reducing the incidence of caries and may be useful in high-risk patients with rampant caries when used twice daily for caries prevention.[6] NaF mouthrinses used twice daily along with traditional fluoride toothpaste have demonstrated that it may also have an effect on the remineralization of incipient caries lesions.[11] Fluoride mouthrinses have also been found to inhibit the formation of the biofilms on the tooth structure.[12]

Home Care

With school activities now emerging as a major influence in the daily schedule of the child, routine personal hygiene must be scheduled. The development of a routine ideally has been reinforced with the routines established during the preschool period. Unfortunately, it is not only school activities that fill the daily schedule for children in this age group. Internet surfing and social media use on electronic devices, as well as activities such as music lessons, sports activities, dance lessons, homework, religious instruction, daily chores, babysitting, and television, all begin to influence the daily schedule and the time remaining for personal hygiene.

Although brushing after all meals is ideal, such a schedule may be unrealistic. A compromise should be worked out. An appropriate recommendation would be for a thorough brushing of the teeth with fluoride toothpaste and massaging of the gingiva before bed, with additional brushing at the start of each day.[7] Brushing after lunch at school is impractical because many children do not have the time or accommodations to brush their teeth at school. Swishing vigorously with water after lunch helps to dislodge any large particles of food remaining and neutralizes any acid that may be present. Brushing after dinner should also be encouraged.

Parents should remain active in supervising oral care during this period. Periodic inspection of the mouth by the parent is appropriate. Because fine motor activity is further developing during this period, parental assistance may be required to remove all plaque, especially on the buccal surfaces of the posterior maxillary molars and the lingual surfaces of the mandibular posterior molars. Brushes of the appropriate size and contour should be selected to meet the child's needs.[13] With increasing oral dimensions and numbers of teeth, larger brushes should be considered. Soft nylon bristled brushes are recommended over other varieties.

TOOTHBRUSH INNOVATIONS

M. Catherine Skotowski

Billions of dollars are spent on oral health care products each year. The toothbrush is the most commonly used oral health care product for removing plaque and delivering toothpaste to the teeth. For many years, toothbrushes designed for children varied only slightly from those designed for adults, primarily by size, colors, and designs on the toothbrush. However, nowadays a consumer can stroll down any oral health care aisle of a grocery store, pharmacy, or department store and find several types of toothbrushes in many shapes and sizes, designed specifically for children. Toothbrush handles have been ergonomically designed for better grip control and the varying levels of a child's manual dexterity development. Toothbrush bristles are usually soft but are often arranged in various heights to optimize plaque removal on all sides of the teeth. Although some manufacturers have added longer bristles at the tip of the brush head to facilitate plaque removal on the distal surfaces of the most posterior teeth, others have extended bristle lengths at the outer portions of the brush head to aid in cleansing buccal and lingual surfaces. Bristles can be multicolored merely for appearances; however, in one manufacturer's case, a small section of colored bristles have been added to "indicate" when it is time to replace the toothbrush.

Toothbrushing apps for electronic device use have also become popular, assisting children with various oral health concepts in innovative and fun ways.

One of the most noticeable advances to the toothbrush market is the advent of power toothbrushes designed specifically for children. Although power toothbrushes were first introduced in the 1960s, it has only been in the past few decades or so that manufacturers have targeted the children's power toothbrush market. Smaller brush heads, the use of brighter colors, popular cartoon characters, and built-in timers (some with musical tunes) are some of the features designed to make power brushes more appealing to children and adolescents. Some of the power toothbrushes have rechargeable stands that require electricity, whereas others on the less expensive end are battery operated. In terms of plaque removal, power toothbrushes appear to be as effective as, if not better than, manual toothbrushes.[14,15]

The novelty toothbrushes, both manual and power, may provide some extra motivation for those who use them because they are unique, fun to use, and possibly more appealing. The ultimate desired outcome of their use is improved oral hygiene efforts on the part of children and adolescents (the wish of many dedicated oral health professionals).

Although mechanical toothbrushes have been available for some time, there has recently been a dramatic increase in their development and promotion. All types, shapes, head size variations, rotations, and vibrations (oscillating and ultrasonic powered) are now available. Some are modified and promoted for children, others only for adults. Some studies show dramatic improvements in plaque removal and gingival health; others report results that are not so impressive.[14,15] The novelty of the device may increase children's compliance with daily brushing. It is important to consider the initial cost and the cost of brush head replacements when recommending a mechanical brush. For patients with special health care needs, especially those with limited motor activity, these power bushes can be beneficial.

With the increased size and independence of the child, the bathroom becomes the ideal location for cleaning. The previously recommended supine position which increases visibility and stability in the very young child is no longer appropriate. A well-lit bathroom with a wall mirror or hand mirror greatly aids the cleaning process.

Use of disclosing tablets or solutions helps the child and parent to evaluate the thoroughness of the cleaning (Fig. 32.1). At least weekly, the teeth should be disclosed, and with the parent's supervision, the child's mouth should be inspected. Areas of disclosed plaque should be noted with instructions on modification of technique so that it will be removed daily.

With the exfoliation of primary teeth and the eruption of permanent teeth, the gingiva may be tender and even swollen, causing the child to hesitate to do a thorough cleaning. Careful wiping of this area with the brush should maintain the health of the tissues. As the permanent teeth erupt, the alignment may be irregular and the gingival tissue may lose its "knife edge" anatomy with the tooth. Instead, a ledge of gingival tissue may emerge that allows plaque to accumulate (Fig. 32.2). Careful manipulation of the brush is necessary until the gingival contour assumes a smooth margin with the tooth. In mouths with a developing discrepancy between arch length and tooth size, the malalignment of the teeth causes retention of food and plaque. Until orthodontic correction, additional brushing by both child and parent may be necessary.

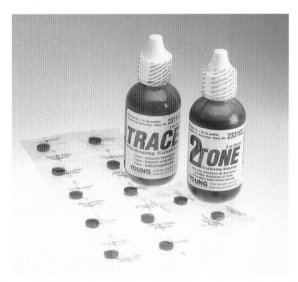

• **Figure 32.1** Disclosing solution and tablets used to evaluate the thoroughness of cleaning. (Pictured: Young's cherry-flavored Trace Disclosing Solution, 2-Tone Disclosing Solution, and Disclosing Tablets. Courtesy Practicon Dental, Greenville, NC.)

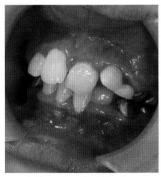

• **Figure 32.2** Mixed dentition. Note crowding of teeth and ledge of gingiva and areas of gingivitis.

Toward the end of this period the child may have developed enough fine motor activity to be able to floss. Like any other motor activity, this skill must be learned and practiced frequently. Parents can be helpful in assisting the child. Inappropriate use of the floss by "snapping" it into the interproximal surfaces can injure the gingiva. Once passed through the contact, the floss must be carefully manipulated along one surface of the tooth and then the opposite surface, making sure that it reaches the area just under the gingival crevice. One of the many commercially available floss holders may greatly assist in the process (Fig. 32.3).

As the child extends his or her social activities, overnight, weekend, or extended periods away from home occur. As they "pack their bags," toothbrushes, dentifrices, and floss will probably be thought of last, if at all. Again, parents must ensure that the appropriate tools are available; whether they will be used is another question.

Children with developmental disabilities may require partial or total assistance in oral care, depending on their mental and physical capabilities. If a parent must help with or be totally responsible for mouth care, a mouth prop may be helpful (Fig. 32.4). With good head stability and mouth propping, the cleaning process is enhanced. Children with severe mobility limitations may require more than one person to assist in activities like toothbrushing. Modifications to oral hygiene devices may also be needed. For instance, a three-headed toothbrush may be useful. Stabilization and proper positioning may be necessary, and if so, the bathroom may be an inappropriate location. Use of the bedroom or other living area with available floor space, beds, or couches allows the child to be placed in a supine position and stabilized. In these situations the use of a dentifrice further complicates the process because of the foaming and the need to expectorate; however, there are toothpastes that do not contain sodium lauryl sulfates (the foaming agents) and still contain fluoride.

Diet

According to prevalence data from 2013 to 2014, 17.4% of school-aged children were considered obese, and there are many factors responsible, including diet and physical activity.[16] Diet also may play a role in the dental caries process.[17] Sugar-sweetened beverages (SSBs) are defined as soda, fruit drinks (including sweetened bottled waters and fruit juices and nectars with added sugars), sports and energy drinks, and sweetened coffees and teas. Consumption of SSBs in 6- to 11-year-olds increased daily from an average of 17.4 ounces in 1994 to 20.5 ounces in 2004.[18] Currently 64.5% of boys and 61% of girls aged 2 to 19 years of age consume at least one SSB daily.[19] Milk consumption declined from 81% to 77% of children having at least one serving per day.[18] Added sugar consumption increased from 275 kcal/day in 1977 to 1978 to a peak of 387 kcal/day in 2003 to 2004 and declined to 326 kcal/day in 2011 to 2012.[20] This change was a 51-kcal/day increase from the 1970s, and added sugar intakes of children continue to exceed recommendations.[20] Although per capita consumption of sweeteners was approximately 142 pounds annually in 2008, up 19% since 1970,[21] there has been a substantial decrease in the use of ordinary refined table sugar. Forty-three percent of the sweeteners used currently are refined sugar from sugarcane and beets; 57% are from corn sweeteners. Beverages (not milk or 100% fruit juice) account for almost half (47%) of all added sugars consumed by the US population, and SSBs account for 39% of these sugars (25% soft drinks, 11% fruit drinks, and 3% sport/energy drinks).[22] The high daily rates of SSB consumption and between-meal intake of sugars remain a risk factor for children susceptible to proximal caries even though caries development is now declining in the United States.[23] Caries rates have dramatically reduced during the last 20 years, even as dramatic changes have taken place in our dietary practices. Data have demonstrated that those children with a higher SSB content have a higher prevalence of dental caries even when adjusting for socioeconomic and maternal oral health characteristics.[24] The use of SSBs also differs according to race/ethnicity and geographic region.[25] It is important that dentists stay aware of dietary practices and changes taking place and monitor

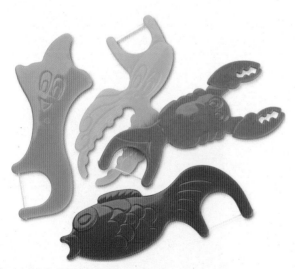

• **Figure 32.3** Disposable flossers designed especially to make flossing easier for children. (Pictured: SmileGoods FlosSeas Flossers. Courtesy Practicon Dental, Greenville, NC.)

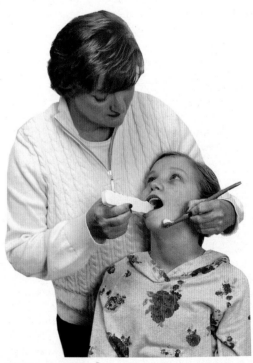

• **Figure 32.4** A mouth prop and a three-headed toothbrush can be used to facilitate oral health care in a child with special health care needs. (Pictured: Open Wide Mouth Rest and Surround toothbrush. Courtesy Specialized Care Co., Inc., Hampton, NH.)

their patients' dietary habits, as well as their weight gains, between appointments.

Although children are introduced to a variety of new foods during the preschool years, the real challenge is to develop good dietary habits during this age group. At this age, there is exposure to a full day in school with frequent treats and school lunches, either from home or purchased at school; vending machines[26]; and a multitude of after-school activities, usually associated with food.[27] All of these factors influence children's dietary habits, as well as the habits that are formed at home regarding modeling healthy food choices.[27] In addition, children in this age group are heavily influenced by the commercial media, especially television. The effect of food choices and purchases has been carefully studied, and although advocacy organizations have attempted to influence the number of commercials related to food shown during the daytime hours, it remains common for the school-aged child to be exposed to many enticements during a period of television, radio, and social media entertainment. If children accompany parents to the market, the purchases they request are frequently related to commercials they have encountered. The more that children eat food outside the home, the higher the likelihood their diet is to be unhealthy.[28] School-aged children are getting foods with little nutritional value not only from fast food restaurants, but also from convenience stores and schools.[27] Although some dramatic changes have occurred recently in food selection and dietary practices, we know that a large percentage of a family's meals are eaten on the run, whether they are from fast food restaurants or in the form of prepackaged meals.

For children with severe caries, the dentist must evaluate all etiologic factors, including diet and dietary practices. A dietary history may be helpful in determining diet practices. Every exposure to a food containing a refined carbohydrate, especially one that adheres to the teeth and dissolves slowly, produces acid in and around the plaque and this may help to identify areas of concern to help a family make small changes in diet. However, the key concepts to diet recommendations are limiting meals and snacks to three to six defined meals or snacks a day, limiting SSB consumption, and eating according to the Choose MyPlate guidelines from the US Department of Agriculture (USDA).[29] It is unrealistic to recommend to a parent of a 6- to 12-year-old child to cut out all candy and sweets. It is better to advise them of possible substitutes, such as a chocolate candy instead of a caramel, or that consumption of candy and sweets should take place only after meals have been eaten rather than before or between meals. Children can learn appropriate eating habits, but they must be realistic, and the parents must be enthusiastic about the change.[30] Families that encourage a home food environment that models healthy eating, by helping to provide some limits on food (while not being too restrictive) and having healthy food at home, will fare much better in helping to maximize the likelihood of a child's healthy weight and eating.[27]

Regarding meals at school, parents must work with school authorities to provide wholesome and nutritious meals that also have eye appeal for the child. In addition, parents should work with specific teachers to encourage the use of appropriate snacks and party foods for special occasions. More than 100,000 schools and 31 million children are participating in free and reduced-cost meals as part of the USDA National School Lunch/Breakfast Programs. There are a set of strict guidelines that now encourage healthy, reduced calorie and sodium meals that also provide fruits and vegetables through the schools. The most recent guidelines recommend only unflavored 1% or nonfat milk and flavored nonfat milk. Children may have access to vending machines at school,

and it is important to recognize the role these may play in the diet of school-aged children. As dentists, it is important to advocate for nutritional and healthy school choices, such as bottled water, and collaborate with other community health leaders in maintaining appropriate choices.[26]

A favorite activity of many school-aged children is gum chewing. Although frowned on by school officials and parents, it may have anticaries effect. Studies have reported an increase in salivary flow and mechanical pumping of saliva to interproximal sites. This results in a neutralization of interproximal acids. These studies have used both sugarless and sugar-containing gums. All studies agree on the beneficial effects of sugarless gums, but a difference of opinion exists on the effect of sugar-containing gums.[31–33] Xylitol-containing gums have been shown to decrease *Streptococcus mutans* levels in saliva and plaque when used routinely.[34] Reduction in caries incidences is reported in all age groups, and when the xylitol-containing gum is used by mothers, it may decrease the transmission of *S. mutans* from mother to child.[35] However, it is important to recognize that therapeutic doses of xylitol and high frequency may be difficult to achieve. Systemic reviews regarding the effectiveness show only a small effect of caries prevention in the pediatric population.[36]

The diets of children with developmental disabilities may be modified for a number of reasons. To increase caloric requirements, supplements are frequently added to routine foods. Unfortunately, these supplements are frequently refined carbohydrates, which increase the risk of acid production. Foods may be altered, minced, pureed, or mashed to assist the child in swallowing and to meet the need for less chewing. Due to chewing and swallowing difficulties, fresh fruits and vegetables are often withheld from the diet and substituted with pastries, canned fruits, puddings, and gelatin desserts, which contain a high percentage of refined carbohydrates. The dentist and their staff must be aware of these modifications and be realistic in providing alternative dietary recommendations to parents of children with developmental disabilities.

Sealants

Sealants are recommended for children to reduce caries risk on the occlusal surface of permanent teeth. This age group is particularly vulnerable to dental decay due to the changes in diet, the independence in oral hygiene practices, and newly erupting teeth. Evidence continually supports that sealants reduce the risk of dental decay in pit and fissures.[37] This age group would benefit from sealants due to the fact that first and second molars will be erupting. This is the age group frequently targeted for school-based sealant programs (see Chapter 33).

References

1. O'Mullane DM, Baez RJ, Jones S, et al. Fluoride and oral health. *Community Dent Health*. 2016;33:66–99.
2. Groeneveld A, Van Eck AA, Backer Dirks O. Fluoride in caries prevention: is the effect pre- or post-eruptive? *J Dent Res*. 1990;69(special issue):751–755.
3. American Academy of Pediatric Dentistry. Guideline on fluoride therapy. *Pediatr Dent*. 2016;38(6):181–184.
4. Hunt CE, Navia JM. Pre-eruptive effects of Mo, B, Sr, and F on dental caries in the rat. *Arch Oral Biol*. 1975;20:497–501.
5. Rozier RG, Adair S, Graham F, et al. Evidence-based clinical recommendations on the prescription of dietary fluoride supplements for caries prevention: a report of the American Dental Association Council on Scientific Affairs. *J Am Dent Assoc*. 2010;141:1480–1489.

6. Weyant RJ, Tracy SL, Anselmo TT, et al. Topical fluoride for caries prevention: executive summary of the updated clinical recommendations and supporting systemic review. *J Am Dent Assoc*. 2013;144:1279–1291.

7. Recommendations for using fluoride to prevent and control dental caries in the United States. Centers for Disease Control and Prevention. *MMWR Recomm Rep*. 2001;50(RR–14):1–42.

8. Centers for Disease Control and Prevention. Community water fluoridation: other fluoride products; 2016. https://www.cdc.gov/fluoridation/basics/fluoride-products.html. Accessed August 16, 2017.

9. Adair SM. Evidence-based use of fluoride in contemporary pediatric dental practice. *Pediatr Dent*. 2006;28:133–142.

10. Crall JJ, Bjerga JM. Fluoride uptake and retention following combined applications of APF and stannous fluoride in vitro. *Pediatr Dent*. 1984;6:226–229.

11. Songsiripradubboon S, Hamba H, Trairatvorakul C, et al. Sodium fluoride mouthrinse used twice daily increased incipient caries lesion remineralization in an in situ model. *J Dent*. 2014;42:271–278.

12. Hannig C, Gaeding A, Basche S, et al. Effect of conventional mouthrinses on initial bioadhesion to enamel and dentin in situ. *Caries Res*. 2013;47:150–161.

13. Nowak AJ, Skotowski MC, Widmer R, et al. A practice based evaluation of a range of children's manual toothbrushes: safety and acceptance. *Compend Contin Educ Dent*. 2002;23(3 suppl 2):17–24.

14. Grossman E, Proskin H. A comparison of the efficacy and safety of an electric and manual children's toothbrush. *J Am Dent Assoc*. 1997;128:469–474.

15. Nowak AJ, Skotowski MC, Cugini M, et al. A practice based study of a children's power toothbrush: efficacy and acceptance. *Compend Contin Educ Dent*. 2002;23(3 suppl 2):25–32.

16. U.S. Department of Health and Human Services. Prevalence of obesity among adults and youth: United States, 2011-2014. *NCHS Data Brief*. 2015;(219).

17. Ogden CL, Carroll MD, Lawman HG, et al. Trends in obesity prevalence among children and adolescents in the United States, 1988-1994 through 2013-2014. *JAMA*. 2016;315(21):2292–2299.

18. Turner L, Chaloupka FJ. Wide availability of high-caloric beverages in US elementary schools. *Arch Pediatr Adolesc Med*. 2011;165(3):223–228.

19. Rosinger A, Herrick K, Gahche J, et al. U.S. Department of Health and Human Services. Sugar-sweetened beverage consumption among US youth, 2011-2014. *NCHS Data Brief*. 2017;(271).

20. Powell ES, Smith-Tallie LP, Popkin BM. Added sugars intake across the distribution of US children and adult consumers: 1977-2012. *J Acad Nutr Diet*. 2016;116:1543–1550.

21. Wells HW, Buzby JC: Dietary assessment of major trends in U.S. food consumption, 1970-2005, Economic Information Bulletin No. (EIB-33), March 2008.

22. U.S. Department of Health and Human Services and U.S. Department of Agriculture. 2015-2020 dietary guidelines for Americans, 8th ed; 2015. http://health.gov/dietaryguidelines/2015/guidelines/.

23. Marshall TA, Broffitt B, Eichenberger-Gilmore J, et al. The roles of meal, snack, and deaily total food and beverage exposures on caries experience in young children. *J Public Health Dent*. 2005;65:166–173.

24. Wilder J, Kaste LM, Handler A, et al. The association between sugar-sweetened beverages and dental caries among third-grade students in Georgia. *J Pub Health Dent*. 2016;76:76–84.

25. Centers for Disease Control and Prevention. Get the facts: sugar-sweetened beverages and consumption; 2017. https://www.cdc.gov/nutrition/data-statistics/sugar-sweetened-beverages-intake.html. Accessed August 16, 2017.

26. American Academy of Pediatric Dentistry. Policy on beverage vending machines in schools. *Pediatr Dent*. 2016;38(special issue):60–61.

27. Couch SC, Glanz K, Zhou C, et al. Home food environment in relation to children's diet quality and weight status. *J Acad Nutr Diet*. 2014;114:1569–1579.

28. Vepasäläinen H, Mikkilä V, Erkkola M, et al. Association between home and school food environments and dietary patterns among 9-11-year-old children in 12 countries. *Int J Obes Suppl*. 2015;5(suppl 2):S66–S73.

29. US Department of Agriculture. Choose my plate; 2017. https://www.choosemyplate.gov/. Accessed August 16, 2017.

30. Singleton JC, Achterberg L, Shannon B. Role of food and nutrition in the health perceptions of young children. *J Am Diet Assoc*. 1992;92:67–70.

31. Beiswanger BB, Elias A, Crawford JL, et al. The effects of sugarless chewing gum use after meals on dental caries. *J Dent Res*. 1996;75(special edition):1003.

32. Jensen ME. Responses of interproximal plaque pH to snack foods and effect of chewing sorbitol-containing gum. *J Am Dent Assoc*. 1986;113:262–266.

33. Jensen ME, Wefel JS. Human plaque pH responses to meals and the effects of chewing gum. *Br Dent J*. 1989;167:204–208.

34. Deshpande A, Jadad AR. The impact of polyol-containing chewing gums on dental caries: a systematic review of original randomized controlled trails and observational studies. *J Am Dent Assoc*. 2008;184:1602–1614.

35. Nakai Y, Shinga-Ishihara C, Kaji M, et al. Xylitol gum and maternal transmission of mutans streptococci. *J Dent Res*. 2010;89:56–60.

36. Marghalani A, Guinto E, Phan M, et al. Effectiveness of Xylitol in reducing dental caries in children. *Ped Dent*. 2017;39:103–110.

37. Wright JT, Tampi MP, Graham L, et al. Sealants for preventing and arresting pit-and-fissure occlusal caries in primary and permanent molars, a systematic review of randomized controlled trials—a report of the American Dental Association and the American Academy of Pediatric Dentistry. *J Am Dent Assoc*. 2016;147:631–645.

33

Pit and Fissure Sealants: Scientific and Clinical Rationale

MARTHA H. WELLS

CHAPTER OUTLINE

In the past several decades, "the power of prevention" perspective has been permeating health care, as we have begun to focus on the burdens that chronic diseases leave in their wake—decreased life expectancy, reduced quality of life, and escalating health care costs. Of particular interest to the dental profession is dental caries, a chronic disease affecting more than 90% of adults aged 20 to 64.[1] Although chronic diseases are among the most common and costly of all health problems, they are also among the most preventable. One of the most powerful prevention tools that the dental health profession has is the dental sealant.

Epidemiology of Pit and Fissure Caries

In the past several decades, dramatic improvements in the prevention of caries have occurred due to a multitude of factors: fluoride exposure, enhanced awareness of the benefits of early care, increased access to dental care, and increased financial coverage by insurance companies, group plans, and government-funded programs of preventive and restorative dental procedures for children.

Despite these efforts, dental caries is still the single most common chronic disease of childhood, more common than asthma and hay fever.[2] The facts from the most recent National Health and Nutrition Examination Survey (NHANES) for the years 2011 to 2012 are alarming[3,4]:

- Approximately 56% of children aged 6 to 8 had dental caries in their primary teeth, and 21% of children aged 6 to 11 had experienced caries in their permanent teeth.
- The prevalence of caries continues to rise with age, as 67% of adolescents aged 16 to 19 had experienced tooth decay.

- The progressive and cumulative effects of caries continue into adulthood, with 91% of adults experiencing caries. Just over 33% of adults aged 20 to 39 had experienced some tooth loss (not including third molars), and 19% of seniors were edentulous.
- Approximately 20% of children aged 6 to 8 had untreated primary tooth decay, and 15% of adolescents had untreated caries in the permanent dentition.

While dental caries is common, the distribution of caries is unequal, with certain subgroups of the population experiencing a disproportionately greater burden of dental disease. According to the National Institute for Dental and Craniofacial Research, 20% of the population bears at least 60% of the caries.[5] Dental caries is more prevalent among children living in poverty,[5a] with poor children experiencing five times more untreated dental caries than children in higher income families.[6] Minority populations are also vulnerable, as children of Mexican American and non-Hispanic black ethnicities are more likely to experience severe and untreated caries.[4,7] Moreover, the pattern of caries involving specific tooth surfaces has changed. In the early 1970s, smooth surface lesions accounted for almost 25% of the Decayed, Missing, Filled Surfaces (DMFS) index. Recent data indicate that approximately 90% of caries in permanent teeth of children occur in pits and fissures, and approximately two-thirds of caries are on the occlusal surface alone.[8] Like permanent teeth, the pits and fissures of primary teeth are also at risk, as roughly 44% of carious lesions in the primary teeth affect the occlusal surfaces of molars.[8]

The occlusal surface is prone to caries for several reasons. First, newly erupted, immature tooth enamel has a relatively high organic content and is more permeable, which makes it more susceptible to caries attack. Second, the pit and fissure morphology provides an environment for plaque retention and bacteria proliferation. The enamel is thinner in pits and fissures and may experience accelerated demineralization. In addition, the molars take a relatively long time to fully erupt (1.5 to 2.5 years compared with just several months for premolars).[9] This prolonged eruption time may interfere with adequate oral hygiene, as toothbrush bristles have difficulty reaching the occlusal surface when it is out of the plane of occlusion, and the operculum covering the distal portion of the tooth may increase plaque retention.[10] In addition, fluoride is less effective in preventing caries on the occlusal surfaces compared with smooth surfaces,[11] and data from fluoridated communities show significantly higher reductions in interproximal lesions compared with pit and fissure lesions.[12] Hence targeting preventive efforts at the occlusal surfaces of molars is appropriate for attempting to decrease the caries experience for US children.

Dental caries has afflicted the human population for centuries, and before the early 1970s, treatment consisted of removing the carious tooth structure. However, in 1955, Buonocore revolutionized dentistry with the first research on adhesive dentistry. From his research came the idea that dentists might have the ability to bond a physical barrier over susceptible pits and fissures and, in effect, "seal" out caries, preventing the carious process. In 1971 the first dental sealant, Nuva-Seal (L.D. Caulk), was introduced, and since that time many studies have examined various products' ability to seal the occlusal surfaces of teeth to maximize "the power of prevention."

Sealant Effectiveness

Unquestionably, dental sealants prevent pit and fissure caries in both primary and permanent teeth. The long-term benefit

of caries reduction from using sealants on permanent teeth has been well documented, as decades worth of research has shown clear evidence of a reduction in caries, and clinical practice guidelines have been developed.[8,11] Wright et al. provide a summary of the evidence of sealant efficacy in caries reduction[13]:

> The results of this systematic review suggest that children and adolescents who receive sealants in sound occlusal surfaces or in noncavitated pit-and-fissure carious lesions in their primary or permanent molars (compared to a control without sealants) experience a 76% reduction in the risk of developing new carious lesions after 2 years of follow up. Even after 7 or more years of follow-up, children and adolescents with sealants had a caries incidence of 29%, whereas those without sealants had a caries incidence of 74%.

In addition, compared with teeth without sealants, teeth that receive sealants are less likely to receive subsequent restorative treatment. If restorative treatment is required, the time until the first restorative treatment is greater than that for unsealed molars, and the restoration is likely to be less extensive.[14]

The effectiveness of sealants in preventing caries is so well recognized in the literature that a study design with a "sealant-free" control group is no longer considered ethically acceptable.[15] The 2016 Clinical Practice Guidelines of the American Dental Association (ADA) recommend the use of sealants compared with nonuse in permanent molars, and the strength of the recommendation was strong, meaning that the evidence of caries reduction by sealants was of moderate to high quality.[11] Given the long clinical history and ample available literature as to their effectiveness, the expectation would be that sealants would have been widely adopted by the dental profession and utilized to their fullest preventive effect. However, even with 50 years' worth of scientific knowledge, sealants are still underused.

Current Sealant Utilization

In 1974, when sealants were new technology, the initial ADA sealant utilization survey found that only 39% of dentists were placing sealants.[16] While adhesive dentistry was making great strides in acceptance for restorative procedures, utilizing sealants for prevention was still low, and thus by 1981 the ADA's Council on Dental Materials, Instruments, and Equipment sponsored a major conference with the title, "Pit and Fissure Sealants: Why Their Limited Usage?" By the late 1980s and 1990s, regional and national surveys indicated large increases in sealant utilization among dentists.[17,18] Survey data suggest that 79% of dentists utilize sealants in their practice "very often" or "often" in permanent teeth, while 53% "rarely" or "never" use sealants in primary teeth.[19] Regional surveys indicate that most pediatric dentists (up to 96%) and most recent graduates (90% of dentists in practice for 10 years or less) utilize sealants.[18,20,21] However, despite the reported increased incorporation of sealants into dentists' practices, the number of children receiving sealants is unexpectedly low.

Data from the NHANES for the years 2011 to 2012 suggest that the prevalence of dental sealants on permanent teeth in children aged 6 to 11 years was 41% and was 43% for adolescents aged 12 to 19 years.[3] Both of these figures are an increase from the 1999 to 2004 prevalence at 30% and 38%, respectively. However, in the low-income population, sealant use rates still remain low and have been found to be 22% or lower.[22] Sealant rates were also lowest in non-Hispanic black (30%) compared with non-Hispanic white (47%), Hispanic (40%), or non-Hispanic Asian (43%) adolescents.[3] With the knowledge that by age 19 nearly 70% of adolescents have experienced tooth decay and that 90% of these caries occur in the pits and fissures, one might expect much higher utilization rates.

Low utilization has been attributed to a lack of confidence in the bonding of sealants to enamel, concern for sealing over caries, and the difficulty of achieving isolation.[23] Survey data indicate that dentists are apprehensive about sealing over incipient caries, as 80% of respondents indicate that they choose not to seal over incipient caries.[24] Fear of placing a sealant over caries was one of the most frequently voiced concerns in the survey's comments section. This topic will be discussed in detail later in this chapter.

Another significant reason cited for limiting sealant usage is the lack of reimbursement for sealant placement. Surveys reveal that lack of insurance reimbursement for both initial placement and reapplication is a frequently reported reason for limiting sealant usage.[12,19] Concerning the lack of reimbursement, insurance companies provide the following reasons[25,26]: (1) concerns about cost-effectiveness of sealants; (2) sealants excluded in the original or current contract; (3) guidelines for sealant placement are not defined; and (4) potential for inappropriate usage and fees. However, these reasons are not well founded. Of the insurance companies that do provide sealant coverage, approximately two-thirds define certain clinical conditions for reimbursement such as age limitations and restriction of sealant placement to permanent teeth, with some specifying molars only.[12] Medicaid programs have made significant strides in making sealants a covered benefit. In 1991 only 58% of Medicaid programs provided reimbursement, but by 1994 all 50 states included sealants in their Medicaid programs.[21,27] However, only 12% provide reimbursement for sealants on premolars, and 30% reimburse sealant application only once per tooth per lifetime (thus not covering reapplication as necessary). Many studies are providing evidence that sealant application in any teeth at risk for caries (primary and permanent molars and premolars) is cost-effective and worthy of reimbursement.[28–31]

How Sealants Work

Three types of materials are utilized as sealants: resin, glass ionomer (traditional and resin-modified), and polyacid-modified resins. The most commonly accepted material is the resin-based sealant, as it has shown superior retention rates compared with glass ionomer sealants.[32–35] The resin-based sealant utilizes the principles of adhesive dentistry as it is retained by micromechanical retention. For the adhesion of the sealant to the enamel to be successful, the tooth must be clean and remain dry because the resin is hydrophobic. The tooth enamel is etched with 35% to 37% phosphoric acid, which creates surface irregularities in which the sealant material flows and forms resin tags (Fig. 33.1). The resin is polymerized (usually by visible light but there are also autopolymerizing resins) and forms a thin, plastic coating over the pits and fissures of the occlusal surface. This physical barrier is essential in preventing the carious process (Fig. 33.2).

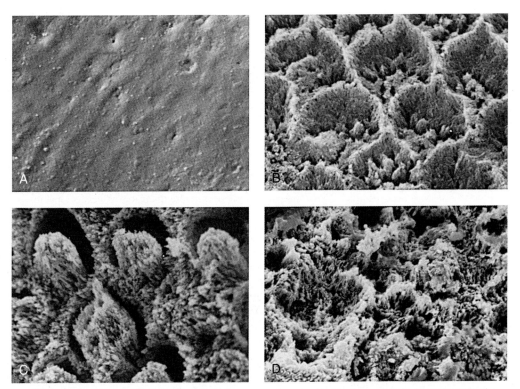

• **Figure 33.1** Effects of the acid-etch technique on surface morphology (scanning electron microscopy). (A) The surface of sound enamel is relatively smooth, with occasional depressions representing terminations of enamel prisms. Several different patterns of etching can occur: (B) the loss of prism cores following etching; (C) the loss of prism peripheries following etching; (D) surface porosities occur, but without a distinct prism morphologic appearance.

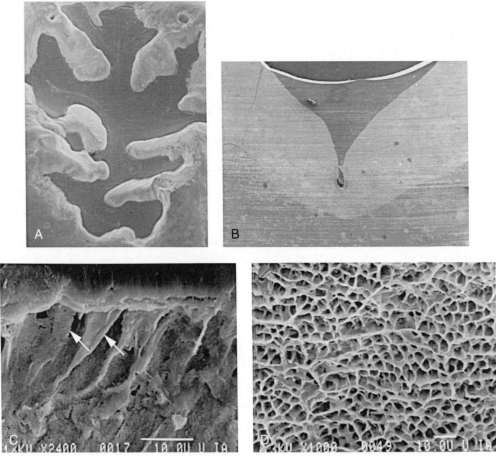

• **Figure 33.2** The enamel-resin interface (scanning electron microscopy). (A) Following sealant placement, the pits and fissures on this occlusal surface are protected from cariogenic challenges by the physical barrier of the sealant. (B) The interface between the enamel forming the fissure and the sealant appears to be an intimate one, with no apparent space between the etched enamel and sealant. (C) Following partial demineralization of enamel that has been sealed, resin tags *(arrows)* may be seen in the etched enamel. (D) Complete demineralization of enamel that has been sealed allows one to visualize the appearance of the acid-resistant resin tags.

Glass ionomer sealants have a different bonding mechanism. They adhere to the enamel through both mechanical retention and chemical bonding, known as chelation. However, the chemical bond alone is weak. Glass ionomers are hydrophilic and can withstand some minimal moisture. For the glass ionomer sealant, the tooth is cleaned, and a tooth conditioner of polyacrylic acid is applied. The tooth is rinsed and dried, and the glass ionomer is placed on the occlusal surface. If it is a resin-modified glass ionomer, it is light cured.

Types of Sealants

Sealant products come in a variety of materials, colors, and viscosities. Resin-based sealants are available as unfilled, filled, clear, colored, visible-light polymerized, autopolymerizing (chemically cured), and fluoride-releasing materials. The earliest sealants were autopolymerizing but have largely been replaced by visible-light curing sealants, though studies have shown similar retention rates and similar strengths.[15,36–38]

Color

Sealants are often available as clear or opaque white. The advantages to an opaque sealant are that it is easy to see during application and easy to monitor its retention at a recall visit. Assessment of a clear sealant requires tactile exploration of the sealed surface. One study examining the visibility of clear and opaque sealants found that the error rate for identifying an opaque sealant was less than 2%, while for clear resin it was nearly 23%. The most common error for the examiners was to incorrectly state that a clear resin sealant was present on a tooth that had never been treated.[39] No apparent difference in the clinical efficacy of either type of sealant has been reported. However, as will be discussed later, sealant retention is critical for the caries preventive effect; hence being able to quickly and correctly assess sealant retention is clinically important.

One additional sealant material is available with color-changing properties. Clinpro (3M ESPE, St. Paul, MN) is a sealant that is pink upon application and turns white when cured. This color change is not correlated with ensuring that the sealant is adequately cured and provides no clinical advantage. Thus the color-changing property has been described as a "perceived marketing benefit."[40] However, this material has similar properties to and is as caries-protective as other resin-based sealants, and thus may be chosen for its other properties (unfilled, fluoridated).[41,42]

Filler Content

Sealants also are available with various filler content. For the most part, the filler content dictates the sealant's physical characteristics regarding viscosity, flow ability, and resistance to wear. Unfilled sealants have some advantages. Unfilled sealants have lower rates of microleakage[43,44] and better penetration into the fissures.[45,46] The theory is that unfilled sealants penetrate deeper into the fissures due to their low viscosity, create longer resin tags, and therefore are better retained. However, unfilled and filled sealants have similar retention rates.[47,48] Another clear advantage of the unfilled sealant is that occlusal adjustment is not necessary. Due to the lack of filler, the unfilled sealant will abrade rapidly if left in occlusion. On the other hand, filled sealants require occlusal adjustment, as individuals are not able to abrade occlusal interferences caused by filled sealants to a comfortable level.[49] The necessity to adjust the occlusion may increase the time and cost of the procedure and may also prevent delegation of sealant placement to auxiliaries.[40,50] On the other hand, filled materials have greater wear resistance and less porosity. In fact, several studies have examined flowable composite as a sealant material. Flowable composite requires the use of a bonding agent that improves fissure penetration and decreases microleakage.[51,52] For clinical retention, flowable composite is equal to[53] and possibly superior to conventional sealant materials.[54] However, the superiority of any type of sealant material remains inconclusive.[13] The dentist should understand the properties of sealant materials and choose a material for its clinical advantages.

Fluoride-Releasing Sealants[55]

Based on the knowledge of the benefits of fluoride release from glass ionomer materials, dental manufacturers have also developed fluoride-releasing resin sealants (FRS). However, studies have shown that salivary fluoride levels are the same before and after sealant placement, and there is no long-lasting release of fluoride to plaque and saliva.[56,57] One should not consider fluoride-containing sealants as a fluoride reservoir with long-term release of fluoride into the immediately adjacent environment.[38] Clinical studies have not demonstrated significant caries prevention of FRS over the benefits obtained from conventional sealants.[58] Only one randomized controlled trial has shown a cariostatic effect of FRS on the distal surface of adjacent primary molars[59]; however, the percentage of new decayed or filled surfaces at 30 months follow-up was so small that it may not indicate a true clinical significance.[60] Studies are contradictory as to the inferiority of retention rates of FRS compared with those of conventional sealants.[38,58,61] Given that the evidence is inconclusive as to the benefit of sealants containing fluoride, dentists should not choose a sealant material based on this property.

Glass Ionomer

Glass ionomer cement sealants were introduced as an alternative to resin-based sealants based on their fluoride releasing and recharging ability, their higher moisture toleration, and their easy application. It is generally accepted that the effectiveness of sealants depends on long-term retention,[62] and in clinical studies, retention is considered the principal evaluation criteria, as it is used as a surrogate measure of effectiveness in preventing caries.[38] When compared with resin-based sealants, patients who receive glass ionomer sealants have a five times greater chance of experiencing sealant loss at 2 to 3 years.[13] However, studies have shown that while glass ionomer sealants are not retained as well, the caries preventive effect is similar or superior to resin-based sealants.[13,63–65] Hence the panel of experts convened to write the 2016 Clinical Practice Guidelines was unable to determine the superiority of one type of sealant material over another due to low quality of evidence.[11]

If glass ionomer sealants have poor retention, how can they still protect against caries? The theories for the protective benefit of glass ionomer material despite its poor retention rates are that (1) the glass ionomer material remains in the deepest parts of the fissures, still providing a physical barrier, even though it is not clinically evident, or (2) the glass ionomer imparts a long-term benefit to the tooth such that the fissures are more resident to demineralization. Studies suggest that the residual cariostatic property of glass ionomer sealant is most likely due to a physical barrier of remaining glass ionomer in the fissures rather than a chemical effect on demineralization inhibition.[66–68]

Glass ionomer sealants are widely used in countries with limited access to dentistry as part of the atraumatic restorative treatment (ART) technique. (See Chapter 22 for a discussion of ART.) Several studies have shown the caries-preventive effect of ART sealants.[69–71] The technique for ART sealants is to apply a conventional, high viscosity glass ionomer with "finger pressure" on a clean, dry tooth that has been conditioned with polyacrylic acid.[70] High-viscosity materials are better retained than those of low to medium viscosity.[71]

The panel of experts convened for the 2016 Clinical Practice Guidelines were not able to provide specific recommendations for the effectiveness of different sealant materials, since the evidence of the head-to-head comparisons was of low quality. The panel recommends choosing the type of material most appropriate for particular clinical scenarios. For instance, when a child is cooperative and the tooth can be adequately isolated, a resin-based sealant will be better retained. However, if isolation is difficult or the tooth is not fully erupted, or the child would benefit from sealant placement but has less than ideal cooperation, a glass ionomer may be more appropriate.[11]

Polyacid-Modified Resin Composites (Compomers)

Polyacid-modified resin composites were introduced in the 1990s as a new class of materials that aimed to combine the esthetic property of composite with the fluoride-releasing property and adhesion of glass ionomer. These materials have been nicknamed "compomers." They are similar to composite in that they contain no water and are hydrophobic, set by a polymerization reaction, lack the ability to bond to tooth structure, and require bonding agents of the type used with conventional composite resins.[72] Like glass ionomers, they do release fluoride; however, their fluoride release levels are significantly lower than those of glass ionomer cements.[72] As a sealant material, polyacid-modified resin composites underperform glass ionomer cements in terms of fluoride release and underperform conventional resin composite materials in terms of retention.[73–75]

Who Really Needs Sealants?

Caries Risk Assessment

Caries management emphasizes the need for caries risk assessment, which is the likelihood of the incidence of caries during a certain time period. It is important to analyze the risk of caries for an individual during the decision-making process for sealants. Placing fissure sealants should not be considered "routine" for all children, as low-risk teeth receive little benefit from sealant placement,[76,77] and it is not cost-effective.[29,78] Not only should the patient be evaluated for caries risk, but the tooth itself should be evaluated as well. Heller and colleagues studied caries progression in sound teeth with and without sealants and in teeth with incipient carious lesions (defined by dark staining of the grooves, chalky appearance, or a slight explorer catch; Fig. 33.3) with and without sealants. These researchers found that the preventive benefit for sealing sound teeth was only 4.5%, while sealing over incipient caries lowered the caries incidence by 41%, almost a 10-fold difference.[77] Therefore sealants are indicated when the dentist determines that the tooth or the patient is at risk of experiencing caries.[8]

Sealant Versus Fluoride Varnish: Which Is More Likely to Reduce Occlusal Caries?

Fluoride varnish reduces caries in permanent teeth.[79] Along with reducing the incidence of smooth surface lesions, varnish has also been shown to reduce pit and fissure caries.[80,81] Fluoride varnish may be effective for pit and fissure caries because it adheres to the deeper part of the fissures for a long period of time allowing a high uptake of fluoride ions.[80] However, when compared against each other, sealants are more effective in reducing the incidence of caries. When compared with varnish, sealants would still reduce the incidence of caries by 34%.[11] Hence the 2016 Clinical Practice Guideline recommends the use of sealants compared with varnish.[11]

Age at Placement

Previous studies from the 1950s and 1960s showed a peak in caries incidence occurring shortly after eruption and then tapering.

The theory was that the occlusal surface was most vulnerable to caries within the first few years after eruption and that the risk of developing caries after this time period dropped dramatically. However, longitudinal data from the postfluoridation era show new carious lesions develop yearly.[82,83] In 1988 Ripa et al. analyzed data from nearly 2000 children aged 10 to 13 years who were examined annually for 3 years to determine caries activity. The authors found that the occlusal surfaces of molars suffered relatively constant attack between ages 10 and 16, at a rate of 10.4% per year.[82] New information indicates that fluorides may have caused a delay in pit and fissure caries, resulting in occlusal surfaces that decay at a later age.[84] Hence the nature of primary caries is changing from a rapidly progressing disease of childhood to a slowly progressing disease that commences in childhood but progresses steadily in adulthood.[84] In accordance, the evidence-based recommendations endorse that adults as well as children should receive sealants when the tooth or the patient is at risk of experiencing caries.[8] The question of whether to place a sealant over a fissured surface should not be based on how long ago the tooth erupted but on the clinical impression of whether a sealant is necessary to prevent caries. Fig. 33.4 is a decision-making tree for sealant placement and can be utilized to help dentists decide when to apply sealants.

Which Teeth Should Be Sealed?

Traditionally, noncarious first and second permanent molars with deep fissures were the candidates for sealants; however, recommendations have been extended to any tooth at risk of developing caries, including primary teeth; permanent molars with incipient, noncavitated lesions; and/or premolars.[8] At-risk primary teeth benefit from sealant placement, as resin-based sealants are retained well on primary molars, with retention rates in the 70% to 95% range at approximately 3 years.[85,86] Glass ionomer cements are not retained well and are not recommended for use as sealant material on primary teeth.[87] Given the preventive benefit to the primary molar, when the child is able to cooperate for sealant placement, sealants should be utilized.[8]

The indications for sealant placement include: (1) deep, retentive pits and fissures, which may cause wedging or catching of an

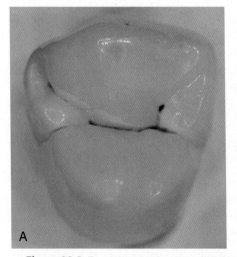 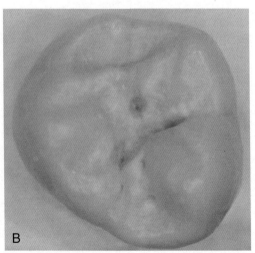

• **Figure 33.3** Examples of early, noncavitated incipient caries. The premolar exhibits distinct, dark brown early caries (A), while the molar exhibits white demineralization around the pits and fissures and light brown discoloration within the pits and fissures (B). Both of these teeth would be candidates for sealants and would not require mechanical preparation prior to sealant placement.

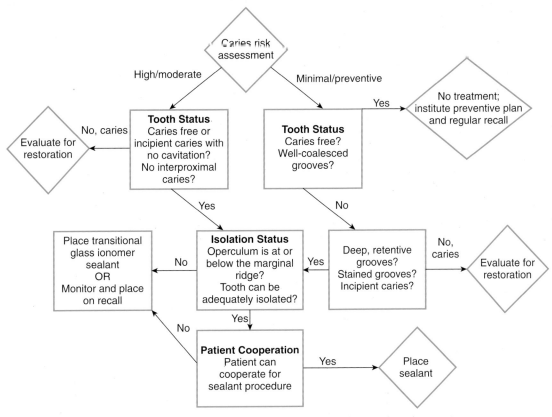

• **Figure 33.4** Flow chart to aid in making decisions about sealant placement.

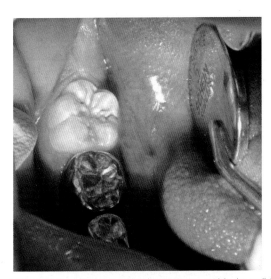

• **Figure 33.5** Molar with deep, retentive grooves, an ideal candidate for sealant placement—especially since the patient has existing stainless steel crown restorations that indicate a high caries risk assessment.

explorer (Fig. 33.5); (2) stained pits and fissures with minimal appearance of decalcification or opacification (i.e., incipient caries with no cavitation; see Fig. 33.3); (3) no radiographic or clinical evidence of interproximal caries in need of restoration on teeth to be sealed; (4) use of other preventive treatment, such as fluoride therapy, to inhibit interproximal caries formation; and (5) the

possibility of adequate isolation from salivary contamination. Thus if placing a sealant is clinically indicated on any tooth with pit and fissures, a sealant should be utilized to prevent caries development.

Contraindications for sealant placement include: (1) well-coalesced, self-cleaning pits and fissures; (2) radiographic or clinical evidence of interproximal caries in need of restoration; (3) the presence of many interproximal lesions or restorations with no preventive plan/treatment to inhibit caries formation; (4) limited life expectancy of the primary tooth; and (5) no possibility of adequate isolation from salivary contamination either due to eruption status or patient behavior.

Diagnosing Occlusal Caries

Diagnosing occlusal caries can be difficult, and research has shown that dentists correctly diagnosis occlusal caries in only 42% of cases.[88] In 2005 Stookey challenged the long-held belief that probing an occlusal groove with an explorer was necessary to diagnose a carious lesion.[89] He summarized the evidence, which suggests that the use of an explorer does not increase dentists' ability to make a correct diagnosis, and forceful use of an explorer can damage the tooth. Dentists are just as likely to make a correct diagnosis of a dry tooth in terms of the presence or absence of caries using only visual inspection as they are when utilizing an explorer.[88] Proponents of eliminating the use of an explorer raise the concern that not only is tactile examination unreliable, but forceful explorer usage can cause enamel defects, resulting in possible caries development or progression by causing cavitation of a previously non-cavitated lesion.[90–92] In one study, a dentist was asked to gently probe a sample of third molars, half of which had initial carious lesions and half of which had sound occlusal surfaces.[92] The teeth were then extracted and the fissures were examined with a scanning electron microscope. Enamel defects were noted for all of the teeth with initial caries and for two of the sound surfaces. Forceful use of an explorer in demineralized fissures can, in essence, cause cavitation by creating an entrance through which cariogenic microorganisms can penetrate into the softened substructure.[91] Opponents of the explorer do not endorse eliminating the explorer altogether. They recommend that the explorer be used differently, mainly to eliminate plaque in the fissures and to determine surface roughness of incipient lesions[89]: "The tip of the explorer should be moved gently across the surface of any non-cavitated area to determine the presence or absence of surface roughness as an indication of whether the underlying demineralized area reflects an active lesion."

The concept of using moderate, firm pressure to find a "catch" in the fissure is no longer the most contemporary approach to caries diagnosis and management. The use of explorers is not necessary for the detection of early lesions, since it does not improve the validity of the diagnosis of fissure caries, and visual examination of a clean, dry tooth is sufficient to detect early lesions.[8,88] Several new technologies have shown promise to aid in caries diagnosis and in caries monitoring over time: light-induced and infrared laser fluorescence devices, the electronic caries detector, quantitative laser fluorescence, and transillumination. However, to date, no technology can substitute for a thorough visual exam and clinical judgment based on experience.

Sealing Over Incipient Caries

A paradigm shift has occurred in the management of carious lesions. One hundred and fifty years ago, complete removal of all traces of caries was the gold standard; however, advances in the field of cariology have challenged this perspective. In 2015, a group of cariology experts from around the world convened for the International Caries Consensus Collaboration (ICCC), which reported the group's clinical recommendations for carious tissue removal and cavity management. The experts agree that a tooth should not be restored surgically until the lesion is cavitated and into dentin. Hence early lesions—ones that are in enamel or just into dentin and are noncavitated—should be managed through biofilm removal (i.e., toothbrushing) and/or remineralization or by sealing over them.[93]

What is the science behind this decision? If sealants are applied properly and are monitored periodically, caries arrest beneath a sealant, as demonstrated by numerous studies.[42,94–98] Oong et al. found that sealing over noncavitated lesions reduced the probability of lesion progression by more than 70%.[99] What is the scientific rationale for this finding? Sealants significantly reduce the bacteria levels in lesions because (1) acid etching alone eliminates 75% of the viable microorganisms[100] and (2) retained sealant deprive bacteria of access to nutrients; bacteria which persist under sealants cannot produce acid when isolated from carbohydrate substrate, and thus progression of the lesion is unlikely.[99] In a recent review of six studies that addressed the reduction in viable bacteria after sealant placement, the authors found that sealing caries was associated with a 100-fold reduction in mean total viable bacteria counts.[99]

Despite the recommendation by experts to seal over noncavitated occlusal surfaces,[11,93] many dentists in the United States are reluctant to seal carious teeth, as they are concerned that the caries will progress underneath the sealant.[101,102] Fontana et al. addressed this barrier to sealant utilization in a recent a study in which the authors sealed noncavitated lesions with a clear sealant and monitored these lesions with visual inspection, radiography, and laser fluorescence.[42] The use of radiography and laser fluorescence added objective ways to measure caries progression, since visual inspection can be subjective. After almost 4 years of follow-up, sealants that were reapplied yearly as needed and were 98% effective in preventing progression of lesions (Fig. 33.6). This study is part of the rapidly growing body of high-quality evidence emphasizing the power of the sealant.

However, practitioners who are concerned about sealing over caries will often decide to take an invasive approach by prepping the tooth "just in case." Some will erroneously call this a "preventive resin restoration" (PRR) when, in fact, it is most likely a fissurotomy or enameloplasty procedure. The PRR is more appropriately termed the conservative adhesive resin restoration. (See Chapter 22 for a detailed discussion of conservative adhesive restorations.) The most contemporary definition of a PRR (conservative adhesive restoration) is that one area (pit/fissure) of the occlusal surface has a lesion that is cavitated and extends to dentin while the rest of the surface remains noncavitated or caries-free. An example of this would be a permanent maxillary first molar where the distal pit of the occlusal surface is carious but the central pit and radiating fissures remain caries-free. In this instance, the distal

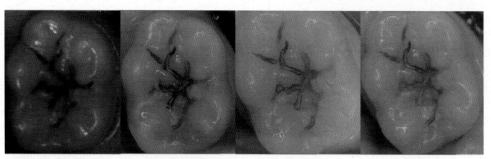

| Baseline Pre-Sealant (0-months) ICDAS 4; x-ray D1 Diagnodent 52 (Taken with Suni camera) | Post-Sealant (12-months) ICDAS 4; x-ray D1 Diagnodent 45 (Taken with Digidoc camera) | Post-Sealant (24-months) ICDAS 4; x-ray D1 Diagnodent 59 (Taken with Digidoc camera) | Post-Sealant (44-months) ICDAS 4; x-ray D1 Diagnodent 52 (Taken with Digidoc camera) |

• **Figure 33.6** Sealed carious permanent molars monitored over 44 months. *ICDAS*, International Caries Detection and Assessment System. (From Fontana M, Platt JA, Eckert GJ, et al. Monitoring of sound and carious surfaces under sealants over 44 months. *J Dent Res*. 2014;93:1070–1075.)

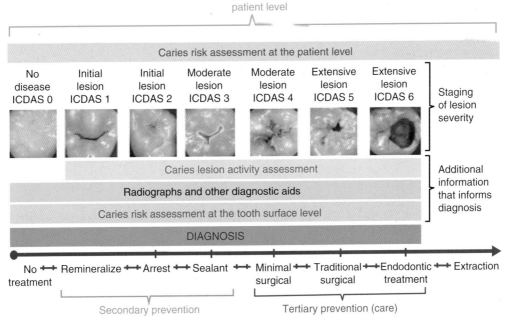

• **Figure 33.7** Caries diagnosis and management system continuum. *ICDAS*, International Caries Detection and Assessment System. (From Zero DT, Zandona AF, Vail MM, Spolnik KJ. Dental caries and pulpal disease. *Dent Clin North Am.* 2011;55:29–46.)

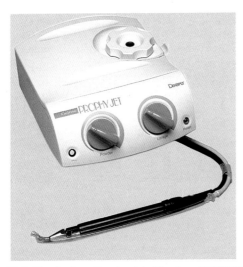

• **Figure 33.8** The Cavitron Prophy Jet. (Courtesy DENTSPLY Professional, York, PA.)

pit is opened, caries is removed, and intact pit and fissures are not opened with a bur. A restorative material (composite, glass ionomer, amalgam) is placed in the distal pit cavity prep, and sealant is utilized over the remaining intact pits and fissures. Hence the "preventive" portion of the "PRR" is placing sealant over intact but susceptible pits and fissures. The PRR (conservative adhesive restoration), when utilized as discussed previously, is an excellent restoration, especially if the sealant is reapplied as needed. However, it cannot be overemphasized that mechanical preparation of a noncavitated lesion is not necessary. Once a permanent tooth has been restored, it begins the cycle of restoration. The restoration will likely be replaced several times during that person's life, and repeated restorations may compromise the survival of the tooth itself. Fig. 33.7 is a diagram of the continuum of caries and the

recommended clinical management.[41] As one can appreciate, surgical intervention is much further down the continuum than likely indicated by the training of many practitioners in the United States. In summary, unless the lesion is a cavitated, dentin carious lesion, it should be sealed.[93]

Preparing the Tooth for a Sealant

Cleaning the Tooth

For a resin-based sealant to flow into the fissures of the tooth, the fissures must be free of debris. Several methods have been suggested for cleaning the fissures. Historically it has been advocated to clean the tooth with pumice slurry and a prophy cup or bristle brush; however, other cleaning methods have been shown to be effective. Debris can be cleaned using an explorer through the fissures and forcefully rinsing with air-water spray[38] or with a dry bristle toothbrush.[103] A recent clinical study showed improved retention with the pumice slurry and rubber cup cleaning method.[104] Complete debridement of the fissures is very difficult, and as a result complete penetration of the sealant rarely occurs with conventional cleaning methods.[105,106] A superior cleaning method is the utilization of an air-polishing system such as a Prophy Jet, as it removes more debris than conventional methods (Fig. 33.8).[107,108] This in turn allows greater sealant penetration and an increased number of resin tags for micromechanical retention.[109–111] Despite these advantages, air-polishing most likely never became the standard for pit and fissure sealant application, due to the increased equipment cost and complexity of the procedure without significantly improved retention rates.[40,112]

Mechanical Preparation

Minimally invasive techniques have been described to improve the penetration and retention of fissure sealants. The fissurotomy and enameloplasty techniques involve utilizing a small bur to remove any residual debris and/or dubious enamel tissue as well as to widen the fissure, leading to increased enamel surface and improved penetration of the sealant into the fissure.[113] In lab studies, the enameloplasty allows deeper sealant penetration and better adaptation as well as increases the surface area for acid etching,[114,115] but studies conflict as to whether the technique decreases microleakage.[43] While one recent systematic review concluded that a preparation method before fissure sealant application can increase sealant retention, the review included a number of different preparation methods besides a bur, including cleaning the fissure with a rubber cup, air abrasion, and the use of a carbon dioxide laser.[113] When examining the use of a bur only, the literature is conflicting regarding any clinical benefit from mechanical preparation. Several studies have reported increased retention of sealants after mechanical preparation of the fissures,[116–119] while other studies have not shown a superior retention rate or enhanced performance of the sealant.[120–123] A limited number of studies have shown that air abrasion in combination with acid-etching results in improved retention of sealants[124–126]; however, air abrasion alone cannot be a substitute for acid etching.[127–129]

Other disadvantages to invasive techniques are that mechanical preparation limits the delegation of sealant placement to auxiliaries, which decreases cost-effectiveness, and opening the fissures by bur preparation can predispose the teeth to caries after sealant loss.[113] The European Academy of Pediatric Dentistry summarizes the evidence well in its guidelines that state: "purposeful removal of enamel or enameloplasty just to widen the base of a fissure in a sound tooth is an invasive technique, which disturbs the equilibrium of the fissure system and exposes a child unnecessarily to the use of a handpiece or air abrasion."[130] They conclude that plaque should be removed in order to obtain sufficient bonding, but that the removal of tooth structure by a bur is unnecessary and undesirable.

In addition, as discussed earlier, sealant can be placed over incipient, noncavitated lesions without removal of tooth structure. There is a significant volume of evidence of high sealant retention without the use of a bur.

Effect of a Recent Professionally Applied Fluoride Treatment

Dentists might note the need for sealant placement or sealant repair at a patient's dental exam and would like to complete the procedures the same day. However, many patients receive a prophylaxis and fluoride application prior to their dental exam. Hence the concern that fluoride might inhibit or decrease sealant bond strength has been explored. Multiple studies confirm that sealant bond strengths and retention rates are not affected by a topical fluoride gel or foam treatment prior to sealant application.[131–133] If a patient has had a gel or foam application, the practitioner need not delay sealant application or repair. However, many offices exclusively use fluoride varnish. For these practitioners, the teeth should be examined and sealed prior to the application of varnish (Box 33.1).

Factors Affecting Sealant Success

Etchant

Etchants are available as separate phosphoric acid etchants, self-etching systems, liquids, and gels. Historically the clinical sealant procedure involved an etching time of 60 seconds and a rinsing time of at least 10 seconds. However, multiple studies have shown similar bond strengths for both permanent and primary teeth, with lower etching times of 15 to 30 seconds.[134–137] Etching time should be increased for fluorotic teeth. The usual recommendation

---

• BOX 33.1 **The Clinical Procedure**

Isolation

Isolation should be achieved by any of the methods previously mentioned. The most common method of isolation is the cotton roll method, as described by Waggoner and Siegal[140]:

The patient is in a supine position with the head extended back and the chin up because this improves visibility and moisture control.

For maxillary isolation: a triangular buccal isolation shield, such as a Dri-Angle (Fig. 33.12), is placed against the buccal mucosa over the Stensen duct with the apex of the triangle directed posteriorly. A cotton roll may be placed in the maxillary vestibule to hold the tissue away from the tooth. The mouth mirror is used throughout the entire procedure and should be left in position throughout the procedure until polymerization of the sealant is achieved. Besides providing indirect vision, this will also act as a shield for the tongue.

For mandibular isolation: Cotton rolls are placed on both the buccal and lingual sides of the teeth. A cotton roll holder may be utilized or the rolls may be held in place with the fingers. Waggoner and Siegal advocate utilizing a triangular isolation shield as a tongue shield by bending the apex of the triangular shield at a right angle (Fig. 33.13). This bend is placed between the lingual cotton roll and the alveolar ridge so that the larger portion of the shield rests on the tongue. This prevents the tongue from pushing saliva over the lingual cotton roll. Changing cotton rolls or adding additional cotton rolls is unnecessary. Excess moisture can be evacuated from the area with the high volume evacuation suction. Utilizing a four-handed delivery method will increase the success of achieving adequate isolation.

Etching

Once isolated, the tooth is etched, most commonly with 37% phosphoric acid. The etchant can be applied liberally and should flow onto all of the susceptible pits and fissures, including lingual grooves of maxillary molars and buccal pits of mandibular molars (Fig. 33.14). The etchant should extend up the cuspal line angles, 2 to 3 mm beyond the anticipated margin of the sealant. The etchant should remain on the surface for 15 to 20 seconds.

Rinsing and Drying

The tooth should be rinsed utilizing the air-water spray and high volume suction. The goal of rinsing is to remove all of the etchant from the tooth surface. The tooth should then be thoroughly dried until the surface appears chalky or frosted (see Fig. 33.9A and B). Unlike dentin bonding, in which the collagen fibrils should remain moist to prevent collapsing, the enamel keeps its crystalline structure. This means that the enamel should be thoroughly dried or desiccated to maximize the penetration of the hydrophobic sealant. The tooth must remain dry and uncontaminated from this point forward.

Sealant Application and Polymerization

If a bonding agent is to be used, it should be applied with a microbrush. The bonding agent should be lightly dried and cured. The sealant should be applied to all pits and fissures, including the lingual grooves of maxillary molars and the buccal pits of mandibular molars (Fig. 33.15). The sealant may be applied with a variety of instruments: an explorer tip, a PICH instrument (a calcium

• BOX 33.1   The Clinical Procedure—cont'd

hydroxide, or Dycal, placer), or a small brush. Many manufacturers offer their own delivery system, which may consist of a preloaded syringe with a small tip so that the sealant can be applied directly from the syringe to the tooth. The sealant should not be overfilled, to ensure that the sealant material does not extend past the etched area, to limit the amount of occlusal interference created, and to ensure optimal depth of cure. If overfilling occurs, the excess material may be removed with a small brush. If small bubbles form within the sealant material, these should be teased out before polymerization. Once the sealant has been satisfactorily placed, the curing light tip should be placed as closely as possible to the surface, and the sealant should be cured for the amount of time recommended by the manufacturer, which is usually 20 seconds with an light-emitting diode curing light that has an output of 800 to 1000 mW/cm^2. The operator should understand which type of curing light is being used and how its energy output can affect the exposure time. As mentioned previously, very short curing times are insufficient to achieve optimal cure, especially of opaque sealants.

Evaluating the Sealant

Once the sealant has been cured, the operator should visually and tactilely examine the sealant before removing the isolation materials. If the operator discovers bubbles, voids, or areas of deficient material, material can be directly added at this time because the oxygen inhibited layer has not been disturbed. The sealant's retention should also be evaluated by attempting to dislodge the sealant with an explorer. If material de-bonds, the fissure should be inspected for remaining debris. The area should be re-etched, rinsed, dried, and new sealant material applied. If some of the sealant pooled over the distal

marginal ridge, a ledge may have been created that should be removed. Also, if any sealant material was misplaced into the interproximal areas, it should be removed. Most likely the excess material can be removed with an explorer or scaler. The unpolymerized layer should be removed by rubbing the surface with pumice on a cotton roll or by rinsing the surface for 30 seconds to limit the patient's exposure to bisphenol-A.

Depending on the sealant material type, the occlusion may require adjustment. Filled sealants and flowable composite used as sealant require adjustment, whereas unfilled sealants abrade quickly and are considered to be "self-adjusting." The occlusion can be adjusted with the use of a round composite finishing bur in the high-speed handpiece or with a stone or round bur in the slow speed handpiece.

Periodic Evaluation

Sealants should be evaluated at every recall visit. Retention of the sealant material is critical to its success. Partial or complete loss of a sealant results in a surface that is equally at risk for caries as one that had never been sealed. One-time sealant placement does not impart any long-term protection unless the physical barrier over the fissure, the sealant, remains intact. Loss of the sealant in any groove or pit renders that pit or fissure susceptible to caries attack. Therefore sealants should be maintained and repaired or replaced as needed. If a sealant partially remains, attempts can be made to try to dislodge the remaining material with an explorer. If it remains intact, there is no need to remove the material with a handpiece. The tooth may be cleaned with pumice and a rubber cup, and the usual sealant application steps can be followed, etching both the enamel and remaining sealant and then applying additional material.

---

for rinsing is 20 to 30 seconds. A few studies have shown that a shorter rinse time yields similar enamel bond strengths as a 20-second rinse time.[138,139] Hence the exact rinse time is not as important as ensuring that the rinse is thorough enough to remove all of the etchant from the surface.[140]

The different forms of etchant (i.e., gel or liquid) have been shown to perform similarly in regard to penetration, bond strength, and clinical retention.[135,141,142] On the other hand, different types of etchants do not provide similar results. Self-etching systems yield significantly lower bond strengths than separate etch systems and exhibit much lower retention rates in clinical trials, as reported in a recent systematic review (highest level of evidence).[143] Self-etching systems have decreased bond strengths on uncut enamel.[144] Utilizing a self-etching bonding system without the use of a separate etch step is not recommended.[8,143]

Drying Agents and Time

Given the hydrophobic nature of resins, drying agents such as alcohol or acetone have been explored as possible treatments after the etchant step, before sealant placement. However, a laboratory study showed that the use of drying agents did not decrease microleakage or increase sealant penetration.[145] Furthermore, one clinical investigation showed no significant improvements of retention rates with the use of drying agents.[146] There is no recommended drying time. Rather, a specific result should be obtained. The occlusal surface should have a chalky or frosted appearance (Fig. 33.9). If this result is not obtained after thorough drying, the tooth should be re-etched.

Curing

The polymerization process begins when photoinitiators, most commonly camphoroquinone, absorb energy from blue light with a wavelength in the region of 470 nanometers.[147] This absorption facilitates the conversion of low-viscosity monomer units into a polymer matrix. A sealant must be adequately cured in order for it to obtain its purported physical properties. If the curing time is insufficient, the bonding is poor, and decreases in hardness may result, leading to subsequent sealant failure.[148]

Several types of curing lights are available (see Chapter 21). The traditional unit is the quartz tungsten halogen (QTH) curing light unit. These units require a fan for cooling, are relatively low-cost, are easy to maintain and repair if a bulb needs replacement, and deliver energy density outputs of 400 to 800 mW/cm^2. They have largely been replaced by light-emitting diode (LED) curing lights. LED curing lights have changed dramatically in the past decade, and units continue to offer increasing intensity.[149] In general, higher energy output means that curing time can be shortened (from 40 seconds for QTH to 20 seconds with a higher powered LED for 2 mm of composite).[150,151] Some of the highest powered LEDs on the market offer outputs of 1000 to more than 3000 mW/cm^2 of energy and usually have "turbo," "boost," or "plasma" modes that offer very high energy outputs in very small increments of time, like 5 seconds.

Not much literature has been published either confirming or challenging recommended curing times for sealants. Most manufacturers recommend a 20-second exposure time. However, one must consider which kind of curing light is being utilized, as not all perform equally. One study has found that 20 seconds of curing

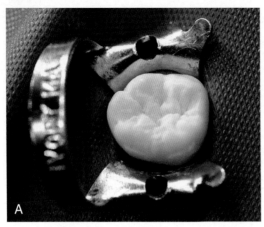 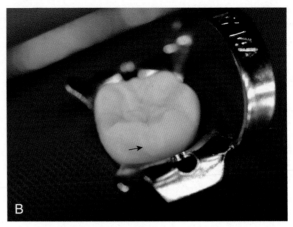

• **Figure 33.9** (A) Etched enamel displaying frosted appearance. (B) Note the demarcation between the chalky, etched enamel *(arrow)* and the shiny unetched enamel of the buccal surface.

with a traditional QTH light is insufficient to cure resin-based sealants to a clinically adequate depth.[147] Two in vitro studies have examined the depth of cure of dental sealant with LED units that offer high energy and very short curing times, and found these very short curing times to be inadequate to optimally cure dental sealant, especially opaque material.[152,153] Several factors affect the level of cure, including shade of the material, the filler content, the thickness of the material, the intensity of the curing light, and the distance of the light source from the material.[154] Opaque shades, though white in color, behave more like materials in the dark shade range because they are not translucent, so light does not pass through them easily to cure deeper areas of the material. Hence clear sealants can be cured to a deeper level than opaque sealants given similar curing times.[147,153] More research is necessary to determine the appropriate balance between saving chair time with faster curing and still obtaining clinically sufficient physical properties of resin materials. Clinicians should ensure optimal curing by using a high-intensity light source, placing the light tip as close as possible to the sealant and maximizing the curing duration.

In addition to ensuring an optimal cure, a practitioner might be able to improve retention of the sealant by delaying polymerization for several seconds after sealant application, assuming scrupulous isolation can be maintained. A study by Chosack and Eidelman found that the longer sealants were allowed to remain on the etched surface before polymerization (20 seconds vs. 5 or 10 seconds), the more sealant material penetrated into microporosities, creating longer resin tags, which are critical for micromechanical retention.[155]

Isolation

Resin-based sealants are moisture-sensitive. Saliva contamination significantly lowers bond strengths because it prevents the formation of resin tags that alter mechanical retention and thus results in decreased retention.[156–158] At times, practitioners who are placing sealants will notice that a small amount of saliva seeps onto the tooth from the tongue or the cotton roll, and the practitioner erroneously believes that if the tooth is rinsed and dried well, the sealant retention will not be affected. However, even minimal exposure to saliva results in the formation of a surface coating that

---

• **BOX 33.2** **Troubleshooting Sealant Placement**

Sealant placement is very technique-sensitive. If sealant material de-bonds upon immediate evaluation, one of the following three causes is the most likely culprit:

1. Debris remains in the fissure. The tooth must be clean. If plaque or organic debris remains in the fissure, the resin cannot flow into the fissure to form tags and micromechanically bond to the enamel. Clean the fissures with a rubber cup and pumice, re-etch, and complete the application steps again.
2. Saliva contaminated the enamel. If isolation was not meticulously maintained and saliva contacted the occlusal surface, then saliva pooled in the microporosities created by the etchant step. Even if the operator noticed the saliva contamination and decided to dry the tooth again, the viscous saliva cannot be removed by rinsing alone. Thus the resin sealant will "float" on the saliva and cannot form resin tags. In this case, the tooth should be re-etched, dried, and resealed with no saliva contamination.
3. The tooth was not completely dry after the rinsing step. If the tooth does not appear chalky after an adequate etching time, it is most likely not dry. Enamel bonding is different from dentin adhesion. In restorative dentistry, one is advised not to desiccate the dentin; however, enamel needs to be absolutely dry prior to sealant application. If water remains in the etched enamel pores, the hydrophobic resin will "float" on top of the water and not form resin tags. Again, no micromechanical bonding will occur, and the sealant will de-bond when evaluated with an explorer.

---

cannot be completely removed by rinsing.[159] The acid etch step creates microporosities in the enamel, and if saliva touches the tooth, these porosities are occluded so the sealant cannot form resin tags to micromechanically bond to the tooth. Achieving adequate isolation is a critical step to the success of the sealant and is considered a key concept in the clinical procedure (Box 33.2).[160]

Several studies have shown that cotton roll isolation is comparable to rubber dam isolation.[116,161,162] However, a recent systematic review has shown that retention is increased when rubber dam isolation is utilized (Fig. 33.10).[38] In addition, vacuum systems such as the Vac-Ejector and Isolite have been shown to produce sealant retention rates comparable to those placed under cotton roll and rubber dam isolation.[163–166] (See Chapter 22 for a discussion of isolation systems.) Whenever possible, especially if concurrent operative

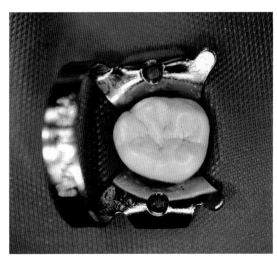

• **Figure 33.10** Rubber dam isolation can be single tooth or quadrant depending on the needs of the patient and will assist the practitioner in keeping saliva from contaminating any of the fissures once they have been etched.

treatment is provided, rubber dam isolation should be used. However, given the discomfort that can be associated with rubber dam placement on nonanesthetized tissues, rubber dam isolation is not imperative as long as the operator can maintain a dry field with alternative techniques.

Timing of Sealant Placement

The timing of sealant placement has been known to correlate with the overall retention of the sealant, as studies have shown that partially erupted teeth require repair or replacement more often than fully erupted teeth.[167] Dennison et al. concluded that when the operculum of the gingiva extended over the distal marginal ridge of the tooth, more than 50% of the teeth had to be resealed due to sealant loss within 36 months; when the operculum was at the level of the marginal ridge, retreatment fell to 26%.[168] Except for high-risk children, sealant placement should be delayed until the gingival tissues are at or below the marginal ridge.[140] For partially erupted teeth, which are at high risk for experiencing caries, the best practice is to place a sealant and repair or replace it as necessary. Utilizing a bonding agent for these teeth under the sealant may be beneficial.[169] Alternatively, the sealant in this scenario may be a glass ionomer sealant if the practitioner has difficulty achieving adequate isolation.[8]

Not only should tooth eruption be considered when deciding when to place a sealant, but a child's level of cooperation must also be considered. The child must be able to tolerate the isolation method and the length of the procedure to place a successful sealant. If the child is unable or unwilling to cooperate for the procedure, placing sealants should be delayed until the level of cooperation is adequate, or if the child has high caries risk, an ART sealant with a glass ionomer could be used as a transitional sealant.

Use of Intermediate Bonding Agent

Resin-based dental sealants are hydrophobic. Due to this property, they cannot stand even slight moisture contamination. Dentinal bonding agents have hydrophilic properties so that they can infiltrate wet dentin. Utilizing a layer of bonding agent between the enamel and hydrophobic resin sealant has been studied to determine if this additional step could enhance retention rates. Numerous laboratory studies have found decreased microleakage and enhanced penetration of sealant material into the fissures with the adjunct of a bonding agent.[170–174] A recent systematic review and meta-analysis (highest level of evidence) examined five studies that met inclusion criteria. Results of the meta-analysis indicated that adhesive systems beneath fissure sealants had a significant positive benefit on retention and thus caries prevention.[175] The authors note that the positive effect was seen in studies that used fifth-generation bonding agents (those that require a separate etch and rinse step but have the "prime" and "bond" together as one step). It seems that the smaller molecular size of the adhesive components, compared with the sealant components, penetrate better into enamel porosities, and this improves bond strength. Not only do permanent teeth benefit from the adjunct of a bonding agent, but studies are also favorable for primary teeth; they also show similar laboratory results to that of permanent teeth with increased bond strengths and decreased microleakage when a bonding agent is utilized.[176,177] The use of a bonding agent should only be utilized with hydrophobic resin-based sealant materials. Glass ionomers chemically bond to the enamel, so utilizing a bonding agent under this material is not logical.

Another advantage of utilizing a bonding agent is noted for hypomineralized permanent molars, which often present a challenge for the dentist regarding adhesive dentistry. These teeth often have enamel defects and are at higher risk for eventually needing restorative treatment compared with "normal" teeth.[178] Hence these teeth are excellent candidates for preventive efforts. However, research has shown that hypomineralized teeth need to be retreated with sealant application after a much shorter time period than teeth in the control group.[179] The addition of a bonding agent with sealant application in hypomineralized teeth can increase fissure sealant retention compared with acid etching alone.[180]

Even though recent systematic review shows a positive effect for the use of a bonding agent, there are two main disadvantages to this technique. Utilizing a bonding agent increases the cost of the procedure and increases chair time.[40] Several studies have found this step to be unnecessary,[47,181–183] and they highlight the importance of proper sealant placement technique: fastidious isolation and proper placement negate the need for this additional step. However, a bonding agent should be used when "in the opinion of the dental professional, the bonding agent would enhance sealant retention in the clinical situation."[8]

Auxiliary Application

Well-trained dental auxiliaries are proficient at the application of pit and fissure sealants. As early as 1976, Stiles et al. reported "no difference in the retention of the sealant when applied by a dentist or a trained dental auxiliary."[184] Since then, several studies have examined sealant placement by auxiliaries and found high retention rates.[185–188] In addition, delegating sealant application is cost-effective and results in increased sealant usage.[185] In studies addressing sealant longevity by operator, researchers found that proper education of personnel and following up on each individual's aptitude in sealant placement are essential, as "individual operator rather than provider type is highly sensitive to sealant success or failure."[189,190] Hence both dental assistants and dental hygienists are as proficient in sealant application as the dentist, and the literature supports the delegation of sealant application to qualified personnel.

Four-Handed Delivery

No clinical trials have addressed the two-handed versus four-handed delivery on the retention of pit and fissure sealants. However, expert opinion supports the use of a trained dental assistant or auxiliary during sealant placement.[191] Having an assistant during sealant application may improve the quality and efficiency of sealant placement, improve isolation, shorten placement time, reduce operator fatigue, and enhance patient care.[191] Griffin et al. found a positive association for four-handed delivery and increased retention rates; however, this is considered indirect evidence and is weaker than randomized controlled trials.[191] Nevertheless, given this positive association, when possible, sealants should be applied with the assistance of trained personnel.[8]

School-Based Sealant Programs

School-based sealant programs have been developed to increase sealant usage to reduce caries and to provide prevention services to children less likely to receive dental care, such as those children from minority or low-income backgrounds. In 2001, the Centers for Disease Control and Prevention (CDC) created a Task Force to review the scientific evidence of the efficacy of school-based programs. Based on findings that the median caries reduction was 60% for children aged 6 through 17 years, the Task Force endorsed school-based sealant programs in 2002.[192] School-based sealant programs can (1) help serve low-income children who are at high risk of developing caries and are less likely than their higher-income counterparts to have a dental visit, (2) connect participating students with sources of dental care in the community, and (3) enroll eligible children in public insurance programs.[193] However, despite the CDC's Task Force endorsement, in 2013 only 15 states had programs in more than half of schools where most students were low income.[194] A recent economic analysis reported that providing sealants in school programs to 1000 children would prevent 485 fillings, toothaches for a year in 133 children, and 1.59 disability-adjusted life-years. School-based sealant programs save society money and remain cost-effective.[194] They are "an important and effective public health approach that complements clinical care systems in promoting the oral health of children and adolescents."[193]

Other Uses for Sealant

Interproximal Dental Sealant

Two techniques can be utilized for sealing interproximal lesions, which have been termed "microinvasive" interventions. The first is to use fissure sealant material with the etch and rinse technique. If the lesion is visible, such as the mesial of a permanent first molar when the second primary molar exfoliates, the sealant can be directly applied. Otherwise, orthodontic separators are placed, and the material is applied at a later date when the teeth are separated and the lesion is visible. The second technique is to utilize a resin infiltration system, such as ICON (DMG America, Englewood, NJ). (See Chapter 40 for a more detailed discussion of the technique.) A recent Cochrane systematic review concluded that microinvasive treatments (i.e., interproximal sealants) arrest noncavitated enamel and early dentinal lesions (limited to the

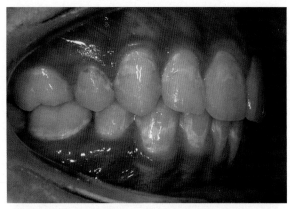

• **Figure 33.11** Generalized demineralization after orthodontic treatment. (From Cobourne MT, DiBiase AT. *Handbook of Orthodontics*. Edinburgh: Mosby; 2010.)

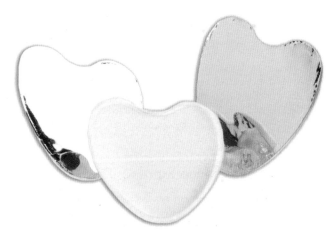

• **Figure 33.12** Dri-Angle isolation shield. (Courtesy Dental Health Products, Inc., Niagara Falls, NY.)

outer third of dentin). These treatments are significantly more effective at arresting lesions compared with other preventive methods like fluoride varnish or recommending flossing.[195]

Sealing Restorations

Given the caries preventive effect of sealant application, researchers have examined other uses for sealants, such as increasing restoration longevity by sealing over the restoration, repairing the margins of restorations, and preventing enamel demineralization ("white spot lesions") around orthodontic brackets (Fig. 33.11). Several studies have shown that restoration longevity can be increased by sealant application along the margins of both composite and amalgam restorations.[94,196,197] In 1998, Mertz-Fairhurst et al. compared conventional amalgams to both sealed amalgam restorations and to sealed composite restorations placed over frank caries without caries removal (only a 1-mm bevel was placed around the lesion in intact enamel).[94] In the 10-year follow-up, they found that the conventional amalgam restorations had the highest occurrence of open margins and the highest rate of recurrent caries, while the sealed amalgams had the best outcomes with only one clinical failure noted in the entire group. Considering that sealing over restorations significantly reduces microleakage, one would expect sealed restorations to show decreased incidences of recurrent caries.[198]

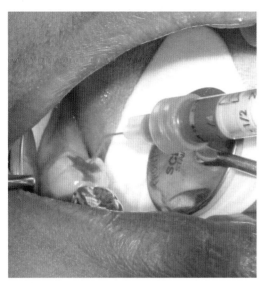

• **Figure 33.13** Isolation of a mandibular molar utilizing a cotton triangle to shield the tongue. Note that when sealant is applied with four-handed delivery, the operator has extra help in maintaining adequate isolation (in this case, the operator is able to retract the cheek while the assistant retracts the tongue with mirrors).

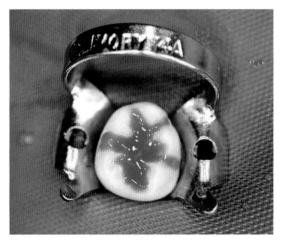

• **Figure 33.14** Etchant application to a mandibular molar. Note how the etchant extends onto the buccal and lingual grooves.

In addition to preventing recurrent caries, sealants can increase the longevity of restorations through repair of marginal defects.[199] Several studies have shown success in repairing marginal defects with sealant.[196,199,200] Serious consideration should be given to repairing marginal defects over replacement of the restoration, because repair is the most conservative treatment option, as it does not result in any further loss of tooth structure and it also lowers the cost of replacement.[199] Practitioners should seal restorations immediately after they are placed[201] and repair margins with a sealant whenever possible.[202] Sealed restorations are superior to unsealed restorations in conserving sound tooth structure, protecting margins, preventing recurrent caries, and prolonging the clinical survival of the restorations.

Preventing White Spot Lesions

A complication of poor oral hygiene during orthodontic treatment is the development of demineralized enamel around the orthodontic

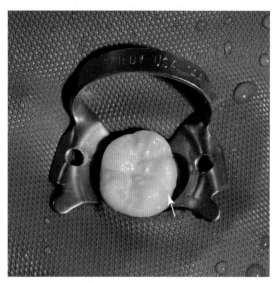

• **Figure 33.15** Sealed mandibular molar. Note how the sealant extends into all susceptible fissures, including the buccal groove (arrow).

brackets, commonly called "white spot lesion" (WSL) (see Fig. 33.11). The literature regarding the efficacy of dental sealants in preventing these lesions is conflicting. Several laboratory studies have found that utilizing a filled sealant around the orthodontic bracket is more effective at decreasing demineralization compared with unfilled products and fluoride.[203–205] In addition, others have reported reduced severity and significant reductions in demineralization around brackets when sealant is used.[206–208] In contrast, other authors report no difference between the decalcification rates of treatment groups versus controls and conclude that sealants alone do not suffice as a stand-alone method to prevent WSL,[209] and the additional time and expense of using sealant to prevent decalcification is not justified.[209–212] Further research is required to determine the effectiveness of sealant application to prevent enamel decalcification.

Sealant Safety

In 1996 Olea and colleagues released an article that started a controversy about the safety of dental sealants, as they confirmed the estrogenicity of a sealant containing bisphenol-A diglcidylether methacrylate (bis-GMA) and found free bisphenol-A (BPA) in saliva samples of subjects after sealant placement.[213] BPA is a synthetic chemical resin used in the production of plastic products. Human exposure is to BPA is widespread: in one study, CDC scientists found BPA in the urine of nearly all of the 2517 people tested.[214] Exposure to BPA is of concern because some animal studies report deleterious effects in fetuses and newborns exposed to BPA.[215] Given that the National Toxicology Program has concluded that there is "some concern" for adverse effects on the brain, behavior, and prostate gland in fetuses, infants, and children at current human exposure levels to BPA, the question arises: Are there any adverse events when using dental sealants that contain resin?

The evidence suggests that exposure to BPA from dental sealants is transient[216] and that patients are not at risk.[217] Moreover, clinicians can limit the amount of patient exposure to BPA (Table 33.1).[218] Resin-based sealants improve children's oral health, and since BPA exposure from dental materials appears transient and can potentially

TABLE 33.1	Recommendations to Limit Patient Exposure to Bisphenol-A From Resin-Based Dental Sealant	
Recommendation	**Rationale**	
Select a product that is BPA-free or one that contains bis-GMA instead of BPA dimethacrylate (bis-DMA)	Saliva can hydrolyze bis-DMA into free BPA	
Utilize rubber dam isolation	Ideal isolation will limit exposure	
After light curing, rub the surface with pumice on a cotton roll or rinse the sealant for 30 s	The most significant exposure to BPA occurs immediately after sealant placement because residual monomer remains in the unpolymerized, oxygen inhibited layer	

bis-DMA, Bisphenol-A diglycidylether methacrylate; *bis-GMA,* bisphenol-A glycidyldimethacrylate; *BPA,* bisphenol-A.

be controlled, the concern about the estrogenicity of sealants should not deter their usage.[11]

Future Advances

As noted earlier, since dental sealants must be applied in a moisture-free environment or they will fail, so much attention is focused on developing moisture-tolerant sealants. At least three resin dental sealants with hydrophilic chemistry have been developed: Embrace WetBond (Pulpdent, Watertown, MA), UltraSeal XT hydro (Ultradent, South Jordan, UT), and Smartseal and Loc (Detax Gmbh & Co, Ettlingen, Germany). In laboratory studies, hydrophilic sealants have shown similar physical properties to other commercially available sealants and more intimate marginal adaptation to the fissure than a traditional resin sealant.[219–221] However, the clinical data for these products are limited, are primarily reported for Embrace WetBond, and are conflicting. In clinical studies, at 1-year follow-up, Embrace compared with conventional sealants has shown better retention rates,[222] poorer retention rates,[223] and no difference in retention.[224] More research is needed to determine caries preventive effects of these new products. Boksman warns that the dental professional must be cautious about claims of new techniques and materials, as only one in five dental products lives up to manufacturers' claims.[225] Some practitioners have switched to newer products and been disappointed when, owing to their poor clinical performance, they were removed from the market. Dental professionals should select dental products based on the best available science.

Summary

The abundance of published data leaves little room for skepticism regarding sealant success, yet some practitioners report that sealants "fall off" or that previously sealed teeth still require treatment. Acknowledging these concerns, Liebenberg emphasizes the importance of diligently following the correct clinical technique, choosing the appropriate cases, and maintaining the integrity of the sealant with reapplication as necessary in order to assist the practitioner in achieving sealant success.[226] The technique is demanding and unforgiving, yet when applied per evidence-based recommendations, dental sealants can dramatically improve

the oral health and quality of life of our children, adolescents, and adults.

References

1. Dye BA, Tan S, Smith V, et al. Trends in oral health status: United States, 1988-1994 and 1999-2004. *Vital Health Stat 11.* 2007;248:1–92.
2. Benjamin RM. Oral health: the silent epidemic. *Public Health Rep.* 2010;125(2):158–159.
3. Dye BA, Thornton-Evans G, Li X, et al. Dental caries and sealant prevalence in children and adolescents in the United States, 2011-2012. *NCHS Data Brief.* 2015;191:1–8.
4. Dye B, Thornton-Evans G, Li X, et al. Dental caries and tooth loss in adults in the United States, 2011-2012. *NCHS Data Brief.* 2015;197:197.
5. National Institutes of Health. NIH Consensus Statement. Diagnosis and Management of Dental Caries Throughout Life. *NIH Consens Statement.* 2001;18(1):1–23. http://www.dentalwatch.org/basic/nih.pdf. Accessed August 17, 2017.
5a. Federal Poverty Level: Yearly income of $24,600 for a family of 4; US Department of Health and Human Services. Annual Update of the HHS Poverty Guidelines. *Fed Regist.* 2017;82(19):8831–8832. https://www.federalregister.gov/documents/2017/01/31/2017-02076/annual-update-of-the-hhs-poverty-guidelines. Accessed August 17, 2017.
6. U.S. General Accounting Office. *Report to Congressional Requesters. Oral Health: Dental Disease Is a Chronic Problem Among Low-Income Populations.* Washington, DC: 2000. http://www.gao.gov/new.items/he00072.pdf. Accessed August 17, 2017.
7. Tomar SL, Reeves AF. Changes in the oral health of US children and adolescents and dental public health infrastructure since the release of the Healthy People 2010 Objectives. *Acad Pediatr.* 2009;9(6):388–395.
8. Beauchamp J, Caufield PW, Crall JJ, et al. Evidence-based clinical recommendations for the use of pit-and-fissure sealants: a report of the American Dental Association Council on Scientific Affairs. *J Am Dent Assoc.* 2008;139(3):257–268.
9. Ekstrand KR, Christiansen J, Christiansen ME. Time and duration of eruption of first and second permanent molars: a longitudinal investigation. *Community Dent Oral Epidemiol.* 2003;31(5):344–350.
10. Antonson SA, Wanuck J, Antonson DE. Surface protection for newly erupting first molars. *Compend Contin Educ Dent.* 2006;27(1):46–52.
11. Wright JT, Crall JJ, Fontana M, et al. Evidence-based clinical practice guideline for the use of pit-and-fissure sealants: a report of the American Dental Association and the American Academy of Pediatric Dentistry. *J Am Dent Assoc.* 2016;147(8):672–682e12.
12. Hicks JFC. Pit and fissure sealants and conservative adhesive restorations: scientific and clinical rationale. In: Pinkham JR, et al, eds. *Pediatric Dentistry: Infancy Through Adolescence.* 4th ed. St. Louis: Elsevier; 2005.
13. Wright JT, Tampi MP, Graham L, et al. Sealants for preventing and arresting pit-and-fissure occlusal caries in primary and permanent molars: a systematic review of randomized controlled trials—a report of the American Dental Association and the American Academy of Pediatric Dentistry. *J Am Dent Assoc.* 2016;147(8):631–645e18.
14. Bhuridej P, Damiano PC, Kuthy RA, et al. Natural history of treatment outcomes of permanent first molars: a study of sealant effectiveness. *J Am Dent Assoc.* 2005;136(9):1265–1272.
15. Ripa LW. Sealants revisted: an update of the effectiveness of pit-and-fissure sealants. *Caries Res.* 1993;27(suppl 1):77–82.
16. Gift HC, Frew RA. Sealants: changing patterns. *J Am Dent Assoc.* 1986;112(3):391–392.
17. Call RL, Mann J, Hicks J. Attitudes of general practitioners towards fissure sealant use. *Clin Prev Dent.* 1988;10(2):9–13.

18. Hicks MJ, Flaitz CM, Call RL. Comparison of pit and fissure sealant utilization by pediatric and general dentists in Colorado. *J Pedod*. 1990;14(2):97–102.
19. Seale NS, Casamassimo PS. Access to dental care for children in the United States: a survey of general practitioners. *J Am Dent Assoc*. 2003;134(12):1630–1640.
20. Faine RC, Dennen T. A survey of private dental practitioners' utilization of dental sealants in Washington state. *ASDC J Dent Child*. 1986;53(5):337–342.
21. Siegal MD, Garcia AI, Kandray DP, et al. The use of dental sealants by Ohio dentists. *J Public Health Dent*. 1996;56(1):12–21.
22. Dye BA, Li X, Beltran-Aguilar ED. Selected oral health indicators in the United States, 2005-2008. *NCHS Data Brief*. 2012;96:1–8.
23. Horowitz AM, Frazier PJ. Issues in the widespread adoption of pit-and-fissure sealants. *J Public Health Dent*. 1982;42(4):312–323.
24. Primosch RE, Barr ES. Sealant use and placement techniques among pediatric dentists. *J Am Dent Assoc*. 2001;132(10):1442–1451, quiz 61.
25. Glasrud PH. Insuring preventive dental care: are sealants included? *Am J Public Health*. 1985;75(3):285–286.
26. Glasrud PH, Frazier PJ, Horowitz AM. Insurance reimbursement for sealants in 1986: report of a survey. *ASDC J Dent Child*. 1987;54(2):81–88.
27. Palmer C How many will have sealants in 2000? *ADA News*; 1992.
28. Chi DL, van der Goes DN, Ney JP. Cost-effectiveness of pit-and-fissure sealants on primary molars in Medicaid-enrolled children. *Am J Public Health*. 2014;104(3):555–561.
29. Quinonez RB, Downs SM, Shugars D, et al. Assessing cost-effectiveness of sealant placement in children. *J Public Health Dent*. 2005;65(2):82–89.
30. Goldman AS, Chen X, Fan M, et al. Cost-effectiveness, in a randomized trial, of glass-ionomer-based and resin sealant materials after 4 yr. *Eur J Oral Sci*. 2016;124(5):472–479.
31. Dennison JB, Straffon LH, Smith RC. Effectiveness of sealant treatment over five years in an insured population. *J Am Dent Assoc*. 2000;131(5):597–605.
32. Forss H, Halme E. Retention of a glass ionomer cement and a resin-based fissure sealant and effect on carious outcome after 7 years. *Community Dent Oral Epidemiol*. 1998;26(1):21–25.
33. Forss H, Saarni UM, Seppa L. Comparison of glass-ionomer and resin-based fissure sealants: a 2-year clinical trial. *Community Dent Oral Epidemiol*. 1994;22(1):21–24.
34. Boksman L, Gratton DR, McCutcheon E, et al. Clinical evaluation of a glass ionomer cement as a fissure sealant. *Quintessence Int*. 1987;18(10):707–709.
35. Raadal M, Utkilen AB, Nilsen OL. Fissure sealing with a light-cured resin-reinforced glass-ionomer cement (Vitrebond) compared with a resin sealant. *Int J Paediatr Dent*. 1996;6(4):235–239.
36. Shapira J, Fuks A, Chosack A, et al. Comparative clinical study of autopolymerized and light-polymerized fissure sealants: five-year results. *Pediatr Dent*. 1990;12(3):168–169.
37. Houpt M, Fuks A, Shapira J, et al. Autopolymerized versus light-polymerized fissure sealant. *J Am Dent Assoc*. 1987;115(1):55–56.
38. Muller-Bolla M, Lupi-Pegurier L, Tardieu C, et al. Retention of resin-based pit and fissure sealants: a systematic review. *Community Dent Oral Epidemiol*. 2006;34(5):321–336.
39. Rock WP, Potts AJ, Marchment MD, et al. The visibility of clear and opaque fissure sealants. *Br Dent J*. 1989;167(11):395–396.
40. Simonsen RJ. Pit and fissure sealant: review of the literature. *Pediatr Dent*. 2002;24(5):393–414.
41. Zero DT, Zandona AF, Vail MM, et al. Dental caries and pulpal disease. *Dent Clin North Am*. 2011;55(1):29–46.
42. Fontana M, Platt JA, Eckert GJ, et al. Monitoring of sound and carious surfaces under sealants over 44 months. *J Dent Res*. 2014;93(11):1070–1075.
43. Hatibovic-Kofman S, Wright GZ, Braverman I. Microleakage of sealants after conventional, bur, and air-abrasion preparation of pits and fissures. *Pediatr Dent*. 1998;20(3):173–176.
44. Duangthip D, Lussi A. Variables contributing to the quality of fissure sealants used by general dental practitioners. *Oper Dent*. 2003;28(6):756–764.
45. Irinoda Y, Matsumura Y, Kito H, et al. Effect of sealant viscosity on the penetration of resin into etched human enamel. *Oper Dent*. 2000;25(4):274–282.
46. Montanari M, Pitzolu G, Felline C, et al. Marginal seal evaluation of different resin sealants used in pits and fissures. An in vitro study. *Eur J Paediatr Dent*. 2008;9(3):125–131.
47. Boksman L, McConnell RJ, Carson B, et al. A 2-year clinical evaluation of two pit and fissure sealants placed with and without the use of a bonding agent. *Quintessence Int*. 1993;24(2):131–133.
48. Barrie AM, Stephen KW, Kay EJ. Fissure sealant retention: a comparison of three sealant types under field conditions. *Community Dent Health*. 1990;7(3):273–277.
49. Tilliss TS, Stach DJ, Hatch RA, et al. Occlusal discrepancies after sealant therapy. *J Prosthet Dent*. 1992;68(2):223–228.
50. Simonsen RJ, Neal RC. A review of the clinical application and performance of pit and fissure sealants. *Aust Dent J*. 2011;56(suppl 1):45–58.
51. Kakaboura A, Matthaiou L, Papagiannoulis L. In vitro study of penetration of flowable resin composite and compomer into occlusal fissures. *Eur J Paediatr Dent*. 2002;3(4):205–209.
52. Gillet D, Nancy J, Dupuis V, et al. Microleakage and penetration depth of three types of materials in fissure sealant: self-etching primer vs etching: an in vitro study. *J Clin Pediatr Dent*. 2002;26(2):175–178.
53. Dukic W, Glavina D. Clinical evaluation of three fissure sealants: 24 month follow-up. *Eur Arch Paediatr Dent*. 2007;8(3):163–166.
54. Corona SA, Borsatto MC, Garcia L, et al. Randomized, controlled trial comparing the retention of a flowable restorative system with a conventional resin sealant: one-year follow up. *Int J Paediatr Dent*. 2005;15(1):44–50.
55. Kuşgöz A, Tüzüner T, Ulker M, et al. Conversion degree, microhardness, microleakage and fluoride release of different fissure sealants. *J Mech Behav Biomed Mater*. 2010;3:594–599.
56. Rajtboriraks D, Nakornchai S, Bunditsing P, et al. Plaque and saliva fluoride levels after placement of fluoride releasing pit and fissure sealants. *Pediatr Dent*. 2004;26(1):63–66.
57. Jensen OE, Billings RJ, Featherstone JD. Clinical evaluation of Fluroshield pit and fissure sealant. *Clin Prev Dent*. 1990;12(4):24–27.
58. Carlsson A, Petersson M, Twetman S. 2-year clinical performance of a fluoride-containing fissure sealant in young schoolchildren at caries risk. *Am J Dent*. 1997;10(3):115–119.
59. Cagetti MG, Carta G, Cocco F, et al. Effect of fluoridated sealants on adjacent tooth surfaces: a 30-mo randomized clinical trial. *J Dent Res*. 2014;93(7 suppl):59S–65S.
60. Elkhadem A, Wanees S. Fluoride releasing sealants may possess minimal cariostatic effect on adjacent surfaces. *Evid Based Dent*. 2015;16(1):12.
61. Boksman L, Carson B. Two-year retention and caries rates of UltraSeal XT and FluoroShield light-cured pit and fissure sealants. *Gen Dent*. 1998;46(2):184–187.
62. Ahovuo-Saloranta A, Hiiri A, Nordblad A, et al. Pit and fissure sealants for preventing dental decay in the permanent teeth of children and adolescents. *Cochrane Database Syst Rev*. 2008;(4):CD001830.
63. Mickenautsch S, Yengopal V. Caries-preventive effect of glass ionomer and resin-based fissure sealants on permanent teeth: an update of systematic review evidence. *BMC Res Notes*. 2011;4(1):22.
64. Yengopal V, Mickenautsch S, Bezerra AC, et al. Caries-preventive effect of glass ionomer and resin-based fissure sealants on permanent teeth: a meta analysis. *J Oral Sci*. 2009;51(3):373–382.
65. Beiruti N, Frencken JE, van't Hof MA, et al. Caries-preventive effect of a one-time application of composite resin and glass ionomer sealants after 5 years. *Caries Res*. 2006;40(1):52–59.

66. Frencken JE, Wolke J. Clinical and SEM assessment of ART high-viscosity glass-ionomer sealants after 8-13 years in 4 teeth. *J Dent.* 2010;38(1):59–64.
67. Smith NK, Morris KT, Wells M, et al. Rationale for caries inhibition of debonded glass ionomer sealants: an in vitro study. *Pediatr Dent.* 2014;36(7):464–467.
68. Sundfeld D, Machado LS, Franco LM, et al. Clinical/photographic/scanning electron microscopy analysis of pit and fissure sealants after 22 years: a case series. *Oper Dent.* 2017;42(1):10–18.
69. Zhang W, Chen X, Fan MW, et al. Do light cured ART conventional high-viscosity glass-ionomer sealants perform better than resin-composite sealants: a 4-year randomized clinical trial. *Dent Mater.* 2014;30(5):487–492.
70. Liu BY, Xiao Y, Chu CH, et al. Glass ionomer ART sealant and fluoride-releasing resin sealant in fissure caries prevention–results from a randomized clinical trial. *BMC Oral Health.* 2014;14:54.
71. de Amorim RG, Leal SC, Frencken JE. Survival of atraumatic restorative treatment (ART) sealants and restorations: a meta-analysis. *Clin Oral Investig.* 2012;16(2):429–441.
72. Nicholson JW. Polyacid-modified composite resins ("compomers") and their use in clinical dentistry. *Dent Mater.* 2007;23(5):615–622.
73. Pardi V, Pereira AC, Ambrosano GM, et al. Clinical evaluation of three different materials used as pit and fissure sealant: 24-months results. *J Clin Pediatr Dent.* 2005;29(2):133–137.
74. Pardi V, Pereira AC, Mialhe FL, et al. Six-year clinical evaluation of polyacid-modified composite resin used as fissure sealant. *J Clin Pediatr Dent.* 2004;28(3):257–260.
75. Pereira AC, Pardi V, Mialhe FL, et al. Clinical evaluation of a polyacid-modified resin used as a fissure sealant: 48-month results. *Am J Dent.* 2000;13(6):294–296.
76. Leskinen K, Salo S, Suni J, et al. Comparison of dental health in sealed and non-sealed first permanent molars: 7 years follow-up in practice-based dentistry. *J Dent.* 2008;36(1):27–32.
77. Heller KE, Reed SG, Bruner FW, et al. Longitudinal evaluation of sealing molars with and without incipient dental caries in a public health program. *J Public Health Dent.* 1995;55(3):148–153.
78. Griffin SO, Griffin PM, Gooch BF, et al. Comparing the costs of three sealant delivery strategies. *J Dent Res.* 2002;81(9):641–645.
79. Guideline on fluoride therapy. *Pediatr Dent.* 2016;38(6):181–184.
80. Bravo M, Llodra JC, Baca P, et al. Effectiveness of visible light fissure sealant (Delton) versus fluoride varnish (Duraphat): 24-month clinical trial. *Community Dent Oral Epidemiol.* 1996;24(1):42–46.
81. Tewari A, Chawla HS, Utreja A. Comparative evaluation of the role of NaF, APF & Duraphat topical fluoride applications in the prevention of dental caries–a 2 1/2 years study. *J Indian Soc Pedod Prev Dent.* 1991;8(1):28–35.
82. Ripa LW, Leske GS, Varma AO. Longitudinal study of the caries susceptibility of occlusal and proximal surfaces of first permanent molars. *J Public Health Dent.* 1988;48(1):8–13.
83. Vehkalahti MM, Solavaara L, Rytomaa I. An eight-year follow-up of the occlusal surfaces of first permanent molars. *J Dent Res.* 1991;70(7):1064–1067.
84. Whelton H. Overview of the impact of changing global patterns of dental caries experience on caries clinical trials. *J Dent Res.* 2004;83(SpecC):C29–C34.
85. Vrbic V. Retention of a fluoride-containing sealant on primary and permanent teeth 3 years after placement. *Quintessence Int.* 1999;30(12):825–828.
86. Hotuman E, Rolling I, Poulsen S. Fissure sealants in a group of 3-4-year-old children. *Int J Paediatr Dent.* 1998;8(2):159–160.
87. Chadwick BL, Treasure ET, Playle RA. A randomised controlled trial to determine the effectiveness of glass ionomer sealants in pre-school children. *Caries Res.* 2005;39(1):34–40.
88. Lussi A. Validity of diagnostic and treatment decisions of fissure caries. *Caries Res.* 1991;25(4):296–303.
89. Stookey G. Should a dental explorer be used to probe suspected carious lesions? No–use of an explorer can lead to misdiagnosis and disrupt remineralization. *J Am Dent Assoc.* 2005;136(11):1527, 29, 31.
90. Ekstrand K, Qvist V, Thylstrup A. Light microscope study of the effect of probing in occlusal surfaces. *Caries Res.* 1987;21(4):368–374.
91. van Dorp CS, Exterkate RA, ten Cate JM. The effect of dental probing on subsequent enamel demineralization. *ASDC J Dent Child.* 1988;55(5):343–347.
92. Kuhnisch J, Dietz W, Stosser L, et al. Effects of dental probing on occlusal surfaces–a scanning electron microscopy evaluation. *Caries Res.* 2007;41(1):43–48.
93. Schwendicke F, Frencken JE, Bjorndal L, et al. Managing carious lesions: consensus recommendations on carious tissue removal. *Adv Dent Res.* 2016;28(2):58–67.
94. Mertz-Fairhurst EJ, Curtis JW Jr, Ergle JW, et al. Ultraconservative and cariostatic sealed restorations: results at year 10. *J Am Dent Assoc.* 1998;129(1):55–66.
95. Swift EJ Jr. The effect of sealants on dental caries: a review. *J Am Dent Assoc.* 1988;116(6):700–704.
96. Griffin SO, Oong E, Kohn W, et al. The effectiveness of sealants in managing caries lesions. *J Dent Res.* 2008;87(2):169–174.
97. Handelman SL, Leverett DH, Espeland M, et al. Retention of sealants over carious and sound tooth surfaces. *Community Dent Oral Epidemiol.* 1987;15(1):1–5.
98. Chapko M. A study of the intentional use of pit and fissure sealants over carious lesions. *J Public Health Dent.* 1987;47(3):139–142.
99. Oong EM, Griffin SO, Kohn WG, et al. The effect of dental sealants on bacteria levels in caries lesions: a review of the evidence. *J Am Dent Assoc.* 2008;139(3):271–278, quiz 357–358.
100. Jensen OE, Handelman SL. Effect of an autopolymerizing sealant on viability of microflora in occlusal dental caries. *Scand J Dent Res.* 1980;88(5):382–388.
101. Tellez M, Gray SL, Gray S, et al. Sealants and dental caries: dentists' perspectives on evidence-based recommendations. *J Am Dent Assoc.* 2011;142(9):1033–1040.
102. O'Donnell JA, Modesto A, Oakley M, et al. Sealants and dental caries: insight into dentists' behaviors regarding implementation of clinical practice recommendations. *J Am Dent Assoc.* 2013;144(4):e24–e30.
103. Gillcrist JA, Vaughan MP, Plumlee GN Jr, et al. Clinical sealant retention following two different tooth-cleaning techniques. *J Public Health Dent.* 1998;58(3):254–256.
104. Hegde RJ, Coutinho RC. Comparison of different methods of cleaning and preparing occlusal fissure surface before placement of pit and fissure sealants: an in vivo study. *J Indian Soc Pedod Prev Dent.* 2016;34(2):111–114.
105. Garcia-Godoy F, Gwinnett AJ. An SEM study of fissure surfaces conditioned with a scraping technique. *Clin Prev Dent.* 1987;9(4):9–13.
106. Jasmin JR, van Waes H, Vijayaraghavan TV. Scanning electron microscopy study of the fitting surface of fissure sealants. *Pediatr Dent.* 1991;13(6):370–372.
107. Garcia-Godoy F, Medlock JW. An SEM study of the effects of air-polishing on fissure surfaces. *Quintessence Int.* 1988;19(7):465–467.
108. Strand GV, Raadal M. The efficiency of cleaning fissures with an air-polishing instrument. *Acta Odontol Scand.* 1988;46(2):113–117.
109. Brocklehurst PR, Joshi RI, Northeast SE. The effect of air-polishing occlusal surfaces on the penetration of fissures by a sealant. *Int J Paediatr Dent.* 1992;2(3):157–162.
110. Brockmann SL, Scott RL, Eick JD. The effect of an air-polishing device on tensile bond strength of a dental sealant. *Quintessence Int.* 1989;20(3):211–217.
111. Scott L, Greer D. The effect of an air polishing device on sealant bond strength. *J Prosthet Dent.* 1987;58(3):384–387.
112. Scott L, Brockmann S, Houston G, et al. Retention of dental sealants following the use of airpolishing and traditional cleaning. *Dent Hyg (Chic).* 1988;62(8):402–406.
113. Bagherian A, Sarraf Shirazi A. Preparation before acid etching in fissure sealant therapy: yes or no? A systematic review and meta-analysis. *J Am Dent Assoc.* 2016;147(12):943–951.

114. Garcia-Godoy F, de Araujo FB. Enhancement of fissure sealant penetration and adaptation: the enameloplasty technique. *J Clin Pediatr Dent*. 1994;19(1):13–18.

115. Xalabarde A, Garcia-Godoy F, Boj JR, et al. Fissure micromorphology and sealant adaptation after occlusal enameloplasty. *J Clin Pediatr Dent*. 1996;20(4):299–304.

116. Lygidakis NA, Oulis KI, Christodoulidis A. Evaluation of fissure sealants retention following four different isolation and surface preparation techniques: four years clinical trial. *J Clin Pediatr Dent*. 1994;19(1):23–25.

117. Shapira J, Eidelman E. Six-year clinical evaluation of fissure sealants placed after mechanical preparation: a matched pair study. *Pediatr Dent*. 1986;8(3):204–205.

118. Geiger SB, Gulayev S, Weiss EI. Improving fissure sealant quality: mechanical preparation and filling level. *J Dent*. 2000;28(6):407–412.

119. Feldens EG, Feldens CA, de Araujo FB, et al. Invasive technique of pit and fissure sealants in primary molars: a SEM study. *J Clin Pediatr Dent*. 1994;18(3):187–190.

120. De Craene GP, Martens C, Dermaut R. The invasive pit-and-fissure sealing technique in pediatric dentistry: an SEM study of a preventive restoration. *ASDC J Dent Child*. 1988;55(1):34–42.

121. Le Bell Y, Forsten L. Sealing of preventively enlarged fissures. *Acta Odontol Scand*. 1980;38(2):101–104.

122. Francescut P, Lussi A. Performance of a conventional sealant and a flowable composite on minimally invasive prepared fissures. *Oper Dent*. 2006;31(5):543–550.

123. Blackwood JA, Dilley DC, Roberts MW, et al. Evaluation of pumice, fissure enameloplasty and air abrasion on sealant microleakage. *Pediatr Dent*. 2002;24(3):199–203.

124. Ellis RW, Latta MA, Westerman GH. Effect of air abrasion and acid etching on sealant retention: an in vitro study. *Pediatr Dent*. 1999;21(6):316–319.

125. Chan DC, Summitt JB, Garcia-Godoy F, et al. Evaluation of different methods for cleaning and preparing occlusal fissures. *Oper Dent*. 1999;24(6):331–336.

126. Yazici AR, Kiremitci A, Celik C, et al. A two-year clinical evaluation of pit and fissure sealants placed with and without air abrasion pretreatment in teenagers. *J Am Dent Assoc*. 2006;137(10):1401–1405.

127. Kanellis MJ, Warren JJ, Levy SM. Comparison of air abrasion versus acid etch sealant techniques: six-month retention. *Pediatr Dent*. 1997;19(4):258–261.

128. Kanellis MJ, Warren JJ, Levy SM. A comparison of sealant placement techniques and 12-month retention rates. *J Public Health Dent*. 2000;60(1):53–56.

129. Roeder LB, Berry EA 3rd, You C, et al. Bond strength of composite to air-abraded enamel and dentin. *Oper Dent*. 1995;20(5):186–190.

130. Welbury R, Raadal M, Lygidakis NA. EAPD guidelines for the use of pit and fissure sealants. *Eur J Paediatr Dent*. 2004;5(3):179–184.

131. Koh SH, Chan JT, You C. Effects of topical fluoride treatment on tensile bond strength of pit and fissure sealants. *Gen Dent*. 1998;46(3):278–280.

132. Koh SH, Huo YY, Powers JM, et al. Topical fluoride treatment has no clinical effect on retention of pit and fissure sealants. *J Gt Houst Dent Soc*. 1995;67(2):16–18.

133. Warren DP, Infante NB, Rice HC, et al. Effect of topical fluoride on retention of pit and fissure sealants. *J Dent Hyg*. 2001;75(1):21–24.

134. Tandon S, Kumari R, Udupa S. The effect of etch-time on the bond strength of a sealant and on the etch-pattern in primary and permanent enamel: an evaluation. *ASDC J Dent Child*. 1989;56(3):186–190.

135. Guba CJ, Cochran MA, Swartz ML. The effects of varied etching time and etching solution viscosity on bond strength and enamel morphology. *Oper Dent*. 1994;19(4):146–153.

136. Sadowsky PL, Retief DH, Cox PR, et al. Effects of etchant concentration and duration on the retention of orthodontic brackets: an in vivo study. *Am J Orthod Dentofacial Orthop*. 1990;98(5):417–421.

137. Wang WN, Lu TC. Bond strength with various etching times on young permanent teeth. *Am J Orthod Dentofacial Orthop*. 1991;100(1):72–79.

138. Summitt JB, Chan DC, Burgess JO, et al. Effect of air/water rinse versus water only and of five rinse times on resin-to-etched-enamel shear bond strength. *Oper Dent*. 1992;17(4):142–151.

139. Summitt JB, Chan DC, Dutton FB, et al. Effect of rinse time on microleakage between composite and etched enamel. *Oper Dent*. 1993;18(1):37–40.

140. Waggoner WF, Siegal M. Pit and fissure sealant application: updating the technique. *J Am Dent Assoc*. 1996;127(3):351–361, quiz 91–92.

141. Rock WP, Weatherill S, Anderson RJ. Retention of three fissure sealant resins. The effects of etching agent and curing method. Results over 3 years. *Br Dent J*. 1990;168(8):323–325.

142. Brown MR, Foreman FJ, Burgess JO, et al. Penetration of gel and solution etchants in occlusal fissures. *ASDC J Dent Child*. 1988;55(4):265–268.

143. Botton G, Morgental CS, Scherer MM, et al. Are self-etch adhesive systems effective in the retention of occlusal sealants? A systematic review and meta-analysis. *Int J Paediatr Dent*. 2016;26(6):402–411.

144. Rosa WL, Piva E, Silva AF. Bond strength of universal adhesives: a systematic review and meta-analysis. *J Dent*. 2015;43(7):765–776.

145. Duangthip D, Lussi A. Effects of fissure cleaning methods, drying agents, and fissure morphology on microleakage and penetration ability of sealants in vitro. *Pediatr Dent*. 2003;25(6):527–533.

146. Rix AM, Sams DR, Dickinson GL, et al. Pit and fissure sealant application using a drying agent. *Am J Dent*. 1994;7(3):131–133.

147. Yue C, Tantbirojn D, Grothe RL, et al. The depth of cure of clear versus opaque sealants as influenced by curing regimens. *J Am Dent Assoc*. 2009;140(3):331–338.

148. Strang R, Cummings A, Stephen KW. Laboratory studies of visible-light cured fissure sealants: setting times and depth of polymerization. *J Oral Rehabil*. 1986;13(4):305–310.

149. Kramer N, Lohbauer U, Garcia-Godoy F, et al. Light curing of resin-based composites in the LED era. *Am J Dent*. 2008;21(3):135–142.

150. Schattenberg A, Lichtenberg D, Stender E, et al. Minimal exposure time of different LED-curing devices. *Dent Mater*. 2008;24(8):1043–1049.

151. Ernst CP, Meyer GR, Muller J, et al. Depth of cure of LED vs QTH light-curing devices at a distance of 7 mm. *J Adhes Dent*. 2004;6(2):141–150.

152. Kitchens B, Wells M, Tantbirojn D, et al. Depth of cure of sealants polymerized with high-power light emitting diode curing lights. *Int J Paediatr Dent*. 2015;25(2):79–86.

153. Branchal CF, Wells MH, Tantbirojn D, et al. Can increasing the manufacturer's recommended shortest curing time of high-intensity light-emitting diodes adequately cure sealants? *Pediatr Dent*. 2015;37(4):E7–E13.

154. Rueggeberg FA, Caughman WF, Curtis JW Jr, et al. Factors affecting cure at depths within light-activated resin composites. *Am J Dent*. 1993;6(2):91–95.

155. Chosack A, Eidelman E. Effect of the time from application until exposure to light on the tag lengths of a visible light-polymerized sealant. *Dent Mater*. 1988;4(5):302–306.

156. Barroso JM, Torres CP, Lessa FC, et al. Shear bond strength of pit-and-fissure sealants to saliva-contaminated and noncontaminated enamel. *J Dent Child (Chic)*. 2005;72(3):95–99.

157. Feigal RJ, Hitt J, Splieth C. Retaining sealant on salivary contaminated enamel. *J Am Dent Assoc*. 1993;124(3):88–97.

158. Fritz UB, Finger WJ, Stean H. Salivary contamination during bonding procedures with a one-bottle adhesive system. *Quintessence Int*. 1998;29(9):567–572.

159. Silverstone LM, Hicks MJ, Featherstone MJ. Oral fluid contamination of etched enamel surfaces: an SEM study. *J Am Dent Assoc*. 1985;110(3):329–332.

160. Locker D, Jokovic A, Kay EJ. Prevention. Part 8: the use of pit and fissure sealants in preventing caries in the permanent dentition of children. *Br Dent J.* 2003;195(7):375–378.

161. Eidelman E, Fuks AB, Chosack A. The retention of fissure sealants: rubber dam or cotton rolls in a private practice. *ASDC J Dent Child.* 1983;50(4):259–261.

162. Straffon LH, Dennison JB, More FG. Three-year evaluation of sealant: effect of isolation on efficacy. *J Am Dent Assoc.* 1985;110(5):714–717.

163. Collette J, Wilson S, Sullivan D. A study of the Isolite system during sealant placement: efficacy and patient acceptance. *Pediatr Dent.* 2010;32(2):146–150.

164. Wood AJ, Saravia ME, Farrington FH. Cotton roll isolation versus Vac-Ejector isolation. *ASDC J Dent Child.* 1989;56(6):438–441.

165. Lyman T, Viswanathan K, McWhorter A. Isolite vs cotton roll isolation in the placement of dental sealants. *Pediatr Dent.* 2013;35(3):E95–E99.

166. Alhareky MS, Mermelstein D, Finkelman M, et al. Efficiency and patient satisfaction with the Isolite system versus rubber dam for sealant placement in pediatric patients. *Pediatr Dent.* 2014;36(5):400–404.

167. Rock WP, Bradnock G. Effect of operator variability and patient age on the retention of fissure sealant resin: 3-year results. *Community Dent Oral Epidemiol.* 1981;9(5):207–209.

168. Dennison JB, Straffon LH, More FG. Evaluating tooth eruption on sealant efficacy. *J Am Dent Assoc.* 1990;121(5):610–614.

169. Feigal RJ, Musherure P, Gillespie B, et al. Improved sealant retention with bonding agents: a clinical study of two-bottle and single-bottle systems. *J Dent Res.* 2000;79(11):1850–1856.

170. Koyuturk AE, Akca T, Yucel AC, et al. Effect of thermal cycling on microleakage of a fissure sealant polymerized with different light sources. *Dent Mater J.* 2006;25(4):713–718.

171. Symons AL, Chu CY, Meyers IA. The effect of fissure morphology and pretreatment of the enamel surface on penetration and adhesion of fissure sealants. *J Oral Rehabil.* 1996;23(12):791–798.

172. Borsatto MC, Corona SA, Alves AG, et al. Influence of salivary contamination on marginal microleakage of pit and fissure sealants. *Am J Dent.* 2004;17(5):365–367.

173. Hevinga MA, Opdam NJ, Frencken JF, et al. Microleakage and sealant penetration in contaminated carious fissures. *J Dent.* 2007;35(12):909–914.

174. Asselin ME, Fortin D, Sitbon Y, et al. Marginal microleakage of a sealant applied to permanent enamel: evaluation of 3 application protocols. *Pediatr Dent.* 2008;30(1):29–33.

175. Bagherian A, Sarraf Shirazi A, Sadeghi R. Adhesive systems under fissure sealants: yes or no? A systematic review and meta-analysis. *J Am Dent Assoc.* 2016;147(6):446–456.

176. Marquezan M, da Silveira BL, Burnett LH Jr, et al. Microtensile bond strength of contemporary adhesives to primary enamel and dentin. *J Clin Pediatr Dent.* 2008;32(2):127–132.

177. Swanson TK, Feigal RJ, Tantbirojn D, et al. Effect of adhesive systems and bevel on enamel margin integrity in primary and permanent teeth. *Pediatr Dent.* 2008;30(2):134–140.

178. Chawla N, Messer LB, Silva M. Clinical studies on molar-incisor-hypomineralisation part 1: distribution and putative associations. *Eur Arch Paediatr Dent.* 2008;9(4):180–190.

179. Kotsanos N, Kaklamanos EG, Arapostathis K. Treatment management of first permanent molars in children with molar-incisor hypomineralisation. *Eur J Paediatr Dent.* 2005;6(4):179–184.

180. Lygidakis NA, Dimou G, Stamataki E. Retention of fissure sealants using two different methods of application in teeth with hypomineralised molars (MIH): a 4 year clinical study. *Eur Arch Paediatr Dent.* 2009;10(4):223–226.

181. Mascarenhas AK, Nazar H, Al-Mutawaa S, et al. Effectiveness of primer and bond in sealant retention and caries prevention. *Pediatr Dent.* 2008;30(1):25–28.

182. Marks D, Owens BM, Johnson WW. Effect of adhesive agent and fissure morphology on the in vitro microleakage and penetrability of pit and fissure sealants. *Quintessence Int.* 2009;40(9):763–772.

183. Pinar A, Sepet E, Aren G, et al. Clinical performance of sealants with and without a bonding agent. *Quintessence Int.* 2005;36(5):355–360.

184. Stiles HM, Ward GT, Woolridge ED, et al. Adhesive sealant clinical trial: comparative results of application by a dentist or dental auxiliaries. *J Prev Dent.* 1976;3(3 Pt 2):8–11.

185. Foreman FJ, Matis BA. Retention of sealants placed by dental technicians without assistance. *Pediatr Dent.* 1991;13(1):59–61.

186. Foreman FJ, Matis BA. Sealant retention rates of dental hygienists and dental technicians using differing training protocols. *Pediatr Dent.* 1992;14(3):189–190.

187. Ismail AI, King W, Clark DC. An evaluation of the Saskatchewan pit and fissure sealant program: a longitudinal followup. *J Public Health Dent.* 1989;49(4):206–211.

188. Nilchian F, Rodd HD, Robinson PG. The success of fissure sealants placed by dentists and dental care professionals. *Community Dent Health.* 2011;28(1):99–103.

189. Holst A, Braune K, Sullivan A. A five-year evaluation of fissure sealants applied by dental assistants. *Swed Dent J.* 1998;22(5–6):195–201.

190. Folke BD, Walton JL, Feigal RJ. Occlusal sealant success over ten years in a private practice: comparing longevity of sealants placed by dentists, hygienists, and assistants. *Pediatr Dent.* 2004;26(5):426–432.

191. Griffin SO, Jones K, Gray SK, et al. Exploring four-handed delivery and retention of resin-based sealants. *J Am Dent Assoc.* 2008;139(3):281–289, quiz 358.

192. Truman BI, Gooch BF, Sulemana I, et al. Reviews of evidence on interventions to prevent dental caries, oral and pharyngeal cancers, and sports-related craniofacial injuries. *Am J Prev Med.* 2002;23(1 suppl):21–54.

193. Gooch BF, Griffin SO, Gray SK, et al. Preventing dental caries through school-based sealant programs: updated recommendations and reviews of evidence. *J Am Dent Assoc.* 2009;140(11):1356–1365.

194. Griffin S, Naavaal S, Scherrer C, et al. School-based dental sealant programs prevent cavities and are cost-effective. *Health Aff (Millwood).* 2016;35(12):2233–2240.

195. Dorri M, Dunne SM, Walsh T, et al. Micro-invasive interventions for managing proximal dental decay in primary and permanent teeth. *Cochrane Database Syst Rev.* 2015;(11):CD010431.

196. Gordan VV, Shen C, Riley J 3rd, et al. Two-year clinical evaluation of repair versus replacement of composite restorations. *J Esthet Restor Dent.* 2006;18(3):144–153, discussion 54.

197. Moncada G, Fernandez E, Martin J, et al. Increasing the longevity of restorations by minimal intervention: a two-year clinical trial. *Oper Dent.* 2008;33(3):258–264.

198. dos Santos PH, Pavan S, Assuncao WG, et al. Influence of surface sealants on microleakage of composite resin restorations. *J Dent Child (Chic).* 2008;75(1):24–28.

199. Moncada G, Martin J, Fernandez E, et al. Sealing, refurbishment and repair of class I and class II defective restorations: a three-year clinical trial. *J Am Dent Assoc.* 2009;140(4):425–432.

200. Moncada GC, Martin J, Fernandez E, et al. Alternative treatments for resin-based composite and amalgam restorations with marginal defects: a 12-month clinical trial. *Gen Dent.* 2006;54(5):314–318.

201. Donly KJ, Garcia-Godoy F. The use of resin-based composite in children: an update. *Pediatr Dent.* 2015;37(2):136–143.

202. Green D, Mackenzie L, Banerjee A. Minimally invasive long-term management of direct restorations: the '5 Rs.' *Dent Update.* 2015;42(5):413–416, 19–21, 23–26.

203. Hu W, Featherstone JD. Prevention of enamel demineralization: an in-vitro study using light-cured filled sealant. *Am J Orthod Dentofacial Orthop.* 2005;128(5):592–600, quiz 70.

204. Buren JL, Staley RN, Wefel J, et al. Inhibition of enamel demineralization by an enamel sealant, Pro Seal: an in-vitro study. *Am J Orthod Dentofacial Orthop.* 2008;133(4 suppl):S88–S94.

205. Salar DV, Garcia-Godoy F, Flaitz CM, et al. Potential inhibition of demineralization in vitro by fluoride-releasing sealants. *J Am Dent Assoc.* 2007;138(4):502–506.

206. Benham AW, Campbell PM, Buschang PH. Effectiveness of pit and fissure sealants in reducing white spot lesions during orthodontic treatment. A pilot study. *Angle Orthod.* 2009;79(2):338–345.

207. Heinig N, Hartmann A. Efficacy of a sealant: study on the efficacy of a sealant (Light Bond) in preventing decalcification during multibracket therapy. *J Orofac Orthop.* 2008;69(3):154–167.

208. O'Reilly MT, De Jesus Vinas J, Hatch JP. Effectiveness of a sealant compared with no sealant in preventing enamel demineralization in patients with fixed orthodontic appliances: a prospective clinical trial. *Am J Orthod Dentofacial Orthop.* 2013;143(6):837–844.

209. Hammad SM, Knosel M. Efficacy of a new sealant to prevent white spot lesions during fixed orthodontic treatment: a 12-month, single-center, randomized controlled clinical trial. *J Orofac Orthop.* 2016;77(6):439–445.

210. Leizer C, Weinstein M, Borislow AJ, et al. Efficacy of a filled-resin sealant in preventing decalcification during orthodontic treatment. *Am J Orthod Dentofacial Orthop.* 2010;137(6):796–800.

211. Wenderoth CJ, Weinstein M, Borislow AJ. Effectiveness of a fluoride-releasing sealant in reducing decalcification during orthodontic treatment. *Am J Orthod Dentofacial Orthop.* 1999;116(6):629–634.

212. Farrow ML, Newman SM, Oesterle LJ, et al. Filled and unfilled restorative materials to reduce enamel decalcification during fixed-appliance orthodontic treatment. *Am J Orthod Dentofacial Orthop.* 2007;132(5):578e1–578e6.

213. Olea N, Pulgar R, Perez P, et al. Estrogenicity of resin-based composites and sealants used in dentistry. *Environ Health Perspect.* 1996;104(3):298–305.

214. Calafat AM, Ye X, Wong LY, et al. Exposure of the U.S. population to bisphenol A and 4-tertiary-octylphenol: 2003-2004. *Environ Health Perspect.* 2008;116(1):39–44.

215. Wolstenholme JT, Rissman EF, Connelly JJ. The role of bisphenol A in shaping the brain, epigenome and behavior. *Horm Behav.* 2011;59(3):296–305.

216. Fung EY, Ewoldsen NO, St Germain HA Jr, et al. Pharmacokinetics of bisphenol A released from a dental sealant. *J Am Dent Assoc.* 2000;131(1):51–58.

217. Azarpazhooh A, Main PA. Is there a risk of harm or toxicity in the placement of pit and fissure sealant materials? A systematic review. *J Can Dent Assoc.* 2008;74(2):179–183.

218. Fleisch AF, Sheffield PE, Chinn C, et al. Bisphenol A and related compounds in dental materials. *Pediatrics.* 2010;126(4):760–768.

219. Kane B, Karren J, Garcia-Godoy C, et al. Sealant adaptation and penetration into occlusal fissures. *Am J Dent.* 2009;22(2):89–91.

220. O'Donnell J. A moisture tolerant resin based pit and fissure sealant: research results. *Inside Dentistry.* 2008;4(9):108–110.

221. Bagherian A, Ahmadkhani M, Sheikhfathollahi M, et al. Microbial microleakage assessment of a new hydrophilic fissure sealant: a laboratory study. *Pediatr Dent.* 2013;35(7):194–198.

222. Khatri SG, Samuel SR, Acharya S, et al. Retention of moisture-tolerant and conventional resin-based sealant in six- to nine-year-old children. *Pediatr Dent.* 2015;37(4):366–370.

223. Schlueter N, Klimek J, Ganss C. Efficacy of a moisture-tolerant material for fissure sealing: a prospective randomised clinical trial. *Clin Oral Investig.* 2013;17(3):711–716.

224. Bhat PK, Konde S, Raj SN, et al. Moisture-tolerant resin-based sealant: a boon. *Contemp Clin Dent.* 2013;4(3):343–348.

225. Boksman L. Have recent advances in adhesives and materials dictated a change in sealant protocols? *Oral Health J.* 2006;96(10):69–78.

226. Liebenberg WH. The fissure sealant impasse. *Quintessence Int.* 1994;25(11):741–745.

34

Pulp Therapy for the Young Permanent Dentition

ANNA B. FUKS AND EYAL NUNI

CHAPTER OUTLINE

The Dentin-Pulp Complex Concept

The most important, and most difficult, aspect of pulp therapy is determining the health of the pulp or its stage of inflammation. Consequently, an intelligent decision regarding the best form of treatment can be made. Permanent teeth in children and adolescents have a more cellular pulp and a rich vascular supply with better healing potential than in adults,[1] and their degree of root development will affect the treatment plan.

Immature permanent teeth are those in which root development and apical closure have not been completed. These teeth can be present in children from 6 years of age until 3 years after the eruption of the third molars. After apical closure, these teeth are classified as mature teeth. It should be kept in mind that the apposition of secondary dentin in the pulp chamber and the root canal is a continuous process. Physiologic secondary dentinogenesis represents the deposition of dentin after completion of the crown and root formation. It continues, at a much slower rate, throughout the life of the tooth.[2] It is extremely important to maintain pulp vitality whenever possible, because young permanent teeth have wide root canals, and dentin apposition can prevent fracture. Root fracture is a common finding after traumatic injury in endodontically treated teeth with wide root canals.[3] The aim of all treatment planning for young permanent teeth is to preserve pulp vitality, providing conditions for continuous root development and physiologic dentin apposition. The pulp and the dentin are closely related and are usually looked upon as one unit, the pulp-dentin complex.[4,5] All procedures performed in the dentin will have an effect on the pulp.

Reactions to Caries and Operative Procedures

The molecular and cellular changes that take place during primary dentinogenesis are mimicked during the dentin-pulp reactions to injury. Kuttler[6] proposed the concept of tertiary dentin formation, encompassing a wide range of responses, from the secretion of a regular, tubular dentin to a very dysplastic atubular dentin. These responses are the result of different cellular and molecular processes, and they express reactions ranging from mild to severe stimulus. Tertiary dentin has been classified as either reactionary or reparative dentin, the former being secreted by surviving postmitotic odontoblasts in response to a mild stimulus. Reparative dentin is secreted by a new generation of odontoblast-like cells differentiated after the death of the original postmitotic odontoblasts.[2]

The dentin matrix is considered to be a reservoir of growth factors and cytokines sequestered during dentinogenesis. During caries progression, these molecules may be released from the dentin degraded by bacterial acids with other components of the extracellular matrix, inducing the formation of reactionary dentin.[6] Members of the transforming growth factor (TGF) superfamily, specifically TGF-βs, have received considerable attention in effecting mesenchymal cells and inducing dentin regeneration.

These chemotactants are hypothesized to provide the signals involved in the recruitment, proliferation, and differentiation of the cells to the site of pulp injury to initiate tissue regeneration and dentin bridge formation.

Reparative dentinogenesis encompasses a complex sequence of biological events involving stem/progenitor cells recruitment and differentiation before matrix secretion at the site of the injury. It was demonstrated in a few in vivo studies that ethylenediamine tetraacetic acid (EDTA) solubilized dentin matrix components, shows morphogenetic activity, and can induce reparative dentinogenesis.[7]

In addition to the caries process, various factors associated with the method of cavity preparation and restoration can influence the tertiary dentin response. The size of the cavity, the residual dentin thickness (RDT), the etching of the cavity, and the type and method of application of the restorative material have an effect on the type and quality of the tertiary dentin. Several studies have reported that the alterations in the pulp related to the previously mentioned factors are more important than those related to the restorative materials.[8–11] RDT is apparently the most significant factor determining the secretion of reactionary dentin. Maximal reactionary dentin was observed in a study where the RDT in the cavities was between 0.5 and 0.25 mm. Reduced reactionary dentin and reduced odontoblastic survival were observed in teeth with an RDT less than 0.25 mm.[11] In these deep cavities, little more than 50% of the odontoblasts survived, whereas in shallow cavities, odontoblastic survival was about 85% or greater. Despite the cutting of the odontoblastic process, the cells responded by secreting reactionary dentin.

Pulp exposure in young permanent teeth is mainly the consequence of caries or trauma. In carious exposures, the pulp and the dentin are infected, whereas in iatrogenic exposures during operative procedures, only the dentin may be infected; the pulp may sometimes not even be inflamed. In traumatic pulp exposures, the dentin is not infected, and the pulp tissue may remain vital and uninfected if treated soon after the injury.

Clinical Pulpal Diagnosis

Patient History

The medical and dental history should always be carefully documented. In order to make the most accurate diagnosis, information must be obtained from several sources, with thorough clinical and radiographic examinations. Belanger refers to the importance of assessing the type of pain described by the child, whether it is spontaneous or is precipitated by a stimulus.[12] Sensitivity to pressure may indicate that the pulpal inflammation has extended to the periodontal ligament (PDL). However, this sensitivity may also be the result of a much more innocuous situation such as a sealant placed in excess or a high restoration causing hyperocclusion.[12] Children often complain of "toothaches" during the eruption of the first permanent molars. In these cases the dentist should carefully ascertain whether the complaint is due to a pericoronitis or to biting on an operculum, rather than to pain resulting from a pulp condition. Food impaction can also mimic the symptoms of an irreversible pulp condition. In cases of trauma, both patient and parents should be asked about the timing and nature of the injury, and whether previous treatment or traumatic incidents have occurred.

Clinical Examination

Both extraoral and intraoral examinations are important for the detection of the pulpally involved tooth. Extraoral examination

should focus on swelling, local lymphadenopathy, and extraoral sinus tract. Intraoral examination should focus on the tooth suspected as the origin of pain, but all the teeth on the same side should be inspected carefully, because referred pain can occur. The examination includes observation of the soft tissues for redness, swelling, or sinus tract.

Tooth discoloration is also an important finding, especially in traumatized teeth. Examining tissues by palpation and percussion, determining periodontal involvement, and assessing tooth mobility should follow. Special attention should be paid to fractured restorations or those with marginal breakdown, as these may also be indicators of pulp involvement.[13] Additional tests should include thermal and electric pulp test (EPT) of the involved tooth and of an appropriate control tooth. As in primary teeth, sensibility tests, sometimes called vitality or pulp tests, such as thermal and EPT have limited reliability in young permanent teeth, and do not reflect the extent of pulp inflammation.[14,15] Studies concluded that until innervation is completed (after 4 to 5 years in function), the EPT is not a reliable means of determining tooth vitality.[16] Cold test has been found more reliable in immature permanent teeth.[14,15] Reliability of sensibility tests in traumatized teeth, especially in the period adjacent to the traumatic incident is limited, because of possible damage to the pulp innervation system.[17,18]

The presence of extraoral or intraoral sinus tract requires the performance of a tracing radiograph in order to trace the origin of the infection.[19,20] When the originating tooth is detected, root canal treatment should be performed. Sensitivity to palpation in the vestibule may be indicative of an acute apical pathologic process. Emphasis should be placed on soft tissue swelling or bony expansion in the area, which may indicate the presence of Garré osteomyelitis.[21]

Pain to percussion does not indicate the state of the pulp inflammation; rather, it is an indication of inflammation in the PDL. This inflammation is most often a result of pulp inflammation that extended into the PDL or a sequel of dental trauma.[22] Periodontal probing is part of the intraoral examination; bone loss can be a consequence of reversible (treatable) or irreversible (untreatable) pulpitis.[20] Diagnosis of reversible pulpitis indicates that the inflammation should resolve and vital pulp therapy is a potential treatment option. Treatment options range from indirect pulp treatment (IPT), to direct pulp capping, to partial or cervical pulpotomy. It depends on the progress of the inflammatory process within the pulp and the degree of root development. Clinically the difference between reversible and irreversible pulpitis is frequently determined on the basis of the duration and intensity of the pain. Prolonged response to cold stimuli, spontaneous pain, or referred pain will lead to a diagnosis of irreversible or untreatable pulpitis. Although in primary teeth pulpectomy is the treatment of choice in these cases, immature permanent teeth should be carefully considered for pulpotomy, apexogenesis, or regenerative treatment, in an attempt to enable further tooth development.[18]

Radiographic Examination

Radiographs should follow a careful clinical examination. Performing bitewing radiographs is necessary to assess the depth of the caries, the morphology of the pulp chamber, the height of the pulp horns, the integrity and depth of restorations, and the level of bone support. Bitewing views can also demonstrate the presence of a calcified bridge in the pulp chamber, indicating the formation of tertiary dentin by a vital pulp in response to caries or pulp treatment.

On each periapical radiograph, inspection of the PDL continuity should be done to diagnose inflammatory and resorptive lesions. The interpretation of radiographs of young, immature permanent teeth can be difficult because of their normally large and open apex and radiolucent dental papilla. Less experienced dentists treating these teeth should avoid confusing pathologic changes with normal apical anatomy. In a young child, a vertical bitewing with a small size radiograph can be used instead of a periapical radiograph in order to see the periapical area of posterior teeth. Treatment decisions should not be made based on a single radiograph, so an additional radiograph of the antimeres should be taken for comparison. The degree of root development of the affected tooth and the amount of dentin apposition along the canal should be compared with those of the contralateral tooth. It is important to remember that the root canals of permanent teeth are wider in the buccolingual plane than the mesiodistal. Therefore it is difficult to determine the extent of apical closure in a regular radiograph showing only the mesiodistal plane. In the anterior region, radiographs of each central incisor should be obtained separately from a distal angulation to prevent overlapping of the PDL of the central incisor over the lateral incisor. Performing radiography in this manner is mandatory in teeth after traumatic injuries. Lateral external inflammatory root resorption is a common finding in necrotic young teeth after trauma. External replacement root resorption can also be seen after traumatic injuries.[18]

In recent years the use of cone beam computed tomography (CBCT) in endodontics has significantly increased. CBCT is a technique that produces undistorted three-dimensional digital imaging of the teeth and their surrounding tissues at reduced cost and with less radiation for the patient than traditional CT scans. The American Association of Endodontics (AAE) and the American Academy of Oral and Maxillofacial Radiology (AAOMR) state that the use of CBCT is justified in cases in which the benefits to the patient outweigh the potential risks of exposure to x-rays, especially in the case of children or young adults. CBCT should only be used when the question for which imaging is required cannot be answered adequately by lower dose conventional dental radiography or alternate imaging modalities.[19]

Direct Pulp Evaluation

In some instances, during the clinical treatment, a final diagnosis can only be reached by direct visualization of the pulp tissue. The quality (color) and the amount of bleeding from a direct exposure of the pulp tissue must be assessed; profuse or deep purple-colored bleeding or pus exudate indicates irreversible pulpitis. Based on these observations, the treatment plan may be confirmed or changed.

Vital Pulp Therapy for Teeth Diagnosed With Normal Pulp or Reversible Pulpitis *Without Pulp Exposure*

Complete removal of all carious tissue followed by "extension for prevention," to place the margins of the restoration in areas less vulnerable to caries, was considered the gold standard 150 years ago.[23] A paradigm shift in carious lesions treatment has occurred, and in 1997 Fusyama[24] suggested that the superficial layer, grossly denatured *infected* dentin, should be removed, while the underlying layer, partially demineralized caries *affected* dentin (containing intact, undenatured collagen fibrils amenable to remineralization), should be preserved during caries excavation.[25,26] These terms are

now considered outdated—particularly the term *infected*, which conveys the idea that dental caries is an infectious disease that can be cured solely by removing bacteria (as opposed to managing the causative factors: fermentable carbohydrates and the bacterial dental biofilm).[27] Presently, managing a carious lesion includes several options, from the complete surgical excision, where no visible carious tissue is left prior to placement of the restoration, to the opposite extreme, where no caries is removed and noninvasive methods are used to prevent progression of the lesion.[28,29]

In describing the clinical manifestation of caries, a group of cariology experts (International Caries Consensus Collaboration [ICCC]) agreed that it would be ideal to relate the visual, clinical appearance of the lesion directly to what is taking place histopathologically.[30] However, as histologic terms are less helpful when communicating with dentists in the clinical setting, and for practical purposes, when trying to describe which carious tissue should be removed, the ICCC[23] described the different physical properties associated with the different statuses of dentin, as follows:

Soft dentin: This will deform when a hard instrument is pressed onto it and can be easily scooped up (e.g., with a sharp excavator) with little force being required.

Leathery dentin: Although this dentin does not deform when an instrument is pressed on it, it can still be lifted without much force. There might be little difference between *leathery* and *firm* dentin, while *leathery is a transition in the spectrum between soft and firm dentin.*

Firm dentin: This dentin is physically resistant to hand excavation, and some pressure needs to be exerted through an instrument to lift it.

Hard dentin: A pushing force needs to be used with a hard instrument to engage the dentin. Only *a sharp cutting-edge instrument or a bur will lift it. A scratchy sound or "cri dentinaire" can be heard when a straight probe is taken across the dentin.* (For details, see Chapter 23.)

To remove carious tissue in teeth with vital pulps and without signs of irreversible pulp inflammation, several strategies are available, based on the above-mentioned level of hardness of the remaining dentin.[28] The decision among these strategies will be guided by the depth of the lesion and by the dentition (primary or permanent).

Nonselective removal to hard dentin (complete excavation or complete caries removal): This uses the same criteria for carious tissue removal both peripherally and pulpally, and only hard dentin is left. This is considered overtreatment and is no longer advocated (ICCC).

Selective removal to firm dentin: This leaves "leathery" dentin pulpally while the cavity margins are left hard after removal. This is the treatment of choice for both dentitions in shallow or moderately cavitated dentinal lesions (radiographically extending less than the pulpal third or quarter of dentin).

Selective removal to soft dentin: This is recommended in deep cavitated lesions (radiographically extending into the pulpal third or quarter of dentin). Soft carious tissue is left over the pulp to avoid exposure and further injury to the pulp, while peripheral enamel and dentin are prepared to hard dentin, to allow a tight seal and a durable restoration. Selective removal to soft dentin reduces the risk of pulp exposure significantly when compared with nonselective removal to hard or selective removal to firm dentin.

Stepwise removal: This is carious tissue removal in two stages. Soft carious tissue is left over the pulp on the first step and the tooth is sealed with a provisional restoration that should be durable to last up to 12 months to allow changes in the dentin and pulp to take place. In reentering, after removing the restoration, as the dentin is drier and harder, caries removal is continued. There is some evidence that in such deep lesions the second step might be omitted, as it increases the risk of pulp exposure.[31–34]

The second step also adds additional cost, time, and discomfort to the patient; there is also enough evidence that is not considered necessary for primary teeth, and selective removal to soft dentin should be carried out.[32]

Selective Caries Removal to Firm or Leathery Dentin and Protective Liner

The progress of a carious lesion into the dentin begins with acid demineralization produced by bacteria, followed by a more extensive tissue breakdown caused by bacterial enzymatic activity. The demineralized dentin, previously referred to as "affected dentin" and amenable to remineralization, should be left untouched, and the broken-down part, previously known as "infected dentin" should be removed.[26,28,29] Clinically it is difficult to differentiate between the different layers of carious dentin. As a practical approach, the remaining dentin should feel hard when examined with an explorer.

A chemomechanical approach to caries excavation using dyes has been developed. With this method, sound and carious dentin are clinically separated, and only carious dentin can be removed, resulting in a more conservative preparation. When a bur is used, healthy tissue is frequently removed. It has also been reported that this method contributes to patient comfort, as it has been said to be painless, requiring less drilling and local anesthesia. The main drawback of this technique is the time needed to complete the procedure, because it is much more time-consuming than the use of a bur.[35]

Another chemomechanical product has been developed in Brazil under the commercial name of Papacarie (Fórmula & Ação, São Paulo, Brazil). This product is a gel containing papain, an enzyme similar to human pepsine that acts as a debriding agent with no harm to healthy tissue. No statistical difference was observed in a clinical study after 6 to 18 months when papain was used, compared with conventional caries removal in primary teeth.[36]

The American Academy of Pediatric Dentistry (AAPD)[37] recommends the placement of a protective barrier on the floor of the preparation between the restorative material and the pulp-dentin complex. A protective barrier is recommended in deep preparations, and the preferred materials are glass ionomer cements or calcium hydroxide liners. There is sufficient evidence to show that pulp reaction to dental materials is transitory, and overt inflammation occurs only after bacteria or their by-products have reached the pulp.[38–40] When bacteria and bacteria-produced irritants have been removed by caries excavation, and a bacteria-tight restoration has been placed, new bacteria are prevented from reaching the deeper portion of the dentin, and the inflamed pulp will have a great opportunity to heal.

Selective Caries Removal to Soft Dentin—Indirect Pulp Treatment

The main objective of IPT is to maintain the vitality of teeth with reversible pulp injury or teeth with deep caries that might otherwise need endodontic therapy if the decay was completely removed (AAPD).[37] The rationale for this treatment is based on the observation that postmitotic odontoblasts can be induced to upregulate their secretory activities in response to reduced infectious challenge.[41] This results in the deposition of tertiary dentin, which increases the distance between the firm (formerly called "affected") dentin and the pulp, and in the deposition of peritubular (sclerotic) dentin, which results in decreased dentin permeability.

Clinically, IPT is defined as the procedure in which nonmineralizable carious tissue is removed and a thin layer of caries is left at the deepest site of the cavity to prevent pulp exposure.[37,42] It is important to remove the carious tissue completely from the dentinoenamel junction and from the lateral walls of the cavity to achieve optimal interfacial seal between the tooth and the restorative material, thus preventing microleakage. Several clinical studies have demonstrated a high percentage of success utilizing this technique.[2,31,33,43] The indication for Selective Caries Removal to Soft Dentin (IPT) should be limited to teeth without signs of irreversible pulpitis. In this procedure, the deepest layer of the remaining carious dentin should be covered with a liner. The materials used for these procedures are calcium hydroxide liners and glass ionomer liners, with good results in clinical studies.[32–43]

Until recent years, the dentist's dilemma lay in the assessment of how much caries to leave at the pulpal or axial floor. It was generally believed that the carious tissue that could remain at the end of the cavity preparation was the quantity that, if removed, would result in overt exposure.[44,45] In case of doubt, deep carious lesions may be managed by stepwise excavation performed in two visits that may result in fewer pulp exposures compared with direct complete excavation. At 1-year follow-up, there was a statistically significant higher success rate with stepwise excavation than with one-visit treatment.[34,46] At present, there is enough evidence of good clinical and radiographic success without reentering, if the restoration is maintained leakage free.[31,47–49] Both approaches require knowledge of tooth anatomy, clinical experience, and a good understanding of the process of caries progression. If the tooth is too broken down to allow for a proper restoration, placement of a crown should be considered. Fig. 34.1 demonstrates the (Selective Caries Removal to Soft Dentin) IPT technique using a calcium hydroxide liner.

The preferred tool for caries excavation is a large carbide round bur (no. 6 or 8), because the bur allows better control of the "partial removal caries step" than spoon excavators do.[50] Use of a bur also results in a significant reduction in viable counts of both *Streptococcus mutans* and lactobacilli.[51]

Vital Pulp Therapy for Teeth Diagnosed With Normal Pulp or Reversible Pulpitis *With Pulp Exposure*

Direct Pulp Capping

Guidelines published by the AAPD (2016 to 2017)[37] state that direct pulp capping may be performed when a small exposure of the pulp is encountered during cavity preparation in teeth with a normal pulp or reversible pulpitis. Direct capping may also be used after a recent clean fracture due to a traumatic injury. The aim of this treatment is to maintain pulp vitality by forming a calcified barrier to wall off the exposure, keeping in mind that in teeth affected by caries there is an inflammatory response of the pulp to bacteria or bacterial products.[52–55]

When direct pulp capping is indicated, it should be performed immediately after the exposure to prevent contamination of the pulp. Because the extent of the inflammatory process in the pulp cannot be accurately assessed by clinical tests, the diagnosis of reversible (treatable) pulpitis may be sometimes incorrect. In some

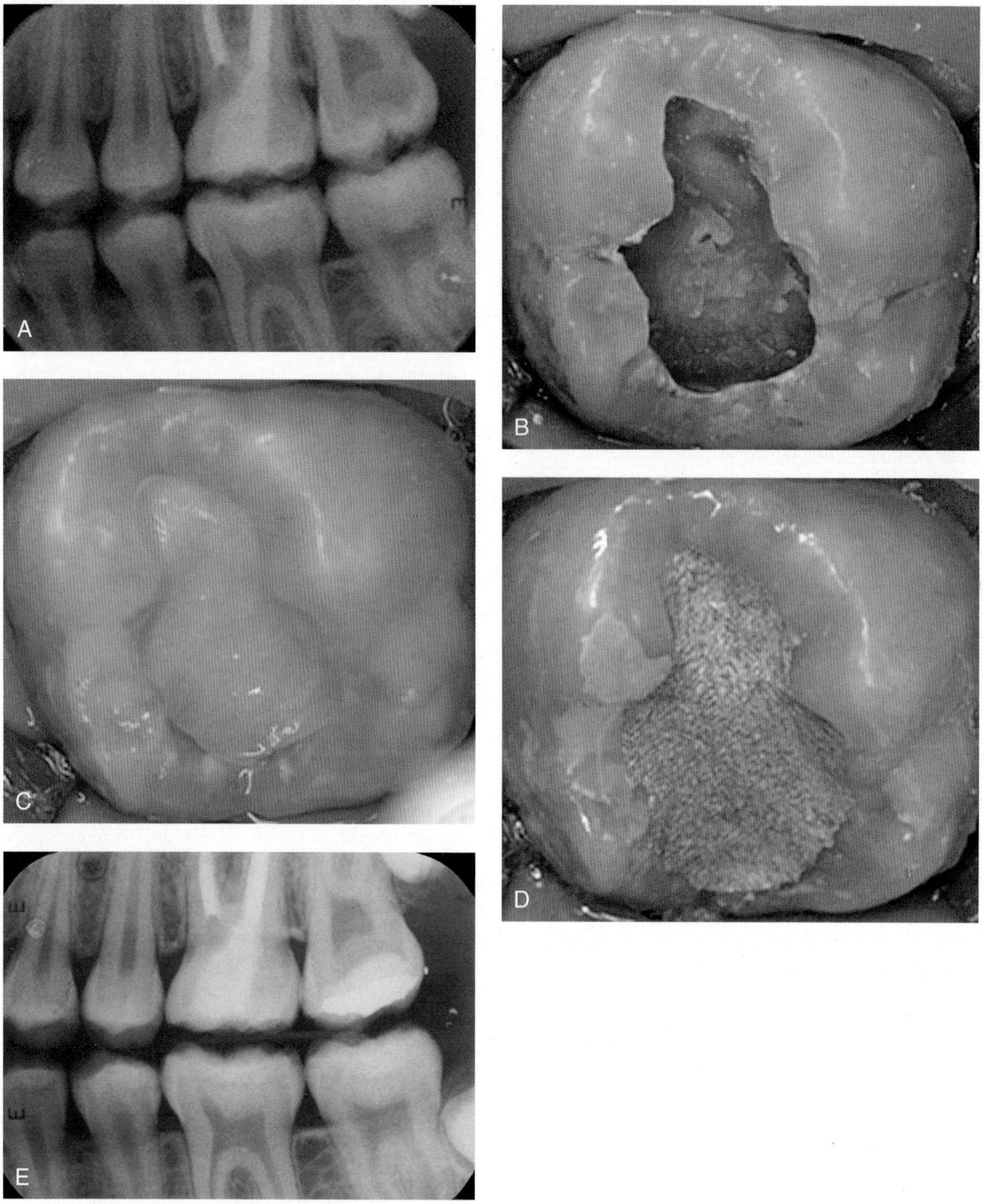

• **Figure 34.1** (A) Maxillary permanent second molar with deep caries almost reaching the pulp. (B) Clinical view of the tooth after incomplete caries removal. (C) The cavity was capped with a calcium hydroxide liner and covered with glass ionomer. (D) The tooth was filled with amalgam. (E) Postoperative radiograph; notice the layers of the different materials used and the remaining affected caries. (Courtesy Dr. A. Kupietsky.)

teeth affected by deep caries, pulp inflammation might have reached the stage of irreversible pulpitis without showing clinical signs.

The characteristics of the pulp-capping material are very important. Ideally it should be biocompatible, nonresorbable, able to establish and maintain a good seal to prevent bacterial contamination, and able to promote pulp repair and dentin bridge formation. Ideally the dentin bridge formed after direct pulp capping should be without tunnel defects that could allow the penetration of bacteria into the pulp at a later stage.[56]

Mineral trioxide aggregate (MTA) and calcium hydroxide are the most frequently recommended capping materials. The mechanism of action of the two materials in vital pulp treatment are similar, as the main soluble component of MTA is calcium hydroxide.[57] Calcium hydroxide dissolves in an aqueous environment into calcium and hydroxyl ions, creating a high pH in the close environment (~12). This alkaline pH is responsible for the antibacterial activity of these materials.[58] The initial effect of calcium hydroxide applied to exposed pulp tissue is the development of a superficial necrosis as a result of the high pH. This necrosis causes low-grade irritation to the tissue and stimulates the pulp to defense and repair. Contrary to calcium hydroxide, MTA causes mild inflammatory and necrotic changes in the subjacent pulp. Thus it is less caustic than the traditional calcium hydroxide preparations.[59] Calcium ions are released from the capping material, forming inorganic precipitations that have been associated with the mechanism controlling cytological and functional changes in the interacting pulpal cells.[60]

The high pH and low solubility of calcium hydroxide prolongs its antibacterial effect. However, being water soluble, it might dissolve under leaky restorations and be washed out, leaving an empty space under the filling material. Hard-setting calcium hydroxide cements can induce dentin bridge formation, but they do not provide an effective long-term seal against bacteria or their by-products.[61,62]

Recent studies suggest that the mechanisms by which calcium hydroxide or MTA stimulate the wound-healing process are related to the solubilizing effect of calcium hydroxide on the dentin matrix component. Growth factors and other bioactive molecules, sequestered within the dentin matrix during dentinogenesis (e.g., TGF-βs), may be released by the action of calcium hydroxide and mediate the changes in cell behavior observed during reparative dentinogenesis.[4,63]

MTA presents some advantages over calcium hydroxide as the material of choice for direct pulp capping. It is a hard-setting, biocompatible material with an antibacterial effect that provides a biologically active substrate for cell attachment. These features make this material effective in preventing microleakage, improving the treatment outcome. As previously mentioned, MTA stimulates reparative dentin formation with negligible pulpal necrosis and minimal inflammatory reaction in the exposed pulp.[59] Tziafas et al. demonstrated that after direct pulp capping with MTA in dogs, the underlying pulp tissue was consistently normal, and only at a later stage was some hemorrhage in the pulp core observed. The beginning of a hard tissue barrier was observed after 2 weeks, and reparative dentinogenesis was disclosed after 3 weeks, associated with a firm fibrodentin matrix.[64] It was also demonstrated that, compared with calcium hydroxide, MTA consistently induces the formation of a dentin bridge at a greater rate with a superior structural integrity. Therefore MTA appears to be more effective than calcium hydroxide for maintaining long-term pulp vitality after direct pulp capping.[59]

However, MTA presents a major drawback by staining tooth material, for both the gray and white versions (Fig. 34.2).[65–68] Hence its use in vital pulp therapy procedures (pulp capping, pulpotomy) is not recommended in teeth where there is an esthetic concern. In these teeth, alternatives to MTA (such as calcium hydroxide) should be considered. New generations of bioceramic materials with similar characteristics of MTA are available in the dental market. Direct pulp capping should always be followed by an immediate and definitive restoration.

A practice-based, randomized clinical trial evaluated and compared the success of direct pulp capping in permanent teeth with MTA or CaOH (calcium hydroxide). Thirty-five practices in the northwest dental practice-based research network were randomized to perform direct pulp caps with either CaOH (16 practices) or MTA (19 practices). A total of 367 individuals received a direct pulp cap with CaOH ($n = 181$) or MTA ($n = 195$). They were followed for up to 2 years at regular recall appointments, or as dictated by tooth symptoms. The primary outcomes were the need for extraction or root canal therapy. Teeth were also evaluated for

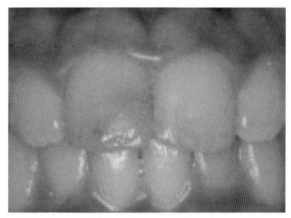

• **Figure 34.2** Right permanent central incisor 1.5 years after partial pulpotomy using white mineral trioxide aggregate. Notice the gray discoloration of the crown. (Courtesy Dr. E. Nuni.)

pulp vitality, and radiographs were taken at the dentist's discretion. The probability of failure at 24 months was 31.5% for CaOH versus 19.7% for MTA (permutation log-rank test, $P = .046$). This large randomized clinical trial provided confirmatory evidence for a superior performance with MTA as a direct pulp-capping agent, as compared with CaOH when evaluated in a practice-based research network for up to 2 years.[69]

Direct Pulp Capping Technique

The tooth should be isolated with a rubber dam and disinfected with sodium hypochlorite (NaOCl). After cavity preparation with high-speed burs under constant water spray and caries removal with slow-speed burs, the cavity should be rinsed with NaOCl (every 3 to 4 minutes), which disinfects the cavity and removes the blood clot, if present, from the pulp exposure site. If the bleeding cannot be stopped within 1 to 10 minutes, it suggests that the pulp inflammation has progressed deeper into the tissue, and the treatment procedure should be modified, for example, by shifting to partial pulpotomy.[70–72]

MTA should be prepared according to the manufacturer's instructions and placed directly over the exposed pulp tissue (1.5 to 2 mm thick). The material should then be covered with a glass ionomer liner followed by a permanent restoration.[73]

The Pulpotomy Procedure

Although use of direct pulp capping and pulpotomy in cariously exposed pulps of mature teeth remains a controversial issue, these procedures are universally accepted in young immature permanent teeth. The pulpotomy procedure involves removing pulp tissue that has inflammatory or degenerative changes, leaving intact the remaining appearing vital noninflamed tissue, which is covered with a pulp-capping agent to promote healing at the amputation site.[71–73]

The only difference between pulpotomy and pulp capping is that in pulpotomy, additional tissue is removed from the exposed pulp. Traditionally, pulpotomy implied the removal of the entire coronal pulp up to the cervical area. Today the depth of tissue removal is based on clinical judgment: only tissue with profuse bleeding, judged to be inflamed or infected, should be removed, because the capping material should be placed on healthy tissue. Although many materials and drugs have been used as capping agents after pulpotomy, MTA seems to be the treatment of choice to stimulate dentin bridge formation in young permanent teeth with exposed pulps.[63] New generation bioceramic materials can also be used.[69]

In esthetic areas, MTA is not recommended because of its discoloration effect. Calcium hydroxide may be used, as its outcomes are similar in some studies.[73,74]

Aguilar and Linsuwanont reported that partial pulpotomy and full (cervical) pulpotomy provide a more predictable outcome than direct pulp capping in teeth with carious exposure.[72]

Partial (Cvek) Pulpotomy Technique

The tooth should be isolated with a rubber dam and disinfected with NaOCl solution. In traumatically exposed pulps, only tissue judged to be inflamed should be removed (~2 mm). Cvek[75] has shown that, in exposures resulting from traumatic injuries, pulpal changes are characterized by a proliferative response, with inflammation extending only a few millimeters into the pulp. Care should be taken to remove all the tissue coronal to the amputation site to prevent continuation of bleeding, contamination, and discoloration of the tooth. In teeth with carious exposure, it might be necessary to remove tissue to a greater depth in order to reach noninflamed pulp. Cutting of the tissue with an abrasive high-speed diamond bur with water cooling has been shown to be the least damaging to the underlying tissue.[76] After pulp amputation, the preparation is thoroughly washed with NaOCl to disinfect and control hemorrhage. If hemorrhage persists, amputation should be performed at a more apical level.[72] Once hemorrhage has been controlled and the blood clot removed, a dressing of MTA (or calcium hydroxide in an esthetic area) is gently placed over the amputation site. Care should be taken not to push the material into the pulp.[77]

The MTA should be covered with a glass ionomer liner, and a permanent restoration should be placed (Fig. 34.3). If the pulpotomy is successful, a tertiary dentin bridge will be formed; occasionally, obliteration of the pulp may occur.

Cervical Pulpotomy

Pulpotomy in mature teeth is performed only when irreversible pulpitis is diagnosed, and it should be considered an emergency treatment. In these teeth, root canal treatment will follow at the next appointment. In immature permanent teeth, cervical pulpotomy is performed to allow maturation of the root. This procedure is performed in teeth in which it is assumed that healthy pulp tissue, with a potential to produce a dentin bridge and complete the formation of the root, still remains in the root canal. The technique for cervical pulpotomy in immature permanent teeth is similar to that for primary teeth, and the dressing material should maintain pulp vitality and function. Care should be taken to remove the blood clot before placing the dressing material over

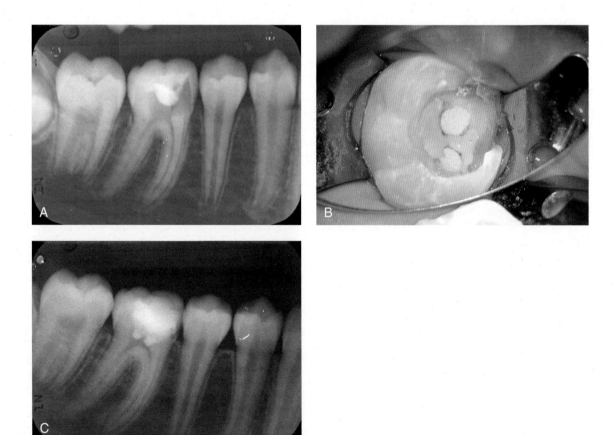

• **Figure 34.3** Partial pulpotomy technique: (A) Mandibular first permanent molar with a broken temporary filling and extensive caries. (B) Clinical view of the tooth showing two amputation sites covered with white mineral trioxide aggregate. (C) The same tooth after 2 months. No symptoms are present, and no pathologic process is evident in the radiograph. It is recommended that the composite temporary filling be replaced by a more definitive restoration (crown), to prevent failure of the treatment due to microleakage. (Courtesy Dr. E. Nuni.)

the pulp stumps, as its presence may compromise the treatment outcome. It has been demonstrated that leaving the blood clot may result in the formation of dystrophic calcifications and internal resorption. A blood clot may also interfere with dentin bridge formation and serve as a substrate for bacteria in leaky restorations.[78] Cervical pulpotomy is frequently performed in teeth in which the histopathologic status of the pulp stumps is not clear. If the symptoms continue and pulpectomy is needed, the MTA may be removed using an ultrasonic instrument and an operative microscope.

There is a controversy as to the indications for performing root canal treatment after root maturation, before obliteration of the root canal space occurs that will prevent performing root canal treatment in the future. Prophylactic endodontic treatment is not recommended because of the low percentage of pulp necrosis.[79,80]

Root canal treatment can be considered in posterior teeth, where apicectomy is difficult to perform in cases of treatment failure, especially in children.[18]

Clinical and radiographic follow-up of these teeth is essential to ensure that pulpal or periapical pathosis is not developing. The roots should show continued normal development and maturogenesis. It is of the utmost importance to perform a permanent restoration as soon as possible to prevent bacterial leakage and ensure the success of the treatment.[81]

Apexogenesis

Apexogenesis is indicated in immature teeth when only part of the pulp tissue inside the root canal remains vital and apparently healthy. This procedure allows continued physiologic development and formation of the root apex apically to the dressing material.[37] The root formed may be irregular but nevertheless provides additional support for the tooth. Apexogenesis can be regarded as a very deep pulpotomy. MTA, another type of bioceramic material, or calcium hydroxide is placed over the vital pulp stump after hemostasis control with NaOCl but before the formation of a blood clot (Fig. 34.4). The use of the operative microscope is recommended in order to execute this meticulous procedure correctly.

It is difficult to determine the status of the pulp deep in the root canal or to predict the formation of a calcified barrier and continued root development. Radiographic and clinical follow-up is mandatory, and if signs and symptoms of pathology appear, apexification or pulp regenerative procedure should follow. The use of MTA (bioceramics) as a dressing material should be carefully considered because of the difficulty in removing the material from deep inside the root canal.

Nonvital Pulp Treatment for *Immature* Teeth

Apexification

Apexification is a method of treatment for immature permanent teeth in which root growth and development ceased due to pulp necrosis. Its purpose is to induce root end closure with no canal wall thickening or continuous root lengthening. It can be achieved in two ways: (1) as a long-term procedure using calcium hydroxide dressing to allow the formation of a biologic hard tissue barrier, or (2) as a short-term (more recent) procedure, creating an artificial apical plug of MTA or other bioceramic material. Apexification is most often performed in incisors that lost vitality because of traumatic injury, after carious exposures, and in teeth with anatomic variations such as dens invaginatus with an immature root.

The apex in immature teeth may present two morphologic variations: divergent with flaring apical foramen (blunderbuss apex) or parallel to convergent. This morphology is difficult to determine because of the two-dimensional image obtained by dental radiographs. In both forms, conventional endodontic treatment cannot be performed, because it is difficult if not impossible to achieve an apical seal that will prevent extrusion of the filling material. When apexification is carried out successfully in teeth with radiographic signs of rarefying osteitis, healing of the bone will be observed gradually. The tooth should continue to erupt, and the alveolar bone should continue to grow in conjunction with the adjacent teeth. Follow-up should be performed to ensure the absence of adverse posttreatment clinical and radiographic signs.

For more than a decade, an alternative treatment to apexification has been available in the form of pulp regenerative therapy, even in cases of infected necrotic immature teeth. This will be discussed shortly.

Long-Term Apexification With Calcium Hydroxide

This mode of treatment requires compliance of both the patient and the parent because of its long duration. Calcium hydroxide apexification is a predictable procedure, and an apical barrier will

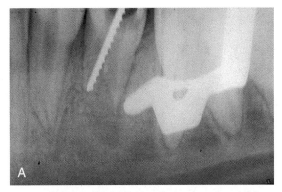
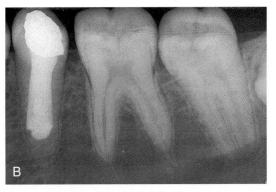

• **Figure 34.4** (A) Mandibular premolar with incomplete root development due to partial pulp necrosis. Apexogenesis with calcium hydroxide was instituted. (B) Two years later, apical closure was evident in the radiograph. Root canal treatment was completed using gutta-percha with a root canal sealant. (Courtesy Dr. E. Galon.)

be formed in 74% to 100% of cases.[82] The most common complication is cervical root fracture due to the thin walls of the cervical part of the tooth, which may fracture easily.[3]

It has been reported that calcium hydroxide significantly increases the risk of root fracture after long-term application (more than 1 month) as a result of structural changes in the dentin. Therefore, to reduce this risk in immature teeth, it is advisable to minimize the time needed for apical barrier formation.[83,84]

Apexification is traditionally performed using a calcium hydroxide dressing that disinfects the root canal and induces apical closure. The high pH and low solubility of calcium hydroxide keeps its antimicrobial effect for a long period of time.[85–87]

Calcium hydroxide assists in the debridement of the root canal, because it increases the dissolution of necrotic tissue when used alone or in combination with NaOCl.[88]

The mechanism of action of calcium hydroxide in induction of an apical barrier is still controversial, although it is formed by cells originating from the adjacent connective tissue. The calcified barrier, even when appearing radiographically and clinically complete, is histologically porous and may be composed of cementum, dentin, bone, or osteodentin.[89]

This procedure requires multiple visits and could take a year or more to achieve a complete apical barrier that would allow root canal filling using gutta-percha (GP) and sealer.[90]

It is unclear whether the stage of root development at the beginning of the treatment or the presence of a pretreatment infection affects the time required for barrier formation.[89]

Calcium Hydroxide Apexification Technique

After isolation with rubber dam, coronal access preparation should be wide enough to include the pulp horns to prevent future contamination and discoloration. Gates-Glidden drills can be used in anterior teeth to remove the lingual eminence in the cervical portion of the root canal, facilitating cleaning of all aspects of the canal. The length of the root canal should be determined radiographically with a large GP point, because an electronic apex locator is not reliable in teeth with open apices. Inserting a large paper point to the point of bleeding may also assist in length determination. The working length should be approximately 1 mm short of the radiographic root end. Debridement of the root canal is mainly achieved by irrigations with NaOCl solution. The irrigation should be done without pressure, verifying that the needle is loose inside the root canal and short of the working length. Minimal or no instrumentation is advised to prevent damage to the thin dentin walls. In order to facilitate disinfection and debris removal from these wide canals, passive ultrasonic irrigation with NaOCl solution is recommended.[91]

A calcium hydroxide dressing in a creamy consistency can then be applied with a Lentulo spiral mounted in a low-speed engine, with specially designed syringes, or with files.

The second visit is scheduled from 2 weeks to 1 month later. The goal in the second visit is to complete the debridement and remove the tissue remnants denatured by the calcium hydroxide dressing that could not be removed mechanically in the first appointment. In addition, the canal should be further disinfected. After disinfection, a thick paste of calcium hydroxide is packed in the root canal to a level apical to the cemento-enamel junction (CEJ) using endodontic pluggers; this will reduce dentin weakening in this fracture-sensitive area.[92] The coronal access should be restored with a filling that will provide a long-term coronal seal.

The tooth should be monitored clinically and radiographically at 3-month intervals to examine the formation of an apical hard

tissue barrier and to confirm the absence of pathology such as root resorption and apical periodontitis. If a calcified barrier is not evident and the calcium hydroxide has been washed out, it should usually be replaced. When a calcified barrier can be seen on the radiograph, the tooth is reopened and the calcium hydroxide is removed by copious irrigations. The apical area should be gently examined using a GP point and/or through the operative microscope to determine the completeness of the apical barrier. If the barrier is incomplete and the patient feels the touch of the GP point, the apexification procedure is reestablished until a complete barrier is formed. The frequency in which the calcium hydroxide dressing should be replaced is controversial. Some authors support a single application of the material and claim that it is only required to initiate the healing reaction, while others propose to replace the calcium hydroxide only when symptoms develop or if the material appears to have been washed out of the canal when viewed radiographically.[89]

When a completed apical barrier can be traced, the canal is obturated with a permanent root canal filling material (e.g., thermoplasticized GP) and sealer.

Fig. 34.5 shows an immature maxillary central incisor with a necrotic pulp and acute apical abscess treated with calcium hydroxide apexification. The bony lesion healed, and the endodontic treatment was properly completed.

When a calcified barrier is formed coronal to the apex, it should not be perforated in order to fill the tooth to the apical end; the tissue forming the apical barrier should be regarded as healthy tissue, and root canal filling should be placed up to this point.

As noted earlier, immature teeth with thin dentin walls, especially after calcium hydroxide apexification, are at high risk of fracture. The stage of root development seems to be a key factor.[3,84] In order to reduce this risk, a short-term calcium hydroxide dressing and a permanent restoration with an intracanal placement of bonded composite resin is recommended.[93]

Short-Term Apexification With Mineral Trioxide Aggregate (One-Visit Apexification)

For more than a decade, MTA has been commonly used as an artificial apical barrier in a short-term apexification. MTA reduces the time needed for completion of the root canal treatment and for restoration of the tooth. The apical barrier is achieved in one visit, and the whole treatment is completed in just a few visits.[94]

MTA characteristics such as low solubility, excellent sealability, biocompatibility, release of calcium hydroxide, high pH, and radiopacity are responsible for its preferable clinical results and popularity as an apical plug material.[95] Other bioceramic materials with similar characteristic can also be utilized, like Biodentine (Septodont, Saint-Maur-des-Fosses, France), NuSmile NeoMTA (NuSmile, Houston, TX), MTA Angelus (Angelus, Londrina, PR, Brazil), EndoSequence root repair material (Brasseler Savannah, GA), or iRoot BP Plus (Innovative Bioceramix Inc., Vancouver, Canada).[69]

Disinfection of the root canal is done in the first visit as in the long-term apexification procedure. At the second visit, MTA can be placed in the apical portion of the immature root and will act as an apical plug after setting. It is very difficult to remove the MTA from within the canal after it sets; if retreatment is necessary, it can be done by apical surgery. Therefore complete debridement and disinfection of the root canal and of the dentin walls are mandatory. This technique has a number of advantages: (1) patient compliance is less crucial, (2) cost and clinical time are reduced,

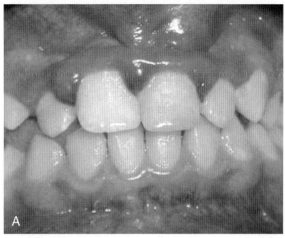

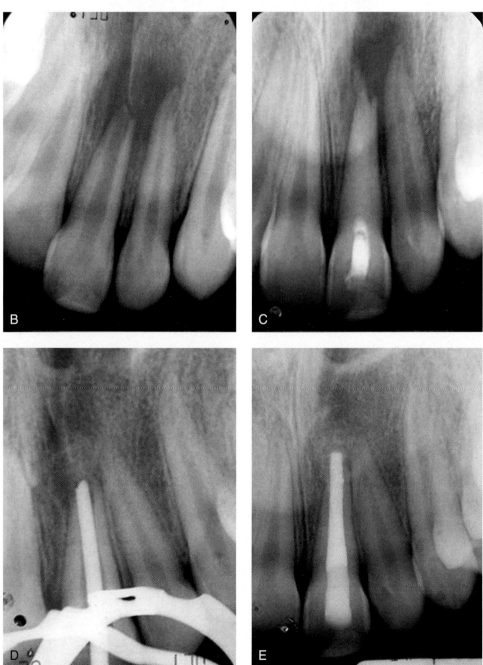

• **Figure 34.5** (A) Clinical photograph of a traumatized left central incisor with an acute apical abscess (notice the vestibular swelling). (B) Radiograph of the same tooth showing an incompletely formed root, an open apex, and periapical bone destruction. (C) Radiograph of the tooth filled with a calcium hydroxide paste to achieve apexification. (D) Radiograph showing the completeness of the apical barrier checked with a gutta-percha point. (E) The tooth after root canal filling with gutta-percha and sealer. (Courtesy Dr. Z. Elazary.)

(3) the dentin will not lose its physical properties, and (4) it allows for earlier restoration with bonded composite resin within the root canal, thus minimizing the likelihood of root fracture.

Mineral Trioxide Aggregate Apexification Technique

Disinfection of the root canal is achieved as described in the first visit of the long-term apexification. Calcium hydroxide dressing is also indicated in order to raise the low pH of the inflamed periapical tissue before the MTA placement. Lee et al. have demonstrated that an acidic environment has an adverse effect on the setting and micro hardness of MTA.[18,96]

In the second visit, after rubber dam placement, the canal is irrigated and dried. After mixing according to the manufacturer's instructions, a plug of MTA is compacted into the apical 4 to 5 mm of the canal, about 1 mm short of the radiographic apex (Fig. 34.6). Placement of MTA in the apical part is more complicated than the use of calcium hydroxide. The material is introduced into the apical area using special carriers or endodontic pluggers and compacted using hand condensation with indirect ultrasonic activation.[97]

Placement of a resorbable material at the root end (e.g., calcium sulfate; CollaCote, Zimer Dental, Carlsbad, CA) against which the MTA can be compacted, keeping it within the confines of the canal space, has been suggested but does not seem necessary.[98,99]

Proper placement of the material is verified by a radiograph (see Fig. 34.6A). A wet cotton pellet or paper point is placed over the MTA, providing moisture for its setting, and the tooth is sealed with a temporary filling.

After a few days the tooth is reentered and the hardness of the MTA is examined with an endodontic instrument. In cases where the MTA is not set, its placement should be repeated the same way described. After setting, the root canal filling can be completed using thermoplasticized GP and sealer. The tooth is then permanently restored with a bonded composite resin extending into the canal space in an attempt to strengthen the root.[93] In short roots, the composite resin can be placed in direct contact with the MTA plug (see Fig. 34.6).[18]

Using new generation bioceramic materials (e.g., Biodentine Allington Maidstone, Kent, UK) can shorten the treatment period even further. The short setting time of this material (~10 minutes) will allow the placement of a permanent root filling and tooth restoration at the same visit of the apical plug placement.[18]

Revascularization and Regeneration

This approach, introduced more than a decade ago, for treatment of immature necrotic and infected permanent teeth is based on the observation of spontaneous revascularization that occasionally

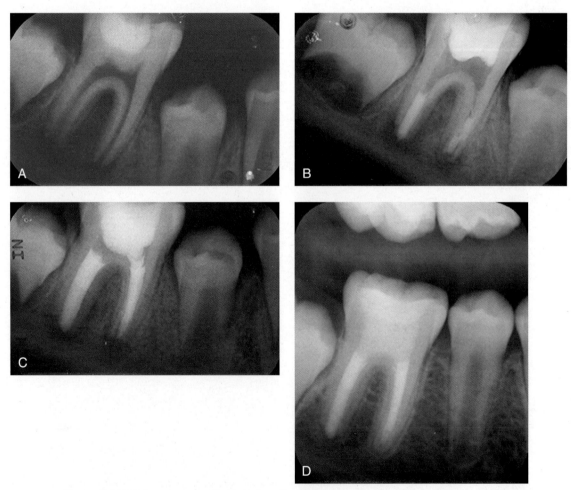

• **Figure 34.6** (A) Immature mandibular molar with periapical pathologic radiolucent areas. (B) Apical plugs with mineral trioxide aggregate (MTA). (C) Warm gutta-percha filling over the hardened MTA plugs. (D) Successful follow-up after 15 months showing healing of the periapical lesions. (Courtesy Dr. E. Nuni.)

occurs in immature teeth after traumatic injury.[100–103] When this treatment is successful, root lengthening and apical closure with thickening of the canal walls (maturogenesis) are expected, thus improving the long-term prognosis of the young tooth. A few factors are necessary for a successful endodontic regeneration. These factors include absence of infection within the root canal space, a physical scaffold, stem cells, signaling molecules, and an effective coronal seal.[104,105]

The nature of the hard and soft tissue formed as a result of revascularization is not clear. Radiographic evidence of changes in root length and wall thickness does not necessarily indicate a regeneration of functional pulp tissue and the formation of new dentin and cementum. Histologic studies in dogs and humans suggest that in some cases these radiographic changes may be a result of deposition of cementum-like and bone-like tissues, meaning an ingrowth of PDL tissue instead of pulp tissue.[18,105–109]

Technique

The first step of the treatment is disinfection of the root canal space using irrigation solutions (like NaOCl) and an intracanal dressing (with a mix of antibiotics in a paste or calcium hydroxide).

After disinfection, bleeding is introduced into the canal space through the apical foramen to create a scaffold on which a new tissue will grow and repopulate the canal space. Alternatives such as platelet-rich plasma (PRP), platelet-rich fibrin (PRF), or autologous fibrin matrix (AFM) can also be used. Application of MTA or bioceramics and a good coronal seal is the last step of the treatment (see Chapter 35).[110]

Advances in the field of material sciences, stem cell biology, and dental tissue engineering have raised the possibility of using biology-based treatment strategies to regenerate functional dental tissues. In the short-term future, regeneration of an individual tooth structure is a more realistic approach than a regeneration of an entire tooth.[111]

Nonvital Pulp Treatment for *Young Mature* Teeth

Root Canal Treatment in Young Mature Permanent Teeth

Special Considerations

Root canal treatment in mature teeth of children and adolescents is basically similar to that performed in adults. However, because of their wider canals and thinner dentin walls in comparison with those of adult patients, special precautions are needed, described as follows.

Access

The coronal access should be wide enough to include the pulp horns to prevent future contamination and discoloration. During opening of the access cavity, care should be taken to remove only a minimal amount of dentin in the canal orifices. Removing too much dentin will weaken anterior teeth and may cause perforation in molars.

Instrumentation

The length of the root canal should be determined carefully using radiographs; an electronic apex locator or paper points can also be used. Though the root canals are larger, they may be curved, so instrumentation should be done with precurved instruments in anticurvature filing motions. The use of nickel titanium (NiTi) rotatory instruments will ease the preparation of the root canal.

Irrigation

Irrigation during root canal treatment should be done only after making sure that the rubber dam is placed properly and that leakage of fluids into the mouth cannot occur accidentally. The needle of the irrigation syringe is placed loosely in the root canal to avoid pushing the irrigation solution beyond the apex. NaOCl is used in various concentrations (0.5% to 5.25%) as the preferred irrigation solution.[112]

Intracanal Dressing

In teeth with infected root canals, the emphasis is on disinfection and removal of tissue remnants. Because effective mechanical preparation of wide canal walls is difficult, it is recommended that treatment be done in two sessions, with placement of an antiseptic dressing between visits. Calcium hydroxide paste is the preferred dressing material because it dissolves tissue remnants.[88]

The placement of the dressing material can be accomplished using a Lentulo spiral shorter than the length of the root canal, specially designed syringes, or files.

The Isthmus

The isthmus is a thin communication between two or more root canals in the same root that contains pulp tissue. Any root containing two canals or more has a high incidence of isthmi.[113]

An isthmus is formed when a root projection cannot close itself, and it will be larger in children where root formation is not fully complete. These web-like connections between root canals are part of the root canal system. They can function as a reservoir for bacteria and therefore should be cleaned and obturated during root canal treatment.[113]

Obturation

The apical foramen in young teeth is large, and adaptation of a master cone should be done carefully to avoid extrusion of filling materials that can easily occur during obturation. Lateral condensation requires more accessory GP points; initial points should be placed such that they will not block access to the canal. Filling with warm GP or using warm condensation techniques should be done cautiously to avoid overfilling.

In some cases fabrication of a customized master cone is favorable. A GP point is fitted several millimeters short of the apex; the apical 2 to 3 mm are softened (with a solvent or a heat source) and tamped gradually into place. The completed customized cone represents an impression of the apical portion of the canal preventing extrusion of filling material during obturation.[18]

References

1. Mjor AI, Heyeraas KJ. Pulp-dentin and periodontal anatomy and physiology. In: Orstavik D, Pitt Ford TR, eds. *Essential Endodontology.* London: Blackwell; 1998.
2. Smith AJ. Dentin formation and repair. In: Hargreaves KM, Goodis HE, eds. *Seltzer and Bender's Dental Pulp II.* Carol Stream, IL: Quintessence; 2002.
3. Cvek M. Prognosis of luxated non-vital maxillary incisors treated with calcium hydroxide and filled with gutta-percha. A retrospective clinical study. *Endod Dent Traumatol.* 1992;8:45–55.

4. Graham L, Cooper PR, Cassidy N, et al. The effect of calcium hydroxide on solubilisation of bio-active dentine matrix components. *Biomaterials*. 2006;27(14):2865–2873.

5. Massagué J. The transforming growth factor-beta family. *Annu Rev Cell Biol*. 1990;6:597–641.

6. Kuttler Y. Classification of dentin into primary, secondary and tertiary. *Oral Surg*. 1959;12:996–999.

7. Howard C, Murray PE, Namerow KN. Dental pulp stem cell migration. *J Endod*. 2010;36:1963–1966.

8. Cox CF, White KC, Ramus DL, et al. Reparative dentin: factors affecting its deposition. *Quintessence Int*. 1992;23:257–270.

9. Lee SJ, Walton RE, Osborne JW. Pulp response to bases and cavity depths. *Am J Dent*. 1992;5:64–68.

10. Murray PE, About I, Lumley PJ, et al. Postoperative pulpal and repair responses. *J Am Dent Assoc*. 2000;131:321–329.

11. Murray PE, About I, Lumley PJ, et al. Cavity remaining dentin thickness and pulpal activity. *Am J Dent*. 2002;15:41–46.

12. Belanger GK. Pulp therapy for young permanent teeth. In: Pinkham JR, ed. *Pediatric Dentistry: Infancy Through Adolescence*. Philadelphia: Saunders; 1999.

13. Fuks AB, Heling I, Nuni E. Pulp therapy for the young permanent dentition. In: Casamassimo P, Fields H, McTigue D, et al, eds. *Pediatric Dentistry: Infancy Through Adolescence*. 5th ed. Elsevier Saunders; 2013:490–502.

14. Fuss Z, Trowbridge H, Bender IB, et al. Assessment of reliability of electrical and thermal pulp testing agents. *J Endod*. 1986;12:301–305.

15. Fulling HJ, Andreasen JO. Influence of maturation status and tooth type of permanent teeth upon electrometric and thermal pulp testing. *Scand J Dent Res*. 1976;84(5):286–290.

16. Johnsen DC, Harshbarger J, Rymer HD. Quantitative assessment of neural development in human premolars. *Anat Rec*. 1983;205:421–429.

17. Perez R, Berkowitz R, McIlveen L, et al. Dental trauma in children: a survey. *Endod Dent Traumatol*. 1991;7(5):212–213.

18. Nuni E. Pulp therapy for the young permanent dentition. In: Fuks AB, Peretz B, eds. *Pediatric Endodontics*. Switzerland: Springer International Publishing AG; 2016:117–148.

19. Special Committee to Revise the Joint AAE/AAOMR Position Statement on use of CBCT in Endodontics. AAE and AAOMR Joint position statement: use of cone beam computed tomography in endondontics; 2015/2016 update. http://www.aae.org/uploadedfiles/clinical_resources/guidelines_and_position_statements/conebeamstatement.pdf. Accessed August 17, 2017.

20. Slutzky-Goldberg I, Tsesis I, Slutzky H, et al. Odontogenic sinus tracts: a cohort study. *Quintessence Int*. 2009;40:13–18.

21. Kadom N, Egloff A, Obeid G, et al. Juvenile mandibular chronic osteomyelitis: multimodality imaging findings. *Oral Surg Oral Med Oral Pathol Oral Radiol Endod*. 2011;111:38–43.

22. Berman LH, Hartwell GR. Diagnosis. In: Cohen S, Hargreaves KM, eds. *Pathways of the Pulp*. St Louis: Mosby; 2006.

23. Innes NPT, Frencken JE, Bjorndal L, et al. Managing carious lesions: consensus recommendations on terminology. *Adv Dent Res*. 2016;28(2):49–57.

24. Fusyama T. The process and results of revolution in dental caries treatment. *Int Dent J*. 1997;47(3):157–166.

25. Yoshiyama M, Tay FR, Doi J, et al. Bonding of self-etch and total etch adhesives to carious dentin. *J Dent Res*. 2002;81:556–560.

26. Ten Cate JM. Remineralization of caries lesions extending into dentin. *J Dent Res*. 2001;80(5):1407–1411.

27. Schwendicke F, Dörfer CE, Paris S. Incomplete caries removal: a systematic review and meta-analysis. *J Dent Res*. 2013;92:306–314.

28. Ricketts D, Lamont T, Innes NPT, et al. Operative caries management in adults and children. *Cochrane Database Syst Rev*. 2013;(3):CD003808.

29. Green D, Mackenzie L, Banerjee A. Minimally invasive long term management of direct restorations; the '5rs.' *Dent Update*. 2015;42(5):413–426.

30. Ogawa K, Yamashita Y, Ichijo T, et al. The ultrastructure and hardness of the transparent human carious dentin. *J Dent Res*. 1983;62(1):7–10.

31. Maltz M, Garcia R, Jardim JJ, et al. Randomized trial of partial *vs.* stepwise caries removal. *J Dent Res*. 2012;91:1026–1031.

32. Schwendicke F, Frencken JE, Bjorndal L, et al. Managing carious lesions: consensus recommendations on carious tissue removal. *Adv Dent Res*. 2016;28(2):58–67.

33. Corralo D, Maltz M. Clinical and ultrastructural effects of different liners/restorative materials on deep carious dentin: a randomized clinical trial. *Caries Res*. 2013;47:243–250.

34. Orhan AI, Oz FT, Orhan K. Pulp exposure occurrence and outcomes after 1- or 2-visit indirect pulp therapy vs complete caries removal in primary and permanent molars. *Pediatr Dent*. 2010;32:347–355.

35. Ericson D, Zimmerman M, Raber H, et al. Clinical evaluation of efficacy and safety of a new method for chemo-mechanical removal of caries: a multi-centre study. *Caries Res*. 1999;33:171–177.

36. Motta LJ, Bussadori SK, Campanelli AP, et al. Randomized controlled clinical trial of long-term chemo-mechanical caries removal using Papacarie gel. *J Appl Oral Sci*. 2014;22:307–313.

37. American Academy of Pediatric Dentistry. Pulp therapy for primary and immature permanent teeth. *Pediatr Dent*. 2017;39:325–333.

38. Brannstrom M. Communication between the oral cavity and the dental pulp associated with restorative treatment. *Oper Dent*. 1984;9:57–68.

39. Browne RM, Tobias RS, Crombie IK, et al. Bacterial microleakage and pulpal inflammation in experimental cavities. *Int Endod J*. 1983;16:147–155.

40. Cox CF, Keall CL, Keall HJ, et al. Biocompatibility of surface-sealed dental materials against exposed pulps. *J Prosthet Dent*. 1987;57:1–8.

41. Tziafas D, Kodonas K. Differentiation potential of dental papilla, dental pulp, and apical papilla progenitor cells. *J Endod*. 2010;36:781–789.

42. McDonald RE, Avery DR. Treatment of deep caries, vital pulp exposure, and pulpless teeth. In: McDonald RE, Avery DR, eds. *Dentistry for the Child and Adolescent*. Philadelphia: Saunders; 1994.

43. Straffon LH, Corpron RL, Bruner FW, et al. Twenty-four-month clinical trial of visible-light-activated cavity liner in young permanent teeth. *ASDC J Dent Child*. 1991;58:124–128.

44. Levin LG, Law AS, Holland GR, et al. Identify and define all diagnostic terms for pulpal health and disease states. *J Endod*. 2009;35:1645–1647.

45. Massler M, Pawlak J. The affected and infected pulp. *Oral Surg Oral Med Oral Pathol*. 1977;43:929–947.

46. Bjørndal L, Reit C, Bruun G, et al. Treatment of deep caries lesions in adults: randomized clinical trials comparing stepwise vs. direct complete excavation, and direct pulp capping vs. partial pulpotomy. *Eur J Oral Sci*. 2010;118:290–297.

47. Bjørndal L, Larsen T, Thylstrup A. A clinical and microbiological study of deep carious lesions during stepwise excavation using long treatment intervals. *Caries Res*. 1997;31:411–417.

48. Bjørndal L, Thylstrup A. A practice-based study on stepwise excavation of deep carious lesions in permanent teeth: a 1-year follow-up study. *Community Dent Oral Epidemiol*. 1998;26:122–128.

49. Mertz-Fairhurst EJ, Adair SM, Sams DR, et al. Cariostatic and ultraconservative sealed restorations: nine-year results among children and adults. *ASDC J Dent Child*. 1995;62:97–107.

50. Falster CA, Araujo FB, Straffon LH, et al. Indirect pulp treatment: in vivo outcomes of an adhesive resin system vs calcium hydroxide for protection of the dentin-pulp complex. *Pediatr Dent*. 2002;24:241–248.

51. Orhan AI, Oz FT, Ozcelik B, et al. A clinical and microbiological comparative study of deep carious lesion treatment in deciduous and young permanent molars. *Clin Oral Investig*. 2008;12:369–378.

52. Bergenholtz G. Effect of bacterial products on inflammatory reactions in the dental pulp. *Scand J Dent Res*. 1977;85:122–129.

53. Bergenholtz G. Inflammatory response of the dental pulp to bacterial irritation. *J Endod.* 1981;7:100–104.
54. Bergenholtz G, Cox CF, Loesche WJ, et al. Bacterial leakage around dental restorations: its effect on the dental pulp. *J Oral Pathol.* 1982;11:439–450.
55. Warfvinge J, Dahlen G, Bergenholtz G. Dental pulp response to bacterial cell wall material. *J Dent Res.* 1985;64:1046–1050.
56. Kitasako Y, Murray PE, Tagami J, et al. Histomorphometric analysis of dentinal bridge formation and pulpal inflammation. *Quintessence Int.* 2002;33:600–608.
57. Parirokh M, Torabinejad M. Mineral trioxide aggregate: a comprehensive literature review—Part I: chemical, physical, and antibacterial properties. *J Endod.* 2010;36(1):16–27.
58. Tronstad L, Andreasen JO, Hasselgren G, et al. pH changes in dental tissues after root canal filling with calcium hydroxide. *J Endod.* 1981;7(1):17–21.
59. Witherspoon DE. Vital pulp therapy with new materials: new directions and treatment perspectives-permanent teeth. *Pediatr Dent.* 2008;30(3):220–224.
60. Schröder U. Effects of calcium hydroxide-containing pulp-capping agents on pulp cell migration, proliferation, and differentiation. *J Dent Res.* 1985;64:541–548.
61. Tziafas D. Basic mechanisms of cytodifferentiation and dentinogenesis during dental pulp repair. *Int J Dev Biol.* 1995;39:281–290.
62. Fuks AB, Heling I, Nuni E. Pulp therapy for the young permanent dentition. In: Casamassimo PS, Fields HW, McTigue DJ, et al, eds. *Pediatric Dentistry: Infancy Through Adolescence.* 5th ed. Philadelphia: Saunders; 2013:490–502.
63. Tziafas D, Smith AJ, Lesot H. Designing new treatment strategies in vital pulp therapy. *J Dent.* 2000;28(2):77–92.
64. Tziafas D, Pantelidou O, Alvanou A, et al. The dentinogenic effect of mineral trioxide aggregate (MTA) in short-term capping experiments. *Int Endod J.* 2002;35(3):245–254.
65. Boutsioukis C, Noula G, Lambrianidis T. Ex vivo study of the efficiency of two techniques for the removal of mineral trioxide aggregate used as a root canal filling material. *J Endod.* 2008;34(10):1239–1242.
66. Belobrov I, Parashos P. Treatment of tooth discoloration after the use of white mineral trioxide aggregate. *J Endod.* 2011;37(7):1017–1020.
67. Bogen G, Kim JS, Bakland LK. Direct pulp capping with mineral trioxide aggregate: an observational study. *J Am Dent Assoc.* 2008;139:305–315.
68. Hilton TJ, Ferracane JL, Mancl L, et al. Comparison of CaOH with MTA for direct pulp capping: a PBRN randomized clinical trial. *J Dent Res.* 2013;92(suppl 7):16S–22S.
69. Wang Z. Bioceramic materials in Endodontics. *Endod Topics.* 2015;32(1):3–30.
70. Camp JH, Fuks AB. Pediatric endodontics: endodontic treatment for the primary and young permanent dentition. In: Cohen S, Hargreaves KM, eds. *Pathways of the Pulp.* St Louis: Mosby; 2006.
71. Fuks AB. Pulp therapy for the primary and young permanent dentitions. *Dent Clin North Am.* 2000;44:571–596.
72. Aguilar P, Linsuwanont P. Vital pulp therapy in vital permanent teeth with cariously exposed pulp: a systematic review. *J Endod.* 2011;37(5):581–587.
73. Mente J, Geletneky B, Ohle M, et al. Mineral trioxide aggregate or calcium hydroxide direct pulp capping: an analysis of the clinical treatment outcome. *J Endod.* 2010;36:806–813.
74. Qudeimat MA, Barrieshi-Nusair KM, Owais AI. Calcium hydroxide vs mineral trioxide aggregates for partial pulpotomy of permanent molars with deep caries. *Eur Arch Paediatr Dent.* 2007;8(2):99–104.
75. Cvek M. A clinical report on partial pulpotomy and capping with calcium hydroxide in permanent incisors with complicated crown fracture. *J Endod.* 1978;4:232–237.
76. Granath LE, Hagman G. Experimental pulpotomy in human bicuspids with reference to cutting technique. *Acta Odontol Scand.* 1971;29:155–163.
77. Tziafas D, Molyvdas I. The tissue reactions after capping of dog teeth with calcium hydroxide experimentally crammed into the pulp space. *Oral Surg Oral Med Oral Pathol.* 1988;65(5):604–608.
78. Schröder U. Effect of an extra-pulpal blood clot on healing following experimental pulpotomy and capping with calcium hydroxide. *Odontol Revy.* 1973;24:257–268.
79. Oginni AO, Adekoya-Sofowora CA, Kolawole KA. Evaluation of radiographs, clinical signs and symptoms associated with pulp canal obliteration: an aid to treatment decision. *Dent Traumatol.* 2009;25(6):620–625.
80. Heide S, Kerekes K. Delayed partial pulpotomy in permanent incisors of monkeys. *Int Endod J.* 1987;20(2):65–74.
81. Heling I, Gorfil C, Slutzky H, et al. Endodontic failure caused by inadequate restorative procedures: review and treatment recommendations. *J Prosthet Dent.* 2002;87:674–678.
82. Sheehy EC, Roberts GJ. Use of calcium hydroxide for apical barrier formation and healing in non-vital immature permanent teeth: a review. *Br Dent J.* 1997;11:183.
83. Andreasen JO, Farik B, Munksgaard EC. Long-term calcium hydroxide as a root canal dressing may increase risk of root fracture. *Dent Traumatol.* 2002;18:134–137.
84. Hatibović-Kofman S, Raimundo L, Zheng L, et al. Fracture resistance and histological findings of immature teeth treated with mineral trioxide aggregate. *Dent Traumatol.* 2008;24(3):272–276.
85. Fava LR, Saunders WP. Calcium hydroxide pastes: classification and clinical indications. *Int Endod J.* 1999;32:257–282.
86. Kim D, Kim E. Antimicrobial effect of calcium hydroxide as an intracanal medicament in root canal treatment: a literature review—Part I. In vitro studies. *Restor Dent Endod.* 2014;39(4):241–252.
87. Kim D, Kim E. Antimicrobial effect of calcium hydroxide as an intracanal medicament in root canal treatment: a literature review—Part II. in vivo studies. *Restor Dent Endod.* 2015;40(2):97–103.
88. Hasselgren G, Olsson B, Cvek M. Effects of calcium hydroxide and sodium hypochlorite on the dissolution of necrotic porcine muscle tissue. *J Endod.* 1988;14:125–127.
89. Rafter M. Apexification: a review. *Dent Traumatol.* 2005;21(1):1–8.
90. Kleier DJ, Barr ES. A study of endodontically apexified teeth. *Endod Dent Traumatol.* 1991;7:112–117.
91. van der Sluis LW, Versluis M, Wu MK, et al. Passive ultrasonic irrigation of the root canal: a review of the literature. *Int Endod J.* 2007;40(6):415–426.
92. Metzger Z, Solomonov M, Mass E. Calcium hydroxide retention in wide root canals with flaring apices. *Dent Traumatol.* 2001;17:86–92.
93. Seghi RR, Nasrin S, Draney J, et al. Root fortification. *J Endod.* 2013;39(3 suppl):S57–S62.
94. Giuliani V, Bacccetti T, Pace R, et al. The use of MTA in teeth with necrotic pulps and open apices. *Dent Traumatol.* 2002;18:217.
95. Abouqal R, Rida S. Apexification of immature teeth with calcium hydroxide or mineral trioxide aggregate: systematic review and meta-analysis. *Oral Surg Oral Med Oral Pathol Oral Radiol Endod.* 2011;112(4):e36–e42.
96. Lee YL, Lee BS, Lin FH, et al. Effects of physiological environments on the hydration behavior of mineral trioxide aggregate. *Biomaterials.* 2004;25(5):787–793.
97. Yeung P, Liewehr FR, Moon PC. A quantitative comparison of the fill density of MTA produced by two placement techniques. *J Endod.* 2006;32:456–459.
98. Trope M. Treatment of immature teeth with non-vital pulps and apical periodontitis. *Dent Clin North Am.* 2006;54(2):313–324.
99. Patino MG, Neiders ME, Andreana S, et al. Collagen as an implantable material in medicine and dentistry. *J Oral Implantol.* 2002;28(5):220–225.
100. Andreasen JO, Borum MK, Andreasen FM. Replantation of 400 avulsed permanent incisors. 3. Factors related to root growth. *Endod Dent Traumatol.* 1995;11:69–75.

101. Banchs F, Trope M. Revascularization of immature permanent teeth with apical periodontitis: new treatment protocol? *J Endod*. 2004;30:196–200.

102. Iwaya SI, Ikawa M, Kubota M. Revascularization of an immature permanent tooth with apical periodontitis and sinus tract. *Dent Traumatol*. 2001;17:185–187.

103. Kling M, Cvek M, Mejare I. Rate and predictability of pulp revascularization in therapeutically reimplanted permanent incisors. *Endod Dent Traumatol*. 1986;2(3):83–89.

104. Hargreaves KM, Giesler T, Henry M, et al. Regeneration potential of the young permanent tooth: what does the future hold? *J Endod*. 2008;34(suppl 7):S51–S56.

105. Huang GT. Apexification: the beginning of its end. *Int Endod J*. 2009;42(10):855–866.

106. Wang X, Thibodeau B, Trope M, et al. Histologic characterization of regenerated tissues in canal space after the revitalization/revascularization of immature dog teeth with apical periodontitis. *J Endod*. 2010;36(1):56–63.

107. Thibodeau B, Teixeira F, Yamauchi M, et al. Pulp revascularization of immature dog teeth with apical periodontitis. *J Endod*. 2007;33(6):680–689.

108. Becerra P, Ricucci D, Loghin S, et al. Histologic study of a human immature permanent premolar with chronic apical abscess after revascularization/revitalization. *J Endod*. 2014;40(1):133–139.

109. Nazzal H, Duggal MS. Regenerative endodontics: a true paradigm shift or a bandwagon about to be derailed? *Eur Arch Paediatr Dent*. 2017;18(1):3–15.

110. American Association of Endodontists. Guide to clinical endodontics. http://www.nxtbook.com/nxtbooks/aae/guidetoclinicalendodontics6/index.php#/12. Accessed February 12, 2018.

111. Nor JE, Cucco C. The future: stem cells and biological approaches for pulp regeneration. In: Fuks AB, Peretz B, eds. *Pediatric Endodontics*. Swizerland: Springer International Publishing AG; 2016:117–148.

112. Mohammadi Z. Sodium hypochlorite in endodontics: an update review. *Int Dent J*. 2008;58(6):329–341.

113. Estrela C, Rabelo LE, de Souza JB, et al. Frequency of root canal isthmi in human permanent teeth determined by cone-beam computed tomography. *J Endod*. 2015;41(9):1535–1539.

35

Managing Traumatic Injuries in the Young Permanent Dentition

DENNIS J. MCTIGUE

CHAPTER OUTLINE

Injuries to the primary dentition are discussed in Chapter 16. Also covered there are the following fundamental areas relevant to managing trauma in children of any age:
- Classification of traumatic injuries to teeth
- Medical and dental history
- Clinical and radiographic examinations
- Common reactions of teeth to trauma

This chapter deals with injuries to the young permanent dentition, but the reader is strongly advised to review the fundamental areas just noted in Chapter 16. Frequent reference will be made to them.

The reader is encouraged to review and use an excellent online resource, "The Dental Trauma Guide" (www.dentaltrauma guide.org),[1] to assist in diagnosing and treating tooth injuries. This guide, developed by Dr. Jens O. Andreasen and sponsored in part by the University Hospital, Copenhagen, and the International Association of Dental Traumatology, contains updated guidelines on a broad array of injuries and is easy to use.

Etiology and Epidemiology of Trauma in the Young Permanent Dentition

Falls during play account for most injuries to young permanent teeth. Children engaging in contact sports are at greatest risk for dental injury, though the use of mouth guards greatly reduces their frequency (see Chapter 41). In the teenage years, automobile accidents cause a significant number of dental injuries when occupants not wearing seat belts hit the steering wheel or dashboard. As noted in Chapter 16, children with seizure disorders also injure their permanent teeth more frequently. In contrast to the primary dentition, permanent teeth suffer crown fractures more frequently than luxation injuries. The lower crown/root ratio and denser alveolar bone in the permanent dentition contribute to this phenomenon. Maxillary central incisors are again most commonly injured, and protruding incisors are at greatest risk (Fig. 35.1).[2]

Classification of Injuries to Young Permanent Teeth

Classification of tooth fractures and luxation injuries is discussed in Chapter 16 (see Fig. 16.1).

History

The essential elements of the medical and dental history are discussed in Chapter 16. The use of a trauma assessment form to help organize the gathering of historical and clinical data is emphasized (see Fig. 16.8). The reader is reminded to determine the status of the child's tetanus prophylaxis and to consult the child's physician if there is any question about its adequacy.

Another issue worthy of review relates to the potential for injury to the central nervous system. Older children are likely to suffer harder blows at play, and thus the dentist should find out if the child lost consciousness or became disoriented or nauseated after the injury. Positive findings indicate immediate medical consultation. As noted in Chapter 16, significant head injuries can lead to symptoms many hours after the initial trauma, and parents should be cautioned to watch for the signs noted previously for 24 hours, including waking the child every 2 to 3 hours throughout the night.[3–5]

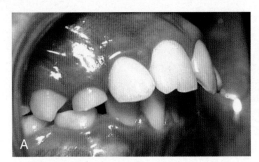 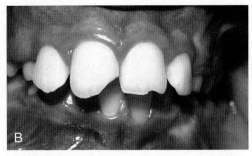

• **Figure 35.1** (A) Lateral view showing large horizontal overjet. (B) Same patient with fractured central incisors. (From McTigue DJ. Management of orofacial trauma in children. *Pediatr Ann.* 1985;14: 125–129.)

Clinical Examination

Refer to Chapter 16 for a thorough discussion of the clinical examination. An important difference between the primary and permanent dentition exists in respect to "vitality" or sensibility testing. Whereas it is not routinely performed in the primary dentition, sensibility testing can be a useful diagnostic aid in the permanent dentition. The dentist should be aware that pulp testing might not elicit reliable responses from erupting permanent teeth and from those with open apices. Furthermore, recently traumatized teeth may not respond to any sensibility test for several months. Positive findings immediately following a traumatic injury are thus more valuable for assessing pulp vitality than are negative responses.

Cold testing with agents like difluorodichloromethane or carbon dioxide snow yields the most reliable results,[6] although the thermal shock of the low temperature applied can cause infraction lines in the enamel.[7] Some clinicians prefer electrical vitality testing because it uses a stimulus that can be gradually increased and precisely recorded. Using both cold tests and electric pulp tests provided the best sensitivity and specificity in a group of adult patients.[8]

Pulp tests that use cold or electrical impulse do not actually measure "vitality" because that requires confirmation of uninterrupted blood flow through the pulpal tissue. Instead, these tests measure neural response, which serves as a proxy for vascular health. Laser Doppler flowmetry has potentially great clinical value because this technique directly measures blood flow and does not rely on sensory nerve response.[9] This technique is also painless and is reliable in teeth with immature apices.[10] However, modifications in this instrument's design and a significant reduction in its cost are necessary for it to achieve widespread use. Another noninvasive technique that has potential diagnostic value is pulse oximetry, which measures blood oxygen saturation in the vessels monitored.[11,12] Although there is currently no commercial product available, future technological advances will enable development of affordable devices that attach to teeth and will give the clinician a better measure of tooth vitality.

Principles of radiographic diagnosis for permanent teeth do not differ from those for primary teeth. A common error made by dentists in diagnosing traumatic injuries is to take an insufficient number of radiographs. Additional views taken from slightly different angles both vertically and horizontally can significantly improve the accuracy of diagnosis.[13]

It is important to note the urgency of follow-up radiographs after injury. Reviewing radiographs at 1 month after injury will detect signs of pulpal necrosis and rapidly progressing

(inflammatory) resorption. At 2 months, replacement resorption can be detected.[13]

Cone beam computed tomography (CBCT) enables the clinician to view a three-dimensional image of a dental injury.[14] The increased radiation, complexity, and cost of this procedure, however, contraindicate its use in children for most dentoalveolar injuries. CBCT should be used only when the patient's history and a clinical examination demonstrate that the benefits to the patient outweigh the potential risks. The clinician should use CBCT only when the need for imaging cannot be met by lower dose two-dimensional radiography.

Pathologic Sequelae of Traumatized Teeth

Refer to Chapter 16 for a discussion of the pathologic sequelae of traumatized teeth.

Treatment of Traumatic Injuries to the Permanent Dentition

The dentist treating a traumatic injury follows essentially the same principles of gathering historical information and completing a clinical examination, regardless of the child's age. Furthermore, the pathologic sequelae of injuries to teeth are similar for both primary and permanent teeth. However, there are many significant differences in the way that injuries to permanent teeth are treated. As in the primary dentition, a complete diagnostic workup (described in Chapter 16) should precede all treatment. Even though a blow may cause little if any obvious injury to a permanent tooth, it may lead to pulp necrosis as a result of disruption of the neurovascular bundle at the apex of the tooth. Posttreatment evaluation is indicated for all traumatic injuries.

Enamel Fractures

In some cases, minor enamel fractures can be smoothed with fine disks. Larger fractures should be restored using an acid-etch/composite resin technique (see Chapter 40 for restorative techniques).

Enamel and Dentin Fractures

The primary issue in managing fractures that expose dentin is to prevent bacterial irritants from reaching the pulp. Standard care in the past called for covering exposed dentin with calcium hydroxide

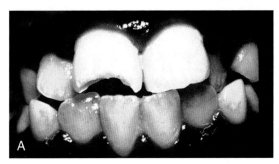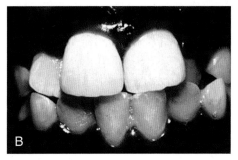

• **Figure 35.2** A fractured incisor (A) can quickly be restored using an acid-etch/composite resin technique (B).

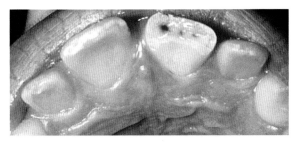

• **Figure 35.3** Crown fracture exposing the pulp.

(CaOH) or glass ionomer cement to seal out oral flora. Sealing exposed dentin with a bonding agent enables the unexposed pulp to form reparative dentin. Some clinicians have then advocated simultaneous acid etching of dentin and enamel, followed by dentin and enamel bonding without placement of CaOH or glass ionomer.[15] However, a review of pulp capping with dentin adhesive systems reported that these systems are not indicated owing to increased inflammatory reactions, delay in pulp healing, and failure of dentin bridge formation.[16] This author recommends covering the deepest portion of dentin fractures with glass ionomer cement, followed by a dentin-bonding agent (see Chapters 22 and 40). The tooth can then be restored with an acid-etch/composite resin technique (Fig. 35.2). If adequate time is not available to restore the tooth completely, an interim covering of resin material (a resin "patch") can temporize the tooth until a final restoration can be placed. Some dentists routinely place such a partial restoration to ensure an appropriate posttreatment evaluation when the patient returns for the final restoration. This is a reasonable strategy, provided that care is taken to ensure an adequate seal. Another option may be to immediately re-bond a fractured segment to the injured tooth. Refer to Chapter 40 for a description of this technique.

Fractures Involving the Pulp

The management of crown fractures that expose the pulp is particularly challenging (Fig. 35.3). Pertinent clinical findings that dictate treatment include the following:
1. Vitality of the exposed pulp
2. Time elapsed since the exposure
3. Degree of root maturation of the fractured tooth
4. Restorability of the fractured crown

The objective of treatment in managing these injuries is to preserve a vital pulp in the entire tooth (see Chapter 34). This allows for physiologic closure of the root apex in immature teeth.

It is important to note that root end closure does not signal completion of root maturation. Progressive deposition of dentin normally continues in roots through adolescence, making them stronger and more resistant to traumatic insult. Maintaining a vital pulp in the tooth crown allows the clinician to monitor the tooth's vitality periodically.

It is not always possible to maintain vital tissue throughout the tooth. Three treatment alternatives are available, based on the clinical findings just noted:
1. Direct pulp cap
2. Pulpotomy
3. Pulpectomy

Direct Pulp Cap

The direct pulp cap is only indicated in small exposures that can be treated within a few hours of the injury. The chances for pulp healing decrease if the tissue is inflamed, has formed a clot, or is contaminated with foreign materials. The objective, then, is to preserve vital pulp tissue that is free of inflammation and physiologically walled off by a calcific barrier.

A rubber dam is applied, and the tooth is gently cleaned with water. Commercially available CaOH paste or mineral trioxide aggregate (MTA) is applied directly to the pulp tissue and to surrounding dentin.[17] It is essential that a restoration be placed that is capable of thoroughly sealing the exposure to prevent further contamination by oral bacteria. As in the management of dentin fractures, it is acceptable to use an acid-etch/composite resin system for an initial restoration. A calcific bridge stimulated by the capping material should be evident radiographically in 2 to 3 months. While MTA for direct pulp caps has been reported to be as successful as CaOH,[18] significant discoloration of the tooth crown can occur with its use (see Fig. 34.2).[19]

In fractures exposing pulps of immature permanent teeth with incomplete root development, a direct cap is no longer the treatment of choice. Failure in these cases leads to total pulpal necrosis and a fragile, immature root with thin dentinal walls. Thus the preferred treatment in pulp exposures of immature permanent teeth is pulpotomy.

Pulpotomy

The objectives of the pulpotomy technique are to remove only the inflamed pulp tissue and to leave healthy tissue to enhance physiologic maturation of the root. As previously noted, this technique is favored for immature permanent teeth with exposed pulps. It is also indicated in large exposures or for pulps exposed for more than a few hours. Owing to its higher success rate, many clinicians have totally abandoned the direct pulp cap in favor of pulpotomy.

It is difficult to determine clinically how far the inflamed pulp extends. The tooth shown in Fig. 35.4 had been fractured for 4 days with a pulp exposure approximately 3 mm in diameter. The dentist elected to remove all tissue in the pulp chamber, with obvious success. Fig. 35.4B demonstrates complete maturation of the root, including apical closure and dentinal wall thickening, as well as a calcific barrier at the amputation site. However, maintaining some pulp tissue in the crown allows the dentist to monitor the vitality of the tooth and thus is preferable when possible.

In 1978, Cvek noted that in most cases of pulps exposed for more than a few hours, the initial biological response is pulpal hyperplasia.[20] Inflammation in these cases rarely extends beyond 2 mm. In his study involving 60 teeth with pulps exposed from 1 hour to 90 days, Cvek removed only 2 mm of the pulp and the surrounding dentin. He covered the pulp stumps with CaOH and reported a success rate of 96%. The long-term success reported by Fuks and colleagues confirms these findings and indicates that this conservative removal of tissue is the treatment of choice (Figs. 35.5 and 35.6).[21]

Absolute isolation to prevent contamination of the pulp with oral bacteria is essential. The inflamed pulp is gently removed to a level approximately 2 mm below the exposure site with a sterile diamond bur at high speed. Copious irrigation is mandatory to avoid pulp injury. The preparation should provide adequate space for the CaOH or MTA pulp dressing and a glass ionomer seal. Attaining a bacteria-tight coronal seal is essential for the success of this technique. The tooth can then be esthetically restored with composite resin.

MTA has been shown to perform well in pulpotomies, causing dentinal bridge formation while maintaining normal pulpal histologic features.[22,23] As noted previously, however, its tendency to stain teeth is a clinical concern.[19] See Chapter 34 for details on its use.

Pulpectomy

A pulpectomy involves complete pulp tissue removal from the crown and root and is indicated when no vital tissue remains. It is also indicated when root maturation is complete and the permanent restoration requires a post buildup. In the absence of rapidly progressing (inflammatory) root resorption, treatment is to obturate the canal with gutta-percha. The reader is referred to standard endodontic textbooks for more information on this technique.

One of the greatest challenges facing the clinician is the treatment of a nonvital immature permanent tooth with an open apex. Physiologic root maturation cannot occur without the presence of vital pulp tissue, apical papilla stem cells, odontoblasts, and the Hertwig epithelial root sheath.[74] Traditional treatment for these cases was an apexification procedure wherein CaOH was carried to the root apex to contact vital tissues directly. The CaOH stimulated the formation of a cementoid barrier against which gutta-percha could subsequently be condensed. Multiple visits over a period of 9 to 18 months were required, however, and the outcome was a shortened root with thin walls (Fig. 35.7).[25] In addition, long-term CaOH therapy has been shown to weaken the tooth root and increase the likelihood of root fractures.[26]

An alternative to the CaOH apexification technique for managing devitalized immature incisors is the apical barrier technique using MTA.[27] The material is condensed into the apical area and allowed

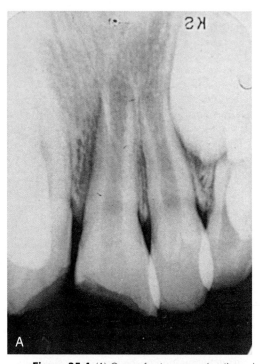
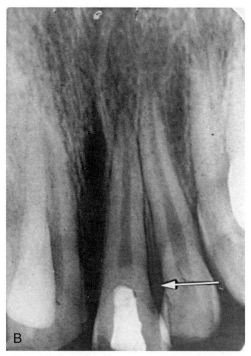

• **Figure 35.4** (A) Crown fracture exposing the pulp in an immature permanent incisor. Note the open apex and thin dentinal walls in the root. (B) A calcium hydroxide pulpotomy stimulated the formation of a calcific barrier *(arrow)* and enabled the root to mature, demonstrating apical closure and root wall thickening.

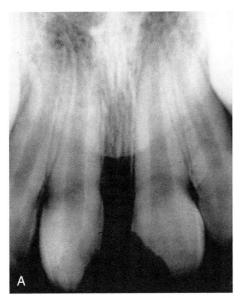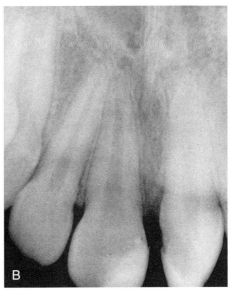

• **Figure 35.5** (A) Maxillary right permanent central incisor suffered crown fracture with pulp exposure. (B) One-year postoperative radiograph of the same tooth successfully treated with a calcium hydroxide partial pulpotomy. Note completion of root development both apically and laterally.

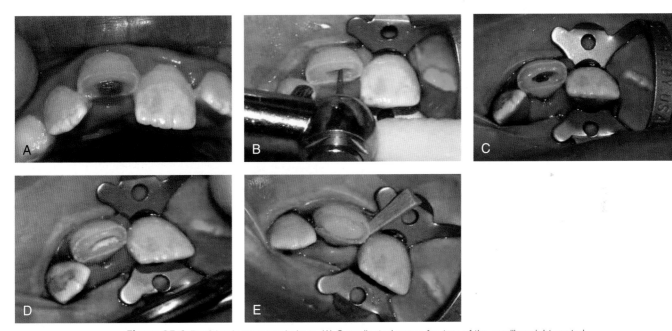

• **Figure 35.6** Partial pulpotomy technique. (A) Complicated crown fracture of the maxillary right central incisor, exposing the pulp. (B) Removing pulp to a depth of 2 mm with sterile diamond bur. (C) Blood clot after pulp amputation. (D) Calcium hydroxide base on pulp stump. (E) Glass ionomer seal. (Courtesy Dr. Ashok Kumar.)

to set. Gutta-percha is then condensed against the MTA barrier at a subsequent appointment (Fig. 35.8). Though overall treatment time is greatly reduced, the shortened root and thin walls continue to place the tooth at risk for subsequent cervical root fracture.

Regenerative Endodontics

Iwaya, Hoshino, and others reported a dramatic alternative to apexification of necrotic immature teeth termed revascularization or "regenerative" endodontics.[28–30] These procedures seek to replace damaged dentin, root structures, and pulp cells with live tissues that restore normal physiologic function.[31] The concept is to

thoroughly disinfect the root canal system and then stimulate bleeding from the apical papilla to fill the root chamber with a blood clot. A host of growth factors in the area then act on dental stem cells, primarily from the apical papilla, to use the clot as a scaffold and differentiate into healthy cells of the pulp-dentin complex that can complete physiologic root maturation.

The technique (Fig. 35.9) is to first cleanse the canal by copious irrigation with sodium hypochlorite or ethylenediaminetetraacetic acid (EDTA).[32] Owing to the immature status of the root and thin radicular walls, instrumentation is kept to a minimum and used mainly to agitate the irrigant. The irrigant is also activated by placing an ultrasonic tip about 3 mm short of the working length in the canal to facilitate better debridement of the pulp tissue remnants and to minimize the substrate for microbial proliferation. The canal space is then dried using sterile paper points. A low concentration triple antibiotic paste of ciprofloxacin, metronidazole, and minocycline is carefully placed into the canal with a Lentulo spiral up to the cementoenamel junction (CEJ).[29] Owing to its tendency to stain teeth, minocycline is often replaced with clindamycin.[33,34] CaOH is also sometimes used in lieu of the antibiotic paste, again to avoid tooth discoloration.[35] The access cavity is sealed with a sterile cotton pellet and glass ionomer cement.

The patient is scheduled for a follow-up appointment after 3 to 4 weeks. At the follow-up appointment, the area is anesthetized with local anesthetic containing no epinephrine. The antibiotic paste or CaOH is rinsed out, and a sterile endodontic file is placed beyond the apex to initiate bleeding. A clot is allowed to form as close to the CEJ as possible to facilitate root thickening at the tooth cervix. MTA is then placed against the clot, and the tooth is temporarily sealed with glass ionomer cement. The final restoration is placed at a subsequent appointment. Root maturation should be apparent radiographically within several months (Fig. 35.10).

Regenerative endodontics is still an emerging field and no evidence-based guidelines are available to inform the clinician about its precise indications or technique. More research will refine the technique and will undoubtedly lead to its greater use in the future.

Criteria for Success

Criteria to judge success of the techniques used to manage pulpal insult in fractured teeth include the following:
- Completion of root development in immature teeth
- Absence of clinical signs such as pain, mobility, or fistula
- Absence of any radiographic signs of pathologic processes, such as periapical radiolucency of bone or root resorption

Posterior Crown Fractures

Posterior crown fractures in the permanent dentition pose a restorative challenge for the clinician. These fractures usually occur secondary to hard blows to the underside of the chin, and vertical crown fractures may result (Fig. 35.11). Although bonding with posterior composite resins is sometimes possible, full coverage with stainless steel or cast metal crowns is often the only restorative alternative. The reader is reminded to watch for mandibular fractures and cervical spine injuries in these cases.[36]

Root Fractures

The prognosis for root fractures is best when the fracture occurs in the apical one-third of the root. The prognosis worsens progressively with fractures that occur more cervically in the root. Bender and Freedland reported that more than 75% of teeth with intraalveolar root fractures maintain their vitality.[37]

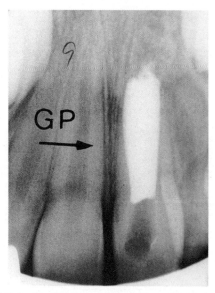

• **Figure 35.7** An apexification procedure allowed this immature permanent tooth to be obturated successfully with gutta-percha (GP). The root, however, remains fragile and at increased risk of future trauma because no further dentinal wall apposition can occur.

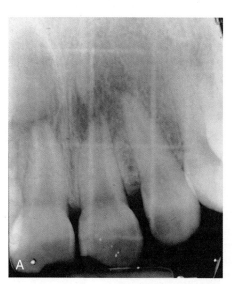 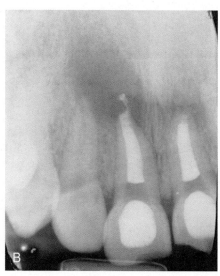 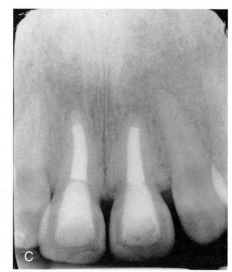

• **Figure 35.8** Apexification using apical barrier technique. (A) Preoperative view. (B) Four-week postoperative view. (C) Twenty-seven-month postoperative view.

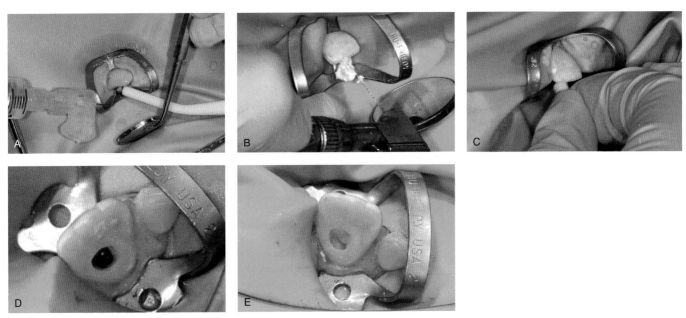

• **Figure 35.9** Regenerative endodontic technique. (A) Copious irrigation of pulp canal with sodium hypochlorite. (B) Spinning triple antibiotic paste. (C) Stimulating bleeding by extending file 2 to 3 mm beyond tooth apex. (D) Blood clot at cervix of tooth. (E) Mineral trioxide aggregate placed on blood clot.

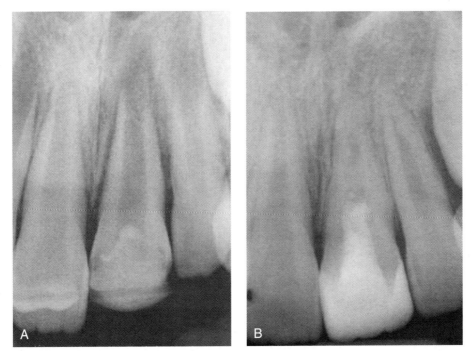

• **Figure 35.10** Successful revascularization of necrotic immature permanent left maxillary central incisor. (A) Preoperative radiograph of immature incisor with complicated crown fracture, open apex, and apical periodontitis. (B) Twenty-seven-month postoperative view. Note apical closure and root wall thickening.

A tooth with a fractured root is usually mobile, and its coronal fragment is often displaced. Several baseline radiographs should be taken from various angulations to verify the extent of the fracture. Optimal results are obtained if the coronal fragment is repositioned as soon as possible.[13] The tooth position should be verified radiographically, and the pulp sensitivity should be tested. Accurate repositioning of the tooth enhances the likelihood of both hard tissue healing of the root fracture and pulp healing.[38] Immature teeth with incompletely formed root apices and positive pulp sensitivity at the time of injury are also significantly related to pulp healing and hard tissue repair of the fracture.

Tooth splinting techniques are detailed later in this chapter; however, current evidence indicates that teeth with roots fractured in the apical and middle thirds heal better if splinted for only 3 to 4 weeks with a functional splint that allows for some mobility of the teeth.[13,39] Teeth sustaining cervical third root fractures should be stabilized with a flexible splint for 3 to 4 months.

Root canal therapy should not be initiated until clinical and radiographic signs of necrosis or resorption are apparent. Even in those cases, treatment can often be limited to the coronal fragment, because in most instances the apical fragments maintain their vitality.

Managing Sequelae to Dental Trauma

In Chapter 16, common reactions of the teeth to trauma are described. Three of the most challenging sequelae include pulp canal obliteration (PCO), rapidly progressing (inflammatory) resorption (both external and internal), and replacement resorption. These pathologic processes can occur following crown fractures or luxation injuries.

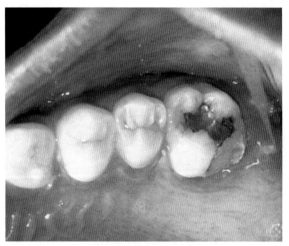

• **Figure 35.11** A vertical crown fracture of the distolingual cusp of this maxillary molar occurred secondary to a blow to the underside of this child's chin.

Pulp Canal Obliteration

PCO is a degenerative pathologic process that ultimately leads to obliteration of the pulp canal (Figs. 35.12 and 35.13B). Andreasen showed that its occurrence depends on the type of luxation injury sustained and the stage of root development.[40] Thus immature teeth with open apices suffering moderate to severe injuries are likely to undergo PCO. It was noted previously that most primary teeth with PCO resorb normally, and thus treatment is usually not indicated. A conservative approach is also recommended for PCO in the permanent teeth. Current evidence indicates that pulp necrosis is an uncommon sequela of PCO, reportedly as low as 1%[40] or as high as 33%.[41] Crown discoloration may occur more frequently. Endodontic procedures can be successfully completed in a great majority of obliterated canals if necessary.[7] The dentist is advised, then, to closely monitor PCO in permanent teeth and to initiate endodontic procedures only in response to periapical changes or for prevention of coronal discoloration in fully mature teeth.

Rapidly Progressing (Inflammatory) Resorption

Rapidly progressing (inflammatory) resorption can occur externally, internally, or both (see Fig. 35.13). It commonly arises following luxation injuries when the periodontal ligament (PDL) is inflamed and the pulp is necrotic.[42] Odontoclastic activity can occur so rapidly that the teeth are destroyed in a matter of weeks. Rapidly progressing resorption can be prevented by prompt extirpation (within 3 weeks) of the pulp in mature teeth that have suffered luxation injuries. Luxated teeth with open apices should be observed closely, and their pulps should be extirpated at the first sign of resorption. Regenerative endodontic or apical barrier techniques are then indicated to complete treatment.

Immediate management of rapidly progressing resorption is essential. As soon as this process is detected radiographically, the pulp tissue in the tooth is thoroughly extirpated. Copious irrigation with sodium hypochlorite assists in the dissolution of organic debris in the canal. In permanent teeth, CaOH is placed in the

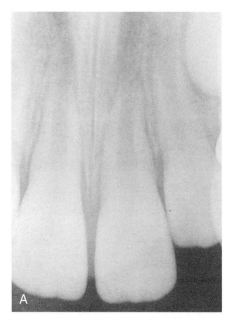
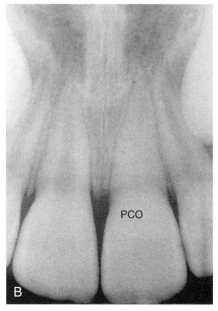

• **Figure 35.12** (A) Ten-day postoperative view of immature maxillary left central incisor in 7-year-old child that had been extruded and repositioned. (B) Sixteen-month postoperative view demonstrating pulp canal obliteration (PCO).

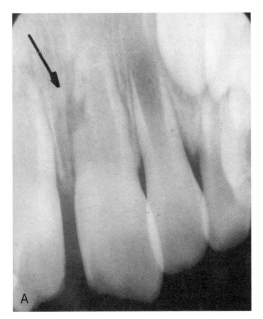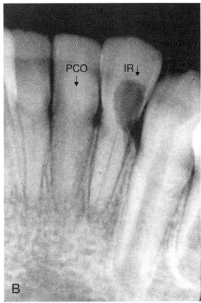

• **Figure 35.13** (A) External rapidly progressing resorption *(arrow)*. (B) Internal resorption *(IR)* of the lateral incisor; pulp canal obliteration *(PCO)* of the permanent central incisor. ([B] From McTigue DJ. Management of orofacial trauma in children. *Pediatr Ann.* 1985;14:125–129.)

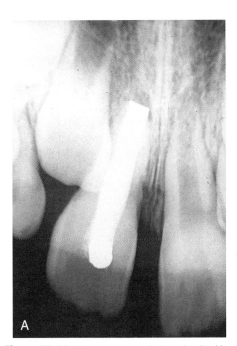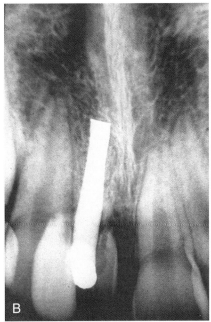

• **Figure 35.14** (A) A permanent incisor that had been avulsed and stored dry for 3 hours was filled with gutta-percha before reimplantation. (B) Three years later, replacement resorption has completely destroyed the root.

canal with a technique identical to that used to induce apexification (see Chapter 34). Here the objective is not to induce apical closure but to create an environment unfavorable for the resorptive process. It is theorized that CaOH has antiseptic properties because of its extreme alkalinity. This medicament apparently percolates through the dentinal tubules to the areas of resorption at the PDL and halts its progress.

CaOH should be retained in the tooth until radiographic signs of healing are apparent. This may take several months, and repeated applications of CaOH may be necessary if the resorption progresses.

When radiographs confirm that the process has stopped, gutta-percha is placed as the final filling material.

Replacement Resorption (Ankylosis)

Replacement resorption occurs most commonly following severe luxation injuries like avulsions or intrusions, in which PDL cells are destroyed. Alveolar bone directly contacts cementum on the involved tooth and fuses with it. Then, as the bone undergoes its normal physiologic, osteoclastic, and osteoblastic activity, the root is resorbed or replaced with bone (Fig. 35.14). In young children with rapid bone turnover, roots are completely resorbed in 3 to 4 years. In adults, the process may take up to 10 years. Replacement resorption can be prevented by prompt and appropriate management of luxation injuries.

Treating Luxation Injuries in the Permanent Dentition

The reader is referred to Chapter 16 for the definition of the various types of luxation injuries. Luxation injuries damage the supporting structures of the teeth—that is, the PDL and alveolar bone. In addition, in mature teeth with closed apices, the pulp frequently becomes necrotic. Pulp necrosis occurs less frequently when immature teeth with open apices are luxated, but, as noted earlier, PCO is a common finding in these cases.

Vitality of the PDL is far more important than pulp vitality in determining the prognosis of luxated teeth. The primary objective of treatment in these injuries is to maintain PDL vitality.

Concussion

Concussion injuries in permanent teeth must be followed closely. Although the prognosis is normally good, pulp necrosis and root resorption have been reported. Involved teeth can be carefully taken out of occlusion if the child complains of pain.

Subluxation

Pulp necrosis occurs far more commonly in subluxated permanent teeth than in primary teeth. These teeth should be monitored closely with radiographs for at least 1 year, and root canal therapy should be instituted at the first sign of pathologic change. Immature teeth with open apices are less likely to undergo pulpal necrosis. Splinting of subluxated teeth should be limited to a maximum of 2 weeks with a flexible splint and then only when the patient requires it for comfort.[13]

Intrusive Luxation

The prognosis for intruded permanent teeth is not good. These teeth frequently undergo pulpal necrosis, root resorption, and alveolar bone loss. Treatment for intruded teeth is controversial, owing to the lack of research in this area.[43] Guidelines published by the International Association for Dental Traumatology recommend different strategies, depending on the apical development of the intruded tooth.[13]

The treatment of choice for immature teeth intruded less than 7 mm is to allow them to reemerge spontaneously. If no movement is noted within 3 weeks, orthodontic repositioning using light forces should be employed (Fig. 35.15). Immature teeth intruded more than 7 mm should be orthodontically or surgically repositioned.

Mature permanent teeth intruded less than 3 mm should be allowed to reemerge without intervention. If no movement is noted within 3 weeks, they should be repositioned surgically or orthodontically before they ankylose. Those teeth intruded beyond 7 mm should be repositioned surgically. Evidence is not available to clearly indicate whether orthodontic or surgical repositioning is preferable for mature teeth intruded between 3 and 7 mm. The pulp in mature intruded teeth will likely become necrotic and lead to rapidly progressing resorption, so it should be extirpated within 3 weeks following the injury, and CaOH should be placed in the root canal using the same technique as described for apexification in Chapter 34. Radiographic monitoring of the tooth should occur for at least 1 year, and the CaOH in the canal should be replaced if signs of root resorption persist.

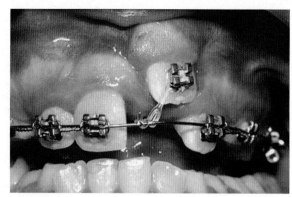

• **Figure 35.15** Orthodontic repositioning of intruded permanent incisor prevents replacement resorption (ankylosis) and alveolar bone loss.

Extrusion

Extruded permanent teeth (Fig. 35.16A) should be repositioned as soon as possible and splinted for 2 to 3 weeks. It normally takes the PDL fibers this period of time to reanastomose. Extruded permanent teeth with closed apices will undergo pulpal necrosis; therefore root canal therapy should be initiated after the teeth are splinted. Extruded teeth with open apices have a chance to revascularize and maintain their vitality, so the decision to initiate therapy should be delayed until clinical or radiographic signs indicate necrosis.

Lateral Luxation

Alveolar bone fractures frequently occur in lateral luxation injuries and can complicate their management (see Fig. 35.16B). In the most severe cases, PDL and marginal bone loss occur. Treatment is to reposition the teeth and alveolar fragments as soon as possible. A splint should then be applied for 3 to 6 weeks, depending on the degree of bone involvement. The author's current protocol includes prescribing a 0.12% chlorhexidine mouthrinse. If the apices are closed, the pulps will likely become necrotic; therefore endodontic therapy should be instituted soon after the teeth are splinted. Again, teeth with open apices should be monitored until signs of necrosis are evident.

Avulsion

The prognosis for long-term retention of an avulsed permanent tooth worsens the longer the tooth is out of its socket.[44] The primary therapeutic concern is to maintain the vitality of PDL fibers, and the longer they are out of the mouth, the worse the prognosis for their survival. It is thus imperative that the avulsed tooth be immediately reimplanted by the first capable person, whether that person is a parent, teacher, or sibling (Fig. 35.17).

Owing to a variety of circumstances, it is sometimes not possible to reimplant a tooth immediately. Research has shown that the best transport medium for avulsed teeth is cell culture media such as ViaSpan (DuPont Merck Pharmaceutical Company, Wilmington, DE) or Hanks balanced salt solution (HBSS; United Biochemicals, Sanborn, NY).[45] ViaSpan is not readily available for clinical use, but HBSS is commercially available as EMT Tooth Saver (Biochrom AG, Berlin, Germany). Use of HBSS significantly increases the likelihood of PDL cell survival for several hours.[46]

The best alternative storage medium if culture media is not available is milk.[47,48] It is readily available, relatively aseptic, and its osmolality is more favorable to maintaining the vitality of the PDL cells than is saline solution or tap water. Cool milk has

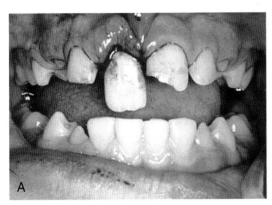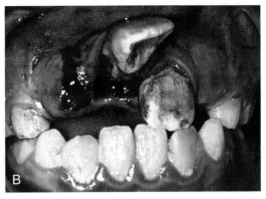

• **Figure 35.16** (A) Extrusion injury of maxillary right central incisor and crown fracture of maxillary left central incisor. (B) Laterally luxated tooth.

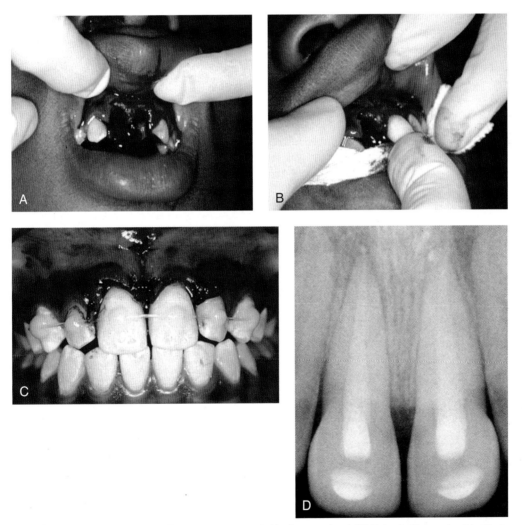

• **Figure 35.17** (A) Both maxillary permanent central incisors avulsed. (B) Reimplanting avulsed teeth with finger pressure. (C) Aesthetic, flexible splint fabricated using 50-pound test monofilament fishing line retained with composite resin. (D) Calcium hydroxide pulpectomies completed to prevent rapidly progressing resorption. (Courtesy Dr. Jeff Hays.)

been shown to maintain the ability of PDL precursor cells to reproduce for twice as long as room temperature milk.[49] Though some studies have indicated that storing the tooth in the patient's mouth (saliva) may be favorable toward PDL survival, the danger of an alarmed child swallowing, aspirating, or chewing on the tooth eliminates this option in the author's opinion. Water is not a good transport medium because it is a hypotonic solution and causes PDL cells to swell and rupture. Thus in these cases, with the tooth stored in cold milk, the patient should be taken to the dentist as soon as possible.

Because root resorption is so closely correlated with the extraoral period, the dentist should reimplant the tooth in its socket as soon as possible after the child arrives. Adequate evidence exists, however, to support the immediate placement of the avulsed tooth into HBSS while the patient is brought to the dental operatory and appropriate informed consent is being obtained from the parent.[6] Soaking the tooth may reduce ankylosis and help debride necrotic cells, foreign bodies, and bacteria. The author's current protocol is again to prescribe an oral mouthrinse of 0.12% chlorhexidine used empirically to reduce the likelihood of bacterial invasion of the PDL space. Controversy exists regarding the benefit of systemic antibiotics for pulp or periodontal healing.[50–52] Given the evidence that systemic antibiotics can prevent bacterial invasion of the necrotic pulp,[53] Andreasen recommends a 1-week course of doxycycline for tooth avulsion patients.[1] Doxycycline is preferred, owing to its antiresorptive properties[54]; however, tetracycline is known to stain developing teeth. Therefore penicillin V is the antibiotic of choice for children age 8 years and younger.

When immature teeth with open apices are avulsed, the ideal treatment objective is spontaneous revascularization of the pulp in addition to maintenance of PDL health. This would enable physiologic maturation of the immature root, including apexogenesis and root wall thickening. The tooth should be splinted for approximately 1 to 2 weeks. Success in these cases has been reported; therefore dentists should await clinical or radiographic signs of necrosis before initiating regenerative endodontic therapy. When the splint is removed, the dentist may note that the tooth is quite mobile. This mobility is preferable to long-term rigid splinting, because the latter has been correlated with an increased incidence of replacement resorption. The mobility of the tooth physiologically interrupts areas of incipient resorption/ankylosis on the PDL, allowing it to heal normally.

In *mature* teeth with closed apices, a splint that affords the tooth functional mobility should be applied for 7 to 14 days. The necrotic pulp should be extirpated and replaced with CaOH after 1 week to prevent the initiation of rapidly progressing root resorption (see Fig. 35.17D). Importantly, root canal therapy should not be performed in the hand before reimplantation. This extends the extraoral period and places the PDL at greater risk to injury as a result of the additional manipulation of the tooth. The CaOH can be removed and a gutta-percha pulpectomy performed after 2 weeks. In those cases where the pulp was not removed within

2 to 3 weeks of the reimplantation, or when rapidly progressing resorption is evident radiographically, the CaOH should be maintained in the tooth until radiographic signs of healing are apparent.

PDL cells on avulsed teeth that have been stored dry for more than 1 hour are necrotic, and these teeth will eventually ankylose and resorb. There is some evidence that the pace of this resorption can be reduced if these teeth are soaked in fluoride for approximately 20 minutes before reimplantation.[55]

In summary, the procedure for reimplantation of a mature tooth is as follows:
1. Hold the tooth by the crown to prevent damage to the PDL.
2. Gently rinse the tooth with tap water. No attempt should be made to scrub or sterilize the tooth.
3. Manually reimplant the tooth in the socket as soon as possible.
4. Apply a light, functional splint for 1 to 2 weeks.
5. Complete CaOH pulpectomy after 1 week and then remove splint.

Splinting Technique

Various methods of splinting teeth have been advocated, but it is apparent that the ideal splint should possess the following characteristics:
1. Be passive and not cause trauma
2. Be flexible and allow functional movement of the tooth
3. Allow for vitality testing and endodontic access
4. Be easy to apply and remove

Many splints can meet these criteria, and several good commercial products are available. To allow for flexibility, a light orthodontic arch wire or a 30- to 60-pound test monofilament fishing line can be used (see Fig. 35.17C).

Summary

Advances in dental research have greatly improved the ability of dentists to ensure long-term retention of traumatized teeth in children. It is the dentist's responsibility to stay abreast of this new information and to be available to patients who need urgent treatment. As noted in the beginning of this chapter, www.dentaltraumaguide.org is an excellent resource for up-to-date information on the management of dental injuries.

PREVENTIVE/INTERCEPTIVE ORTHODONTIC TREATMENT

Henry Fields

There are relationships between malocclusion, orthodontics, and the dental trauma patient. Certain types of malocclusion are more prone to trauma, and following trauma, orthodontics can play a role in treatment. The data are clear that patients with protrusive teeth (excess overjet) and incompetent lips are most at risk for traumatic dental injuries (TDI)—as are children with previous primary dentition TDI or permanent dentition TDI prior to 9 years of age.[1–3]

If this is the case, why not just provide early phase I orthodontic treatment for children with significant class II malocclusion? Information from the two early treatment randomized prospective clinical trials combined with experience from Britain do not make the case based on an analysis of

the benefits of treatment.[4] This is especially true if we recognize that most TDI are enamel and dentin fractures with moderate long-term sequelae compared with those with periodontal type injuries (intrusion, extrusion, avulsion, and luxation) that have significant long-term consequences. It can be reasonably concluded that the benefits of treatment for this latter group can have an impact, but predicting who is most at risk is not easy.

Given this fact, early orthodontic treatment for those who have increased overjet, incompetent lips, and a history of permanent dentition TDI prior to 9 years old makes some sense if the treatment is limited to retraction of the incisors (not early class II growth modification) and then definitive orthodontics later. This, combined with a mouth guard that is worn consistently, can greatly reduce TDI.

PREVENTIVE/INTERCEPTIVE ORTHODONTIC TREATMENT—cont'd

Orthodontic Treatment for Immediate Trauma

There is a place for orthodontics, as mentioned in this chapter, following TDI for patients who have experienced intrusion, avulsion, and lateral luxation injuries. Contemporary thought is that both immature intruded less than 7 mm and mature teeth intruded less than 3 mm should have a chance to re-erupt for approximately 3 weeks.[13] For those that do not actively or completely re-erupt following observation, and those with mature roots intruded 3 to 7 mm, orthodontic traction can be useful. Orthodontics as an alternative to surgical repositioning appears to have better supporting tissue outcomes,[5] but may be impractical in terms of treatment time and appointments required as the intrusion approaches or exceeds 7 mm. Although there are many methods to extrude teeth, using a light flexible overlay wire like .012 or .014 NiTi, supported by a heavier base wire (.016 or .018 steel), is relatively simple and effective (Fig. 35.18). Conversely, when avulsed teeth are not completely reimplanted or extruded teeth are encountered, achieving good positioning can be aided by using a light continuous archwire to intrude them (Fig. 35.19).

Teeth that have been laterally luxated in any direction can be immediately repositioned and splinted. If this cannot be accomplished and they have consolidated in a new position without occlusal interference, ideally waiting for 3 months, as one would with a transplanted tooth before orthodontic movement is attempted, is recommended.[6] In the case of lingually displaced maxillary teeth, they are often in traumatic occlusion, which prevents complete jaw closure. For these patients, immediate movement with light continuous orthodontic forces is best to better align the teeth and eliminate the occlusal interferences.

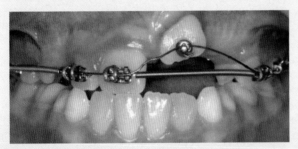

• **Figure 35.18** Extrusion using a base wire and a flexible overlay wire. Remember that the method works by having the overlay wire slide through the brackets, so loose steel ties are recommended. Probably extending the overlay wire through one bracket on either side of the intruded tooth is adequate, since the more brackets, the more friction that is incurred and the slower the movement.

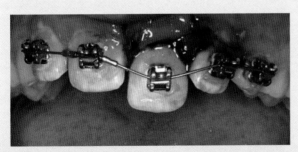

• **Figure 35.19** Intrusion or alignment can sometimes be accomplished by a continuous flexible wire, while monitoring any negative reactive side effects.

Orthodontic Treatment for Patients With Traumatic Dental Injuries

There is often a question of when to start orthodontic treatment for patients with TDI. Should treatment begin immediately, or should there be a period of healing before starting orthodontic tooth movement? Current recommendations suggest delaying orthodontic treatment for 3 months for minor dental trauma such as concussion, subluxation, and crown fractures. If the patient sustains major dental trauma (avulsion, root fracture, severe luxation), orthodontic treatment should possibly be delayed for up to 1 year to allow healing and determine the status of the injured teeth.[7]

Patients who have experienced orthodontic treatment and trauma are more at risk for root resorption and pulpal necrosis of the injured teeth than those who have had either orthodontics or trauma alone.[8-10] Those teeth with completed endodontic treatment are usually less prone to root resorption than normal teeth.[11]

Orthodontics can also be helpful following traumatic injury when teeth are missing and spaces need to be closed or teeth repositioned for subsequent restorative treatment. The advent of temporary anchorage devices (TADS) has altered the possibilities for tooth movement dramatically in these cases.

References

1. Bauss O, Freitag S, Rohling J, et al. Influence of overjet and lip coverage on the prevalence and severity of incisor trauma. *J Orofac Orthop*. 2008;69:402–410.
2. Goettems ML, Brancher LC, da Coasta CT, et al. Does dental trauma in the primary dentition increases the likelihood of trauma in the permanent dentition? A longitudinal study. *Clin Oral Investig*. 2017;21:2415–2420.
3. Glendor U, Koucheki B, Halling A. Risk evaluation and type of treatment of multiple dental trauma episodes to permanent teeth. *Endod Dent Traumatol*. 2000;16:205–210.
4. Thiruvenkatachari B, Harrison JE, Worthington HV, et al. Orthodontic treatment for prominent upper front teeth (Class II malocclusion) in children. *Cochrane Database Syst Rev*. 2013;(11):CD003452.
5. Andreasen JO, Bakland LK, Andreasen FM. Traumatic intrusion of permanent teeth: part 3—a clinical study of the effect of treatment variables such as treatment delay, method of repositioning, type of splint, length of splinting and antibiotics on 140 teeth. *Dent Traumatol*. 2006;22:99–111.
6. Paulsen HU, Andreasen JO, Schwartz O. Pulp and peiodontgal healing, root development and root resortpiuon subsequent to transplantation and orthodontic rotation: a long-term study of autotransplanted premolars. *Am J Orthod Dentofacial Orthop*. 1995;108:630–640.
7. Kindelan SA, Day PF, Kindelan JD, et al. Dental trauma: an overview of its influence on the management of orthodontic treatment: part 1. *J Orthod*. 2008;35:68–78.
8. Brin I, Ben-Bassat Y, Heling I, et al. The influence of orthodontic treatment on previously traumatized permanent incisors. *Eur J Orthod*. 1991;13:372–377.
9. Bauss O, Scheafer W, Sadat-Khonsari R, et al. Influence of orthodontic extrusion on pulpal vitality of traumatized maxillary incisors. *J Endod*. 2010;36:203–207.
10. Bauss O, Reohling J, Sadat-Khonsari R, et al. Influence of orthodontic intrusion on pulpal vitality of previously traumatized maxillary permanent incisors. *Am J Orthod Dentofacial Orthop*. 2008;134:12–17.
11. Spurrier SW, Hall SH, Joondeph DR, et al. A comparison of apical root resorption during orthodontic treatment in endodontically treated vital teeth. *Am J Orthod Dentofacial Orthop*. 1990;97:130–134.

References

1. Andreasen JO, ed. *The Dental Trauma Guide*. San Diego: International Association of Dental Traumatology; 2012.

2. Jarvinen S. Incisal overjet and traumatic injuries to upper permanent incisors. A retrospective study. *Acta Odontol Scand*. 1978;36(6):359–362.

3. Palchak MJ, Holmes JF, Vance CW, et al. A decision rule for identifying children at low risk for brain injuries after blunt head trauma. *Ann Emerg Med*. 2003;42(4):492–506.

4. Tecklenburg FW, Wright MS. Minor head trauma in the pediatric patient. *Pediatr Emerg Care*. 1991;7(1):40–47.

5. Pandor A, Goodacre S, Harnan S, et al. Diagnostic management strategies for adults and children with minor head injury: a systematic review and an economic evaluation. *Health Technol Assess*. 2011;15(27):1–202.

6. Trope M. Clinical management of the avulsed tooth: present strategies and future directions. *Dent Traumatol*. 2002;18(1):1–11.

7. Andreasen JO, Andreasen FM, Andersson L. *Textbook and Color Atlas of Traumatic Injuries to the Teeth*. 4th ed. Copenhagen: Blackwell Munksgaard; 2007:891.

8. Weisleder R, Yamauchi S, Caplan DJ, et al. The validity of pulp testing: a clinical study. *J Am Dent Assoc*. 2009;140(8):1013–1017.

9. Alghaithy RA, Qualtrough AJ. Pulp sensibility and vitality tests for diagnosing pulpal health in permanent teeth: a critical review. *Int Endod J*. 2017;50(2):135–142.

10. Mesaros SV, Trope M. Revascularization of traumatized teeth assessed by laser Doppler flowmetry: case report. *Endod Dent Traumatol*. 1997;13(1):24–30.

11. Caldeira CL, Barletta FB, Ilha MC, et al. Pulse oximetry: a useful test for evaluating pulp vitality in traumatized teeth. *Dent Traumatol*. 2016;32(5):385–389.

12. Pozzobon MH, de Sousa Vieira R, Alves AM, et al. Assessment of pulp blood flow in primary and permanent teeth using pulse oximetry. *Dent Traumatol*. 2011;27(3):184–188.

13. Diangelis AJ, Andreasen JO, Ebeleseder KA, et al. International Association of Dental Traumatology guidelines for the management of traumatic dental injuries: 1. Fractures and luxations of permanent teeth. *Dent Traumatol*. 2012;28(1):2–12.

14. Palomo L, Palomo JM. Cone beam CT for diagnosis and treatment planning in trauma cases. *Dent Clin North Am*. 2009;53(4):717–727, vi–vii.

15. White KC, Cox CF, Kanka J, et al. Histologic pulpal response of acid etching vital dentin. *J Dent Res*. 1992;71(1 suppl):188.

16. Costa CA, Hebling J, Hanks CT. Current status of pulp capping with dentin adhesive systems: a review. *Dent Mater*. 2000;16(3):188–197.

17. Hilton TJ, Ferracane JL, Mancl L. Northwest Practice-based Research Collaborative in Evidence-based Dentistry. Comparison of CaOH with MTA for direct pulp capping: a PBRN randomized clinical trial. *J Dent Res*. 2013;92(7 suppl):16S–22S.

18. Schwendicke F, Brouwer F, Schwendicke A, et al. Different materials for direct pulp capping: systematic review and meta-analysis and trial sequential analysis. *Clin Oral Investig*. 2016;20(6):1121–1132.

19. Felman D, Parashos P. Coronal tooth discoloration and white mineral trioxide aggregate. *J Endod*. 2013;39(4):484–487.

20. Cvek M. A clinical report on partial pulpotomy and capping with calcium hydroxide in permanent incisors with complicated crown fracture. *J Endod*. 1978;4(8):232–237.

21. Fuks AB, Gavra S, Chosack A. Long-term followup of traumatized incisors treated by partial pulpotomy. *Pediatr Dent*. 1993;15(5):334–336.

22. Schmitt D, Lee J, Bogen G. Multifaceted use of ProRoot MTA root canal repair material. *Pediatr Dent*. 2001;23(4):326–330.

23. Salako N, Joseph B, Ritwik P, et al. Comparison of bioactive glass, mineral trioxide aggregate, ferric sulfate, and formocresol as pulpotomy agents in rat molar. *Dent Traumatol*. 2003;19(6):314–320.

24. Karabucak B, Li D, Lim J, et al. Vital pulp therapy with mineral trioxide aggregate. *Dent Traumatol*. 2005;21(4):240–243.

25. Rafter M. Apexification: a review. *Dent Traumatol*. 2005;21(1):1–8.

26. Rosenberg B, Murray PE, Namerow K. The effect of calcium hydroxide root filling on dentin fracture strength. *Dent Traumatol*. 2007;23(1):26–29.

27. Shabahang S, Torabinejad M. Treatment of teeth with open apices using mineral trioxide aggregate. *Pract Periodontics Aesthet Dent*. 2000;12(3):315–320, quiz 322.

28. Iwaya SI, Ikawa M, Kubota M. Revascularization of an immature permanent tooth with apical periodontitis and sinus tract. *Dent Traumatol*. 2001;17(4):185–187.

29. Hoshino E, Kurihara-Ando N, Sato I, et al. In-vitro antibacterial susceptibility of bacteria taken from infected root dentine to a mixture of ciprofloxacin, metronidazole and minocycline. *Int Endod J*. 1996;29(2):125–130.

30. Banchs F, Trope M. Revascularization of immature permanent teeth with apical periodontitis: new treatment protocol? *J Endod*. 2004;30(4):196–200.

31. Murray PE, Garcia-Godoy F, Hargreaves KM. Regenerative endodontics: a review of current status and a call for action. *J Endod*. 2007;33(4):377–390.

32. Trevino EG, Patwardhan AN, Henry MA, et al. Effect of irrigants on the survival of human stem cells of the apical papilla in a platelet-rich plasma scaffold in human root tips. *J Endod*. 2011;37(8):1109–1115.

33. Kim JH, Kim Y, Shin SJ, et al. Tooth discoloration of immature permanent incisor associated with triple antibiotic therapy: a case report. *J Endod*. 2010;36(6):1086–1091.

34. McTigue DJ, Subramanian K, Kumar A. Case series: management of immature permanent teeth with pulpal necrosis: a case series. *Pediatr Dent*. 2013;35(1):55–60.

35. Bose R, Nummikoski P, Hargreaves K. A retrospective evaluation of radiographic outcomes in immature teeth with necrotic root canal systems treated with regenerative endodontic procedures. *J Endod*. 2009;35(10):1343–1349.

36. Bertolami CN, Kaban LB. Chin trauma: a clue to associated mandibular and cervical spine injury. *Oral Surg Oral Med Oral Pathol*. 1982;53(2):122–126.

37. Bender IB, Freedland JB. Clinical considerations in the diagnosis and treatment of intra-alveolar root fractures. *J Am Dent Assoc*. 1983;107(4):595–600.

38. Cvek M, Andreasen JO, Borum MK. Healing of 208 intra-alveolar root fractures in patients aged 7-17 years. *Dent Traumatol*. 2001;17(2):53–62.

39. Andreasen JO, Andreasen FM, Mejare I, et al. Healing of 400 intra-alveolar root fractures. 2. Effect of treatment factors such as treatment delay, repositioning, splinting type and period and antibiotics. *Dent Traumatol*. 2004;20(4):203–211.

40. Andreasen FM. Pulpal healing after luxation injuries and root fracture in the permanent dentition. *Endod Dent Traumatol*. 1989;5(3):111–131.

41. Oginni AO, Adekoya-Sofowora CA, Kolawole KA. Evaluation of radiographs, clinical signs and symptoms associated with pulp canal obliteration: an aid to treatment decision. *Dent Traumatol*. 2009;25(6):620–625.

42. Tronstad L. Root resorption—etiology, terminology and clinical manifestations. *Endod Dent Traumatol*. 1988;4(6):241–252.

43. Tsilingaridis G, Malmgren B, Andreasen JO, et al. Intrusive luxation of 60 permanent incisors: a retrospective study of treatment and outcome. *Dent Traumatol*. 2012;28(6):416–422.

44. Andreasen JO, Hjorting-Hansen E. Replantation of teeth. I. Radiographic and clinical study of 110 human teeth replanted after accidental loss. *Acta Odontol Scand*. 1966;24(3):263–286.

45. Hiltz J, Trope M. Vitality of human lip fibroblasts in milk, Hanks balanced salt solution and Viaspan storage media. *Endod Dent Traumatol*. 1991;7(2):69–72.

46. Krasner P, Person P. Preserving avulsed teeth for replantation. *J Am Dent Assoc.* 1992;123(11):80–88.

47. Blomlof L. Storage of human periodontal ligament cells in a combination of different media. *J Dent Res.* 1981;60(11):1904–1906.

48. Sigalas E, Regan JD, Kramer PR, et al. Survival of human periodontal ligament cells in media proposed for transport of avulsed teeth. *Dent Traumatol.* 2004;20(1):21–28.

49. Lekic PC, Kenny DJ, Barrett EJ. The influence of storage conditions on the clonogenic capacity of periodontal ligament cells: implications for tooth replantation. *Int Endod J.* 1998;31(2):137–140.

50. Hinckfuss SE, Messer LB. An evidence-based assessment of the clinical guidelines for replanted avulsed teeth. Part II: prescription of systemic antibiotics. *Dent Traumatol.* 2009;25(2):158–164.

51. Andreasen JO, Borum MK, Jacobsen HL, et al. Replantation of 400 avulsed permanent incisors. 2. Factors related to pulpal healing. *Endod Dent Traumatol.* 1995;11(2):59–68.

52. Andreasen JO, Borum MK, Andreasen FM. Replantation of 400 avulsed permanent incisors. 3. Factors related to root growth. *Endod Dent Traumatol.* 1995;11(2):69–75.

53. Hammarstrom L, Pierce A, Blomlof L, et al. Tooth avulsion and replantation—a review. *Endod Dent Traumatol.* 1986;2(1):1–8.

54. Sae-Lim V, Wang CY, Trope M. Effect of systemic tetracycline and amoxicillin on inflammatory root resorption of replanted dogs' teeth. *Endod Dent Traumatol.* 1998;14(5):216–220.

55. Coccia CT. A clinical investigation of root resorption rates in reimplanted young permanent incisors: a five-year study. *J Endod.* 1980;6(1):413–420.

36

Treatment Planning and Management of Orthodontic Problems

JOHN R. CHRISTENSEN, HENRY FIELDS, AND ROSE D. SHEATS

When considering treatment for problems during the mixed-dentition years, the precise problem and the goals of treatment must be clearly in mind. Few problems will receive definitive or complete treatment at this stage of development, although some simple and isolated dental problems may be resolved. As described in previous chapters, information regarding the patient's problems is gathered through an interview of the patient and the parents and a clinical examination. The clinician reviews the information and develops a list of goals for treatment. The goals should address functional and esthetic concerns of the patient and the clinician. After the goals of treatment have been established, a list of orthodontic problems is generated from the clinical database and the problems are ranked in order from most to least severe.[1]

After the problem list has been generated and each problem has been ranked in order of severity, possible solutions to each problem should be listed. The solution list should be comprehensive; that is, all reasonable solutions should be considered for each specific problem without regard for the other problems. After the solution list has been constructed, the clinician looks for similar solutions listed for more than one problem. In some cases the best solution for one problem is the best solution for all problems, and

the treatment plan is easily derived. Unfortunately, in most cases a solution for one problem is not the solution for the others and, worse, may magnify the second problem. The treatment plan should reflect the goals of treatment established by the clinician. Treatment planning is not entirely scientific and clinical wisdom is needed to determine a plan in these cases.

The clinician is trained to identify functional and esthetic problems, so the problem list does not always match the concerns of the parent and child. When the clinician presents the problem list and treatment plan, these concerns should be listened to carefully because they may dictate treatment direction and treatment satisfaction outcomes. Often the motivation for treatment can be elicited from these concerns. If the child patient desires to have treatment, cooperation will usually be good during treatment and little parental support will be necessary. This is called internal motivation. External motivation, motivation supplied by the parent for treatment, will require continuous parental support to successfully complete treatment. If the chief complaint or reason for seeking treatment ranks low on the treatment priority list or will be addressed later in the treatment plan, an explanation should be provided to the child and parent to justify this situation.

Skeletal Problems

Orthodontic problems in the preadolescent patient are generally thought of as either dental or skeletal in origin. The complexity of these problems varies tremendously. Many dental problems are well within the treatment domain of the general practitioner. Skeletal problems, as diagnosed from the facial profile analysis and confirmed by supplemental means, are best managed by a specialist. However, the general practitioner should understand how skeletal discrepancies are treated.

There are three basic alternatives for treating skeletal discrepancies: growth modification, camouflage, and orthognathic surgery. Growth modification is a means to change skeletal relationships by using the patient's remaining growth to alter the size or position of the jaws. Camouflage and orthognathic surgery usually are considered for adolescent patients with minimal or no growth remaining or nongrowing adult patients. Camouflage orthodontic treatment is aimed at hiding a mild skeletal discrepancy by moving teeth within the jaws so the teeth fit together. The skeletal discrepancy still exists, but it is disguised by a compensated occlusion and acceptable facial esthetics. Orthognathic surgery places the jaws and teeth in a normal or near-normal position using surgical procedures and presurgical and postsurgical orthodontic treatment.[2] For the mixed-dentition patient, only growth modification or no treatment is a reasonable choice for skeletal intervention.

Growth modification during the early mixed-dentition years rests on several assumptions that are not as clear as many would presume. First, a child must be growing for the growth to be modified. Most normal children in the 6- to 12-year age group are actively growing, and their faces are also growing. Furthermore, clinicians have thought that it is easiest to correct skeletal problems if a child is undergoing maximal facial growth during treatment. Although the data to support this contention are not voluminous or clear,[3] clinicians have long sought to predict maximum somatic growth and maximal facial growth from other indicators. There appears to be wide variation in the amount of facial growth occurring at one time and an equally wide variation in the correlation of facial growth with overall body growth and other indicators that have been chosen.[4-6] Because of this state of inaccuracy, the clinician should use as many indicators as possible (personal growth history, skeletal growth maturation, secondary sexual characteristics, onset of menarche) to make an educated decision about whether the child is growing at an acceptable rate. Girls tend to enter the adolescent growth spurt as defined by obvious somatic growth at approximately 10 years and boys at approximately 12 years.

The data are not totally clear that one must treat children when they are at a certain rate of facial growth to be successful, and experience has shown most skeletal and dental problems can be managed in one phase during the transition from the mixed to permanent dentitions. For these reasons a single stage of orthodontic treatment is most popular and adequately effective. This enables practitioners to successfully manage most problems in a more mature patient who is both reasonably cooperative and compliant. Asynchrony between dental development and rapid facial growth may create a situation in which the patient may be ready for growth modification but not for orthodontic dental treatment, or vice versa. These patients must be handled individually by balancing the dental and skeletal interventions. Similarly, some patients have compelling problems that demand earlier treatment, as described later.

The second assumption made when growth modification is undertaken is that the practitioner can accurately diagnose the source of the skeletal discrepancy and design treatment that will apply the appropriate amount and direction of force to correct the discrepancy. Diagnosis is not an exact science and may be confusing even with the use of cephalometric measures,[7] and the discrepancy may be due to several small skeletal problems rather than one easily identified discrepancy. It is important to remember that not all class II or class III malocclusions are created equal or have only one skeletal feature at fault. Force delivery to dental and skeletal structures also is inexact, and the clinical impression and treatment response may dictate alteration in the amount and direction of force applied to modify growth. Certainly orthodontic treatment for skeletal problems is not just a "see it" and "fix it" situation.

Third, growth modification is usually only one portion of a treatment plan. Most appliances used to modify growth (e.g., headgears and functional appliances) are designed to alter skeletal structures rather than precisely move teeth. Although the appliances can cause tooth movement, they are not as precise as fixed orthodontic appliances (braces) and usually are used before or in conjunction with fixed appliances. Therefore most growth modification treatments are followed immediately or later by traditional fixed orthodontic appliances to move the teeth into a final position.

There are several theories offered to explain how growth modification works to achieve the desired results. The first theory suggests that growth modification appliances change the absolute size of one or both jaws. For example, a class II skeletal profile may be treated by making a deficient mandible larger to fit a normal-sized maxilla or by limiting the size of an oversized maxilla. Some clinical data show dramatic size changes, but there appears to be large variability in patient response to growth-modifying appliances, with modest changes in various structures being the rule rather than the exception.

Alternatively, growth modification may work by accelerating the desired growth but not changing the ultimate size or shape of the jaw. A deficient mandible may not end up larger than it ultimately would have been, but it may achieve its final size sooner. This requires the clinician to make some final dentoalveolar changes or compensations to establish an ideal occlusion following growth modification. This type of growth modification response also shows large individual variability. There is support for this interpretation of growth modification based on recent randomized clinical trials that demonstrate little difference between an early- and a late-treatment group of patients with skeletal class II malocclusion.[8]

A third possibility is that growth modification may work by changing the spatial relationship of the two jaws. The ultimate size of the jaw and its rate of growth are not changed, but by modifying the orientation of the jaws to each other a more balanced profile may result. For example, a convex profile and an increased lower facial height could be made more proportional to each other if the vertical growth of the maxilla could be inhibited and the mandible allowed to rotate upward and forward. The profile would then become less convex and the vertical relations more ideal. Jaw reorientation would be successful in a concave class III patient with a short face if the mandible could be rotated downward and backward (more vertical) to create a more acceptable profile. Reorientation does not work well in class II short faces or class III long faces because correcting one problem (e.g., the vertical) makes the other problem (e.g., the anteroposterior) worse. A recent meta-analysis review offered the following conclusions on growth modification with functional appliances: (1) functional appliances can accelerate forward growth of the mandible in the prepubertal and adolescent growth stages, (2) functional appliances restrain maxillary growth, and (3) functional appliances correct class II malocclusion with dental and skeletal changes.[9]

As you can see, growth modification is at best inexact. From the best available data, it appears that if a patient is growing, on average, modest skeletal changes can be accomplished during the mixed-dentition years. These are reasonably comparable if attempted early or late in this period of development. It may be advisable to attempt these changes during the earlier mixed-dentition years if patients have esthetic complaints or if they are trauma prone.

A number of studies have demonstrated early orthodontic treatment has a positive benefit on a patient's self-esteem and a reduction in negative social encounters.[10,11] However, there are some questions about early treatment and patient quality of life. Although it appears that orthodontic treatment has been found to enhance some aspects of quality of life (especially esthetics), it does not necessarily change social acceptance. In addition, treatment does not seem to improve oral health status or oral function compared with untreated populations.[12]

A Cochrane review on early orthodontic treatment and trauma prevention indicated there was a reduction in dental trauma, although there was a great deal of uncertainty regarding this finding.[13] Other studies question whether early treatment provides a protective benefit to incisal trauma.[14] A prudent approach may be to consider each individual patient and assess their psychosocial well-being and their risk factors for trauma. Otherwise, conventional late mixed-dentition treatment appears to be just as sensible.

Growth Modification Applied to Anteroposterior Problems

Anteroposterior skeletal problems are class II and class III in nature. However, these descriptions are not very informative because the source of the discrepancy may be the maxilla, the mandible, or a combination of the two. Therefore the first step in patient evaluation is to identify the source of the problem and then design a treatment plan to resolve the problem. Although this approach appears to indicate that these problems are clearly identifiable and treatable with concise approaches, the previous discussion makes it clear that this is not the case. In many moderately severe cases of anteroposterior problems, a number of approaches may work that rely more on patient compliance than clinical expertise.

Class II Growth Modification

A class II malocclusion is the result of maxillary protrusion, mandibular retrusion, or a combination of both. Class II maxillary protrusion has been managed by headgear therapy to restrict or redirect maxillary growth on the basis of retrospective studies and randomized clinical trials.[8,9] Headgear places a distal force on the maxillary dentition and the maxilla (Fig. 36.1). Theoretically, the relative movement of dental and skeletal structures depends on the amount and time of force application. In actual practice, it is probably not possible to move selectively only teeth or bones.[9] In general, skeletal and tooth movement are greater with higher forces, but tooth movement can occur with either heavy or light forces. One approach is to apply forces ranging from 12 to 16 ounces per side for 12 to 14 hours and monitor the skeletal and dental changes and adjust accordingly. The skeletal and dental response varies according to the type of headgear chosen and the resultant direction of force exerted by the headgear. The most common varieties, cervical and high pull, provide predominantly distal and

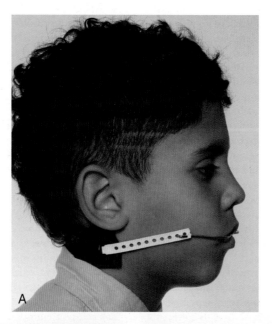

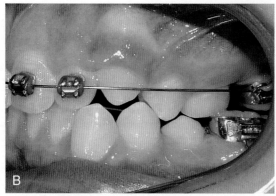

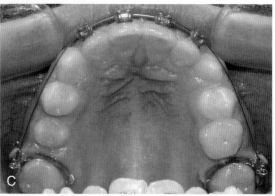

• **Figure 36.1** The class II maxillary–protrusive patient is best treated by headgear therapy to restrict or redirect maxillary growth. (A) This patient is being treated with cervical headgear that places a distal and extrusive force on both maxillary skeletal and dental structures. The force is provided by a neck strap attached to the outer bows of the headgear. (B) The molar relationship is beginning to approach a class III dental position. (C) Space is beginning to open up between the second primary molar and the first permanent molar. This type of change is not apparent for every patient because the amount of growth and the amount of cooperation can vary from patient to patient.

occlusal and distal and apical forces, respectively. Traditionally, one avoids using a headgear that tends to extrude posterior teeth in a person with a long face or a limited overbite. On the other hand, a headgear that extrudes the molars is often useful in a patient with a short face and a deep bite.

Class II maxillary protrusion can also be managed with a removable functional appliance of the activator, bionator, or twin block type (Fig. 36.2). Although a functional appliance is primarily designed to stimulate mandibular growth, studies have indicated there are secondary effects of restricting forward maxillary skeletal and dental movement.[8,15,16] This happens because the mandible, which is postured forward, tends to return to a more distal position as a result of the distal muscle and soft tissue forces. The distal force is transmitted through the appliance to the maxilla and the maxillary teeth. The maxillary teeth tend to tip lingually rather than to move bodily while the mandibular teeth tip facially.

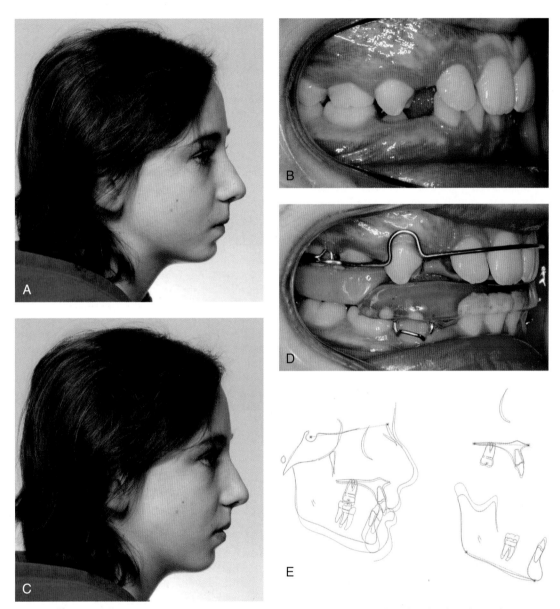

• **Figure 36.2** The class II mandibular–deficient patient is usually treated with a functional appliance that positions the mandible forward in an attempt to stimulate, accelerate, or redirect mandibular growth. (A) This patient has a class II mandibular–deficient profile. (B) The patient's molar and canine relationships reflect the skeletal class II relationship. (C) The profile is immediately improved when the functional appliance is in place because the mandible is pushed forward into a class I relationship. (D) Because functional appliances (a twin block in this case) position the mandible forward using the upper and lower dental arches, there may be movement of the upper and lower teeth. Dental aspects of the malocclusion must be considered during treatment planning. (E) In this case the patient wore an appliance similar to that shown in (D) for approximately 1 year. In the overall superimposition the blue lines show there was slightly more change in the anteroposterior position of the mandible than in the maxilla. The maxillary superimposition shows the vertical position of the teeth was well controlled. In the mandibular superimposition, it is evident the patient grew favorably. In addition, the mesial and vertical eruption of the lower molar helped to change the dental relationship to class I.

Another functional appliance is the Herbst appliance, which is a fixed appliance used to reposition the mandible forward. It is held in place with bands, stainless steel crowns, bonding, or a cemented cast framework (Fig. 36.3). A pin and tube apparatus forces the mandible forward and places constant force on the maxilla and maxillary and mandibular teeth as the mandible attempts to return to a normal and more distal posture. Maxillary teeth tend to move distally and mandibular anterior teeth move forward. This appliance has shown changes similar to those of functional appliances in randomized clinical trials.[17] The use of temporary anchorage devices (TADs) combined with the Herbst appliance may reduce some of the lower incisor tooth movement.[18]

If the class II malocclusion is due to a mandibular deficiency, treatment options focus on changing the mandibular position. The mandibular-deficient patient is usually treated with a removable or fixed functional appliance that positions the mandible forward in an attempt to stimulate or accelerate mandibular growth. Retrospective clinical studies have shown that these appliances can produce a small average increase in mandibular projection (2 to 4 mm/year).[19,20] This has been confirmed by randomized clinical trials.[8,21] Patient response varies greatly, and in many cases the increased growth does not totally correct the class II skeletal problem for several reasons. First, the amount of growth is not enough to overcome the discrepancy. Second, all the available growth would have to be specifically directed to produce anteroposterior change. This is usually not the case because some dental eruption and vertical growth occurs. This interaction between anteroposterior and vertical dimensional changes decreases ultimate mandibular projection and class II correction because the mandible grows downward and forward and not straight forward. The rest of the anteroposterior discrepancy is managed by restricting maxillary growth, tipping the maxillary teeth back, and tipping the mandibular teeth forward. Different appliances can be designed that exaggerate the secondary responses of maxillary restriction and dental movement if desired. The Herbst appliance, mentioned previously, also has been used with mandibular-deficient patients. Some studies also indicate that headgear treatment may cause an increase in mandibular growth.[21,22] In general, a review of class II treatments shows headgears and functional appliances are equally effective in treating the class II malocclusion.[23] It appears a headgear has a small restrictive influence on maxillary position, whereas functional appliances move B point forward leading to an ANB improvement of approximately 1 degree with either approach. A large portion of the change is dental in nature; headgears influence maxillary molar position distal, whereas functional appliances tend to move the lower molar mesial and procline the lower incisors.

Class III Growth Modification

Similar to class II malocclusions, a change in the position of the maxilla, the mandible, or both results in a class III malocclusion. The first possibility is a small maxilla. True midface deficiency can be treated by using a reverse-pull headgear or facemask to exert anteriorly directed force on the maxilla (Fig. 36.4).[24] The facemask applies force to the maxilla through an appliance (either a removable splint or fixed appliance) attached to the teeth; tooth movement also occurs. Some clinicians use the facemask with maxillary expansion (either rapid or slow) to enhance the transverse coordination of the arches and to facilitate anterior movement of the maxilla due to alteration of the bony interfaces with other skeletal structures. A comparison of clinical studies found that less maxillary incisor movement occurs when expansion accompanies protraction.[25] One prospective study found no difference between the expansion and nonexpansion approaches.[26]

Another approach is to use a facemask with miniplates attached to the maxilla. This method can be used in the late mixed dentition, probably at approximately 10 to 11 years of age, and shows greater skeletal change and movement in the zygomatic area as well.[27] Finally, miniplates can be attached to the maxilla and mandible, and intraoral elastics can be used at approximately the same age. This has the effect of substantial change with no need for an extraoral appliance, which means the elastic force can be used continuously.[28]

Timing of this treatment has been controversial. Some authors believe that the ideal time to attempt this treatment is soon after eruption of the permanent incisors, whereas others have waited a bit longer. Clearly, postpubertal treatment is not indicated for growth modification.[29] Data indicate that there is little anteroposterior difference in treatment effect whether treatment is applied early or late, if the treatment is completed before 10 to 11 years of age.[30,31] Unfortunately, the long-term success of maxillary protraction is not clear. One fact appears to be emerging: mistaken diagnosis or treatment in patients whose class III malocclusion is the result of mandibular protrusion will usually fail. Even with those who are correctly diagnosed, one in four will require additional treatment to correct the skeletal malocclusion.[32]

Functional appliances designed to stimulate maxillary growth do not seem to be effective. The improvement in facial profile obtained by using these appliances in patients with very minor class III problems is usually the result of a downward and backward rotation of the mandible. The occlusion improves because of facial tipping of the maxillary incisors and lingual tipping of the lower incisors.

Class III mandibular protrusion has been historically managed with chin cup therapy (Fig. 36.5). The theory of chin cup therapy is to apply a distal and superior force through the chin that inhibits or redirects growth at the condyle. Again, studies in animals have

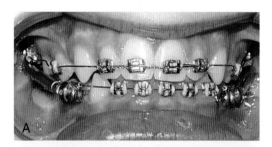
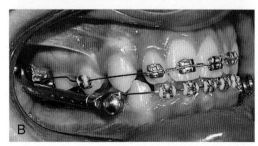

• **Figure 36.3** The Herbst appliance is a fixed appliance that uses a pin and tube apparatus to reposition the mandible into a more forward position. (A) This class II patient demonstrates correction to a near class I occlusion. (B) Used in conjunction with fixed appliances, some of the dental effects can be more readily controlled.

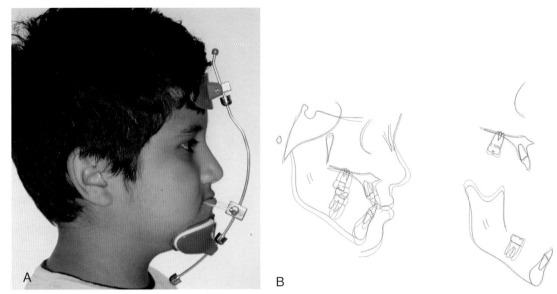

• **Figure 36.4** (A) The class III maxillary–deficient patient is treated by using a reverse pull headgear or facemask to exert anteriorly directed force on the maxilla. The force is provided by rubber bands extending from the facemask to intraoral hooks or wires. (B) These superimpositions show a successful case in treating a case of class III maxillary deficiency. The overall superimposition shows the maxilla has been moved forward to a greater extent than the mandible. The mandible was rotated down and backward somewhat, which helped with the anteroposterior change in the skeletal relations. There was little change in tooth position in both the maxillary and mandibular superimpositions, which suggests most of the change was skeletal in nature.

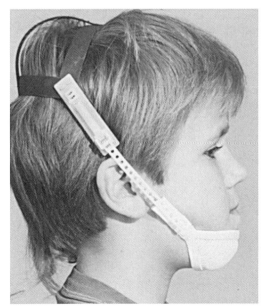

• **Figure 36.5** The class III mandibular–protrusive patient has historically been treated with chin cup therapy. The chin cup was designed to apply a distal and superior force through the chin to inhibit growth at the condyle. In clinical practice, this device has not been proven to be routinely successful, although chin cup therapy does cause a distal rotation of the mandible. Therefore the chin cup may be useful for managing mild mandibular protrusion in which the vertical proportions are short to normal.

shown some change in absolute mandibular size, but clinical application in humans routinely has been less successful.[33,34] The typical short-term treatment response to chin cup therapy is a distal rotation of the mandible and lingual tipping of the lower incisors. Therefore chin cup therapy is well tolerated in patients with mild mandibular protrusion and short to normal vertical proportions. However, it is contraindicated in a person with a long lower face, because the anteroposterior correction would come at the expense of an increased vertical dimension. The long-term results of chin cup therapy indicate that, although a transient positive change can occur, the long-term results are difficult to differentiate from those in untreated patients.[31]

In summary, treatment of class III malocclusion in the mixed dentition is based on the diagnosis of maxillary deficiency or mandibular excess. In cases of mandibular excess the clinician can choose between a chin cup or a class III type functional appliance. Both have been shown to restrict mandibular growth but have little influence on maxillary position.[35] Treatment is recommended before age 10. In maxillary deficient patients a reverse pull headgear can move the maxilla forward. If the headgear is attached to the maxillary teeth, there is some proclination of the upper incisors as well as downward and backward rotation of the mandible. This results in an increased lower anterior facial height.[35] If treatment is delayed until the late mixed dentition when permanent teeth have erupted to a point where bone miniplates can be placed, a combination of upper and lower miniplates with continuous intermaxillary elastic traction has been shown to stimulate upper jaw growth and restrain lower jaw growth without dental compensations.[28] The issue seems to be the variable response from patient to patient. It is very difficult to predict how one individual will react to class III growth modification.

Growth Modification Applied to Transverse Problems

The most common transverse problem in the preadolescent is maxillary constriction with a posterior crossbite. Management of maxillary constriction can begin as soon as the problem is discovered if the child is mature enough to accept treatment. Treatment has the potential to eliminate crossbites of the permanent teeth, increase arch length, and simplify future diagnostic decisions complicated by functional shifts. Most clinicians agree with the philosophy of early correction if there is a mandibular shift. In general, it is believed that long-term facial asymmetry attributable to soft tissue enlargement and in some cases mandibular asymmetry can result from untreated mandibular shifts.[36] Regardless of philosophy, treatment before adolescence and midpalatal suture bridging is recommended.

Three appliances can be used to correct the constriction, but the appliances are not interchangeable. In Chapter 28 the quad helix and the W arch for management of maxillary constriction are described. The appliances provide both skeletal and dental movement in the 3- to 6-year-old child.[37] As the patient gets older, more dental change and less skeletal change occur. This is true because the midpalatal suture, which was open at an early age, has developed bone interdigitation that makes it difficult to separate. More force is required to separate the suture after initial interdigitation of the suture to obtain true skeletal correction than a quad helix or W arch can deliver.

In the older preadolescent patient, in whom there is a chance that the midpalatal suture is closed, an appliance that can deliver large amounts of force is necessary to correct the skeletal constriction.[38] Rapid palatal expansion is the term given to the procedure in which an appliance cemented or bonded to the teeth is opened 0.5 mm/day to deliver 2000 to 3000 g of force (Fig. 36.6). In the active phase of treatment, there is a change in the inclination of the anchor teeth but little dental movement because the periodontal ligament has been hyalinized, which limits dental movement, and the force is transmitted almost entirely to the skeletal structures. However, during retention, the skeletal structures begin to relapse toward the midline. Because the teeth are held rigidly by the appliance, they move relative to the bones. Depending on the amount of expansion needed, active treatment normally takes 10 to 14 days. Another approach to skeletal expansion is slow rather than rapid palatal expansion.[39] Essentially the same appliance is used as in rapid palatal expansion, although force levels are calibrated to provide only 900 to 1300 g of force. Coupled with a slower activation rate, slow palatal expansion widens the palate by dental and skeletal movement. Although the final position of the teeth and supporting structures is approximately the same in rapid and slow expansion, proponents of slow expansion maintain that slower expansion is more physiologic and stable. There is some evidence that both rapid and slow maxillary expansion can result in loss of buccal bone (height and thickness).[40] These findings are from cone beam computed tomography (CBCT) and should be viewed with some caution due to the resolution of the image.

Transverse growth modification also can be accomplished by means of acrylic or wire buccal shields attached to functional appliances or lip bumpers. The buccal shields relieve the teeth and alveolar structures from the resting pressure of the cheek muscles and soft tissues. Transverse expansion of 3 to 5 mm can be achieved, although the changes vary considerably. Whether the movement is dental or skeletal and whether it will remain stable are still in

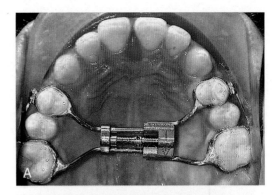

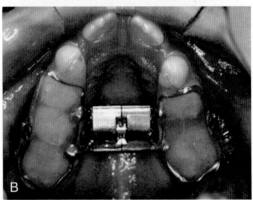

• **Figure 36.6** Rapid palatal expansion is used to treat maxillary constriction and posterior crossbite when there is a chance that the midpalatal suture is partially closed. The jackscrew in the appliance provides approximately 2000 to 3000 g of force when it is opened 0.5 mm/day. Depending on the amount of expansion needed, the appliance is normally activated two times each day for 10 days to 2 weeks. The appliance can be either cemented on the teeth with orthodontic bands (A) or bonded to the teeth (B).

question because there are no controlled experimental studies to provide answers.

Transverse expansion is accomplished by passive or active movement of teeth. Acrylic or wire buccal shields remove lip and cheek pressure to allow movement of both maxillary and mandibular teeth. Active expansion is performed with either a W arch–type appliance or a screw-type appliance. The decision to use one appliance or another is based on the age of the patient (an indirect measure of the interdigitation of the palatal suture) and the amount of expansion required. Studies seem to indicate there is less risk for buccal alveolar bone change if the movement is completed at a younger age rather than the complete permanent dentition.

Growth Modification Applied to Vertical Problems

Vertical skeletal problems are manifested as long and short facial heights and usually are located below the palatal plane.[41] The short-faced person has a reduced mandibular plane angle and undererupted teeth. In the long-faced patient the mandibular plane angle, lower facial height, and amount of dental eruption are increased in comparison with the patient with a normal face. Vertical skeletal problems can be managed with growth modification techniques, and some can be managed successfully; however, even when the treatment has been successful, maintaining the correction is extremely difficult. The face grows vertically for a long time, and there is a tendency for the original growth pattern and problem to recur.

Vertical Excess

Vertical skeletal excess may be managed with extraoral force or intraoral force. Extraoral force is delivered by means of a high-pull headgear through the maxillary first molars. The force is applied in a superior and distal direction and is designed to inhibit vertical development of the maxilla and eruption of the posterior maxillary teeth (Fig. 36.7).[42] Because no force is applied to the mandibular teeth, they are free to erupt and compensate for the reduced vertical development in the maxilla. In some cases, this compensatory eruption can eliminate all the positive effects of the high-pull headgear and lead to downward and backward rotation of the mandible instead of forward mandibular projection.

An alternative method for controlling vertical development is to block the eruption of the maxillary and mandibular teeth. A functional appliance can be designed that will force the mandible open to an increased vertical rest position. The force of the mandible attempting to return to its original vertical rest position is transmitted to the maxilla and the teeth in both arches. This results in mandibular growth being directed forward because no dental eruption has occurred to increase the vertical dimension with less growth in lower and total face height (Fig. 36.8).[43] TADs may prove to be of value in restricting vertical facial development. TADs are small-diameter titanium screws placed into cortical bone. They do not osseointegrate, so they can be removed after use. TADs provide the clinician with an anchor to apply force to teeth without causing other teeth to move because the screw is in bone. In theory, the screws should not move, although it appears they do move with force application. In cases of vertical excess, TADs are placed to provide an intrusive force to the maxillary posterior teeth.[44] However, placing TADs in the mixed dentition patient is more difficult because there are unerupted teeth in the way of insertion and the cortical bone does not hold the implant as well

before approximately 12 years of age. An alternative is to place the TADs in the palate, where there is better retention of the TAD. Regardless of the means used to manage vertical excess, excellent patient cooperation is necessary because treatment must be continued or retained as long as the patient is growing.

Vertical Deficiency

Vertical skeletal deficiencies can be managed with either headgear or functional appliances, depending on the accompanying antero-posterior relationships. The force vector from the headgear should direct the maxilla distally and extrude the maxillary posterior teeth, which would require cervical pull headgear. Because functional appliances are typically designed to inhibit eruption of upper and lower anterior teeth and promote eruption of the posterior teeth, they can also increase vertical facial height (Fig. 36.9). In addition, because there is a component of forward or mesial movement of teeth as they erupt, an astute clinician will encourage lower molar eruption in class II cases (lower molar moves forward into class I) and upper molar eruption in class III cases. As in vertical skeletal excess, the original growth pattern tends to recur until growth is complete, and retention should be designed to prevent this recurrence.

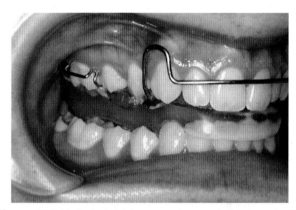

• **Figure 36.8** Vertical skeletal excess also can be managed with a functional appliance designed to inhibit eruption of the maxillary and mandibular teeth. The appliance is constructed so that the mandible is placed in an open posture at an increased vertical position. The force of the mandible attempting to return to its normal, more closed vertical position is transmitted to the maxilla and to the teeth in both arches.

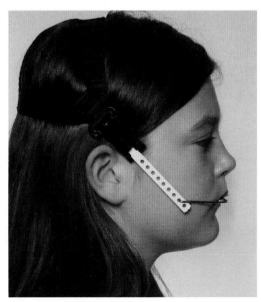

• **Figure 36.7** The patient with vertical skeletal excess is often treated with high-pull headgear. The force, generated by the strap resting on the head, is applied in a superior and distal direction and is intended to inhibit vertical development of the maxilla and eruption of the maxillary posterior teeth.

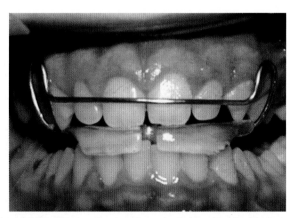

• **Figure 36.9** This functional appliance is designed to allow the posterior teeth to erupt and, in this class II patient, drift anteriorly and aid in correction of the dental relationship. This type of appliance can open the bite and increase the dental and skeletal vertical dimensions.

SLEEP DISORDERED BREATHING

Rose D. Sheats

Children 6 to 12 years old should sleep 9 to 12 hours per day to promote optimal health.[1] One condition to be considered in children who sleep less than this amount is pediatric sleep disordered breathing (SDB). SDB consists of partial or complete obstruction of the upper airway during sleep which manifests itself as increased respiratory effort, fragmented sleep, oxygen desaturation, and hypercapnia. It comprises a spectrum of conditions ranging from snoring, hypoventilation, and obstructive sleep apnea. The diagnosis must be made by a physician, but pediatric dentists can aid in the recognition of and screening for this medical condition. Children suspected of suffering from SDB should be referred to their pediatrician, a pediatric sleep specialist, or an otolaryngologist.

Pediatric SDB occurs in 1%–5% of children,[2–4] but the increasing prevalence of childhood overweight and obesity is likely to portend an increase in the incidence of pediatric SDB.[5] In addition to obesity, other risk factors for pediatric SDB include snoring, preterm birth, African American race, male gender, and the presence of enlarged tonsils and adenoids.[6] Specific craniofacial features such as narrow maxillary width and mandibular retrognathia have also been associated with pediatric SDB, although such findings are not consistently supported by data.

Several syndromes with craniofacial components are associated with increased risk for SDB. Children with Down syndrome have an especially high risk, with an estimated prevalence of 50%–80%.[7,8] Approximately one-third (34%) of syndromic children with cleft palate have SDB, whereas nonsyndromic cleft palate children have half that prevalence (17%).[9] Other conditions associated with increased risk for SDB include Pierre Robin sequence, Prader-Willi syndrome, sickle cell diseases, cerebral palsy, Chiari malformation, and neuromuscular conditions such as Duchenne muscular dystrophy, Guillain-Barré syndrome, and myotonic dystrophy.

SDB has been associated with pediatric nocturnal enuresis.[10–12] A proposed mechanism postulates that release of brain or atrial natriuretic peptides is increased because of cardiac wall distension secondary to the negative intrathoracic pressure caused by snoring or increased upper airway resistance. Other possible mechanisms include diminished arousal response or changes in bladder pressure as a consequence of SDB.

Signs and symptoms of SDB overlap those of attention-deficit/hyperactivity disorder (ADHD) and thus often result in misclassification of the disease or inappropriate management of the condition.[13] Classic signs and symptoms of SDB include snoring, difficulty waking up in the morning, inability to concentrate, irritability, and hyperactivity. Unlike adults, children do not often present with excessive daytime sleepiness.

Many cases of pediatric SDB remain undiagnosed or untreated. Risks of untreated pediatric SDB include adverse impacts on the neurocognitive, cardiovascular, and metabolic systems.[14,15] Childhood snoring was at one time considered benign, but evidence has been accumulating to suggest that it too is associated with cardiovascular and neurocognitive impairment.[16,17]

Findings from the Childhood Adenotonsillectomy Trial reveal spontaneous remission of SDB at the 7-month follow-up in nearly half of the 203 children aged 5 to 9 years assigned to the Watchful Waiting group (nontreatment).[18] However, it is important to note that in this study, children diagnosed with severe SDB were excluded from enrollment. As in other studies, the investigators identified obesity and African American race, as well as severity of baseline SDB, as risk factors for SDB at follow-up.

Screening for pediatric SDB should begin in the early mixed dentition years and should start with a careful medical history. Childhood obesity and reports of medication to manage attention-deficit disorder (ADD) or ADHD should alert the clinician to the possible risk of undiagnosed SDB. Clinicians should inquire about childhood snoring, nocturnal enuresis, and other behavioral features associated with both ADD/ADHD and SDB. Poor academic performance and disruptive behavior at school or at home may also be clues to the presence of pediatric SDB.

Questionnaires have been developed to screen for risk of pediatric SDB.[19] The most psychometrically rigorous questionnaire is the Pediatric Sleep Questionnaire which has been validated for children 2 to 18 years.[20] It consists of 22 questions that examine three domains: snoring, sleepiness, and behavior. A single global score suggests that the child is at either "low risk" or "high risk" for SDB. A "high-risk" score merits referral to medical colleagues for further evaluation.

Clinical examination should include an evaluation of the posterior airway space, especially with respect to tonsillar presence and size. Pediatric dentists are particularly well trained to assess and record tonsillar size using the Brodsky scale.[21] The presence of enlarged tonsils associated with signs or symptoms of SDB should initiate a referral to a pediatric sleep specialist or otolaryngologist for evaluation.

First line treatment for pediatric SDB is adenotonsillectomy (AT), but this does not lead to cure in all cases.[22] In otherwise healthy children, AT normalizes SDB in 74% of children, but success rates decrease in obese children and African American children.[18,23] Thus it is important to consider additional treatment options to resolve this condition in children with residual sleep disordered events. Although positive airway pressure is often the second line of treatment, poor adherence plagues this effective therapeutic modality. In addition, data suggest that positive airway pressure may have an adverse impact on craniofacial growth. A recent case-control study of positive airway pressure in syndromic children demonstrated a deleterious effect on maxillary growth.[24]

Pediatric dentists, in collaboration with the child's sleep physician, may be a valuable adjunct to the medical team managing SDB in the pediatric patient. The pediatric dentist's knowledge of craniofacial growth and development in this population is critical for examining potential treatment options. The clinician should monitor jaw growth in children undergoing treatment for SDB and discuss future treatment options, including potential need for orthognathic surgery.

Rapid maxillary expansion (RME) has been demonstrated to improve signs and symptoms of pediatric SDB,[25,26] but this treatment thus far has only been explored in those children with SDB who required expansion to correct maxillary transverse deficiency. In addition RME has also been demonstrated to ameliorate nocturnal enuresis.[27,28] However, caution should be exercised in recommending RME for children younger than 8 years, because anecdotal reports suggest this procedure may lead to nasal deformity.[29] Data are currently lacking to demonstrate the risks and benefits of offering maxillary expansion to young children, especially to those whose arch widths are coordinated.

Mandibular advancement devices have routinely been used in adults with obstructive sleep apnea to prevent the tongue from collapsing into the posterior airway space during sleep. Such appliances are used in orthodontics to manage skeletal and dental class II malocclusions in growing children but are not commonly used to treat SDB in children. Evidence is too limited and of poor quality to support their use at this time in the management of SDB in children in the mixed dentition.[30–33] Concerns include the unknown impact on craniofacial growth in class I and class III children, as well as the difficulty in device retention and treatment adherence during the tooth exchange period. Further research is needed to clarify the risks and benefits of mandibular advancement devices in the management of pediatric SDB in 6- to 12-year-olds.

SDB in the child patient has the potential to not only disrupt optimal sleep but can also to lead adverse neurocognitive, cardiovascular, and metabolic problems. Pediatric dentists are well positioned to screen for SDB in patients 6 to 12 years old, to make appropriate referrals when indicated, and to participate in the management of this condition when feasible.

References

1. Paruthi S, Brooks L, D'Ambrosio C, et al. Consensus Statement of the American Academy of sleep medicine on the recommended amount of

SLEEP DISORDERED BREATHING—cont'd

sleep for healthy children: methodology and discussion. *J Clin Sleep Med.* 2016;12:1549–1561.

2. Bixler E, Vgontzas A, Lin H, et al. Sleep disordered breathing in children in a general population sample: prevalence and risk factors. *Sleep.* 2009;32:731–736.

3. Rosen C, Larkin E, Kirchner H, et al. Prevalence and risk factors for sleep-disordered breathing in 8- to 11-year-old children: association with race and prematurity. *J Pediatr.* 2003;142:383–389.

4. Lumeng J, Chervin R. Epidemiology of pediatric obstructive sleep apnea. *Proc Am Thorac Soc.* 2008;5:242–252.

5. Arens R, Muzumdar H. Childhood obesity and obstructive sleep apnea syndrome. *J Appl Physiol.* 2010;108:436–444.

6. Katz E, D'Ambrosio CM. Pediatric obstructive sleep apnea syndrome. *Clin Chest Med.* 2010;31:221–234.

7. Southall D, Stebbens V, Mirza R, et al. Upper airway obstruction with hypoxaemia and sleep disruption in Down syndrome. *Dev Med Child Neurol.* 1987;29:734–742.

8. Maris M, Verhulst S, Wojciechowski M, et al. Sleep problems and obstructive sleep apnea in children with Down syndrome, an overwiew. *Int J Pediatr Otorhinolaryngol.* 2016;82:12–15.

9. Muntz H, Wilson M, Park A, et al. Sleep disordered breathing and obstructive sleep apnea in the cleft population. *Laryngoscope.* 2008;118:348–353.

10. Sans Capdevila O, Crabtree V, Kheirandish-Gozal L, et al. Increased morning brain natriuretic peptide levels in children with nocturnal enuresis and sleep-disordered breathing: a community-based study. *Pediatrics.* 2008;121:e1208–e1214.

11. Jeyakumar A, Rahman S, Armbrecht E, et al. The association between sleep-disordered breathing and enuresis in children. *Laryngoscope.* 2012;122:1873–1877.

12. Umlauf M, Chasens E. Sleep disordered breathing and nocturnal polyuria: nocturia and enuresis. *Sleep Med Rev.* 2003;7:403–411.

13. Owens J. Neurocognitive and behavioral impact of sleep disordered breathing in children. *Pediatr Pulmonol.* 2009;44:417–422.

14. Tan H, Gozal D, Kheirandish-Gozal L. Obstructive sleep apnea in children: a critical update. *Nat Sci Sleep.* 2013;5:109–123.

15. Amin R, Somers V, McConnell K, et al. Activity-adjusted 24-hour ambulatory blood pressure and cardiac remodeling in children with sleep disordered breathing. *Hypertension.* 2008;51:84–91.

16. Kennedy J, Blunden S, Hirte C, et al. Reduced neurocognition in children who snore. *Pediatr Pulmonol.* 2004;37:330–337.

17. Li A, Au C, Ho C, et al. Blood pressure is elevated in children with primary snoring. *J Pediatr.* 2009;155:362–368.e361.

18. Marcus C, Moore R, Rosen C, et al. A randomized trial of adenotonsillectomy for childhood sleep apnea. *N Engl J Med.* 2013;368:2366–2376.

19. De Luca Canto G, Singh V, Major M, et al. Diagnostic capability of questionnaires and clinical examinations to assess sleep-disordered breathing in children: a systematic review and meta-analysis. *J Am Dent Assoc.* 2014;145:165–178.

20. Chervin RD, Hedger K, Dillon JE, et al. Pediatric sleep questionnaire (PSQ): validity and reliability of scales for sleep-disordered breathing, snoring, sleepiness, and behavioral problems. *Sleep Med.* 2000;1:21–32.

21. Brodsky L. Modern assessment of tonsils and adenoids. *Pediatr Clin North Am.* 1989;36:1551–1569.

22. Brietzke S, Gallagher D. The effectiveness of tonsillectomy and adenoidectomy in the treatment of pediatric obstructive sleep apnea/hypopnea syndrome: a meta-analysis. *Otolaryngol Head Neck Surg.* 2006;134:979–984.

23. Friedman M, Wilson M, Lin H, et al. Updated systematic review of tonsillectomy and adenoidectomy for treatment of pediatric obstructive sleep apnea/hypopnea syndrome. *Otolaryngol Head Neck Surg.* 2009;140:800–808.

24. Roberts S, Kapadia H, Greenlee G, et al. Midfacial and dental changes associated with nasal positive airway pressure in children with obstructive sleep apnea and craniofacial conditions. *J Clin Sleep Med.* 2016;12:469–475.

25. Pirelli P, Saponara M, Guilleminault C. Rapid maxillary expansion in children with obstructive sleep apnea syndrome. *Sleep.* 2004;27:761–766.

26. Villa M, Rizzoli A, Miano S, et al. Efficacy of rapid maxillary expansion in children with obstructive sleep apnea syndrome: 36 months of follow-up. *Sleep Breath.* 2015;15:179–184.

27. Bazargani F, Jonson-Ring I, Neveus T. Rapid maxillary expansion in therapy-resistant enuretic children: an orthodontic perspective. *Angle Orthod.* 2016;86:481–486.

28. Schutz-Fransson U, Kurol J. Rapid maxillary expansion effects on nocturnal enuresis in children: a follow-up study. *Angle Orthod.* 2008;78:201–208.

29. Proffit WR, Fields HW, Sarver DM. *Contemporary Orthodontics.* 5th ed. St Louis: Mosby–Year Book; 2012.

30. Carvalho FR, Lentini-Oliveira DA, Prado LB, et al. Oral appliances and functional orthopaedic appliances for obstructive sleep apnoea in children. *Cochrane Database Syst Rev.* 2016;(10):CD005520.

31. Nazarali N, Altalibi M, Nazarali S, et al. Mandibular advancement appliances for the treatment of paediatric obstructive sleep apnea: a systematic review. *Eur J Orthod.* 2015;37:618–626.

32. Villa MP, Bernkopf E, Pagani J, et al. Randomized controlled study of an oral jaw-positioning appliance for the treatment of obstructive sleep apnea in children with malocclusion. *Am J Respir Crit Care Med.* 2002;165:123–127.

33. Huynh NT, Desplats E, Almeida FR. Orthodontics treatments for managing obstructive sleep apnea syndrome in children: a systematic review and meta-analysis. *Sleep Med Rev.* 2016;25:84–94.

Dental Problems

Space Maintenance

A philosophy for space maintenance and the appliances recommended for the primary dentition are discussed in Chapter 26. The same philosophy and appliances apply to space maintenance in the 6- to 12-year-old age group. However, treatment for early loss of primary teeth in the mixed dentition requires some additional thought and consideration. Loss of posterior teeth in the primary dentition is a nearly universal indication for space maintenance therapy. In the mixed dentition the timing of permanent tooth eruption, timing of tooth loss, presence of permanent teeth, and extent of crowding must also be taken into account.

Premature loss of a primary molar at a very early age delays the eruption of the permanent tooth. On the other hand, premature loss of a primary molar at an age near the time of normal eruption of the permanent tooth may accelerate the eruption of the permanent tooth and make space maintenance unnecessary. In general, eruption of the permanent premolar will be delayed if the primary molar is lost before age 8 years, whereas the premolar will tend to erupt earlier than normal if the primary molar is lost after age 8 years. A more accurate method of determining delayed or accelerated eruption of permanent teeth is to examine the amount of root development and alveolar bone overlying the unerupted permanent tooth from panoramic or periapical films. The permanent tooth begins to erupt when root development is approximately one-half to two-thirds completed. In terms of alveolar bone coverage, approximately 6 months should be anticipated for every millimeter of bone that covers the permanent tooth. If it is apparent that the tooth will be delayed in erupting and the space is adequate, space maintenance is absolutely indicated. Because space loss usually occurs within the first 6 months after the premature loss of a primary molar, space maintenance should be undertaken unless the tooth is expected to erupt within 6 months or unless there is enough space in the arch that a 1- or 2-mm space reduction will not compromise eruption of the permanent tooth.

A second factor to consider is the amount of time that has elapsed since the primary tooth was lost. At one extreme is the case of a primary molar scheduled for extraction. At the other extreme is a primary molar already missing for 6 months or longer. In the first case, space maintenance is certainly indicated to prevent space loss when the tooth is extracted. In the second case the majority of space loss has already occurred, and space maintenance may not be indicated. The clinician should complete space and profile analyses and decide based on those findings. If there is excess space in the arch or if so much space has been lost that extraction of permanent teeth is inevitable, space maintenance is contraindicated. A space maintainer is indicated to prevent any more space loss if the space remaining is only marginally adequate to allow the permanent tooth to erupt. As always, there is little if any rationale for maintaining inadequate space.

Another way to look at space maintenance in the mixed dentition is by what tooth is lost prematurely. In general, after the first permanent molar erupts, there is more space lost when the primary second molar is lost than the primary first molar. A systematic review of early loss of the primary first molar indicated that there is an immediate loss of 1.5 mm of space in the mandibular arch and 1.0 mm of loss in the maxillary arch.[45] Thereafter there is little space loss. Many use this information to question whether space maintainers should be used in the mixed dentition to replace missing primary first molars. Second primary molar loss seems to be completely different. Northway et al. report there are significant space loss and continued space loss when the second primary molar is lost prematurely.[46] Unless there are unusual circumstances such as missing teeth (see later), space maintenance is indicated when second primary molars are lost.

The absence of a permanent successor complicates space maintenance in the mixed dentition. The second premolar is the most commonly missing posterior tooth in the permanent dentition, excluding the third molars. If the primary second molar is lost prematurely, the clinician must decide about the space that would have been occupied by the missing second premolar. Two choices can be made. One alternative is to maintain space in the arch and eventually construct a fixed prosthesis or have an implant placed and restored. This is most feasible if the skeletal and dental relationships are class I, there is no crowding, and there is good interarch occlusion. This is an even more inviting alternative if only one of the premolars is missing (i.e., a unilateral missing premolar). The advent of resin-bonded bridges and intraosseous implants has made this option more popular. Another alternative is to allow or encourage the space to close. Factors that favor this solution include crowding in the arch, protrusive incisors and lips, bilateral missing premolars, and possibly other missing teeth. This topic is addressed in more detail later in this chapter.

The amount of crowding in the arch is an important factor in the decision about space maintenance, and it is predicted from the space analysis and put in perspective by the facial form analysis. If the incisor position is normal and there is adequate

space or minor crowding in the arch, space maintenance should be initiated. However, early loss of a primary molar in an arch with substantial crowding must be considered carefully. Space maintainers alone will not solve a problem of this magnitude. Either permanent teeth will be extracted or the arches will have to be expanded. Expansion is possible only if the incisor position is normal or retrusive and the periodontium is healthy enough to allow the incisors to be moved facially. If expansion is contemplated, space maintainers should be placed. However, in some cases, crowding of this magnitude is managed by extracting two first premolars and closing the remaining space with orthodontic appliances.

If no space maintenance is implemented and tooth movement results from drifting before first premolar extractions, less space remains to be closed later. Consultation with a specialist is desirable before this type of decision is made. If the crowding approaches 10 mm/arch, space maintainers may be needed even though permanent tooth extraction is inevitably required. The average width of a premolar is approximately 7 mm; therefore the extraction of two premolars would effectively result in a gain of 14 mm of arch length. If more space is lost in an arch that is already severely crowded, a two-premolar extraction may not resolve all the crowding. Space maintainers would ensure that no further decrease in arch length occurs. In some instances, timed extraction (called serial extraction) can alleviate the crowding and relieve the demands of subsequent orthodontic treatment.

Probably the most significant difference between space maintenance strategy in the mixed dentition and that in the primary dentition is bilateral loss of teeth in the mandibular arch. In the primary dentition, two band and loop appliances are indicated; in the mixed dentition the lingual arch is preferred if all lower incisors have erupted. Primary second molars or permanent first molars may be used as abutment teeth. If oral hygiene is a problem, it is recommended that primary second molars be banded. This is done so that if decalcification under bands occurs because of poor oral hygiene, it occurs on teeth that will eventually exfoliate.

Space maintenance in the mixed dentition requires close supervision as permanent teeth erupt and primary teeth exfoliate. When primary abutment teeth exfoliate, an appliance may have to be remade using permanent teeth as abutments. Space-maintaining appliances should be removed when the permanent tooth erupts into its proper position.

Potential Alignment and Space Problems

Ectopic Eruption

Problems associated with ectopic eruption of the permanent first molar have been discussed previously in Chapter 31. A 3- to 6-month observation period usually is the best initial therapy if the resorption is not too severe, because there is a possibility that the molar will self-correct spontaneously or "jump" distally and erupt into its normal position (Fig. 36.10). Intervention is necessary if the molar is still blocked from erupting at the end of the observation period or if the permanent molar is severely impacted.[47] The goal of treatment is to move the ectopically erupting tooth away from the tooth it is resorbing, allow it to erupt, and retain the primary second molar.

If a small amount of movement is needed and little or none of the permanent molar is clinically visible, a piece of 20- to 22-mm brass wire can be passed around the contact between the permanent molar and the primary second molar. The brass wire is tightened every 2 weeks. When the wire is tightened, the periodontal ligament space is compressed and the molar is forced distally until it can slip past the primary molar and erupt (Fig. 36.11). In some cases a steel spring clip separator may be used to dislodge the molar, but only in cases in which there is minimal

resorption of the primary molar. It may be difficult to seat the spring if the contact point between the molars is below the cementoenamel junction of the primary molar. Some authors advocate elastomeric separators, but they must be carefully supervised because they can dislodge in an apical direction and bury in the sulcus causing a periodontal abscess. Some elastomeric separators are not radiopaque and can be difficult to locate.

Another method of moving the permanent molar distal is to band the primary second molar and apply a distal force to the permanent molar through a helical spring or elastomer (Fig. 36.12). In fact, a type of band and spring appliance can be constructed at chairside using the orthodontic archwire tube on a molar band; the appliance is easily activated intraorally at subsequent appointments. These methods require that the occlusal surface of the permanent molar be visible so that force can be applied to move the tooth distally. A small ledge of resin or a metal button can be bonded to the occlusal surface to serve as the point of force application, or the end of the spring can be bonded directly to the impacted tooth. However, salivary contamination of the occlusal surface sometimes makes bonding a frustrating and difficult procedure. An even more cost-effective technique is to bond a permanent first molar bracket on the primary second molar and a permanent second molar bracket on the permanent first molar; then a self-retained helical spring is constructed between the two teeth to move the permanent first molar distally. This can all be accomplished chairside in a few minutes by a proficient wire bender. Such a band and spring appliance should be evaluated every 2 weeks and

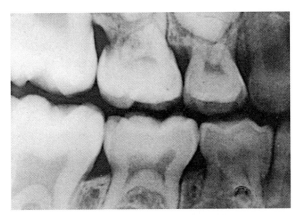

• **Figure 36.10** This radiograph illustrates the ability of an ectopically erupting permanent first molar to self-correct spontaneously. Note that the distal root of the primary maxillary second molar has been resorbed. Usually this type of resorption is the result of an erupting permanent molar that is caught on the distal aspect of the primary molar. If the resorption does not progress too far, the permanent molar usually "jumps" past the resorptive defect in 3 to 6 months.

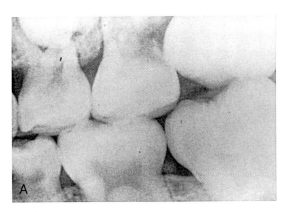

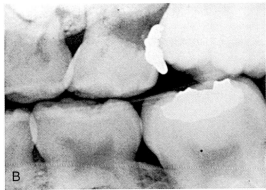

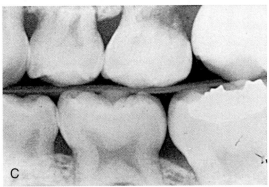

• **Figure 36.11** (A) This radiograph shows an ectopically erupting permanent maxillary left first molar. (B) Because only a small amount of movement is required to correct the ectopic eruption, a piece of 20-mm brass wire is slipped around the contact point between the permanent molar and the primary second molar and is tightened. (C) After the wire has been tightened 3 times at 2-week intervals, the molar is dislodged and begins to erupt into a normal position. (From Fields HW, Proffit WR. Orthodontics in general practice. In: Morris AL, Bohannan HM, Casullo DP, eds. *The Dental Specialties in General Practice.* Philadelphia: Saunders; 1983.)

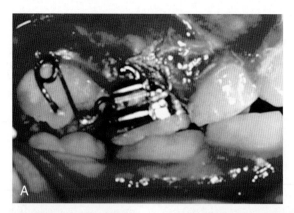

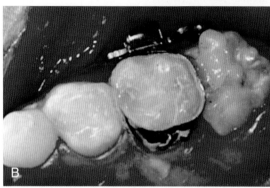
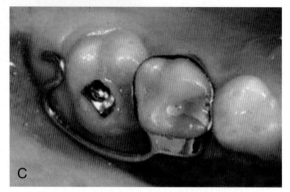

• **Figure 36.12** (A and B) A band and helical spring appliance is used to treat an ectopically erupting permanent molar that requires a large amount of movement. The primary second molar is banded, and a helical spring is soldered to the band. A small ledge of composite resin, a metal button bonded to the occlusal surface of the permanent molar, or a small preparation can serve as a point of force application. The spring is reactivated at monthly intervals until the permanent molar is dislodged. (C) Another band and spring design with a metal button bonded to the occlusal surface of the erupting permanent molar. Elastomeric chain or thread is attached from the button to the distal hook on the wire and changed monthly to provide the distal force to dislodge the molar. ([A and B] From Fields HW, Proffit WR. Orthodontics in general practice. In: Morris AL, Bohannan HM, Casullo DP, eds. *The Dental Specialties in General Practice.* Philadelphia: Saunders; 1983.)

can work effectively in a short time because of the minimal root development on the permanent molar.

Occasionally, the primary second molar must be removed if the permanent molar has caused extensive resorption of the primary root structure. In these cases, loss of arch length is certain, and some plan of treatment for the impending space deficiency should be considered in advance (Fig. 36.13). If there is a congenitally missing second premolar or premolar extraction is being considered because of the crowding, then reduction in arch length by mesial movement of the molars is advantageous. To manage the space after extraction of the primary molar, a distal shoe can be placed to guide eruption of the permanent molar. A distal shoe maintains space but does not regain space that was lost before the primary molar extraction. An alternative plan is to allow the permanent molar to erupt and then use the appropriate appliance to regain the space (described subsequently). After the space is regained, a space maintainer should be placed.

Ectopic eruption of lateral incisors is usually an early indication of crowding but may only be the result of aberrant tooth positioning. If a primary canine exfoliates prematurely as a result of ectopic eruption, the lower incisors typically drift to that side of the arch, creating a midline discrepancy. If the laterals cause resorption and exfoliation of both primary canines, the incisors usually tip lingually

and decrease arch length. When this happens and the incisors align, it appears that the space problem is corrected because the incisor alignment usually improves, but this is only temporary, and the space shortage will become apparent again when the permanent canines begin to erupt. Whether the loss of primary canines is unilateral or bilateral, the clinician should determine whether there is an arch length inadequacy and assess anteroposterior lip and incisor position. This information helps to determine whether space maintenance, space regaining, or more extensive treatment is needed.

The goal of treatment should be to manage the space according to the long-term plan. Past recommendations for treatment of crowding and lateral incisor ectopic eruption have included placing a lingual arch with a soldered spur distal to the lateral incisor to hold the midline. If the midline has already shifted, it has been recommended to remove the contralateral primary canine to promote spontaneous midline correction. If space loss cannot be tolerated because of lingual incisor tipping, a lingual arch should be placed following extraction. However, there is no evidence in the literature that removal of the contralateral primary canine will result in spontaneous midline correction. There is also no evidence that the midline shift is progressive if the primary canine is not removed. A recent study of growth study data confirmed there is no significant

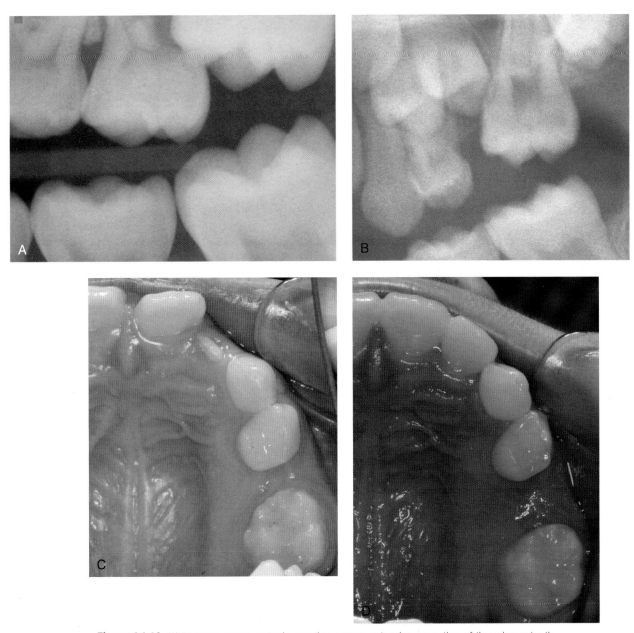

• **Figure 36.13** (A) In some cases, ectopic eruption causes extensive resorption of the primary tooth root and the tooth is lost prematurely. In some cases the tooth may abscess due to communication with the oral environment. (B) When the primary second molar is lost, the clinician should anticipate mesial movement of the permanent molar and a reduced arch length. (C) This space loss occurred within the first 6 months of tooth removal. (D) The space was opened with braces and a coil spring. Space maintenance was necessary to hold space for the unerupted second premolar.

difference in the position of the lower dental midline after unilateral loss of a primary canine or normal exfoliation of both canines.[48] There are studies to show that removal of the mandibular primary canines will result in an improved irregularity index (a measure akin to crowding) compared with those that do not have primary canine removal. However, this tooth removal comes at the expense of nearly 3 mm in arch perimeter decrease.[49] Based on this evidence, the clinician should carefully consider whether to remove the contralateral canine when there is ectopic eruption of the lower lateral incisor. Further discussion on lower anterior crowding and premature canine loss will occur later. If there is sufficient crowding

so that space maintenance is contraindicated, or if the incisors are considered too protrusive to be maintained in this position, no lingual arch should be placed following the extraction of the contralateral primary canine. In situations in which both canines exfoliate prematurely because of ectopic eruption, similar treatment decisions should be made, although the clinician does not normally have to worry about a midline shift.

Transposition

Early transposition can be addressed during the mixed dentition and provides an opportunity to intercept a developing problem.

As mentioned earlier, the type of transposition amenable to early treatment is most commonly encountered in the mandibular arch. The lateral incisors resorb either the primary canine or primary canine and first molar (Fig. 36.14A). They rotate as they erupt, so treatment includes repositioning them mesially and derotating them (see Fig. 36.14B). If this is accomplished before canine eruption, transposition can be prevented (see Fig. 36.14C).

Impacted Teeth

The most common site of impacted teeth in the mixed dentition is in the maxillary canine region. These teeth often erupt in a mesial direction and become impacted in the palate or resorb the permanent lateral incisor roots.[50] This problem is often diagnosed because there is no bulge on the facial alveolus in the canine area at approximately 9 or 10 years of age.[51] Some type of radiograph is indicated to locate the canine. In most cases this is a panoramic radiograph. This may even merit the use of a small field of view CBCT image (see Chapter 31 for details). If the permanent canine overlaps less than half of the lateral incisor root on a panoramic radiograph, there is a greater than 90% chance of redirecting the canine distally simply by timely extraction of the primary canines

(Fig. 36.15).[52] If there is more than this amount of overlap, the chance of normal eruption diminishes. Other treatments have been proposed to prevent the maxillary canine from erupting into the palate. Besides removal of the primary canine, others have suggested palatal expansion and primary canine removal,[53] headgear treatment, and removal of both the primary canine and primary first molar.[54]

Missing Permanent Teeth

The absence of permanent teeth creates many treatment problems for the clinician, and most treatment decisions of this nature are best made by a specialist. The maxillary lateral incisor and the mandibular second premolar are the most common congenitally missing teeth in the permanent dentition, whereas anterior teeth, specifically the incisors, are often lost to trauma. Treatment decisions are based not only on which tooth is missing but also on arch length, adjacent tooth morphology and color, incisor position, and lip and profile esthetics.

Treatment of congenitally missing maxillary lateral incisors varies depending on whether one or both incisors are absent and on the

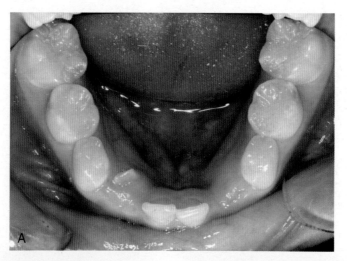

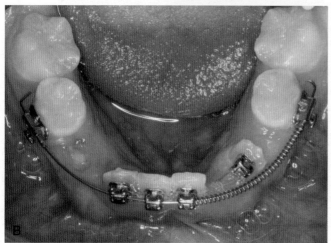

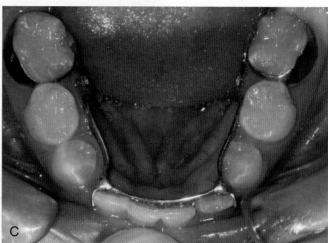

• **Figure 36.14** (A) Early transposition can cause loss of the primary canine or primary canine and first molar. In this patient the lower left first primary molar was removed to allow the lateral incisor to erupt. (B) Often the lateral incisor will require mesial movement and rotation. (C) Correction with banded and bonded appliances has prevented true transposition.

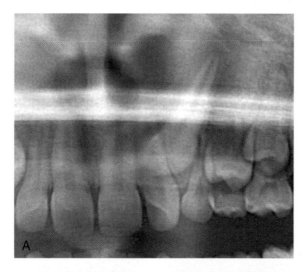

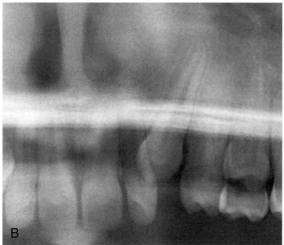

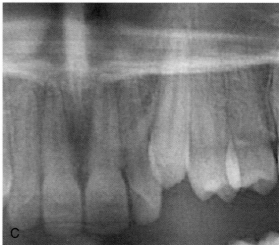

• **Figure 36.15** (A) Even though this patient has considerable mesial migration of the permanent maxillary left canine and it overlaps the entire lateral root, the primary canine was extracted in an attempt to redirect its eruption path. (B) Note the distal and occlusal movement of the permanent left canine with reduced overlap of the lateral incisor. (C) Nearly 1 year later the permanent left canine will erupt into relatively normal position.

position of the permanent canine when it erupts into the arch. The canine either erupts into the normal canine position or resorbs the primary lateral incisor and spontaneously substitutes for the missing lateral incisor. If the canine erupts into its proper position, the primary lateral incisor will eventually have to be removed because it does not make an esthetically pleasing substitute for the permanent lateral incisor and because the root will eventually resorb. The missing lateral incisor can be replaced with a resin-bonded bridge or an implant. In general, prosthetic replacement of the missing lateral incisor is preferred when the occlusion, incisor position, and profile are nearly ideal (Fig. 36.16).[55] This approach should always be considered when the contralateral lateral incisor is present and has excellent size and shape. Until recently, this approach was also favored when the occlusion was near ideal because it was difficult to close the space without creating a midline discrepancy or retracting the incisors. The use of TADs has made space closure much easier and more predictable.

The clinician must also consider the long-term consequences of treatment. If the patient and clinician elect to open the space

for prosthetic replacement of the lateral incisor, the placement of an implant or resin-bonded bridge has to be delayed until the patient has stopped growing. This is often greater than 5 years between the finish of orthodontic treatment and a definitive restoration. Retention must be well planned, and the patient must be very compliant with retention so the teeth remain in the ideal position for restorations. Even with good retention, studies have shown there is a 1 in 10 chance the roots of the central incisor and canine will converge and prevent implant placement.[56] Another long-term consequence of implant-supported restoration of the lateral incisor is the implant itself. Though the implant has a high success rate, there are implant failures. In addition, resorption of labial bone around the implant, a normal finding over time, causes the gingiva to appear blue. Lastly, the implant may show infraocclusion after several years. Because the implant does not erupt like teeth, any vertical growth change will result in a change in the vertical relationship of the implant and adjacent teeth.[57]

If the permanent canine erupts into the lateral incisor position, the primary canine can be extracted. Depending on the situation,

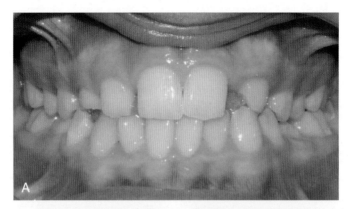

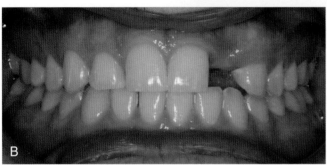

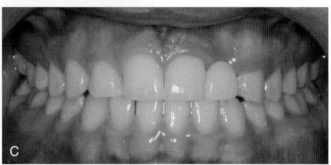

• **Figure 36.16** (A) This patient is missing the maxillary left lateral incisor. Because the patient has class I molars and relatively good alignment, a decision was made to replace the missing lateral incisor prosthetically. (B) At the end of treatment, a space identical in size to the right lateral incisor was created to replace the left lateral incisor. (C) A dental laboratory created a left lateral incisor pontic with thin abutment wings. The abutment teeth were etched and composite resin was used to bond the abutment wings to each tooth. This type of restoration does not work with a deep bite because of the shearing force of occlusion on the lingual surface.

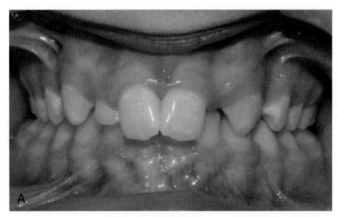

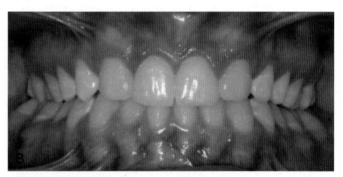

• **Figure 36.17** (A) This patient was congenitally missing both upper lateral incisors. A decision was made to substitute the canines into the lateral position. (B) The central incisors and canines have been recontoured by adding resin and using a dental bur. If the first premolar is too small in shape, it is possible to recontour the first premolar with composite resin to mimic a canine.

the permanent canine can be moved back to the correct position, and a prosthetic solution for the missing lateral incisor can be determined as discussed previously. There are several factors to consider in canine substitution. The existing malocclusion, crowding, patient profile, crown shape and color of the canine, and smiling gingival display all influence whether this approach should be considered (Fig. 36.17). These canines require recontouring by enamel removal, bleaching to lighten the color, and resin addition to improve the esthetic appearance of the teeth. The recommended treatment is to extrude the canine and intrude the first premolar to create gingival margins that match normal occlusions. The ideal case for canine substitution is a nice profile, a class II dental relationship, no crowding in the lower arch, and small canines with color that matches the central incisors.[57] Canine substitution cases are considered difficult to treat well. A normal pretreatment occlusion favors canine retraction and prosthetic replacement, as does short or wide canine crown morphology and dark canine color. These elements reduce the chances of providing an esthetic canine substitution for the lateral incisor. Even if the canine must be retracted, this is not without some virtue. The canine brought bone with it during its eruption, and this bone will enhance future esthetics and potential implant placement in the lateral incisor position. The clinician should discuss all treatment options with the patient in missing lateral incisor cases. It is especially important when studies show patients are more satisfied with natural tooth replacement (canine substitution) than prosthetic replacement.[58,59]

When incisors are lost to trauma, the clinician must study the existing situation in a manner similar to congenitally missing lateral incisors. The age and growth status of the patient, the amount of crowding, and the skeletal relationship must be considered. The number of teeth lost, the status of the periodontium, and the injuries to adjacent teeth further complicate decisions. Not only is the clinician faced with the normal questions of conventional orthodontics, but the clinician is making decisions on teeth with uncertain prognoses and diminished or missing bony support. Traditional management of replacing incisors lost to trauma usually involves prosthetic tooth replacement or natural tooth replacement through substitution of teeth.

Another possibility is the use of transplanted posterior teeth, usually a premolar, into the position of the missing maxillary central incisor. With reshaping and either resin or veneer restoration, this option can be quite successful. Although not widely adopted in North America, posterior tooth transplantation is a real option in Scandinavian countries.[60]

Arch length, incisor position, and facial appearance must be thoroughly evaluated before a treatment plan is generated when a premolar is congenitally missing. Unlike primary canines and laterals, a primary molar may be a reasonable substitute for a missing premolar. The size, shape, and restorative status of the primary molar give some indication of the possibility of maintaining the tooth for a period of time (Fig. 36.18). Ankylosis and advanced root resorption indicate that the primary molar should be removed. Most clinicians favor removing the primary

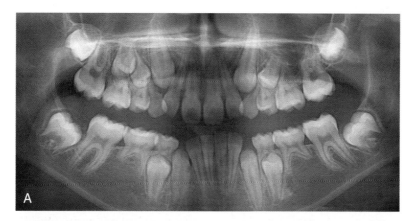

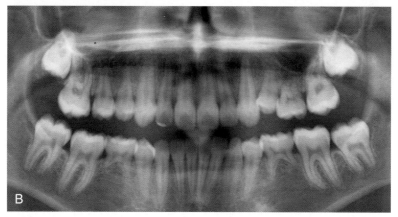

• **Figure 36.18** In some cases, retaining primary molars as an interim replacement for missing premolars is acceptable. Usually, the primary molars ultimately will require replacement. (A) Patient with missing maxillary left second premolar and both mandibular second premolars. (B) The parents and patient did not want prosthetic replacement of teeth, so the orthodontic treatment was directed to the anterior teeth only.

molar and closing the space orthodontically (Fig. 36.19); but in certain situations a resin-bonded bridge, conventional bridge, or implant may be a more ideal treatment (Fig. 36.20). Prosthetic replacement is more likely in class I skeletal and dental patients with ideal or nearly ideal occlusions or when a tooth is missing unilaterally. Again, the introduction of TADs allows the clinician to determine if space closure is appropriate in a case where prosthetic replacement used to be automatic, such as when it would be difficult to move teeth without affecting the occlusion and relationship of the remaining teeth. The TAD can be used to move a posterior segment forward without causing the anterior teeth to shift (creating a midline deviation), because the movement of the teeth is pitted against the stability of the TAD within the bone and not the teeth. As a general guideline, use of TADs is contraindicated in children younger than 12 years because of bone

density, the presence of unerupted teeth, and the inability to hold the miniscrew.

If the arch is so crowded that teeth must be extracted, or if the incisors are too protrusive or the profile too full, the retained primary molar should be removed and the case treated in a manner similar to that for a four-premolar extraction case. Typically, first premolars are removed in an extraction case, but the majority of congenitally missing premolars are second premolars. If it can be determined that the second premolar is missing and that extractions are necessary to resolve the arch length inadequacy, the primary molar can be removed early, allowing the space to close by mesial drifting of the permanent first molar and distal drifting of the anterior teeth. Unfortunately, congenital absence of the second premolar may not be definitively determined at an early age, and this delays the extractions. The longer the extractions are delayed,

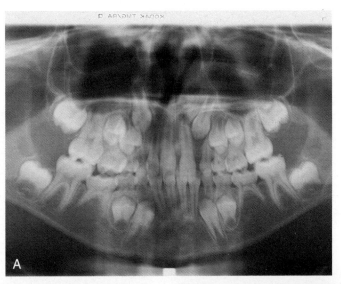

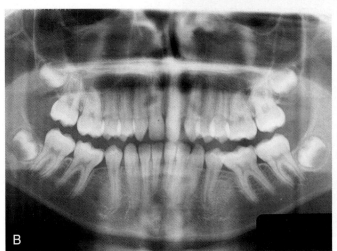
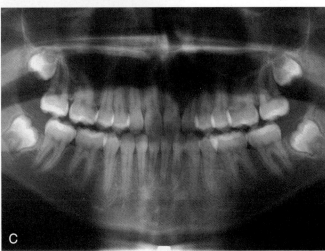

• **Figure 36.19** Closing the spaces that accompany missing teeth and avoiding prosthetic replacements are sometimes advantageous. (A) This patient is missing maxillary lateral incisors and mandibular second premolars. (B) The remaining primary teeth were extracted and allowed to drift. (C) Orthodontics was completed, and the teeth were finally positioned.

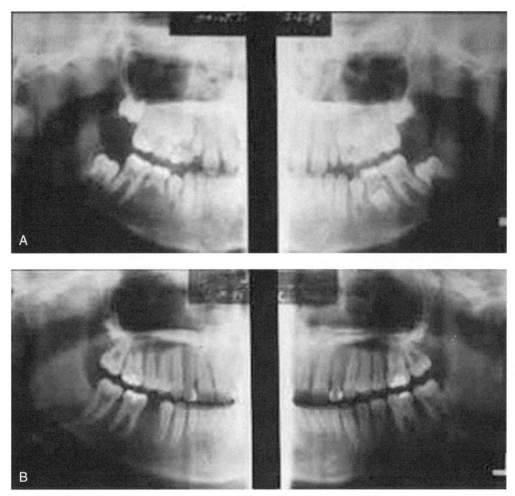

• **Figure 36.20** When permanent teeth are missing, often unilaterally, the best solution is to adjust the space and plan for prosthetic replacement. (A) Because of the short roots and restorative status, the primary mandibular right second molar was extracted. (B) The space was adjusted to accommodate a prosthetic replacement.

the less drifting and spontaneous space closure will occur. Using the space of the missing second premolars to reduce protrusion is much more complicated and requires the teeth to be retracted into the space of the missing teeth. This precludes dental drifting and should be planned by the specialist.

One further word of caution. If the primary molars are ankylosed and the permanent successor missing, then the primary molars should be extracted before the vertical bony discrepancy of the alveolus becomes too great (Fig. 36.21). This may require subsequent space maintenance. Studies show that loss of bony ridge will be minimal, and the maintenance of good bony contours for the adjacent teeth without periodontal defects will be improved. There is a reduction of alveolar bone width of 25% to 30%, but the authors show that implant placement is still feasible without bone grafting.[61] Later, implants or restorations can be placed, and in some cases the space can be closed orthodontically. Some have suggested using decoronation of the ankylosed primary molar to maintain alveolar width, but there are no data to support this claim.

Supernumerary Teeth

A supernumerary tooth may create space and eruption problems. It can cause permanent teeth to erupt into malalignment or even prevent eruption. Treatment is directed at minimizing the effect of the supernumerary tooth by immediate removal or observation and later removal. Management of the supernumerary varies depending on the size, shape, number of supernumeraries, and the dental development of the patient. Typically, the supernumerary is detected on a panoramic radiograph or an anterior occlusal film unless there is clinical evidence of an extra tooth at an earlier age. If the supernumerary is conical and is not inverted, there is a reasonable chance that it will erupt, at which time it should be removed (Fig. 36.22). If the supernumerary is inverted, it may migrate superiorly away from the teeth and possibly into the nose. A tubercular-shaped tooth will not migrate but may, as with any supernumerary tooth, significantly impede eruption of the adjacent teeth. When multiple supernumerary teeth are present or if the supernumerary tooth fails to erupt, there is an increased chance of impeding the eruption of at least one tooth. In these cases,

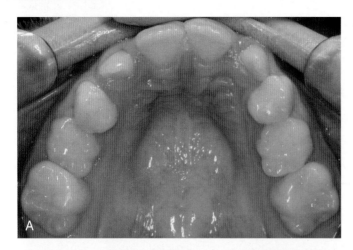

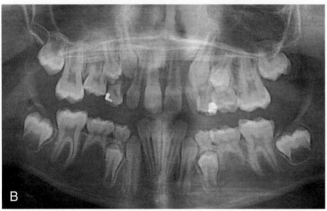

• **Figure 36.21** (A) This patient has an ankylosed primary maxillary right second molar, as illustrated by the more apical marginal ridges of the tooth. (B) The panoramic radiograph shows that the maxillary right and mandibular second premolars are missing. Because of the developing vertical discrepancy in the bone levels, the primary molars should be removed as atraumatically as possible and the space either maintained or closed.

surgical removal makes sense. Ideally, the surgery is timed so that removal of the supernumerary tooth does not interfere with permanent tooth development. However, the earlier the supernumerary can be removed, the more likely it is that the permanent teeth will erupt normally. Surgery to remove a supernumerary is often complicated, especially if there are multiple supernumerary teeth or if access to the supernumerary tooth is limited. These patients are appropriately referred to a specialist.

Tooth Size Discrepancies

Isolated tooth size discrepancies can cause alignment problems. The maxillary lateral incisor commonly creates this type of problem because it is undersized or has a pegged shape. Occasionally the lateral incisor can be restored to its normal size with composite resin and requires no other treatment. As discussed in Chapter 31, sometimes the pegged lateral needs a combination of tooth movement and restorative dentistry to achieve normal occlusion. Depending on the size of the discrepancy, the pegged lateral can be treated in one of three ways.

If the lateral incisor is only slightly smaller than normal, the entire space can be closed. An alternative method for a marginally small incisor is to move the lateral incisor orthodontically until it contacts the central incisor and leave space distal to the lateral. This solution is generally not esthetically pleasing unless only a small space is left distal to the lateral. It also requires retention to hold the space. The canine usually is not brought forward to close the space because this would put the canine in an end-to-end relationship and disrupt the previously normal occlusion. An alternative to this approach is to use interproximal tooth reduction in the lower arch to make those anterior teeth narrower, so the upper space can be fully closed. A third solution, usually reserved for incisors that are considerably undersized, is a combination of orthodontic tooth movement and resin bonding to reshape the crown (Fig. 36.23). The lateral incisor should be positioned so that the resin addition will be cosmetically pleasing and will restore near-normal crown anatomy. This type of treatment is best performed by a specialist who has completed a diagnostic setup as described in Chapter 38 to plan the tooth movement and restorative requirements.

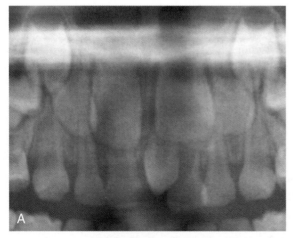

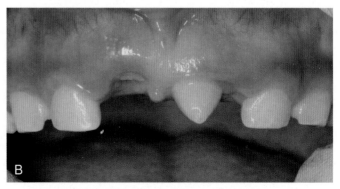

• **Figure 36.22** (A) A conical supernumerary in the maxillary central incisor region was detected during a radiographic examination. This supernumerary was not interfering with the normal eruption of the permanent incisors. (B) The supernumerary was allowed to erupt before it was removed.

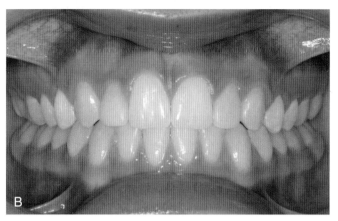

• **Figure 36.23** (A) One possible solution to a small lateral incisor is a combination of orthodontic tooth movement and resin bonding to reshape the crown of the tooth. (B) This patient had bilateral small lateral incisors. The laterals were positioned so resin addition would make the teeth esthetically pleasing, restore near-normal crown anatomy, and provide good functional occlusion.

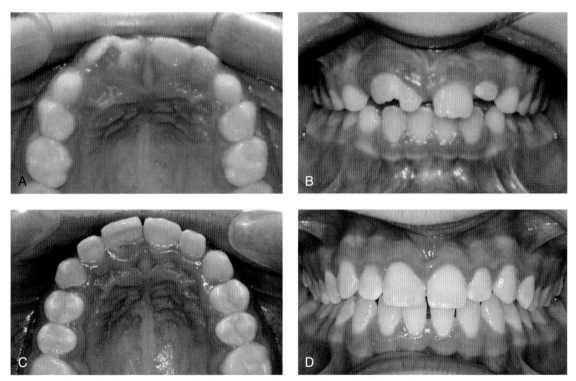

• **Figure 36.24** (A and B) The right central incisor was fused to a supernumerary tooth creating a single large incisor. In addition to the unappealing appearance, there was no room for the lateral incisor to erupt. The tooth was sectioned after careful review of the canal anatomy with a cone beam computed tomography radiograph. After sectioning, the tooth was moved into correct position with orthodontics (C) and restored on the mesial surface (D).

Occasionally a single tooth will be extremely large, which will result in crowding and malpositioning of the teeth. In these cases the tooth often can be reduced to match the contralateral tooth and repositioned.

Fusion and gemination in the permanent dentition are even more difficult to treat and should also be referred to a specialist. It is possible in some cases to divide fused permanent teeth, move one or both of the resulting teeth into good position, and then restore the remaining tooth or teeth.[62] Often endodontic treatment is required because the division violated the pulpal space (Fig. 36.24).

Dens evaginatus and incisor talon cusps provide interesting challenges in securing an ideal occlusion (see Fig. 31.16). In most cases of dens evaginatus a fine, threadlike pulp extends from the main pulp chamber into the evagination, and the location of this pulp tissue extension should be determined radiographically. Most such teeth in the posterior region do not require treatment because the force of mastication slowly wears the evagination down, and reparative dentin is formed. However, in the anterior region the attrition must be accomplished mechanically with a handpiece and bur. A small amount of tooth structure is removed at each appointment, and after each session calcium hydroxide paste is applied to the exposed dentin to stimulate the reparative process. Usually the tooth can be treated at monthly appointments without permanent injury to the pulp. When treatment is complete, the exposed dentin is covered with a calcium hydroxide base and a resin restoration is placed.

Alignment Problems

Anterior and posterior tooth irregularities with adequate space should be regarded as different from anterior and posterior space shortages. Tooth irregularity alone consists simply of rotated and tipped teeth in which there is no shortage of arch length when the leeway space is considered. Arch length discrepancies (i.e., a true lack of space) also result in tooth irregularities but are a different situation and require different management and timing.

Appliance Considerations

Tooth irregularities can be managed with either fixed or removable appliances. If a simple tipping force and no rotation are required to align the tooth, a removable appliance with a finger spring is an appropriate choice. A great variety of removable appliances exist; however, several essential components must be included in the design. The appliance must be retentive so the force applied to the tooth will not dislodge the appliance. Adams clasps are often prescribed and are very retentive, although they require careful adjustment and may interfere with the occlusion. Other types of clasps, such as ball clasps and "C" clasps, are also popular but provide distinctly less retention and flexibility. Multiple clasps should be used to enhance the retention. Additional retention and stability are gained from the palatal acrylic in maxillary appliances. A helical finger spring made of 0.022-inch stainless steel wire incorporated into the palatal acrylic delivers a light, continuous force. The spring should be activated 2 mm to move the tooth approximately 1 mm/month (Fig. 36.25).

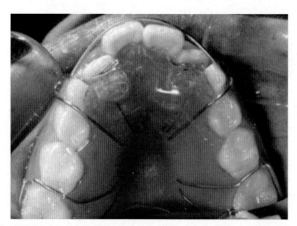

• **Figure 36.25** Removable appliances can be used to manage alignment problems but are more effective for some problems than for others. Notice that the maxillary right lateral incisor can easily be tipped facially, but it is more difficult to rotate the left lateral incisor and requires use of the lingual finger spring and the labial bow in concert to create a movement. In general, this type of movement is more efficient with a fixed banded and bonded appliance.

Fixed appliances (braces) can be used to correct irregularities and are indicated when bodily movement of teeth or rotational control is necessary. Orthodontic appliances have evolved to a point in which specific brackets are designed for specific teeth. The brackets are constructed to provide proper crown and root positioning when they are precisely placed on the teeth. The bracketing process is described in Fig. 36.26.

There are several ways in which brackets can be bonded to teeth. The traditional phosphoric acid etch, rinse, dry, and application of a primer is still used in orthodontic practice. As companies have developed all-in-one etch and prime technology, the traditional technique has been replaced with a one-step etch and prime conditioner. This reduces the number of steps required, makes isolation easier, and decreases the time to place brackets. The method is described in Fig. 36.27.

Another method to reduce bonding time and to theoretically be more accurate with bracket placement is indirect bonding. The method is considered a more accurate way to place braces because the clinician may mark and measure each tooth, has unlimited working time, and complete access to each tooth. This method is described in Fig. 36.28. Intraoral scanners are replacing the traditional impression so the clinician can scan the teeth and feed the data directly to a computer (see Fig. 36.28C).

The clinician should understand the physical properties of orthodontic wires. An initial archwire must be selected that is strong enough to withstand the force of occlusion in the posterior segments yet flexible enough in the anterior region to be deflected into the brackets and deliver a light, continuous force. The initial wire is normally made of a nickel titanium (NiTi) alloy of an appropriate diameter to provide ample strength and flexibility. Other wires can be selected, such as small-diameter stainless steel or braided stainless steel, based on the amount of irregularity of the teeth. If posterior wire strength is critical, loops can be bent into the archwire to produce anterior flexibility. Retention is essential after tooth movement in the mixed dentition because the teeth have a strong propensity to relapse.

Most retention problems are due to stretching and compression of gingival fibers during tooth movement. Gingival fibers reorganize very slowly following tooth movement, and in some cases irregularity returns even if retention is well conceived. Some clinicians have suggested that if the periodontium is healthy, a circumferential supracrestal fiberotomy may be performed to reduce relapse.

When treatment is complete or nearly complete, the supracrestal gingival fibers are cut with a scalpel using a 12B blade, under local anesthesia. Theoretically, the stretched gingival fibers will not need to reorganize but will reattach in a new position after being cut. Extreme care should be taken in patients with a thin gingival biotype.

Crowding Problems

The first sign of crowding in the mixed dentition usually coincides with eruption of the permanent incisors. Arch length insufficiency may manifest in several ways, ranging from slight incisor rotation and irregularity to gross incisor malalignment. The first step should be to perform a space analysis and determine the extent of the arch length inadequacy. This finding is then placed in the context of the facial profile analysis and posterior dental relationships.

Mild to Moderate Spacing

Many children have a midline diastema in the mixed dentition, and this is considered a normal stage of development. Occasionally, a large midline diastema is present that is due to a mesiodens or other midline intrabony pathologic process, protruding incisors, or a tooth size problem. A diastema caused by a midline supernumerary tooth or abnormality is managed by removal of the supernumerary tooth or the abnormality. The supernumerary tooth should be removed as early as possible without causing injury to the adjacent permanent teeth. Early removal of the mesiodens allows the permanent teeth to erupt normally, and the space usually closes spontaneously.

In some cases a large diastema may be due to faciolingual rather than mesiodistal positioning of the incisors. Flared incisors are cosmetically unappealing and are at greater risk of traumatic injury.[63] If the teeth can be tipped back into an ideal position to close the diastema and if the overbite will not hinder tooth movement, a removable appliance may be selected. The appliance is designed to include at least two clasps for retention, palatal acrylic, and a

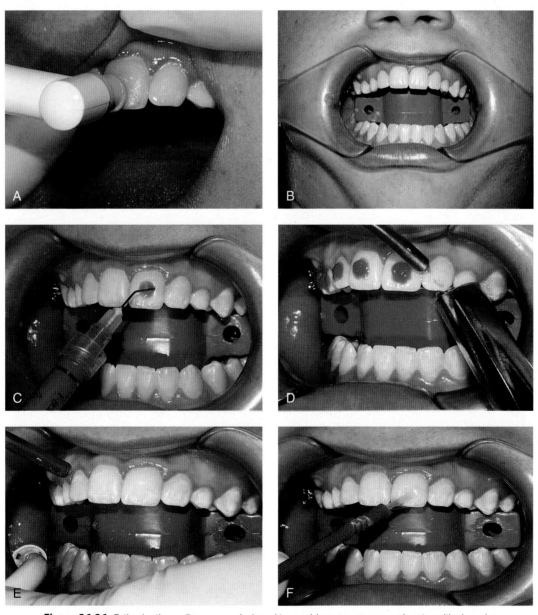

• **Figure 36.26** Orthodontic appliances are designed to provide proper crown and root positioning when they are precisely placed on the teeth. Therefore it is imperative to follow the appropriate sequence when placing the appliances. This is the sequence of steps when using an acid-etched and light-cured resin. (A) Before the appliances are placed, the teeth selected for treatment must be thoroughly cleaned, preferably with pumice. (B) After the teeth have been cleaned, they are isolated to provide a field free of salivary contamination. (C) An etching solution or gel as shown here is painted on the facial surface of the teeth. The tooth is rinsed with water (D) and dried (E). (F) The tooth is painted with a bonding agent.

Continued

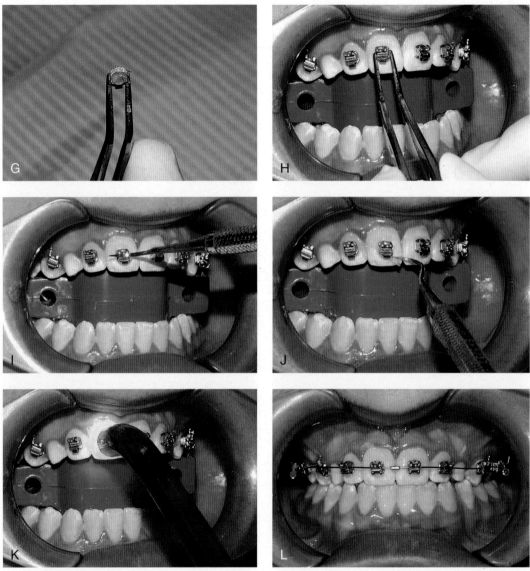

• **Figure 36.26, cont'd** (G) A small amount of resin is placed on the bracket pad. (H) The bracket is placed on the tooth. (I) The bracket is adjusted to the proper orientation with the tooth based on the long axis of the crown and root and height from the incisor edge. (J) The excess resin is cleaned up. (K) The resin is light cured. (L) An archwire is placed in the bracket and ligated with steel ligature ties or elastomeric ties.

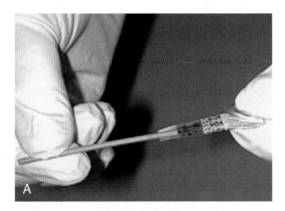

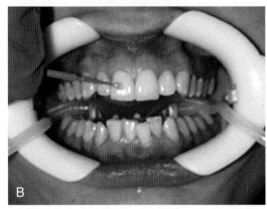

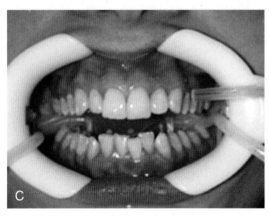

• **Figure 36.27** One-step tooth preparation has been developed to save time in the bonding process. This replaces the etch, rinse, and dry steps. After the tooth is cleaned and dried, an etch/primer is used. (A) The etch/primer is combined in a special bubble "pop" dispenser. (B) The one-step liquid etch/primer is rubbed on the tooth for several seconds. (C) The preparation is lightly air-dried. The tooth is now ready for the bracket and bonding resin to be applied.

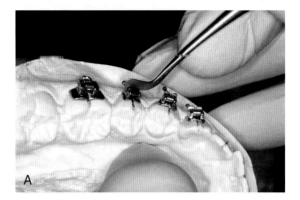

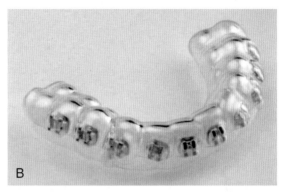

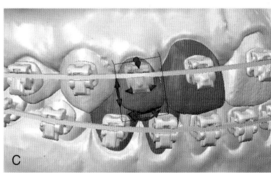

• **Figure 36.28** (A) After the patient has had an impression, a stone model is poured. A separating medium is painted on the model and the clinician marks the teeth with a pencil to indicate the long axis of the tooth. The braces are placed on the model with some type of stable adhesive. Unlike a patient, the model can be turned whatever way the clinician needs to place the bracket in the optimal position. (B) Next, an indirect bonding tray is constructed that includes the brackets that are to be transferred to the patient's teeth. The patient's teeth are prepared in a similar manner to direct bonding, and a small amount of resin is placed on each bracket. After the adhesive has set, the tray is peeled away from the teeth and a wire is inserted in the brackets. (C) The advent of scanned models makes indirect bonding even easier. This model was constructed from a digital scan of the patient's teeth. Virtual brackets are placed on the teeth, and the clinician can manipulate bracket placement until the bracket is in the optimal position. The design allows the clinician to move the bracket freely in all three dimensions. From this virtual setup, an indirect bonding tray is fabricated. ([A] Courtesy Dr. Linwood Long, Jr; [B and C] Courtesy Dr. Michael Mayhew.)

0.028-inch labial bow with adjustment loops (Fig. 36.29). The labial bow is activated to tip the incisors lingually by closing the adjustment loops. At the same time, acrylic must be removed from the lingual side of the appliance to permit tooth movement and accommodate excess gingival tissue. The labial bow is activated approximately 2.0 mm/month until the diastema is closed and the teeth are in ideal position.

Fixed orthodontic appliances are suggested if incisors are so protrusive that bodily movement is required to close the diastema or if the teeth are rotated. The molars are banded or bonded and the incisors are bonded with orthodontic brackets. The first step is to align teeth with small, round archwires. After initial alignment, the teeth are retracted via a larger rectangular wire with closing loops or elastomeric chain (Fig. 36.30). Rectangular archwires are necessary to provide full control of tooth position during retraction.

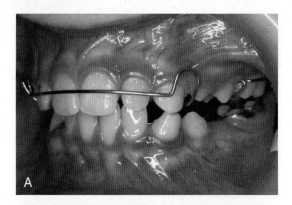

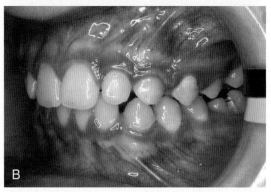

• **Figure 36.29** (A and B) A Hawley retainer with an active labial bow, and appropriate posterior retentive clasps can be used to tip anterior teeth lingually and reduce overjet if there is room available in the arch and the overbite and overjet are not prohibitive. This appliance is not good at controlling rotations. (From Proffit WR, Fields HW Jr, Sarver DM. *Contemporary Orthodontics*. 5th ed. St Louis: Elsevier; 2013.)

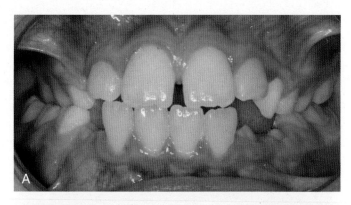

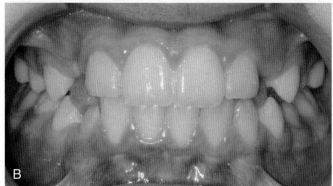

• **Figure 36.30** (A) When rotations are present or bodily movement is required to close space and retract incisors, the best alternative is a fixed appliance. This patient required both transverse expansion and diastema closure to make room for the permanent canines. (B) The space closure was completed using fixed appliances and elastomeric chain.

Headgear may be necessary to reinforce the molar anchorage at the same time because the molars have a strong tendency to come forward while the incisors are retracted. It is important to determine if teeth should be tipped or bodily moved in the treatment planning phase. At the same time, a decision on headgear is based on initial molar position, the amount of space to close, and vertical dimensions of the face.

If the diastema is due to a discrepancy in size between the upper and lower anterior teeth (the mandibular teeth are relatively larger than the maxillary), treatment usually requires the addition of resin to the interproximal surfaces of the maxillary incisors. Closing the space using orthodontics only will result in reduced overjet and overbite and possible anterior occlusal trauma. In addition, relapse is common because the occlusion will force the space open again.

Treatment to close a midline diastema not associated with an anteroposterior position or a tooth size problem is usually initiated if the diastema is greater than 2 mm and one of the following three situations exist. The first is if the diastema inhibits or disturbs the eruption of the lateral incisors. In general, treatment is started to coincide with the normal eruption time of the lateral incisor. If the diastema is large enough to be esthetically objectionable, a clinician can consider treatment if the patient is being teased or suffering psychological problems due to appearance. If the diastema is still present after eruption of the permanent canines, treatment can be considered. The diastema is due to faulty mesiodistal positioning of the incisors, but the choice of appliance is still based on the tooth

movement required to close the space. If the central incisors can be tipped together to close the diastema, a removable appliance can be used. Finger springs are either incorporated into the palatal acrylic or soldered to the labial bow to engage the distal edge of the incisor crown (Fig. 36.31). The springs are activated at a rate of 2 mm/month, and closure should not take more than 2 months.

Brackets are bonded on the facial surface of the central incisors if the teeth require bodily mesiodistal movement or rotational control to close the diastema. After initial alignment, a large segmental or full rectangular archwire is placed in the brackets, and the teeth are moved together via elastomeric chain (Fig. 36.32). No matter which type of treatment is used to close a midline diastema, retention can be a problem and should be planned. In most cases a removable appliance maintains the space closure. The appliance should be adjusted periodically if the diastema is closed before the lateral incisors and canines have erupted fully. If the diastema reopens during or following retention and the clinician determines the frenal attachment is contributing to the continued opening of the diastema, a surgical procedure, frenectomy, can be performed. The frenectomy is completed after space closure because the scar tissue created by the procedure may actually impede closure if the surgery is accomplished first. If the diastema again reopens following retention and the frenectomy, a small orthodontic wire can be bonded to the lingual surface of the incisors to keep the teeth together (Fig. 36.33). The only contraindications to a bonded wire retainer are an excessively deep bite (occlusion will dislodge the bonded wire) and poor oral hygiene.

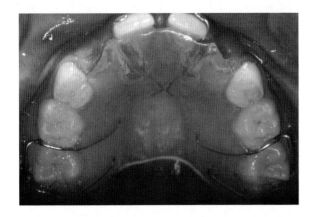

• **Figure 36.31** In this case a midline diastema is due to the mesiodistal positioning of the maxillary central incisors. A removable appliance with finger springs incorporated into the palatal acrylic closes the space, tipping the teeth together. (From Proffit WR, Fields HW, Jr, Sarver DM. *Contemporary Orthodontics.* 5th ed. St Louis: Elsevier; 2013.)

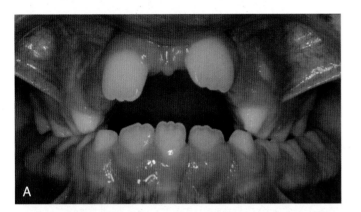

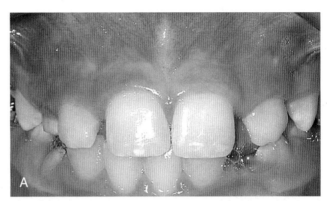

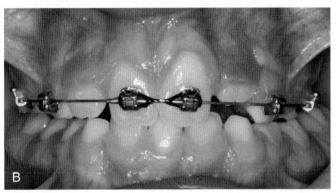

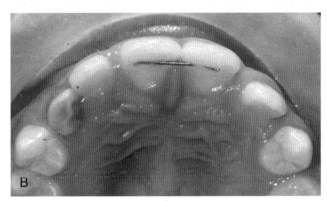

• **Figure 36.32** (A) If bodily mesiodistal movement is needed to close a diastema, fixed appliances are placed on the teeth. (B) After initial alignment, either a segmental or a full archwire is placed in the brackets, and the teeth are moved together with an elastomeric chain.

• **Figure 36.33** (A) Following diastema closure, retention is required. (B) One method that reduces the need for patient cooperation is the light, multistranded bonded wire. The wire must be placed far enough gingivally to prevent occlusal interferences. In addition, the patient must clean the area carefully and avoid direct contact with hard foods.

Mild Crowding

As mentioned earlier, children can have various amounts of irregularity without any real arch length shortage when the leeway space is included. Mild irregularity is even considered normal in patients who have no arch length discrepancy. Longitudinal studies of persons with ideal occlusions show that there is a period when up to 2 mm of transitional irregularity occurs early in the mixed dentition and eventually resolves.[64] Observation is usually the best course. Some patients have little or no overall arch length shortages and demonstrate noticeable crowding during incisor eruption. This is due to the larger permanent incisors and the transitional crowding they cause during the transition from the primary to

mixed dentitions. Gianelly[65] has described these conditions and noted that a large percentage of patients with irregularity can be treated simply by protecting the leeway space with a lingual arch. On the other hand, if the leeway space is left unattended, the molars will move anteriorly into the leeway space and a true arch length shortage will exist.

The clinical management of irregularity without a true arch length shortage can take several forms depending on the amount of irregularity. In general, if the irregularity is minor, no treatment is indicated. If the irregularity is slightly more severe, interproximal stripping or disking of the primary teeth (usually the canines) can be accomplished to provide temporary space (Fig. 36.34). Disking

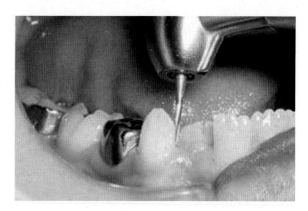

• **Figure 36.34** When the arch length discrepancy is determined to be 2 mm or less and the lateral incisor is erupting lingual to its proper position, the primary canine can be disked with either a high- or low-speed handpiece or a handheld strip. In this case a tapered fissure bur in a high-speed handpiece is being used to disk the mesial surface of the primary canine.

WHITE SPOT LESIONS

John R. Christensen

Tooth movement with fixed appliances (braces) carries some risk for teeth. One unfortunate consequence of fixed appliance therapy is the development of white spot lesions (WSLs). WSLs are defined as "the first sign of caries-like lesion on enamel that can be detected with the naked eye."[1] Practically, a WSL is a thin white line around the periphery of an orthodontic bracket that appears more white and chalky when the teeth are dried. The white appearance is due to demineralization of the surface and subsurface enamel.

WSLs have been demonstrated as early as 4 weeks after the placement of orthodontic appliances.[2] The development of WSLs is reported to be very rapid in the first 6 months of orthodontic treatment and then begins to slow after 12 months.[3] The prevalence for WSLs has been reported to be from 2% to 96% of orthodontic cases. The wide disparity is due to the different methods used to define a WSL. For example, the use of quantitative light-induced fluorescence yields a higher number of WSLs compared with a visual examination.[4] Regardless of the definition, it is apparent that WSLs do develop during orthodontic treatment. One report showed 62% of patients develop a least one WSL on one of the maxillary anterior teeth and that an average of 3.9 teeth of the 6 had WSLs.[5]

These statistics provide a dilemma for the clinician. First, orthodontic treatment is initiated to not only improve the function of the masticatory system but to improve the esthetics of a patient's smile. A prudent clinician would know there is a high likelihood of white spot development during orthodontic treatment. The presence of a WSL detracts from the esthetics of a finished case. Therefore it is important for the clinician to identify those patients at greatest risk for white spot development and to create a plan to prevent the occurrence of such lesions. Heymann and Grauer developed a risk assessment analysis to differentiate patients into high- and low-risk candidates for WSL prior to orthodontic treatment.[4] If a patient exhibited two of the following characteristics they were deemed to be high risk for white spot development. The characteristics were existing WSL, poor oral hygiene, high dietary sugar exposure, long treatment time, labial appliances, and a high DMFT score. Although these characteristics seem reasonable and rather easy to determine, the next step is more difficult. In other words, if a patient is classified as high risk, what preventive measures should be taken?

Prevention can be divided into four approaches. The first is diet. The second is oral hygiene. The third is chemotherapeutic agents. The last is the design and delivery of the orthodontic appliance itself. Diet counseling has been studied extensively in preventing dental caries, but there is a paucity of articles looking at dietary recommendations and WSL development during orthodontic treatment. It appears that dietary counseling has minimal influence on the development of WSLs.[6] This does not mean the clinician should not discuss diet with a prospective orthodontic patient, but it appears that other factors have more influence on WSL development.

Oral hygiene instruction prior to orthodontic treatment is critical to help a patient maintain excellent oral hygiene during treatment. The change in the local environment (brackets, adhesive, and wires) makes cleaning more time consuming and more difficult. There are no statistically significant findings on oral hygiene and reduction in WSLs, but there are tendencies one can point to. The first is a prospective study on orthodontic patients that found the level of visible plaque around the appliance shortly after bonding was the best predictor for WSLs at appliance removal.[7] Another divided the study group into good, medium, and poor compliance groups for oral hygiene. The good compliance group developed 1.0 WSLs during treatment, the medium compliance 1.4, and the poor compliance group 3.3 lesions. Although these numbers were not statistically significant, it appears that good compliance with oral hygiene measures influences white spot development.[6]

These findings are rather distressing for the clinician. If neither diet nor oral hygiene influences the development of WSLs during orthodontic treatment, what should a clinician do? The most recent focus is on chemotherapeutic agents to influence the effect of plaque and bacteria on the enamel surface or to make the enamel surface more resistant to breakdown. Fluoride exposure is probably the most popular and widely tested chemotherapeutic agent. Fluoride can be delivered via toothpaste, rinses, professional application, and release from the orthodontic appliance (adhesive and elastomeric ties). However, there are no studies that have shown fluoride release from the orthodontic appliance has a significant influence on enamel demineralization.

There are many studies promoting the use of fluoride during orthodontic treatment to prevent or reduce WSLs, but these studies are not rigorous enough to avoid potential bias under close examination. A recent Cochrane review suggested a professionally applied fluoride varnish delivered at every orthodontic appointment may reduce WSLs by 70%.[8] Because fluoride delivery from toothpaste and over-the-counter rinses is highly dependent on patient cooperation, a professionally applied fluoride varnish at every orthodontic appointment may be the best way to protect a patient against demineralization.

Other chemotherapeutic agents used to promote oral hygiene have been investigated to see if they decrease decalcification. The use of an essential oil mouthrinse reduced plaque and gingivitis scores in orthodontic patients.[9] The study did not look at reduction of WSLs. A second study did report a decrease in WSLs with the use of MI Paste Plus (GC America, Alsip, IL) during orthodontic treatment.[10]

Often demineralization becomes apparent during orthodontic treatment. When discovered, the clinician has several choices. The first is to inform the patient (and parents) of the condition. The clinician can review risk factors and begin more aggressive fluoride therapy or add additional therapies such as amorphous calcium phosphate (ACP). MI Paste is a product that contains casein phosphopeptide ACP, a milk-derived protein that helps to promote enamel remineralization. Studies are equivocal about whether the effect of MI Paste on remineralization of WSLs is greater than fluoride products, but it has been shown to enhance remineralization similar to fluoride products.[11] ACP is contraindicated in patients with milk protein allergies.

WHITE SPOT LESIONS—cont'd

The other choices for the clinician in cases of severe demineralization is to accelerate the finish of treatment, finish with less than ideal results, or discontinue treatment all together. This is a difficult situation for patients, parents, and doctors. The decision should be made after all meet to discuss the advantages and disadvantages of each possible alternative. After orthodontic treatment is completed or discontinued, postorthodontic treatment of WSLs can be initiated.

Treatment of WSLs or demineralization after orthodontic treatment is unpredictable. Many variables such as the size and depth of the lesion and whether the lesion is active (porous enamel) or arrested (nonporous enamel) make treatment outcomes successful in some and fail in others. Postorthodontic treatment of WSLs can be divided into three or four strategies. The first is recognition of the problem and resumption of good oral hygiene practices at home. These practices are no different from normal hygiene recommendations, such as twice daily brushing with fluoride toothpastes.

A second strategy is to apply some type of remineralizing solution on the affected teeth. This can include professional application of fluoride, ACP, or a combination of the two. These applications can be applied at a predetermined interval to help with the natural resolution of WSLs.

Alteration of the enamel surface can also improve the appearance of WSLs. The most common alteration of the surface has been microabrasion. In microabrasion, the teeth are isolated with a rubber dam to protect the patient's soft tissues and a slurry of acid and abrasive material is rubbed or applied on the enamel surface. Many acids have been used; hydrofluoric, hydrochloric, citric, nitric, and phosphoric acids have all been tested. The abrasive material has been dental pumice, synthetic diamond dust, aluminum oxides, and silicon carbide.[12] The procedure removes 25 to 200 µm of enamel and improves WSLs if they are shallow. Many clinicians use a tooth-bleaching regimen following the microabrasion to give better results.

In some cases, bleaching of the teeth may provide desired results. The bleaching procedure may be done in the dental office, or the bleaching material may be delivered with trays at home. The bleaching material may be a hydrogen peroxide–based material or a carbamide peroxide material of varying percentage. It appears bleaching will lighten both the white spot and the unaffected healthy enamel, with the healthy enamel lightening more than the white spot.[13] This difference in color change helps to disguise the difference between the WSLs and healthy enamel.

Restorative procedures can be used to treat WSLs. The most conservative restorative procedure is called resin infiltration. The resin infiltration procedure consists of placing acid etch on the facial surface of the tooth to create porosities in the enamel. An unfilled or low viscosity resin is applied to the facial surface and allowed to penetrate the porous enamel surface to fill the WSL. This technique is relatively new during the writing of this chapter, and long-term data on effectiveness are difficult to find. It appears there is promise for improvement of WSLs with this treatment.[14,15]

Finally, the clinician can restore WSLs with a traditional restorative approach. The affected areas of enamel are removed with an appropriate dental bur and handpiece. The preparation may be beveled and the tooth restored with a traditional acid etch, primer, and color-matched composite resin. The obvious issue with restoration is that tooth structure is removed and replaced with a composite resin. This procedure is not reversible and will require additional care and treatment for the lifetime of the tooth.

The presence of a WSL at the end of orthodontic treatment is at best a frustration and at worst an esthetic failure for the patient and clinician. Based on available literature, the clinician should implement a sound oral hygiene plan and apply fluoride varnish during treatment to avoid or minimize white spot development. At the end of treatment, the clinician can choose from several treatment options based on the size, number, and appearance of WSLs on the teeth. One can safely say there is no one treatment to completely eliminate or disguise this problem.

References

1. Fejerskov O, Nyvad B, Kidd EAM. *Dental Caries: The Disease and Its Clinical Management*. Copenhagen: Blackwell Munksgaard; 2003.
2. Reilly MM, Featherstone JD. Decalcification and remineralization around orthodontic appliances: an in vivo study. *J Dent Res*. 1985;64:301.
3. Tufekci E, Dixon JS, Gunsolley JC, et al. Prevalence of white spot lesions during orthodontic treatment with fixed appliances. *Angle Orthod*. 2011;81:206–210.
4. Heymann GC, Grauer D. A contemporary review of white spot lesions in orthodontics. *J Esthet Restor Dent*. 2013;25:85–95.
5. Behrents RG. Offense or defense? *Am J Orthod Dentofacial Orthop*. 2016;149(3):303–304.
6. Hadler-Olsen S, Sandvik K, El-Agroudi MA, et al. The incidence of caries and white spot lesions in orthodontically treated adolescents with a comprehensive caries prophylactic regimen—a prospective study. *Eur J Orthod*. 2011;34:633–639.
7. Øgaard B, Larsson E, Henriksson T, et al. Effects of combined application of antimicrobial and fluoride varnishes in orthodontic patients. *Am J Orthod Dentofacial Orthop*. 2001;120:28–35.
8. Benson PE, Parkin N, Dyer F, et al. Fluorides for the prevention of early tooth decay (demineralised white lesions) during fixed brace treatment. *Cochrane Database Syst Rev*. 2013;(12):CD003809.
9. Tufekci E, Casagrande ZA, Lindauer SJ, et al. Effectiveness of an essential oil mouthrinse in improving oral health in orthodontic patients. *Angle Orthod*. 2008;78(2):294–298.
10. Robertson MA, Kau CH, English JD, et al. MI Paste Plus to prevent demineralization in orthodontic patients: a prospective randomized controlled trial. *Am J Orthod Dentofacial Orthop*. 2011;140(5):660–668.
11. Li J, Xie X, Wang Y, et al. Long-term remineralizing effect of casein phosphopeptide-amorphous calcium phosphate (CPP-ACP) on early caries lesions in vivo: a systematic review. *J Dent*. 2014;42(7):769–777.
12. Sundfeld RH, Croll TP, Briso AL, et al. Considerations about enamel microabrasion after 18 years. *Am J Dent*. 2007;20(2):67.
13. Knösel M, Attin R, Becker K, et al. External bleaching effect on the color and luminosity of inactive white-spot lesions after fixed orthodontic appliances. *Angle Orthod*. 2007;77(4):646–652.
14. Senestraro SV, Crowe JJ, Wang M, et al. Minimally invasive resin infiltration of arrested white-spot lesions: a randomized clinical trial. *J Am Dent Assoc*. 2013;144(9):997–1005.
15. Knösel M, Eckstein A, Helms HJ. Durability of esthetic improvement following Icon resin infiltration of multibracket-induced white spot lesions compared with no therapy over 6 months: a single-center, split-mouth, randomized clinical trial. *Am J Orthod Dentofacial Orthop*. 2013;144(1):86–96.

may be accomplished with a handheld strip, a sandpaper disk in a low-speed handpiece, or a tapered bur in a high-speed handpiece. The enamel-reducing instrument must be held vertically to reduce the true mesiodistal dimension of the tooth even subgingivally to be successful. The procedure is performed without anesthesia so that the child can indicate any discomfort. Extreme discomfort usually indicates that sufficient enamel has been removed to cause the pulpal tissues to react. Careful disking can yield 2 to 4 mm of space. A professional-strength topical fluoride preparation can be applied to the canines after disking and may reduce postoperative sensitivity. Note that in the mixed dentition, interproximal reduction of permanent teeth before the eruption of the permanent canines and evaluation of the patient's tooth size is contraindicated. If teeth are prematurely reduced, an iatrogenic tooth size problem may be created.

If it is apparent that disking will not alleviate the anterior irregularity, it may be appropriate to extract the primary canines and place a lingual arch so that the available space can be used by the larger incisors for alignment, and the smaller premolars can erupt later in the remaining space. For the most part, this therapy is undertaken in the mandibular arch, although there are a few situations in which it is indicated in the maxilla. A lingual arch is necessary because the lower incisors tend to tip lingually without the support of the primary canines. This results in shortening of arch length and some reduction in dental alveolar bone. In this situation the lingual arch is placed in a passive state (i.e., the arch exerts no force to move the incisors and increase the space). The clinician should communicate to the parent that this treatment requires close supervision and the primary first molars may have to be disked or extracted when the permanent canines erupt. The lingual arch remains in place until the second premolars have erupted or until it is evident there will be sufficient space for all the permanent teeth to erupt. Essentially, one is using the leeway space and controlling all available arch length to achieve alignment of the teeth (Fig. 36.35). In some cases, this means the molars (those that are end to end) will not achieve a class I relationship because the mandibular mesial molar shift has been prevented. Either headgear or interarch mechanics such as elastics will need to be used to achieve the correct occlusal relationships. In other situations a class I molar relationship may have already been present and this is not a concern.

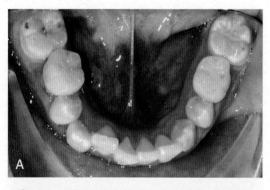
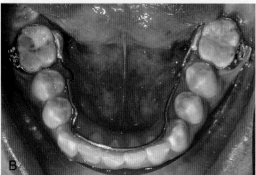

• **Figure 36.35** Space that is available in the arches (leeway) can be used to alleviate crowding by maintaining space when crowding is present and allowing alignment when the larger primary second molars exfoliate or are extracted. (A) This patient shows some crowding with the primary second molars in place. (B) A lower lingual arch was placed so the leeway space could be used for spontaneous alignment.

A true arch length discrepancy of 0 to 2 mm may not be apparent or may be manifested as a mild irregularity, most likely in the incisor region. Treatment may be indicated for these children if the lateral incisors erupt lingual to their proper position or in very irregular positions. If treatment is deemed necessary, interproximal stripping of primary teeth as described earlier may be used. With true, small arch length shortages, ultimately minor crowding will either be accepted, permanent teeth will have to be reduced in the mesiodistal dimension, or the arch will have to be expanded with fixed or removable appliances, as described in the next section.

Moderate Crowding

Treatment for a moderate arch length discrepancy of less than 5 mm is based on the facial profile, incisor position, crowding, and the amount of facial keratinized tissue. If the profile is straight, with good anteroposterior or slightly retrusive position of the lips and incisors, a small amount of expansion can be tolerated to accommodate all the teeth. Expansion is not a good treatment option if the incisors are already protrusive. The clinician should always keep in mind the interaction between crowding, incisor position, and profile because they are essentially all part of the same problem just expressed in a different way.

Moderate crowding may be localized or generalized. Localized crowding may be the result of space loss after extraction or premature exfoliation of a primary tooth. If space loss is 3 mm or less, the adjacent tooth usually can be tipped into proper position with a removable appliance, an active lingual arch, or a fixed banded and bonded appliance. For example, a removable appliance with a finger spring can tip a permanent maxillary or mandibular first molar distally after removal of a primary second molar compromised by ectopic eruption. Numerous other fixed appliances such as lingual holding arches or a Nance lingual arch supporting segmental arches with compressed coil springs can be used (Fig. 36.36A). Alternatively, a Nance arch with compressed helical springs can be used to move posterior teeth distally (Fig. 36.36B). Regardless of the appliance configuration, the method is basically the same, and these appliances can be used either unilaterally or bilaterally. For arch perimeter increases in the maxillary arch, the distal molar movement is accompanied by an anterior movement of the anchor or anterior segment.[66,67] Without additional anchorage, the anterior teeth move facially in a ratio of approximately one-third anterior and two-thirds posterior (Fig. 36.37). With additional anchorage, such as TADs in the anterior palate, distal molar movement of approximately 1 mm/month has been demonstrated with no change in the position of the anterior teeth.[68] The challenge then is to preserve the distal molar movement and retract and align the remaining teeth.

Alternatively, headgear can be used if bilateral space regaining is desired. After the space has been regained, arch length should be near ideal and should be maintained. A band and loop appliance or a lingual archlike appliance can be placed to maintain the space.

If localized crowding is not due to terminal molars drifting anteriorly but is in the anterior or midportions of the arch, permanent tooth impaction is likely. Orthodontic tooth movement is necessary to increase the space and allow room for eruption (Fig. 36.38). Fixed orthodontic appliances are placed on a portion or the entire arch, and the teeth are aligned with light, flexible archwires. After alignment, a heavy archwire is placed to maintain good arch form during space-regaining movements. A compressed coil spring is the simplest means to open space and provides adequate force to open the space. After the space has been opened, the clinician should allow the tooth up to 6 months to erupt. If the tooth

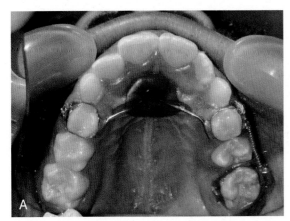
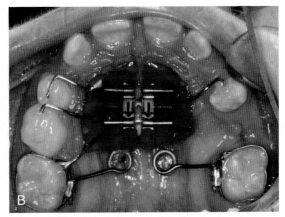

• **Figure 36.36** A fixed appliance can be used to distalize molars in either arch. In the maxillary arch (A), a modified Nance palatal arch and nickel titanium springs on an archwire, or a Nance arch and helical springs can be used to distalize molars (B). Some anterior incisor movement also occurs.

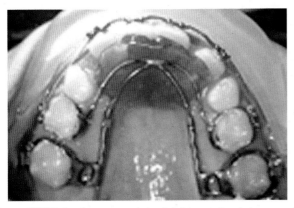

• **Figure 36.37** Another approach to distalizing molars is to use palatal forces and springs supported by teeth and the palate. Even with this method, some anterior tooth movement is observed unless the appliance is supported with temporary anchorage devices.

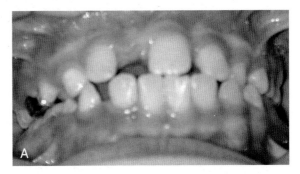
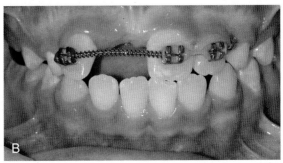

• **Figure 36.38** Many situations rely on the same principles for treatment of crowding in the anterior segment. In general, the first step is to align and open space. (A) This patient lost the maxillary right central incisor to trauma and subsequently space redistributed. (B) The teeth were aligned with a segmental arch in the first phase of treatment, and then a coil spring was used to open the space for the prosthetic replacement.

does not erupt within that time period, it may be necessary to surgically expose the tooth. There are two surgical methods to expose a tooth. The first is a closed exposure. In a closed exposure a flap is elevated and the tooth is located. An orthodontic attachment, often a bracket pad with a soldered gold chain, is bonded to the tooth. The gold chain is tied to the existing orthodontic appliances, and the flap is replaced. The clinician applies force to the gold chain by elastomeric thread, auxiliary wires, or loops from a continuous archwire to bring the tooth into position. Closed exposure is preferred when the tooth crown is located beyond the mucogingival junction. The other type of surgical exposure is an open exposure. In this type of exposure, the soft tissue is elevated and repositioned around the crown to provide adequate keratinized tissue around the impacted tooth. Open exposure is considered when the crown is below the mucogingival junction and minimal repositioning is required. Adequate attached gingiva is essential for good periodontal support and esthetic appearance. Closed exposure simulates the actual eruption of the tooth and usually results in better hard and soft tissue esthetics. If the clinician is not well versed in surgical exposure, the patient is best referred to a specialist. In an open exposure the tooth can be allowed to erupt or an orthodontic attachment is bonded to the crown and the

tooth is moved into the arch (Fig. 36.39). Several methods can be used to generate the force to move the tooth occlusally, but using an overlay flexible wire (usually NiTi) is simple and effective. The overlay wire technique is an especially applicable technique for extruding traumatically intruded incisors so that they can be assessed and/or accessed for endodontic treatment. The method is simple, does not impinge on the adjacent tissue, permits easy cleaning, and allows reasonably efficient movement of teeth (Fig. 36.40).

Patients characterized by anterior or generalized crowding of less than 5 mm present difficult treatment decisions. As stated

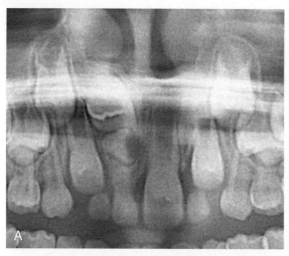

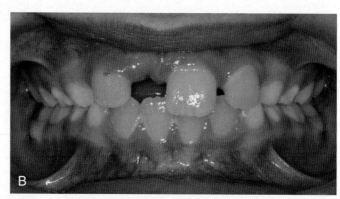

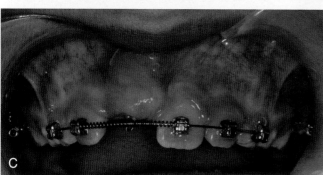

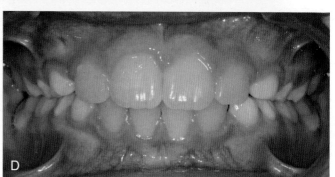

• **Figure 36.39** (A) A panoramic radiograph was obtained on a patient who had an unerupted right central incisor. The radiograph showed that a supernumerary tooth was blocking the eruption of the central incisor. (B) The primary incisors and the supernumerary were removed to see if the central incisor would erupt. It was determined the central incisor would need to be exposed and a bonded bracket and chain attached so the tooth could be brought into alignment. (C) The space was opened for the unerupted central incisor and it was brought into position with elastic thread tied to a base archwire. (D) The tooth in final position. Note the more gingival attachment on the extruded tooth. These levels should approximate one another with time.

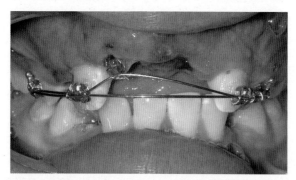

• **Figure 36.40** Extrusion with overlay wires can be used successfully following traumatic intrusion injuries. The overlay archwire, which is a light and flexible wire and now usually nickel titanium, is ligated with a stiffer supporting archwire, usually stainless steel. The light wire is engaged in the bracket and provides light continuous forces over a large range to rapidly and physiologically extrude the tooth.

earlier, incisor and lip position provide important guides to whether arch length can be created by expansion as does the presence of adequate facial keratinized tissue. Upright or lingually inclined incisors may be moved facially into correct alignment if the lips are retrusive. However, the risk associated with generalized arch expansion is instability of the new position.[69,70] Movement of teeth facially may upset the existing equilibrium and cause relapse after the appliances are removed. Relapse does not occur in all cases; some patients maintain increased arch dimensions and remain stable after treatment is complete. However, there does not seem to be a good method for predicting stability.[71] Unfortunately, clinical judgment and long-term retention must be relied on in many cases.

If the clinician elects to alleviate arch length inadequacy by expansion (because the leeway space is inadequate), several approaches can be taken. An active lower lingual arch can be constructed with adjustment loops to tip the incisors facially if the overbite is not prohibitively deep to prevent movement of the incisors (Fig. 36.41); the lower lingual arch may also move the

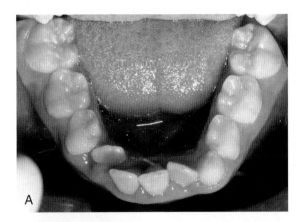

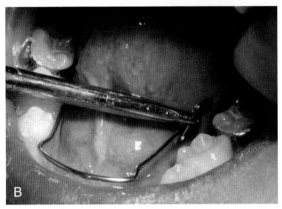

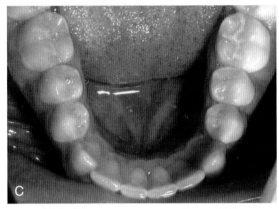

• **Figure 36.41** (A) Generalized crowding of less than 5 mm is occasionally managed with an adjustable lingual arch if the overbite is not too deep to prevent facial movement of the mandibular incisors. (B) The appliance is activated on several occasions by opening the adjustment loops. (C) The same patient after treatment.

molars distally a small amount. The adjustment loops, located mesial to the molars, should not be activated beyond 1 mm because the activation of such a large wire (0.036 inches) places extremely large forces on the teeth. When the appliance is properly activated, the wire contacts the tooth high on the cingulum of the incisors. The direction of force is apical, but it tips the incisors facially because of the inclination of the lingual surface of the teeth. In 4 to 6 weeks the appliance can be activated another millimeter. This process is repeated until arch length is adequate for the permanent dentition. Primary canines may have to be disked or removed as discussed previously if the crowding is in the anterior region.

A lip bumper, a wire appliance inserted in tubes on the lower molars, may be used to decrease lower lip pressure and achieve generalized arch expansion in the incisor, canine, and premolar regions (Fig. 36.42). The location of the expansion depends on the location of the lip bumper. The lip bumper removes resting pressure of the lips and cheeks from these teeth. The teeth move facially as a result of lack of lip pressure and the force of resting tongue pressure. The pressure from the lower lip may tip the molar distally.[72] Remember that ultimately both arches must be coordinated.

Arch expansion may also be accomplished via a functional appliance with buccal shields in the vestibule.[73] The buccal shields disrupt the equilibrium between the tongue and the cheek and allow the teeth to move facially (Fig. 36.43). Some investigators claim that properly constructed buccal shields stretch the underlying periosteum of the bone and cause skeletal remodeling in the transverse dimension. Although this claim has not been substantiated

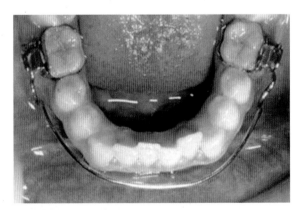

• **Figure 36.42** A lip bumper is also used to treat generalized crowding of less than 5 mm. The lip bumper is designed to decrease lower lip pressure on the teeth and to allow generalized expansion by facial movement of the teeth.

by careful investigation, there is no doubt that enough expansion can be created in this manner to relieve minor to moderate crowding.

Like removable appliances, fixed (banded and bonded) appliances can be used to tip teeth. Fixed orthodontic appliances are necessary to increase arch length when bodily movement of teeth is required to alleviate crowding and align the teeth. Banded and bonded appliances also offer the opportunity to efficiently control rotational problems of teeth. A variety of archwire designs can be used to expand the arch, depending on the number of teeth with attachments (Fig. 36.44). Clearly, any dimension of the arch can be altered with this method. After the expansion has been completed, a lower lingual arch is placed to retain the expansion.

In most cases, further treatment is necessary to align the remaining permanent teeth when they erupt (Fig. 36.45). In addition, distal movement of the maxillary molars may be required if some of the leeway space was used to align the mandibular teeth and cannot be used for the mesial molar shift. When a class I molar relationship is present initially, this is not an issue. Therefore multibonded appliances should be used sparingly in the lower arch, generally only in cases in which the molars are already class I and there is some increased overjet, unless one is prepared to complete the case appropriately by adjusting the interarch relationships. Regardless of which appliance is selected, expansion influences incisor position and profile.

Severe Crowding

Crowding of more than 5 mm is considered severe. This amount of crowding is managed either with generalized arch expansion or with removal of selected permanent teeth. This degree of generalized arch expansion can be accomplished with different appliances but usually requires bodily tooth movement with fixed appliances.

Achieving considerable expansion often is difficult. Incisor position, profile, and periodontal status all influence whether the patient should be treated without extraction. Patients with this degree of crowding are most appropriately referred to a specialist.

The decision to extract teeth is based on the factors listed previously and is further influenced by the location of the crowding, the position of the dental midline, and the dental and skeletal relationships of the patient. After careful case analysis, appropriate

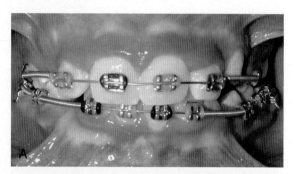

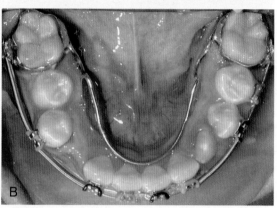

• **Figure 36.44** Expansion of the dental arches to reduce crowding can be accomplished with fixed appliances and is usually indicated when there are rotations or bodily tooth movement is required. (A) Expansion during the mixed dentition using fixed appliances. (B) The mechanics often are a combination of coil springs and elastomeric chains to move teeth and increase arch dimensions. A lingual arch can be used for maintenance of the intermolar dimension. (From Proffit WR, Fields HW, Jr, Sarver DM. *Contemporary Orthodontics*. 5th ed. St Louis: Elsevier; 2013.)

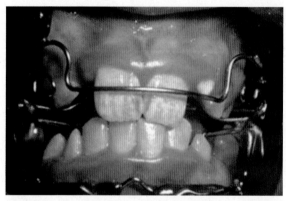

• **Figure 36.43** Generalized arch expansion can also be accomplished via a functional appliance with buccal shields. The buccal shields disrupt the equilibrium between the facial musculature and the tongue and allow the teeth to move facially.

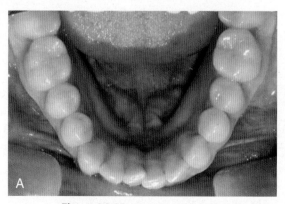

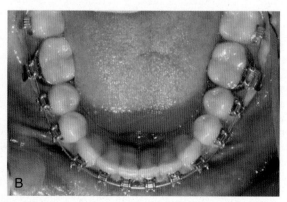

• **Figure 36.45** (A) Arch expansion can be accomplished during the permanent dentition years too. (B) The anterior irregularities, mostly rotations, were managed with a fixed appliance. (From Proffit WR, Fields HW, Jr, Sarver DM. *Contemporary Orthodontics*. 5th ed. St Louis: Elsevier; 2013.)

teeth may be removed to make subsequent tooth movement easier to accomplish and to minimize the effects of extraction on the profile. The permanent first premolar is most often selected for extraction because it is located at a midpoint in the arch and because the space it occupies can be used to correct midline problems, incisor protrusion, molar relationship problems, or crowding. Other teeth can be removed depending on the specifics of the case and the type of therapy used. Management of extraction cases is best performed by a specialist.

In some children, crowding is so severe in the mixed dentition that expansion is not feasible, and extractions are necessary to obtain a suitable occlusion that is in harmony with the supporting structures and the facial profile. In these cases a planned sequence of extractions of primary and permanent teeth can benefit the patient by reducing incisor crowding and irregularity in the early mixed dentition, which will make subsequent orthodontic treatment easier and quicker. The extractions also make room for teeth to erupt within the alveolus and through keratinized tissue rather than being forced buccally or lingually into positions that may affect the periodontal health of the teeth. Guidance of eruption and serial extraction are terms used to describe this sequence of extractions.[74,75] Guidance of eruption was originally developed to manage severe crowding without orthodontic appliances but now is viewed as the first step in treatment culminating in fixed orthodontic appliance therapy. For this reason the clinician should consult with a specialist before embarking on a planned extraction sequence.

Guidance of eruption should be considered an option when crowding is greater than 10 mm per arch, a measurement that should be confirmed by space analysis after the permanent lateral incisors have erupted. In addition, the patient should have a class I dental and skeletal pattern with good lip and incisor position (unless one is prepared to address these problems) because guidance of eruption does not correct skeletal problems. Guidance of eruption begins in the early mixed dentition with the eruption of the lateral incisors (Fig. 36.46A). If a significant arch length discrepancy is predicted, the primary canines should be removed. This allows the incisors ample room to erupt and align (see Fig. 36.46B). Typically, the incisors also tip lingually and upright, causing the bite to deepen. Faciolingual incisor displacement usually improves, but rotations are more resistant to spontaneous correction.

The child is observed for 2 years or until it appears that the canines and premolars are ready to erupt. At that time, another space analysis should be completed to ensure that the arch length deficiency is still great enough to warrant permanent tooth extraction, and a radiograph should be obtained to determine the position of the unerupted teeth. The goal of treatment is to encourage the eruption of the permanent first premolar so that it can be extracted before the permanent canine erupts (see Fig. 36.46C). Unfortunately, the mandibular canine erupts first nearly half the time in the mandibular arch. If it appears that the canine is ahead of the premolar and will erupt facially, the primary first molar should be removed when half to two-thirds of the first premolar root is formed. At this stage of root development, premolar eruption will be accelerated, and the premolar will erupt before the canine enters the arch. This makes removal of the first premolar much easier. In the maxillary arch the first premolar normally erupts before the canine, and this is not a problem. In some cases the primary first molar is removed, but the permanent canine still erupts before the first premolar. This can lead to impaction of the first premolar,

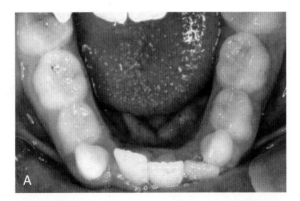

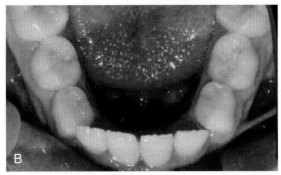
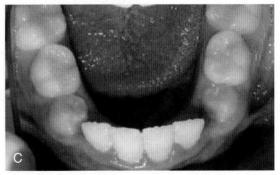

• **Figure 36.46** The initial stages of serial extraction are described here. (A) Due to severe crowding and substantial overall arch length deficiencies, the primary canines require extraction. (B) This allows incisor alignment. (C) Extraction of the primary first molars speeds up the eruption of the first premolars that can then be extracted prior to permanent canine eruption.

requiring surgical removal. Similarly, it may become apparent that the permanent canine will erupt before the first premolar regardless of the extraction sequence. In this situation the primary first molar and first premolar are removed at the same time. This procedure is called *enucleation* because the premolar is removed from within the alveolar bone.

Surgical removal of teeth from within the alveolar bone should be avoided if possible because it carries the potential for creating bone and soft tissue defects. These occur if the alveolar bone is fractured or removed. New alveolar bone will not be stimulated to form because no tooth will erupt through this area. Surgical soft tissue defects resolve infrequently.

An alternative extraction sequence has been advocated to prevent lingual tipping of the lower incisors and the subsequent increase in overbite, but this sequence is recommended only when incisor crowding is limited. The primary canine is not removed when the lateral incisor erupts. Instead, the primary canine is retained, and the primary first molar is extracted to accelerate the eruption of the permanent first premolar. This allows some anterior crowding to resolve. The premolar is extracted when it erupts into the arch. The primary canine is often extracted at the same time as the premolar or is left to exfoliate when the permanent canine erupts. The drawback of this alternative is that substantial incisor crowding is not readily resolved, which somewhat defeats the goal of selective tooth removal to encourage good dental alignment.

Anteroposterior Dental Problems

Anterior Crossbite

Anterior crossbite in the mixed dentition is not an uncommon finding. The clinician should determine whether the crossbite is skeletal or dental in origin from the profile analysis and intraoral findings. Skeletal problems should be referred to a specialist, whereas dental problems can be addressed immediately. The most common cause of nonskeletal crossbite is a lack of space for the permanent maxillary incisors to erupt. A space analysis verifies the space shortage. Anterior crossbite develops because the permanent tooth buds form lingual to the primary teeth. When space is inadequate, the incisors are forced to erupt on the lingual side of the arch. If it is apparent that the permanent incisors are beginning to erupt lingually, the adjacent primary teeth should be disked or removed to provide space for the permanent incisors. If space is provided as the incisors are just beginning to erupt, they will migrate facially out of crossbite, and appliance therapy may not be necessary.

If the incisor fails to erupt facially or if the anterior crossbite is not diagnosed early in the mixed dentition, appliance therapy is needed to correct the crossbite. Space for the incisors is gained by disking, extracting the adjacent primary teeth, or increasing the arch perimeter. At this point a decision must be made as to whether the teeth should be tipped into position or moved bodily into place. If tipping will accomplish treatment goals the dentist can use either a removable appliance or a fixed appliance to correct the crossbite. As described earlier a removable appliance can be used to tip one or more teeth into proper alignment. The appliance is constructed of palatal acrylic with at least two Adams clasps for retention and a finger spring to move the teeth (Fig. 36.47). The spring is a double helix design that provides a physiologic amount of force over an extended range of action. The spring is activated 2 mm to provide 1 mm of tooth movement per month. As with most removable appliances, full-time wear (except for eating and brushing) is necessary to accomplish the desired tooth movement.

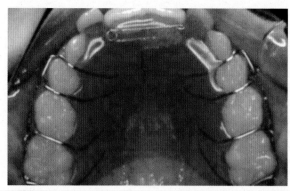

• **Figure 36.47** If an anterior crossbite can be corrected by tipping the teeth facially, a removable appliance will accomplish this goal. In this case a single finger spring is tipping both maxillary central incisors out of crossbite.

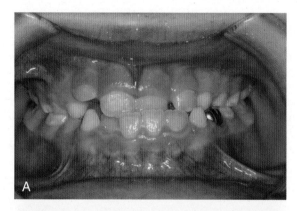

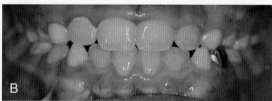

• **Figure 36.48** (A) Fixed appliances also can be used to tip teeth out of anterior crossbite. In this patient, both maxillary lateral incisors were in anterior crossbite. (B) After the brackets were placed, progressively larger round wires were used to tip the teeth out of crossbite. A rectangular archwire will be used to achieve proper crown and root position.

An anterior crossbite with an accompanying deep overbite does not necessarily require a bite plane or bite-opening device during treatment. Most persons habitually keep the mandible open and occlude only during swallowing and parafunctional movements. If the crossbite has not improved after 3 months of active treatment, it may be necessary to open the bite by adding acrylic to the appliance to cover the occlusal surfaces of the posterior teeth. This limits closure and keeps the anterior teeth apart, which allows uninhibited incisor movement. In most cases the crossbite will correct quickly and the bite plane can be removed. Extended use of a bite plane is discouraged because the teeth not in contact with the appliance will continue to erupt, creating a vertical occlusal discrepancy.

Fixed appliances also can tip teeth out of crossbite and do not require as much cooperation from the child. A fixed appliance also provides precise control of tooth movement in all three planes of space by using rectangular wires (Fig. 36.48). The disadvantage of either a labial or a lingual fixed appliance is the patient's inability to clean around the teeth and appliance thoroughly, which can result in marginal gingivitis and caries. A maxillary lingual arch is a suitable appliance to correct an anterior crossbite if the teeth require tipping. The maxillary arch is constructed of 0.036-inch wire and has adjustment loops like those used in a lower lingual arch. Finger springs made of 0.022-inch wire provide the tooth-moving force. The springs are usually soldered on the opposite side of the arch from the tooth being moved to increase the length and range of the spring (Fig. 36.49). The springs are activated approximately 3 mm before the appliance is cemented in place. During cementation, the springs are tied with steel ligatures to the lingual arch so that they will not interfere with the seating of the appliance. After the excess cement has been cleaned away, the ligature is cut away to activate the springs. In some cases the spring slips over the incisal edge of an incisor that is not fully erupted. In these cases, additional retention is needed to keep the spring in place. The retention can come from bonding a stainless steel button or a composite ledge to the lingual surface of the tooth. Conversely, a stainless steel guidewire can be soldered to the lingual arch at the midline to prevent the spring from slipping incisally. Three millimeters of activation provides 1 mm of tooth movement per month. The appliance should be removed, reactivated, and recemented at 4- to 6-week intervals until the crossbite is corrected.

In older patients, space may need to be created for crossbite correction by arch expansion because there are no primary teeth to disk or extract. In this situation the permanent molars should be banded and the incisors bonded with orthodontic brackets.

An anterior crossbite that requires bodily movement of teeth to correct the problem is best managed with bonded brackets and a planned sequence of archwires. Initially, teeth can be tipped out of crossbite. Usually an archwire is selected that is strong enough to withstand the force of occlusion in the posterior segments yet flexible enough in the anterior region to engage the brackets of the malaligned teeth. If posterior strength is a requirement, a stainless steel archwire with loops bent mesial and distal to the tooth in crossbite is placed. Loops in the anterior region are designed to provide horizontal or vertical tooth movement and exert optimal force to move the teeth out of crossbite while stabilizing those

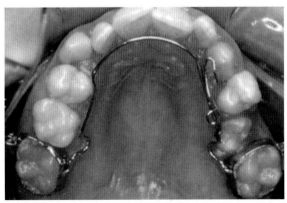

• **Figure 36.49** Fixed lingual appliances can be used to tip the teeth out of anterior crossbite. This patient required facial movement of the maxillary left canine to correct the crossbite. A small finger spring was soldered to the base lingual arch and was activated to provide the force necessary to move the tooth.

that are in the correct position. Alternatively, a flexible titanium alloy wire can be used for alignment. This requires no wire bending or loop forming but moves both the teeth in crossbite and those not in crossbite.

After alignment is completed by either method, a rectangular archwire is inserted into the brackets that can deliver a root-positioning force to the tooth previously in crossbite. The purpose of such a force is to move the root into proper position so the entire tooth essentially moves forward out of crossbite and the angulation of anterior teeth is similar.

Retention must be planned in all cases, regardless of the appliance selected. Active tooth movement is usually continued until the crossbite is slightly overcorrected. The correction should be retained with a passive fixed or removable appliance for 2 months if there is a positive overbite. If there is not adequate overbite, retention should be continued until adequate overbite develops. Circumferential supracrestal fiberotomy can be considered if rotational movement was made during treatment. In a small number of cases the anterior crossbite is caused by excessive spacing and flaring of the mandibular incisors. A removable appliance can be constructed with an adjustable 0.028-inch labial bow to retract the lower incisors and close the space. The appliance is activated 2 mm/month and acrylic removed from the lingual surface. Treatment should be continued until the space is closed and there is positive overbite and overjet. The tooth movement can be retained with the same removable appliance, which is made passive.

Incisor Protrusion

Incisor protrusion in the mixed dentition is a serious esthetic problem for the preadolescent patient. Spaced, protrusive incisors are not only unattractive but also more prone to dental injury than incisors with a normal angulation. For these reasons, treatment is usually undertaken to move the incisors lingually into a more suitable position if the overbite is not prohibitively deep and the overjet will allow lingual movement. This treatment is used for a dental problem, not a skeletal problem. Skeletal problems should be referred to a specialist for growth modification.

Treatment of incisor protrusion has already been discussed in the earlier section on management of diastemas in the mixed dentition (see Figs. 36.29 and 36.30). To summarize, teeth that can be tipped back into ideal alignment can be treated with a removable appliance that incorporates an active labial bow. The bow is activated by means of an adjustment loop to provide a lingual tipping force to the flared incisors. One to 2 mm of palatal acrylic is removed from the appliance to allow the crown to move lingually and to accommodate the palatal tissue that tends to bunch up behind the tooth being moved. The retention schedule should be full-time wear for 3 months.

If bodily movement of teeth is necessary to correct incisor protrusion, the maxillary first molars should be banded and brackets bonded to the anterior permanent teeth. A small, round, flexible archwire is placed in the brackets to align the teeth initially. Anterior tooth retraction is accomplished by either a round or rectangular archwire with a closing loop or elastomeric chain, depending on whether tipping or bodily tooth movement is required. A headgear or a transpalatal arch is usually used during retraction to supplement anchorage. The choice between cervical, combination, or high-pull headgear is based on the patient's vertical facial dimensions, although this is not as simple as one might imagine. Cervical headgear is generally used when the patient has normal vertical facial proportions, whereas high-pull headgear is indicated when the patient has increased lower facial height. The clinician should follow cases of incisor retraction carefully to prevent problems associated with retraction. A complication encountered during incisor retraction is movement of the root of the permanent lateral incisor into the path of the unerupted permanent canine. The lateral incisor root either impedes eruption of the canine or may be resorbed. To avoid this complication, the wire should be bent or the bracket placed so that the lateral incisor root is upright or even tipped slightly to the mesial.

Transverse Dental Problems

Posterior crossbite correction in the mixed dentition can be difficult and confusing. The clinician must rely on a well-documented database to determine whether skeletal or dental correction is necessary. The presence of a mandibular shift also is an important finding. A posterior crossbite with an associated mandibular shift should be managed as soon as possible to prevent soft tissue, dental, and skeletal compensation. Crossbites can be corrected with a W arch or a quad helix in the primary and early mixed dentitions. Both skeletal and dental movements occur with these appliances, and it is difficult to affect only one or the other. In the late mixed dentition the midpalatal suture may be more interdigitated, and the clinician can make primarily dental or skeletal changes depending on the appliance selected to treat the patient. Skeletal problems should be referred to a specialist for treatment with a rapid palatal expander (RPE; see Fig. 36.6), but dental problems usually can be managed without referral. It is infrequent that a patient requires skeletal crossbite correction and has no other orthodontic issues.

Posterior dental crossbites are either generalized or localized. Generalized crossbites of dental origin are usually bilateral and are corrected with a W arch or a quad helix (Fig. 36.50). If the crossbite is due to a unilateral dental constriction, an unequal (asymmetric) W arch (made of 0.036-inch wire) or a quad helix (0.038-inch wire) can be used to expand the arch. Alternatively, a lower lingual arch can be used to stabilize the lower teeth, and cross-elastics can be worn to the maxillary arch to correct the crossbite unilaterally. These appliances have been discussed in previous sections. Localized crossbites are usually due to displacement of single teeth in one or both arches. For example, a maxillary lingual crossbite involving the permanent first molars is usually the result of lingual displacement of the maxillary molar or the facial displacement of the mandibular

molar. If teeth in opposing arches are both at fault, it is easy to correct the problem using a simple crossbite elastic. The offending teeth are fitted with orthodontic bands without attachments. After the bands are fitted, they are removed, and a button is welded to the opposite surface of the band from the direction in which the tooth is to be moved. Another method is to bond the teeth with buttons attached to bondable pads. There is a greater risk of bond failure than band loosening. Whether the buttons are bonded or banded, the technique to correct the crossbite is identical.

In the example just noted, a button is welded to the lingual surface of the maxillary band and to the buccal surface of the mandibular band. After the bands have been welded and cemented, a medium weight ($\frac{3}{16}$-inch, 6-ounce elastic) is attached from button to button through the occlusion (Fig. 36.51). The elastic should be worn full time, except when the patient is eating, and should be changed at every meal. The elastic should be worn until the crossbite is slightly overcorrected. It may be prudent to leave the bands in place and discontinue the use of elastic for 1 month to ensure that the teeth do not relapse into crossbite. When the occlusion is stable after 4 to 6 weeks without elastic force, the bands can be removed.

Vertical Dental Problems

Vertical problems in the mixed dentition are primarily open bite or deep bite malocclusions. Vertical problems are difficult to diagnose. Treatment is based on which teeth should be encouraged or discouraged to erupt and a specialist should be consulted. Dental open bite is most often the result of an active digit habit that has impeded eruption of the anterior teeth. In some cases the digit habit has been discontinued but the open bite has been maintained because the tongue rests between the teeth and prevents eruption. Treatment is essentially the same as that described for digit habits in the late primary and early mixed dentitions. If therapy without an appliance is unsuccessful, a palatal crib (see Fig. 27.7) is effective if the patient desires to stop the habit. The crib reminds the child to refrain from the habit and blocks the tongue from being placed forward. Therapy is successful in most cases, unless the child is unwilling to abandon the habit.

In some cases of open bite and minimal incisal display, the anterior teeth are encouraged to erupt. This is accomplished by

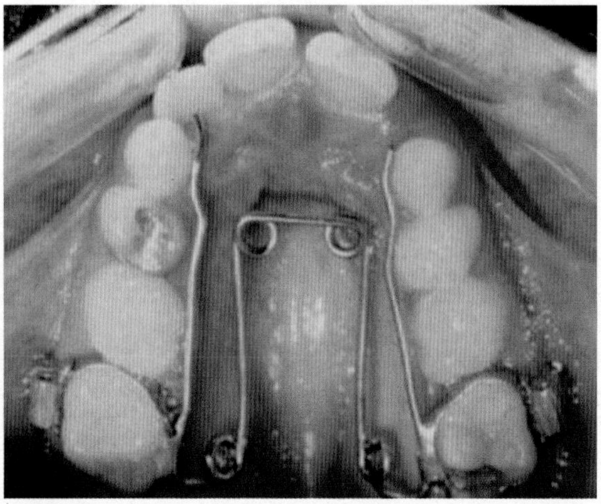

• **Figure 36.50** Posterior crossbites of dental origin in the mixed dentition can be treated with either a W arch or a quad helix. In this patient a quad helix is being used to correct a bilateral posterior crossbite.

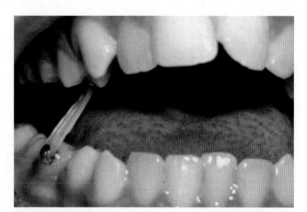

• **Figure 36.51** If teeth are at fault in both arches, a simple crossbite elastic is used to correct the crossbite. Bands can be placed on both permanent right first molars, and buttons can be welded to the lingual side of the maxillary band and to the facial side of the mandibular band. A medium-weight (4- to 6-ounce) elastic is attached from one button to the other to provide the force required to correct the crossbite.

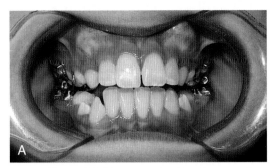
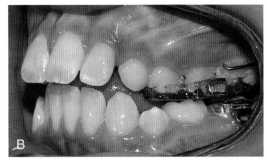

• **Figure 36.52** A removable bite plane can allow eruption of posterior teeth or anterior teeth to increase or reduce overbite. (A) This bite plane prevents eruption of posterior teeth while encouraging anterior teeth to erupt. (B) The bite plane is retained with the clasps around the molar tubes. For posterior eruption to occur, the acrylic would open the bite and be placed between the anterior teeth.

opening the bite and preventing the posterior teeth from erupting with acrylic stops between the teeth, while allowing the anterior teeth to erupt (Fig. 36.52). Skeletal open bite treatment has been described previously, and these patients should be referred to a specialist.

Dental deep bite is caused by overeruption of the anterior teeth or undereruption of the posterior teeth. It should be distinguished from skeletal deep bite, which is characterized by a flat mandibular plane angle and a short vertical dimension, as well as by overerupted and undererupted teeth. In a normal incisor-to-lip relationship, 2 mm of the maxillary central incisor is exposed when the lip is at rest. If more than 2 mm of incisor is exposed, maxillary anterior overeruption should be considered. In the mandibular arch, overeruption is difficult to diagnose; however, the curve of Spee may provide some clue. An excessive curve of Spee (2 mm or more) suggests mandibular incisor overeruption.

Management of deep bite in a growing patient can usually be incorporated into comprehensive orthodontic treatment. Occasionally, treatment in the mixed dentition is aimed at preventing further anterior eruption and encouraging or allowing posterior eruption. This is usually only indicated when the mandibular anterior teeth are impinging on the maxillary lingual gingiva and causing tissue irritation or gingival recession. In these cases the incisor teeth are placed in contact with a bite plane, and the appliance is constructed so that acrylic touches the upper and lower incisors but allows the posterior teeth to erupt. This is a variation of the appliance shown in Fig. 36.52. The appliance must be worn full time to enable correction and then must be worn as a retainer to maintain the correction until the patient stops growing vertically.

If the deep bite is deemed to be the result of maxillary incisor overeruption or a combination of maxillary and mandibular incisor overeruption, fixed orthodontic appliances are placed on the teeth. An intrusion arch, a wire that connects the permanent first molars to the incisors, is constructed to exert a light intrusive force on the incisors (Fig. 36.53). An alternative is a continuous archwire with a V bend near the molars and a 2 × 4 appliance. Because there is an equal and opposite reaction to every force placed on the teeth, the molars experience an extrusive force by either means. Specifically, the molar erupts and tips distally and facially. Facial movement of the molars can be counteracted by a transpalatal arch or a lower lingual arch, but neither will prevent distal crown tipping. In the maxillary arch, headgear that delivers distal root tip to the molars can offset the extrusive and distal crown tipping forces of intrusion arches. Often overbite reduction is the first

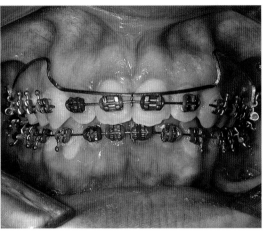

• **Figure 36.53** The intrusion arch can be used to lift the maxillary teeth and reduce overbite. The auxiliary arch, shown here extending from the molars to the incisors gingival to the brackets, is inserted in the auxiliary molar tube. The molar is tied to the segmental archwires so it uses the anchorage of the molars, premolars, and canines.

phase of comprehensive orthodontic treatment, and consultation with a specialist is appropriate.

References

1. Proffit WR, Fields HW, Sarver DM. *Contemporary Orthodontics*. 5th ed. St Louis: Mosby–Year Book; 2012.
2. Proffit WR, White RP, Sarver DM. *Contemporary Treatment of Dentofacial Deformity*. St Louis: Mosby–Year Book; 2003.
3. Hagg U, Pancherz H, Taranger J. Pubertal growth and orthodontic treatment. In: Carlson DS, Ribbens KA, eds. *Craniofacial Growth During Adolescence, Monograph 20*. Craniofacial Growth Series. Ann Arbor, MI: Center for Human Growth and Development, University of Michigan; 1987.
4. Baccetti T, Franchi L, McNamara JA Jr. An improved version of the cervical vertebral maturation (CVM) method for the assessment of mandibular growth. *Angle Orthod*. 2002;72(4):316–323.
5. Chertkow S. Tooth mineralization as an indicator of the pubertal growth. *Am J Orthod Dentofacial Orthop*. 1980;77:79–91.
6. Thompson GW, Popovich F, Anderson DL. Maximum growth changes in mandibular length, stature, and weight. *Hum Biol*. 1976;48:285–293.
7. Anderson G, Fields HW, Beck FM, et al. Development of cephalometric norms using a unified facial and dental approach. *Angle Orthod*. 2006;76:557–563.

8. Tulloch JFC, Phillips C, Proffit WR. Benefit of early class II treatment: progress report of a two-phase randomized clinical trial. *Am J Orthod Dentofacial Orthop.* 1998;113:62–72.

9. De Clerk H, Proffit W. Growth modification of the face: a current perspective with emphasis on class III treatment. *Am J Orthod Dentofacial Orthop.* 2015;148:37–46.

10. O'Brien K, Wright J, Conboy F, et al. Effectiveness of early orthodontic treatment with the twin-block appliance: a multicenter, randomized, controlled trial. Part 2: psychosocial effects. *Am J Orthod Dentofacial Orthop.* 2003;124(5):488–494.

11. Liu Z, McGrath C, Hägg U. The impact of malocclusion/orthodontic treatment need on the quality of life: a systematic review. *Angle Orthod.* 2009;79(3):585–591.

12. Kiyak HA. Does orthodontic treatment affect patients' quality of life? *J Dent Educ.* 2008;72(8):886–894.

13. Thiruvenkatachari B, Harrison J, Worthington H, et al. Early orthodontic treatment for class II malocclusion reduces the chance of incisal trauma: results of a Cochrane systematic review. *Am J Orthod Dentofacial Orthop.* 2015;148:47–59.

14. Koroluk LD, Tulloch JF, Phillips C. Incisor trauma and early treatment for class II division 1 malocclusion. *Am J Orthod Dentofacial Orthop.* 2003;123:117–126.

15. Baumrind S, Korn EL, Isaacson RJ, et al. Quantitative analysis of the orthodontics and orthopedic effects of maxillary traction. *Am J Orthod Dentofacial Orthop.* 1983;84:384–398.

16. Bookstein FL. On the cephalometrics of skeletal change. *Am J Orthod Dentofacial Orthop.* 1982;82:177–198.

17. O'Brien K, Wright J, Conboy F, et al. Effectiveness of treatment for class II malocclusion with the Herbst or twin-block appliances: a randomized, controlled trial. *Am J Orthod Dentofacial Orthop.* 2003;124:128–137.

18. Luzi C, Luzi V, Melsen B. Mini-implants and the efficiency of Herbst treatment: a preliminary study. *Prog Orthod.* 2013;14(1):21.

19. McNamara JA, Bookstein FL, Shaughnessy TG. Skeletal and dental changes following functional regulator therapy on class II patients. *Am J Orthod Dentofacial Orthop.* 1985;88:91–110.

20. Remmer HR, Manandras AN, Hunter WS, et al. Cephalometric changes associated with treatment using the activator, the Frankel appliance, and the fixed appliance. *Am J Orthod Dentofacial Orthop.* 1985;88:363–372.

21. Keeling SD, Wheeler TT, King GJ, et al. Anteroposterior skeletal and dental changes after early class II treatment with bionators and headgear. *Am J Orthod Dentofacial Orthop.* 1998;113:40–50.

22. Baumrind S, Korn EL. Patterns of change in mandibular and facial shape associated with the use of forces to retract the maxilla. *Am J Orthod Dentofacial Orthop.* 1981;80:31–47.

23. Southard T, Marshall S, Allareddy V, et al. An evidence-based comparison of headgear and functional appliance therapy for the correction of class II malocclusions. *Semin Orthod.* 2013;19:174–195.

24. Turley PK. Orthopedic correction of class III malocclusion with palatal expansion and custom protraction headgear. *J Clin Orthod.* 1988;22:314–325.

25. Kim JH, Viana MA, Graber TM, et al. The effectiveness of protraction facemask therapy: a meta-analysis. *Am J Orthod Dentofacial Orthop.* 1999;115:675–685.

26. Vaughn GA, Mason B, Moon HB, et al. The effects of maxillary protraction therapy with or without rapid palatal expansion: a prospective, randomized clinical trial. *Am J Orthod Dentofacial Orthop.* 2005;128:299–309.

27. Sar C, Arman-Özçırpıcı A, Uçkan S, et al. Comparative evaluation of maxillary protraction with or without skeletal anchorage. *Am J Orthod Dentofacial Orthop.* 2011;139:636–649.

28. Nguyen T, Cevidanes L, Cornelis MA, et al. Three-dimensional assessment of maxillary changes associated with bone anchored maxillary protraction. *Am J Orthod Dentofacial Orthop.* 2011;139:790–798.

29. Cha KS. Skeletal changes of maxillary protraction in patients exhibiting skeletal class III malocclusion: a comparison of three skeletal maturation groups. *Angle Orthod.* 2003;73:26–35.

30. Baik HS. Clinical results of the maxillary protraction in Korean children. *Am J Orthod Dentofacial Orthop.* 1995;108:583–592.

31. Merwin D, Ngan P, Hagg U, et al. Timing for effective application of anteriorly directed orthopedic force to the maxilla. *Am J Orthod Dentofacial Orthop.* 1997;112:292–299.

32. Wells AP, Sarver DM, Proffit WR. Long-term efficacy of reverse pull headgear therapy. *Angle Orthod.* 2006;76:915–922.

33. Sakamoto T, Iwase I, Uka A, et al. A roentgenocephalometric study of skeletal changes during and after chin cap treatment. *Am J Orthod Dentofacial Orthop.* 1984;85:341–350.

34. Sugawara J, Asano T, Endo N, et al. Long-term effects of chincup therapy on skeletal profile in mandibular prognathism. *Am J Orthod Dentofacial Orthop.* 1990;98:127–133.

35. Jamilian A, Cannavale R, Piancino M, et al. Methodological quality and outcome of systematic reviews reporting on orthopaedic treatment for class III malocclusion: overview of systematic reviews. *J Orthod.* 2016;43:102–120.

36. Kilic N, Kiki A, Oktay H. Condylar asymmetry in unilateral posterior crossbite patients. *Am J Orthod Dentofacial Orthop.* 2008;133:382–387.

37. Bell R, LeCompte E. The effects of maxillary expansion using a quad helix appliance during the deciduous and mixed detentions. *Am J Orthod Dentofacial Orthop.* 1981;79:152–161.

38. Haas AJ. The treatment of maxillary deficiency by opening the midpalatal suture. *Angle Orthod.* 1965;35:200–217.

39. Hicks E. Slow maxillary expansion: a clinical study of the skeletal versus the dental response to low magnitude force. *Am J Orthod Dentofacial Orthop.* 1978;73:121–141.

40. Brunetto M, Andriani Jda S, Ribeiro GL, et al. Three-dimensional assessment of buccal alveolar bone after rapid and slow maxillary expansion: a clinical trial study. *Am J Orthod Dentofacial Orthop.* 2013;143(5):633–644.

41. Fields HW, Proffit WR, Nixon WL, et al. Facial pattern differences in long-faced children and adults. *Am J Orthod Dentofacial Orthop.* 1984;85:217–223.

42. Firouz M, Zernik J, Nanda R. Dental and orthopedic effects of high-pull headgear in treatment of class II, division 1 malocclusion. *Am J Orthod Dentofacial Orthop.* 1992;102:197–205.

43. Iscan HN, Sarisoy L. Comparison of the effects of passive posterior bite-blocks with different construction bites on the craniofacial and dentoalveolar structures. *Am J Orthod Dentofacial Orthop.* 1997;112:171–178.

44. Yao CC, Lai EH, Chang JZ, et al. Comparison of treatment outcomes between skeletal anchorage and extraoral anchorage in adults with maxillary dentoalveolar protrusion. *Am J Orthod Dentofacial Orthop.* 2008;134(5):615–624.

45. Tunison W, Flores-Mir C, ElBadrawy H, et al. Dental arch space changes following premature loss of primary first molars: a systematic review. *Pediatr Dent.* 2008;30(4):297–302.

46. Northway WM, Wainwright RL, Demirjian A. Effects of premature loss of deciduous molars. *Angle Orthod.* 1984;54(4):295–329.

47. Kennedy DB, Turley PK. The clinical management of ectopically erupting first permanent molars. *Am J Orthod Dentofacial Orthop.* 1987;92:336–345.

48. Christensen R, Fields H, Casamissimo P, et al. Lower dental midline stability: effect of primary canine loss, AAPD 2017 Annual Meeting Poster Presentation (56), 2017.

49. Kau CH, Miotti FA, Harzer W. Extractions as a form of interception in the developing dentition: a randomized controlled trial. *J Orthod.* 2004;31:107–114.

50. Ericson S, Kurol J. Incisor resorption caused by maxillary cuspids: a radiographic study. *Angle Orthod.* 1987;57:332–346.

51. Kurol J. Early treatment of tooth-eruption disturbances. *Am J Orthod Dentofacial Orthop.* 2002;121:588–591.

52. Ericson S, Kurol J. Early treatment of palatally erupting maxillary canines by extraction of primary canines. *Eur J Orthod.* 1988;10:283–295.
53. Sigler LM, Baccetti T, McNamara JA Jr. Effect of rapid maxillary expansion and transpalatal arch treatment associated with deciduous canine extraction on the eruption of palatally displaced canines: a 2-center prospective study. *Am J Orthod Dentofacial Orthop.* 2011;139(3):e235–e244.
54. Bonettia GA, Zanarinib M, Parentic SI, et al. Preventive treatment of ectopically erupting maxillary permanent canines by extraction of deciduous canines and first molars: a randomized clinical trial. *Am J Orthod Dentofacial Orthop.* 2011;139(3):316–323.
55. Kokich VO, Kinzer GA, Janakievski J. Congenitally missing maxillary lateral incisors: restorative replacement. *Am J Orthod Dentofacial Orthop.* 2011;139:435–445.
56. Olsen T, Kokich V. Postorthodontic root approximation after opening space for maxillary lateral incisor implants. *Am J Orthod Dentofacial Orthop.* 2010;137:158e1–158e8.
57. Zachrisson B, Rosa M, Sverker T. Congenitally missing maxillary lateral incisors: canine substitution. *Am J Orthod Dentofacial Orthop.* 2011;139:434–445.
58. Schneider U, Moser L, Fornasetti M, et al. Esthetic evaluation of implants vs canine substitution in patients with congenitally missing maxillary lateral incisors: Are there any new insights? *Am J Orthod Dentofacial Orthop.* 2016;150(3):416–424.
59. De-Marchi LM, Pini NI, Ramos AL, et al. Smile attractiveness of patients treated for congenitally missing maxillary lateral incisors as rated by dentists, laypersons, and the patients themselves. *J Prosthet Dentistry.* 2014;112(3):540–546.
60. Czochrowska EM, Stenvik A, Bjercke B, et al. Outcome of tooth transplantation: survival and success rates 17–41 years posttreatment. *Am J Orthod Dentofacial Orthop.* 2002;121:110–119.
61. Ostler M, Kokich V. Alveolar ridge changes in patients congenitally missing mandibular second molars. *J Prosthet Dent.* 1994;71:144–149.
62. Tsurumachi T, Kuno T. Endodontic and orthodontic treatment of a cross-bite fused maxillary lateral incisor. *Int Endod J.* 2003;36:135–142.
63. Andreasen JO, Andreasen FM, Andersson L. *Traumatic Injuries to the Teeth.* Munksgaard Denmark: Blackwell; 2007.
64. Moorrees CFA, Gron AM, Lebret LML, et al. Growth studies of the dentition: a review. *Am J Orthod Dentofacial Orthop.* 1969;55:600–616.
65. Gianelly AA. Treatment of crowding in the mixed dentition. *Am J Orthod Dentofacial Orthop.* 2002;121:569–571.
66. Bussick TJ, McNamara JA Jr. Dentoalveolar and skeletal changes associated with the pendulum appliance. *Am J Orthod Dentofacial Orthop.* 2000;117:333–343.
67. Byloff FK, Darendeliler MA. Distal molar movement using the pendulum appliance. Part 1: clinical and radiological evaluation. *Angle Orthod.* 1997;67:249–260.
68. Antonarakis GS, Kiliaridis S. Maxillary molar distalization with noncompliance intramaxillary appliances in class II malocclusion. A systematic review. *Angle Orthod.* 2008;78:1133–1140.
69. Little RM, Riedel RA, Artun J. An evaluation of changes in mandibular anterior alignment from 10 to 20 years postretention. *Am J Orthod Dentofacial Orthop.* 1988;93:423–428.
70. Little RM, Riedel RA, Stein A. Mandibular arch length increase during the mixed dentition: postretention evaluation of stability and relapse. *Am J Orthod Dentofacial Orthop.* 1990;97:393–404.
71. Little R. The effects of eruption guidance and serial extraction on the developing dentition. *Pediatr Dent.* 1987;9:65–69.
72. Nevant CT, Buschang PH, Alexander RG, et al. Lip bumper therapy for gaining arch length. *Am J Orthod Dentofacial Orthop.* 1991;100:330–336.
73. Owen AH III. Morphologic changes in the transverse dimension using the Frankel appliance. *Am J Orthod Dentofacial Orthop.* 1983;83:200–217.
74. Hotz RP. Guidance of eruption versus serial extraction. *Am J Orthod Dentofacial Orthop.* 1970;58:1–20.
75. Kjellgren B. Serial extraction as a corrective procedure in dental orthopedic therapy. *Trans Eur Orthod Soc.* 1947;8:134–160.

PART 5

Adolescence

Adolescence represents an extremely important time in the dental care of the pediatric patient because it is a time of unprecedented change. It is the transitional period between puberty and maturity where accelerated physical growth and dynamic hormonal change are accompanied by heightened self-awareness and social maturity. As adolescents begin to develop more independence, the responsibility of dental home care should be managed effectively by themselves rather than by their parents, and this section will address the specific preventive needs of adolescents. The dentist is in a unique position among health care professionals to guide the adolescent's oral health because of the frequent recall examinations. In turn, the adolescent should have more opportunities to discuss some of the physical, psychosocial, and risky behavioral issues that may impact his or her oral health. The practitioner must have the requisite knowledge of adolescent oral health concerns and be able to apply the principles of anticipatory guidance to the adolescent's dental care. In addition, the dentist needs to be an excellent clinician as well as an exceptional educator and communicator in providing information that is clinically relevant and psychologically sensitive to meet the teenager's needs. This section will provide guidance on managing the restorative and esthetic needs of adolescents. Also, as the risk for traumatic injuries increases in this age group, the section will conclude with a discussion of trauma prevention and sports dentistry.

37

The Dynamics of Change

DEBORAH STUDEN-PAVLOVICH AND ADRIANA MODESTO VIEIRA

CHAPTER OUTLINE

Physical Changes

Body

Adolescence in some societies is a very short transitional period that marks the arrival of a child to full citizenship within his or her respective tribe and culture. In today's technology-focused age, adolescence is a time of enormous transition and is certainly not of short duration. The current adolescent has never known a world without the internet and has received music only through downloads. No longer children but not quite adults, adolescents confront a combination of physical and mental health issues that may result in long-term problems in adulthood, ranging from obesity, to hypertension, substance abuse, and depression. Certainly, adolescence is an in-between age in our society and must be understood as something separate from childhood or adulthood.

Critical to the definition of adolescence, regardless of culture, and to the understanding of the adolescent physically is the concept of puberty. Puberty is the landmark in physical development when an individual becomes capable of sexual reproduction. In common law, this has been established historically in our society as age 14 years for boys and age 12 years for girls. The advent of puberty is paralleled by the development of genital tissue and secondary sexual characteristics, such as the development of hair in the genital area.

It is also a time when there is an increase in the mass of muscles, a redistribution of body fat, and an increase in the rate of skeletal growth. A growth spurt is associated with this time of life. This growth spurt follows two different forms, depending on gender. It appears earlier in females than in males. The average onset in males is 2 years later than that in females. The fact that males experience their growth spurt later than females and therefore have a longer maturation period before the growth period is one of the reasons why the height of males generally exceeds the height of females. The earlier growth spurt of females also accounts for the period of time during which mean height of a group of young female adolescents may exceed that of males. It is also important to realize that in females menarche serves as a signal that growth is ending, but for males no such marker exists. The magnitude of the velocity of change during the growth spurt also differs between the sexes. In 1975, Tanner and colleagues[1] concluded that the growth spurt in females peaks at a 9-cm change per year at age 12 years, and that in males it peaks at just over 10 cm at age 14 years.

Craniofacial Changes

During and following adolescence, continued changes in the skeletal growth of the face and skull take place because the facial sutures are still open and viable[2] and mandibular growth can potentially continue. These changes not only cause variation and individuality in facial appearance[3] but also affect the dental structures. The continued changes make a final and unchanging dentition and occlusion a difficult concept to imagine, much less attain. There is a slow increase in facial height accompanied by an increase in prognathism in males.[4,5]

Profile changes occur as changes in specific locations take place. The brow area becomes larger as a result of pneumatization of the frontal sinuses and apposition on the glabella.[6] Also, appositional changes during adolescence and early adult life in the frontal bone area and brow result in this area becoming more prominent.[4] In adolescence, the nose and chin also become more prominent. The tip of the nasal bone lies well ahead of the basal bone of the premaxilla. Soft tissue changes also contribute to the growth in the length of the nose and can affect the harmony existing between the nose, lips, and chin. The mandible shows a greater prognathism than the maxilla because of the circumpubertal growth spurt, which has more effect on the mandible than on the maxilla, especially in males. The chin also becomes more prominent owing to local bone deposition. Lip prominence is reduced by these changes in adjacent structures.

Underlying maxillary changes also occur. The maxillary sinuses, which have expanded laterally and vertically since birth, occupy the space left by the permanent teeth as they erupt. By puberty, the sinuses are usually fully developed, although they may continue to enlarge. Considerable individual variation in the size of the maxillary sinuses occurs, and they often lack symmetry. Lowering of the palatal vault continues because of remodeling. In 1966, Björk[7] concluded that sutural growth as well as appositional growth of the maxilla contributed significantly to the increase in the height of the maxillary body (Fig. 37.1). This can be an example of sexual dimorphism in skeletal growth (Table 37.1). Vertical maxillary facial growth is often greater in females. Because the mandible does not continue to grow as much in females, marked vertical changes in the maxilla can result in downward and backward positioning of the mandible and an increase in facial convexity (Fig. 37.2).[4]

Mandibular growth contributes more than profile changes. This growth may be sufficient to provide room for the third molars. In many cases growth is inadequate, and these molars become impacted (Fig. 37.3). The marked mesial inclination of the posterior permanent teeth diminishes somewhat as the mandible completes its growth from under the maxilla, and the lower incisors tend to become upright. Often this is accompanied by crowding of the lower incisors.[2]

Late mandibular growth imparts an increase in the vertical height of the mandibular ramus, which becomes more upright. The elongation of the ramus accommodates the massive vertical expansion of the nasal region and the lowering of the palate, which is accompanied by dental eruption. Usually the maxillary growth and mandibular growth are compatible and coordinated. If they are not, significant orthodontic problems may result. Particularly in males, there may be late anterior growth that is undesirable.[4]

Dental Changes

All of the permanent teeth generally have erupted by age 12 years, except possibly the four second molars, which may erupt as late as age 13 years, and the third molars, which usually erupt between the ages of 17 and 21 years.

Except for the third molars, the dentist should be concerned about any unerupted permanent tooth after age 13 years and should examine the area in question radiographically.

The roots of all teeth are considered to have been completed by age 16 years except for those of the third molars, which can achieve completion as late as age 25 years.

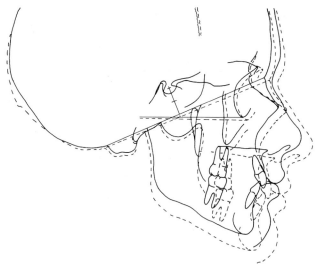

• **Figure 37.1** This anterior cranial base superimposition of the Bolton standard 12- and 18-year-olds (*solid line* and *broken line*, respectively) demonstrates the magnitude of anteroposterior and vertical skeletal growth during this period as well as the soft tissue change. (Redrawn from Broadbent BH Sr, Broadbent BH Jr, Golden WH. *Bolton Standards of Developmental Growth*. St Louis: Mosby; 1975.)

TABLE 37.1	Growth of the Aging Skeleton: Sexual Dimorphism in Craniofacial Growth	
	Females	**Males**
Circumpubertal growth spurt	10–12 years	12–14 years
Mature size	Growth plateaus at age 14 years with increases to 16 years	Active growth to 18 years
Supraorbital ridges	Absent	Well developed
Frontal sinuses	Small	Large
Nose	Small	Large
Zygomatic prominences	Small	Large
Mandibular symphysis	Rounded	Prominent
Mandibular angle	Rounded	Prominent lipping
Occipital condyles	Small	Large
Mastoid processes	Small	Large
Occipital protuberance	Insignificant	Prominent

From Behrents RG. *Growth in the Aging Craniofacial Skeleton.* Ann Arbor, MI: Center for Human Growth and Development, University of Michigan; 1985.

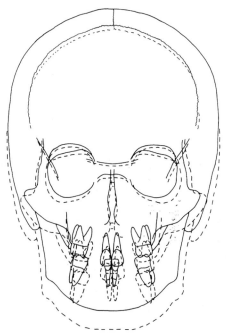

• **Figure 37.2** This anterior cranial base superimposition of the Bolton standard 12- and 18-year-olds (*solid line* and *broken line*, respectively) demonstrates the magnitude of transverse and vertical skeletal growth during this period. (Redrawn from Broadbent BH Sr, Broadbent BH Jr, Golden WH. *Bolton Standards of Developmental Growth*. St Louis: Mosby; 1975.)

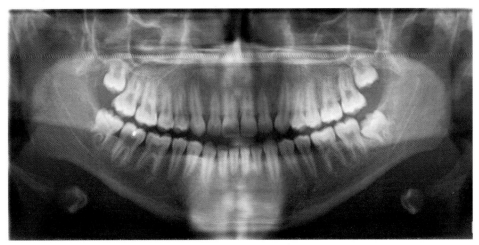

• **Figure 37.3** This panoramic radiograph shows a complete permanent dentition of a 17-year-old patient. All four third molars are present.

Cognitive Changes

According to Piaget, adolescents go through the Formal Operations stage in their cognitive development, and by middle to late adolescence are capable of extremely sophisticated intellectual tasks. High ability at abstract thinking allows the adolescent to deal with complex and difficult vocational and educational challenges. Formal operational thinking and the ability to store information in the memory after perceiving it are hallmarks of the maturation of cognitive ability in adolescents.

The new information available to the adolescent, along with more sophisticated ways of analyzing this information, often makes him or her appear to be a rebel, a complainer, or an accuser. Persons of this age often ascertain the possible and become discontented, even angry, with the real. Kiell[8] pointed out in 1967 that Aristotle, more than 2000 years ago, concluded that adolescents "are passionate, irascible, and apt to be carried away by their impulses." It has been noted that the thoughts of adolescents are both introspective and analytic. They are also egocentric. This dwelling on one's self may make an individual overly self-conscious. Clothes, cars, hairstyles, tastes in music, and identification with certain people or groups probably reflect the adolescent's involvement in self-consciousness.

In summary, by mid- to late adolescence, most young people are capable of formal operational thinking, and can, both in and out of school, master subject material that is extensive, difficult, and abstract. These measures of cognitive development correlate with age and experience. Adolescents are able to plan effectively, have increased reasoning ability, and are able to exhibit inhibitory control. These aspects of brain maturation continue to develop even after adolescence is over. Many have matured into skillful, enthusiastic communicators and conversationalists. Many are also opinionated and perhaps argumentative. These last two characteristics may make for some challenging times for parents, teachers, and dentists. Hopefully, parents will continue to guide their children with a light but steady hand, staying connected yet allowing increasing independence.

Emotional Changes

The very rapid and dramatic changes that occur in adolescents may be paralleled by many emotional circumstances. The self-confidence and personal identity of an adolescent may be compromised if his or her feelings about body image are negative. In 1984, Mussen and colleagues[9] noted that the following issues create the possibility of misinterpretation and anxiety for this age group:

- Being attractive or unattractive
- Being loved or unloved
- Being strong or weak
- Being masculine or feminine

For females, the onset of menstruation may also present circumstances that can be anxiety provoking. This is not necessarily the rule, but the chances of anxiety rise if there is a prevailing negative reaction to the menstrual process by family and peers, if the child is showered with sympathy, or if there is considerable pain before and during menses. Reassurance that menstruation is a normal bodily function sometimes accompanied with emotional swings due to hormonal fluctuations may alleviate the adolescent's anxiety.

The advent of puberty and the hormones associated with puberty lead to sexual feelings and urges. The timing of this process, its nature and magnitude, and the choice of what to do about these feelings and urges is handled differently from one adolescent to another. Family guidance, the adolescent's own values, the values of peers, and the value system of the person that the adolescent first loves are just a few of the factors that ultimately predict how he or she will deal with these new feelings.

One last emotion is critical to understanding adolescents. This is the emotion of love. Adolescents are capable of great commitment to one another, and some of these relationships can become long-term commitments. Unfortunately, many such relationships do not last, as one partner becomes uninterested. This can lead to genuine depression for the abandoned partner. Often parents do not take these romantic bonds seriously and refer to them in belittling terms.

Social Changes

Adolescence represents the final transition socially from childhood to adulthood. When it is over, if everything proceeded as it should, the emerging young adult will be able to establish and maintain loving and sexual relationships with a partner, be independent of the parents, be capable of working with peers, and be self-directed.

There is no other period in human development distinguished by psychosocial changes of the same magnitude as those experienced during adolescence. These are formidable social challenges, and some adolescents cannot master them. Bullying, attempted or successful suicide, alcohol and substance abuse, running away from home, sexual promiscuity, and dropping out of school are some of the frequently cited instances of adolescent failure to socialize properly.

Peers are important social agents in large technologic societies, in which children of the same age group are often kept together. It can be argued that as relationships and dependencies on parents start to decline, the importance of peers escalates. This shift in relationships contributes to the development of intimacy by increasing comfort with peers and encouraging openness and self-disclosure with others. Increasingly, the adolescent may find that it is difficult to share secrets, thoughts, and fantasies with his or her parents. In these situations, the close friend becomes the adolescent's confidant. The superficial sharing of activities with friends that sufficed during childhood is replaced during adolescence by concern, loyalty, reliability, and respect between adolescent friends.

Despite the obvious value of peers, there are peer relationships that are not so fortunate for the involved adolescent. For example, to avoid rejection or ridicule from peers an adolescent may experiment with drugs, participate in criminal acts, or defy authority.

Another important social change in the adolescent is an increase in the size and range of acquaintances. Children younger than adolescents tend to limit their friends to those of their neighborhood, school, and perhaps church. Adolescents, on the other hand, may have individual friends, belong to a circle of friends, and can identify with larger groups such as an Explorer troop, soccer team, or "friends" from social media. An adolescent's ability to sustain relationships with all three of these groups indicates good social skills and is a sign that the socialization process is going well.

Popularity is an important desire in adolescents. There are few adolescents who are not preoccupied with acceptance by peers. The following qualities in an adolescent seem to correlate with social acceptance by peers:
- Friendly, likes other people
- Energetic and enthusiastic
- Flexible and forgiving
- Laughs, good sense of humor
- Outgoing
- Self-confident but not conceited
- Appears natural
- Tolerant of the shortcomings of others
- Shows leadership qualities
- Others feel good when this person is around

The adolescent who gets along with his or her peer group seems to relate successfully to adults. Those who do not achieve peer acceptance seem to have more difficulty with adults and grow up to have a variety of social and emotional difficulties.[10] Some of the issues facing adolescents will be discussed as follows.

Bullying

Bullying in youth is an intentional negative behavior that typically occurs repeatedly and where there is an imbalance of power, with a more powerful person or group attacking a less powerful one.[11] Bullying is defined as having three elements: aggressive or deliberately harmful behavior (1) between peers that is (2) repeated and over time and (3) involves an imbalance of power, for example,

related to physical strength or popularity, making it difficult for the victim to defend himself or herself.[12]

Behavior falls into four categories: direct-physical (e.g., assault, theft), direct-verbal (e.g., threats, insults, name-calling), indirect-relational (e.g., social exclusion, spreading rumors), and cyberbullying. Cross-sectional findings indicate that there is an increased risk of suicidal ideation and/or suicide attempts associated with bullying behavior and cyberbullying.[13]

Bullying predicts future mental health problems. Studies have shown that bullying behavior in childhood or adolescence is a predictor of antisocial behavior and antisocial personality disorder (PD) in adulthood. Studies have focused on three groups: those who were victims, those who were bullies, and those who were both victims and bullies (bully/victims). Children and adolescents involved in bullying behavior had the worst outcomes when they were both bullies and victims, leading to depression, anxiety, and suicidality (suicidality only among males) as adults.[14] More recently, it was found that female victims of bullying have an almost fourfold likelihood of developing a PD later in life compared to adolescents with no involvement in bullying behavior. Most of the females had borderline PD. Female adolescents diagnosed with anxiety disorder during adolescence had more than a threefold risk of developing a PD during late adolescence or early adulthood.[15]

Pediatric dentists can identify a range of health conditions that affect not only adolescents' functioning and opportunities, but also the quality of their adult live. Assessment for adolescents with psychopathology, other signs of emotional distress, or unusual chronic complaints should also include screening for participation in bullying as victims or bullies.

Suicide

Suicide among young people continues to be a serious problem. For some teens, suicide may appear to be a solution to their problems and stress. Each year in the United States thousands of teenagers commit suicide.[16]

Suicide has replaced murder/homicide as the second leading cause of death for adolescents 15 to 19 years old. Suicide rates may have increased due to the stresses and anger levels induced by electronic media and a reluctance to use antidepressant medication. Fewer antidepressants have been prescribed since 2004 when the US Food and Drug Administration (FDA) required "black box warning" labels on antidepressants to warn health care providers of increased risks of suicidal thinking and behavior among children and adolescents being treated with such medications.[17]

Suicide is especially high among teens because of the severe stressors of adolescence and the immaturity of the adolescent brain.[18] Any attempt to categorize adolescence is destined to fall woefully short of the complexity of today's reality. The best we can do as pediatric dentists is to keep pace with the emerging scientific evidence and assimilate that information with our own experiences and foundational knowledge. The goal of this approach goes beyond the mere exercise of intellectual curiosity; it reaches for an understanding of the world of the next adolescent who sits in your dental chair.

The American Academy of Pediatrics (AAP) updated its guidelines for screening patients for suicidal thoughts, identifying risks factors for suicide, and assisting at-risk young people.[17] The AAP recommends that pediatricians look for risk factors linked to teen suicide, which include a history of physical or sexual abuse, mood disorders, substance abuse, and teens who may be lesbian, gay, or bisexual.

Additionally, according to the American Foundation for Suicide Prevention (AFSP)—the nation's largest suicide prevention network—since the risk of suicide is heightened by a convergence of multiple risk factors, with the most common being depression and other mental health conditions, screening for these risks is the first critically important step in preventing suicide death.

As pediatric dentists it is our professional responsibility to help identify those adolescents who may be at higher risk for suicide. Positive youth development suggests that a good interpersonal relationship between the adolescent patient and the pediatric dentist may influence an improvement in the adolescent's oral health and at the same time, serve as a good role model. Because dental health professionals frequently encounter adolescents in their practices over time as well as in their communities, we may have several potential opportunities to observe changes in behavior and to ask appropriate questions to identify adolescents at high risk for psychological problems. Referral should be made when the treatment needs are beyond the treating dentist's scope of practice, and consultation with nondental professionals or a team approach may be indicated.[19]

The first step to appropriately identify these adolescents at risk is a thorough medical history that includes both systemic conditions as well as behavioral issues. Routine history taking should include questions about mood disorders, antidepressant medications, school problems, and stressful life events. Asking open-ended questions may elicit more than a "yes" or a "no" response. If the adolescent appears to be sad at the dental appointment, allow your responses to reflect the patient's mood. This approach may allow the adolescent to feel understood, and a dialogue may follow. Adolescents at risk for suicide can be identified through direct questioning or screening by self-report accompanied by knowledge of the risk factors. It is important for the pediatric dentist to maintain a nonjudgmental and open approach in questioning the adolescent.

A second step in identification occurs while performing the comprehensive oral examination. Be alert to teens whose appearances and/or behaviors are beyond normal self-expression. Signs that may be indicative of inner turmoil include self-injury and increased risk-taking behavior. Extensive body art and/or branding are some examples of risky behaviors that may manifest during adolescence. The devastating oral effects associated with "meth mouth" are of increasing concern in this age group. Regularly weigh your patient at recall examinations. A significant increase or decrease in weight or appetite could be a characteristic of depression or eating disorders. Ask if the patient is experiencing any energy loss, sleep problems, or lack of interest in daily activities. Adolescents in crisis may exhibit one or more of these behaviors, and the dental health professional should be aware of these indicators.

Finally, familiarize yourself with local, state, and national resources for treatment of psychopathology and suicide prevention. A list of telephone numbers of mental health agencies, family and children services, crisis hotlines, and intervention agencies should be available in the dental office for possible referral of your adolescent patients and their parents. Severe moodiness in a teenager may not be something that will be outgrown; it may be a behavior that requires our recognition and appropriate referral for proper intervention.

Risky Behaviors

Smoking/Vaping

The use of tobacco products by adolescents is widespread and may not only result in chronic systemic effects but also contribute to oral soft tissue damage. In addition to oral malodor and stained teeth, adolescents who smoke experience impaired gingival health as well as delayed wound healing. Cigarette smoking also is a significant contributing factor for the development and subsequent life-threatening effects caused by oral, pharyngeal, and laryngeal carcinomas.

Currently, the use of electronic-cigarettes (e-cigarettes) and vaporizers appears to be replacing the traditional cigarette. A new survey sampling 40,000 US students indicated that US teenagers are more likely to use e-cigarettes than traditional cigarettes. The authors reported that its use is driven by the belief that e-cigarettes are less harmful.[20] Many adolescents surveyed believed that e-cigarettes were a harmless form of entertainment and were unaware that they could contribute to nicotine addiction. The Centers for Disease Control and Prevention (CDC) found that although high school students are smoking traditional cigarettes less than ever before, they are using e-cigarettes at more than twice the rate of regular cigarettes.[21] The dentist should be concerned that this type of tobacco use may serve as a new gateway to smoking cigarettes because the products are similar. Even though the e-cigarette market is beginning to face regulatory pressure, its production has little oversight for safety and could account for some of the heavy metals, such as lead and zinc, which have been detected in some e-cigarettes.

Another adolescent smoking trend is the rising use of smoking cigars. Health officials believe several factors are responsible for this upswing. Unlike cigarettes, cigars are promoted with candy, chocolate, and fruit flavors. Cigars are taxed less and can be sold in single lots, unlike cigarettes that must be sold in packs of 20 and are more expensive. In addition, cigars are marketed more heavily in black neighborhoods than in other urban areas. The CDC reported that cigar use among African American adolescents has more than doubled since 2009, whereas traditional cigarette smoking has declined significantly.[21]

Sexual Activity

Many adolescents engage in sexual activity that may directly or indirectly affect their oral health. These adolescent sexual behaviors include a range of activities from kissing and fondling, to oral, anal, and vaginal sex. The most recent Youth Risk Behavior Survey of US high school students reports:

- 41% had sexual intercourse.
- 30% had sexual intercourse during the previous 3 months, and, of these
  - 43% did not use a condom the last time they had sex.
  - 14% did not use any method to prevent pregnancy.
  - 21% had drunk alcohol or used drugs before their last sexual intercourse.[21]

Risky sexual behaviors place adolescents at risk for unplanned pregnancies and sexually transmitted infections (STIs), including HIV.

Certain behaviors place the adolescent at higher risk for developing STIs. These include (1) early age at sexual debut; (2) lack of condom use; (3) multiple partners; (4) prior STI; (5) history of STI in a partner; and (6) sex with a partner who is 3 or more years older. Other adolescent risk-taking behaviors that are associated with STIs are: (1) alcohol use; (2) depression; (3) dropping out of school; (4) illicit drug use; (5) pregnancy; and (6) smoking.[21]

Adolescents contract STIs at a higher rate than adults because of sexual risk taking and possible barriers to health care access.[22] During the teen's dental examination, sexually active adolescents may present with herpes simplex virus (HSV)-2 lesions in the oral and perioral regions. According to a recent national survey, more than two-thirds of US teenagers have engaged in oral sex—including nearly 25% who have never experienced intercourse.[21] Consequently, STIs are spreading faster among teens than any other age group. In addition, females are more likely than males to contract HSV-2 from a single act of unprotected sex.[21] Palliative treatment is recommended and may include analgesics (e.g., acetaminophen) and antiviral medications (e.g., acyclovir) to alleviate the symptoms. Recurrent herpes labialis may be treated with topical penciclovir cream for vesicular perioral lesions.[23] The cream may have a small, favorable effect on the duration of symptoms if applied at the onset of the infection. Thus, it is important for the pediatric dentist to address the adolescent's sexual activity and use this opportunity to discuss risk reduction as a component of the overall medical history.

By building a trusting relationship with the adolescent over time, the dentist may be able to obtain an honest, detailed health history to ascertain the teen's sexual activity. Since sexuality is an expected stage in the development of adolescents and young adults, pediatric dentists have a professional responsibility to be knowledgeable in initial screening and management/referral of common sexual health issues. The dental health professional's ability to listen to adolescents' concerns and to help them access necessary community resources will allow the pediatric dentist to serve his or her teenage patients effectively.

Gender Identity

Along with sexual activity, sexual identity develops and may solidify during adolescence. Gender identity and subsequent discussions with the patient are relatively recent to medical and dental providers. In 1983, the AAP issued its first report on sexual minority teens, and then made revisions in 1993 and 2004.[24] Since the last update, research on this subject has expanded rapidly with numerous publications about lesbian, gay, bisexual, transgender, and questioning (LGBTQ) youth. In 2011, the Institute of Medicine published a report documenting the health of the LGBTQ people.[25] They stated that being a member of this group of adolescents is not, itself, a risky behavior. In addition, sexual minority youth should not be considered abnormal.[25]

Typically, a young person's sexual orientation emerges before or early in adolescence.[26] In fact, many teens are in conflict with their sexual attractions and some may refer to themselves as "questioning."[26] In the United States, the exact prevalence of adolescent homosexuality and same-sex experiences is unknown. A study of 9th to 12th graders from Massachusetts reported 3% as gay, lesbian, or bisexual.[27] Another 1% reported as "questioning."[27] In the National Survey of Family Growth, 13.4% of females and 4.0% of males self-reported of having sex with someone of the same gender.[28] So, the pediatrician and the pediatric dentist need to be cognizant that some of the concerns their patients may have are regarding their sexual orientation. Over the years, the pediatric dentist has probably developed lasting relationships with his or her patients, and these patients may be comfortable in discussing their concerns with the pediatric dentist. The dentist should be able to provide current and nonjudgmental information in a confidential manner. In addition, the dental professional should assist the adolescent with the names of other health care professionals and agencies for possible referral. Pediatric health care providers are important in facilitating a healthy transition from adolescence to adulthood so the pediatric dentist needs to be knowledgeable about the issues facing sexual minority youth.

Health care issues and disparities exist among LGBTQ teens, and unfortunately, many of the public health systems have ignored them. From a psychological standpoint, the disclosing of one's sexual orientation may result in significant stress for the adolescent and their families. The family may reject or disapprove this disclosure, resulting in a lack of social support from families and friends. Some sexual minority youth may experience physical or emotional abuse; therefore as mandated reporters, the pediatric dentist needs to be aware of the probable root cause of the abuse and the perpetrator. As a result, LGBTQ adolescents also appear to be overrepresented among runaway and homeless youths in the United States.[29]

By knowing an adolescent patient's sexual orientation, the pediatric dentist can become more knowledgeable and sensitive to the teen's medical and dental needs.

Summary

Adolescence is the transitional period between puberty and maturity associated with accelerated physical growth and dynamic hormonal changes, contradictions in self-awareness, and the conflicting demands of modern society. All of these factors contribute to the persona of the turbulent teenager. Adolescent dental patients have distinct oral needs that require enhanced understanding by dental professionals in order to provide high-quality dental services to this age group. However, for many adolescents, these years may be an emotional period and a time when dental and medical needs are neglected. The intent of the following chapters is to present clinically relevant information that will assist the dental team in providing optimal care to their adolescent patients.

References

1. Tanner JM, Whitehouse RH, Marshall WA, et al. *Assessment of Skeletal Maturity and Prediction of Adult Height: TW2 Method*. New York: Academic Press; 1975.
2. Kokich VG. Age changes in the human frontozygomatic sutures from 20 to 95 years. *Am J Orthod*. 1976;60:411–430.
3. Enlow DH. *Handbook of Facial Growth*. Philadelphia: Saunders; 1990.
4. Behrents RG. *Growth in the Aging Craniofacial Skeleton. Monograph 17, Craniofacial Growth Series*. Ann Arbor, MI: Center for Human Growth and Development; 1985.
5. Björk A. The face in profile. *Sven Tandlak Tidskr*. 1947;40(suppl 5B).
6. Ranly DM. *A Synopsis of Craniofacial Growth*. New York: Appleton-Century-Crofts; 1980.
7. Björk A. Sutural growth of the upper face studied by the implant method. *Acta Odontol Scand*. 1966;24:109–127.
8. Kiell N. *The Universal Experience of Adolescence*. Boston: Beacon; 1967.
9. Mussen PH, Conger JJ, Kagan J, et al. *Child Development and Personality*. 6th ed. New York: Harper & Row; 1984.
10. Hartup WW. The peer system. In: Mussen PH, ed. *Handbook of Child Psychology*. Vol. 4. 4th ed. Hetherington EM, volume ed. *Socialization, Personality, and Social Development*. New York: John Wiley; 1983.
11. Nansel TR, Overpeck M, Pilla RS, et al. Bullying behaviors among US youth: prevalence and association with psychosocial adjustment. *JAMA*. 2001;285(16):2094–2100.
12. Olweus D. Bullying at school: basic facts and effects of a school based intervention program. *J Child Psychol Psychiatry*. 1994;35(7):1171–1190.
13. Brunstein KA, Sourander A, Gould M. The association of suicide and bullying in childhood to young adulthood: a review of cross-sectional and longitudinal research findings. *Can J Psychiatry*. 2010;55(5):282–288.

14. Copeland WE, Wolke D, Angold A, et al. Adult psychiatric outcomes of bullying and being bullied by peers in childhood and adolescence. *JAMA Psychiatry*. 2013;70(4):419-426.
15. Antila H, Arola R, Hakko H, et al. Bullying involvement in relation to personality disorders: a prospective follow-up of 508 inpatient adolescents. *Eur Child Adolesc Psychiatry*. 2017;26(7):779–789.
16. American Academy of Child and Adolescent Psychiatry. Suicide in children and teens; 2017. http://www.aacap.org/AACAP/Families_and_youth/Facts_for_Families/FFF-Guide/Teen-Suicide-010.aspx. Accessed February 1, 2018.
17. Shain BN. Suicide and suicide attempts in adolescents. *Pediatrics*. 2016;120(3):669–676.
18. Romer D. Adolescent risk taking, impulsivity, and brain development: implications for prevention. *Dev Psychobiol*. 2010;52(3):263–276.
19. American Academy of Pediatric Dentistry. Guideline on adolescent oral health care. *Pediatr Dent*. 2016;38(6):155–162.
20. Arrazola RA, Singh T, Corey CG, et al. Tobacco use among middle and high school students—United States, 2011-2014. *Morb Mortal Wkly Rep*. 2015;64(14):381–385.
21. Kann L, McManus T, Harris WA, et al. Youth risk behavior surveillance—United States, 2015. *MMWR Surveill Summ*. 2016;65(6):1–174.
22. Alexander SC, Fortenberry D, Pollak KI, et al. Sexuality talk during adolescent health maintenance visits. *JAMA Pediatr*. 2014;168(2): 163–169.
23. Opstelten W, Knuistingh A, Eekhof J. Treatment and prevention of herpes labialis. *Can Fam Physician*. 2008;54:1683–1687.
24. American Academy of Pediatrics, Committee on Adolescence. Homosexuality and adolescence. *Pediatrics*. 2004;113(6):1827-1832.
25. Institute of Medicine, Committee on Lesbian, Gay, Bisexual, and Transgender Health Issues and Research Gaps and Opportunities. *The Health of Lesbian, Gay, Bisexual, and Transgender People: Building a Foundation for Better Understanding*. Washington, DC: National Academies Press; 2011.
26. Spigarelli MG. Adolescent sexual orientation. *Adolesc Med State Art Rev*. 2007;18(3):508–518.
27. Garofalo R, Wolf RC, Wisslow LS, et al. Sexual orientation and risk of suicide attempts among a representative sample of youth. *Arch Pediatr Adolesc Med*. 1999;153:487–493.
28. Chandra A, Mosher WD, Copen C, et al. Sexual behavior, sexual attraction, and sexual identity in the United States: data from the 2006-2008 National Survey of Family Growth. *Natl Health Stat Report*. 2011;36:1–36.
29. National Youth Coalition for Housing. LGBT young people. http://www.youthhomelessnessmatters.info/lgbt-young-people. Accessed June 13, 2017.

38

Examination, Diagnosis, and Treatment Planning for General and Orthodontic Problems

ERICA BRECHER, THOMAS R. STARK,[a] JOHN R. CHRISTENSEN, ROSE D. SHEATS, AND HENRY FIELDS

CHAPTER OUTLINE

The classic portrayal of adolescence as a time of rising hormones, rebelliousness, and fads contrasts vividly with the way dentistry has viewed adolescent oral health. Dentistry for children ends abruptly with eruption of the permanent premolars and canines. Adult dentistry begins with consideration of what to do with the third molars. For many dental professionals, the first intervention that comes to mind for the adolescent is orthodontic care, which is often initiated during the preadolescent transitional period.

Entirely opposite to the prevailing beliefs about the quiescence of the teenage years is the reality of a rapidly changing patient challenging his or her environment head-on and learning to cope in the process. The implications of these changes for dentistry[1] are summarized as follows:

1. *Rapid, unpredictable, and irregular skeletal and dental growth.* The adolescent growth spurt is associated with accompanying

facial growth of up to 35% of total height of the face. More than a dozen teeth, primary and permanent, exfoliate and erupt between the ages of 10 and 13 years. Immunologic changes, hormonal shifts, and other subtle and not so subtle physical developments alter the oral cavity.

2. *The environmental challenges, with their obstacles and pitfalls.* Few adults would choose to return to adolescence. Today's adolescents encounter many challenges at home, school, and among their peers. They are navigating the path of their future education and careers while learning to cope with the peer pressures of sex, drugs, alcohol, and smoking. Perhaps the most poignant statement on this aspect of the teenage years is that accidental death is the leading cause of mortality. Dental professionals see trauma, oral manifestations of sexual activity, hormonal gingivitis, smokeless tobacco-induced hyperkeratosis, noncompliance with dental recommendations, and drug-related behaviors, to mention a few examples.

3. *The need to learn to cope, make decisions, and become independent.* It is not surprising that primitive cultures associated emerging adulthood with rituals and great significance. Adolescence has always been a time to make decisions, seek independence from

---

[a]The views expressed in this chapter are those of the author and do not reflect the official policy or position of the Department of the Army, Department of Defense, or the US Government.

families, deal with sexuality, and choose a career. The dentist may see this turmoil reflected in poor compliance with oral hygiene or refusal to accept treatment.

The Patient History

The health history of the adolescent is constantly changing and must be kept current. An adult history format captures both of these elements. Perhaps more important from the standpoint of accuracy is the process of obtaining information from the teenager. The following are some of the topics that should be considered when taking a history from an adolescent patient.

The health history should address the issues of smoking, recreational drugs and alcohol, birth control, pregnancy, and sexually transmitted diseases. The controversy over inclusion of these issues is easily quieted by the simple realities of adolescent life in the United States. Consider these facts:

- Every day, approximately 3000 teenagers start smoking. Ninety percent of smokers begin before age 18.[2]
- In 2014, the live birth rate in 15- to 19-year-old women was 24.2 per 1000.[3] Although teenage pregnancies have steadily declined over the past 20 years, pregnancy status should be considered because radiation and dental medications can be dangerous to a fetus.
- The majority of adolescents now try drugs or alcohol before leaving high school. Untoward interactions between prescribed and illicit medications can be fatal.
- Sexually transmitted diseases are epidemic in the adolescent age group. Half of all new infections occur in 15- to 24-year-olds.[4]

Both the dentist and the patient are at risk if there is inadequate surveying of these elements in the health history. These issues can be addressed forthrightly by including them as choices interspersed with others on a health history form. A less threatening approach is to phrase these questions in the past tense or to associate a risk with them in order to alert the patient to their importance.

The history-taking process should allow privacy and encourage disclosure. Taking an accurate history may mean allowing the adolescent to assume greater participation in the process, yielding information that might not be available from or known to a parent. The dentist may be caught in a double bind by providing an environment that fosters disclosure if pregnancy or illicit drug use is uncovered and the parents are unaware of it. Unfortunately, the adolescent may see this as betrayal or breach of confidence and the relationship between the dentist and patient may be jeopardized. There is no easy way to deal with this type of problem, but the dentist who treats adolescents should be aware of the responsibilities of the situation. It also may mean delaying treatment until the problem is resolved. In general, the Health Insurance Portability and Accountability Act (HIPAA) permits disclosure of a minor's medical information between provider and guardian.[5] However, many states have specific minor consent and privacy laws, which may grant exceptions for conditions such as pregnancy, substance abuse, or treatment of sexually transmitted diseases, among others. Dentists should consult their state-specific laws for further information concerning the applicability of HIPAA to the disclosure of information concerning the treatment of minors. The dentist's responsibility is to help direct the family to address the issue.

The dentist can take some actions that both facilitate an accurate history and deal consistently with identified problems of a serious nature:

- Encourage parents to complete histories with adolescents, not for them.
- Allow the adolescent the opportunity to contribute to the history alone, which can be done in the context of a final check before treatment at chairside.
- Never treat an adolescent without a consenting parent available. Dental care would be considered nonurgent care and most jurisdictions require adult consent.
- Explain suspicions or concerns to both the parent and adolescent.
- Establish a policy on deferring treatment and dealing with identified problems of a serious nature that is medicolegally consistent and sound.
- Have resources available if consultation with a specialist is needed.

The Examination

The techniques of clinical examination remain the same for the adolescent, but closer attention is paid to the identification of problems specific to this group, such as occlusal disharmonies, periodontal conditions, and temporomandibular joint disorders (TMDs). Table 38.1 lists some of the clinical findings peculiar to adolescent patients.

Behavioral Assessment

The access to dental care available to most healthy Americans has made it unlikely that a teenager will present for a first dental appointment, although first visits during adolescence are possible. Personality changes and other behavioral aberrations can suggest problems for the adolescent. Extremes in behavior, such as depression or overt sexual behavior, may indicate sexual abuse, especially if the child demonstrates a reluctance to allow oral examination. Depression, manifested by severe introversion, can also be a sign of suicidal tendency, family dysfunction, or even drug use. As a health care provider, it is the dentist's responsibility to be aware of the impact of the problem on the child and comment to parents about noticeable changes in behavior. Although few behavioral problems preclude delivery of care, exceptions do occur. The following are situations that may require behavioral management:

1. *Sexual abuse.* The young adolescent girl or boy who has been sexually abused with oral penetration may be reluctant to accept dental care from a dentist of the same sex as the perpetrator. Aids in uncovering this situation are a good history of previous compliance, behavioral cues, such as depression, and overt refusal of care when oral contact is made. Nonetheless, confirmation is difficult because the parents may be unaware of the abuse. If sexual abuse is suspected, dentists are mandated reporters and must report suspicion of abuse to the appropriate local agency.

2. *Rampant caries.* Clinicians have noted that rampant caries, a condition of rapid onset and progression of decay in an adolescent (more often a girl), is often associated with personality problems (Fig. 38.1). The typical manifestation is a shy, reluctant, introverted person who is passive about treatment. The behavioral signs can be varied, with the girl crying silently or not saying a word during the appointment. In some cases, appointments can degenerate as the child whimpers and finally loses her composure. Time and engagement in conversation are often the most successful behavioral management keys in dealing with these adolescents. Dramatic changes in behavior can occur with the dentist's verbal reinforcement of improved

TABLE 38.1	Possible Clinical Findings in Examination of the Adolescent		
Structure	Finding	Comment	
Extraoral Evaluation			
Skin	Acne	May be painful locally	
		Adolescent may take antibiotics	
		May appear as radiopacity on some radiographs if calcification occurs	
	Cosmetic use	Can complicate evaluation of the skin	
		Can cause local allergic response	
Neck	Hematoma	From suction; indicates sexual activity	
Ears	Healing or scarred punctures	Multiple ear piercings common in both sexes	
Hair	Coloring and preparation	Can complicate examination of the scalp	
Intraoral Examination			
Mucosa	Generalized erythema	Effect of smoking	
		Sexually transmitted disease	
Buccal mucosa	Erythema, hyperkeratosis	Use of smokeless tobacco	
Tongue	Coating, odor	Smoking; poor hygiene; fungal overgrowth from medication	
Breath	Acetone; alcohol	Excessive dieting, alcohol abuse, metabolic disorders (e.g., diabetes)	
Gingiva	Inflammation	Hormonal changes (e.g., puberty gingivitis)	
		Poor oral hygiene	
	Pregnancy tumor	Use of oral contraceptives	
		Pregnancy	
Teeth	Erosion	Bulimia	
	Wear facets	Temporomandibular joint disorders/bruxism	
	Excessive stain	Tobacco use	
		Coffee or tea use	
	Discoloration	Existing pulpal pathosis from trauma	

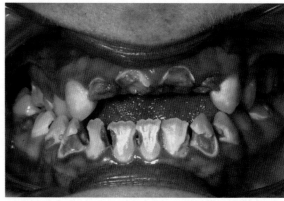

• **Figure 38.1** This 14-year-old girl has rampant caries, which is a distinct clinical entity with rapidly progressing decay, multiple pulpally involved teeth, and short onset. Patients may give a history of minimal caries before the development of overt signs of decay.

hygiene and provision of temporary esthetic anterior restorations that allow the patient to smile and experience a more positive self-image.

3. *Extreme anxiety.* Pinkham and Schroeder[6] described the behavioral management of the child who shows extreme anxiety at the prospect of dental treatment. Desensitization by psychological intervention may be the key to the development of acceptable clinical behavior in such children. Tools available to the dentist are the use of noninvasive therapies at first, reinforcement of positive accomplishments, positive peer interaction, and involvement with a psychologist. The poorly treated or untreated adolescent phobic may become the adult dental phobic.

4. *Eating disorders.* Treatment of the child with an eating disorder can be difficult. Eating disorders are a type of psychiatric disorder and require appropriate medical intervention. Experience indicates that these patients, disproportionately girls, tend to develop dependency on a male authority figure.

5. *Illicit drug use.* Clinicians have noted bizarre behavior on the part of adolescents and young adults who present for treatment after taking nonprescription medications. A number of untoward reactions to dentist-administered medications have been associated with prior ingestion of drugs or alcohol by a young patient. Manifestations of drug ingestion may vary from a slight mental dissociation or drifting to outright verbal aberrations or extreme changes in personality.

Another common drug used by adolescents is nicotine, in the form of cigarettes, smokeless tobacco, and e-cigarettes. This drug is addictive and has cardiovascular, respiratory, and oral consequences. It is important to educate adolescents that e-cigarettes are not approved for smoking cessation, and contain nicotine, toxins, and carcinogens.[7] Although difficult, cessation programs combining motivated participants, nicotine replacement therapy, and behavioral support seem to have the best chances of extinguishing the habit.

Management of behavioral problems in the adolescent can be complex and often involves parents and other professionals. Most practitioners treating adolescents try to treat these patients alone rather than in a setting in which other peers are present. This one-on-one relationship provides the necessary attention to the patient and prevents disruptive interactions. Any dentist who has worked with a group of seventh- or eighth-grade students will appreciate this recommendation. The teenager who is acting up but is simply expressing healthy emotions should respond to reason and provide compliance.

An important part of behavior management in this age group involves the simple transfer of information. A good communicator is aware of the characteristics of adolescence, which enhances his or her ability to relate to teenagers. These characteristics are as follows:

1. *Peers are important.* The adolescent's relationship to those outside the nuclear and extended family becomes important. Friends, classmates, teammates, and popular persons of similar age are all involved in the life of the teenager. A dentist can enhance his or her ability to communicate with adolescents by asking

about peer interaction and by knowing who is involved in the teen's life.

2. *Fads and experimentation are part of adolescence.* Successful adolescent practitioners are those who are aware of the trends, popular fads, and celebrities that are of interest to teens. The dentist who knows the trends and interests of the adolescent has an edge in establishing communication and in reaching the teen on a nonauthoritarian basis. These are an entree into the teen's world that can be fostered and can lead to discussion of more significant issues with a sense of relationship. Contrast that access to the barrier that arises when both teen and dentist see themselves as worlds apart.

3. *Teens are trying to establish independence, searching for identity, making educational or career choices, and experimenting with sexuality.* All of these involve a certain degree of stress. Within that stressful period are times of anxiety, satisfaction, anger, excitement, and a host of other emotions. How the practitioner fosters the healthy development of personality in a child and counsels him or her toward independence and career may be important in terms of both the teen's life and his or her dental health. In talking with teens, it is helpful to remember their "problem list" and to empathize about the stress of their lives, which is real to them. The office visit should provide a respite from pressures and be a cameo of the role that the adolescent plays as an adult patient. The relationship that the dentist would like to have with the adolescent as an adult should be fostered.

4. *The basis of success in adolescent-adult interactions is a good relationship.* The most significant factor in successful compliance and communication is the quality of the relationship between the dentist and the adolescent. In earlier periods of life, the child could be successfully motivated with reason, praise, or other approaches. The changing values and their short-term intensity in adolescence belie the use of these approaches in fostering long-term motivation. A feeling of trust, good communication, and a perception by the teenager of the dentist's sincere interest provide a strong motivation for compliance.

General Appraisal

The general appraisal of the adolescent is confounded by the timing of physical growth changes, especially in the early teenage years. Within a group of young teenagers, girls can tower over boys and look far more like adults than male peers. Similarly, within a group of boys, variations in voice tone, skin condition, amount and distribution of fat, and skeletal proportion are often remarkable. Differentiation of growth disorders is difficult at best.

Determination of Developmental Status

Patients in the preadolescent stages are growing rapidly and many clinicians prefer to attempt orthodontic growth modification then. If that can be tied to the transition to the permanent detention, then one stage of orthodontic treatment can be sufficient to complete the care. For others, growth modification must start before the eruption of all permanent teeth so there are two phases of treatment; growth modification is followed by a final phase of comprehensive treatment. After peak growth, statural and facial growth decrease dramatically. At that point, the only logical options for care of a skeletal discrepancy are camouflage or surgical orthodontic care.

The most important question is whether patients have remaining facial growth. It determines when surgical care can be instituted for those with excess growth issues like mandibular protrusion or vertical facial excess. The most reliable and sensible method, which speaks directly to this issue, is taking serial cephalometric radiographs and superimposing their tracings (see Fig. 31.53). The Cervical Vertebral Maturation method is a useful guide to assess peak adolescent growth and utilizes information obtained from a cephalometric radiograph (see Fig. 31.4). These methods are helpful not only for orthodontic treatment planning but also for determining when implant placement is feasible.

Head and Neck Examination

The principles of the head and neck examination of the teenager are similar to those applied to the adult or child. Variations from normal can be caused by a variety of factors, the most notable of which are growth and developmental changes and the effects of the adolescent's environment.

The physical changes and habits in the teen require modification of the procedures used in children. On the positive side, the loss or redistribution of body fat and the elongation of the neck allow one to perform a better lymph node evaluation. These changes facilitate a thorough head and neck and cancer examination.

Facial Examination

In the facial examination the dentist analyzes the soft tissue profile and the frontal face. During adolescence the face is beginning to assume adult-like features, and treatment decisions can be based more on current rather than projected facial appearance. This does not mean that growth is complete—only that it has slowed considerably from its previous pace during the early adolescent growth spurt. The adult profile tends to be straighter than the adolescent's because of continued mandibular skeletal growth. In addition, the soft tissue of the chin increases slightly in thickness. The nose continues to grow in horizontal and vertical directions. Most of this growth is horizontal but the nasal tip tends to drop a small amount. The lips are less protrusive in the adult because of these nasal and chin changes combined with a slight thinning of the soft tissue thickness of the lips.

For patients with class I skeletal and dental characteristics, the facial profile examination should provide an adequate basis for analysis when minor orthodontic treatment is considered. For the patient with a skeletal problem, additional information (e.g., a cephalometric radiograph and analysis) is required to diagnose the problem definitively and prescribe treatment.

Treatment of skeletal orthodontic problems during preadolescence or early adolescence, when the adolescent growth spurt is still active, can result in growth modification. The preadolescent patient is assumed to be growing and is expected to experience a pubertal growth spurt. The young adolescent, especially the male, still has enough growth remaining to allow significant skeletal changes to occur with treatment. Once the adolescent has experienced the pubertal growth spurt, growth remains but is significantly slower, and equal to the down side of the growth rate curve. Adults have such limited facial growth it is of little therapeutic potential.

These differences in growth potential have a large impact on how skeletal malocclusion is managed in the adolescent. As the individual becomes more skeletally mature, less skeletal growth modification can be accomplished. Therefore, as noted earlier, it is essential to establish the growth or developmental status of the patient in order to plan sensible treatment.

Intraoral Examination

The larger size of the adolescent oral cavity permits good visualization. Normal intellectual status and reasonable behavior provide cooperation in functional assessment of the occlusion and the temporomandibular joint (TMJ). There are more teeth to evaluate and gingival and periodontal issues are present that were not critical in early childhood. The clinician should approach the adolescent as an adult, especially in the later teen years. For the first visit, the dentist may choose to "walk" the adolescent through the examination, using a hand mirror or computer images to explain procedures and normal findings.

Periodontal Evaluation

In the adolescent more emphasis is placed on the periodontal examination. The prevalence of periodontal disease begins to increase in this age group.[8] Although usually minor, loss of periodontal support due to periodontitis is common in the teenage population.[9] Therefore a thorough evaluation of the supporting structures is an absolute necessity. A periodontal probe is used to measure pocket depths, the width of keratinized gingiva, and the amount of attached gingiva and to establish a bleeding index (Fig. 38.2). Periodontal probing should be confined to fully erupted teeth. Mobility tests may reveal slightly increased mobility in erupted

teeth without complete root formation. The use of disclosing agents to reveal plaque may be helpful. If a panoramic radiograph is used for diagnosis, selected periapical films may be needed if the clinical examination exposes any unusual periodontal findings. Referral to a specialist is suggested if significant periodontal disease is evident. During orthodontic treatment, gingival, plaque, and bleeding indices should be established at regular intervals to detect newly active periodontal disease. With the increase in childhood and adolescent obesity there has been an increase in the number of adolescents with diabetes mellitus type 2 (noninsulin-dependent diabetes).[10] Approximately one-third of children and adolescents are now categorized as overweight or obese, so we are likely to see adolescent patients exhibit many of the comorbidities associated with diabetes, such as periodontal disease and bone loss. Studies support a strong correlation between glycemic control and severity of periodontitis.[11] Dentists should include periodontal evaluation as a part of the adolescent examination.

Related Hard and Soft Tissue Problems

A number of pathologic conditions may occur in adolescence and may be first noticed in this period. One is TMD, described in more detail later in this chapter. An eating disorder can manifest as enamel erosion of all teeth if vomiting is a regular component of this psychiatric disorder.[12] *Bulimia* is the term given to characterize those

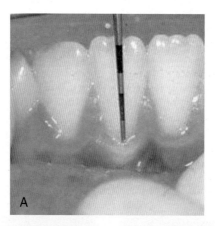

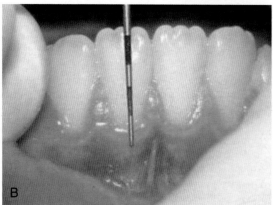
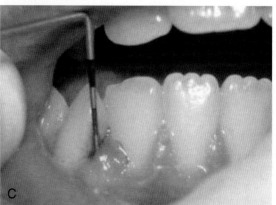

• **Figure 38.2** The prevalence of periodontal disease begins to increase in the adolescent patient; therefore a thorough evaluation of the periodontium is absolutely necessary. A periodontal probe is used to measure pocket depth (A) and the width of the keratinized gingiva (B). Probing is also done to establish a bleeding index (C). The amount of attached gingiva is determined by subtracting the pocket depth from the width of the keratinized gingiva.

who vomit regularly to purge themselves of food in a misdirected attempt to control their weight. Bulimia affects far more girls than boys, but boys can exhibit similar behavior. The regurgitated stomach contents, which are highly acidic, erode the enamel of teeth in a process called perimolysis (Fig. 38.3). Dentin is exposed, making teeth sensitive and encouraging decay. Enamel flakes off, leaving sharp edges. Restorations may appear to have grown out of their preparations as enamel and dentin dissolve around them. In the early bulimic, these clinical signs may be absent. Pulpal pathosis, elongated clinical crowns, gingival recession, and loss of vertical dimension are a few of the treatment issues noted in bulimia. Unless the vomiting is stopped, extensive treatment may be futile. The dentist should work with a psychotherapist to deal with this problem. Dental erosion may have a variety of etiologies aside from bulimia in this age group, such as sports and carbonated beverage intake[13] or gastroesophageal reflux.[14] The dentist should investigate the cause of erosion carefully before making treatment recommendations and referrals.

Another pathologic problem is dental trauma. The clinical and radiographic examinations should address tooth crazing, chips, or discoloration with adjunctive radiographs to clarify the status of teeth. Not all teeth that appear sound are clinically healthy (Fig. 38.4), and not all trauma is to hard tissues. It is important to obtain a thorough trauma history during the patient interview process. The effects of smoking and oral sexual activity (Fig. 38.5) may also be identified during the examination. Oral piercing has become popular in teenagers and young adults. It is associated with risks of systemic infection and tissue damage during placement, as well as tooth fracture, gingival recession, and localized infection while the item is being worn[15] (Fig. 38.6).

Evaluation of third molars is usually completed during mid- to late adolescence. Parents commonly ask about treating these teeth. The reasons for extraction of third molars include but are not limited to impaction or failure to erupt, periodontal disease, cysts or tumors, decay, posteruption malposition, nonfunction as a result of an absent opposing tooth, difficulty with hygiene, and recurrent pericoronitis. If any of these conditions are present, the clinician should discuss removal with the parent and patient. The American Association of Oral and Maxillofacial Surgeons has conducted trials on third molars and oral health.[16] They have recommended advising patients and parents about the odds of a third molar remaining free of symptoms and pathology and then make a decision about removal. The discussion must also include the risks of surgery to remove the third molars.

The concept of anterior crowding as the result of forward pressure from third molars is currently unproven and is not a reason to extract. Surgical access and root development are important issues in determining when to extract. Some root development is desired to stabilize teeth, but complete root development can make extraction more difficult and may increase the likelihood of root fractures. Smokers, and females using oral contraceptives, may also run a high risk of postsurgical dry socket.

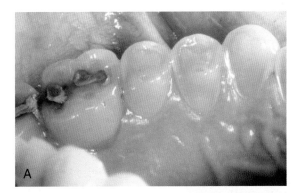

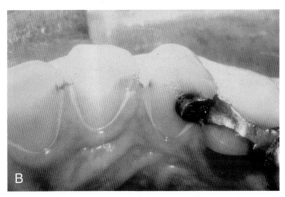
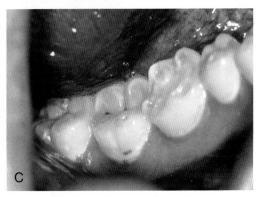

• **Figure 38.3** Common intraoral findings for a bulimic patient. (A) The loss of occlusal enamel with fractures of both the enamel and restorations is seen. (B) Progressive loss of enamel as witnessed here with posterior teeth progressively more eroded the longer they are present in the oral cavity. (C) Lingual exposure of dentin highlighted by outlines of remaining enamel and exposed surfaces of restorations. (From Casamassimo P, Castaldi C. Considerations in the dental management of the adolescent. *Pediatr Clin North Am.* 1982;29:648.)

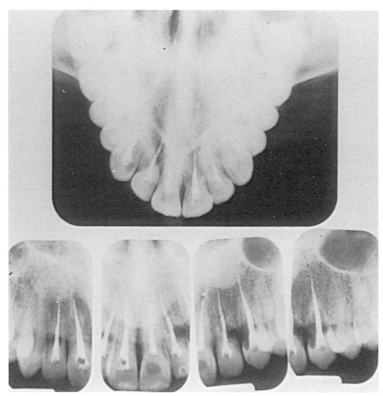

• **Figure 38.4** Severe resorption of roots secondary to trauma is evident on radiographic examination. These teeth were remarkably clinically stable despite the amount of root resorption.

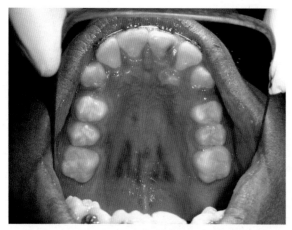

• **Figure 38.5** This patient exhibits palatal hematomas secondary to oral sex. Negative intraoral pressures cause blood to be pulled to the surface of the palatal tissue.

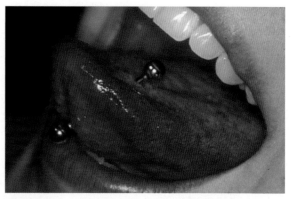

• **Figure 38.6** An example of a tongue piercing, known as a dumbbell, which is common among teenagers and young adults. It has been shown to fracture enamel.

Occlusal Evaluation

The anteroposterior, transverse, and vertical components of the occlusion should be evaluated as described in Chapter 31. The major difference is that arch length deficiencies are no longer predicted from space analyses but are measured directly from the casts because all permanent teeth have erupted by this age (Fig. 38.7).

Careful attention should be paid to teeth adjacent to edentulous areas because the adjacent teeth may need to be repositioned with orthodontics prior to restorative treatment. The position of the teeth, the amount of supporting bone, the health of the teeth, and the number of missing teeth will determine the direction of treatment.

Once again, the interaction between the facial profile and dental crowding should be considered. Committing the patient to treatment based solely on dental characteristics can have a disastrous effect on the facial profile. The nose and chin will continue to grow and the lips thin over time so the clinician must factor these changes into decisions on how to manage the crowding.

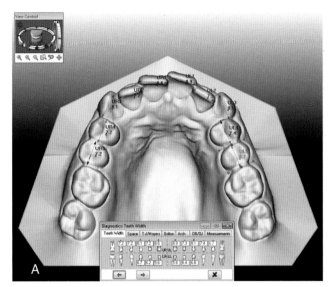
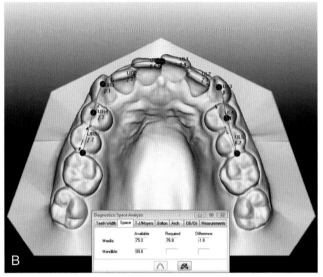

• **Figure 38.7** (A) Arch length analysis in the adolescent patient is measured directly from casts rather than by using prediction tables of mixed dentition space analysis because all permanent teeth usually have erupted by this age. The first step is to measure the mesiodistal width of each individual permanent tooth. Depending on the software, the tooth widths are added together to get a sum of the mesiodistal widths in the arch. (B) Next, the arch circumference is determined by digital placement of the measuring tool from the mesial of the permanent first molar to the mesial of the contralateral first molar. The difference between the arch circumference and the sum of the mesiodistal width indicate the amount of crowding or spacing within the arch. If one or two primary teeth have not exfoliated, the width of the contralateral erupted permanent tooth can be substituted for the unerupted permanent tooth.

Radiographic Evaluation

The adolescent radiographic examination ranges from a transitional to an adult multifilm survey, depending on the child's dentition. The issues surrounding radiographic examination in the adolescent are related to the type and frequency of exposure. The types of films used in adolescent radiography should be determined by the number of teeth present, the assessment of closed contacts not clinically visible, and the reason for radiographic examination. For the new adolescent patient with no apparent major dental needs, an individualized exam of posterior bitewings with a panoramic film or selected periapical films should suffice. For the adolescent patient with major dental care needs, a full mouth intraoral exam is preferred. The number of films is dictated by the size of the examination area and the information required to make a proper diagnosis.[17]

The radiographic examination in this age group should address mainly growth and development issues: the eruption status of unerupted premolars and canines. Later in adolescence, a final issue is third molar development. The development of these teeth can be evaluated by using periapical radiographs or a panoramic radiograph.

The adolescent should be able to tolerate no. 2 size intraoral films. For the child with a small oral cavity, techniques to aid in positioning are described in the radiographic section of Chapter 31.

Multiple or serial periapical radiographs are required for diagnosis of pathosis or for management of conditions that require significant follow up, such as endodontic therapy for traumatized incisors.

Bitewing radiography during early adolescence is affected by the developing occlusion and lack of contacts. A thorough clinical exam should determine if posterior surfaces can be adequately visualized until the premolars have fully erupted. The benefit of exposing bitewing films to examine two or four interproximal surfaces should be weighed against the risk of radiation exposure. In these cases, the caries risk assessment and a current clinical examination help to determine whether films are necessary.

The panoramic film has a role in adolescent dentistry as a full-mouth radiographic survey for a new patient who does not have major treatment needs. The panoramic film reveals bone pathosis and orients the examiner to the presence and position of third molars. The panoramic film also grossly displays sinuses and the TMJ (Fig. 38.8), which may be less well displayed on a multifilm intraoral survey. Table 38.2 summarizes the issues that apply to radiography of the adolescent patient.

Treatment Planning for Nonorthodontic Problems

In the adolescent patient, attention must be paid to the long-term consequences of treatment. Decisions made for the adolescent will influence their care for the rest of their lives. The clinician should develop goals for the treatment and develop a treatment plan that will serve the patient not only as an adolescent but also as an adult. The decisions may be as simple as a choice of restorative material to as complex as the delivery and timing of prosthetic replacement of teeth.

All phases of treatment planning should be addressed. The adolescent depicted in Fig. 38.9 illustrates the complexity of problems requiring preventive, periodontal, restorative, surgical, and orthodontic management.

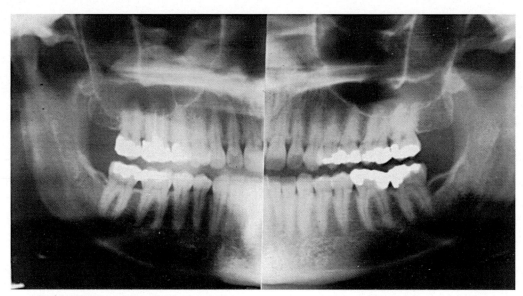

• **Figure 38.8** A large mucosal cyst in the sinus is evident in this panoramic radiograph of a 21-year-old patient. The cyst is possibly a reaction to pulpal pathosis in the permanent maxillary first and second molars.

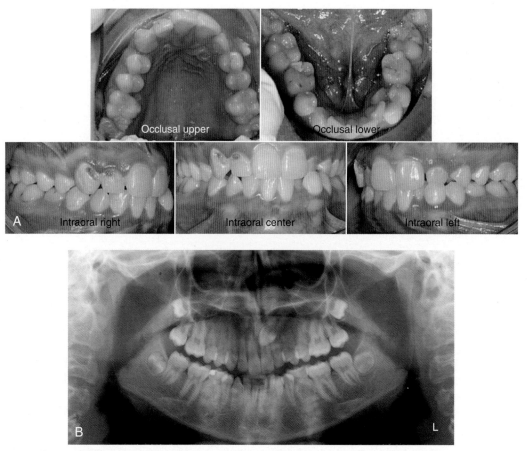

• **Figure 38.9** This adolescent patient has multiple problems that required interdisciplinary cooperation to solve. (A) Note the caries, periodontal disease, crowded teeth, midline discrepancy and malocclusion, and retained primary teeth. (B) The patient also has an impacted maxillary canine.

TABLE 38.2 Radiographic Issues in the Adolescent

Aspect	Recommendation
Frequency	
Full mouth survey	No suggested frequency or interval Determined by patient age, dental development, and caries risk assessment Preferred when clinical evidence of generalized dental disease
Bitewing radiographs	No suggested frequency or interval Determined by patient age, dental development, and caries risk assessment Should be taken if clinical caries noted Should be taken if multiple interproximal restorations present and are being followed Should be taken if incipient caries are noted on previous films and are being monitored Interval for these situations should be individualized and re-evaluated at each periodic examination
Periapical radiographs	No suggested frequency or interval Pathosis or treatment needs should dictate frequency To evaluate dental trauma To determine developmental status of third molars
Panoramic radiographs	Possible component of a full mouth survey for a disease-free new patient Evaluate the mesiodistal position of maxillary canines "Third molar" panoramic radiograph to determine the developmental status of third molars
Type	

Full mouth survey	Number of films included to be based on tissue coverage needed
	Early adolescence (12–15 years):
	    Maxillary and mandibular periapicals (no. 1 size)
	    Canine periapicals (no. 1 or 2 size)
	    Bitewings (two films, no. 2 size)
	    Four posterior quadrant periapicals (no. 2 size) to include premolars and erupted molars
	Late adolescence (16–21 years):
	    Complete set (21-film) survey

Bitewing radiographs	Size determined by oral access, but no. 2 size used if possible One film sufficient until eruption of second molars Position varies with the location and number of posterior contacts
Periapical radiographs	Should be adult no. 1 size films rather than no. 2 size; used as occlusal film as in primary tooth survey An exception would be use of no. 2 film as initial trauma screen size
Panoramic radiographs	Can be used with bitewings for a full mouth survey and is desirable in caries-free and pathosis-free patients after a clinical examination "Third molar" panoramic radiograph can be used to determine developmental status of third molars

All adolescents should receive the benefit of a preventive plan that addresses the needs of the adult dentition. Proper toothbrush positioning and flossing technique should be reviewed. In addition, the preventive plan should address environmental concerns, such as smoking, diet, trauma prevention, and the effect of medications on the periodontium and teeth.

Periodontal and gingival concerns are solidly tied to restorative care. In the child, the minor inflammation around a stainless steel crown on a primary tooth that is due to grossly adjusted margins is tolerated. In the adolescent with a cast crown, the tissues must be completely healthy.

Restorative treatment planning for the teen is characterized by a number of issues.[18]

1. Pulp size is large, affecting the choice of coronal coverage.
2. Anterior teeth continue to erupt, requiring consideration of various types of esthetic restorations for traumatized or defective teeth to prevent exposure of margins.
3. Esthetic awareness by the patient may force the dentist to undertake management of congenital or acquired discoloration or may require repeated treatment of teeth if transitional procedures are used.
4. Partially erupted posterior teeth may not serve as good abutments for prostheses.
5. Decreased chewing efficiency resulting from loss of a posterior tooth may force interim replacement with a removable appliance, although this may not be the treatment of choice.
6. Planned or active orthodontic treatment may delay restoration of missing teeth.

The use of acid-etch composite resins and porcelain veneers has greatly improved the management of adolescent restorative problems by providing esthetically acceptable, reasonably priced, conservative interim and permanent restorations. Their consideration as treatment options in restorative treatment planning is a must (see Chapter 40).

The two remaining elements of importance in adolescent treatment planning are interrelated. They are consent and compliance. Treatment of adolescents under the age of majority requires parental consent. Payment for services also demands clarification of consent. The proposed treatment is best explained with both parent and adolescent present, although the actual delivery of care can occur with the adolescent alone in the operatory. Good one-on-one dialogue during active treatment helps to ensure compliance. Some general guidelines for communication to maximize success include the following:

1. Show the adolescent the same respect and interest as you would an adult.
2. Be sincere.
3. Treat the adolescent in privacy as an adult, separate from younger children.
4. Outline the procedures and explain the reasons for them.
5. Minimize or eliminate authoritarian posturing, using your knowledge rather than age as a reason for your role as a dentist.
6. Be flexible enough to adapt to a changing relationship.

Treatment Planning and Treatment for Orthodontic Problems

Adolescent orthodontic problems create difficult treatment decisions for the general practitioner and the specialist. The nature of the malocclusion heavily influences how the problem will be managed.

Skeletal Problems

If the malocclusion is skeletal, treatment is aimed at altering the relationship or orientation of the jaws and teeth. This can be accomplished by growth modification, camouflage, or orthognathic surgery. Because the physical maturity of the adolescent patient varies among persons of the same age, any one of three treatments may be appropriate. If the developmental assessment of the patient suggests that the patient is actively growing, growth modification is a viable treatment alternative. Growth modification, previously discussed in Chapter 36, attempts to change the actual size, shape, or orientation of the jaws to obtain an acceptable occlusion. Functional appliances and extraoral traction are used to secure these changes. The clinician may lean toward more noncompliant appliances in this age group because the remaining growth potential is so small there can be no wasted time not wearing appliances.

In the nongrowing, physically mature adolescent, which is most likely the case, skeletal malocclusion is appropriately treated by camouflage or orthognathic surgery. Camouflage is the orthodontic movement of teeth without changing the underlying skeletal malocclusion. Camouflage should be considered only when the soft tissue profile is acceptable and when tooth movement will not change or compromise the profile. Teeth are tipped or bodily moved on the denture base to positions considered less than ideal but acceptable for normal occlusion. For example, a mild class II mandibular deficiency with a relatively prominent bony pogonion can be managed by camouflage (Fig. 38.10). To camouflage this type of problem, the upper teeth are moved backward and the lower teeth are tipped forward to bring the teeth together and disguise the skeletal problem. In conjunction with the tipping of teeth for camouflage, often teeth in the maxillary arch are extracted to provide space in which to move the upper teeth backward. Although a small amount of soft tissue change may occur and the final position of the mandibular incisors may be less than ideal,

functional occlusion can be achieved without surgery. Traditionally, camouflage of class II skeletal problems has been considered more acceptable in women and camouflage of class III problems more acceptable in men because the respective convex and straight profiles are more acceptable for these groups. Recent data indicate more acceptance among laypeople.[19] The esthetic results in males with moderately class II problems were judged to be as acceptable as those in females with class II problems, whereas the results in males with moderate class III problems remained more esthetically acceptable than those in females with class III problems. Camouflage of class III problems usually is addressed with lingual tipping of mandibular anterior teeth to obtain an acceptable overbite and overjet while at the same time moving the upper dentition anteriorly. Often, mandibular tipping is more easily accomplished when extractions are performed in the lower arch. At least for class II patients, most consider treatment by camouflage extremely acceptable even though they realize they have somewhat smaller or more retrusive chin points.[20]

With the maturity of the alveolar bone, temporary anchorage devices (TADs) have a place in orthodontic treatment planning for the adolescent, as do other skeletal anchorage methods, such as bone plates. TADs are germane to camouflage treatment. Patients who previously could not lose any anchorage can now be treated with near absolute anchorage when TADs are placed. This opens new dimensions of treatment in many planes of space, especially for the anteroposterior and vertical. The direction of space closure can be carefully controlled as can absolute intrusion (Fig. 38.11). Usually age 12 years is a safe time to begin skeletal anchorage considerations due to bone maturation.

Skeletal malocclusion in the nongrowing patient can also be managed with orthognathic surgery.[21] The specialist works with an oral and maxillofacial surgeon to surgically reposition one or both jaws into proper alignment (Fig. 38.12). Typically, the orthodontic treatment plan calls for a presurgical period of orthodontic tooth movement to align teeth in both arches and position the teeth over the bony bases so that they will fit together following surgery. Orthognathic surgery is performed under general anesthesia, and the maxilla, mandible, or both jaws are repositioned and held in the new position by surgical screws or bone plates and screws. It is possible to move the entire jaw or individual segments of the jaw in almost any direction within the constraints of the soft tissue covering. There is some restriction on the amount of change that can be achieved, and some types of change are more stable than others. Following the surgical procedure, jaw function is reduced with elastic traction. After healing is demonstrated, a short period of postsurgical orthodontic tooth movement is necessary to settle the teeth into the final occlusion.

Dental Problems

If the orthodontic problem in the adolescent is strictly dental, conventional orthodontic treatment can be used to manage the malocclusion. Identification and management of dental orthodontic problems have already been discussed and basically do not change with the age of the patient. However, there are several aspects of dental orthodontic treatment that have not been discussed and should be mentioned here. Despite the preventive efforts of the dental profession, some persons continue to lose permanent teeth to decay or trauma. Other patients lose primary teeth during adolescence and have no successors. When this occurs, a combination of orthodontic tooth movement and restorative dentistry is recommended to obtain optimal esthetic and functional results.

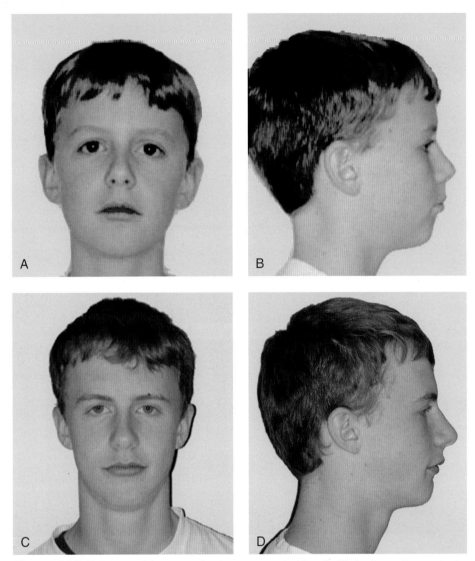

• **Figure 38.10** (A) This preadolescent patient has a convex facial profile (B) due to maxillary protrusion. Because the facial profile is acceptable even though the skeletal relationships are not ideal, the teeth were moved to reduce the overjet and obtain a functional occlusion by retracting the maxillary teeth and proclining the mandibular teeth. (C) At the adolescent posttreatment stage, the facial profile (D) remains convex but acceptable with continued maxillary protrusion.

In the anterior region, orthodontic treatment is often designed to move teeth to simplify restorative or prosthetic treatment. To provide precise control of tooth movement, orthodontic brackets should be placed on the anterior teeth and the permanent first molars. Treatment must be carefully planned so that only the teeth that require movement are affected, and the other teeth remain stationary. This means that molar, canine, and midline relationships should be carefully studied and controlled during treatment.

In cases of missing or small teeth, a diagnostic setup is performed so final tooth position and dental relationships can be defined for the best result. Multiple setups might be required for a single patient to represent different treatment approaches. Digital study casts can be manipulated so several treatment alternatives can be examined by the patient and dentist (Fig. 38.13).

Coil springs, elastomeric chains, and intraoral elastics can be used to open and close space for the best potential result. It is also an excellent opportunity to consider the use of a TAD, because the adolescent has bone dense enough to support this type of anchorage. These opportunities can be used for solutions to anterior problems (Fig. 38.14) and posterior problems (Fig. 38.15). Once the space has been established and is nearly ideal, a closed coil spring or loops bent into the archwire are used to hold or maintain the space until the restorative or prosthetic treatment is completed. Although this type of treatment sounds simple, close attention to detail is necessary. Uncontrolled tooth movement can result in unanticipated changes in the midline, overjet, and overbite.

In certain cases, treatment can be accomplished with clear aligners. This is a relatively new approach to tooth movement, and was initially considered when there was generalized malalignment and good skeletal relations. The development of new materials and a more complete understanding of how aligners move teeth has expanded the types of cases being treated. The clinician uses a removable tray to exert force on the tooth to move it rather than using traditional orthodontic brackets and wires. An accurate

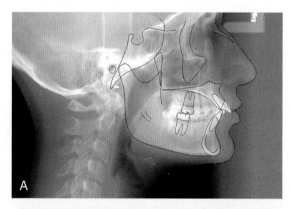

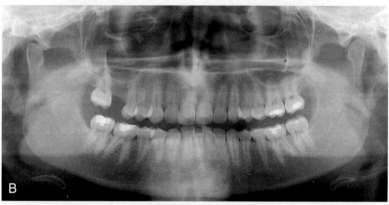

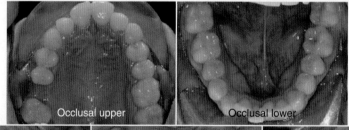

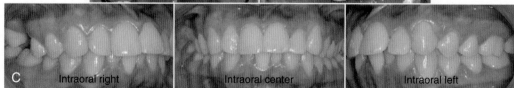

• **Figure 38.11** (A–C) This patient has a class II malocclusion, increased overjet, and missing teeth. In an attempt to reduce the malocclusion and the class II skeletal tendency, she was treated with extractions and space closure.

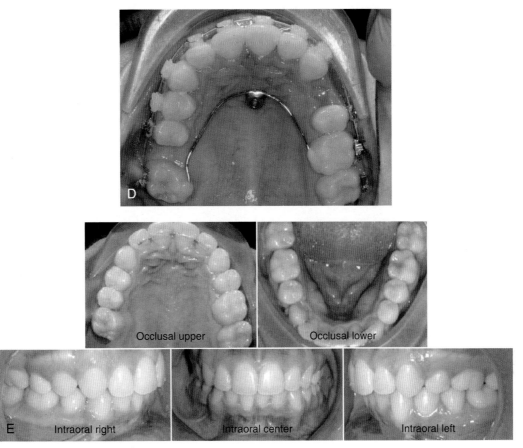

• **Figure 38.11, cont'd** (D) An osseointegrated implant was placed in the palate and used to control the space closure and retraction. (E) The problems were successfully addressed using this implant-supported camouflage treatment. Subsequently, the implant was removed.

impression or intraoral scan is made of the patient and is sent to a dental lab making aligners. The result is a digital representation of the malocclusion. Computer software has been designed to move the teeth individually in approximately 0.25 mm increments (Fig. 38.16). A series of aligners is constructed to move the teeth into position as determined by the doctor. The aligners are sent to the clinician for delivery and the patient wears one tray after another until the tooth movement is complete. The aligners are considered to be much more esthetic than traditional braces and more comfortable; however, there is still discomfort associated with tooth movement. The major drawback to removable aligners is that certain precise tooth movements are not as easy to make as with braces, so tooth movement can be less predictable. Obviously, to be successful, the patient must be thoroughly cooperative to wear the appliances as instructed. Clear aligner therapy continues to evolve and more and more challenging cases are being successfully treated.

Adolescent orthodontic treatment is a challenging exercise in problem solving. A good database and growth assessment are necessary to allow the proper decisions about treatment alternatives. Unless the orthodontic problem is obviously the result of dental malalignment, the patient should be referred to a specialist because of the difficulty in managing skeletal discrepancies in patients of this age. The unknowns of how much more a patient may grow and the direction the growth will occur make treatment decisions very difficult. It is not an overstatement to say decisions made at

this time can impact how an individual will look the rest of his or her life.

Temporomandibular Disorders in Children and Adolescents

TMDs collectively describe a group of painful and nonpainful musculoskeletal and neuromuscular conditions involving the muscles of mastication, the TMJ, and all associated structures.[22] While some TMDs are asymptomatic and do not require any interventions beyond education and reassurance, painful TMDs may require therapeutic and symptomatic care. Since pain is the most common reason that patients seek treatment,[23–25] it is vital that TMDs are understood in the broader perspective of orofacial pain conditions.[26] Orofacial pain is a general term that includes TMDs and other pain syndromes of the head and neck.[22] Chronic pain conditions, such as TMDs, frequently present during adolescence.[27] Pain conditions that last from days to weeks are generally referred to as acute while chronic pain conditions tend to persist for months to years.[28] Dentists are certainly well versed in treating acute dental pain; however, diagnosing and managing chronic pain in an adolescent population can be a challenging endeavor. Acute pain may resolve spontaneously or with minimal interventions, while chronic pain tends to be resistant to conventional treatment and may require a multidisciplinary approach to management.[27,29] An

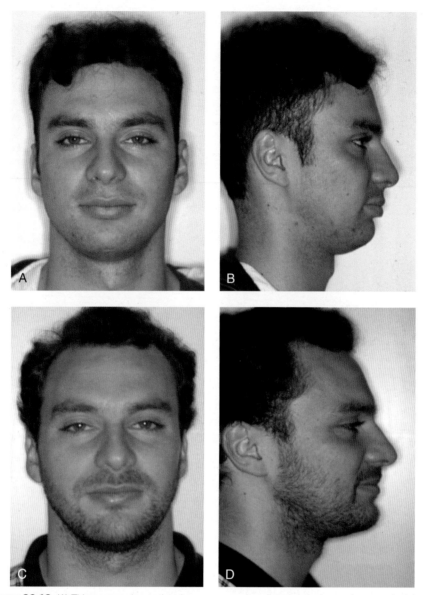

• **Figure 38.12** (A) This nongrowing patient has a severe class II malocclusion and convex facial profile (B) due to mandibular retrusion. The teeth cannot be moved together to provide a stable, functional occlusion, so orthognathic surgery was performed to advance the mandible. (C) After surgery the patient demonstrated more mandibular prominence (D) and facial height.

in-depth description of pain medicine is beyond the scope of this text; however, as a general rule, the longer pain persists the more challenging it becomes to manage due to neuroplasticity and sensitization at the level of the central nervous system.[28,29]

The American Academy of Orofacial Pain (AAOP) has established clinical guidelines that can be useful for diagnosing TMD in a clinical setting; however, critically evaluating TMD in a research setting is often bewildering. There is considerable variation in the epidemiologic data due to differences in study design, populations, and diagnostic criteria.[30] It is important to recognize that population-based research, and particularly surveys, have the potential to either under- or overestimate TMD findings.

The Diagnostic Criteria for Temporomandibular Disorders (DC-TMD) offers a validated, objective methodology for research purposes.[31] The DC-TMD protocol consists of a clinical exam with specific interview questions to aid in identifying individuals with TMDs. This tool was developed as part of an international consortium, and studies using this methodology should be considered to have met an appropriate level of scientific rigor. The DC-TMD also provides a helpful protocol for objectively classifying nonpainful and painful TMDs into subgroups. TMDs are divided into two main categories: (1) myogenous (muscle related) and (2) arthrogenous (joint related). Following this diagnostic paradigm is an important step toward reviewing the available data and understanding the various types of TMDs.

Epidemiologic studies reveal that TMDs are a sizable public health concern affecting 5% to 12% of the total population with an estimate of 5% to 7% requiring treatment.[22,31] Although uncommon in young children, signs and symptoms of TMD often initially present during adolescence.[25,32,33] Fortunately, the prevalence of severe TMD is low in the adolescent population.[34] The only study to date using the DC-TMD demonstrated an 11.9% prevalence

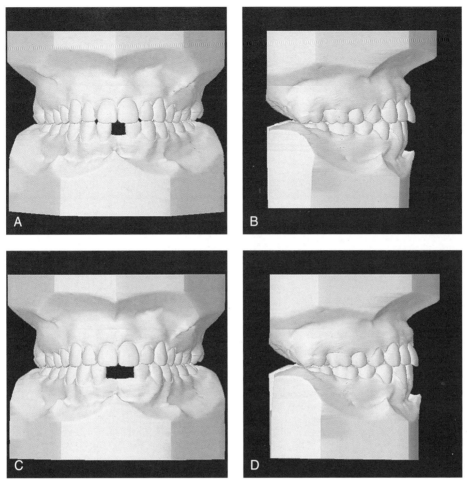

• **Figure 38.13** It is now possible to produce digital casts and manipulate the images to simulate setups. This series of images demonstrates options for this patient with missing lower central incisors using this technology. (A) An alternative is to make space for one incisor implant. (B) This solution positions the anterior teeth with more overbite and overjet than a setup with space for two mandibular central incisors implants (C), which reduces the overbite and overjet when the posterior dental relationships are identical (D). (Courtesy OrthoCAD by Cadent, Inc., Carlstadt, NJ.)

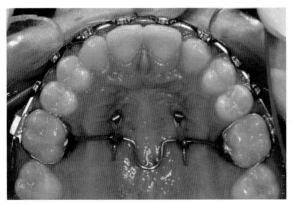

• **Figure 38.14** This patient had missing maxillary lateral incisors, and the canines were substituted for them. The canines have already been recontoured to mimic a lateral incisor, and further reduction is anticipated. Palatal temporary anchorage devices (TADs) were placed before space closure. A transpalatal arch with hooks was constructed so elastomeric chains could be stretched from the hooks to the TADs. This allows the posterior teeth to come forward without lingual movement of the upper incisors.

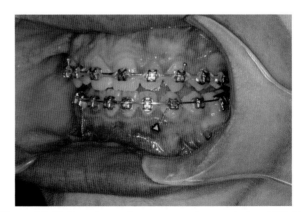

• **Figure 38.15** The advent of temporary anchorage devices (TADs) has made closure of posterior space feasible when posterior permanent teeth are missing. In this case, the patient was missing both second premolars, and the clinician elected to close all the space without prosthetic replacement of teeth. The TADs anchor the anterior segment and the posterior teeth to move forward with minimal posterior movement of the lower incisors. This is an example of indirect anchorage. In some cases, the TAD is used to directly bring the posterior teeth forward, in which case it is called direct anchorage.

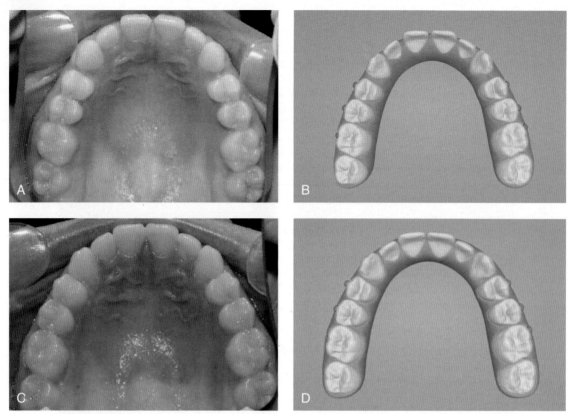

• **Figure 38.16** Orthodontic treatment for adolescents can be accomplished with removable aligners. The clinician submits a polyvinylsiloxane impression of the original malocclusion (A) to the dental laboratory to create a digital representation of the malocclusion (B). A series of aligners is created by the software and then constructed on actual models. The series is sent to the clinician who monitors the progress of the case and compares the actual tooth movement with the predicted movement. At the end of treatment, the clinician can compare the actual tooth movement (C) with the predicted movement (D).

of TMD in adolescents.[35] A recent systematic review of studies using previous methodologies determined the prevalence of TMD signs to be 16% in the adolescent population.[30] TMD symptoms tend to fluctuate with time,[32,36] and it is estimated that approximately 2% of symptomatic patients seek treatment.[25] The incidence of TMD-related pain increases from early adolescence to young adulthood,[32,33,37] and, similar to the adult population, TMDs tend to be more common in females than males.[32,33,35] The reason for this disparity is unknown; however, it is likely related to hormonal differences.[38–40] Numerous studies demonstrate the impact that TMD and orofacial pain have on activities of daily living (ADL),[41] quality of life,[42] psychosocial distress,[43] and sleep quality.[44]

Prior to considering factors related to TMDs, it is important to recognize the signs and symptoms commonly associated with the diagnosis. Signs are clinically observable findings. There is a wide range of clinical signs that have been studied in patients with TMD. Often, the signs of TMD are also common in asymptomatic children who have no complaints about pain. They may reflect normal variations or transient changes consistent with normal findings and have no clinical significance.[32] The following are examples of signs that should be documented:
• TMJ sounds (upon palpation)
• Occlusal wear
• Occlusal interferences
• Limitation in mandibular range of motion (ROM; <40 mm)
• Mandibular deviation or deflection on opening
• Tenderness to palpation and/or manipulation

Symptoms are based on subjective information gathered from interviewing the patient and caregiver. Most adolescents are capable of describing what they are feeling; therefore a structured approach to interviewing the patient is recommended. The following should be considered when evaluating for TMD symptoms:
• Pain
• Headaches
• Dizziness
• Nausea
• Jaw tightness
• Jaw instability
• Sleep bruxism

The relationship between signs and symptoms remains unclear. Symptoms, such as pain and dysfunction, are not consistently associated with clinical signs. The clinician is cautioned not to predict a future diagnosis of a severe TMD based on clinical signs and symptoms. Although risk and perpetuating factors may be identified, none consistently lead a patient to a lifetime of a pain. Asymptomatic TMDs in adolescence are benign and tend to be self-limiting, only rarely progressing to a more serious condition.[34]

There is no unique theoretical model or single etiologic factor that can explain the onset of TMD.[22] Therefore it is not possible to foresee who will develop a significant TMD and more importantly who will experience a transition from acute to persistent or recurrent pain. Since studies do not point to absolute etiologic factors for TMD, it is not possible to reliably predict those who will require invasive or advanced treatment. The focus on etiology should be determining the initiating, predisposing, and perpetuating factors.[22,45] Initiating factors are related to onset; predisposing factors are related to risk; and perpetuating factors are factors that interfere with recovery. Like other domains of TMD, there is considerable individual variability. Degenerative disease, developmental abnormalities, trauma, and other conditions usually have a clear and obvious relationship to TMD while other factors have weak or conflicting associations. In fact, the cause of TMDs in some individuals may be unknown (Box 38.1).

Bothersome TMJ sounds are often noticed due to the proximity of the TMJs to the ears. Clicking, popping, snapping, scraping, and grinding sounds associated with jaw function are commonly reported in both adolescent and adult populations.[36] Dislocation and subsequent reduction of the articular disk upon jaw movements is a frequent source of TMJ sounds.[26,45] A magnetic resonance image (MRI) study demonstrated that 35% of asymptomatic adults have a displaced disk.[46] Unique TMJ anatomy, degenerative changes, and temporary sticking of the disk also account for TMJ sounds.[45] In the adolescent population, the incidence of TMJ sounds has been reported to be as high as 17%, and data suggest TMJ clicking may come and go during this timeframe.[45] TMJ noises are common in both adult and adolescent populations, and treatment for asymptomatic TMJ sounds do not typically require any management beyond education and reassurance.[22,26]

Parafunctional activity refers to nonfunctional oromandibular movements, such as jaw clenching, tooth grinding, or tooth gnashing

---

• BOX 38.1   Some Established Causes of Temporomandibular Joint Dysfunction in Children and Adolescents

Inherited
Hemifacial Microsomia
Hemifacial atrophy
Juvenile rheumatoid arthritis
Ankylosis
Cleft related

Acquired
Infectious (Septic Arthritis)
Traumatic (sports injury)
Iatrogenic (cortisone damage, surgical displacement, irradiation)
Factitial (habits, hobbies)
Neoplastic (tumors)
Idiopathic

---

or tapping.[45] Parafunction also includes lip biting, cheek biting, and biting of other tissues or objects. These parafunctional activities may occur alone or in combinations.

Sleep bruxism or nocturnal bruxism, a common form of parafunction, is classified by the *International Classification of Sleep Disorders,* 3rd Edition (ICSD-3) as a sleep-related movement disorder involving stereotyped, rhythmic masticatory muscle activity along with grinding and clenching of the teeth.[47] It is regarded as an involuntary behavior and the pathophysiology is thought to involve a complex process involving the regions of the brain responsible for motor function.[48] On the other hand, bruxing while awake (diurnal bruxism) is considered to be a voluntary condition.

Bruxism is common in children and adolescents; however, it is difficult to interpret in literature due to the variability of age groups and diagnostic strategies.[49] The majority of studies are surveys that rely on recall of the patient or parents,[50,51] and most do not use polysomnography (PSG) or electromyography (EMG) to confirm the presence of sleep bruxism.[49,50] Available data suggest sleep bruxism occurs in 14% to 38% of children[48,51] and approximately 13% to 22% of the adolescent population.[48,52] Although the incidence of sleep bruxism decreases from adolescence to adulthood, longitudinal studies in adolescents have demonstrated that self-reports of both sleep bruxism and diurnal bruxism in childhood predict the same parafunctional activity during adulthood.[53] No apparent gender differences are present.

The paradigm of sleep bruxism as a primary versus secondary condition should also be considered. Primary sleep bruxism is a normal phenomenon that occurs without a known cause, while secondary sleep bruxism is related to nocturnal parafunctional activity related to a specific condition or substance. Sleep bruxism has been associated with a variety of medical conditions such as gastroesophageal reflux disease (GERD),[54] cerebral palsy, and other neurologic conditions.[55] Although a causal relationship has not been established, sleep bruxism frequently presents in patients with obstructive sleep apnea.[56] Recent studies have demonstrated that in the adolescent population sleep bruxism may be associated with behavioral problems and psychosocial disorders.[55,57] It should be noted that several medications and substances have been associated with sleep bruxism. Antidepressants such as selective serotonin reuptake inhibitors (SSRIs) and selective norepinephrine reuptake inhibitors (SNRIs)[58] and stimulants such as methylphenidate, caffeine, and nicotine should be considered as potential secondary causes of sleep bruxism.[59,60]

Bruxism is not consistently associated with pain.[48] However, sleep bruxism should be suspected as a contributing factor if a patient complains of jaw pain upon waking. Similarly, if a patient complains of masticatory pain toward the end of the day, habitual daytime parafunctional activity may be a perpetuating factor.

SLEEP DISORDERED BREATHING

Rose D. Sheats

The natural history of sleep disordered breathing (SDB) in the pediatric patient is not well understood, although data are beginning to accrue. One would anticipate that as the child matures, tonsillar and adenoidal tissue would regress, and airway space would enlarge with growth, leading to a decrease in the prevalence of SDB in adolescents. However, a longitudinal study of 319 children from age 8.5 years to 13.7 years revealed a 71% remission rate, suggesting persistence of SDB in nearly 30% of preadolescents diagnosed with SDB.[1] In addition, a 10% incidence rate in the adolescent group was also demonstrated. Risk factors for persistent or incident SDB in this adolescent sample consisted of obesity and male gender, mimicking the risk factors in adult populations.

Another study suggested that the prevalence of SDB in a cohort of children studied from middle childhood (8–11 years) to late adolescence (16–19 years) remained approximately 4.5%, despite the fact that 91% of middle childhood cases in the study remitted over time, and late adolescent cases were likely incident cases.[2] Obesity in middle childhood was a risk

Continued

SLEEP DISORDERED BREATHING—cont'd

factor for the development of SDB in late adolescence, as was male gender, African American race, increased body mass index (BMI), and a history of adenotonsillectomy. Half of the habitual snorers in middle childhood remained habitual snorers in late adolescence.

These studies highlight the need for early recognition of childhood obesity and timely intervention to manage this trend. Pediatric dentists should alert families to the risk of SDB development as one of the consequences of obesity and assist in facilitating referral for the medical or behavioral management of obesity.

There is a controversy about the role of orthodontic premolar extractions as a risk factor for the development of SDB. The theory is that premolar extractions reduce the volume of the airway. Most studies examined the changes in the volume of the posterior airway space before and after orthodontic treatment (premolar extractions) using both two-dimensional and three-dimensional images.[3] However, they failed to demonstrate an association between the dimensions of the posterior airway space and SDB. Another study analyzed over 5000 electronic medical records from a population of adults aged 40 to 70 years—the age range at which SDB is most prevalent. The study was strengthened with the inclusion of overnight sleep studies to confirm or exclude the presence of obstructive sleep apnea.[4] The investigators compared a group of adults who had undergone extraction of four premolars with those who had intact dentitions (other than missing third molars). They found no difference in the prevalence of obstructive sleep apnea between the two groups, and concluded that orthodontic extraction of premolars does not pose an increased risk for SDB. This is the strongest evidence to date refuting orthodontic extractions as a risk factor for the development of SDB in the future.

The adolescent patient diagnosed with SDB may be a candidate for one of the mandibular advancement devices commonly used to manage adult SDB.[5,6] These appliances function by preventing the tongue from collapsing into the posterior airway during sleep and should be prescribed in collaboration with the physician managing the SDB. Because these appliances are similar to those used to manage class II dental and skeletal malocclusions, the dentist must be cautious in recommending such an appliance for class I or class III growing patients, as their impact may be unfavorable on the growth of the craniofacial skeleton. Furthermore, it has

been clearly demonstrated these appliances cause changes in the occlusion over time, resulting in posterior open bites, reduced overjet and overbite, retroclined maxillary incisors, and proclined lower incisors.[7] Patients, parents, and dentists must give careful consideration to the risks and benefits of mandibular advancement appliances in the management of SDB before proceeding.

Given the prevalence of SDB in the adolescent population, further elucidation of the role dentists play in screening and referring these patients for management of SDB bears investigation. Much research is still needed to identify the most appropriate strategies and optimal time for intervention.

References

1. Goodwin JL, Vasquez MM, Silva GE, et al. Incidence and remission of sleep-disordered breathing and related symptoms in 6- to 17-year old children—the Tucson Children's Assessment of Sleep Apnea Study. *J Pediatr.* 2010;157:57–61.
2. Spilsbury JC, Storfer-Isser A, Rosen CL, et al. Remission and incidence of obstructive sleep apnea from middle childhood to late adolescence. *Sleep.* 2015;38:23–29.
3. Hu Z, Yin X, Liao J, et al. The effect of teeth extraction for orthodontic treatment on the upper airway: a systematic review. *Sleep Breath.* 2015;19:441–451.
4. Larsen AJ, Rindal DB, Hatch JP, et al. Evidence supports no relationship between obstructive sleep apnea and premolar extraction: an electronic health records review. *J Clin Sleep Med.* 2015;11:1443–1448.
5. Scherr S, Dort L, Almeida F, et al. Definition of an effective oral appliance for the treatment of obstructive sleep apnea and snoring: a report of the American Academy of Dental Sleep Medicine. *J Dent Sleep Med.* 2014;1:39–50.
6. Schütz TCB, Dominguez GC, Hallinan MP, et al. Class II correction improves nocturnal breathing in adolescents. *Angle Orthod.* 2011;81:222–228.
7. Pliska BT, Nam H, Chen H, et al. Obstructive sleep apnea and mandibular advancement splints: occlusal effects and progression of changes associated with a decade of treatment. *J Clin Sleep Med.* 2014;10:1285–1291.

Malocclusion and orthodontic treatments have been implicated as precursors of painful TMDs; however, neither have shown a clear and consistent relationship when closely scrutinized.[61,62] In fact, some reported precursors, such as an anterior open bite, may actually be the result of TMD rather than the cause.[26] Furthermore, there is no reported relationship between malocclusion and nonpainful TMDs including asymptomatic disk displacements.[63] Preventive orthodontic therapy to eliminate risk factors has not withstood scientific scrutiny, nor has orthodontic therapy to manage existing TMDs.

Some have proposed a class II skeletal or dental relationship may cause a TMD. However, full-time anterior repositioning occlusal splint therapy to change the occlusal scheme has not been validated in the literature.[22] In fact, full-time wear of an anterior re-positioning appliance to "re-capture" the articular disk may result in a permanent posterior open bite.

Nonworking and working occlusal interferences have little consistency in predicting TMD. However, one study demonstrated that patients with preexisting TMDs seem to be more vulnerable to artificial occlusal interferences.[64] A majority agree that prophylactic removal of occlusal interferences is contraindicated.[26,29,65] No single occlusal factor has been isolated as a source for TMD; however, an unstable occlusal scheme or orthopedic position coupled with excessive parafunction may increase the risk for developing a TMD.

A history of trauma has a modest relationship with TMD in the adolescent population.[66] Jaw injuries and iatrogenic trauma from

third molar removal have been found to be potential initiating events for TMDs.[67] However, a controlled prospective study of third molar removal demonstrated no statistical difference at 6 months between the control group and the wisdom tooth extraction group.[68] Ankylosis, a rare but serious manifestation of TMJ trauma, occurs when there is fusion of the mandible to the cranial base or zygoma.[69] Given the variability of traumatic injuries to the masticatory system and the differing levels of individual response to injury, it is reasonable to screen for trauma in patients with a history of TMD.

It is important to rule out any secondary conditions as the true source of the pain and/or dysfunction in TMD. Potential secondary causes include systemic diseases, such as juvenile idiopathic arthritis, Ehlers-Danlos syndrome, or Marfan syndrome.[45,70,71] Congenital conditions, such as hemifacial microsomia and Treacher Collins syndrome,[72] or local structural factors such as hyper- or hypoplasia of the mandibular condyle or a bifid condyle may also contribute to TMDs.[73] Tumors and pseudotumors are rare but should be considered.[74]

Pain in the masticatory structures may be due to referred pain from another structure.[75] Examples include masticatory pain secondary to headaches,[27] salivary gland pain,[76] lymph node pain,[77] ear pain,[78,79] and dental pain. Resolution or symptom improvement of perceived temporomandibular problems can occur when efforts are directed toward the true source of the pain.

Diagnosis of Temporomandibular Disorder

The clinician interested in TMD management should recognize that overdiagnosis and subsequent overtreatment are perhaps the most consistent aspects of dealing with this disorder in adolescents. The AAOP guidelines and the DC-TMD provide criteria for categorizing TMDs into two main subgroups: (1) myogenous (muscle related) and (2) arthrogenous (joint related). Painful extracapsular (muscular) TMDs are commonly subdivided into myalgia and myofascial pain conditions. Intracapsular (joint related) conditions are categorized as inflammatory (capsulitis), disk displacement disorders (reducing and nonreducing), degenerative disorders (osteoarthritis), and subluxation.[22]

The interview and examination should identify the patient's chief complaint and classify it as either a primarily muscular or a primarily joint-related pain condition. A thorough understanding of the relevant anatomy is essential to provide an accurate diagnosis and to provide meaningful treatment recommendations. The human TMJs are complex structures classified as ginglymoarthrodial joints. Capable of both rotation (hinging) and translation (gliding), these unique joints are composed of the mandibular condyles, glenoid fossae of the temporal bones, and interposing articular disks (Fig. 38.17). Unique to the TMJs, the articular disks are chiefly composed of dense fibrous connective tissue. Although the disks do not contain nerves or vessels, their posterior attachments are highly innervated and vascular and are a potential source of intracapsular (joint) pain. The articular surfaces of the condyles and fossae are lined with fibrocartilage. This feature is likely responsible for the durability and healing capacity of the TMJs.[22]

The paired muscles of mastication muscles (masseters, medial pterygoids, and temporalis) function to close the jaw while the lateral pterygoids function to open the mouth and protrude the mandible. The digastric muscles are also classified as jaw-depressing muscles. Accessory cervical musculature including the supra and infra hyoid muscles and sternocleidomastoid also may activate during mastication, swallowing, and other complex jaw movements.[80–82] A detailed description of the anatomy and physiology of jaw function is beyond the scope of this textbook and the reader is referred to a book dedicated to TMJs.

Dentists who treat adolescents should include a TMD screening examination to establish baseline function. The patient interview must include a thorough medical, dental, and social history. Identifying stressors and screening for psychological conditions can be useful as somatic complaints and behavioral problems have been associated with TMD in adolescent populations.[83,84] A history of recent or past trauma to the masticatory and cervical structures also should be obtained. In addition to checking for potential etiologic factors, it is important to ask about other chronic pain conditions, such as low back pain, stomach aches, neck pain, or primary headache syndromes because they are frequently associated with TMD in adolescents.[84,85] Headache disorders are common during adolescence and often precede pain in the masticatory system.[27] Primary headaches, such as migraine and tension-type headaches, frequently present as pain in the temporal region and may be misinterpreted as a TMD. If a bothersome primary headache is suspected, a referral to a primary care provider or neurologist is warranted.

It is critical for the clinician to understand the patient's symptoms, especially if the chief complaint is suggestive of a TMD. The patient may complain about pain, tightness, or instability of the jaw, or even a stuffy or ringing sensation in the ears. Since symptoms are subjective, it is helpful to use a systematic approach when interviewing the patient. The mnemonic OPQRSTU aids the practitioner when interviewing the adolescent patient with pain complaints (Table 38.3). It is important to identify the onset, provoking and palliating factors, quality or character, region, severity, timing, and impact of pain to provide a more objective means of quantifying a pain complaint. The natural history of the pain complaint as well as past treatments and results of those treatments also should be obtained.

The clinical examination confirms the information gathered from the detailed history. Clinical signs of TMD include TMJ sounds, tenderness to palpation, and alterations in mandibular ROM. The clinical examination should assess posture and signs of parafunction.

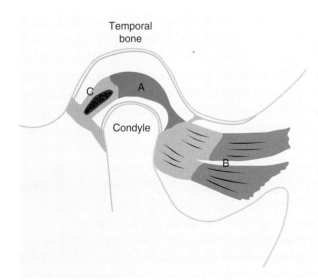

• **Figure 38.17** Articular disk (A) is interposed between the mandibular condyle and the glenoid fossa of the temporal bone. The lateral pterygoid muscles (B) are located anterior to the disk while the posterior attachment (C) contains tissue that is richly innervated and highly vascular.

TABLE 38.3	"OPQRSTU" Mnemonic for Evaluating Pain Symptoms	
Onset	When did pain first begin? What was associated with pain initiation? (Trauma, eating, stress)
Provoking and **P**alliating factors	What makes it pain worse? (Eating, poor sleep) What makes pain better? (Heat, ice, rest)
Quality	What does pain feel like? (Ache, throb, tight)
Region	Where is the pain? (Point with 1 finger)
Severity	How intense is the pain (0–10/10, mild, moderate, severe)
Timing	Is pain intermittent or constant? How long does pain last? When does pain occur? (Time of day, during school, during jaw function, at rest)
U—"You"	How does pain impact the patient? (Interferes with school, activities, sleep)

The most important aspect of the clinical exam is to reproduce the patient's "familiar pain" by palpation of the masticatory and cervical structures. Functional manipulation of the TMJs and masticatory muscles is also recommended. A systematic palpation of the cervical and masticatory structures is critical for uncovering potential pain generators as well as evaluating for any soft tissue masses. Pain or tenderness upon palpation or discovery of taut, fibrous bands of the musculature may indicate overuse. Parafunction, such as jaw clenching, grinding or bracing, may result in symptomatic masticatory muscles. A forward head posture with rounded shoulders may result in pain in the cervical muscles (Fig. 38.18).

Proper palpation technique involves standing directly in front or behind the patient and using the pads of the index fingers to apply light, steady pressure. The lateral capsules of the TMJs should be palpated at rest and while the patient opens and closes the mouth and while moving the mandible from side to side (Fig. 38.19). This can help detect any irregular movement of the condyles as well as joint noises or pain. During the exam the patient is asked whether it feels the same on both sides, if one side feels different, or if either side feels sore. The presence or absence of pain with palpation, clicking, or crepitus should be documented.

The palpation technique for masticatory muscles is similar (Fig. 38.20). A slight increase in finger pressure is acceptable when palpating muscles. The superior and inferior aspects of the masseter muscles and posterior, middle, and anterior aspects of the temporalis muscles should be palpated. The temporalis tendon may be palpated intraorally by placing the index finger in the vicinity of the insertion of the temporalis muscle on the coronoid process. The clinician may appreciate taut bands or discrete nodules within the musculature that are painful to palpation. The lateral pterygoid muscles are

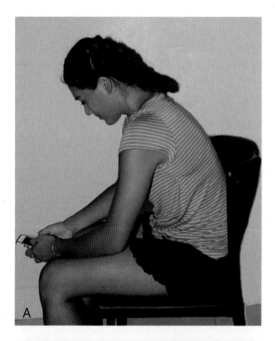

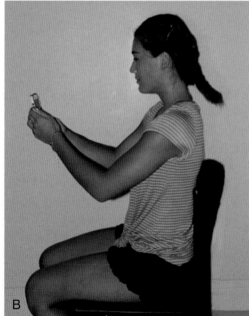

• **Figure 38.18** (A) Patient demonstrates a forward head posture and rounding of the shoulders while using a mobile device. This posture puts strain on the cervical musculature. (B) An improved cervical posture will put less strain on the head and cervical muscles.

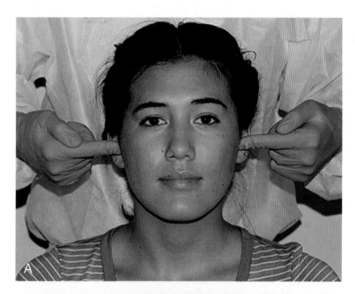

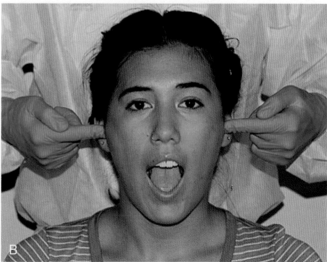

• **Figure 38.19** (A) Temporomandibular joint palpation during rest. Pain with palpation is a sign of a joint-related problem. (B) The joint is palpated during motion to detect any irregular movement of the condyles as well as joint noises or pain.

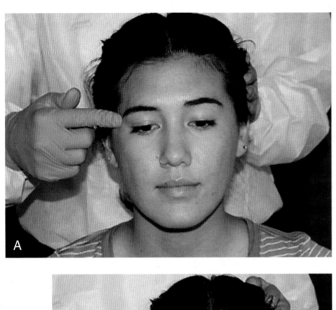
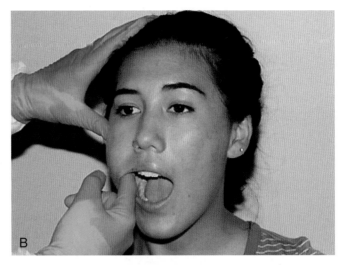
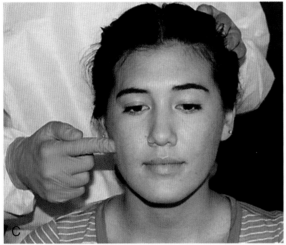
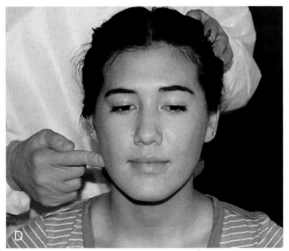

• **Figure 38.20** A systematic approach to facial muscle palpation allows the clinician the ability to identify the areas of muscular involvement. (A) The clinician can start with palpating the anterior aspect of the temporalis muscle followed by (B) intraoral palpation of the temporalis tendon. (C) Following examination of the temporalis muscle, the superior and (D) inferior aspects of the masseter muscle are palpated.

difficult to palpate intraorally and are best tested by having the patient protrude against chin resistance, which generally produces pain if the lateral pterygoid is symptomatic (Fig. 38.21). The medial pterygoid muscles are difficult to palpate or test.

Cervical structures may refer pain to the orofacial region and are frequently problematic in myofascial pain syndromes where they may be the primary cause of facial pain and headaches. The cervical muscles may be palpated in a similar manner to the masticatory muscles. Muscles, such as the trapezius and sternocleidomastoid, may be palpated by gently gripping the musculature between the thumb and index or middle finger (Fig. 38.22).

Mandibular function and ROM should be recorded. The vertical position of the mandible should be noted when various joint noises occur. Clicking when opening and closing is usually a sign of an anteriorly or anteriomedially displaced disk. Crepitus is usually a sign of joint degeneration. The amount of mandibular movement is measured with a millimeter gauge placed between an upper and lower anterior tooth. The amount of overbite is added because that is actually the distance the mandible opens. If there is an

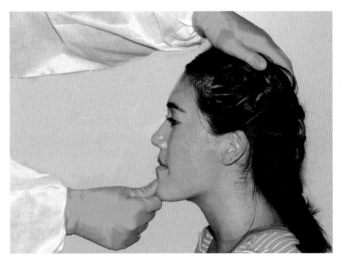

• **Figure 38.21** It is best to test lateral pterygoid muscles by having patient protrude the lower jaw against resistance.

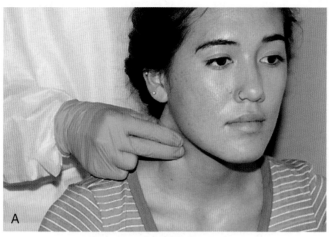
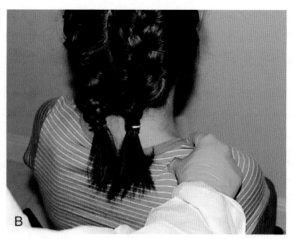

• **Figure 38.22** Palpate the cervical muscles to determine their contribution to the temporomandibular disorder. (A) Palpate the sternocleidomastoid and (B) trapezius muscles using a pincher grasp.

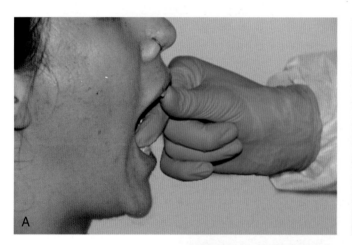
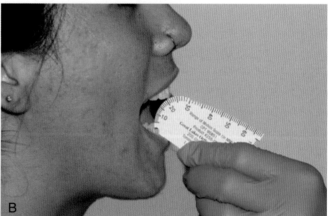
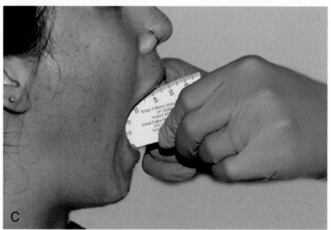

• **Figure 38.23** (A) To assess passive range of motion (ROM) in a patient with temporomandibular joint disorder, the clinician should provide slow, steady pressure with the thumb and index finger. (B) The pain-free mandibular ROM was only 21 mm. (C) Assisted or passive mandibular ROM increases to 43 mm.

open bite, the amount is subtracted from the maximal measurement. The same teeth should be measured to provide consistent readings. Mandibular ROM of less than 40 mm should be considered to be limited mobility.[26,86] Passive range of motion or assisted opening can be assessed by placing gentle downward mandibular pressure with the thumb and index finger (Fig. 38.23). Muscle pain may also limit mandibular ROM and the limited opening can commonly be overcome with this passive maneuver. If opening limitation persists and firm resistance is encountered during assisted opening, it is possible that there is an intracapsular disorder, such as a nonreducing disk displacement. Mandibular opening deviation (movement away from midline that returns to midline) or deflection (persistent movement away from midline) may also be observed. Deflection is commonly associated with an intracapsular disorder, such as disk displacement without reduction or TMJ ankylosis. Deviations can be caused by either an intracapsular interference or muscle engrams (muscle memory). Lateral movement of the mandible is measured and can determine if there is unilateral translation of the condyles. The amount of lateral movement is measured in millimeters of change in the maxillary and mandibular dental midlines. Less than 8 mm is considered to be limited mobility. The amount of protrusive movement is also recorded and less than 5 mm is considered limited.[86] Alterations in movement may indicate a deviation in form or a reducing disk displacement. Severely decreased movement may indicate a permanently dislocated disk. Excessive movement may indicate focal or systemic ligamentous laxity, like that found in Ehlers-Danlos syndrome.[71]

Systematic review of other adjunctive diagnostic and treatment therapies, such as kinesiology, thermography, and jaw tracking, are shown to have limited efficacy in management of TMD in children.[26]

Imaging and Temporomandibular Disorder

The role of imaging in TMD diagnosis relies on the basic principles of selection criteria. Imaging should be considered when there is a history of, or the clinician suspects there is, a symptomatic intracapsular condition. Asymptomatic joint sounds alone do not merit imaging. A panoramic radiograph is generally regarded as an appropriate screening radiograph. The selection criteria for initial TMJ imaging include a:

1. Recent trauma or history of progressive pathologic joint condition
2. Significant dysfunction and alteration in range of motion
3. Significant occlusal change (open bite, mandibular shift)

The practitioner is cautioned not to rely solely on imaging, as radiographic changes may be a result of adaptive remodeling.[22] For example, one study of symptomatic and asymptomatic children demonstrated that 10% of asymptomatic children had osteoarthritic changes in the mandibular condyles.[87] TMJ imaging also has the limitations of poor specificity and sensitivity in addition to higher financial costs and radiation burden. When more complex imaging is required, open and closed mouth MRI is usually chosen for good hard and soft tissue detail. Intravenous contrast may be added to improve visualization; however, a recent study demonstrated that asymptomatic pediatric patients often show incidental joint effusion.[87] Computed tomography (CT) or cone beam computed tomography (CBCT) shows excellent hard tissue detail but generally requires more radiation than conventional radiographs.[88]

Management of Temporomandibular Disorder

Dentists are in a favorable position to treat adolescent patients using the basic principles of TMD management. The clinician should determine whether to address a specific TMJ problem based on training and experience or to seek assistance from specialists in TMD therapy and orofacial pain management. Dentists managing TMD should have established referral sources; physical therapists, behavioral health providers, and primary care providers should all be part of the team.

Patients with nonpainful TMDs, such as asymptomatic TMJ sounds, usually do not require treatment. If the patient presents with painful TMDs, therapeutic and symptomatic care may be required.[22,26,29] After appropriate records are obtained to provide a diagnosis, supportive therapy and elimination of perpetuating factors often result in resolution. Conservative treatment options are appropriate for most painful TMDs. The patient is counseled about daytime clenching and conservative treatment approaches, such as soft diet, warm or cold compresses, and a brief course of clock-regulated analgesics, are suggested. Additional conservative treatment options, such as abdominal breathing entrainment, physical self-regulation, and biofeedback training, can be considered to supplement initial treatment strategies.[22,26,29]

Acute TMDs may resolve with little to no interventions. Chronic TMDs tend to be more challenging and a biopsychosocial approach to pain management may be appropriate. This approach includes simultaneous management of biological, psychological, and social factors related to the patient's persistent pain (see online Case Study).[22]

It is important to eliminate or modify contributing factors causing TMJ problems. There are many and varied factors the clinician must consider. Parafunction, gum chewing, nail biting, and substance abuse (nicotine, caffeine, 3,4-methylenedioxymethamphetamine [MDMA], others) should be reviewed. Other health-related factors contributing to the problem may be stress, primary headaches, systemic disease, poor diet, and poor sleep hygiene.[22,26,28,29,89]

The adolescent stage of development introduces many new problems for treating TMDs. Untreated behavioral health comorbidities, such as depression, anxiety, and posttraumatic stress disorder (PTSD), will also likely interfere with recovery. Catastrophic thinking, including rumination, magnification, and hopelessness, is a well-established barrier to symptom improvement.[28] Adolescent adjustment problems may trigger TMD. Since psychosocial issues may not be readily discussed with parents or dentists, it is important to refer patients to a primary care or behavioral health provider trained in adolescent development.

After the patient has been educated about TMD and conservative therapies have not proven successful, the clinician may move to a second level of therapy. Custom-designed, full coverage, removable appliances are generally recommended if self-care measures are ineffective. These appliances are typically used at nighttime and are designed to allow for eruption and positioning of teeth if the patient is in the mixed dentition. A recent randomized, controlled trial demonstrated that occlusal appliance therapy at night was more effective than relaxation therapy alone.[89]

Pharmacologic management can be considered depending on the diagnosis. Acute inflammatory joint pain may be managed with nonsteroidal antiinflammatory drugs (NSAIDs) or corticosteroids. More complex pharmacologic management may be indicated in cases of chronic myofascial pain and headaches.

As with all dental problems, a dentist may determine that referral to another dental specialist is in the patient's best interest. In some cases, a team approach is best because pharmacotherapy, counseling, and physical therapy may be indicated to treat the problem. Different providers will bring different and unique skills. This approach is considered after conservative and reversible therapies are exhausted. Advanced treatment may be required, and different experts can prescribe topical and systemic medications, perform specialized injections, and provide targeted exercises. Patients with temporomandibular problems or facial pain, who are resistant to these treatments, may consider arthrocentesis or TMJ surgery.

References

1. Casamassimo PS. Dental and oral health problems: prevention and services. In: *Congress of the United States, Office of Technology Assessment:*

Adolescent Health. Vol. 11. Background and the Effectiveness of Selected Prevention and Treatment Services, OTA-H-466. Washington, DC: US Government Printing Office; 1991.

2. U.S. Department of Health and Human Services. *The Health Consequences of Smoking—50 Years of Progress: A Report of the Surgeon General.* Atlanta: U.S. Department of Health and Human Services, Centers for Disease Control and Prevention, National Center for Chronic Disease Prevention and Health Promotion, Office on Smoking and Health; 2014.

3. Hamilton BE, Martin JA, Osterman MJK, et al. Births: final data for 2014. *Natl Vital Stat Rep.* 2015;64(12):1–64.

4. Centers for Diseases Control and Prevention. *Sexually transmitted disease surveillance 2013.* Atlanta: US Department of Health and Human Services; 2014.

5. Office for Civil Rights. HHS: Standards for privacy of individually identifiable health information. Final rule. *Fed Regist.* 2002;67(157):53181–53273.

6. Pinkham JR, Schroeder CS. Dentist and psychologist: practical considerations for a team approach to the intensely anxious dental patient. *J Am Dent Assoc.* 1975;90:1022–1026.

7. Youth EC. *US Department of Health and Human Services. A Report of the Surgeon General—Executive Summary.* Atlanta, GA: US Department of Health and Human Services, Centers for Disease Control and Prevention, National Center for Chronic Disease Prevention and Health Promotion, Office on Smoking and Health; 2016.

8. Poulsen S. Epidemiology and indices of gingival and periodontal disease. *Pediatr Dent.* 1981;3:82–88.

9. Jenkins WM, Papapanou PN. Epidemiology of periodontal disease in children and adolescents. *Periodontol 2000.* 2001;26(1):16–32.

10. Kumar S, Kelly AS: Review of childhood obesity. From *Epidemiology, Etiology, and Comorbidities to Clinical Assessment and Treatment,* Mayo Clinic Proceedings, January 5, 2017.

11. Khanuja PK, Narula SC, Rajput R, Sharma RK, Tewari S. Association of periodontal disease with glycemic control in patients with type 2 diabetes in Indian population. *Front Med.* 2017;11(1):110–119.

12. Brady WF. The anorexia nervosa syndrome. *Oral Surg Oral Med Oral Pathol.* 1980;50:509–513.

13. Salas MM, Nascimento GG, Vargas-Ferreira F, et al. Diet influenced tooth erosion prevalence in children and adolescents: results of a meta-analysis and meta-regression. *J Dent.* 2015;43(8):865–875.

14. Ganesh M, Hertzberg A, Nurko S, et al. Acid rather than nonacid reflux burden is a predictor of tooth erosion. *J Pediatr Gastr Nutr.* 2016;62(2):309–313.

15. Plessas A, Pepelassi E. Dental and periodontal complications of lip and tongue piercing: prevalence and influencing factors. *Aust Dent J.* 2012;57(1):71–78.

16. White R, Proffit W. Evaluation and management of asymptomatic third molars: lack of symptoms does not equate to lack of pathology. *Am J Orthod Dentofacial Orthop.* 2011;140:10–18.

17. American Academy of Pediatric Dentistry. Guideline on prescribing dental radiographs for infants, children, adolescents, and persons with special health care needs. *Reference Manual.* 2016;38(6):355–357.

18. Castaldi CR, Brass GA. *Dentistry for the Adolescent.* Philadelphia: Saunders; 1980.

19. Raj M. *The perception of facial attractiveness by providers and consumers.* Master's thesis. The Ohio State University, College of Dentistry, Section of Orthodontics; 2002.

20. Mihalik CA, Proffit WR, Phillips C. Long-term follow-up of class II adults treated with orthodontic camouflage: a comparison with orthognathic surgery outcomes. *Am J Orthod Dentofacial Orthop.* 2003;123(3):266–278.

21. Proffit WR, White RP, Sarver DM. *Contemporary treatment of dentofacial deformity.* St Louis: Mosby–Year Book; 2003.

22. American Academy of Orofacial Pain. De Leeuw R, Klasser GD, eds. *Orofacial Pain. Guidelines for Assessment, Diagnosis, and Management.* Hanover Park, IL: Quintessence Publishing; 2013.

23. Nilsson IM, Willman A. Treatment and self-constructed explanations of pain and pain management strategies among adolescents with temporomandibular disorder pain. *J Oral Facial Pain Headache.* 2016;30(2):127–133.

24. Ohrbach R, Vir E, Fillingim RB. Clinical orofacial characteristics associated with risk of first-onset TMD: the OPPERA prospective cohort study. *J Pain.* 2013;14(12 suppl):T33–T50.

25. Hirsch C, John T, Schaller HG, et al. Pain related impairment and health care utilization in children and adolescents: a comparison of orofacial pain with abdominal pain, back pain, and headache. *Quintessence Int.* 2006;37:381–390.

26. Okeson JP. *Management of Temporomandibular Disorders and Occlusion.* 7th ed. St Louis: Elsevier; 2013.

27. Nilsson IM, List T, Drangsholt M. Headache and co-morbid pains associated with TMD pain in adolescents. *J Dent Res.* 2013;92(9):802–807.

28. Sessel BJ. *Orofacial Pain: Recent Advancements in Assessment, and Understanding of Mechanisms.* Washington, DC: International Association for the Study of Pain; 2014.

29. Sharav Y, Benoliel R. *Orofacial Pain and Headache.* 2nd ed. Hannover Park, IL: Quintessence Publishing; 2015.

30. da Silva CG, Pacheco-Pereira C, Porporatti AL, et al. Prevalence of clinical signs of intra-articular temporomandibular disorders in children and adolescents. *J Am Dent Assoc.* 2016;147(1):10–18.

31. Schiffman E, Ohrbach R, Truelove E. Diagnostic criteria for temporomandibular disorders (DC/TMD) for clinical and research applications: recommendations of the International RDC/TMD Consortium Network and Orofaical Pain Special Interest Group. *J Oral Facial Pain Headache.* 2014;28(1):6–27.

32. Nilsson IM, List T, Drangsholt M. Incidence and temporal patterns of temporomandibular disorder pain among Swedish adolescents. *J Oralfac Pain.* 2007;21(2):127–132.

33. Hongxing L, Astrøm N, List T, et al. Prevalence of temporomandibular disorder pain in Chinese adolescents compared to an age-matched Swedish population. *J Oral Rehab.* 2016;43:241–248.

34. Kohler AA, Helkimo AN, Magnusson T, et al. Prevalence of symptoms and signs indicative of temporomandibular disorders in children and adolescents. A cross-sectional epidemiological investigation covering two decades. *Eur Arch Paediatr Dentistry.* 2009;10(1):16–25.

35. Graue AM, Jokstad A, Assmus J, et al. Prevalence among adolescents in Bergen, Western Norway, of temporomandibular disorders according to the DC/TMD criteria and examination protocol. *Acta Odontol Scand.* 2016;74(6):449–455.

36. Magnusson T, Egermark I, Carlsson GE. A longitudinal epidemiologic study of signs and symptoms of temporomandibular disorders from 15 to 35 years of age. *J Orofac Pain.* 2000;14(4):310–319.

37. List T, Wablund K, Wenneberg B, et al. TMD in children and adolescents: prevalence of pain, gender differences, and perceived treatment need. *J Orofac Pain.* 1999;13(1):9–20.

38. Vilanova LS, Gonçalves TM, Meirelles L, Garcia RC. Hormonal fluctuations intensify temporomandibular disorder pain without impairing masticatory function. *Int J Prosthodont.* 2015;28(1):72–74.

39. Hassan S, Muere A, Einstein G. Ovarian hormones and chronic pain: a comprehensive review. *Pain.* 2014;155(12):2448–2460.

40. Hirsch C, Hoffman J, Türp JC. Are temporomandibular disorder symptoms and diagnoses associated with pubertal development in adolescents? An epidemiological study. *J Orofac Orthop.* 2012;73(1):6–8.

41. Karibe H, Goodard G, Aoyagi K, et al. Comparison of subjective symptoms of temporomandibular disorders in young patients by age and gender. *Cranio.* 2012;30(2):114–120.

42. Nilsson IM, List T, Willman A. Adolescents with TMD pain—the living with TMD pain phenomenon. *J Orofac Pain.* 2011;25(2):107–116.

43. Bonjardin LR, Gaviliao MG, Pereira LJ, et al. Anxiety and depression in adolescents and their relationship with signs and symptoms of temporomandibular disorder. *Int J Prosthodont.* 2005;18:347–352.

44. Finan P, Goodin BR, Smith MT. The association of sleep and pain: an update and a path forward. *J Pain.* 2013;14(12):1539–1552.

45. Howard JA. Temporomandibular joint disorders in children. *Dent Clin North Am*. 2013;57(1):99–127.

46. Larheim TA, Westesson P, Sano T. TMJ disc displacement: comparison in asymptomatic volunteers and patients. *Radiology*. 2001;218:428–432.

47. American Academy of Sleep Medicine (AASM). *International Classification of Sleep Disorders*. 3rd ed (ICSD-3). Darien, IL: AASM; 2014.

48. Feu D, Catharino F, Abdo Quintao CC, et al. A systematic review of etiological and risk factors associated with bruxism. *J Orthod*. 2013;40:163–171.

49. Manfredini D, Restrepo C, Diaz-Serrano K, et al. Prevalence of sleep bruxism in children: a systematic review of the literature. *J Oral Rehabil*. 2013;40(8):631–642.

50. Paesani DA, Lobbezoo F, Gelos C, et al. Correlation between self-reported and clinically based diagnoses of bruxism in temporomandibular disorders patients. *J Oral Rehabil*. 2013;40(11):803–809.

51. Cheifetz AT, Osganian SK, Allred EN, et al. Prevalence of bruxism and associated correlates in children as reported by parents. *J Dent Child*. 2005;72(2):67–73.

52. Strausz T, Ahlberg J, Lobbezoo F, et al. Awareness of tooth grinding and clenching from adolescence to young adulthood: a nine-year follow-up. *J Oral Rehabil*. 2010;37(7):497–500.

53. Carlsson GE, Egermark I, Magnusson T. Predictors of bruxism, other oral parafunctions, and tooth wear over a 20-year follow-up period. *J Orofac Pain*. 2003;17(1):50–57.

54. Sakaguchi K, Yagi T, Maeda A, et al. Association of problem behavior with sleep problems and gastroesophageal reflux symptoms. *Pediatr Int*. 2014;56(1):24–30.

55. Ortega AO, DosSantos MT, Mendes FM, et al. Association between anticonvulsant drugs and teeth-grinding in children and adolescents with cerebral palsy. *J Oral Rehabil*. 2014;41(9):653–658.

56. Manfredini D, Guarda-Nardini L, Marchese-Ragona R. Theories on possible temporal relationships between sleep bruxism and obstructive sleep apnea events. An expert opinion. *Sleep Breath*. 2015;19(4):1459–1465.

57. De Luca Canto G, Singh V, Conti P, et al. Association between sleep bruxism and psychosocial factors in children and adolescents: a systematic review. *Clin Pediatr*. 2015;54(5):469–478.

58. Patel SB, Kumar SKS. Myofascial pain secondary to medication induced bruxism. *J Am Dent Assoc*. 2012;143(10):e67–e69.

59. Bertazzo-Silveira E, Kruger CM, Porto de Toledo I, et al. Association between sleep bruxism alcohol, caffeine, tobacco, and drug use. *J Am Dent Assoc*. 2016;147(11):859–866.

60. Malki GA, Zawawi KH, Melis M, et al. Prevalence of bruxism in children receiving treatment for attention deficit hyperactivity disorder: a pilot study. *J Clin Pediatr Dent*. 2004;29(1):63–67.

61. Mohlin B. TMD in relation to malocclusion and orthodontic treatment. *Angle Orthod*. 2007;77(3):542–548.

62. Hirsch C. No increased risk of temporomandibular disorders and bruxism in children and adolescents during orthodontic therapy. *J Orofac Orthod*. 2009;70(1):39–50.

63. Manfredini D, Perinetti G, Guarda-Nardini L. Dental malocclusion is not related to temporomandibular joint clicking: a logistic regression analysis in a patient population. *Angle Orthod*. 2014;84(2):310–315.

64. LeBell Y, Niei PM, Jamsa T, et al. Subjective reactions to intervention with artificial interference in subjects with and without a history of temporomandibular disorders. *Acta Odontol Scand*. 2006;64:59–63.

65. Kirveskari P, Jamsa T, Alanen P. Occlusal adjustment and the incidence of demand for temporomandibular disorder treatment. *J Prosth Dent*. 1998;79(4):433–438.

66. Fischer DJ, Mueller BA, Critchlow CW, et al. The association of temporomandibular disorder pain with history of head and neck injury in adolescents. *J Orofac Pain*. 2006;20(3):191–198.

67. Akhter R, Hassan NM, Ohkubo R, et al. The relationship between jaw injury, third molar removal, and orthodontic treatment and TMD symptoms in university students in Japan. *J Orofac Pain*. 2008;22(1):50–56.

68. Juhl GI, Jensen TS, Norholt SE, et al. Incidence of symptoms and signs of TMD following third molar surgery: a controlled, prospective study. *J Oral Rehabil*. 2009;36(3):199–209.

69. Allori AC, Chang CC, Farina R. Current concepts in pediatric temporomandibular joint disorders: part 1 etiology, epidemiology and classification. *Plast Reconstr Surg*. 2010;126(4):1263–1275.

70. Carrasco R. Juvenile idiopathic arthritis overview and involvement of the temporomandibular joint prevalence, systemic therapy. *Oral Maxil Surg Clin*. 2015;27(1):1–10.

71. Hirsch C, John MJ, Stang A. Association between generalized joint hypermobility and signs and diagnoses of temporomandibular disorders. *Eur J Oral Sci*. 2008;116(6):525–530.

72. Wolford LM, Perez DE. Surgical management of congenital deformities with temporomandibular joint malformation. *Oral Maxil Surg Clin*. 2015;27(1):137–154.

73. Ahmad M, Schiffman EL. Temporomandibular joint disorders and orofacial pain. *Dent Clin North Am*. 2016;60(1):105–124.

74. Wei WB, Chen MJ, Yang C, et al. Tumors and pseudotumors at the temporomandibular joint region in pediatric patients. *Int J Clin Exp Med*. 2015;8(11):21813.

75. Okeson JP. *Bell's Oral and Facial Pain*. 7th ed. Chicago: Quintessence Publishing; 2014.

76. Iro H, Zenk J. Salivary gland diseases in children. *GMS Curr Top Otorhinolaryngol Head Neck Surg*. 2014;13:Doc06.

77. Lang S, Kansy B. Cervical lymph node diseases in children. *GMS Curr Top Otorhinolaryngol Head Neck Surg*. 2014;13:Doc08.

78. Brustowicz KA, Padwa BL. Malocclusion in children caused by temporomandibular joint effusion. *Int J Oral Maxillofac Surg*. 2013;42(8):1034–1036.

79. Bast F, Collier S, Chadha P, et al. Septic arthritis of the temporomandibular joint as a complication of acute otitis media in a child: a rare case and the importance of real-time PCR for diagnosis. *Int J Pediatr Otorhi*. 2015;79(11):1942–1945.

80. Clark GT, Browne PA, Nakano M, et al. Co-activation of sternocleidomastoid muscles during maximum clenching. *J Dent Res*. 1993;72(11):1499–1502.

81. Eriksson PO, Häggman-Henrikson B, Nordh E, et al. Co-ordinated mandibular and head-neck movements during rhythmic jaw activities in man. *J Dent Res*. 2000;79(6):1378–1384.

82. Shimazaki K, Matsubara N, Hisano M, et al. Functional relationships between the masseter and sternocleidomastoid muscle activities during gum chewing: the effect of experimental muscle fatigue. *Angle Orthod*. 2006;76(3):452–458.

83. LeResche L, Mancl LA, Drangsholt MT, et al. Predictors of onset of facial pain and temporomandibular disorders in early adolescence. *Pain*. 2007;129(3):269–278.

84. Hirsch C, Turp JC. Temporomandibular pain and depression in adolescents- a case control study. *Clin Oral Investig*. 2010;14:145–151.

85. Headache Classification Committee of the International Headache Society. The international classification of headache disorders (beta version). *Cephalalgia*. 2013;33(9):629–808.

86. Hirsch C, John MT, Lautenschager C, et al. Mandibular jaw movement capacity in 10-17 year old children and adolescents: normative values and and influence of gender, age and TMD. *Eur J Oral Sci*. 2006;114(6):465–470.

87. Cho BH, Jung YH. Osteoarthritic changes and condylar positioning of the temporomandibular joint in children and adolescents. *Imaging Sci Dent*. 2012;42(3):169–174.

88. Kottke R, Saurenmann RK, Schneider MM. Contrast-enhanced MRI of the temporomandibular joint: findings in children without juvenile idiopathic arthritis. *Acta Radiol*. 2015;56(9):1145–1152.

89. Wahlund K, Nilsson IM, Larsson B. Treating temporomandibular disorders in adolescents; a randomized, controlled, sequential comparison of relaxation training and occlusal appliance therapy. *J Oral Facial Pain Headache*. 2015;29(1):41–50.

39
Prevention of Dental Disease

TAD R. MABRY

Adolescence generally denotes the period between childhood and adulthood. It is known for being a phase of life associated with change, rebellion, and friction. It encompasses a time frame when patients may progress from junior high school to senior high school and then go off to college, the workforce, or some other aspect of adult life. Adolescence can be a period of heightened involvement in peer group relationships, often at the expense of social or familial associations.

The period encompasses the completion of physical growth and development in both girls and boys. Typically, all permanent teeth have erupted except for impacted third molars. The occlusion has stabilized either on its own or with orthodontic intervention. A gradual but continuous increase in the incidence of dental caries is often noted during this period.[1] Periodontal disease may manifest itself because of fewer routine or parentally supervised home care sessions. The frequency of dental visits may decline. In addition, the increase in sex hormones in this age group is suspected to alter the subgingival microflora, resulting in an increased incidence of periodontal disease.[2]

Dietary habits undergo dramatic changes during this period. As adolescent girls complete their maximal growth and development, it is not unusual for them to begin dietary experimentation and modification. Some of these modifications can lead to serious pathologic conditions such as anorexia nervosa and bulimia. In adolescent boys, similar modifications in dietary habits occur. During this period the boy's skeletal growth and body weight usually undergo dramatic changes, typically peaking at 16 to 18 years of age. Caloric requirements increase dramatically, and large amounts of protein and carbohydrates are consumed. In both boys and girls, irregular meals, frequent snacking, vending machine purchases, fast food meals, and unusual eating patterns are common practices.

These changes can have profound effects on the oral environment and pose substantial challenges for the provision of professional dental care. The eruption of teeth into an environment of increased plaque secondary to reduced cleansing efforts combined with frequent snacking on foods and beverages high in carbohydrates can pose a significant risk for caries development in the immature enamel of newly erupted teeth.

Besides being a time of increased caries risk, adolescence is also a time when the desire for social acceptance can lead individuals to actions that place them at risk for additional dental complications. Such actions would include tobacco and e-cigarette use, intraoral and perioral piercings, and adolescent pregnancy. Periodic professional visits that emphasize routine home care, optimal use of topical fluorides, dietary management strategies, and counseling on the dental implications of risky behaviors are both the goals and challenges for dentists who treat adolescents.

Risk Assessment

Risk assessment takes on some added dimensions for the adolescent patient. Through the years, these individuals have become increasingly responsible for their own oral hygiene practices. Typically, it is the first time in their lives that they have a say in the decision-making process associated with their dental treatment options. Although treatment decisions are legally still in the hands of the parents or legal guardians, the wills and desires of the adolescent patient should not be discounted by the provider.

The American Academy of Pediatric Dentistry (AAPD) has developed a set of guidelines used to assess the caries risk of patients in the mixed or permanent dentition (Table 39.1). In addition, the AAPD has developed caries management protocols based on these risk assessments (Table 39.2). Although these protocols are useful in determining the direction of patient care, they should be considered as guidelines only, and each adolescent should have an individualized treatment plan that addresses his or her unique preventive, restorative, and counseling needs.

The caries risk assessment comprises just one part of the overall risk assessment for the adolescent patient. Other factors that must be considered when developing a comprehensive treatment plan include the need for, as well as the timing of, referrals for orthodontics or third molar extractions, where indicated. Risk factors such as pathologic dietary conditions, tobacco use, alcohol or drug

TABLE 39.1	Caries Risk Assessment for Patients Older Than 6 Years (for Dental Providers)			
Factors	High Risk	Moderate Risk	Protective	
Biologic				
Patient is of low socioeconomic status	Yes			
Patient has >3 between meal sugar-containing snacks or beverages per day	Yes			
Patient has special health care needs		Yes		
Patient is a recent immigrant		Yes		
Protective				
Patient receives optimally fluoridated drinking water			Yes	
Patient brushes teeth daily with fluoridated toothpaste			Yes	
Patient receives topical fluoride from health professional			Yes	
Additional home measures (e.g., xylitol, MI Paste, antimicrobial)			Yes	
Patient has dental home/regular dental care			Yes	
Clinical Findings				
Patient has ≥1 interproximal lesions	Yes			
Patient has active white spot lesions or enamel defects	Yes			
Patient has low salivary flow	Yes			
Patient has defective restorations		Yes		
Patient wears an intraoral appliance		Yes		

Circling those conditions that apply to a specific patient helps the practitioner and patient/parent to understand the factors that contribute to or protect against caries. Risk assessment categorization of low, moderate, or high is based on preponderance of factors for the individual. However, clinical judgment may justify the use of one factor (e.g., >1 interproximal lesion, low salivary flow) in determining overall risk.

Overall assessment of the dental caries risk: Low ☐ Moderate ☐ High ☐

From American Academy of Pediatric Dentistry. Guideline on caries-risk assessment and management for infants, children, and adolescents. *Pediatr Dent*. 2016;38(Special issue):142–149.

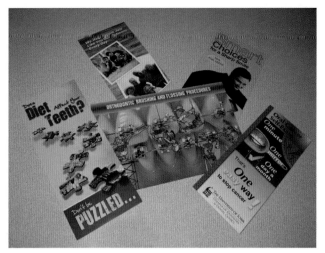

• **Figure 39.1** Brochures useful for guiding discussions with at-risk adolescents.

assessment will typically dictate the focus of education to minimize the odds of development of early childhood caries. For the adolescent patient, anticipatory guidance not only includes caries reduction strategies based on a caries risk assessment but also preventive measures aimed at reducing the likelihood these individuals would choose to participate in behaviors that could jeopardize their oral health. Adolescents often participate in these types of activities without knowing the negative consequences associated with them. The goal of this form of anticipatory guidance is to educate adolescents on the detrimental effects associated with these risky behaviors in hopes that they may elect not to participate in these activities when pressured by their peers.

Several organizations such as the AAPD, as well as the American Academy of Pediatrics (AAP) and the American Dental Association (ADA), have educational materials in the form of pamphlets and brochures that can be used to guide the discussion that a dental professional may have with the at-risk adolescent (Fig. 39.1).

Dietary Management

As with younger age groups, the overall recommendations on dietary management for adolescents should concentrate on balanced intake, reduction of the frequency of snacking, and selection of foods that are not retentive to the teeth and soft tissues. Unfortunately, these recommendations conflict with the typical lifestyles of adolescents. With their newly gained independence, rebellious attitude toward established social systems, and acceptance of media messages and peer group pressure, it is a difficult task for the dentist and his or her staff to communicate recommendations and instill health-promoting behaviors.

Fortunately, owing to the increasing social development that occurs in middle adolescence, there is a strong desire to look attractive. The mouth takes on added importance. The challenge to dental professionals is to somehow make the daily care of teeth, including sound dietary habits, desirable for this patient population.

For the patient who has been at high risk for dental disease during the early years and has had caries in the primary or mixed dentition, dietary management is a major concern. Depending on the patient's present oral status, emotional and psychological maturity, and parental influences, counseling can be performed

abuse, intraoral or perioral piercings, or teenage pregnancy must be factored in when planning treatment care for the adolescent. Counseling that addresses the dental as well as the medical complications associated with these risk factors should be included as part of the comprehensive treatment plan. If a provider is not comfortable or feels that further counseling expertise is warranted, a referral should be made to a professional who could provide such counseling.

Anticipatory guidance is the implementation of preventive strategies based on a risk assessment. It is in the patient's best interest to preemptively provide education that might prevent the development of a pathologic condition rather than treat the condition after it has occurred. For the infant or toddler a caries risk

TABLE 39.2	**Example of a Caries Management Protocol for Patients Older Than 6 Years**				

| | | INTERVENTIONS | | | |
Risk Category	Diagnostics	Fluoride	Diet	Sealants[a]	Restorative
Low risk	• Recall every 6–12 months • Radiographs every 12–24 months	• Twice daily brushing with fluoridated toothpaste[b]	No	Yes	• Surveillance[c]
Moderate-risk Patient/parent engaged	• Recall every 6 months • Radiographs every 6–12 months	• Twice daily brushing with fluoridated toothpaste[b] • Fluoride supplements[d] • Professional topical treatment every 6 months	• Counseling	Yes	• Active surveillance[e] of incipient lesions • Restoration of cavitated or enlarging lesions
Moderate-risk Patient/parent not engaged	• Recall every 6 months • Radiographs every 6–12 months	• Twice daily brushing with toothpaste[b] • Professional topical treatment every 6 months	• Counseling, with limited expectations	Yes	• Active surveillance[e] of incipient lesions • Restoration of cavitated or enlarging lesions
High-risk patient/ parent engaged	• Recall every 3 months • Radiographs every 6 months	• Brushing with 0.5% fluoride • Fluoride supplements[d] • Professional topical treatment every 3 months	• Counseling • Xylitol	Yes	• Active surveillance[e] of incipient lesions • Restoration of cavitated or enlarging lesions
High-risk Patient/parent not engaged	• Recall every 3 months • Radiographs every 6 months	• Brushing with 0.5% fluoride • Professional topical treatment every 3 months	• Counseling, with limited expectations • Xylitol	Yes	• Restore incipient, cavitated, or enlarging lesions

[a]Indicated for teeth with deep fissure anatomy or developmental defects.
[b]Less concern about the quantity of toothpaste.
[c]Periodic monitoring for signs of caries progression.
[d]Need to consider fluoride levels in drinking water.
[e]Careful monitoring of caries progression and prevention program.
From American Academy of Pediatric Dentistry. Guideline on caries-risk assessment and management for infants, children, and adolescents. *Pediatr Dent.* 2016;38(Special issue):142–149.

with the patient only or, if indicated, with both the patient and the parents. At this age the adolescent may enjoy independence from the involvement of his or her parents. Therefore the dentist must decide the extent of parental inclusion in the dietary consultation.

The sense of independence among adolescents often leads to snacking at will. Such poor eating habits are a major factor in the increasing rates of childhood obesity.[3,4] Often these poor eating patterns carry over into adulthood. There has been a notable change in snacking habits of adolescents since the 1970s.[5] Several troubling issues have been identified:

• The number of adolescents who snack on a given day increased from 74% in 1977 to 1978 to 98% in 2005 to 2006.
• The main contributor of snacking calories is desserts.
• Snacking, which accounted for 300 calories a day in 1977 to 1978, accounted for 526 calories a day in 2005 to 2006.[6]
• Children are moving toward constant eating.

The busy lifestyles of adolescents nowadays make the sit-down family meal a rarity. This has a deleterious effect on the dietary patterns of adolescents. Research has shown that parental presence at family evening meals exerts substantial influences in terms of increasing the adolescents' consumption of fruits, vegetables, and dairy products while lowering the consumption of soft drinks.[7]

A growing trend among adolescents is the consumption of sports drinks and energy drinks. Adolescents, as well as their parents,

often fail to recognize the difference between these two.[8] Sports drinks are promoted by the beverage industry as products that optimize athletic performance by replacing fluid and electrolytes lost in vigorous exercise. In contrast, energy drinks purport everything from an increase in energy and a decrease in fatigue to enhanced mental alertness and focus. Many of the ingredients have minimal therapeutic benefit and are not well regulated. Energy drinks typically contain a blend of stimulants that include caffeine, taurine, ginseng, guarana, L-carnitine, and creatine. Some of these energy drinks exceed 500 mg of caffeine in a single serving, which is equivalent to the amount of caffeine found in 14 cans of the typical caffeinated soft drink.[9] Caffeine tends to increase blood pressure, heart rate, gastric secretions, body temperature, cardiac arrhythmias, and diuresis.[10] Studies have shown that, although the consumption of caffeine is poorly correlated with anxiety, it may result in increased anxiety for those individuals prone to anxiety disorders.[11,12] Unfortunately, the sales of energy drinks continue to increase largely due to marketing efforts which target youth under 18 years of age.[13]

Both parents and school systems are recognizing the harmful dental effects of carbonated sodas and similar beverages and are limiting the exposure of adolescents to them. Unfortunately, these carbonated beverages are frequently being replaced with sports drinks. The pH of most sports drinks is in the acidic range (pH 3 to 4), which is well within the range to cause enamel demineralization.[14] It is unfortunate that parents and school administrators are failing to recognize the deleterious effects of sports drinks on the dentition.

The AAP Committee on Nutrition (CON) and the Council on Sports Medicine and Fitness (COSMF) recently published a report with the following recommendations to pediatricians[15]:

- Improve the education to both parents and children on the differences between, as well as the potential health risks of, sports drinks and energy drinks
- Understand the potential health risks that energy drinks pose as a result of their stimulant content
- Counsel at-risk individuals as to the relationship between both obesity and dental erosion to excessive sports drink consumption
- Educate patients and parents on effective hydration management, stressing that water should be the initial beverage of choice for hydration purposes

In 2007 the Institute of Medicine recommended prohibiting energy drink use in children and adolescence, including athletes. According to the commission's report, energy drinks have no place in the diet of adolescents.[16]

Although sports drinks and energy drinks are a somewhat new trend among adolescents, the problem associated with the consumption of high-sugar beverages of any type is long-standing in this age group. Sugar-sweetened beverages have become the largest source of added sugars in the diet of adolescents in the United States.[17] These beverages include nondiet sodas, sweetened fruit juices, sweetened coffee and tea drinks, and the sports and energy drinks. Some studies are attributing the increased caloric intake associated with the consumption of these beverages as a factor that is contributing to the increasing obesity rates among adolescents.[18] In addition, the high sugar content of sugar-sweetened beverages has been shown to increase the risk of type 2 diabetes by increasing the dietary glycemic load, leading to insulin resistance and β cell dysfunction.[19] Data from the 2011 to 2012 and 2013 to 2014 National Health and Nutrition Examination Survey (NHANES) revealed that 62.9% of youth 2 to 19 years of age drank at least one sugar-sweetened beverages daily, and nearly 20% drank two daily.[20] The elevated consumption of these beverages not only affects the overall general health of adolescents in the form of increasing rates of obesity and diabetes but also has deleterious effects on the caries rates of adolescents.

Dental professionals should discuss both the dental and physical risks associated with excessive sugar-sweetened beverage consumption as part of their prevention program targeted toward adolescents. It is critical that this topic be discussed with the parents or legal guardians of those patients with special health care needs because these individuals often possess obstacles that preclude the maintenance of adequate oral hygiene. The addition of sugar-sweetened beverages in such an oral environment places the special needs patient at risk for the development of rampant caries.

For the patient who has active lesions in the developing permanent dentition, dietary management and modifications are definitely indicated along with a comprehensive program of oral cleaning and daily topical fluoride use. Developing a complete understanding of the importance of this approach with the patient and determining his or her willingness to cooperate are critical to achieving a successful outcome. If the patient is interested and willing to cooperate, a dietary history may be indicated. If not, it will be only a paper exercise and a waste of time for both parties involved.

Initially, a 24-hour dietary history is usually sufficient. Based on the history and additional information from patients about their typical daily schedule and academic, athletic, and social obligations, the dentist or staff responsible for counseling can assist in devising an individualized preventive plan.

Having the patient acknowledge problems and commit either orally or in writing to recommended interventions can help to improve compliance. During periodic examinations, the patient's progress or lack of progress can be evaluated. Plans may have to be modified repeatedly depending on the patient's changing needs. Because food preferences, social pressures, and growth changes occur frequently, any plan must allow for flexibility.

Although 24-hour diet histories are helpful, more insight can be obtained from a 5- or 7-day history that includes weekends. For improved accuracy, the patient should complete the first day's record with the dentist, paying particular attention to all liquid and solid foods consumed both at meals and between meals. Information about how much of the food was consumed and where the food was eaten is helpful.

After the dietary history has been completed, a staff person assigned to counseling responsibilities should carefully review it with the patient. Foods high in refined carbohydrates or retentive to the oral tissues should be identified. Intake of fresh fruits and vegetables should be noted and commended. Unusual foods or dietary patterns should be noted, and the overall balance of the diet should be evaluated.

Patients should be asked to list problem areas and categorize them according to the ease with which they can be changed. With problems identified and listed according to perceived ease of modification, the patient then develops a plan. It is important that it be the patient's plan and not the dentist's. It is the dentist's role to guide the patient to develop a realistic plan that will build on successes. Periodic reviews can help to determine the status of the dietary modifications and the need for new strategies. Reinforcements and rewards may be helpful, but in the end the patient's own perception of success will likely prove to be the most rewarding aspect for both dentist and patient.

A referral to a registered dietitian should be considered for the adolescent or parent who desires more intensive or more frequent dietary counseling. Consultation with a dietitian would also be useful for patients whose overall health is compromised by their dietary habits.

Numerous phone apps and web-based diet analysis programs are available that provide the opportunity to track daily food and beverage consumption. These programs typically analyze the overall diet quality and provide a score or grade. Several of the programs address the amounts of saturated fat, trans fat, cholesterol, and sodium consumed in an individual's diet. The score or grade represents compliance with established food consumption guidelines. The most common set of guidelines are those established by the US Department of Agriculture (USDA). The USDA has been establishing dietary guidelines since 1916. In 2011 the USDA's MyPyramid food guidance system was replaced with an updated set of guidelines titled MyPlate (see Fig. 20.2). These guidelines target specific populations that include preschoolers 2 to 5 years of age, children 6 to 11 years of age, and pregnant and breastfeeding women, as well as dieters. Guidelines for adolescents are included in the section for children.

Dietary challenges for patients with developmental disabilities can be substantial. Depending on the severity of the disability, dietary habits may or may not be affected. For the patient with severe neuromuscular involvement, diet and eating methods will already have been modified. Parents or caretakers must be made aware of the potentially devastating oral effects caused by pouching, which is the prolonged holding of food in the mouth, and rumination, which is the regurgitation, rechewing, and reswallowing of food. Some patients with developmental disabilities may suffer from gastrointestinal efflux, which may cause enamel erosion. Many of these patients are on medications that cause xerostomia. If management of the diet is not possible, or if medications are an issue, efforts should be made to ensure more frequent and thorough cleansing of the oral cavity as well as frequent use of topical fluorides and sialagogues, if indicated.

Home Care

Personal hygiene, like any established societal activity, is met with varying responses during adolescence. Nagging by the parent or dentist will often lead to a negative response. When an adolescent patient understands the importance of oral hygiene and is ready to make a daily commitment to it, the dentist can assist him or her in developing a routine that will be acceptable to the patient and maintain a healthy oral environment.

During this period, dental flossing should become a part of the daily oral hygiene routine. Adolescents should have well-developed hand-eye coordination and fine motor activity. Those who have difficulty with the traditional method of flossing may benefit from a floss holder (Fig. 39.2).

The goal for the adolescent should be to perform thorough tooth brushing with a fluoridated toothpaste at least twice each day, ideally at the start of the day and at bedtime. After meals, a vigorous rinse with water should be encouraged. If orthodontic appliances are present, additional time, as well as modifications of the routine, will be necessary to remove not only the plaque but also the debris caught around the brackets and wires (Fig. 39.3). Additional attention to maintain healthy marginal gingiva is also important.

Effective daily home care is essential for the adolescent patient with a developmental disability. Again, depending on the severity of the disability, the patient, the parent, or a caregiver must take responsibility for the care. Mouth props may be necessary for some patients who are unable to keep their mouths open for oral care routines (see Fig. 24.5).

Chemical agents that alter plaque, such as chlorhexidine and xylitol, have become popular adjuncts to daily oral hygiene in select patients. Patients who may benefit from the daily use of these agents include those with special health care needs, as well as those with orthodontic appliances. Studies have confirmed the improvement from the use of various antimicrobial agents in reducing plaque, gingivitis, and gingival bleeding sites.[21-23] Adolescents frequently experience marginal gingivitis secondary to plaque deposits. Consideration should be given to prescribing antimicrobial mouthrinses to complement daily oral hygiene practices for such individuals.[24] For those patients with developmental disabilities or medical conditions that limit their ability to rinse and spit, an alternative application method is to apply chlorhexidine as a varnish or gel. Chlorhexidine varnish, although commonly used for years in European and Scandinavian countries, did not become commercially available in the United States until 2011. Studies have shown that the effectiveness in reducing mutans streptococci levels is greater with the chlorhexidine varnishes than it is with the gels or mouthrinses.[25] Although the benefits of chlorhexidine on gingivitis are readily accepted, the benefits of chlorhexidine as a caries control agent are inconclusive.[25] Newer studies have suggested that probiotic mouthrinses may provide a natural defense against harmful oral bacteria.[21]

Most studies on the effects of xylitol on caries rates focus on mothers and young children. Studies on the effects of xylitol on caries rates in adolescents are limited and have confounding results. Although the AAPD recognizes the benefits of sugar substitutes such as xylitol and advocates their use as a preventive measure for children and adolescents, they do not address a specific application schedule of xylitol for adolescents.[26] More research on the subject is encouraged.

Fluoride Administration

Approach to the Adolescent Patient

Although most adolescents have the ability to carry out effective oral hygiene procedures, many neglect to perform these activities regularly. The key to promoting effective caries prevention during what can be a hectic and trying stage of life often depends on recognizing the predominant motivational factors operating in this age group and adopting an approach that is based on less than ideal compliance. The focus on personal appearance and hygiene in this age group can be used as a powerful motivator for developing preventive activities. Another strategy involves appealing to the adolescent's desire to be viewed as autonomous and capable of taking care of him- or herself.

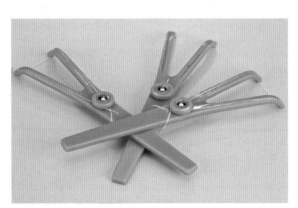

• **Figure 39.2** Floss holders. (Courtesy Practicon Dental, Greenville, NC.)

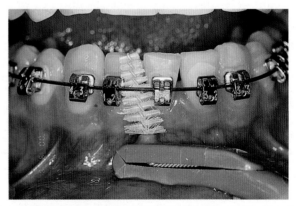

• **Figure 39.3** Use of an interproximal brush to clean around brackets. (From Darby ML, Walsh MW. *Dental Hygiene: Theory and Practice*. 3rd ed. St Louis: Saunders; 2010.)

Regardless of the psychological basis for the motivation, time should be taken to ensure that adolescents understand the nature of the disease processes that the preventive programs are addressing and the general mechanisms by which the prescribed measures are thought to counteract these processes. This emphasis on education is more likely to be accepted and will produce better long-term outcomes than a more authoritarian or condescending approach.

Caries Activity During Adolescence

In spite of a well-documented decline in caries levels in children in the United States and other Western countries over the past 50 years, adolescence still marks a period of significant caries activity. A comparison was made on the data collected by the NHANES from the reporting period of 2011 to 2012 and the reporting period 1988 to 1994. In 2011 to 2012, 50% of 12- to 15-year-olds and 67% of 16- to 19-year-olds had experienced dental caries in their permanent teeth.[27] These numbers reflect a decline in caries experience from the earlier 1988 to 1994 data of 57% (a 7% decline) in the 12- to 15-year-old group and 78% (an 11% decline) in the 16- to 19-year-old group.[28] Despite the significant decline, the 16- to 19-year-olds still had the highest caries rates of any child or adolescent age group evaluated. These older adolescents also had the highest rate of untreated decay, at 19% compared with 12% of those aged 12 to 15.[27] Therefore fluoride administration for the adolescent patient should continue to be an important concern during this stage of continuing caries susceptibility.

Topical fluorides along with occlusal sealants are the primary preventive agents of choice during adolescence because the entire permanent dentition except for third molars have typically erupted by 13 years of age.[29] Most studies have shown that fluorides reduce the incidence of smooth-surface caries to a greater extent than that of occlusal caries.[29] Therefore the combination of fluoride therapy and occlusal sealants (Fig. 39.4) can be used to provide optimal protection for all surfaces of both anterior and posterior teeth.

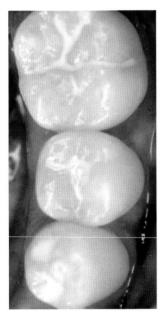

• **Figure 39.4** Occlusal sealant. (Courtesy Dr. Dennis J. McTigue.)

High-Frequency/Low-Concentration Applications

As with younger children, the daily use of a fluoride dentifrice should form the foundation of a sound personal preventive oral health program, regardless of whether the person lives in a fluoridated or a nonfluoridated community. Additional protection can be provided by the daily use of a 0.05% sodium fluoride rinse for those at elevated risk for the development of caries. Although these rinses are not as effective as brushing with an over-the-counter fluoridated dentifrice, they are advisable for those "on-the-go" teenagers who do not take the time to practice thorough plaque removal. Frequent exposures to fluoride may help to suppress the cariogenic potential of the oral flora and can help to establish an environment that may inhibit demineralization or promote remineralization.[30] As noted previously, fluoride mouthrinses also are indicated for persons who have difficulty removing plaque because of the presence of orthodontic appliances or for those with predisposing medical conditions.

Highly Concentrated Fluoride Agents

Frequent applications of highly concentrated fluoride gels, dentifrices, or varnishes may be indicated for adolescents who exhibit poor oral hygiene or other risk-elevating factors, or who continue to exhibit high levels of carious activity at recall examinations. Gels can be applied at home by brushing or by means of customized plastic trays. Custom trays are easily fabricated using vacuum-forming devices that adapt plastic tray material over stone models of the patient's maxillary and mandibular arches. The optimum time to apply the gels is just before bedtime, which prolongs the fluoride contact with the teeth.[30] Professional topical fluoride applications in the form of varnishes, gels, or foams can be applied as frequently as every 3 months for moderate or high caries adolescents. An additional preventive regimen for the high caries risk adolescent with a history of ongoing caries activity is prescribing a highly concentrated fluoride dentifrice (1.1% sodium fluoride, 5000 ppm) for daily use. Individuals who use such highly concentrated fluoride products must be able to expectorate appropriately; therefore their use in some patients with special needs may be limited.

Adolescence is a time of heightened caries activity for many individuals as a result of increased intake of cariogenic substances and inattention to oral hygiene procedures. Because fluorides have been shown to exert a greater anticaries effect in patients with higher baseline levels of caries activity and because the concurrent use of various forms of fluoride often produces greater caries reductions than when the agents are used separately, multiple exposures to a variety of fluoride sources should be encouraged during this period of elevated risk in an attempt to control the caries process.

Risk Factors

Intraoral and Perioral Piercings

A growing interest among adolescents is body modification through intraoral and perioral piercings. This mode of self-expression carries risks and complications not typically experienced with more traditional types of body piercings. The increase in complications is related to the fact that these piercings involve violations of bacteria-rich mucosa that is more sensitive to disruption than would be dermal tissue. Complications can be categorized as immediate or delayed, as well as localized or systemic. Immediate complications occurring at the time of piercing include pain, excessive bleeding, and nerve damage causing immediate paresthesia. It is also possible that infectious diseases, such as hepatitis B and C, and microorganisms responsible for the development of cellulitis and bacterial endocarditis could be introduced at the time of piercing through improper aseptic techniques. Delayed complications include the formation of tissue defects both at the site of the piercing and on tissue adjacent to the jewelry. Ninety-seven percent of patients reported some form of delayed complication.[31] Fractured teeth, allergic reactions to metals, ingestion and aspiration of jewelry parts, dysphasia, masticatory problems, and hypersalivation are additional complications that have been attributed to intraoral and perioral piercings.[32]

Although numerous case reports are available on the subject of complications associated with intraoral piercings, relatively few large studies have investigated the subject. What studies are available reveal a strong correlation between piercings and specific types of dental injuries and pathologic conditions. The most commonly reported dental conditions include fractured teeth and the development of mucogingival defects. Loss of tooth structure due to attrition or fracture has been reported to be as high as 80% in individuals with pierced tongues (Fig. 39.5).[33] Similarly, studies have reported that 19% of individuals with pierced tongues experienced some type of gingival recession.[34]

Because of the high incidence of complications associated with perioral and intraoral piercings, dental professionals should react proactively to those adolescents contemplating piercings. Increasing social acceptance is making it hard to identify those adolescents at risk. Therefore dental professionals should include a discussion of the complications of perioral and intraoral piercings as part of their routine prevention program aimed at all adolescents. Those adolescents who present with existing piercings should be counseled as to their risks and possible complications. Because of the rapid development and progression of tissue defects related to piercings, it may be best to keep individuals with existing piercings on shorter recall schedules than what might otherwise be dictated from their caries risk assessments.

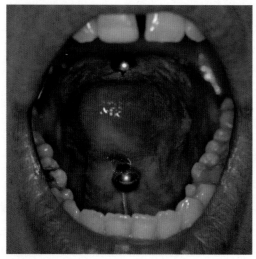

• **Figure 39.5** A fractured lower left first permanent molar associated with an intraoral piercing. (Courtesy Maia Rodrigo.)

Adolescent Pregnancy

In 2015 the birth rate in the United States was 22.3 live births for every 1000 teenagers of ages 15 to 19 years.[35] Although the trend in teenage birth rates has been declining, it is estimated that more than 232,000 teenagers give birth each year.[35] Dentists who treat adolescent patients are likely to encounter pregnant teenagers at some time. When dealing with the pregnant teenager, the dental professional must address a unique set of issues. These would include legal concerns, emotional considerations, and distinct physical and dental problems that would not otherwise be encountered if the patient were not pregnant.

The AAPD recommends that the initial evaluation of a pregnant adolescent takes place during her first trimester.[36] Adolescents who are pregnant are often reluctant to share this information with their dental professional, particularly early on in their pregnancy. This reluctance to divulge information on the pregnancy makes it challenging for the dental professional to provide the anticipatory guidance and treatment that ideally would be initiated at this time.

It is possible that the individual responsible for consenting privileges of an adolescent could change due to a pregnancy. State laws vary widely as to who can consent to treatment for the pregnant adolescent. Treating dentists must be aware of the local statutes that address this situation, as well as those statutes that address the confidentiality of the situation.

Ideally, a dental prophylaxis should be completed during this first trimester. If either adverse periodontal conditions develop or inadequate home hygiene is noted, additional hygiene appointments should also be scheduled during the second and third trimesters. Counseling during this first visit should address dietary considerations, the consequences of hormonal changes on gingival health, and a preventive plan that includes measures to reduce the likelihood of postpartum vertical transmission of mutans streptococci to the newborn. Radiographs with adequate shielding can be taken during this first trimester but are recommended only if they will affect immediate patient care. Nitrous oxide is discouraged at this time. If elective treatment is indicated, it should be completed during the second trimester and only if it is likely to prevent the development of dental complications. Otherwise, it would be best to delay such elective treatment until after delivery. The pregnant patient who is suffering pain or infection should be taken care of immediately, regardless of the trimester of pregnancy. Any administered or prescribed medications should not pose a risk to either the expectant mother or her fetus. Fluoride supplementation is not recommended as a means to provide added protection to the developing teeth of the fetus.

Often these patients will experience nausea and vomiting, which can lead to enamel erosion. An acid-neutralizing rinse should be recommended after episodes of emesis. Rinsing with a teaspoon of sodium bicarbonate mixed in a cup of warm water can provide this neutralizing effect.[37] In addition, immediate toothbrushing should be discouraged.

The dentist who is adequately prepared can be a strong advocate for the health and well-being of both pregnant adolescents and their unborn children. It is imperative that the dental professional who treats adolescents become familiar with the possible complications as well as the recommendations for treating pregnant patients.

Smoking and Smokeless Tobacco

The use of tobacco by minors is a complex issue. The data are clear that tobacco has both systemic and local impacts on the body. Cardiovascular disease (stroke, heart attack, and hypertension), lung disease, and cancer of the oral and respiratory tract are well-known sequelae associated with smoking.[38] Periodontal disease also is more prevalent in smokers.[39] Although most oral cancers occurs after 30 years of age, they can occur earlier.[40] Therefore routine dental examinations on adolescents should include an inspection of all mucosal, tongue, palatal, and oropharyngeal surfaces to rule out the presence of oral cancers.

Smoking cessation is difficult at best. The social and environmental cues that reinforce the smoking habit, combined with the potential nicotine addiction, make this a tough problem to conquer. This may be compounded in adolescents where both the habit and the search for help are often clandestine. Certainly, educating children and adolescents and preventing tobacco use is the preferred approach. When the habit has been acquired, the best cessation results appear to be those in which behavioral support is combined with nicotine replacement therapy (NRT).[41] Clinicians should attempt an intervention because they can potentially cause a great impact on the well-being of an adolescent.[42] Patients willing to try to quit tobacco use should be provided treatments identified as effective, and patients unwilling to quit tobacco use should be provided a brief intervention designed to increase their motivation to quit.[41] The latter can be an unstructured and informal discussion of the reasons to quit and the barriers that the patient might encounter. Working with parents and children in a cessation regimen incorporating NRT requires parental consent because doing so otherwise would be a violation of US Food and Drug Administration regulations, even though those under 18 years of age have ready access to tobacco products on most occasions.[43]

Smokeless tobacco appears to be an increasingly popular alternative to smoking, especially among young males, for whom it increased from 0.7% in 1970 to 7% in 2014.[44] More distressing, the prevalence among male high school students is near 10%.[44] Smokeless tobacco can easily be used to achieve the same effects of nicotine without impinging on family, friends, and smoke-free environments. Whether smokeless tobacco is implicated in oral cancer is important because since 1970 through 2004 the 5-year survival rate of oral cancer victims has increased, but only by 15%.[45] Like smoking, the environment (e.g., certain social situations) can provide behavioral cues that stimulate the desire to use smokeless tobacco.[46]

Aside from the unsightly necessities that accompany some smokeless spit tobaccos, there are other side effects that make it a questionable health practice. The potential for nicotine addiction is high with all types of tobacco products.[47] Certainly long-term use of nicotine in any form carries the risk of hypertension. Blood pressure monitoring indicates that such changes follow tobacco users of any type.[48] Furthermore, it appears that smokeless tobacco is a gateway drug to cigarettes.[49,50]

Smokeless tobacco has several deleterious effects on oral health. There appears to be greater risk of localized periodontal attachment loss in the form of gingival recession in smokeless tobacco users, commonly adjacent to where the tobacco is placed.[51] There also appears to be a greater risk of leukoplakia developing among smokeless tobacco users,[52] including adolescent users.[53] Fortunately, there is good evidence that suggests smokeless tobacco keratosis (Fig. 39.6) is largely reversible.[54] A major area of dispute is whether smokeless tobacco is a likely cause of oral cancer. The evidence is not decisive but points in that direction.[52,55] It is not unreasonable to counsel patients and help them with cessation programs so that they can prevent the transient and possibly more morbid potential

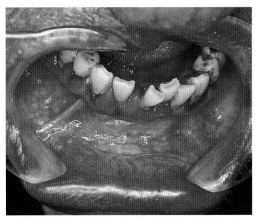

• **Figure 39.6** Clinical appearance of white lesion associated with smokeless tobacco (tobacco pouch keratosis). (From Ibsen OAC, Phelan JA. *Oral Pathology for the Dental Hygienist.* 5th ed. St Louis: Saunders; 2009.)

effects of smokeless tobacco, as well as the potential systemic side effects.

Just as with smokers, cessation programs using a combined behavioral and pharmacologic approach can and should be initiated by dentists for their patients who use smokeless tobacco. These can be self-help programs or those with more personal interactions. Data indicate some substantial success with these types of cessation interventions.[56] Some methods such as NRT may be difficult without parental involvement, given the restrictions for NRT. Enhancing this difficulty is the fact that most smokeless tobacco users do not associate this form of tobacco use with nicotine addiction.

In addition to the long-lasting concerns with smoking and smokeless tobacco use among adolescents is the more recent concerns with the increasing usage of e-cigarettes and marijuana use among adolescents as detailed in Chapter 37.

Transitioning to Adulthood

In 2011 the AAP in conjunction with the American Academy of Family Physicians and the American College of Physicians released a report that provided guidelines on the transitioning of youth from a pediatric medical home to appropriate adult care. A detailed health care transition algorithm was developed that outlined the steps involved to facilitate a smooth transition.[57] The transition of adolescent dental patients to adult dental care is equally if not more complicated than that of medical care. It is a process that is best accomplished with some advance planning.

Borrowing from the medical model, the smooth transition of adolescents from a pediatric dental home to one with an adult focus should involve three key components: provider readiness, family readiness, and adolescent readiness. Provider readiness involves the establishment of an office policy that addresses the age as well as the process for referring an adolescent to an adult dental provider. The AAPD does not require transfer by a specific age yet recommends that it be "at a time agreed upon by the patient, parent, and pediatric dentist."[58] The trend among pediatric dentists is that these transfers are taking place at an early age. Studies have found that, in the majority of pediatric dental practices, less than 10% of patients are between 15 and 21 years of age.[59]

Family readiness describes the practice of informing the parent or legal guardians of the established office policy well in advance of when an actual transfer may occur. The family may need to investigate benefit coverage issues and may elect to do reference checks on potential recipients of the transfer.

Adolescent readiness would be the final key component in the transfer process. It is possible that there could be emotional concerns for the adolescent who, essentially, grew up with and became comfortable with a single pediatric dental provider. Discussion of the transfer would serve the patient best if initiated well in advance of the actual transfer. Doing so could potentially help the provider recognize and address any anxiety associated with the transfer process. In addition, it could allow anxious adolescents to mentally prepare for their new dental home.

It is estimated that 750,000 adolescents with special health care needs reach adulthood each year.[60] These patients pose a unique set of challenges to the transfer process. Although nearly 95% of pediatric dentists routinely see patients with special health care needs, less than 10% of general dentists see these same patients.[61,62] The cooperative abilities of these patients may require some behavior guidance techniques best implemented by a pediatric dentist, but their dental needs may require expertise beyond the skill set of a pediatric dentist. The complexity of these cases is highly varied, and the need for transfer should be considered on an individual basis. Some special needs patients would transition quite well to an adult practice, whereas others may be better served if they remained in a pediatric-based practice their entire life. Often, coordination is needed between multiple dental as well as medical specialties to provide optimum care for these individuals. The key is that these patients have an established dental home through which such care can be coordinated. If a special needs patient is transferred from a pediatric to an adult-based practice, it is imperative that the continued coordination for optimum care be carried out by the newly established dental home.

References

1. Dye BA, Tan S, Smith V, et al. Trends in oral health status: United States, 1988-1994 and 1999-2004. National Center for Health Statistics. *Vital Health Stat 11*. 2007;(248):1–92.
2. Beck JD, Arbes SI Jr. Epidemiology of gingival and periodontal disease. In: Newman MG, Takei H, Klokkevold PR, et al, eds. *Carranza's Clinical Periodontology*. 10th ed. St Louis: Saunders Elsevier; 2006:117–119.
3. Skinner AC, Perrin EM, Skelton JA. Prevalence of obesity and severe obesity in US children 1999-2014. *Obesity J*. 2016;24:1116–1123.
4. Fungwe T, Guenther PM, Juan WJ, et al. *The Quality of Children's Diets in 2003-04 as Measured by the Healthy Eating Index 2005, Nutrition Insight 43*. Washington, DC: Center for Nutrition Policy and Promotion, US Department of Agriculture; 2009 April.
5. Piernas C, Popkin BM. Trends in snacking among US children. *Health Aff*. 2010;20(3):398–404.
6. Food Surveys Research Group. Snacking Patterns of U.S. Adolescents; September, 2010, Dietary Data Brief No. 2.
7. Fulkerson JA, Larson N, Horning M, et al. A review of associations between family or shared meal frequency and dietary and weight status outcomes across the lifespan. *J Nutr Educ Behav*. 2014;49(1):2–19.
8. O'Dea JA. Consumption of nutritional supplements among adolescents: usage and perceived benefits. *Health Educ Res*. 2003;18(1):98–107.
9. Berger AJ, Alford K. Cardiac arrest in a young man following excess consumption of caffeinated "energy drinks." *Med J Aust*. 2003;190(1):41–43.
10. Nawrot P, Jordon S, Eastwood J, et al. Effects of caffeine on human health. *Food Addit Contam*. 2003;20(1):1–30.
11. Bonnett MH, Balkin TJ, Dinges DF, et al. The use of stimulants to modify performance during sleep losss: a review by the sleep deprivation and Stimulant Task Force of the American Academy of Sleep Medicine. *Sleep*. 2005;28(9):1163–1187.
12. Diogo LR. Caffeine, mental health, and psychiatric disorders. *J Alzheimers Disease*. 2010;20:S239–S248.
13. Harris JL, Munsell CR. Energy drinks and adolescents: what's the harm? *Nutr Reviews*. 2015;73(4):247–257.
14. Shaw L, Smith AJ. Dental erosion—the problem and some practical solutions. *Br Dent J*. 1999;186(3):115–118.
15. Committee on Nutrition and the Council on Sports Medicine and Fitness. Sports drinks and energy drinks for children and adolescents: are they appropriate? *Pediatrics*. 2011;127(6):1182–1189.
16. Institute of Medicine. *Nutrition Standards for Foods in Schools: Leading the Way Toward Healthier Youth*. Washington, DC: National Academies Press; 2007.
17. Reed J, Krebs-Smith SM. Dietary sources of energy, solid fats, and added sugars among children and adolescents in the United States. *J Am Diet Assoc*. 2010;110(10):1477–1484.
18. Ludwig DS, Peterson KE, Gortmaker SL. Relation between consumption of sugar-sweetened drinks and childhood obesity: a prospective, observational analysis. *Lancet*. 2001;357(9255):505–675.
19. Malik VS, Popkin BM, Bray GA, et al. Sugar-sweetened beverages and risk of metabolic syndrome and type 2 diabetes: a meta-analysis. *Diabetes Care*. 2010;33(11):2477–2483.
20. Rosinger A, Herrick K, Gahche J, et al. *Sugar-Sweetened Beverage Consumption Among US Youth, 2011-2014. NCHS Data Brief 271*. Hyattsville, MD: National Center for Health Statistics; 2017.
21. Harini PM, Anegundi RT. Efficacy of a probiotic and chlorhexidine mouth rinses: a short-term clinical study. *J Indian Soc Pedod Prev Dent*. 2010;28(3):179–182.
22. Manikandan D, Balaji VR, Niazi TM, et al. Chlorhexidine varnish implemented treatment strategy for chronic periodontitis: a clinical and microbial study. *J Pharm Bioall Sci*. 2016;8(suppl 1):133–137.
23. Brightman LJ, Terezhalmy GT, Greenwald H, et al. The effects of a 0.12% chlorhexidine gluconate mouthrinse on orthodontic patients aged 11 through 17 with established gingivitis. *Am J Orthofac Dentofac Orthop*. 1991;100:324–329.
24. Bhat M. Periodontal health of 14- to 17-year-old U.S. school children. *J Public Health Dent*. 1991;51:5–11.
25. Autio-Gold J. The role of chorhexidine in caries prevention. *Oper Dent*. 2008;33(6):710–716.
26. American Academy of Pediatric Dentistry Council on Clinical Affairs. Policy on the use of xylitol. *Pediatr Dent (special issue)*. 2016;38:47–49.
27. Dye BA, Thornton-Evans G, Xianfen L, et al. *Dental Caries and Sealant Prevalence in Children and Adolescents in the US, 2011-2012, NCHS Data Brief, 191*. Hayttsville, MD: National Center for Health Statistics; 2015.
28. Beltrán-Aguilar ED, Barker LK, Canto MT, et al. Surveillance for dental caries, dental sealants, tooth retention, edentulism, and enamel fluorosis—United States, 1988-1994 and 1999-2002. *MMWR Surveill Summ*. 2005;54(3):1–43.
29. Recommendations for using fluoride to prevent and control dental caries in the United States. Centers for Disease Control and Prevention. *MMWR Recomm Rep*. 2001;50(RR–14):1–42.
30. Castellano JB, Donly KJ. Potential remineralization of demineralized enamel after application of fluoride varnish. *Am J Dent*. 2004;17(6):462–464.
31. Viera EP, Ribeiro AL, Pinheiro Jde J, et al. Oral piercings: immediate and late complications. *J Oral Maxillofac Surg*. 2011;69(12):3032–3037.
32. Titus P, Smily T, Francis G, et al. Ornamental dentistry-An overview. *J Evol Med Dent Sci*. 2013;2(7):666–676.
33. Leichter JW, Monteith BD. Prevalence and risk of traumatic gingival recession following elective lip piercing. *Dent Traumatol*. 2006;22(1):7–13.
34. Campbell A, Moore A, Williams E, et al. Tongue piercing: impact of time and barbell stem length on lingual gingival recession and tooth chipping. *J Periodontol*. 2002;73:289–297.

35. Martin JA, Hamilton BE, Osterman MJK, et al. *Births: Final Data for 2015*. Hyattsville, MD: National Center for Health Statistics; 2017. National Vital Statistics Report, 66(1).

36. American Academy of Pediatric Dentistry. Guideline on oral health care for the pregnant adolescent. *Pediatr Dent*. 2016;38(special issue):163–170.

37. New York State Department of Health. Oral Health Care During Pregnancy and Early Childhood: Practice Guidelines; August 2006.

38. US Department of Health and Human Services (USDHHS). *The Health Consequences of Smoking: A Report of the Surgeon General*. Atlanta: USDHHS, Centers for Disease Control and Prevention, National Center for Chronic Disease Prevention and Health Promotion, Office on Smoking and Health 62; 2004.

39. Bergström J. Tobacco smoking and chronic destructive periodontal disease. *J Odontol*. 2004;92(1):1–8.

40. Howlader N, Noone AM, Miller D, et al, eds. *SEER Stat Fact Sheets: Oral Cavity and Pharynx, 1975–2014*. Bethesda, MD: National Cancer Institute; 2004. http://seer.cancer.gov/statfacts/html/oral/cav.html. Accessed May 24, 2017.

41. Fiore MC, Bailey WC, Cohen SJ, et al. *Treating Tobacco Use and Dependence. Clinical Practice Guideline*. Rockville, MD: US Department of Health and Human Services, Public Health Service; 2000.

42. Demers RY, Neale AV, Adams R, et al. The impact of physicians' brief smoking cessation counseling: a MIRNET study. *J Fam Pract*. 1990;31(6):625–629.

43. Johnson KC, Klesges LM, Somes GW, et al. Access of over-the-counter nicotine replacement therapy products to minors. *Arch Pediatr Adolesc Med*. 2004;158(3):212–216.

44. Centers for Disease Control and Prevention. Smokeless tobacco use in the United States. https://www.cdc.gov/tobacco/data_statistics/fact_sheets/smokeless/use_us/index.htm. Accessed August 17, 2017.

45. National Institute of Dental and Craniofacial Research. Oral cancer 5 year survival rates by race, gender, and stages of diagnosis. http://www.nidcr.nih.gov/datastatistics/. Accessed June 12, 2017.

46. Coffey SF, Lombardo TW. Effects of smokeless tobacco–related sensory and behavioral cues on urge, affect, and stress. *Exp Clin Psychopharmacol*. 1998;6(4):406–418.

47. Benowitz NL. Pharmacology of nicotine: addiction and therapeutics. *Annu Rev Pharmacol Toxicol*. 1996;36:597–613.

48. Bolinder G, de Faire U. Ambulatory 24-h blood pressure monitoring in healthy, middle-aged smokeless tobacco users, smokers, and nontobacco users. *Am J Hypertens*. 1998;11(10):1153–1163.

49. Haddock CK, Weg MV, DeBon M, et al. Evidence that smokeless tobacco use is a gateway for smoking initiation in young adult males. *Prev Med*. 2001;32(3):262–267.

50. Forrester K, Biglan A, Severson HH, et al. Predictors of smoking onset over two years. *Nicotine Tob Res*. 2007;9(12):1259–1267.

51. Robertson PB, Walsh M, Greene J, et al. Periodontal effects associated with the use of smokeless tobacco. *J Periodontol*. 1990;61(7):438–443.

52. Waterbor JW, Adams RM, Robinson JM, et al. Disparities between public health educational materials and the scientific evidence that smokeless tobacco use causes cancer. *J Cancer Educ*. 2004;19(1):17–28.

53. Creath CJ, Cutter G, Bradley DH, et al. Oral leukoplakia and adolescent smokeless tobacco use. *Oral Surg Oral Med Oral Pathol*. 1991;72(1):35–41.

54. Martin GC, Brown JP, Eifler CW, et al. Oral leukoplakia status six weeks after cessation of smokeless tobacco use. *J Am Dent Assoc*. 1999;130(7):945–954.

55. Boffetta P, Hecht S, Gray N, et al. Smokeless tobacco and cancer. *Lancet*. 2008;9(7):667–675.

56. Severson HH, Akers L, Andrews JA, et al. Evaluating two self-help interventions for smokeless tobacco cessation. *Addict Behav*. 2000;25:465–470.

57. American Academy of Pediatrics, American Academy of Family Physicians; American College of Physicians, et al. Supporting the health care transition from adolescents to adulthood in the medical home. *Pediatrics*. 2011;128(1):182–200.

58. American Academy of Pediatric Dentistry. Guideline on adolescent oral health care. *Pediatr Dent*. 2016;38(special issue):155–162.

59. Nowak AJ, Casamassimo PS, Slayton RL. Facilitating the transition of patients with special health care needs from pediatric to adult oral health care. *J Am Dent Assoc*. 2010;141:1351–1356.

60. Seal P, Ireland M. Addressing transition to adult health care for adolescents with special health care needs. *Pediatrics*. 2005;115(6):1607–1612.

61. Nowak AJ. Patients with special health care needs in pediatric dental practices. *Pediatr Dent*. 2002;24(3):227–228.

62. Casamassimo PS, Seale NS, Ruehs K. General dentists' perceptions of educational and treatment issues affecting access to care for children with special health care needs. *J Dent Educ*. 2004;68(1):23–38.

40

Restorative Dentistry for the Adolescent

ELIZABETH VELAN

CHAPTER OUTLINE

Caring for the adolescent dental patient is a rewarding experience. The use of dental techniques and materials to help young people obtain a healthy and beautiful smile is a clinical challenge requiring knowledge, attention to detail, and skill. In return for their efforts, dentists receive the satisfaction of seeing a young person develop a healthy self-image that can have a positive effect on his or her maturation into adulthood.

Fundamentals of Material Selection

The choice of materials is an important consideration for optimizing adolescent dental restorations. When considering which material to choose for a restoration, it is essential to evaluate the tooth to be restored, the patient's caries risk, the location of the restoration, and the forces to which the restoration will be subjected.

Composite resin restorations are a popular choice because they are esthetically pleasing, preserve tooth structure, and contain no mercury. The clinical success of composite resin restoration relies on the adhesive system that provides a durable bond of composite resin to dentin and enamel, effectively sealing restoration margins and microleakage.[1] To achieve this, a contemporary adhesive system should be used (Fig. 40.1). Contemporary adhesive systems include etch-and-rinse or self-etch systems. Etch-and-rinse adhesive systems, although more technique sensitive, have been shown in laboratory studies to have higher bond strength compared with the self-etch systems.[2] The self-etch systems, in addition to being less technique sensitive, may reduce postoperative sensitivity by leaving behind residue that blocks outward fluid flow from dentin tubules.[3] There continues to be controversy and limited clinical studies to identify which adhesive system improves the longevity of composite resin restorations.[2] To optimize the longevity of the restoration, the provider should follow the manufacturer's instructions and confirm the adhesive system is compatible with the composite resin.[4] The selection of composite resin restorations can be confusing because a variety of products are available with slightly different physical properties.[5,6] Essentially there are three types of composite resins that can be used: microfilled, hybrid, and nanofilled. Nanofilled resins have physical properties superior to those of microfills but slightly inferior to hybrids.[7] The mechanical and physical properties of hybrid composite resins are superior to those of microfilled resins because they contain a higher proportion of filler particles. Hybrid resins have traditionally been chosen as a universal restorative material because they can be used in most clinical situations. Microfilled resins are primarily indicated when esthetic restorations are required; because of their particle size, microfilled resins can be polished to an enamel-like luster with more ease and in less time than hybrid resins.

The polymerization of light-activated composite resins is accomplished by using an intense blue light with a peak wavelength of approximately 450 to 470 nm, which corresponds to the absorption peak of camphoroquinone (CQ), the most popular photoinitiator.[8] A typical light-curing polymerization unit uses light-emitting diodes (LEDs) to efficiently produce blue light (Fig. 40.2), although the traditional gun-style units that contain a halogen bulb and cooling fan are still available (see Chapter 21 for a discussion of curing lights).[8] No matter which light is used, light intensity should be periodically checked (via a radiometer) so that a minimal output of 350 mW/cm^2 can be maintained (Fig. 40.3).[8] Eye protection is important when using the curing lights, because direct viewing of the light is detrimental to vision.[9] In the absence of protective amber filters, one should avoid looking directly at the light.

Fundamentals of Clinical Technique

Shade selection is the first step in achieving an esthetically pleasing restoration. The teeth to be matched should be cleaned with a

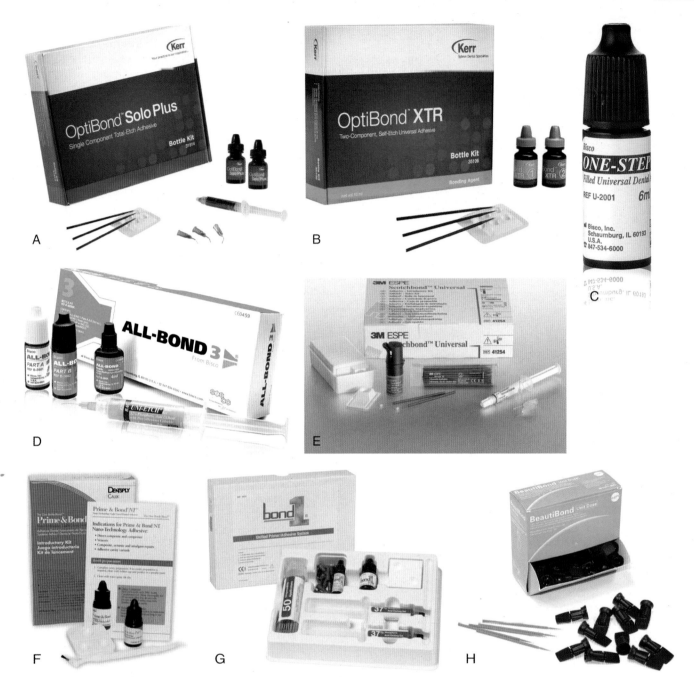

• **Figure 40.1** Representative selection of dentin-enamel adhesive products. ([A and B] Courtesy Kerr Corp., Orange, CA; [C and D] Courtesy Bisco, Inc., Schaumburg, IL; [E] Courtesy 3M ESPE, St. Paul, MN; [F] Courtesy DENTSPLY CAULK, Milford, DE; [G] Courtesy Pentron Clinical, Wallingford, CT; [H] Courtesy Shofu Dental Corp., San Marcos, CA.)

rubber prophylaxis cup and flour of pumice. Tooth dehydration should be prevented because it leads to color change. Moistened shade tabs should be held near the tooth to be matched, only in ambient light or indirect sunlight. One should not use the high-intensity operatory light when selecting shades.

Composite resins come in a variety of shades, which are usually keyed to the VITA shade guide. Unfortunately, a perfect color match between the composite resins and the VITA guide is uncommon, and shades among brands are variable.[10] In recent years the range of shades has been increased to match the shades of teeth that have been whitened or bleached.

To overcome some of the shade-matching pitfalls, many clinicians allow the patient to choose between two similar shades. Another way to verify the shade is to place a small portion of composite resin on the tooth surface, polymerize it, observe the appropriateness of that shade, and then remove it with a hand instrument. It should be noted that one should not etch the tooth before doing this or removal will be difficult.

It is important to maintain an uncontaminated field during the insertion of composite resins. The most reliable and cost-effective way to control moisture is through the use of a well-adapted rubber dam. An alternative product is an intraoral vacuum system. An

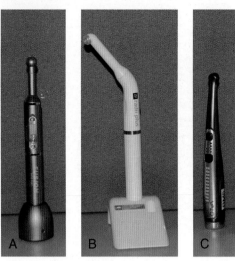

• **Figure 40.2** (A–C) Typical dental composite resin light-curing units. ([A] Courtesy Dentlight LLC, Plano, TX; [B] Courtesy SDI, Bayswater, Australia; [C] Courtesy Ultradent Products, Inc., South Jordan, UT.)

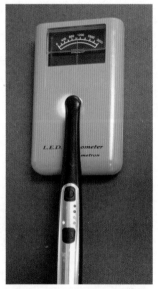

• **Figure 40.3** Light-curing unit showing power output via a radiometer.

example is the Isolite system (Isolite Systems, Santa Barbara, CA), which has a flexible plastic mouthpiece that provides retraction of the soft tissues, a bite block, and constant suction. In limited studies the Isolite system has similar reduction in spatter and humidity levels as a rubber dam (Fig. 40.4).[11,12] Another approach to maintaining a dry field is to use a commercially available lip and cheek retractor (Fig. 40.5). This plastic device, when used with gauze sponges, provides excellent access and good field control.

The use of a base or liner to protect pulp tissue in deep preparations is generally believed to be beneficial. A glass ionomer liner may be used in deep areas of a cavity preparation that is thought to be within 0.5 to 1.0 mm of pulpal tissue (Fig. 40.6). The liner provides chemical adherence to tooth structure and slow release of fluoride.[13]

After adhesive bonding, the photopolymerized composite should be inserted in layers no thicker than recommended by the manufacturer, followed by curing the composite according to the manufacturer's instructions. Appropriately placed layers and adequate time for light exposure help to ensure maximum polymerization and minimize marginal gaps caused by shrinkage.[14] In an effort to mimic the translucency of enamel and the opacity of dentin, manufacturers have produced materials with a variety of opacities. These materials should be placed in increments in which the more opaque materials replace dentin and the more translucent materials replace enamel to produce restorations with similar optical properties to tooth structure.

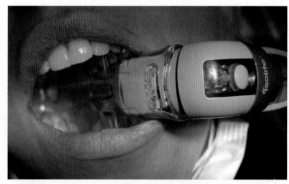

• **Figure 40.4** An example of an intraoral vacuum system.

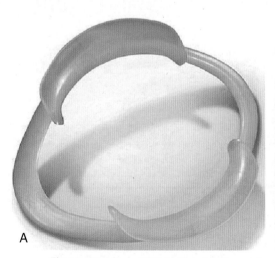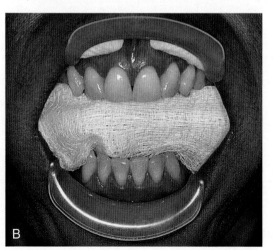

• **Figure 40.5** (A and B) Isolation of teeth may be enhanced through the use of a lip-retracting device. ([A] Courtesy Practicon Dental, Greenville, NC.)

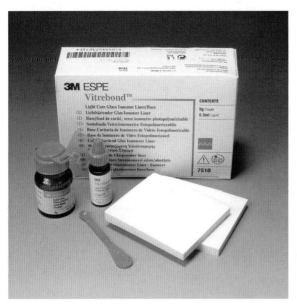

• **Figure 40.6** A light-curable glass ionomer liner. (Courtesy 3M ESPE, St. Paul, MN.)

Plastic or metal instruments are useful for material placement and contouring. Fine sable or camel hair brushes allow the easy contouring and blending of composite resin into the proper form. To prevent composite resin from adhering to the brushes and instruments, they should be lightly touched to the composite resin with a rapid dabbing motion.

After the polymerization process, the contouring and finishing of the restoration is accomplished with carbide finishing burs, ultrafine diamonds, or finishing disks. Fine-pointed burs are helpful for accessing contour areas that are difficult to reach, such as embrasures. Rounded burs may be used on concave surfaces, and disks may be used on flat or convex surfaces. After contouring and finishing, the restoration should be polished with a series of polishing disks or rubber-abrasive instruments. The final finish and polish of proximal areas are best done with abrasive strips.

Restorations for Fractured Anterior Teeth

Trauma to the anterior dentition can often result in tooth fractures involving the enamel; enamel and dentin; and enamel, dentin, and pulp. Injuries such as these can cause pulpal as well as esthetic concerns and should be carefully evaluated by clinical and radiographic means. Clinical findings may range from minimal thermal and pressure sensitivity to the acute distress of a pulp exposure. Radiographs are indicated in diagnosing the presence or absence of root fractures. When indicated, treatment must begin with pulpal therapy and whenever possible preservation of vital pulp tissue. (See Chapter 35 for a discussion of trauma to permanent incisors.)

Clinical Technique: Tooth Fragment

If the tooth fragment is available, is relatively intact, and adapts well to the remaining tooth with no encroachment to the biologic width, the fragment can be bonded to the tooth.[15] This technique allows immediate satisfaction by restoring tooth form and function with excellent esthetics and low cost.[15–18] For the best results, the fragment should be hydrated. Families should be counseled to

place the fragment in saline, Hank's Balanced Solution, or milk while in transit to the dental office. When there is minimal loss of tooth structure, the fragment can be bonded by etching the fragment and tooth and application of a dental adhesive to the fragment and tooth, followed by placement of highly filled flowable composite resin to the fragment and tooth. The fragment is then repositioned and the proximal contacts flossed or a matrix is placed followed by light curing. In this situation the adhesive and flowable composite resin should be light cured together. When there is moderate loss of tooth structure, resin-based composite should be used in lieu of flowable resin. In this situation the adhesive should be cured separately. Following a direct pulp cap or partial pulpotomy, the internal section of the fragment will need to be modified to allow the best fit. In either scenario, after the fragment is bonded, a shallow double chamber should be prepared along the fracture line and restored with composite resin. This procedure will add strength to the rebonding and minimize the risk for stain at the fracture line.[15,18] Families should be cautioned that the longevity of the reattachment is unknown because few clinical studies have evaluated this type of repair.[15] One long-term multicentered clinical study revealed that only 25% of 334 rebonded fragments were retained 7 years after bonding.[19]

Some clinicians consider the class IV composite resin restoration an interim restoration for adolescents until a more permanent ceramic crown can be fabricated.[20] However, with modern materials and techniques, the strength and color stability of composite resin class IV restorations are such that they can be considered final restorations that will provide relatively long service.[21] For early adolescents with severely fractured anterior teeth or caries, these restorations can provide years of service, allowing the teeth to mature so that pulpal injury during crown preparation is less likely.

Clinical Technique: Class IV Restoration

Adhesive dentistry has lessened the need for extensive mechanical retentive features in class IV restorations. The primary retentive feature is a beveled enamel cavosurface margin of a minimum of 1.0 to 2.0 mm in length (Fig. 40.7). Beveling allows maximal bond strength and minimizes leakage by exposing the ends of the enamel rods to etching. Because anterior restorations are sometimes subject to strong shearing forces that can be greater than the bond strength of the restoration to the tooth, features such as grooves or retentive points may be used to gain additional retentive strength.

After administering anesthesia, followed by isolation, the bevel is prepared with a high-speed rotary instrument. Caries is removed if indicated, and a base or liner may be applied to the exposed dentin. Conditioning of the tooth is achieved in accordance with the adhesive system of choice, with adherence to the manufacturer's directions. A wedged celluloid matrix strip can be used to prevent etching and bonding an adjacent tooth. In addition, anterior matrix systems are available to optimize curvature, anatomic form, and contacts when placing direct composite anterior restorations, such as the Garrison Anterior Matrix System or the BioClear Matrix system.[22] After placing, finishing, and polishing the restoration, carefully check the restoration for interferences in all excursive movements (Fig. 40.8). Occlusal stresses on the restoration should be minimized.

Restoration of Diastemas

Many adolescents consider spaces between anterior teeth (diastemas) unattractive.[23] Historically the only restorative treatment to fill

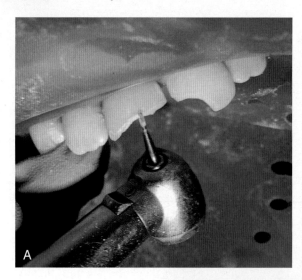
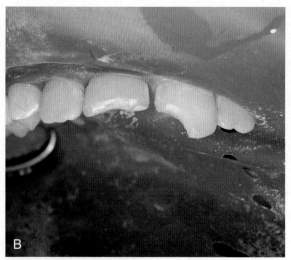
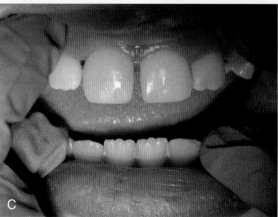

• **Figure 40.7** (A) The incisal edges of the maxillary incisors were fractured as the result of an accident; a beveled enamel cavosurface margin is placed as a retentive feature. (B) Enamel beveled surfaces of teeth shown in (A). (C) Composite resin restorations of fractured teeth shown in (A) and (B).

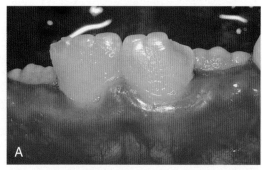
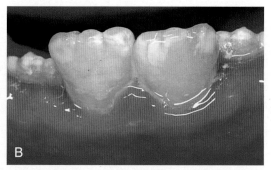

• **Figure 40.8** (A) The incisal edges of the mandibular incisors were fractured as the result of an accident. (B) Composite resin restorations (Filtek Restorative Material, 3M ESPE) of fractured teeth shown in (A).

these spaces has been the fabrication of crowns. Improved composite resin materials and acid-etching technology now allow restoration of diastemas with a method that is nondestructive, reversible, and relatively inexpensive. However, patients should be forewarned that fracture and staining are possible drawbacks of composite resin diastema closure and that replacement is likely to be needed after 5 to 10 years.

When an adolescent patient wants a diastema closure, whether the spaces are the result of natural development or postorthodontic discrepancies, careful evaluation and planning are necessary. If the patient is nearing completion of orthodontic therapy but is still undergoing treatment, the restorative dentist may advise the orthodontist about the optimal arrangement of anterior teeth for diastema closure. The orthodontist may then complete active treatment and place the patient into a retention phase before closing the diastema. The use of diagnostic study casts is recommended for evaluation and treatment planning. A diagnostic waxing of the proposed restorative treatment can aid both the patient and the clinician in envisioning the outcome.

Important pretreatment considerations include the size and location of the space or spaces and the size (length and width) and shape of the teeth to be restored. Normally, composite resin is added to the teeth on both sides of the space. For patients who are undergoing orthodontic treatment, one should determine if the remaining space would best be left in one place, such as the midline between the maxillary central incisors, or distributed over proximal areas throughout the anterior segment. One must also consider the length and width of the teeth to be restored. If the width becomes greater than the length, those teeth appear more square, leading to an unattractive outcome that may be as displeasing as the original diastema. Because of occlusal patterns and chewing stresses, teeth usually cannot be lengthened with composite resin without creating a high probability of resin fracture. However, light reflections can be used to create the illusion of a longer and narrower tooth when the composite resin is extended to cover most or the entire facial surface. To create the illusion of a narrower tooth, one should form mesial and distal line angles in composite resin that are positioned slightly nearer the middle of the tooth and add definite vertical anatomic highlights (developmental depressions). For some patients the best treatment is partial diastema closure, in which an existing space is made smaller by enlarging the teeth with composite resin but not making the teeth so large that they become esthetically displeasing.

Clinical Technique

After cleaning, shade selection, and isolation, treatment should begin one tooth at a time. The space to be eliminated should be carefully measured via a periodontal probe, calipers, or Boley gauge because after one tooth is restored in an effort to eliminate half the space, it is usually difficult to determine how much of the space has actually been restored. The entire labial surface of the tooth should be etched and bonding agent applied because most of the labial surface will be covered with a thin layer of composite resin to allow a subtle color transition from composite resin to tooth. In addition, covering most of the labial surface allows the use of visual illusions that cause the tooth to look narrower or longer, as described previously.

Composite resin (preferably a resin that is viscous and opaque) should be applied, beginning at the gingival margin of the interproximal area. Using instruments and brushes, one should shape the material to allow a smooth-flowing gingival embrasure without creating an overhanging ledge. The entire proximal surface, as well as the labial surface, can be built up and polymerized at once or incrementally. After this buildup, one should finish the proximal area to the proper contour and polish it. Next, the second tooth is restored similarly. A celluloid matrix and wedge are usually inserted after the gingival increment is polymerized to retain the composite resin and to prevent the restorations from bonding together. Upon completion, the matrix is removed, and contouring and polishing are completed (Fig. 40.9).

Anterior teeth that are unusually small, such as peg lateral incisors, may be restored in the same manner as teeth requiring both mesial and distal diastema closure restorations. Again, careful

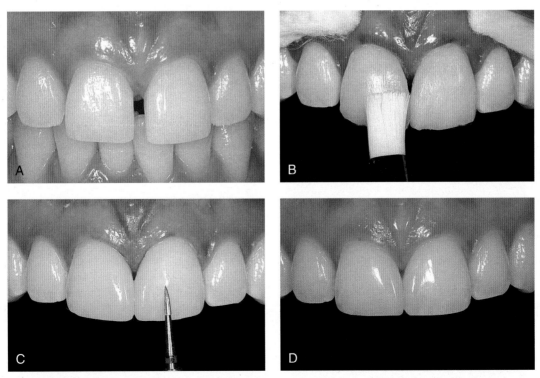

• **Figure 40.9** (A) A preoperative view of a maxillary midline diastema, which the patient found unattractive. (B) The initial increment of composite resin being contoured with a sable brush before polymerization. (C) Contouring and removing excess composite following buildup of the second tooth. (D) A postoperative view of the completed treatment.

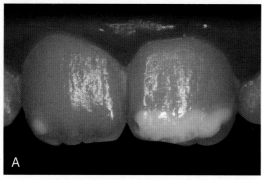
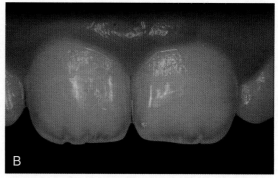

• **Figure 40.10** (A) Preoperatively the maxillary left central incisor is affected with enamel hypoplasia that presents as a large, white lesion. (B) Postoperatively the esthetics of the tooth is greatly improved after HCl acid etching and resin infiltration. (Courtesy Zafer Cehreli.)

treatment planning is advised to determine whether the restorations should be done only on the smaller tooth or on both the small and adjacent teeth for maximal cosmetic benefit. Preoperative diagnosis is necessary to determine whether lengthening is feasible. One should forewarn patients that the possibility of fracturing increases as length increases. In situations where fracturing is a concern, a hybrid resin should be used as a substrate and a microfilled resin placed on the surface. This technique increases the strength and esthetic outcome of the restoration.

Restoration of Discolored Teeth

Although there are many causes of preeruptive tooth discoloration, the most common discolorations result from trauma, enamel hypoplasia (often caused by fluorosis), and the administration of certain types of antibiotics during childhood. These lesions vary from small white or yellowish flecking of the surface enamel, called enamel dysmineralization,[24] to the deep intrinsic bluish gray color often visible in tetracycline staining.

Treatment of Hypoplastic Spots and White Spot Lesions

Discrete hypoplastic white or yellow-brown spots can be improved by the etch-bleach-seal technique, resin infiltration, vital bleaching (which is described later in this chapter), enamel microabrasion, and/or by making shallow saucer-shaped preparations in enamel to remove the intensely colored tooth structure and then restoring the enamel with composite resin. The etch-bleach-seal technique is the least invasive of all approaches.[25] The affected teeth are cleaned with pumice, isolated with a rubber dam, etched for 60 seconds with 37% phosphoric acid, and rinsed. Sodium hypochlorite (5%) is applied and allowed to evaporate. The application process is repeated for 5 to 10 minutes. If improvement is not apparent, the application can continue for 15 to 20 minutes. Some teeth may need to be treated over several appointments. After satisfactory results are achieved, the teeth are sealed with a highly penetrating clear resin.[25] Resin infiltration (Icon, DMG-America, Englewood, NJ) has also been shown to significantly improve the clinical appearance of white spot lesions (Fig. 40.10).[26] Resin infiltration is discussed in more detail later in this chapter. Microabrasion removes enamel but does not necessitate placement of a restoration. The technique for enamel microabrasion involves application of an acidic abrasive paste by a reduced-speed dental handpiece (Fig.

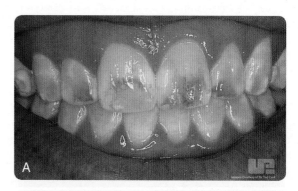
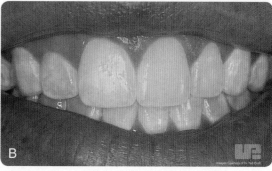

• **Figure 40.11** (A) Preoperative view of maxillary incisors with white and brown enamel dysmineralization defects. (B) After enamel microabrasion and home bleaching. (Courtesy Ultradent Products, Inc., South Jordan, UT.)

40.11).[27] Microabrasion is sometimes used in combination with vital bleaching.[28]

Veneers

Composite resin or porcelain veneers provide a treatment option for patients who have moderate to severe staining of one or more teeth. Patients are most concerned about the appearance of their maxillary teeth as they are more visible in speaking and smiling. In addition, mandibular teeth are often less likely to be successfully veneered because of limited space (insufficient horizontal overlap) and unfavorable forces. For veneer treatment to be successful, the patient must have excellent periodontal health because the placement of veneers will result in contours and margins that require good oral hygiene to maintain gingival health. In addition, patients should be warned that biting on hard objects, such as raw carrots or pencils, may dislodge or break veneers.

Laboratory-Fabricated Veneers

The indirect veneer technique has the advantage of requiring less total chair time because the veneers are fabricated in the laboratory. Excellent esthetically pleasing contours can be achieved with porcelain. Disadvantages include the necessity of two appointments, laboratory expense, and the possibility of creating an excess bulk of restorative material.

The indirect technique usually requires the removal of some enamel (ideally 0.3 to 0.5 mm, but occasionally more in severely stained teeth) from the facial surface to provide space for the veneer (Fig. 40.12). Tooth preparation is best accomplished with a medium-grit diamond rotary instrument (Fig. 40.13), with the goal of producing a long chamfer finish line throughout the surfaces to be covered. This preparation extends to the proximal surfaces to include the contact areas (Fig. 40.14). Gingivally, the preparation

must extend far enough to cover the stained enamel sufficiently to improve the color. For better periodontal health, the finish line should be kept supragingival whenever possible. Following the preparation, an accurate impression of the teeth should be made with an elastomeric impression material such as vinyl polysiloxane or polyether.

At the second appointment, one should isolate the teeth and clean them with pumice. After evaluating (using a try-in paste to help hold the veneers in place) and adjusting the veneers, they should be cleaned with the etching gel and silanated according to the manufacturer's recommendations. The preparations should be acid etched individually or in pairs and the veneers bonded in place, beginning with the central incisors. Celluloid matrices help to protect adjacent teeth. Photopolymerized or dual-polymerized resins of moderate viscosity are preferred for bonding. Excess resin should be removed from margins with brushes before polymerization. Adequate polymerization time (40 to 60 seconds in each area) should be used because the veneers will shield some light transmission. Finishing and polishing are usually necessary only at the margins and may be done with abrasive strips and rubber cups (Fig. 40.15).

Direct Veneers

Veneers made of light-polymerized composite resins can be fabricated directly in the mouth. Compared with the indirect type, direct

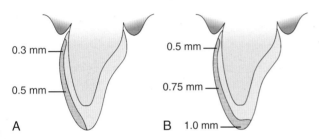

• **Figure 40.12** Cross-sectional views of a laboratory-processed veneer of ideal thickness without incisal coverage (A) and a veneer of greater thickness with incisal coverage (B).

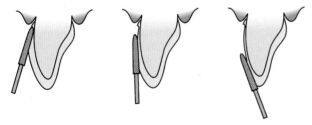

• **Figure 40.13** Cross-sectional view of the steps in diamond instrument placement needed for preparing the facial surface of a maxillary anterior tooth.

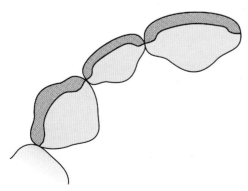

• **Figure 40.14** Incisal view of veneer preparations.

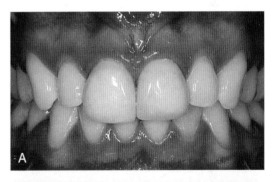

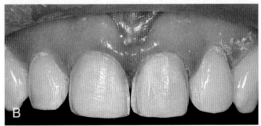

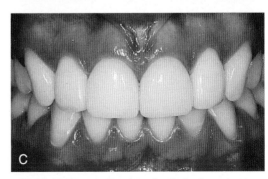

• **Figure 40.15** (A) Preoperative view of esthetically unpleasing maxillary anterior teeth. (B) Central incisors prepared for porcelain veneers. (C) Porcelain veneers in place.

veneers offer the advantages of improved marginal adaptation, placement in one appointment, greater operator control, and no laboratory fee. The disadvantages are that direct veneers require more time, greater skill, and more patience on the part of the clinician. In addition, outcomes are more difficult to predict, and composite resin is more susceptible to staining than porcelain.

The clinical direct technique may be performed with or without any enamel removal. Darkly stained teeth usually require some enamel removal because more composite resin is needed to mask the underlying enamel. The teeth are then pumiced and individually etched, and a bonding agent is applied. Again, celluloid matrices are used between adjacent teeth. Opaquing agents may then be painted on to cover more intensely stained areas or entire surfaces. For the best appearance, opaquing agents should be used minimally and with care. When dark banding is present, an alternative approach is to remove the band with a round bur and then replace the tooth structure with an opaque hybrid composite resin or resin-modified glass ionomer. Next, the composite resin should be applied in a layer 1.0 to 1.5 mm thick and contoured with brushes. The gingival third of the restoration should usually be an opaque yellow shade, and the remaining enamel should be covered with opaque gray or universal composite, overlapping and blending the shades to create a natural-looking, gentle color transition. In many situations a nonopaque shade can be used on the incisal one-fourth to allow a natural, translucent appearance (Fig. 40.16). After all composite resin has been added to a single tooth and contouring with brushes is complete, the material should be polymerized as recommended by the manufacturer. Finishing and polishing are best done with burs and disks, as described previously.

Vital Bleaching

Vital bleaching techniques involve the application of peroxide solutions to increase the value (whiteness) of teeth that are unusually dark. Peroxide bleaching methods appear to work best on teeth that are mildly discolored, predominantly yellow, and from which the discoloration originates in enamel rather than dentin. The basic methods for vital bleaching are: in office power bleaching, custom-fabricated tray bleaching, and over-the-counter bleaching strips.[29]

Power bleaching is an in-office procedure in which a concentrated hydrogen peroxide solution is applied to rubber dam–isolated teeth while heating the teeth, usually with an electric lamp or laser.[30] This method of bleaching may require numerous office visits and often causes temporary tooth sensitivity. Typically, patients who have had this treatment require periodic retreatment to maintain the desired color.

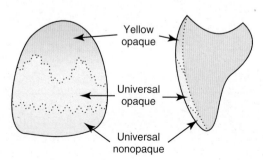

• **Figure 40.16** The use of overlapping shades of composite resin to create a natural-looking directly placed veneer.

Custom tray or over-the-counter vital bleaching is an at-home treatment. This method of vital bleaching uses a milder peroxide solution (usually 10% carbamide peroxide) that the patient applies and wears outside the dental office, often at night during sleep, for approximately 2 to 3 weeks. At-home bleaching appears to work as well as power bleaching and causes less sensitivity. Concerns were initially raised about the potentially hazardous soft tissue effects of applying peroxide solutions in this manner, but long-term studies of the safety and efficacy of this approach are demonstrating no harmful effects.[31] Vital bleaching also appears to cause limited damage to existing restorations, although these may no longer be a color match after the teeth have been whitened.[32] Over-the-counter bleaching strips can achieve similar whitening effects but take longer to accomplish.[29]

Restorations for Posterior Teeth

Fundamentals of Material Selection

There are numerous materials to select from when restoring the young posterior permanent dentition. In the selection process the dentist should consider the size of the caries/defect, the occlusal forces expected to load on the restoration, the patient's caries risk, the ability to isolate the tooth, and the patients' preference.

Resin infiltration (Icon, DMG-America, Englewood, NJ) is a minimally invasive technique used to restore noncavitated proximal caries lesions that radiographically extend from the inner enamel to the outer third of dentin. Studies have suggested this technique is more effective at reducing proximal caries progression compared with noninvasive measures such as fluoride varnish and flossing.[33–35] This technique requires a dry working field and care to protect gingival tissue, such as isolation with a rubber dam. For proximal lesions the teeth must be separated (approximately 50 μm) with a wedge, followed by etching with hydrochloric acid, rinsed for 30 seconds, and then dried to desiccation. The hydrochloric acid removes the hard remineralized outer layer of the lesion, allowing the penetration of the low viscosity resin into the porous enamel. It takes 3 minutes for the resin to penetrate the lesion, excess material is then removed, and the area is light cured from all sides for at least 40 seconds in total. The patient must be followed for caries progression with yearly radiographs; thus preference for this care should be for patients who have established a dental home. Because the lesions remain radiolucent in radiographs, patients should be counseled on the importance of notifying other dental providers of the treatment when they leave the practice.

Composite resin restorations are a popular choice for most patients due to their esthetic nature. However, composite resin restorations in the posterior dentition have several disadvantages to consider. The lifespan of a posterior composite resin restoration is inferior to that of amalgam restorations.[36] Patients with higher caries risk and multisurface restorations are at increased risk for restoration failure.[37] For the clinician the technique for placing composite restorations is more sensitive and requires longer chair time. On the other hand, composite resin restorations preserve tooth structure and manufactures have spent a considerable amount of time improving the material properties of composite. For the most consistent outcome, posterior composite resin restorations should be limited to restorations of appropriate size and careful attention paid to follow the manufacturer's instructions.

Composite resins are sensitive to moisture, and care should be taken to provide adequate isolation. After the preparation is completed, use of a sectional matrix system will provide anatomically correct tight contacts at the height of contour (Fig. 40.17).[38] With the arrival of multiple adhesive systems, care should be taken to confirm that the adhesive system used is appropriate for the clinical situation and the composite is compatible with the adhesive system (see Chapter 21 for a discussion of dental materials). The clinician should carefully follow the manufacturer's recommendations for incremental placement, light-curing, and polishing the composite of their choice.

Amalgam has been successfully used for restoring teeth for the past 150 years. However, with the demand for esthetically pleasing materials and concern over health-related mercury issues, it has been decreasing in popularity despite evidence that the longevity of amalgam restorations is longer than composite resins.[36] A disadvantage to amalgam restorations is the required cavity preparation, because it causes greater loss of tooth structure (depending on size of the lesion) compared with composite resin restorations. For large lesions, difficult-to-isolate areas in nonesthetic zones, and high caries risk patients, amalgam remains an excellent material choice.

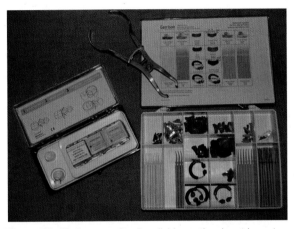

• **Figure 40.17** An example of available sectional matrix systems.

Amalgam is not dependent on absolute isolation, but moisture needs to be controlled. Care should be taken to isolate with either a rubber dam or cotton products. Amalgam is a brittle material in thin sections, thus the cavity design requires more bulk of material to be placed. Amalgam does not bind to the tooth surface, and undercuts/mechanical retention must be added to the cavity design for amalgam to be a stable restoration.[39] In addition, to prevent enamel fracture, all unsupported enamel should be removed while retaining a 90-degree cavosurface angle.

Permanent tooth stainless steel crowns (SSCs) may be indicated as an interim restoration for structurally compromised molars for the following conditions: the tooth is partially erupted, orthodontic treatment is indicated to finalize tooth placement in the arch, teeth with severe developmental defects, and when financial considerations are of concern.[40] There is limited literature reflecting the longevity of permanent SSCs. A recent study suggests a success rate of 88% over a 4-year time period.[41]

Significantly more chair time is indicated for the placement of a permanent tooth SSC compared with a primary tooth SSC. The final preparation is similar to that expected for a cast crown but with less tooth reduction. The occlusal reduction is 1.5 to 2 mm; the proximal walls are left in a slightly tapered position with a smooth feather-edge placed just below the level of the free gingival tissue. Unlike primary SSCs, permanent SSCs cannot be left in hyperocclusion and cannot be overextended into the gingival tissues, because they are more prone to periodontal issues. Hence SSCs for permanent teeth often require trimming. After crimping the SSC, the margins should be thinned and polished to a high shine. A bitewing radiograph is recommended to evaluate the mesial and distal marginal fit prior to cementation with glass ionomer cement (Fig. 40.18B).[40]

Hypoplastic Molar

For the adolescent the second permanent molars may erupt with hypoplastic defects. These hypoplastic molars vary greatly in the severity of the defect, from slightly discolored to abnormal

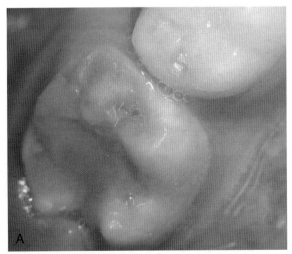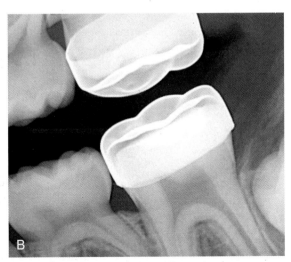

• **Figure 40.18** (A) A hypoplastic 6-year molar with continued sensitivity despite composite restoration treatment. (B) Bitewing radiograph of stainless steel crowns prior to cementation to confirm mesial and distal width of tooth shown in (A).

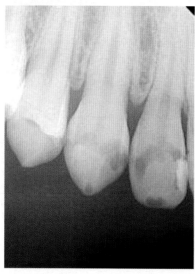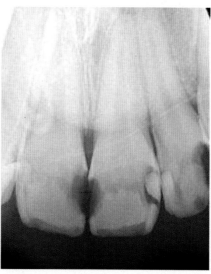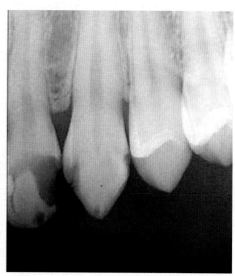

• **Figure 40.19** Radiographs of a 16-year-old with rampant caries.

morphology and/or absence of tooth structure. These teeth are prone to cavities, breakdown, and sensitivity. Restoration of these teeth is dependent on the severity of the defect. When possible, restoring the defect with glass ionomer cement or composite is ideal to minimize the removal of remaining tooth structure (see Fig. 40.18A). When using composite, the margins should be placed on nonaffected enamel because the mechanical bond to affected enamel may fail. When unable to place a resin restoration on unaffected enamel or when unable to obtain ideal restorative conditions (moist environment), a glass ionomer cement is a reasonable option because the chemical bond will still occur on hard but affected enamel. If the tooth continues to be sensitive or the defect is moderate to severe, a permanent tooth SSC can be used as an interim restoration until a cast crown can be placed (see Fig. 40.18B).[42] If morphologically acceptable third molars are present radiographically and the long-term prognoses of the affected teeth are poor, extractions may be considered.

Rampant Caries

Rampant caries has been defined as the "suddenly appearing, widespread, rapidly burrowing type of caries, resulting in early involvement of the pulp and affecting those teeth usually regarded as immune to ordinary decay" (Fig. 40.19).[43] The identification of this disease process in the adolescent can be overwhelming for the child, family, and dentist. The underlying etiology of the disease must be identified. The clinician must determine if the disease process is rampant caries (as defined previously) or long-term dental neglect. For the adolescent a relationship built on trust with his or her dentist will be extremely valuable in identifying the etiology of the disease, especially if the disease is associated with drug use.

While the etiology is being identified and corrected, the progression of the disease should be minimized. Oral health education, diet modification, and the addition of adjunct fluoride products should be initiated. The use of silver diamine fluoride should be discussed to arrest the caries process (at least in nonesthetic zones). Because the financial burden of rampant caries can be substantial, the family should be presented with multiple restorative treatment options. Teeth that are causing pain and localized areas of infections should be addressed immediately. Resin-modified and conventional glass ionomers are well suited for interim caries control therapy. After urgent needs are met, careful treatment considerations for each sextant are planned with the concept that some teeth will require interim restorations to reestablish occlusion and function until definitive restorations can be placed.

References

1. Nedeljkovic I, Teughels W, De Munck J, et al. Is secondary caries with composites a material-based problem? *Dent Mater*. 2015;31(11):e247–e277.
2. Masarwa N, Mohamed A, Abou-Rabii I, et al. Longevity of self-etch dentin bonding adhesives compared to etch-and-rinse dentin bonding adhesives: a systematic review. *J Evid Based Dent Pract*. 2016;16(2):96–106.
3. Hashimoto M, Ito S, Tay FR, et al. Fluid movement across the resin-dentin interface during and after bonding. *J Dent Res*. 2004;83(11):843–848.
4. Soldo M, Simeon P, Matijević J, et al. Marginal leakage of class V cavities restored with silorane-based and methacrylate-based resin systems. *Dent Mater J*. 2013;32(5):853–858.
5. Puckett AD, Fitchie JG, Kirk PC, et al. Direct composite restorative materials. *Dent Clin North Am*. 2007;51(3):659–675, vii.
6. Cramer NB, Stansbury JW, Bowman CN. Recent advances and developments in composite dental restorative materials. *J Dent Res*. 2011;90(4):402–416.
7. da Silva EM, Poskus LT, Guimarães JG. Influence of light-polymerization modes on the degree of conversion and mechanical properties of resin composites: a comparative analysis between a hybrid and a nanofilled composite. *Oper Dent*. 2008;33(3):287–293.
8. Shortall AC, Price RB, MacKenzie L, et al. Guidelines for the selection, use, and maintenance of LED light-curing units—Part 1. *Br Dent J*. 2016;221(8):453–460.
9. Shortall AC, Price RB, MacKenzie L, et al. Guidelines for the selection, use, and maintenance of LED light-curing units—Part II. *Br Dent J*. 2016;221(9):551–554.
10. Barutcigil C, Harorli OT, Yildiz M, et al. The color differences of direct esthetic restorative materials after setting and compared with a shade guide. *J Am Dent Assoc*. 2011;142(6):658–665.
11. Dahlke WO, Cottam MR, Herring MC, et al. Evaluation of the spatter-reduction effectiveness of two dry-field isolation techniques. *J Am Dent Assoc*. 2012;143(11):1199–1204.

12. Kameyama A, Asami M, Noro A, et al. The effects of three dry-field techniques on intraoral temperature and relative humidity. *J Am Dent Assoc*. 2011;142(3):274–280.

13. Weiner R. Liners and bases in general dentistry. *Aust Dent J*. 2011;56(suppl 1):11–22.

14. Souza-Junior EJ, de Souza-Régis MR, Alonso RC, et al. Effect of the curing method and composite volume on marginal and internal adaptation of composite restoratives. *Oper Dent*. 2011;36(2):231–238.

15. Macedo GV, Ritter AV. Essentials of rebonding tooth fragments for the best functional and esthetic outcomes. *Pediatr Dent*. 2009;31(2):110–116.

16. Jagannath-Torvi S, Kala M. Restore the natural—a review and case series report on reattachment. *J Clin Exp Dent*. 2014;6(5):e595–e598.

17. Vaz VT, Presoto CD, Jordão KC, et al. Fragment reattachment after atypical crown fracture in maxillary central incisor. *Case Rep Dent*. 2014;2014:231603.

18. Reis A, Loguercio AD, Kraul A, et al. Reattachment of fractured teeth: a review of literature regarding techniques and materials. *Oper Dent*. 2004;29(2):226–233.

19. Andreasen FM, Norén JG, Andreasen JO, et al. Long-term survival of fragment bonding in the treatment of fractured crowns: a multicenter clinical study. *Quintessence Int*. 1995;26(10):669–681.

20. Krastl G, Filippi A, Zitzmann NU, et al. Current aspects of restoring traumatically fractured teeth. *Eur J Esthet Dent*. 2011;6(2):124–141.

21. Oliveira GM, Ritter AV. Composite resin restorations of permanent incisors with crown fractures. *Pediatr Dent*. 2009;31(2):102–109.

22. Kwon SR, Oyoyo U, Li Y. Influence of application techniques on contact formation and voids in anterior resin composite restorations. *Oper Dent*. 2014;39(2):213–220.

23. Rosenstiel SF, Rashid RG. Public preferences for anterior tooth variations: a web-based study. *J Esthet Restor Dent*. 2002;14(2):97–106.

24. Croll TP. Enamel microabrasion for removal of superficial dysmineralization and decalcification defects. *J Am Dent Assoc*. 1990;120(4):411–415.

25. Wright JT. The etch-bleach-seal technique for managing stained enamel defects in young permanent incisors. *Pediatr Dent*. 2002;24(3):249–252.

26. Senestraro SV, Crowe JJ, Wang M. et.al. Minimally invasive resin infiltration of arrested white-spot lesions: a randomized clinical trial. *J Am Dent Assoc*. 2013;144:997–1005.

27. Croll TP. Enamel microabrasion: the technique. *Quintessence Int*. 1989;20(6):395–400.

28. Pini NI, Sundfeld-Neto D, Aguiar FH, et al. Enamel microabrasion: an overview of clinical and scientific considerations. *World J Clin Cases*. 2015;3(1):34–41.

29. Auschill TM, Hellwig E, Schmidale S, et al. Efficacy, side-effects and patients' acceptance of different bleaching techniques (OTC, in-office, at-home). *Oper Dent*. 2005;30(2):156–163.

30. Lo Giudice R, Pantaleo G, Lizio A, et al. Clinical and spectrophotometric evaluation of LED and laser activated teeth bleaching. *Open Dent J*. 2016;10:242–250.

31. Li Y. The safety of peroxide-containing at-home tooth whiteners. *Compend Contin Educ Dent*. 2003;24(4A):384–389.

32. Attin T, Hannig C, Wiegand A, et al. Effect of bleaching on restorative materials and restorations—a systematic review. *Dent Mater*. 2004;20(9):852–861.

33. Meyer-Lueckel H, Balbach A, Schikowsky C, et al. Pragmatic RCT on the efficacy of proximal caries infiltration. *J Dent Res*. 2016;95(5):531–536.

34. Meyer-Lueckel H, Bitter K, Paris S. Randomized controlled clinical trial on proximal caries infiltration: three-year follow-up. *Caries Res*. 2012;46(6):544–548.

35. Dorri M, Dunne SM, Walsh T, et al. Micro-invasive interventions for managing proximal dental decay in primary and permanent teeth. *Cochrane Database Syst Rev*. 2015;(11):CD010431.

36. Alhareky M, Tavares M. Amalgam vs composite restoration, survival, and secondary caries. *J Evid Based Dent Pract*. 2016;16(2):107–109.

37. Roumanas ED. The frequency of replacement of dental restorations may vary based on a number of variables, including type of material, size of the restoration, and caries risk of the patient. *J Evid Based Dent Pract*. 2010;10(1):23–24.

38. Loomans BA, Opdam NJ, Roeters FJ, et al. A randomized clinical trial on proximal contacts of posterior composites. *J Dent*. 2006;34(4):292–297.

39. Summitt JB, Howell ML, Burgess JO, et al. Effect of grooves on resistance form of conservative class 2 amalgams. *Oper Dent*. 1992;17(2):50–56.

40. Randall RC. Preformed metal crowns for primary and permanent molar teeth: review of the literature. *Pediatr Dent*. 2002;24(5):489–500.

41. Discepolo K, Sultan M. Investigation of adult stainless steel crown longevity as an interim restoration in pediatric patients. *Int J Paediatr Dent*. 2016.

42. Mahoney EK. The treatment of localised hypoplastic and hypomineralised defects in first permanent molars. *N Z Dent J*. 2001;97(429):101–105.

43. Massler J. Teen-age caries. *J Dent Child*. 1945;12:57–64.

41

Sports Dentistry and Mouth Protection

ANDREW SPADINGER

CHAPTER OUTLINE

Background

As a dentist who treats children and adolescents, you will encounter trauma in your office related to sports injuries. Actual numbers of children in the United States participating in sports are difficult to measure due to the lack of a centralized tracking system to collect data from the vast number of sports, leagues, and organizations. In the United States, some 30 million children were estimated to participate in organized sports.[1] If one includes "some form of sports" then the estimate increased to 46 million youths.[2] A survey found 75% of boys and 69% of girls aged 8 to 17 participated in at least one organized sport.[3]

Ten percent to 39% of all dental injuries in children are due to sports accidents.[4] Injury rates vary in studies depending on sample size, location, age of participants, and sports played.[5–8] Children between ages 7 and 11 are the most susceptible to sports-related dental trauma.[9–12] With regulations for mandatory protective equipment in sports like football and lacrosse, basketball and baseball now have the highest incidences of sports-related dental injuries.[12] Males aged 15 to 18 demonstrated the highest incidence of sports-related dental injuries.[8] The greatest number of sports-related dental and orofacial injuries affect the upper lip, maxilla, and maxillary incisors, with 50% to 90% of the injuries affecting the maxillary incisors.[5,6,13]

The consequences of orofacial trauma for child and adolescent athletes include pain, psychological effects, and financial burdens. Dental treatment appointments result in lost time from school and work. The costs associated with all injuries, including orofacial injuries, by young athletes was estimated to be $1.8 billion/year.[1] The patient may have to undergo a lifetime of treatment involving restorative, endodontic, prosthodontic, implant, or surgical procedures.

With the number of children and adolescents playing sports and suffering from orofacial injuries, there arose a need to address these issues. Sports dentistry deals with the prevention and treatment of dental injuries and related oral diseases that result from sports and exercise.[14]

Developmental Evaluation of Child and Adolescent Athletes

Medical Assessment

As part of a thorough medical history, it is advisable to ask parents about their child's athletic activities.[15] A complete medical examination by a physician is necessary for all children and adolescents because a number of medical conditions may limit or preclude them from participating in athletics. The physician can best assess the child's health and suggest appropriate modifications and equipment to reduce the risk of injury. The American Academy of Pediatrics (AAP) lists carditis and fever as two conditions when no sports participation is recommended. The AAP strictly opposes participation in boxing for children, adolescents, and young adults.[16]

Children with attention-deficit/hyperactivity disorder (ADHD) are at higher risk for traumatic injuries.[17] Other children identified at risk for dental trauma include risk-taking children, those being bullied, and obese children.[7] Placing these children in athletic venues puts them at increased risk for traumatic dental injuries.

Participation in sports involves many health hazards for children and adolescents. Parents who allow their children to pursue athletics believe the health benefits gained by sports participation outweigh the risk of injuries. Sports and physical activity are associated with improved physical and emotional health, academic achievement, and quality of life for children. Higher levels of family satisfaction were also reported.[3]

Data from an annual online survey by the Sports and Fitness Industry Association (SIFA) showed some disturbing trends. Although 30.2% of children aged 6 to 12 were engaged in sports in 2008, by 2015 the percentage dropped to 26.6%. Similarly, for adolescents aged 13 to 17, participation was 42.7% in 2008 and only 39.3% in 2015.[18]

Reasons for the decline included lack of interest, specialization in one sport burn out, financial burdens, increased use of video games, and, at the high school level, limitations in roster size.[19]

Intraoral Assessment

Child and adolescent athletes must have a thorough oral and dental examination for the diagnosis and management of dental caries, juvenile periodontal diseases, hard and soft tissue pathology, congenital anomalies, and developing occlusion. Young athletes in the early mixed dentition should be evaluated radiographically according to the AAPD guidelines for the naturally occurring processes of root resorption, exfoliation of primary teeth, and eruption of permanent successors.[20] A class II, division I malocclusion puts the child at risk for sports-related injuries.[21] Inadequate lip seal and excessive overjet place the protruding maxillary incisors at greater risk for injury especially in those playing contact sports (Fig. 41.1). The dentist may be able to reduce these risk factors by initiating orthodontic treatment.[22] The relatively large pulp chambers in immature permanent teeth make them susceptible to pulpal exposures in crown fractures.

An evaluation of the third molars in adolescent athletes is also important. Ideally, referral for extractions, if indicated, should be made so as to avoid in-season problems of pain and acute pericoronitis. To reduce the risk of mandibular angle fractures, extraction of retained third molars should be considered in young athletes who participate in contact sports.[23,24]

The labial mucosa, specifically in the mandibular anterior region of adolescent athletes, should be evaluated for the presence of soft tissue changes such as leukoplakia associated with the habitual use of smokeless tobacco (Fig. 41.2). Snuff dipping is a common habit among athletes, and unfortunately it is occurring at an increasing rate, even among young children. Child and adolescent athletes should be warned at every opportunity about the serious intraoral and systemic dangers of this addictive habit. The use of smokeless tobacco has traditionally been associated most often with baseball. However, male athletes who compete in sports organized according to weight classifications (e.g., wrestling) sometimes dip snuff to suppress appetite and control body weight.

Dietary Assessment

A dietary assessment is another integral part of the evaluation of children and adolescent athletes. Based on the athlete's diet, preventive oral strategies can be suggested. A number of factors influence the specific nutritional needs of athletes, including the type of sport, frequency and intensity of training, fitness levels, and the requirement to achieve physique changes.[25]

Athletes may turn to high-carbohydrate diets to increase bulk or as an energy source for moderate to high intensity exercise. The majority of carbohydrates should come from whole food sources (e.g., grains, fruits, vegetables, milk or yogurt, and legumes). However, some athletes may choose foods less nutrient dense with higher sugar content. Along with increased frequency of ingestion, the high carbohydrate diet may put the athlete at greater risk for caries. The dentist should advise better food choices, provide oral hygiene instruction, and consider fluoride varnish.[25]

Amateur boxers and wrestlers may intentionally become dehydrated or practice aberrant eating behaviors to meet weight classification requirements. This can have a negative impact on strength and performance but also on the cardiovascular system. On exertion in such situations, hyperthermia and even death can result. Gymnasts who practice similar eating behaviors are at risk for these same systemic manifestations.

Adolescent athletes attempting to control weight through dehydration and fasting are vulnerable to hypoglycemic syncope, caused by inadequate glucose reaching the brain. This pathophysiologic event can be brought on by the stress of a dental appointment. Symptoms of hypoglycemia include palpations, sweating, confusion, irritability, headache, and loss of consciousness. The dentist should be alert to these manifestations and have a ready source of sugar available in the office emergency kit.

In female adolescent athletes the dentist should be vigilant for signs of the severe eating disorders of anorexia nervosa and bulimia. Enamel erosion on the lingual surfaces of the teeth (Fig. 41.3), called perimolysis, results from persistent vomiting associated with the binge-purge cycle of eating. Enlargement of the parotid glands may occur.[26] With intensive training, the eating disorders can progress to the female athlete triad of eating disorder, amenorrhea, and osteoporosis.[27] Severe eating disorders signal psychological problems and immediate referral for counseling.

Sports and energy drink consumption should be addressed with pediatric and adolescent athletes. Sports drinks are flavored beverages that may contain carbohydrates, minerals, and nutrients, whereas energy drinks contain stimulants, caffeine, or guarana and may also have varying amounts of carbohydrates and nutrients.[28] Stimulant-containing energy drinks should not be part of the diets of children or adolescents.[29] Pediatric athletes can benefit from

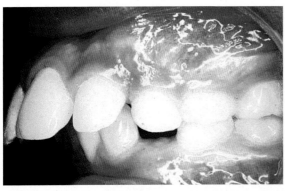

• **Figure 41.1** Excessive overjet and lack of lip protection place these maxillary permanent incisors at risk for traumatic injury during athletic activities.

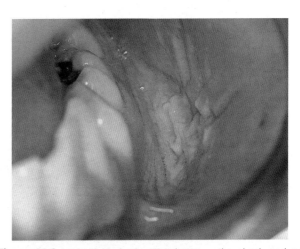

• **Figure 41.2** Leukoplakia in the area between the cheek and gum caused by the placement of smokeless tobacco (snuff dipper's pouch). (From Thibodeau GA, Patton KT. *The Human Body in Health and Disease.* 5th ed. St Louis: Mosby; 2010.)

sports drinks in limited situations.[30] However, water for hydration is the best option. Because most sport and energy drinks have a pH of 3 to 4, they can cause enamel demineralization and dental erosion.[31] For those athletes drinking sports drinks, the dentist should recommend rinsing with water immediately afterward.

After a thorough developmental evaluation of the young athlete has been completed, appropriate advice and recommendations can be given about the prevention of specific sports-related dental and orofacial injuries.

Mouth Protection for Child and Adolescent Athletes

An athletic mouthguard is defined as a resilient device or appliance placed inside the mouth to reduce injuries to the teeth and

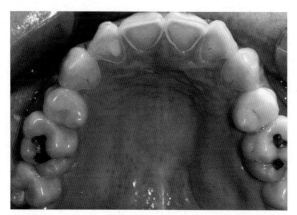

• **Figure 41.3** Lingual erosion in a patient with a history of bulimia. The facial surface of the permanent maxillary central incisors has been covered with veneer restorations. (From Bath-Balogh M, Fehrenbach MK. *Illustrated Dental Embryology, Histology, and Anatomy*. 3rd ed. St Louis: Saunders; 2011.)

surrounding structures. Mouthguards are effective in preventing crown fractures, root fractures, luxations, and avulsions of teeth. To provide protection from both direct and indirect blows, the mouthguard must fit, stay in position during contact to cushion the impact, yet allow the athlete to speak and breathe easily. In most cases the mouthguard is worn on the maxillary arch. However, in athletes with a class III malocclusion, the mouthguard is worn on the mandibular arch. If the mouthguard is strapped to the helmet, as in football or boys' lacrosse, it is recommended that the strap has a feature that allows it to separate with the helmet in the event the helmet gets knocked off the athlete, leaving the mouthguard intact covering the teeth. To date, there is insufficient evidence to determine whether mouthguards offer protection against concussions.[32]

Helmets, facemasks, and mouthguards are effective in reducing the frequency and severity of dental and orofacial trauma.[33] An extensive analysis conducted in 2007 demonstrated the overall risk of an oral facial injury was 1.6 to 1.9 times higher when not wearing a mouthguard compared with when a mouthguard was worn.[32] Multiple epidemiologic surveys and studies have corroborated the protective and positive results of wearing mouthguards.[22]

Types of Mouthguards

The American Society for Testing and Materials (ASTM) recognizes three categories of mouthguards (Fig. 41.4).[34]

Type I: Custom Fabricated

This mouthguard is custom fabricated using a dental cast of the athlete's mouth. In the vacuum process a single layer of thermoplastic material, typically EVA (ethyl-vinyl acetate), is heated and adapted over a dental cast. Vacuum pressure pulls the softened materials over the cast for a retentive appliance. Sometimes the material can be stretched too thin over the incisal edges. Heat-pressure laminated mouthguards typically use two layers of material to better control the thickness of the material. The initial layer of EVA is adapted

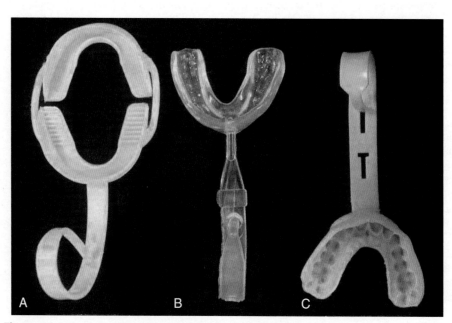

• **Figure 41.4** The three categories of athletic mouthguards include type III, stock (A); type II, mouth formed (B); and type I, custom fabricated (C).

to a cast of the athlete's dentition. An additional layer is adhered to the first layer by using heat and pressure. The result is a mouthguard with the minimum 3-mm thickness in the incisal areas.

Both the vacuum-formed and heat-laminated mouthguards have the best fit and most retention. These appliances allow the athlete to breathe and speak easily. In addition, the fabricator has the ability to make the appliance allow for orthodontic movement of teeth. These mouthguards are the most expensive.

Type II: Mouth Formed/Boil and Bite

This mouthguard is the traditional "boil and bite" mouth-formed mouthguard. Typically the material is placed in boiling water to soften it. The warm, softened material is placed in the mouth and, by a combination of biting force and finger pressure, adapted to the teeth. This mouthguard is available at most sporting goods stores or online websites. There can be a tremendous variety of quality and hence protection, retention, and comfort. In addition, by biting through the material, the 3-mm thickness is not always present.

Type III: Stock

Stock mouthguards are purchased commercially as well. With these mouthguards, there is no attempt to fit the mouthguard to the patient and therefore tend to be uncomfortable. The "retention" comes from biting down during contact. Other shortcomings include difficulty in speaking and breathing with it in the mouth. The stock mouthguard is a cheap alternative and has limited uses in some orthodontic patients.

The Academy for Sports Dentistry (ASD) strongly urges replacing mouthguard with the phrase "a properly fitted mouthguard" to optimally protect the athlete.[35] Furthermore, the ASD establishes the following criteria for a properly fitted mouthguard:

- It should be made on a dental model using an impression of the athlete's mouth.
- It should cover and protect the teeth and surrounding tissues.
- To reduce impact, it should have a minimum of 3 mm in the occlusal/labial area.
- It should be made from an FDA-approved material.
- It should have a retentive fit so as not to be dislodged by a direct or indirect blow.
- It should be fitted by the dentist or under a dentist's supervision. This includes balancing the properly fitted mouthguard for even occlusal contact.
- If necessary, the athlete should be able to speak while the appliance is in place.
- The appliance should be routinely inspected for fit and function. Loss of retention through wear and loss of adequate thickness due to chewing are indications for replacing the mouthguard.

All types of mouthguards should be stored in a plastic container when not in use, to avoid damage from excessive heat and cold.[34] Mouthguards should be rinsed with cold or lukewarm water because hot water may cause distortion. Mouthguards should be inspected regularly during the athletic season to detect distortions, tears, or bite-through problems (Fig. 41.5). When deficiencies are detected, a new mouthguard should be made.

Despite an abundance of studies demonstrating the protective and positive effects of wearing mouthguards, few sports require their use.[22,32] The National Federation of State High School Associations (NFSH) mandates high school athletes wear colored, not white or clear, mouthguards for football, field hockey, ice hockey, lacrosse, and wrestling (if wearing braces).[36] There are no specifications as to what type of mouthguard the athlete must wear. In

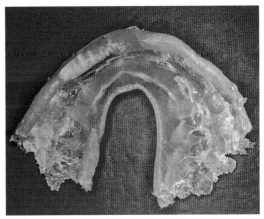

• **Figure 41.5** Distortions, splits, and bite-through problems indicated the need to fabricate a new mouthguard for proper retention, comfort, and maximal protection of the athlete.

addition, wrestlers with braces must wear mouthguards that cover both upper and lower orthodontic appliances. New Hampshire mandated mouthguard use for high school soccer and basketball in 1990.[37] Maine mandated use for high school boys' and girls' soccer in 1999.[37] The National Collegiate Athletic Association (NCAA) requires athletes participating in certain sports to wear mouthguards[38] (Table 41.1). Again, there is no mention as to which type of mouthguard is needed to comply with the rules.

Boxing and mixed martial arts are the only professional sports requiring mouthguards. However, increasing numbers of professional athletes in other sports, hockey and basketball in particular, seem to be wearing mouthguards.

Team Dentist

The Team Dentist is a part of an athletic team's sports medicine group whose role is to ensure the dental health and well-being of the athletes. The ASD developed a course to address specific situations encountered in sports to become a certified Team Dentist. It reviews principles of injury prevention, mouthguard fabrication, doping issues, and the effects of illicit and performance enhancing drugs. Other duties include preseason dental evaluations and on-the-field dental trauma evaluation and treatment.[39]

The Team Dentist must be prepared and ready to provide treatment in a sports facility or athletic field. Informed consent should be obtained prior to examination and treatment. The exam should begin assessing the ABC's (airway, breathing, and circulation), other nondental injuries, and neurologic examination before focusing on the temporomandibular joint, teeth, and oral tissues. Treatment may not be definitive in nature, with the goal being to return the athlete to play when permissible. Team Dentists carry an emergency dental kit to provide on-site, game-time treatment (Box 41.1). These items will allow the practitioner using universal precautions to carry out an examination and perform basic palliative treatment.

Concussions

A concussion is a brain injury and is defined as a complex patho-physiologic process affecting the brain, induced by biomechanical forces.[40] The majority of signs and symptoms of concussions typically resolve in 7 to 10 days, although some cases can linger for weeks

| TABLE 41.1 | NCAA Sports Requiring Mouthguards |

Sport	Position	Mouthguard	Color	Covers All Upper Teeth	When
Field hockey	Field	Mandatory; strongly recommended for goalkeepers	Not specified	Not specified	Regular season competition and NCAA championships
Football	All	Mandatory	Readily visible color (not white or transparent)	Yes	Regular season competition, postseason, and NCAA championships
Women's lacrosse	All	Mandatory	Not specified	Yes	Regular season competition and NCAA championships
Men's lacrosse	All	Mandatory	Yellow or any visible color	Yes	Regular season competition and NCAA championships

NCAA, National Collegiate Athletic Association.
From National Collegiate Athletic Association (NCAA). *2014–2015 NCAA Sports Medicine Handbook.* Indianapolis: NCAA; 2014.

• BOX 41.1 Sample Emergency Dental Kit

2 × 2 gauze	Curing light
Local anesthetics	Bonding agent
Needles/syringe	Theracal
Sutures/scissors	Vitrebond
Cotton rolls	Flashlight
Etchant/bonding agent	Splint materials
Composite/plastic instrument	Gloves/mask
Mirrors/explorers	Wire cutters
Tongue depressors	Canned air
Endo files/broaches	Dremel motor/burrs

---

or months. The long-term effects of concussion are controversial and are still being investigated.

Symptoms are variable and may include temporary loss of consciousness, headache, nausea, amnesia, abnormal behavior, sensitivity to light and noise, fatigue, balance, and vision problems.[41] These symptoms may be immediate or have a delayed onset. Diagnosis of a concussion is difficult because there is no definitive medical test. Brain computed tomography (CT), magnetic resonance imaging (MRI), electroencephalogram (EEG), and blood tests are often normal. Athletes with attention-deficit disorder, learning disabilities, mood disorders, and migraine history are more challenging to assess and diagnose because of the overlap of symptoms.

The Acute Concussion Evaluation (ACE), the Sport Concussion Assessment Tool (SCAT3), and the Child SCAT3 for ages 5 to 12 are examples of standardized tools used by medical professionals and first responders to record symptoms, balance, and cognitive abilities of suspected concussed athletes to aid concussion diagnosis.[42–44]

With the large number of children and adolescents playing sports, there has been an alarming increase in the number of concussions. An estimated 300,000 sports-related concussions occur each year in the United States.[45] Emergency room visits for recreation and sports-related concussions increased 62% from 2001 to 2009.[46] The Centers for Disease Control and Prevention (CDC) created the Heads UP brain injury awareness program as a resource for

parents, coaches, and health care professionals to disseminate information about concussions.[47]

Concussions accounted for an estimated 8.9% of all high school injuries.[48] As expected high-contact sports have higher risks for concussions. In high school athletics, boys' football had the highest risk for concussions. For girls, soccer and basketball had the highest rate of concussion. Rugby, lacrosse, and ice hockey had higher rates of concussions.

The NCAA data show slightly different rates of concussions.[49] Wrestling, football, and ice hockey had the highest concussion rates among men's sports. In women's sports, field hockey presented the highest rate, followed by soccer and ice hockey.

Young, concussed athletes who return to play their sport before proper healing are at risk for a rare, fatal condition called second impact syndrome (SIS). First described in 1984, a second concussive blow to the already injured brain causes severe edema, brain herniation, and death within minutes.[50] According to the CDC in 1997, the true incidence of second impact is unknown.

Return to Play

Under no circumstances should a child or adolescent athlete return to play the same day as their suspected concussion. Determining when an athlete returns to play after a concussion follows a protocol tailored to the individual athlete.[41] Typically, a gradual return to school and social activities that do not trigger symptoms precedes any return to sports. Once asymptomatic at rest, the athlete is guided through a stepwise, mild progression of activities. An athlete can only advance to the next step if his or her symptoms are not exacerbated by the next level of activity. Final clearance to return to play is determined by a physician or his or her trained designee.

Some athletic programs administer a neurocognitive test, the Immediate Post-Concussion Assessment and Cognitive Test (ImPACT) as part of their preseason protocol. Younger athletes, aged 5 to 11, take a similar test, ImPACT Pediatric, to get baseline values.[50] Results from the test taken at baseline (i.e., preseason) are compared with postconcussion test results. When the scores approximate the original scores, the trained physician has a measure of brain function to help make return to play decisions. A number of studies have shown a longer cognitive recovery period for children and adolescent athletes compared with college-aged or professional athletes.[41]

Since 2009 the District of Columbia and all but two states, Arkansas and Wyoming, have passed laws requiring physicians, licensed health care professional, or certified athletic trainers to be trained in concussion management to protect young athletes.[51] Athletes and their parents are required to sign informed consent outlining the dangers of concussions before participating in sports. Often there are strict educational requirements for coaches and trainers to identify concussions. An athlete must be removed from a game if suspected of having been concussed and may not return until being cleared by a licensed health care provider.

The NCAA protects student-athletes by mandating institutions have processes to identify sports-related concussions and return to play. Student-athletes are educated about concussions and must sign a consent to report signs and symptoms of a concussion. Concussed student athletes cannot return to athletic activity for at least that day, and medical clearance is required to return to play.[48]

Professional Activities in Sports Dentistry

The American Dental Association (ADA), the AAPD, and the ASD recommend the use of properly fitted mouthguards to prevent injuries.[22,35,52] Despite all the evidence showing the effectiveness of wearing mouthguards, there is still a lot of work to be done to educate parents, coaches, and athletes. Cost, ranging from $60 to $285 nationwide, may be a barrier to their use.[53] However, in a different study, only 23.2% of children wore a free mouthguard when needed.[54]

Mandates to increase the number of high school sports requiring mouthguards are difficult to enact. Massachusetts made mouthguard use mandatory for boys' and girls' basketball and soccer in 2003 only to rescind them by 2009. Minnesota had a similar experience adding boys' and girls' soccer, baseball, softball, boys' and girls' basketball, and volleyball, with rules mandating mouthguard use in 1992. By 1994, due to strong resistance, the rules in Minnesota were rescinded.[37]

Dentists should be at the forefront using routine dental visits to initiate educational discussions about mouthguards with parents and patients. Dentists may be called upon to help present the case for mouthguards to legislative bodies, school administrators, and sports organizations. Take the Team Dentist to enhance your knowledge and use your skills to help local athletic teams, Special Olympics, or members of the United States Olympic Team.

References

1. Adirim T, Cheng T. Overview of injuries in the young athlete. *Sports Med.* 2003;33(1):75–81.
2. Barron M, Powell J. Fundamentals of injury prevention in youth sports. *J Pediatr Dent Care.* 2005;11(2):10–12.
3. Sabo D, Veliz D. Go out and play-youth sports in America, Women's Sports Foundation Research Report; 2008. files.eric.ed.gov/fulltext/ED539976.pdf. Accessed September 13, 2017.
4. Newsome P, Tran D, Cooke M. The role of the mouthguard in the prevention of sports-related dental injuries. A review. *Int J Paediatr Dent.* 2001;11(6):396–404.
5. Kumamoto D, Maeda Y. Global trends and epidemiology of sports injuries. *J Pediatr Dent Care.* 2005;11(2):15–25.
6. Kumamoto D, Maeda Y. A literature review of sports-related orofacial trauma. *Gen Dent.* 2004;52(3):270–280.
7. Glendor U. Aetiology and risk factors related to traumatic dental injuries: a review of the literature. *Dent Traumatol.* 2009;25(1):19–31.
8. Huang B, Wagner M, Croucher R, et al. Activities related to the occurrence of traumatic dental injuries in 15-18-year-olds. *Dent Traumatol.* 2009;25(1):64–68.
9. Tesini DA, Soporowski NJ. Epidemiology of orofacial sports-related injuries. *Dent Clin North Am.* 2000;44(1):1–18.
10. Rodd HD, Chesham DJ. Sports-related oral injury and mouthguard use among Sheffield school children. *Community Dent Health.* 1997;14(1):25–30.
11. American Dental Association Council on Access, Prevention and Interprofessional Relations and Council on Scientific Affairs. Using mouthguards to reduce the incidence and severity of sports-related oral injuries. *J Am Dent Assoc.* 2006;137(12):1712–1720.
12. Stewart GB, Shields BJ, Fields S, et al. Consumer products and activities associated with dental injuries to children treated in United States emergency departments 1990-2003. *Dent Traumatol.* 2009;25(4):399–405.
13. Takeda T, Ishigami K, Nakajima K, et al. Are all mouthguards the same and safe to use? Part 2. The influence of anterior occlusion against a direct impact on maxillary incisors. *Dent Traumatol.* 2008;24(3):360–365.
14. Academy for Sports Dentistry. Position Statement on The Definition of Sports Dentistry; 2012. www.academyforsportsdentistry.org/position-statement. Accessed September 13, 2013.
15. Ranalli DN. Strategies for the prevention of sports-related oral injuries: a practical guide for the pediatric dentist. *J Southeast Soc Pediatr Dent.* 1997;3:18–19.
16. Rice SG, Council on Sports Medicine and Fitness. Medical conditions affecting sports participation. *Pediatrics.* 2008;121:841–848.
17. Sabuncuoglu O, Irmak MY. The attention-deficit/hyperactivity disorder model for traumatic dental injuries: a critical review and update of the last 10 years. *Dent Traumatol.* 2017;33(2):71–76.
18. Aspen Institute. State of play 2016: trends and developments. https://www.aspeninstitute.org/publications/state-play-2016-trends-developments/. Accessed September 13, 2017.
19. Merkel DL. Youth sport: positive and negative impact on young athletes. *Open Access J Sports Med.* 2013;(4):151–160.
20. American Academy of Pediatric Dentistry Guideline on Prescribing Dental Radiographs for Infants, Children, Adolescents and Persons with Special Health Care Needs. *Pediatr Dent.* 2016-2017;38(special issue):355–357.
21. Fos P, Pinkham JR, Ranalli DN. Prediction of sports-related dental traumatic injuries. *Dent Clin North Am.* 2000;44(1):19–33.
22. American Academy of Pediatric Dentistry. Policy on prevention of sports-related orofacial injuries. *Pediatr Dent.* 2016;38(special issue):76–80.
23. Rahimi-Nedjat RK, Sagheb K, Jacobs C, et al. Association between eruption state of the third molar and the occurrence of mandibular angle fractures. *Dent Traumatol.* 2016;32(5):347–352.
24. Yamuda T, Sawaki Y, Takeuchi M, et al. A study of sports-related mandibular angle fracture: a relation to the position of the third molars. *Scand J Med Sci Sports.* 1998;8:116–119.
25. Broad EM, Rye LA. Do current sports nutrition guidelines conflict with good oral health? *Gen Dent.* 2015;63(6):18–23.
26. Hasler JF. Parotid enlargement: a presenting sign in anorexia nervosa. *Oral Surg Oral Med Oral Pathol.* 1982;53:567–573.
27. Yeager K, Agostini R, Nattiv A, et al. The female triad: disordered eating, amenorrhea, osteoporosis. *Med Sci Sports Exerc.* 1993;25:775–777.
28. American Academy of Pediatrics. Clinical report—sports drinks and energy drinks for children and adolescents: are they appropriate? *Pediatrics.* 2011;127(6):1182–1189.
29. Institute of Medicine. *Nutrition Standards for Foods in Schools: Leading the Way Toward Healthier Youth.* Washington, DC: National Academies Press; 2007.
30. Rodriguez NR, DiMarco NM, Langley S, et al. Position of the American Dietetic Association, Dietitians of Canada, and American

College of Sports Medicine: nutrition and athletic performance. *J Am Diet Assoc.* 2009;109(3):509–527.

31. Shaw L, Smith AJ. Dental erosion: the problem and some practical solutions. *Br Dent J.* 1999;186(3):15–18.

32. Kapnik JJ, Marshal SW, Lee RB, et al. Mouthguards in sports activities: history, physical properties and injury prevention effectiveness. *Sports Med.* 2007;37(2):117–144.

33. Ranalli DN. Sports dentistry in general practice. *Gen Dent.* 2000;48(2):158–164.

34. American Society for Testing and Materials. Standard Practice for the Care and Use of Athletic Mouth Protectors. ASTM F697-00. Philadelphia: American Society for Testing and Materials; Reapproved 2006.

35. Academy for Sports Dentistry. Position statement: a properly fitted mouthguard; 2010. www.academyforsportsdentistry.org/position-statement. Accessed September 13, 2017.

36. National Federation of State High School Associations. Position statement and recommendations for mouthguards in sports; 2014. https://www.nfhs.org/media/1014750/mouthguard-nfhs-smac-position-statement-october-2014.pdf. Accessed September 13, 2017.

37. Mills SM. Mandatory mouthguard rules for high school athletes in the United States. *Gen Dent.* 2015;63(6):35–40.

38. National Collegiate Athletic Association (NCAA). NCAA Sports Medicine Handbook: Guideline 3C Mouthguards. Indianapolis: NCAA; 2014-2015:111-112.

39. McCrory P, Meeuwisse WH, Aubry M, et al. Consensus statement on concussion in sport: the 4th International Conference on Concussion in Sport held in Zurich, November 2012. *Br J Sports Med.* 2013;47:250–258.

40. Halstead ME, Walter KD, Council on Sports Medicine and Fitness. Clinical Report—sport-related concussion in children and adolescents. *Pediatrics.* 2010;126(3):597–615.

41. Gioia G, Collins M. Acute concussion evaluation (ACE); 2006. https://www.cdc.gov/headsup/pdfs/providers/ace-a.pdf. Accessed September 13, 2017.

42. Sport Concussion Assessment Tool (SCAT3). *Br J Sports Med.* 2013;47(5):259.

43. Child Sport Concussion Assessment Tool (Child SCAT3). *Br J Sports Med.* 2013;47(5):263.

44. Thurman DJ, Branche CM, Sniezek JE. The epidemiology of sports-related traumatic brain injuries in the United States: recent developments. *J Head Trauma Rehabil.* 1998;3(2):1–8.

45. Centers for Disease Control and Prevention. Nonfatal traumatic brain injuries related to sports and recreation activities among persons aged <19 years—United States, 2001-2009. *MMWR Morb Mortal Wkly Rep.* 2011;60(39):1337–1342.

46. Centers for Disease Control and Prevention. Heads UP. http://www.cdc.gov/headsup/index.html. Accessed September 13, 2017.

47. Gessel LM, Fields SK, Collins CL, et al. Concussions among United States high school and collegiate athletes. *J Athl Train.* 2007;42(4):495–503.

48. National Collegiate Athletic Association (NCAA). Sports and Medicine Handbook. Guideline 21: Sport-Related Concussion. Indianapolis: NCAA; 2014-2015:56-64.

49. Bey T, Ostick B. Second impact syndrome. *West J Emerg Med.* 2009;10(1):6–10.

50. ImPACT Applications: The Immediate Post-Concussion Assessment and Cognitive Test (ImPACT). https://www.impacttest.com. Accessed September 13, 2017.

51. National Conference of State Legislatures (NCSL). Traumatic brain injury legislation. www.ncsl.org/research/health/traumatic-brain-injury-legislation.aspx. Accessed September 13, 2017.

52. Zenk JK. The ADA Council on Access, Prevention, and Interprofessional Relations. *Northwest Dent.* 2016;95(3):7–8.

53. Walker J. Parents plus: getting mouthguards into kids' mouths. *J Pediatr Dent Care.* 2005;11(2):39–40.

54. Matalon V, Brin I, Moskovitz M, et al. Compliance of children and youngsters in the use of mouthguards. *Dent Traumatol.* 2008;24(4):462–467.

Index

A

AAPD. *see* American Academy of Pediatric Dentistry
ACA. *see* Affordable Care Act
Access to care, dental public health issues and, 161–162
Acero 3S crowns, 316
Acetaminophen, 104, 104*t*
Acid-etch composite resins, for adolescent restorative problems, 571
Acid-etching technology
  for diastemas, 601–602
  effect on enamel surface of, 463, 463*f*
ACLS. *see* Advanced cardiac life support
Acrocephalosyndactyly, airway anomalies in, 90*t*
Actinomycosis, 139
Acute bronchospasm. *see* Asthma
Acute coronary syndrome, 154
  management of, 154
Acute inflammatory lesions, 30*t*–34*t*, 35*f*–39*f*
Acute lymphoid leukemia (ALL), 69
Acute osteomyelitis, 40*t*–42*t*, 43*f*–45*f*
Acute suppurative sialadenitis, 139
Acyclovir, 136
  for primary herpetic gingivostomatitis, 73
Adenomatoid odontogenic tumor, 46*t*, 47*f*
Adhesive materials, resin-based composite, 309
Adhesive systems, 598
Adolescence
  behavior guidance for, 366
  dental disease prevention, 588–597
    dietary management for, 589–592
    fluoride administration for, 592–593
    home care for, 592, 592*f*
    risk assessment in, 588–589, 589*f*, 589*t*–590*t*
    risk factors for, 593–595
    transitioning to adulthood, 595–596
  dynamics of change in, 555–561
    cognitive changes, 557
    craniofacial changes, 555–556, 556*f*–557*f*, 556*t*
    dental changes, 556
    emotional changes, 557
    physical changes, 555–556
    social changes, 557–560
  oral health care in, 164–165
  orthodontic problems in, 562–587
  radiographic issues in, 571*t*
  restorative dentistry for, 598–609
    clinical technique, fundamentals of, 598–601, 600*f*–601*f*
    diastemas, 601–604, 603*f*
    discolored teeth, 604–606

Adolescence *(Continued)*
    fractured anterior teeth, 601, 602*f*
    for hypoplastic molar, 607–608
    material selection, fundamentals of, 598, 599*f*–600*f*
    for posterior teeth, 606–607, 607*f*
    for rampant caries, 608, 608*f*
Adolescent athletes
  developmental evaluation of, 610–612
    dietary assessment in, 611–612, 612*f*
    intraoral assessment in, 611, 611*f*
    medical assessment in, 610
  return to play of, 614–615
Adolescent pregnancy, 594
Adulthood, adolescents to, dental home in, 595–596
Advanced cardiac life support (ACLS), 145–146
AED. *see* Automated external defibrillator
Affordable Care Act (ACA), pediatric dental benefit within, 161–162
Ages 3 to 6 years
  cognitive changes in, 263
  craniofacial changes in, 260–262, 261*f*, 261*t*
  dental changes in, 262–263, 262*f*
  dental disease prevention in, 282–292
    adaptive daily oral hygiene for, 286*b*–288*b*, 286*f*–288*f*, 286*t*–288*t*
    dietary counseling in, 289–291, 290*f*
    dietary management for, 289, 289*b*
    fluoride administration for, 282–286
    home care for, 291, 291*f*
  dental examination for, 266–277
    behavioral assessment for, 266–267
    examination of head and neck in, 268–270, 269*t*–270*t*
    examination of the face in, 270–273
    general appraisal in, 267–268, 268*t*
    history for, 266, 267*t*
    intraoral examination in, 273–277
    occlusal evaluation in, 273–274, 274*f*–277*f*
    patient record for, 265–266
    radiographic evaluation for, 277–280, 278*b*, 278*f*–280*f*, 280*t*
    supplemental orthodontic diagnostic technique for, 277–280
  emotional changes in, 263
  fluoride administration for, 282–286
    cost-benefit considerations for, 284–285
    dietary, 282–283, 283*t*
    method of, 285–286
    professional application of, 283–284, 284*f*

Ages 3 to 6 years *(Continued)*
    prophylaxis before, 285
    topical, 283
  oral habits, 386–393
  physical changes in, 260–263
  social changes in, 263–264
Ages 6 to 12 years
  cognitive changes in, 415
  craniofacial changes in, 411, 412*f*
  dental caries and dietary factors in, 416–417
    dietary counseling and, 417
    importance of, in transitional dentition, 416–417
    sucrose and, 416
  dental changes in, 412–413, 412*f*
  dental disease prevention, 455–460
    diet and, 458–459
    fluoride administration in, 455–456
    home care for, 456–458
    sealants and, 459
  developmental characteristics of, 420*t*
  dynamics of change in, 411–418
  emotional changes in, 415
  examination of, 419–454
    behavioral assessment in, 420
    facial examination in, 423–424, 423*f*–424*f*
    head and neck examination in, 423
    history in, 419–420
    intraoral examination in, 424–435
    occlusal evaluation in, 425–435
    oral hygiene evaluation in, 425
    periodontal evaluation in, 424–425, 425*f*
    radiographic evaluation in, 449–452, 451*f*–452*f*
    supplemental orthodontic diagnostic techniques in, 435–452
  physical changes in, 411–413
  social changes in, 415–416
  treatment planning for, 419–454
    in nonorthodontic problems, 452–453
Aggression, in ages 3 to 6 years, 263
Aggressive periodontitis, 374
Air abrasion, for caries removal, 305
Airway ("A"), in management of medical emergencies, 151–152, 151*f*
Airway anomalies, 88–90
  in specific conditions/diseases, 90*t*
Airway assessment, case study, 96.*e1*, 96.*e1f*–96.*e3f*, 96.*e1t*, 96.*e3t*–96.*e4t*
Airway narrowing, 88–90, 89*f*
Airway obstruction, 88–90, 89*f*

Page number followed by *t, f,* or *b* indicates table, figure, or box, respectively; *e* indicates online-only entries.

617